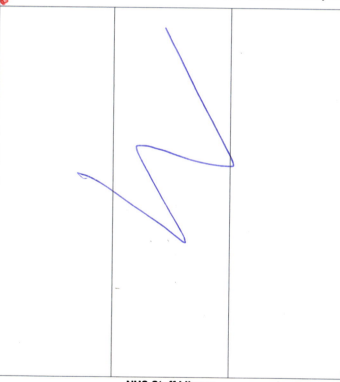

SEVENTH EDITION

SCULLY'S
MEDICAL PROBLEMS IN
DENTISTRY

Content Strategist: Alison Taylor
Content Development Specialist: Barbara Simmons
Project Manager: Julie Taylor
Designer/Design Direction: Miles Hitchen
Illustration Manager: Jennifer Rose
Illustrator: Antbits Ltd

SEVENTH EDITION

SCULLY'S
MEDICAL PROBLEMS IN
DENTISTRY

Professor Crispian Scully CBE

MD, PhD, MDS, MRCS, FDSRCS, FDSRCPS, FFDRCSI, FDSRCSE, FRCPath, FMedSci, FHEA, FUCL, FBS, DSc, DChD, DMed (HC), Dr (hc)

Professor Emeritus, UCL, London, UK; King James IV Professor, Royal College of Surgeons of Edinburgh; Visiting Professor at Universities of Athens, BPP, Edinburgh, Granada, Helsinki, Middlesex, Plymouth and West of England; Consultant at Harley Street Diagnostic Centre, London, UK; Honorary Consultant at University College Hospitals, London, UK; Great Ormond Street Hospital, London; St Savvas Hospital, Athens, Greece, and European Institute for Oncology, Milan, Italy

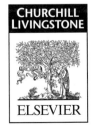

CHURCHILL
LIVINGSTONE

ELSEVIER

EDINBURGH   LONDON   NEW YORK   OXFORD   PHILADELPHIA   ST LOUIS   SYDNEY   TORONTO   2014

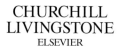

CHURCHILL
LIVINGSTONE
ELSEVIER

Seventh edition © 2014 Elsevier Ltd. All rights reserved.

ISBN: 978-0-7020-5401-3

British Library Cataloguing in Publication Data
A catalogue record for this book is available from the British Library

Library of Congress Cataloging in Publication Data
A catalog record for this book is available from the Library of Congress

Notices
Knowledge and best practice in this field are constantly changing. As new research and experience broaden our understanding, changes in research methods, professional practices, or medical treatment may become necessary.

Practitioners and researchers must always rely on their own experience and knowledge in evaluating and using any information, methods, compounds, or experiments described herein. In using such information or methods they should be mindful of their own safety and the safety of others, including parties for whom they have a professional responsibility.

With respect to any drug or pharmaceutical products identified, readers are advised to check the most current information provided (i) on procedures featured or (ii) by the manufacturer of each product to be administered, to verify the recommended dose or formula, the method and duration of administration, and contraindications. It is the responsibility of practitioners, relying on their own experience and knowledge of their patients, to make diagnoses, to determine dosages and the best treatment for each individual patient, and to take all appropriate safety precautions.

To the fullest extent of the law, neither the Publisher nor the authors, contributors, or editors, assume any liability for any injury and/or damage to persons or property as a matter of products liability, negligence or otherwise, or from any use or operation of any methods, products, instructions, or ideas contained in the material herein.

ELSEVIER your source for books, journals and multimedia in the health sciences
www.elsevierhealth.com

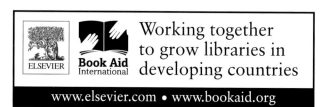

Working together to grow libraries in developing countries

www.elsevier.com • www.bookaid.org

The Publisher's policy is to use **paper manufactured from sustainable forests**

Printed in China

Contents

Preface

The aim of this book is to provide a basis for the understanding of how medical and surgical conditions influence oral health and oral health care, and to help dental health workers (DHWs) keep their patients informed of health risks and respect their choices.

Learning outcomes are for DHWs to be aware of systemic disorders and treatments that may cause complications in dental and oral health care. The reader should thus be able to understand relevant illness identified from the history, physical examination and investigations; be able to present a succinct and, where appropriate, unified list of all problems that could influence oral health care; and formulate a diagnosis/treatment plan for each problem (appropriate to the level of training). The reader should understand that the management of patients with diseases should take into consideration the severity of the condition; the type of operative procedure envisioned and, in particular, the amount of trauma, likely distress and time taken; other risk factors; and the health-care setting (skills/facilities) available. They should appreciate issues of access and informed consent, and the desirability of preventive oral health care and avoidance of harm. The reader should also be able to communicate appropriately and work with other health-care providers; to retrieve medical information using the recommended further reading sections and the Internet, in a manner that reflects an understanding of medical language, terminology, and the relationship between medical terms and concepts; to refine search strategies to improve the relevance and completeness of retrieved items; and to identify and acquire full-text electronic documents available from the Internet sites quoted.

Though dentistry remains largely a technical subject, there are a number of reasons why the education and training of dental professionals should have this basis. Dentistry is a profession and not a trade; medical problems can influence oral health and health care, whilst oral health and health care can influence general health and health care. DHWs need to understand patients and their attitudes to health care; they need to communicate at a reasonable level with other health professionals, with patients and sometimes with the media; they may need to act as advocates for patients; and, finally, they can find themselves in need of health care. It is incumbent upon DHWs to treat their patients in an appropriate way, taking into account both their dental needs and any special considerations related to their medical and drug history. To prevent any implication of negligence, a professional must administer appropriate care, and the patient should agree to it and receive adequate information about it. In general terms, DHWs need to develop strategies to identify patients at risk of medical problems, to assess the severity of those risks and, where necessary, to recognize the need for help and be able to seek advice from a colleague with special competence in the relevant fields.

Since the first edition of this book to this 7th edition, the importance of medicine in dentistry, interactions between medicine and dentistry, and the need for medical knowledge on the part of all members of the dental team have all increased radically – as has the whole of medicine. Increasing evidence supports, but does not prove, an association between oral infection and various systemic diseases. Thus there is interest in the possible associations of oral infection (periodontitis) with conditions such as atherosclerosis, Alzheimer disease, cancers (mouth, pancreas, renal), diabetes, erectile dysfunction, low-birth-weight babies, lung disease and rheumatoid arthritis, although space precludes all but a passing mention. Health-care needs are changing globally as people live longer and medical interventions advance. The populations in many countries are often surviving and ageing with the help of complex treatments. For example, in the UK the proportion of people aged over 65 is predicted to increase from 16% in 2006 to 22% in 2031. Advances in surgical and medical interventions and therapeutics are astounding, raising issues in relation to the understanding of these interventions and therapies, advantages and disadvantages, and the importance of informed consent. The US Federal Drug Administration recognizes this and may now approve new drugs with a Risk Evaluation and Mitigation Strategy (REMS), which consists of a Medication Guide advising patients of important safety information and a communication plan to inform health-care providers about the serious risks associated with their use. Advances in genetics have been equally impressive. During the life of this book, the human genome has been completely catalogued – revealing some 23 000 protein-coding genes. However, these genes were seen to occupy only 1.5% of the genome and, by 2012, the regulatory importance of the remaining DNA became evident. The genetic basis for many disorders has been or is being elucidated, and gene therapy is becoming a reality.

The knowledge base of medicine has thus been extended and effective new technologies, techniques and drugs have been developed, many of which have resulted in complications relevant to oral health care. Many patients who would, in earlier times, have succumbed are alive and live to much greater ages, thanks to advances in drugs, pacemakers and other cardiac devices, radiotherapy, public health and transplants – and they need good oral health and may well need oral health care. A wider range of medical problems has thus become relevant to oral health-care sciences. The world has changed further and the relevance of the book has grown even more, with a greater number of persons who require special care, and with increasing travel, not least by DHWs and trainees to developing countries. This text has become one of the most widely used sources of information for all DHWs who need to contend with the increasing variety of medical problems, particularly as they are aware that they face a growing risk of litigation if they do not keep themselves familiar with current knowledge, in line with the increasing acceptance of the need for continuing professional education and development. Sadly the evidence base in this area is not always strong and clinicians may need to resort to an heuristic approach. Nevertheless they should halt before making decisions when Hungry, Angry, Late or Tired!

In addition to the comments in previous prefaces, I thank Dr Andrew Narendran Robinson sincerely for his help with suggestions and literature searching, and Drs Paes de Almeida, Bagan, Carrozzo, Diz Dios, Malamos and Mosqueda for help with some new illustrations.

This edition has attempted to provide information about the most common diseases, though these, of course, vary depending on the area of the world concerned. The main killing conditions worldwide – trauma, cardiovascular disease, infectious and parasitic diseases, malignant disease, cerebrovascular disease, respiratory infections, AIDS and chronic obstructive pulmonary disease – receive considerable attention. There is detail on the other most common afflictions in resource-rich countries, such as: anaemia, the common cold, diabetes, diarrhoea, hepatitis, lung cancer, sexually shared infections and streptococcal sore throat (http://www.livestrong.com/article/161780-10-most-common-health-diseases/#ixzz25tfVtfQu; accessed 12 June 2013). Less common or rare disorders do not receive so much attention.

Although previous editions have been extremely well received, the new edition has nevertheless been updated throughout and includes several added areas – such as a number of new medications, and comment about anticonvulsant hypersensitivity syndrome, anti-synthetase syndrome, antithrombotic therapy, biological therapies, Brugada syndrome, cosmetic and other implants, darkroom syndrome, dental materials hypersensitivity (chlorhexidine, nickel, titanium), drugs and dietary interactions, E numbers, elder maltreatment, food poisoning, hypnotherapy, implanted cardiac devices, imported infections, long QT syndrome (LQTS), mass gathering medicine, medication-overuse headache, *Mycobacterium abscessus* infections, neuropathic pain, new antiretrovirals, new aspects of alternative medicine, new autoinflammatory disorders (deficiency of the interleukin-1 receptor antagonist [DIRA]; and interleukin-36–receptor antagonist deficiency), new hospital-associated infections, new oral anticoagulants, new substance abuse, *N*-methyl-D-aspartate (NMDA) antagonists such as ketamine, parenteral nutrition, propofol infusion syndrome (PRIS), radiocontrast media, recreational water illnesses, relapsing polychondritis, self-harm, sexual minorities, titanium allergy, transfusion-related immunomodulation (TRIM), vagal nerve stimulation therapy, variably protease-sensitive prionopathy (VPSPr),various newly recognised immunodeficiencies, ventilator-associated pneumonia and vulnerable people. Space precludes more than brief discussion of the association between periodontal infection and various systemic diseases, and there is no examination of forensic issues.

Many data are available nowadays on the Internet, and the explosion in numbers of guidelines means that it is nigh on impossible to summarize all of these in a book, especially avoiding ambiguities and plagiarism at the same time. Increasingly, evidence-based medicine challenges current practice – including that in vital areas such as cardiopulmonary resuscitation. Practitioners should be aware of, and use, the best evidence-based medicine, current teaching and guidance from a responsible body of opinion, which also necessitates access to updated material such as that on the Internet: for example, http://pathways.nice.org.uk/ or http://www.sign.ac.uk/guidelines/published/index.html (accessed 12 June 2013). There is a growing desire in the health-care community for specific practice guidelines but, with advances in the field, guidelines can sometimes restrict diagnostic or therapeutic options; clinician and patient education and discussions are the key, with decisions individualized. Good communication between all health-care professionals (HCPs), and between HCPs and patients, is essential and this is true for DHWs. If contrary advice is received from another HCP, a discussion around the differing opinions is advised with this practitioner.

It is important for the patient not to be compromised in any way. The discussion should be supported by evidence-based written information tailored to the person's needs. Treatment and care, and the information people are given about them, should be culturally appropriate and should take into account people's needs and preferences. It should also be accessible to those with additional needs such as physical, sensory or learning disabilities, and to people who do not speak or read English. Patients should have the opportunity to make informed decisions about their care and treatment, in partnership with their HCPs. If the person agrees, families and carers should be given the option of being involved in decisions about treatment and care. If people do not have the capacity to make decisions, HCPs should follow the UK Department of Health's advice on consent and the code of practice that accompanies the Mental Capacity Act in the UK.

The content of the book is for information and educational purposes only; in no way should it be considered as a substitute for medical consultation with a qualified professional. A physician should always be consulted for any health problem or medical condition. Clinicians are advised always to check the latest guidelines from bodies such as the National Institute for Health and Care Excellence (NICE), the Royal Colleges of Surgeons, the Royal Colleges of Physicians, the British Dental Association (BDA), the General Dental Council (GDC), the Resuscitation Council and the various specialist medical and dental societies or associations (e.g. http://www.sdcep.org.uk/). The spectre of litigation increasingly influences decisions and, although in some instances guidelines may not have led to clarity, clinicians may find their decisions difficult to defend if they fail to record a very good reason for not adhering to the guidelines. Readers should always check the most recent guidelines, drug doses, and potential reactions and interactions before use, discuss management issues with the patient, and never proceed with any intervention without the clear formal informed consent of the patient and consultation with their health-care advisers.

The comments and recommendations herein should be used as guidelines to care, not commandments. Unfortunately, there are very few randomized controlled trials available to provide evidence for the various practices, and so many of the recommendations have to be based on consensus. Any comments or criticisms from readers will, of course, be gratefully received, though I hope that the further significant improvements in this edition, together with the dearth of criticism of previous editions, means that I have fulfilled the aims as best I can. As my now-deceased co-author Professor Rod Cawson said in the preface to one of his other books: 'Some people will criticize this for being too brief, some for being too long but, sad as it may be, this is the best I can do.'

Crispian Scully
London
2014

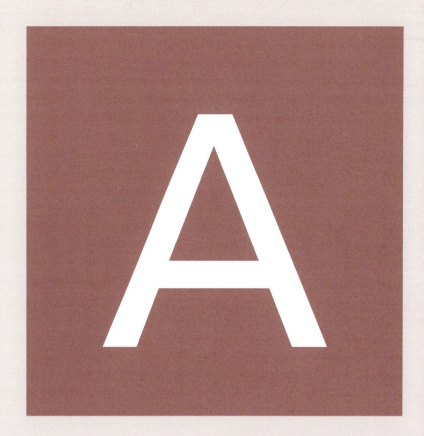

General

Medical emergencies

This chapter is focused on the main diagnostic and management issues in emergency management; fuller discussion of these conditions may be found in the relevant chapters and the controversies in this area are discussed in the references. The expanded knowledge base of medicine, and effective new technologies, techniques and drugs have allowed patients, who in earlier times would have succumbed, to remain alive and live to much greater ages; such patients in particular may be prone to medical emergencies. Collapse and other emergencies are a cause of concern for all involved (Box 1.1).

In general terms, health-care professionals (HCPs) should develop strategies to identify patients at risk of emergencies, assess the severity of those risks and, where necessary, recognize the need for help and be able to seek advice from a colleague with special competence in the relevant fields. All need to contend with the increasing variety of medical problems, particularly as they are aware that they face a growing risk of litigation if they do not keep themselves familiar with current knowledge, in line with the increasing acceptance of the need for continuing professional development (CPD).

There are few randomized controlled trials (RCTs) available to provide evidence for the various practices, and so many of the recommendations have to be based on consensus. The comments and recommendations herein should be used as guidelines to care, not commandments.

Annual theoretical and practical training of all clinical staff is required. Clinical staff have an obligation to be conversant with the current Resuscitation Council (UK) guidelines (2012) (see Further reading). The UK General Dental Council (GDC), in *Standards for the dental team* (2013), states that all dental professionals are responsible for putting patients' interests first and for acting to protect them. Central to this responsibility is the need to ensure that HCPs are able to deal with medical emergencies that may arise. All members of the dental team need to know their roles in the event of an emergency.

The GDC guidance, *Principles of dental team working* (2005), states that dental staff who employ, manage or lead a team should make sure that:

- there are arrangements for at least two people to be available to deal with medical emergencies when treatment is planned to take place
- all members of staff, not just the registered team members, know their role if a patient collapses or there is another kind of medical emergency
- all members of staff who might be involved in dealing with a medical emergency are trained and prepared to deal with such an emergency at any time, and regularly practise simulated emergencies together.

The GDC has stipulated that 10 hours of training and retraining in emergency management is a mandatory requirement of CPD in every 5-year period.

Emergencies are rare. A medical emergency occurring in dental practice is most likely to be the result of an acute deterioration of a known medical condition. It may pose an immediate threat to an individual's life and needs rapid intervention. It is best prevented! The most common medical emergency is the simple faint. Other common emergencies include fitting in an epileptic patient, angina pectoris (ischaemic chest pain), hypoglycaemia in a diabetic patient and haemorrhage. Myocardial infarction and cardiopulmonary arrest are more immediately dangerous (Box 1.2).

PREVENTING EMERGENCIES

Emergency management algorithms are of paramount importance and dental employers are ultimately responsible for the performance of their staff as regards delivery.

Confidence and satisfactory management of emergencies can be improved by the following measures:

- Repeatedly assessing the patient whilst undertaking treatment, noting any changes in appearance or behaviour.
- Never practising dentistry without another competent adult in the room.
- Always having accessible the telephone numbers of the emergency services and nearest hospital accident and emergency

---

Box 1.1 *Common emergencies*

- Collapse
- Fitting
- Chest pain
- Shortness of breath
- Mental disturbances
- Reactions to drugs or sedation
- Bleeding

Box 1.2 *Likely causes of sudden loss of consciousness and collapse*

- Simple faint
- Diabetic collapse secondary to hypoglycaemia
- Epileptic seizure
- Anaphylaxis
- Cardiac arrest
- Stroke
- Adrenal crisis

Table 1.1 *Suggested minimal equipment for emergency use in dentistry*[a]

Equipment	General comments	Detail
Oxygen (O₂) delivery	Portable apparatus for administering oxygen	Two portable oxygen cylinders ('D' size) with pressure reduction valves and flow meters. Cylinders should be of sufficient size to be easily portable but also to allow for adequate flow rates (e.g. 10 L/min), until the arrival of an ambulance or full recovery of the patient. A full 'D' size cylinder contains 340 L of oxygen and should allow a flow rate of 10 L/min for up to 30 min. Two such cylinders may be necessary to ensure the oxygen supply does not fail
	Oxygen face mask (non-rebreathe type) with tube	
	Basic set of oropharyngeal airways (sizes 1, 2, 3 and 4)	
	Pocket mask with oxygen port	
	Self-inflating bag valve mask (BVM; 1-L size bag), where staff have been appropriately trained	
	Variety of well-fitting adult and child face masks for attaching to self-inflating bag	
Portable suction	Portable suction with appropriate suction catheters and tubing (e.g. Yankauer sucker)	
Spacer device for inhalation of bronchodilators		
Automated external defibrillator (AED)	All clinical areas should have immediate access to an AED (collapse-to-shock time <3 min)	
Automated blood glucose measuring device		
Equipment for administering drugs intramuscularly	Single-use sterile syringes (2-mL and 10-mL sizes) and needles (19 and 21 sizes)	Drugs as in Table 1.2

[a]After Resuscitation Council (2012).

department. Details of the patient's general medical practitioner should be recorded in the notes.

- Training staff in emergency service contact protocols and emergency procedures. This should be repeated annually. All clinics should have a defined protocol for how the emergency services are to be alerted. The protocol should include clear directions to enable the emergency services to locate and access the clinic. In a large building, a member of the team should meet the emergency services at the main entrance.
- Having a readily accessible emergency drugs box and equipment that is checked on a weekly basis (Tables 1.1 and 1.2; Figs 1.1–1.3).
- Taking a careful medical history, assessing disease severity, scheduling and planning treatment carefully, and, in some cases, administering medication prior to treatment.
- Using the simple intervention of laying the patient supine prior to giving local analgesia/anaesthesia (LA). This will prevent virtually all simple faints.
- Ensuring that diabetic patients have had their normal meals, medication has been appropriately administered, and treatment is given early in the morning session or immediately after lunch. These measures are likely to prevent most hypoglycaemic collapses.

All this is even more important when conscious sedation (CS) is used, when invasive or painful procedures are planned, or when medically complex individuals are being treated. 'Forewarned is forearmed,' and dental professionals must ensure that medical and drug histories are updated at each visit prior to initiating treatment. It is suggested that disease severity should be assessed using a risk stratification system – for example, the American Society of Anesthesiologists (ASA) classification (Chs 2 and 3) – as this may help identify high-risk individuals.

Few emergencies can be treated definitively in the dental clinic. The role of the dental team is one of support and considered intervention using algorithms that can 'do no harm'. Previously, it has been suggested that 20 or more drugs should be available to the dental professional for the management of emergencies but this is impractical, may

Table 1.2 *Suggested minimal drugs for emergency use in dentistry*[a]

Emergency	Drugs required	Dosages for adults
Anaphylaxis	Adrenaline (epinephrine) injection 1:1000, 1 mg/mL	Intramuscular adrenaline (0.5 mL of 1 in 1000 solution)
		Repeat at 5 min if needed
Hypoglycaemia	Oral glucose solution/tablets/gel/powder (e.g. GlucoGel®, formerly known as Hypostop® gel [40% dextrose])	Proprietary non-diet drink or 5 g glucose powder in water
	Glucagon injection 1 mg (e.g. GlucaGen HypoKit)	Intramuscular glucagon 1 mg
Acute exacerbation of asthma	(β₂ agonist)	Salbutamol aerosol
	Salbutamol aerosol inhaler 100 mcg/activation	Activations directly or up to six into a spacer
Status epilepticus	Buccal or intranasal midazolam 10 mg/mL	Midazolam 10 mg
Angina	Glyceryl trinitrate[b] spray 400 mcg/metered activation	Glyceryl trinitrate, two sprays
Myocardial infarct	Dispersible aspirin 300 mg	Dispersible aspirin 300 mg (chewed)

[a]After Resuscitation Council (2012). No corticosteroid is included.
[b]Do not use nitrates to relieve an angina attack if the patient has recently taken sildenafil, as there may be a precipitous fall in blood pressure; analgesics should be used. Where possible, all emergency equipment should be single-use and latex-free. The kit does not include any intravenous injections.

be a source of confusion and, if a drug is incorrectly administered, may be life-threatening.

The Resuscitation Council recommendations for equipment and drugs are detailed in Tables 1.1 and 1.2. Other agents (e.g. the midazolam antagonist flumazenil) and equipment (e.g. a pulse oximeter) are needed if CS is administered.

General anaesthesia (GA) must be undertaken only by anaesthetists and where advanced life support (ALS) is available.

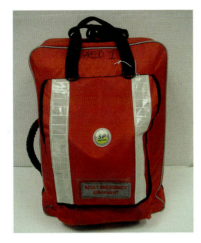

Fig. 1.1 Emergency kit.

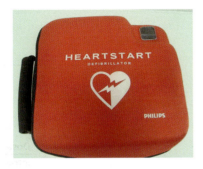

Fig. 1.2 Automatic defibrillator.

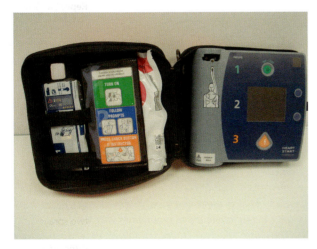

Fig. 1.3 Automatic external defibrillator (AED).

RESUSCITATION AND EMERGENCIES

The GDC does not have any guidelines on resuscitation but would refer registrants to the Resuscitation Council, which does have relevant guidance. Full details are available at http://www.gdc-uk.org/Dentalprofessionals/Standards/Pages/home.aspx (accessed 30 September 2013).

The GDC's *Principles of dental team working* (2005) covers medical emergencies.

MANAGING EMERGENCIES

For all medical emergencies, a structured approach to assessment and reassessment prevents any symptoms and signs being missed and any

Box 1.3 *Assessment in emergencies*	
Airway	Identify foreign body obstruction and stridor
Breathing	Document respiratory rate, use of accessory muscles, presence of wheeze or cyanosis
Circulation	Assess skin colour and temperature, estimate capillary refill time (normally, 2 s with hand above heart), assess rate of pulse (normal is 70 beats/min)
Disability	Assess conscious level using acronym AVPU: • Alert • responds to *Voice* • responds to *Painful* stimulus • *Unresponsive* • Blood glucose
Exposure	Respecting the patient's dignity, try to elicit the cause of acute deterioration (e.g. rash, signs of recreational drug use)

incorrect diagnoses being made. The sequence is best remembered as 'ABCDE' (Box 1.3). 'Drs ABC' highlights the sequence:

- *d*anger (recognizing an emergency)
- *r*espiration (establishing an airway)
- *s*hout for help.
- *A*; airway
- *B*; breathing
- *C*; circulation

People who collapse should be put in the 'recovery position' to maintain a clear airway UNLESS there could be a neck injury, such as after a fall or road traffic accident.

CARDIOPULMONARY RESUSCITATION

Dental staff should be trained in basic cardiopulmonary resuscitation (CPR) so that, in the event of cardiac arrest, they should be able to:

- recognize cardiac arrest (the heart stops beating)
- summon immediate help (dial for the emergency services)
- initiate CPR according to current resuscitation guidelines (evidence suggests that chest compressions can be effectively performed in a dental chair)
- ventilate with high-concentration oxygen via a bag and mask
- apply an automated external defibrillator (AED) as soon as possible after collapse. Follow the machine prompts and administer a shock if indicated, with a maximum collapse-to-shock time of 3 minutes.

Hands-only CPR

- Call the emergency services
- Push hard and fast in the centre of the chest to double a person's chances of survival (the song 'Stayin' Alive' has the right beat for hands-only CPR)
- The method of delivering chest compressions remains the same, as does the rate (at least 100 per minute).

EMERGENCY PROCEDURE

- Call for local assistance
- Assess the patient – ABCDE (as Box 1.3) – and give oxygen if appropriate
- Use the acronym MOVE:
  *M*onitor – reassess ABCDE regularly, attach an AED if appropriate
  *O*xygen – 15 L/min through a non-rebreathe mask
  *V*erify – check that emergency services are coming
  *E*mergency action – correct positioning and drug administration.

Intramuscular (i.m.) injection is used nowadays for giving most emergency drugs. The most accessible site in a clothed patient sitting in a dental chair is the lateral aspect of the thigh. There the vastus lateralis is a large muscle with no large nerves or arteries running through it. In an emergency, the injection can be administered through clothing. The mid-point between the pelvis and the knee is the preferred site.

The Advanced Medical Priority Dispatch System (AMPDS) is a unified system that sends appropriate aid to medical emergencies, including systematized caller interrogation and pre-arrival instructions. AMPDS works on the following response categories:

- A (immediately life-threatening)
- B (urgent call)
- C (routine call).

This may well be linked to a performance targeting system where calls must be responded to within a given time period. For example, in the UK, calls rated as 'A' on AMPDS aim to have a responder on scene within 8 minutes.

The 'ABCDE' approach to the sick patient

The 'ABCDE' approach to the sick patient is outlined at http://www.resus.org.uk/pages/MEdental.pdf by the UK Resuscitation Council (2006, updated 2012; accessed 30 September 2013). Appendix (i), which cannot be bettered, and states:

Dental Practitioners, Dental Care Professionals and their staff should be familiar with standard resuscitation procedures as recommended by the Resuscitation Council (UK). In all circumstances it is advisable to call for medical assistance as soon as possible by dialling 999 and summoning an ambulance.

Early recognition of the 'sick' patient is to be encouraged. Pre-empting any medical emergency by recognising an abnormal breathing pattern, an abnormal patient colour or abnormal pulse rate, allows appropriate help to be summoned, e.g. ambulance, prior to any patient collapse occurring. A systematic approach to recognising the acutely ill patient based on the 'ABCDE' principles is recommended. Accurate documentation of the patient's medical history should further allow those 'at risk' of certain medical emergencies to be identified in advance of any proposed treatment. The elective nature of most dental practice allows time for discussion of medical problems with the patient's general medical practitioner where necessary. In certain circumstances this may lead to a postponement of the treatment indicated or a recommendation that such treatment be undertaken in hospital.

General principles

1. *Follow the Airway, Breathing, Circulation, Disability, and Exposure approach (ABCDE) to assess and treat the patient.*
2. *Treat life-threatening problems as they are identified before moving to the next part of the assessment.*
3. *Continually reassess, starting with Airway, if there is further deterioration.*
4. *Assess the effects of any treatment given.*
5. *Recognise when you need extra help and call for help early. This may mean dialling 999 for an ambulance.*
6. *Use all members of your dental team. This will allow you to do several things at once, e.g. collect emergency drugs and equipment, dial 999.*
7. *Organise your team and communicate effectively.*

8. *The aims of initial treatment are to keep the patient alive, achieve some clinical improvement and buy time for further treatment whilst waiting for help.*
9. *Remember – it can take a few minutes for treatment to work.*
10. *The ABCDE approach can be used irrespective of your training and experience in clinical assessment or treatment. Individual experience and training will determine which treatments you can give. Often only simple measures such as laying the patient down or giving oxygen are needed.*

First steps

- *In an emergency, stay calm. Ensure that you and your staff are safe.*
- *Look at the patient generally to see if they 'look unwell'.*
- *In an awake patient ask, 'How are you?' If the patient is unresponsive, shake him and ask, 'Are you all right?' If they respond normally, they have a clear airway, are breathing and have brain perfusion. If they speak only in short sentences, they may have breathing problems. Failure of the patient to respond suggests that they are unwell. If they are not breathing and have no pulse or signs of life, start CPR according to current resuscitation guidelines.*

Airway (A)

Airway obstruction is an emergency.

1. *Look for the signs of airway obstruction:*
   - *Airway obstruction causes 'paradoxical' chest and abdominal movements ('see-saw' respirations) and the use of the accessory muscles of respiration, e.g. neck muscles. Central cyanosis (blue lips and tongue) is a late sign of airway obstruction. In complete airway obstruction, there are no breath sounds at the mouth or nose.*
   - *In partial airway obstruction, air entry is diminished and usually noisy:*
     Inspiratory 'stridor' is caused by obstruction at the laryngeal level or above.
     Expiratory 'wheeze' suggests obstruction of the lower airways, which tend to collapse and obstruct during expiration. This is most commonly seen in patients with asthma or chronic obstructive pulmonary disease.
     Gurgling suggests there is liquid or semi-solid foreign material in the upper airway.
     Snoring arises when the pharynx is partially occluded by the tongue or palate.
2. *Airway obstruction is an emergency:*
   - *In most cases, only simple methods of airway clearance are needed:*
     Airway opening manœuvres – head tilt/chin lift or jaw thrust.
     Remove visible foreign bodies, debris or blood from the airway (use suction or forceps as necessary).
     Consider simple airway adjuncts, e.g. oropharyngeal airway.
3. *Give oxygen initially at a high inspired concentration:*
   - *Use a mask with an oxygen reservoir. Ensure that the oxygen flow is sufficient (15 litres per minute) to prevent collapse of the reservoir during inspiration.*
   - *If you have a pulse oximeter, titrate the oxygen delivery aiming for normal oxygen saturation levels (94–98%).*

In very sick patients this may not be possible and a lower oxygen saturation (more than 90%) is acceptable for a short period of time.

Breathing (B)

During the immediate assessment of breathing, it is vital to diagnose and treat immediately life-threatening breathing problems, e.g. acute severe asthma.

1. *Look, listen and feel for the general signs of respiratory distress: sweating, central cyanosis (blue lips and tongue), use of the accessory muscles of respiration (muscles of the neck) and abdominal breathing.*
2. *Count the respiratory rate. The normal adult rate is 12 to 20 breaths per minute and a child's rate is between 20 and 30 breaths per minute. A high, or increasing, respiratory rate is a marker of illness and a warning that the patient may deteriorate and further medical help is needed.*
3. *Assess the depth of each breath, the pattern (rhythm) of respiration and whether chest expansion is equal and normal on both sides.*
4. *Listen to the patient's breath sounds a short distance from their face. Gurgling airway noises indicate airway secretions, usually because the patient cannot cough or take a deep breath. Stridor or wheeze suggests partial, but important, airway obstruction.*
5. *If the patient's depth or rate of breathing is inadequate, or you cannot detect any breathing, use bag and mask (if trained) or pocket mask ventilation with supplemental oxygen while calling urgently for an ambulance.*
6. *Hyperventilation and panic attacks are relatively common in general dental practice. In most patients these will resolve with simple reassurance.*

Circulation (C)

Simple faints or vasovagal episodes are the most likely cause of circulation problems in general dental practice. These will usually respond to laying the patient flat and, if necessary, raising the legs (see Appendix (ii) Syncope). The systematic ABCDE approach to all patients will ensure that other causes are not missed.

1. *Look at the colour of the hands and fingers: are they blue, pink, pale or mottled?*
2. *Assess the limb temperature by feeling the patient's hands: are they cool or warm?*
3. *Measure the capillary refill time. Apply cutaneous pressure for five seconds on a fingertip held at heart level (or just above) with enough pressure to cause blanching. Time how long it takes for the skin to return to the colour of the surrounding skin after releasing the pressure. The normal refill time is less than two seconds. A prolonged time suggests poor peripheral perfusion. Other factors (e.g. cold surroundings, old age) can also prolong the capillary refill time.*
4. *Count the patient's pulse rate. It may be easier to feel a central pulse (i.e. carotid pulse) than the radial pulse.*
5. *Weak pulses in a patient with a decreased conscious level and slow capillary refill time suggest a low blood pressure. Laying the patient down and raising the legs may be helpful. In patients who do not respond to simple measures urgent help is needed and an ambulance should be summoned.*

6. *Cardiac chest pain typically presents as a heaviness, tightness or indigestion-like discomfort in the chest. The pain or discomfort often radiates into the neck or throat, into one or both arms (more commonly the left) and into the back or stomach area. Some patients experience the discomfort in one of these areas more than in the chest. Sometimes pain may be accompanied by belching, which can be misinterpreted as evidence of indigestion as the cause. The patient may have known stable angina and carry their own glyceryl trinitrate (GTN) spray or tablets. If they take these, the episode may resolve. If the patient has sustained chest pain, give GTN spray if the patient has not already taken some. The patient may feel better and should be encouraged to sit upright if possible. Give a single dose of aspirin and consider the use of oxygen.*

(See Appendix (ii) Cardiac Emergencies.)

Disability (D)

Common causes of unconsciousness include profound hypoxia, hypercapnia (raised carbon dioxide levels), cerebral hypoperfusion (low blood pressure), or the recent administration of sedatives or analgesic drugs.

1. *Review and treat the ABCs: exclude hypoxia and low blood pressure.*
2. *Check the patient's drug record for reversible drug-induced causes of depressed consciousness.*
3. *Examine the pupils (size, equality and reaction to light).*
4. *Make a rapid initial assessment of the patient's conscious level using the AVPU method: Alert, responds to Vocal stimuli, responds to Painful stimuli or Unresponsive to all stimuli.*
5. *Measure the blood glucose to exclude hypoglycaemia, using a glucose meter. If below 3.0 mmol per litre give the patient a glucose containing drink to raise the blood sugar (e.g. Glucogel; Dextrogel; GSF-syrup or Rapilose gel: see Appendix (ii) Hypoglycaemia) or glucose by other means.*
6. *Nurse unconscious patients in the recovery position if their airway is not protected.*

Exposure (E)

To assess and treat the patient properly loosening or removal of some of the patient's clothes may be necessary. Respect the patient's dignity and minimize heat loss. This will allow you to see any rashes (e.g. anaphylaxis) or perform procedures (e.g. defibrillation).

COMMON EMERGENCIES

See also Appendix 1.1 for the Resuscitation Council guidelines (2012) on dealing with common emergencies.

COLLAPSE (TABLE 1.3)

The cause of sudden loss of consciousness may be suggested by the medical history:

- Collapse at the sight of a needle or during an injection is likely to be a simple faint.
- Following some minutes after an injection of penicillin, collapse is more likely to be due to anaphylaxis.

Table 1.3 *Common emergencies*

Emergency	Recognition	Actions; reassure patient and accompanying people, and			
		1. Call for assistance	2. Give oxygen 15 L/min	3. Other main actions	4. Alert emergency services
Anaphylaxis	Acute Collapse Rash Angioedema Wheezing	Yes	Yes	Adrenaline (epinephrine) 500 mcg for adult i.m. (0.5 mL of 1 in 1000 adrenaline) Legs-up position	Yes
Angina	Severe chest pain, responding to glyceryl trinitrate	Yes	Yes	Glyceryl trinitrate 2 puffs sublingually	Only if no spontaneous recovery after action (3)
Asthma exacerbation	Breathless Wheeze Speechlessness Possible cyanosis	Yes	Yes	Sit patient up and forwards, salbutamol 2 × 100 mcg puffs for adult inhaled via spacer	If no spontaneous recovery after action (3)
Cardiac arrest	Severe chest pain, not responding to glyceryl trinitrate Collapse Pallor Breathlessness Sweating	Yes	Yes	Glyceryl trinitrate 2 puffs and aspirin 300 mg sublingually CPR	Yes
Choking	Inhaled foreign material Coughing Choking	Yes	Yes	Back slap five times, then abdominal thrust five times	Only if no spontaneous recovery after action (3)
Epileptic fit	Collapse Seizures Maybe incontinence	Yes	Yes	Protect patient from harm Consider midazolam 10 mg for adult in buccal mucosa (or i.m. or sublingually)	Only if no spontaneous or other recovery after 5 min, persistent altered conscious state or the fit characteristics are different to those previously described
Faint	Collapse, responding to laying flat Pallor Slow pulse Sweating No chest pain	Yes	No*	Lay patient flat Give glucose orally	Only if no spontaneous recovery after action (3)
Hypoglycaemia	Confusion or aggression, often known diabetes Shake or tremor Collapse	Yes	Yes	Blood glucose assay Give glucose drink, gel or tablets If unconscious, glucagon 1 mg for adult i.m.	Only if no spontaneous recovery after action (3)
Stroke	Face weakness Arm weakness Speech difficulties (Test all above)	Yes	Yes	–	Yes

*Not essential but oxygen may do no harm.

- Collapse of a diabetic at lunchtime, for example, is likely to be caused by hypoglycaemia.
- Collapse of a patient with angina or previous myocardial infarction may be caused by a new or further myocardial infarction.

The clinical features of the episode may also aid diagnosis; for example, severe chest pain suggests a cardiac cause. A structured and systematic assessment, regardless of perceived causative factors, is required to mitigate management errors.

For collapse of uncertain cause, see Table 1.3 and Figure 1.4.

The principles of the *chain of survival*, which applies to emergencies where the patient is not breathing and has no pulse, involve four stages:

- Early recognition and call for help
- Early CPR

- Early defibrillation
- Early ALS.

SIMPLE FAINT

Fainting (syncope) is the most common cause of sudden loss of consciousness. It is associated with a loss of postural tone, and there is spontaneous recovery. Up to 2% of patients may faint before or during dental treatment. Young, fit, adult males in particular are prone to faint, especially before, during and after injections.

Vasovagal (vasodepressor) attack (or pressure on the vagus) is the usual cause of a simple faint. The diagnosis rests on the history, upright posture, an emotional or painful stimulus, gradual not sudden

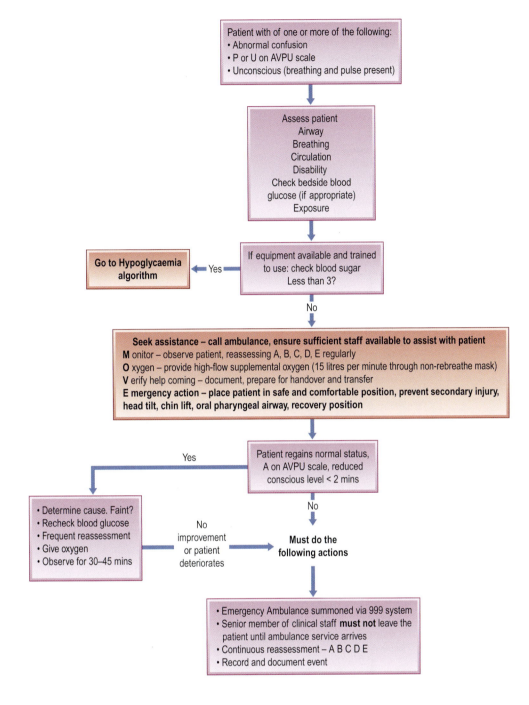

Fig. 1.4 Reduced consciousness algorithm.

fading of consciousness, sweating, nausea, pallor, other manifestations of autonomic activity, and rapid recovery on lying down. Simple faints tend to occur, and recur, in young people.

Other causes of sudden loss of consciousness include:

- situational syncope provoked by coughing, micturition (urination) or postural change
- sudden cardiac syncope due to arrhythmia or circulatory obstruction – typically in older people
- orthostatic hypotension
- neurological disorders.

These should be considered in the differential diagnosis.

Predisposing factors for vasovagal attack include:

- anxiety
- pain
- fatigue

- fasting (rarely)
- high temperature and relative humidity.

Signs and symptoms of a simple faint include:

- premonitory dizziness, weakness or nausea
- pallor
- cold, clammy skin
- dilated pupils
- pulse that is initially slow and weak, then rapid and full
- loss of consciousness.

The simple precaution of laying patients flat *before* giving injections will prevent fainting. Very rarely, patients can suffer *malignant vasovagal syncope* with recurrent, severe and otherwise unexplained syncope; their clinical history is intermediate between that of vasovagal and cardiac syncope, and diagnosis is confirmed by a tilt test.

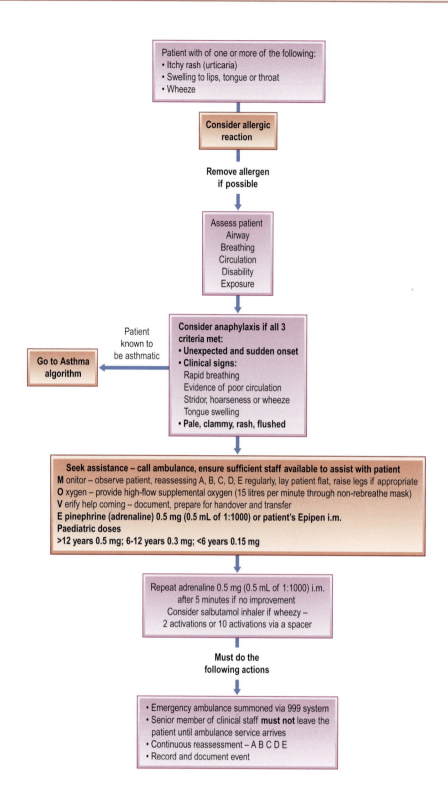

Patient with of one or more of the following:
• Itchy rash (urticaria)
• Swelling to lips, tongue or throat
• Wheeze

Consider allergic reaction

Remove allergen if possible

Assess patient
Airway
Breathing
Circulation
Disability
Exposure

Patient known to be asthmatic

Go to Asthma algorithm

Consider anaphylaxis if all 3 criteria met:
• **Unexpected and sudden onset**
• **Clinical signs:**
Rapid breathing
Evidence of poor circulation
Stridor, hoarseness or wheeze
Tongue swelling
• **Pale, clammy, rash, flushed**

Seek assistance – call ambulance, ensure sufficient staff available to assist with patient
M onitor – observe patient, reassessing A, B, C, D, E regularly, lay patient flat, raise legs if appropriate
O xygen – provide high-flow supplemental oxygen (15 litres per minute through non-rebreathe mask)
V erify help coming – document, prepare for handover and transfer
E pinephrine (adrenaline) 0.5 mg (0.5 mL of 1:1000) or patient's Epipen i.m.
Paediatric doses
>12 years 0.5 mg; 6-12 years 0.3 mg; <6 years 0.15 mg

Repeat adrenaline 0.5 mg (0.5 mL of 1:1000) i.m.
after 5 minutes if no improvement
Consider salbutamol inhaler if wheezy –
2 activations or 10 activations via a spacer

Must do the following actions

• Emergency ambulance summoned via 999 system
• Senior member of clinical staff **must not** leave the patient until ambulance service arrives
• Continuous reassessment – A B C D E
• Record and document event

Fig. 1.5 Anaphylaxis algorithm.

ANAPHYLAXIS

■ Always detail known allergies and the severity of any previous type 1 hypersensitivity reactions.
■ Avoid possible allergens and, when this is not possible, refer the patient for specialist assessment.
■ Life-threatening anaphylaxis may occur, despite no previous history of allergen exposure.
■ Anaphylaxis is the most severe allergic response and manifests with acute hypotension, bronchospasm, urticaria rash and angioedema (Fig. 1.5).

■ The causal agents include:
penicillins – the most common cause, but also other antimicrobials (cephalosporins, sulphonamides, tetracyclines, vancomycin)
latex
muscle relaxants
non-steroidal anti-inflammatory drugs (NSAIDs)
opiates
radiographic contrast media
others – vaccines, immunoglobulins, various foods and insect bites.

- Strict avoidance of the causal agent is essential.
- Where there is a previous history of anaphylaxis, the patient should carry a self-administered i.m. injection device, e.g. EpiPen® (ALK-Abelló, Hungerford, Berkshire, UK) or Twinject® (Verus Pharmaceuticals, San Diego, California, USA) (or less commonly, an adrenaline (epinephrine) aerosol, such as MedihalerEpi). Patients should carry 2 EpiPens® with them because >35% of patients may require more than one adrenaline dose and up to 20% of patients will go on to develop a biphasic anaphylactic response sometimes hours later. The standard dosage of adrenaline supplied by an EpiPen for adults is 0.3 mL of 1 in 1000 (0.3 mg). Child-sized dosages (0.15 mg) are available as the EpiPen JR.
- Diagnosis is as follows:
  facial flushing, itching, paraesthesiae, oedema or sometimes urticaria, or peripheral cold clammy skin
  stridor or wheeze
  abdominal pain, nausea
  loss of consciousness
  pallor progressing to cyanosis
  rapid, weak or impalpable pulse.

Management

Treatment of an anaphylactic reaction should be based on general life-support principles:

- Use the ABCDE approach to recognize and treat problems.
- Call for help early.
- Treat the greatest threat to life first.
- Do not delay initial treatments because of the lack of a complete history or definite diagnosis.

Patients having an anaphylactic reaction in any setting should expect the following as a minimum:

- Recognition that they are seriously unwell
- An early call for help
- Initial assessment and treatments based on an ABCDE approach
- Adrenaline (epinephrine) therapy if indicated
- Investigation and follow-up by an allergy specialist.

CARDIAC ARREST

- Cardiac arrest can occur in a patient with no previous history of cardiac problems, but is more likely in those with a history of ischaemic heart disease, in diabetics and older people.
- Previous angina or myocardial infarction predispose to cardiac arrest.
- Ventricular fibrillation accounts for most sudden cardiac arrests. Causes include myocardial infarction, hypoxia, drug overdose, anaphylaxis, severe infection or severe hypotension.
- After airway and breathing assessment, basic life support (BLS) needs to be initiated immediately to maintain adequate cerebral perfusion until the underlying cause is reversed (Fig. 1.6).
- Basic life support comprises:
  initial assessment
  airway maintenance
  chest compression
  ventilation.

Management

See Figures 1.5 and 1.7.

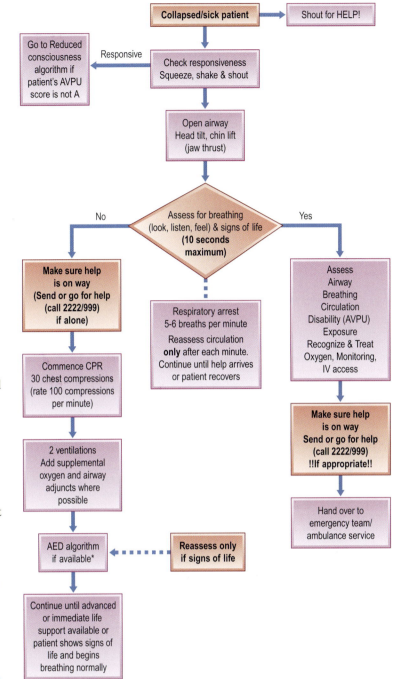

Fig. 1.6 Cardiac arrest – basic life support algorithm (*see Fig. 1.7).

DIABETIC COLLAPSE: HYPOGLYCAEMIA

- Hypoglycaemia is dangerous because the brain becomes starved of glucose.
- Diabetics treated with insulin, those with poor blood glucose control and those with poor awareness of their hypoglycaemic episodes have a greater chance of losing consciousness.
- Remember that a collapse in a diabetic may be caused by other emergencies, e.g. a faint or myocardial infarction. Ischaemic heart disease is common in long-standing diabetes.
- Hypoglycaemia may present as a deepening drowsiness, disorientation, excitability or aggressiveness, especially if it is known that a meal has been missed.
- A management algorithm is provided in Figure 1.8.

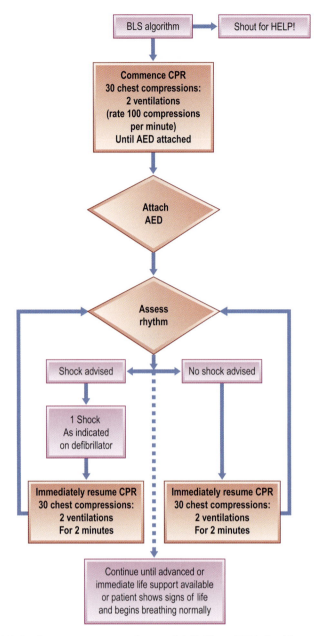

Fig. 1.7 Cardiac arrest – automated external defibrillator (AED) algorithm.

FITTING

- Fits are usually seen in known epileptics.
- Various factors may precipitate a fit, including not eating, cessation of anticonvulsant therapy, menstruation and some drugs, such as alcohol, flumazenil or tricyclic antidepressants.
- Fits may also affect people with no history of epilepsy, especially following hypoxia from loss of consciousness for other reasons or in hypoglycaemia.
- Diagnosis of a tonic–clonic (grand mal) seizure is as follows:
  loss of consciousness with rigid, extended body, which is sometimes preceded by a brief cry
  widespread jerking movements
  possible incontinence of urine and/or faeces
  slow recovery with the patient sometimes remaining dazed (post-ictal).
- A management algorithm for the fitting patient is shown in Figure 1.9.

Guidance from the Resuscitation Council is as follows:

If a patient continues to fit after an ambulance has been called then the emergency administration of buccal midazolam to assist in terminating the seizure is warranted. The dose is 10 mg for adults and an appropriately reduced dose for children. The evidence for using midazolam in this manner and for this indication is strong. It is recommended in the British National Formulary, by the Advanced Paediatric Life Support course, the National Epilepsy organisations and the Royal College of Paediatrics and Child Health. After many years of using midazolam for seizure control as an 'unlicensed' product, the drug has recently acquired a paediatric use marketing authorisation (PUMA) from the European Commission and as such is now classed as a 'licensed' product. 'Buccolam' is available as a 5 mg/ml solution for use in children up to 17 years old. Its use in adults will therefore remain 'off license' but the recommended dose is the same as that for the older child, i.e. 10 mg (2 ml). This 'off license' use is justified in the emergency situation described above. In both the 'licensed' and 'off licensed' setting, the drug does not need to have been prescribed to the patient when used in an emergency. It should, however, be administered by (or under the supervision of) a dental practitioner. There have been concerns regarding the reclassification of midazolam as a 'Schedule 3' Controlled Drug. Such reclassification requires certain legal processes. However, the law for this Schedule 3 drug does NOT require safe custody, i.e. locked cupboard, nor the need to keep a midazolam controlled drug register. Some institutions are encouraging such practices as part of their own Health and Safety protocols but there is no legal obligation to do so. Similarly, concerns have been raised about acquiring stocks of midazolam for use in the emergency setting of seizure control. A dentist can issue a requisition for any licensed product for use within their practice, as appropriate. The dentist will need to use the standardized requisition form, FP10CDF. Dental practitioners who do not use midazolam regularly are permitted to requisition this Schedule 3 Drug under the conditions laid out by the Royal Pharmaceutical Society of Great Britain in their guidance 'Medicines, Ethics and Practice: the professional guide for pharmacists'.

CHEST PAIN

- Acute severe chest pain is usually caused by angina or, less commonly, myocardial infarction.
- Patients with 'unstable' angina and those with a recent history of hospital admission for ischaemic chest pain have the highest risk, and should not be considered for routine dental treatment in primary care.
- Diagnostic features include:
  severe crushing retrosternal pain radiating down the left arm
  breathlessness that may be described as 'heartburn'
  vomiting and loss of consciousness if there is an infarct
  weak or irregular pulse if there is an infarct.
- Management is detailed in Figure 1.10.

SHORTNESS OF BREATH

ACUTE SEVERE ASTHMA

- Anxiety, infection, or exposure to an allergen or drugs may precipitate asthma.
- High-risk asthmatics include those individuals who:
  take oral medication in addition to inhaled β_2 agonists and corticosteroids

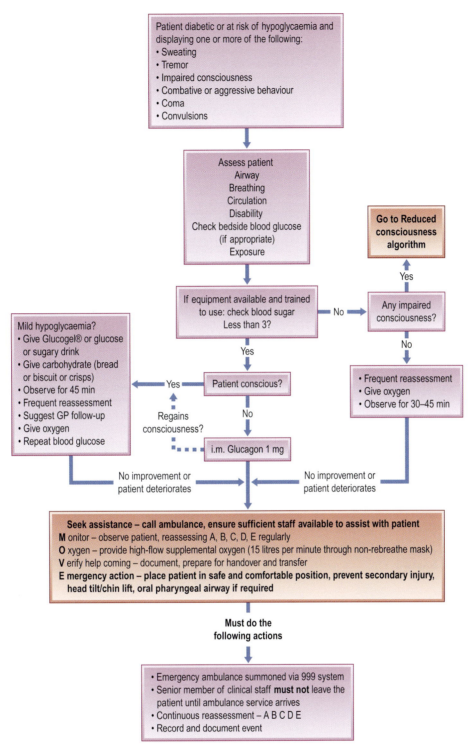

Fig. 1.8 Hypoglycaemia algorithm.

use a nebulizer regularly at home
have required oral steroids for their asthma within the last year
have been admitted to hospital with asthma within the last year.

- Diagnostic features are:
  breathlessness
  expiratory wheeze
  use of accessory muscles – shrugging the shoulders with each
  respiratory cycle with increased severity
  rapid pulse (usually over 110 beats/min) with increasing severity
  but this may slow in life-threatening exacerbation.
- Management is detailed in Figure 1.11.

FOREIGN BODY RESPIRATORY OBSTRUCTION

- Causes of respiratory obstruction include laryngeal spasm and
  foreign body. Although these may occur in any individual, the
  sedated patient poses a significant risk.
- Prevention of inhalation of foreign bodies, including teeth,
  crowns, filling materials or endodontic instruments, is far better
  than the event occurring. At the least, such an event causes
  great embarrassment, at worst respiratory obstruction, lung
  abscess or death.
- Use a rubber dam.

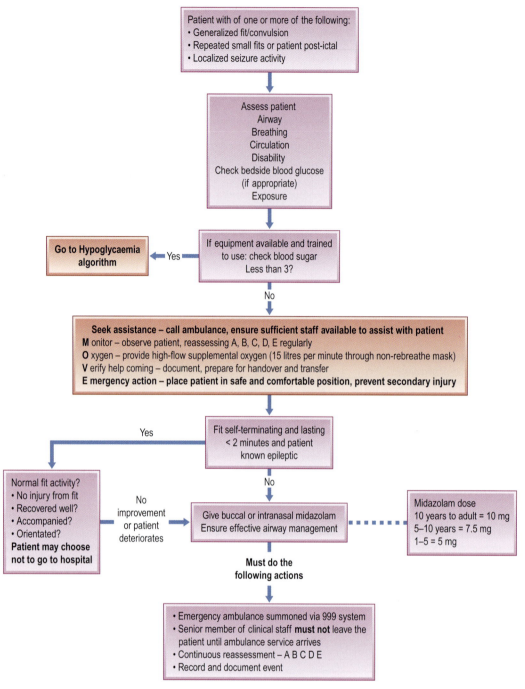

Patient with of one or more of the following:
• Generalized fit/convulsion
• Repeated small fits or patient post-ictal
• Localized seizure activity

Assess patient
Airway
Breathing
Circulation
Disability
Check bedside blood glucose
(if appropriate)
Exposure

Go to Hypoglycaemia algorithm ←Yes— If equipment available and trained to use: check blood sugar Less than 3?

No

Seek assistance – call ambulance, ensure sufficient staff available to assist with patient
M onitor – observe patient, reassessing A, B, C, D, E regularly
O xygen – provide high-flow supplemental oxygen (15 litres per minute through non-rebreathe mask)
V erify help coming – document, prepare for handover and transfer
E mergency action – place patient in safe and comfortable position, prevent secondary injury

Yes — Fit self-terminating and lasting < 2 minutes and patient known epileptic

No

Normal fit activity?
• No injury from fit
• Recovered well?
• Accompanied?
• Orientated?
Patient may choose not to go to hospital

←No improvement or patient deteriorates—

Give buccal or intranasal midazolam
Ensure effective airway management

Midazolam dose
10 years to adult = 10 mg
5–10 years = 7.5 mg
1–5 = 5 mg

Must do the following actions

• Emergency ambulance summoned via 999 system
• Senior member of clinical staff **must not** leave the patient until ambulance service arrives
• Continuous reassessment – A B C D E
• Record and document event

Fig. 1.9 Fitting/convulsions algorithm.

■ Diagnosis is as follows:
irregular breathing with crowing or croaking on inspiration
violent respiratory efforts using accessory muscles
deepening cyanosis.
■ Management is shown in Figures 1.12 and 1.13.

■ Diagnosis varies with the size and site of brain damage but typically includes:
loss of consciousness
unilateral weakness of the arm and leg
facial palsy.
■ Management details are shown in Box 1.4.

LESS COMMON EMERGENCIES

STROKE

■ Stroke may rarely occur in apparently healthy patients, but is more common in older and hypertensive individuals. A history of stroke predisposes to a further event.

ADRENAL CRISIS: COLLAPSE OF A PATIENT WITH A HISTORY OF CORTICOSTEROID THERAPY

■ Collapse in a patient with Addison disease or a history of systemic corticosteroid therapy may be caused by adrenal insufficiency, triggered by general anaesthesia, trauma, infections or other stress, but has never been recorded in primary dental care.

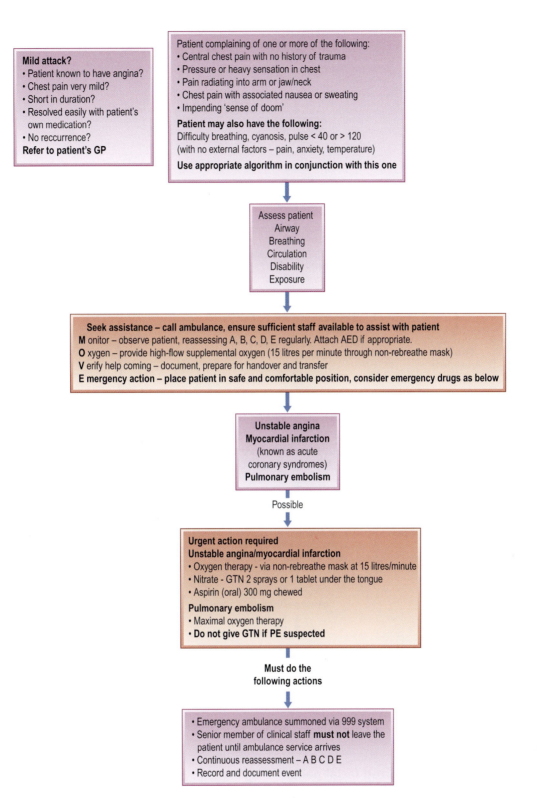

Fig. 1.10 Chest pain algorithm.

- Prevention of this emergency is contentious and will be dealt with in Chapter 6.
- Diagnosis is as follows:
  pallor
  pulse – rapid, weak or impalpable
  loss of consciousness
  rapidly falling blood pressure.
- Management is detailed in Figure 1.14.

REACTIONS TO DRUGS OR SEDATION

Intravascular injection of local anaesthetic agent

- Diagnostic features may include:
  agitation
  confusion
  drowsiness
  fitting
  eventually, loss of consciousness.
- Management is detailed in Box 1.5.

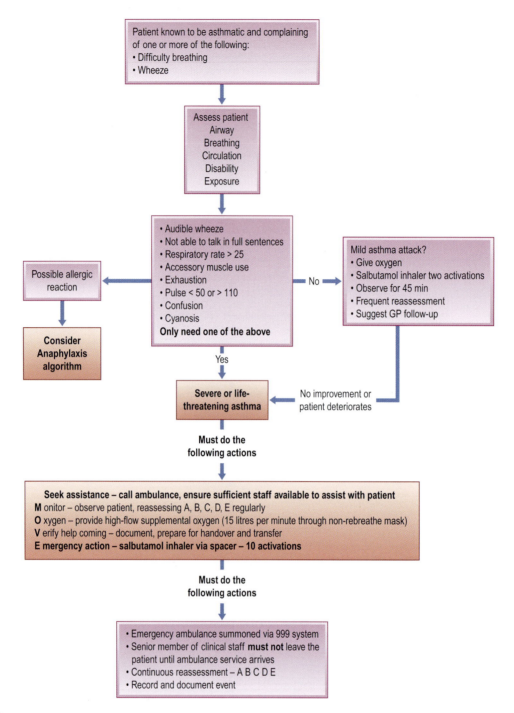

Fig. 1.11 Asthma algorithm.

Temporary facial palsy, diplopia or localized facial pallor

- These occur rarely as a result of action of the anaesthetic agent on the facial nerve or orbital contents; the transient effects resolve.
- If the individual is unable to blink, the eyelids should be taped closed until the anaesthetic abates.

Local anaesthetic allergy

- Allergy to LA is managed as for anaphylaxis, but is very rare.

Cardiovascular reactions to local anaesthetic

- Usually, only palpitations are experienced.
- Identify the likely cause and reassure the patient.

- Await natural subsidence of symptoms.
- If chest pain occurs, treat as above.
- Where possible, defer further immediate dental treatment.

Hypotension resulting from interaction with antihypertensive drugs

- Assess and clear the airway.
- Assess breathing and administer oxygen.
- Assess circulation.
- Lay the patient flat.
- Reassure.
- Summon assistance.
- Where possible, defer further immediate dental treatment.

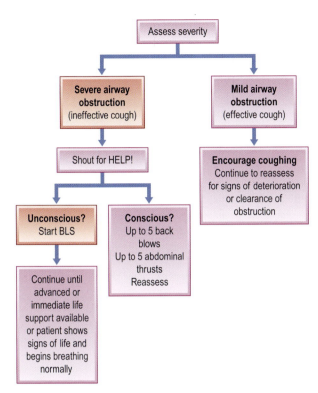

Fig. 1.12 Choking algorithm.

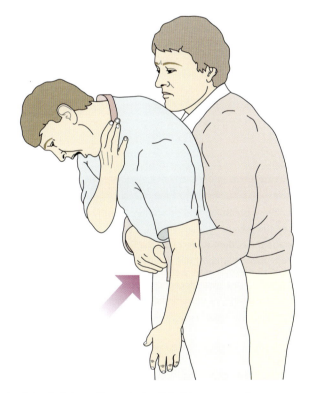

Fig. 1.13 Abdominal thrust (formerly the Heimlich manœuvre).

Box 1.4 *Management of stroke*

- Assess (FAST: *face, arm, speech, time*), clear the airway and check breathing
- Check pulse and capillary refill
- Reassure the patient
- Give high-flow oxygen
- Call an ambulance
- Defer dental treatment

SEDATION EMERGENCIES

Respiratory failure

- Causes include drug overdose or hypoxia.
- Diagnosis is as follows:
  Respiratory rate slows and then stops.
  There is ashen cyanosis.
  Pulse is initially rapid and weak, later irregular or impalpable.
  Cardiac arrest may follow.
- Management is as follows:
  Assess the patient using ABCDE.
  Call an ambulance.
  Administer no further sedation.
  Lay patient flat.
  Commence ventilation with bag and mask containing high oxygen concentration.
  Consider flumazenil administration.
  Defer dental treatment.

Sedative drug overdose or drug interaction

- Accidental overdose or the combination of the sedative agent with another drug used by the patient may be responsible.
- Diagnosis is as follows:
  pallor
  decreased pulse rate
  hypotension
  respiratory depression.
- Management is as follows:
  Stop the drug.
  Give oxygen and ventilate artificially if required.
  For midazolam overdose, give flumazenil.
  If the patient progresses to cardiac arrest, commence CPR.
  Call the emergency services.
  Defer dental treatment.

MENTAL DISTURBANCES

HYPERVENTILATION SYNDROME

- Causes of hyperventilation include:
  anxiety or neurosis
  pain
  cardiovascular disease
  nervous system disease
  acidosis (either metabolic or drug-associated)
  poor respiratory exchange (but in this case it is a compensatory physiological response).
- The clinical features vary widely, but neurological and psychological features may include:
  anxiety
  weakness
  light-headedness
  dizziness
  disturbed consciousness
  perioral and peripheral paraesthesiae
  tetany
  muscle pain or stiffness.
- The most common underlying diagnosis is psychological and is typically seen in a young woman overbreathing secondary to anxiety until carbon dioxide washout results in paraesthesia.

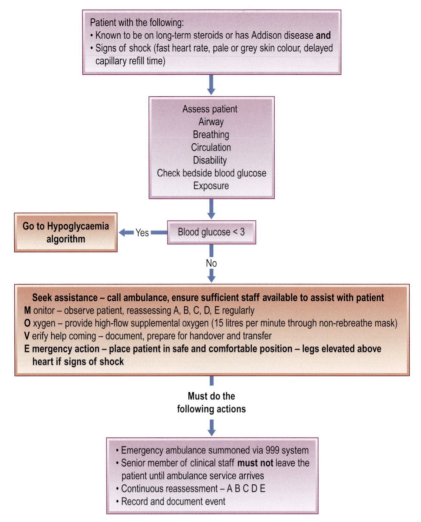

Fig. 1.14 Adrenal insufficiency algorithm.

Box 1.5 *Management of intravascular injection of local anaesthetic*

- Stop the local anaesthetic administration
- Lay the patient flat
- Reassure the patient
- Assess and maintain the airway
- Check breathing and circulation
- Remember that most patients recover spontaneously within half an hour
- Stabilize and defer further dental treatment until another day

Box 1.6 *Management of hyperventilating patients*

- Assess airway, breathing and circulation; identify any disability
- Reassure the patient
- Encourage the patient to decrease the respiratory rate slowly
- If there is obvious sympathetic overactivity, as shown particularly by tachycardia or arrhythmias, a cardiologist's opinion should be obtained, as treatment with a beta-blocker may be necessary
- Defer dental treatment until medical assessment has taken place

■ Cardiovascular and respiratory features may include:
palpitations
chest pain
breathlessness.
■ Management is detailed in Box 1.6.

DISTURBED OR AGGRESSIVE BEHAVIOUR

■ Disturbed or aggressive behaviour may be the result of:
an annoyed patient or underlying psychiatric disorder
drugs, especially barbiturates, alcohol or other drugs of addiction
or drug withdrawal, or corticosteroids
pain or discomfort
infections, particularly in the elderly

hypoglycaemia or other endocrine disorders
temporal lobe epilepsy
cerebral tumours.
■ Management is detailed in Box 1.7.

BLEEDING

■ Post-extraction bleeding causes are usually secondary to local trauma.
■ Haemorrhagic disease, though uncommon, must always be considered (see Box 1.8 and Ch. 8).
Management is detailed in Box 1.8.

Box 1.7 *Management of disturbed or aggressive behaviour*

- Reassure and try to calm the patient, and not to restrain
- Do not sedate, as this may confuse the diagnosis and may occasionally be fatal
- Remember that midazolam or diazepam is likely to worsen the excitement of a psychotic patient
- Call an ambulance
- If the patient is violent and uncontrollable, call the police
- Defer dental treatment

Box 1.8 *Management of the bleeding patient*

- Assess airway, breathing, circulation, disability and exposure
- Reassure the patient. Post-extraction bleeding often worries the patient excessively because a little blood dissolved in saliva gives the impression of a major bleed
- Ask partners or relatives to remain in the waiting room, as their anxiety can prevent early resolution
- Gently clean the mouth
- Locate the source of the bleeding
- Suture the socket under local analgesia
- Enquire into the patient's history, especially family history of abnormal bleeding
- If the bleeding is persistent or severe and there has been an estimated loss of more than about 500 mL, or if the patient is already compromised secondary to severe anaemia, arrange for the patient to be admitted to hospital
- Use tranexamic acid mouthwash 5%, which may help to stabilize the clot in the interim
- If the bleeding is uncontrollable, call an ambulance

KEY WEBSITES

(Accessed 23 May 2013)
A to E Training & Solutions. <http://www.atoetrainingandsolutions.co.uk>.
Advanced Life Support Group. <http://www.alsg.org>.
European Resuscitation Council. <http://www.erc.edu>.
Journal of the American Dental Association. Preparing for medical emergencies: the essential drugs and equipment for the dental office. <http://jada.ada.org/content/141/suppl_1/14S.full>.
National Center for Emergency Medicine Informatics. Common simple emergencies. <http://www.ncemi.org/cse/contents.htm>.
Resuscitation Council (UK). <http://www.resus.org.uk/pages/medental.htm>.
Walsall Healthcare NHS Trust. Medical emergencies in the dental practice. <https://www.walsallhealthcare.nhs.uk/media/133096/walsallmedicalposter.pdf>.

USEFUL WEBSITES

(Accessed 23 May 2013)
Dental Sedations Teachers Group. <http://www.dstg.co.uk>.
Joint Royal Colleges Ambulance Liaison Committee. Clinical practice guidelines 2006 for use in UK ambulance services (version 4.0). <http://jrcalc.org.uk/guidelines.htm>.
SDCEP (Scottish Dental Clinical Effectiveness Programme). <http://www.sdcep.org.uk/>.

REFERENCES AND FURTHER READING

American Academy of Pediatric Dentistry, American Academy of Pediatric Dentistry Committee on Sedation and Anesthesia, 2005–2006. Guideline on the elective use of minimal, moderate, and deep sedation and general anesthesia for pediatric dental patients. Pediatr. Dent. 27 (Suppl. 7), 110.
Aufderheide, T.P., et al. 2011. A trial of an impedance threshold device in out-of-hospital cardiac arrest. NEJM 365, 798.
Balmer, M.C., Longman, L.P., 2008. A practical skill one day medical emergencies course for dentists and DCPs. Br. Dent. J. 204, 453.
Bardy, G.H., 2011. A critic's assessment of our approach to cardiac arrest. NEJM 364, 374.
Boyd, B.C., et al. 2006. The role of automated external defibrillators in dental practice. N. Y. State Dent. J. 72, 20.
Dumas, F., et al. 2013. Chest compression alone cardiopulmonary resuscitation is associated with better long-term survival compared with standard cardiopulmonary resuscitation. Circulation 127 (4), 435.
Dym, H., 2008. Preparing the dental office for medical emergencies. Dent. Clin. North Am. 52, 605.
Fukayama, H., Yagiela, J.A., 2006. Monitoring of vital signs during dental care. Int. Dent. J. 56, 102.
General Dental Council, 2013. Standards for the Dental Team. General Dental Council, London.
Greenwood, M., 2008. Medical emergencies in the dental practice. Periodontol 2000 (46), 27.
Hasegawa, K., et al. 2013. Association of prehospital advanced airway management with neurologic outcome and survival in patients with out-of-hospital cardiac arrest. JAMA 309, 257.
Hostler, D., et al. 2011. Effect of real-time feedback during cardiopulmonary resuscitation outside hospital: prospective, cluster-randomised trial. BMJ 342, d512.
Hüpfl, M., et al. 2010. Chest-compression-only versus standard cardiopulmonary resuscitation: a meta-analysis. Lancet 376, 1552.
Jevon, P., 2012. Updated guidance on medical emergencies and resuscitation in the dental practice. Brit. Dent. J. 212, 41.
JOE Editorial Board, 2008. Medical emergencies and drugs: an online study guide. J. Endod. 34 (Suppl. 5), e201.
Kilgannon, J.H., et al. 2010. Association between arterial hyperoxia following resuscitation from cardiac arrest and in-hospital mortality. JAMA 303, 2165.
Müller, M.P., et al. 2008. A state-wide survey of medical emergency management in dental practices: incidence of emergencies and training experience. Emerg. Med. J. 25, 296.
Resuscitation Council. Medical emergencies and resuscitation: standards for clinical practice and training for dental practitioners and dental care professionals in general dental practice. London, July 2006 revised 2012, with updated Appendix (viii), Resuscitation Council (UK).
Robb, N.D., Leitch, J., 2006. Medical Emergencies in Dentistry. Oxford University Press, Oxford.
Scully, C., Kalantzis, A., 2005. Oxford Handbook of Dental Patient Care. Oxford University Press, Oxford.
Sharma, P.R., Hargreaves, A.D., 2006. Malignant vasovagal syncope. Dent. Update 33 (4), 246, 250.
Stiell, I.G., et al. 2011. Early versus later rhythm analysis in patients with out-of-hospital cardiac arrest. NEJM 365, 787.
Wang, H.E., Yealy, D.M., 2013. Managing the airway during cardiac arrest. JAMA 309, 285.

APPENDIX 1.1 MANAGEMENT OF COMMON EMERGENCIES

The Resuscitation Council guidelines (2012), Appendix ii, deal with common emergencies.

ASTHMA

Patients with asthma (both adults and children) may have an attack while at the dental surgery. Most attacks will respond to a few 'activations' of the patient's own short-acting beta2-adreno-ceptor stimulant inhaler such as salbutamol (100 micrograms/actuation). Repeat doses may be necessary. If the patient does not respond rapidly, or any features of severe asthma are present, an ambulance should be summoned. Patients requiring additional doses of bronchodilator should be referred for medical assessment after emergency treatment. If the patient is unable to use the inhaler effectively, additional doses should be given through a large-volume spacer device. If the response remains unsatisfactory or if the patient develops tachycardia, becomes distressed or cyanosed (blueness around the lips or extremities), arrangements must be made to transfer them urgently to hospital.

Symptoms and signs

Clinical features of **acute severe asthma** in adults include:

- Inability to complete sentences in one breath
- Respiratory rate > 25 per minute
- Tachycardia (heart rate > 110 per minute).

Clinical features of **life-threatening asthma** in adults include:

- Cyanosis or respiratory rate < 8 per minute
- Bradycardia (heart rate < 50 per minute)
- Exhaustion, confusion, decreased conscious level.

Treatment

- Whilst awaiting ambulance transfer, oxygen (15 litres per minute) should be given.
- Assuming the patient's nebuliser is unavailable, up to 10 activations from the salbutamol inhaler should be given using a large-volume spacer device and repeated every 10 minutes if necessary until an ambulance arrives. All emergency ambulances in the UK carry nebulisers, oxygen and appropriate drugs.
- If bronchospasm is part of a more generalized anaphylactic reaction and there are 'life-threatening' signs, an intramuscular injection of adrenaline should be given (see Anaphylaxis).
- The perceived risk of giving patients with chronic obstructive pulmonary disease too much oxygen is often quoted but this should not distract from the reality that ALL sick, cyanosed patients with respiratory difficulty should be given high-flow oxygen until the arrival of the ambulance. This short-term measure is far more likely to be of benefit to the patient than any risks of causing respiratory depression.
- If any patient becomes unresponsive always check for 'signs of life' (breathing and circulation) and start CPR in the absence of signs of life or normal breathing (ignore occasional 'gasps'). For further information about the management of the patient with asthma see http://www.brit-thoracic.org.uk/guidelines/asthma-guidelines.aspx (accessed 30 September 2013).

ANAPHYLAXIS

Anaphylaxis is a severe, life-threatening, generalized or systemic hypersensitivity reaction. It is characterised by rapidly developing life-threatening airway and/or breathing and/or circulation problems usually associated with skin and mucosal changes.

Anaphylactic reactions in general dental practice may follow the administration of a drug or contact with substances such as latex in surgical gloves. In general, the more rapid the onset of the reaction, the more serious it will be. Symptoms can develop within minutes and early, effective treatment may be life-saving. Anaphylactic reactions may also be associated with additives and excipients in medicines. It is wise therefore to check the full formulation of preparations which may contain allergenic fats or oils (including those for topical application, particularly if they are intended for use in the mouth).

Symptoms and signs

The lack of any consistent clinical manifestation and a wide range of possible presentations can cause diagnostic difficulty. Clinical assessment helps make the diagnosis.

Signs and symptoms may include:

- urticaria, erythema, rhinitis, conjunctivitis
- abdominal pain, vomiting, diarrhoea and a sense of impending doom
- flushing is common, but pallor may also occur
- marked upper airway (laryngeal) oedema and bronchospasm may develop, causing stridor, wheezing and/or a hoarse voice
- vasodilation causes relative hypovolaemia leading to low blood pressure and collapse. This can cause cardiac arrest
- respiratory arrest leading to cardiac arrest.

Treatment

- Use an ABCDE approach to recognize and treat any suspected anaphylactic reaction. First-line treatment includes managing the airway and breathing and restoration of blood pressure (laying the patient flat, raising the feet) and the administration of oxygen (15 litres per minute).
- For severe reactions where there are life-threatening airway and/or breathing and/or circulation problems, i.e. hoarseness, stridor, severe wheeze, cyanosis, pale, clammy, drowsy, confusion or coma … adrenaline should be given intramuscularly (anterolateral aspect of the middle third of the thigh) in a dose of 500 micrograms (0.5 mL adrenaline injection of 1:1000); an autoinjector preparation delivering a dose of 300 micrograms (0.3 mL adrenaline injection 1:1000) is available for immediate self-administration by those patients known to have severe reactions. This is an acceptable alternative if immediately available. The dose is repeated if necessary at 5-minute intervals according to blood pressure, pulse and respiratory function. The paediatric dose for adrenaline is based on the child's approximate age or weight. …
- In any unconscious patient always check for 'signs of life' (breathing and circulation) and start CPR in the absence of signs of life or normal breathing (ignore occasional 'gasps').
- In less severe cases any wheeze or difficulty breathing can be treated with a salbutamol inhaler as detailed above in the section on Asthma.
- All patients treated for an anaphylactic reaction should be sent to hospital by ambulance for further assessment, irrespective of any initial recovery.

Antihistamine drugs and steroids, whilst useful in the treatment of anaphylaxis, are not first-line drugs and they will be administered by the ambulance personnel if necessary.

For further information about the management of the patient with an emergency anaphylactic reaction see http://www.resus.org.uk/pages/reaction.pdf (accessed 30 September 2013).

CARDIAC EMERGENCIES

The signs and symptoms of cardiac emergencies include chest pain, shortness of breath, fast and slow heart rates, increased respiratory rate, low blood pressure, poor peripheral perfusion (indicated by prolonged capillary refill time) and altered mental state.

If there is a history of angina the patient will probably carry glyceryl trinitrate spray or tablets (or isosorbide dinitrate tablets) and they should be allowed to use them. Where symptoms are mild and resolve rapidly with the patient's own medication, hospital admission is not normally necessary. Dental treatment may or may not be continued at the discretion of the Dental Practitioner. More severe attacks of chest pain always warrant postponement of treatment and an ambulance should be summoned.

Sudden alterations in the patient's heart rate (very fast or very slow) may lead to a sudden reduction in cardiac output with loss of consciousness. Medical assistance should be summoned by dialling 999.

Myocardial infarction

The pain of myocardial infarction is similar to that of angina but generally more severe and prolonged. There may only be a partial response to GTN.

Symptoms and signs of myocardial infarction

- Progressive onset of severe, crushing pain in the centre and across the front of chest. The pain may radiate to the shoulders and down the arms (more commonly the left), into the neck and jaw or through to the back.
- Skin becomes pale and clammy.
- Nausea and vomiting are common.
- Pulse may be weak and blood pressure may fall.
- Shortness of breath.

Initial management of myocardial infarction

- Call 999 immediately for an ambulance.
- Allow the patient to rest in the position that feels most comfortable; in the presence of breathlessness this is likely to be the sitting position. Patients who faint or feel faint should be laid flat; often an intermediate position (dictated by the patient) will be most appropriate.
- Give sublingual GTN spray if this has not already been given.
- Reassure the patient as far as possible to relieve further anxiety.
- Give aspirin in a single dose of 300 mg orally, crushed or chewed. Ambulance staff should be made aware that aspirin has already been given, as should the hospital. Many ambulance services in the UK will administer thrombolytic therapy before hospital admission. Any dental treatment carried out that might contraindicate this must be brought to the attention of the ambulance crew.
- High-flow oxygen may be administered (15 litres per minute) if the patient is cyanosed (blue lips) or conscious level deteriorates.
- If the patient becomes unresponsive always check for 'signs of life' (breathing and circulation) and start CPR in the absence of signs of life or normal breathing (ignore occasional 'gasps').

EPILEPTIC SEIZURES

Patients with epilepsy must continue their normal dosage of anticonvulsant drugs before attending for dental treatment. Epileptic patients may not volunteer the information that they are epileptic, but there should be little difficulty in recognising a tonic–clonic (grand mal) seizure.

Symptoms and signs

- There may be a brief warning or 'aura'.
- There will be a sudden loss of consciousness, the patient becomes rigid, falls, may give a cry, and becomes cyanosed (tonic phase).
- After a few seconds, there are jerking movements of the limbs; the tongue may be bitten (clonic phase).
- There may be frothing from the mouth and urinary incontinence.
- The seizure typically lasts a few minutes; the patient may then become floppy but remain unconscious.
- After a variable time the patient regains consciousness but may remain confused.
- Fitting may be a presenting sign of hypoglycaemia and should be considered in all patients, especially known diabetics and children. An early blood glucose measurement is essential in all actively fitting patients (including known epileptics).
- Check for the presence of a very slow heart rate (<40 per minute) which may drop the blood pressure. This is usually caused by a vasovagal episode (see Syncope section below). The drop in blood pressure may cause transient cerebral hypoxia and give rise to a brief seizure.

Treatment

- During a seizure try to ensure that the patient is not at risk of injury but make no attempt to put anything in the mouth or between the teeth (in the mistaken belief that this will protect the tongue).
- Do not attempt to insert an oropharyngeal airway or other airway adjunct while the patient is actively fitting.
- Give high-flow oxygen (15 litres per minute).
- Do not attempt to restrain convulsive movements.
- After convulsive movements have subsided place the patient in the recovery position and reassess.
- If the patient remains unresponsive always check for 'signs of life' (breathing and circulation) and start CPR in the absence of signs of life or normal breathing (ignore occasional 'gasps').
- Check blood glucose level to exclude hypoglycaemia. If blood glucose <3.0 mmol per litre or hypoglycaemia is clinically suspected, give oral/buccal glucose (e.g. Glucogel; Dextrogel; GSF-syrup or Rapilose gel), or glucagon (see above and Hypoglycaemia section below).

After the seizure the patient may be confused ('post-ictal confusion') and may need reassurance and sympathy. The patient should not be sent home until fully recovered and they should be accompanied. It may not always be necessary to seek medical attention or transfer to hospital unless the convulsion was atypical, prolonged (or repeated), or if injury occurred. The National Institute for Care and Health Excellence (NICE; formerly the National Institute for Clinical Excellence) guidelines suggest the indications for sending to hospital are:

- status epilepticus
- high risk of recurrence
- first episode
- difficulty monitoring the individual's condition.

Medication should only be given if seizures are prolonged (convulsive movements lasting 5 minutes or longer) or recur in quick succession. In this situation an ambulance should be summoned urgently.

With prolonged or recurrent seizures, ambulance personnel will often administer IV diazepam, which is usually rapidly effective in stopping any seizure. An alternative, although less effective treatment, is midazolam given via the buccal route in a single dose of 10 mg for adults. For children the dose can be simplified as follows: child 1–5 years 5 mg, child 5–10 years 7.5 mg, above 10 years 10 mg. This might usefully be administered while waiting for ambulance treatment, but the decision to do this will depend on individual circumstances.

(See Appendix (viii) Emergency use of buccal midazolam).

HYPOGLYCAEMIA

Patients with diabetes should eat normally and take their usual dose of insulin or oral hypoglycaemic agent before any planned dental treatment. If food is omitted after having insulin, the blood glucose will fall to a low level (hypoglycaemia). This is usually defined as a blood glucose <3.0 mmol per litre, but some patients may show symptoms at higher blood sugar levels. Patients may recognize the symptoms themselves and will usually respond quickly to glucose. Children may not have such obvious features but may appear lethargic.

Symptoms and signs

- Shaking and trembling
- Sweating
- Headache
- Difficulty in concentration/vagueness
- Slurring of speech
- Aggression and confusion
- Fitting/seizures
- Unconsciousness.

Treatment

The following staged treatment protocol is suggested depending on the status of the patient. If any difficulty is experienced or the patient does not respond, the ambulance service should be summoned immediately; ambulance personnel will also follow this protocol. Confirm the diagnosis by measuring the blood glucose.

Early stages – where the patient is co-operative and conscious with an intact gag reflex, give oral glucose (sugar [sucrose], milk with added sugar, glucose tablets or gel [e.g. Glucogel; Dextrogel; GSF-syrup or Rapilose gel]). If necessary this may be repeated in 10–15 minutes.

In more severe cases – where the patient has impaired consciousness, is uncooperative or is unable to swallow safely, buccal glucose gel and/or glucagon should be given.

- Glucagon should be given via the IM route (1 mg in adults and children > 8 years old or >25 kg, 0.5 mg if <8 years old or <25 kg). Remember it may take 5–10 minutes for glucagon to work and it requires the patient to have adequate glucose stores. Thus, it may be ineffective in anorexic patients, alcoholics or some non-diabetic patients.
- Recheck blood glucose after 10 minutes to ensure that it has risen to a level of 5.0 mmol per litre or more, in conjunction with an improvement in the patient's mental status.

- If any patient becomes unconscious, always check for 'signs of life' (breathing and circulation) and start CPR in the absence of signs of life or normal breathing (ignore occasional 'gasps').
- It is important, especially in patients who have been given glucagon, that once they are alert and able to swallow, they are given a drink containing glucose and if possible some food high in carbohydrate. The patient may go home if fully recovered and they are accompanied. Their General Practitioner should be informed and they should not drive.

SYNCOPE

Inadequate cerebral perfusion (and oxygenation) results in loss of consciousness. This most commonly occurs with low blood pressure caused by vagal overactivity (a vasovagal attack, simple faint, or syncope). This in turn may follow emotional stress or pain. Some patients are more prone to this and have a history of repeated faints.

Symptoms and signs

- Patient feels faint/dizzy/light-headed
- Slow pulse rate
- Low blood pressure
- Pallor and sweating
- Nausea and vomiting
- Loss of consciousness.

Treatment

- Lay the patient flat **as soon as possible** and raise the legs to improve venous return.
- Loosen any tight clothing, especially around the neck and give oxygen (15 litres per minute).
- If any patient becomes unresponsive, always check for 'signs of life' (breathing, circulation) and start CPR in the absence of signs of life or normal breathing (ignore occasional 'gasps').

Other possible causes

- **Postural hypotension** can be a consequence of rising abruptly or of standing upright for too long. Several medical conditions predispose patients to hypotension with the risk of syncope. The most common culprits are drugs used in the treatment of high blood pressure, especially the ACE inhibitors and angiotensin antagonists. When rising, patients should take their time. Treatment is the same as for a vasovagal attack.
- Under stressful circumstances, many anxious patients **hyperventilate**. This may give rise to feelings of light-headedness or faintness but does not usually result in syncope. It may result in spasm of muscles around the face and of the hands. In most cases reassurance is all that is necessary.

CHOKING AND ASPIRATION

Dental patients are susceptible to choking with the potential risk of aspiration. They may have blood and secretions in their mouths *for prolonged periods. Local anaesthesia may diminish the normal protective pharyngeal reflexes and 'impression material' or dental equipment is often within their oral cavity and poses additional risks. Good teamwork and careful attention to detail should prevent aspiration episodes and any risk of choking.*

Symptoms and signs

- *The patient may cough and splutter.*
- *They may complain of difficulty breathing.*
- *Breathing may become noisy with wheeze (usually aspiration) or stridor (usually upper airway obstruction).*
- *They may develop 'paradoxical' chest or abdominal movements.*
- *They may become cyanosed and lose consciousness.*

Treatment

- *In cases of aspiration, allow the patient to cough vigorously.*
- *Symptomatic treatment of wheeze with a salbutamol inhaler may help (as for asthma).*
- *If any large pieces of foreign material have been aspirated, e.g. teeth or dental amalgam, the patient should be referred to hospital for a chest X-ray and possible removal.*
- *Where the patient is symptomatic following aspiration they should be referred to hospital as an emergency.*
- *The treatment of the choking patient involves removing any visible foreign bodies from the mouth and pharynx.*
- *Encourage the patient to cough if conscious. If they are unable to cough but remain conscious then sharp back blows should be delivered. These can be followed by abdominal thrusts (Heimlich manœuvre) if the foreign body has not been dislodged. If the patient becomes unconscious, CPR should be started. This will not only provide circulatory support but the pressure generated within the chest by performing chest compressions may help to dislodge the foreign body.*

See Appendix (iv) for the Resuscitation Council (UK) Adult and Child Choking Algorithm.

ADRENAL INSUFFICIENCY

Adrenal insufficiency may follow long-term administration of oral corticosteroids and can persist for years after stopping therapy. A patient with adrenal insufficiency may become hypotensive when under physiological stress. The nature of dental treatment makes this a rare possibility, however, and if a patient collapses during dental treatment other causes should be considered first and managed before diagnosing adrenal insufficiency. Routine enquiry about the current or recent use of corticosteroids as part of the medical history prior to dental treatment should alert the Dental Practitioner to the patient at risk of this condition. Some patients carry a steroid warning card. Acute adrenal insufficiency can often be prevented by administration of an increased dose of corticosteroid prior to treatment.

Dental treatment that requires an increased steroid dose is that which may cause significant physiological stress. Usually, simple dental extractions and restorative procedures, including endodontics, are not a cause for concern, but surgical extractions or implant placement should be considered as a risk. Patients who are systemically unwell from a dentally related infection are also recommended to have a prophylactic increase in steroid dose in addition to any surgical and antimicrobial treatment indicated.

Guidance on the management of those patients with known Addison's disease is available from the Addison's Clinical Advisory Panel (http://www.addisons.org.uk/; accessed 30 September 2013), who recommend doubling the patient's steroid dose before significant dental treatment under local anaesthesia and continuing this for 24 hours.

Medical history, examination, investigations and risk assessment

PROTECTING PATIENTS

Health care aims to improve the health of patients but can itself carry risks. The first principle should be to do no harm (*primum non nocere*). Nevertheless, a UK report estimated that up to 18% of the population believe that they have suffered from a 'medical error', 10% of hospital admissions may result in something going wrong and 5% have had adverse effects from medical care. In a survey of Dutch oral surgeons who had had, on average, 21 years of work experience, 40% of respondents confirmed that they had experienced the death of a patient after oral surgery. Most of these patients had died after a dental extraction, the most important causes of death being postoperative spread of an infection, failure to survive cancer treatment, or heart and/or lung failure.

Operations are now associated with far less morbidity and mortality than formerly but there remains room for improvement. Morbidity and mortality in the dental surgery providing local anaesthesia (LA) and conscious sedation (CS) are rare but greater in patients with medical and/or dental problems; for example, extractions attributed to dental infections were significant predictors for risk factors for myocardial infarction compared with tooth extraction for trauma and other reasons in an Oslo study. Deaths as a result of the use of general anaesthesia (GA) in the dental surgery in the past were few but nevertheless provoked widespread public concern, and it is no longer permissible for a dentist in the UK to act as anaesthetist (this had been the case for some time in some other countries). *GA must only be given in a hospital with critical care facilities – because of the need to have resuscitation equipment available – and must be carried out by a qualified anaesthetist.*

If working in hospital, however, dentists may be required to assess patients for GA and to ensure that essential prerequisites are met before GA, and may need to manage GA patients postoperatively. They must therefore have an understanding of risk assessment and perioperative care.

RISK ASSESSMENT

At the start of a patient's visit, it is essential to:

1. obtain a careful medical, dental, family, social (and sometimes developmental) history, and make a risk assessment

2. assess the patient's needs and agree them with the patient
3. obtain the patient's valid consent to any investigations required
4. obtain the patient's consent to an agreed treatment plan.

Adequate risk assessment is essential and endeavours to anticipate and prevent trouble. The criteria of 'fitness' for a procedure are not absolute but depend on a number of factors, as shown in Box 2.1. Dentistry should be very safe, especially if the procedure is not dramatically invasive and the patient is healthy.

Surgical procedures are generally the most hazardous. The World Health Organization (WHO) recognizes this and grades risks on the basis of severity of the procedure (Table 2.1). WHO also identifies three phases of an operation at each of which, for patient safety, a checklist coordinator must confirm that the surgery team has completed the listed tasks before it proceeds:

- Before anaesthesia induction ('sign in')
- Before skin incision ('time out')
- Before the patient leaves the operating room ('sign out').

Drug use is also potentially dangerous; all agents should be carefully administered, particularly those acting on the neurological system and affecting consciousness and cardiac or respiratory functioning (e.g. sedatives and anaesthetic agents). Most oral care is given under LA and then morbidity is minimal. CS is not as safe as LA, though considerably safer than GA. Even so, CS must be carried out in appropriate facilities, by adequately trained personnel and with due consideration of the possible risks. By contrast, GA with intravenous or inhalational agents is only occasionally required for dental treatment and then only in a hospital setting; control of vital functions is impaired or lost to the anaesthetist. As stated above, GA is only permitted in a hospital with appropriate resuscitation facilities.

A patient attending for dental treatment who is apparently 'fit' may actually have serious systemic disease(s) and be taking drugs (including recreational drugs), either or both of which might influence the health care required. Many patients with life-threatening diseases now survive as a result of advances in surgical and medical care, and either or both can significantly affect the dental management or even the fate of the patient. Though this is most likely when treating hospital patients and other risk groups such as older people, one study showed that 30% of dental patients have a relevant medical condition. The risk is greatest when surgery is needed, and when GA or CS are

Box 2.1 *Factors influencing outcomes of health-care procedures*

- Health of the patient
- Type of procedure
- Duration of the procedure
- Degree of trauma and stress
- Degree of urgency of the procedure
- Skill and experience of the operator
- Skill and experience of the anaesthetist/sedationist
- Facilities and equipment

Table 2.1 *WHO grades of surgery*

Grade	Termed	Includes
1	Minor	Excision of skin lesion; drainage of breast abscess[a]
2	Intermediate	Primary repair of inguinal hernia; excision of varicose vein(s) of leg; tonsillectomy/adenotonsillectomy; knee arthroscopy
3	Major	Total abdominal hysterectomy; endoscopic resection of prostate; lumbar discectomy; thyroidectomy
4	Major+	Total joint replacement; lung operations; colonic resection; radical neck dissection; neurosurgery; cardiac surgery

[a] Includes dentoalveolar surgery.

Table 2.3 *American Society of Anesthesiologists (ASA) classification*

ASA class	Definition
I	Normal, healthy patient
II	A patient with mild systemic disease (e.g. well-controlled diabetes, asthma, hypertension or epilepsy), pregnancy, anxiety
III	A patient with severe systemic disease limiting activity but not incapacitating (e.g. epilepsy with frequent seizures, uncontrolled hypertension, recent myocardial infarct, uncontrolled diabetes, severe asthma, stroke)
IV	A patient with incapacitating disease that is a constant threat to life (e.g. cancer, unstable angina or recent myocardial infarct, arrhythmia or recent cerebrovascular accident)
V	Moribund patient not expected to live more than 24 h with or without treatment

Table 2.2 *Risk assessment and management*

Risks increased by	Risks reduced by
Increasing age	Planned treatment
Medical treatments	Non-invasive procedures
Surgical treatments	Monitoring
Lengthy dental procedures	Reassurance
Drug use – medication or recreational	Competent operator

Table 2.4 *American Society of Anesthesiologists (ASA) grades II and III*

	ASA II	ASA III
Chronic obstructive pulmonary disease (COPD)	Cough or wheeze; well controlled	Breathless on minimal exertion
Angina	Occasional use of glyceryl trinitrate (GTN)	Regular use of GTN or unstable angina
Hypertension	Well controlled on single agent	Poorly controlled; multiple drugs
Asthma	Well controlled with inhalers	Poorly controlled; limiting lifestyle
Diabetes	Well controlled; no complications	Poorly controlled or complications

given – and these problems may be compounded if close medical support is lacking.

Although every care must be taken to identify the medically compromised patient, it must be appreciated that the means to do so in conventional dental settings are limited and by no means always successful. It is impossible to legislate for all possibilities and there have been many cases where apparently fit people have died suddenly within a short time of being declared healthy on medical examination.

The main aims are to ensure that procedures are carried out:

- promptly but safely
- on the correct patient and at the correct site
- with minimal complications and the best possible outcome.

However, although risks arise mainly when the procedure is invasive (tissues are disrupted) and/or the patient is not healthy, they may also be a factor if health-care professionals (HCPs) are overambitious in terms of their skill or knowledge. Clinicians should work only within their field of competence. No interventional procedure is entirely free from risk but care can be improved by making an adequate assessment based on history, clinical signs and, where appropriate, investigations, and by minimizing trauma and stress to the patient (Table 2.2).

Assessment of the risks involved must include the health of the patient, which may be evaluated using a risk-stratification scoring system such as the Physical Status Classification of the American Society of Anesthesiologists (ASA) (Table 2.3). ASA I and II patients can generally be treated in general dental practice or community services. ASA III patients are often best treated in a hospital-based clinic where expert medical support is available. ASA IV and V patients are usually hospitalized or bedridden, and generally are only seeking emergency dental treatment.

Dental treatment must be significantly modified if the patient has an ASA score of III or IV, which is true of a relatively high percentage of patients aged 65–74 years (23.9%) and 75 years or over (34.9%). Controversies can arise in relation to the management of patients with

ASA scores of II and III. Table 2.4 summarizes these scores for some of the more common disorders.

The Prognosis and Assessment of Risk Scale (PARS) is another assessment tool, which is virtually identical to the ASA scale but can be modified by factors such as those shown in Table 2.5; it categorizes patients into groups I–V. Other factors considered in PARS are shown in Table 2.6. The Karnofsky scale, which has been adapted for use in many areas including hospices, cancer clinics and so on, is a quick and easy way to indicate how a patient is feeling on a given day, without going through several multiple choice questions or symptom surveys (Table 2.7). The Medical Complexity classification is another available tool (Table 2.8).

Good communication is essential with both patient and other health professionals. Often, dental treatment in medically compromised patients may have to be delayed until expert advice has been sought and this is always the case for patients undergoing procedures under GA, who must be pre-assessed by the anaesthetist.

INFORMED CONSENT (OTHERWISE KNOWN AS VALID CONSENT)

The patient's autonomy must be respected at all times. Patients can determine what investigations and treatment they are or are not willing to receive. Before they are asked to make a decision, they must be given sufficient information about their condition, suggested treatment(s) (including alternative management if available), any associated risks involved in the proposed treatment, and possible outcomes if nothing is done. They have the right to refuse treatment, even if this could

Table 2.5 *Dental care modifications and the American Society of Anesthesiologists (ASA) scale and Prognosis and Assessment of Risk Scale (PARS)*

ASA	Definition	PARS	Dental care modifications
I	Normal, healthy patient	I	None
II	A patient with mild systemic disease (e.g. well-controlled diabetes, asthma, hypertension or epilepsy), pregnancy, anxiety	II	Dental care should focus on elimination of acute infection before medical/surgical procedure (e.g. prosthetic cardiac valve)
III	A patient with severe systemic disease limiting activity but not incapacitating (e.g. epilepsy with frequent seizures, uncontrolled hypertension, recent myocardial infarct, uncontrolled diabetes, severe asthma, stroke)	III	Dental care should focus on elimination of acute infection and chronic disease before medical/surgical procedure (e.g. organ transplant patients)
IV	A patient with incapacitating disease that is a constant threat to life (e.g. cancer, unstable angina or recent myocardial infarct, arrhythmia or recent cerebrovascular accident)	IV	All potential dental problems should be corrected before medical/surgical procedure (e.g. prior to radiotherapy to head and neck)
V	Moribund patient not expected to live more than 24 h with or without treatment	V	Control of acute dental pain and infection only

Table 2.6 *Prognosis and Assessment Risk Scale*

Factor	Comment
Medical status	Any complicating medical factors
Physical status	
Oral hygiene	
Psychological needs	
Functional ability	
Mental status	Level of understanding
Social environment	Support or significant events planned shortly after treatment
Family environment	
Access issues	Access to dental building, etc.
Financial issues	
Communication needs	Is an interpreter required?
Behaviour	Is behaviour management needed?
Consent	Is patient competent to give consent?

Table 2.7 *Karnofsky scale*

Score	Definition
100	Able to work. Normal, no complaints, no evidence of disease
90	Able to work. Able to carry out normal activity, minor symptoms
80	Able to work. Normal activity with effort, some symptoms
70	Independent, not able to work. Cares for self, unable to carry out normal activity
60	Disabled, dependent. Requires occasional assistance, cares for most needs
50	Moderately disabled, dependent. Requires considerable assistance and frequent care
40	Severely disabled, dependent. Requires special care and assistance
30	Severely disabled. Hospitalized, death not imminent
20	Very sick. Active supportive treatment needed
10	Moribund. Fatal processes are rapidly progressing

Table 2.8 *Medical Complexity classification*

Class	Medical condition	Status	Complications
MC-0	No significant medical problems	MC-0	No complications anticipated
MC-1	Controlled and stable condition/disease	MC-1A	No complications anticipated
		MC-1B	Minor complications anticipated
		MC-1C	Major complications anticipated
MC-2	Poorly controlled and/or unstable condition/disease	MC-2A	No complications anticipated
		MC-2B	Minor complications anticipated
		MC-2C	Major complications anticipated
MC-3	Cardiac or other conditions needing continuous monitoring		

adversely affect the outcome or result in their death. Depending on the situation, time should be allowed for the patient to think about and discuss the proposed treatment with people close to them. Consent is the expressed or implied agreement of the patient to undergo an examination, investigation or treatment. Consent is not an isolated event, but involves a continuing dialogue between clinician and patient (and occasionally their relatives or partner). In order to give informed (valid) consent, the individual concerned must have adequate reasoning faculties and be in possession of all relevant facts at the time consent is given. *Patients who undergo procedures performed without their valid consent may be entitled to claim damages in the civil courts by making a claim of negligence. The clinician is also vulnerable in the criminal courts to a charge of assault and battery following a complaint to the police by the person who received the treatment.*

Information about what the proposed investigations or treatment will involve, the benefits and risks (including adverse effects and complications), and the alternatives available is crucial for patients when they are making up their minds. The courts have stated that patients should be told about 'significant risks which would affect the judgment of a reasonable patient'.

'Significant' has not been legally defined but the General Medical Council (GMC) requires doctors to tell patients about 'serious or frequently occurring' risks. In addition, if patients make it clear that they have particular concerns about certain kinds of risk, the clinician must ensure that they are informed about these risks, even if they are very small or rare. Sometimes, patients may make it clear that they do not want any information about the options, but want the health professional to decide on their behalf. In such circumstances, ensure that the patient receives at least some very basic information about what is proposed. Where information is refused, this should be documented in the patient's notes and/or on a consent form. The important thing is for the clinician to record sufficient details of the consent process in order to be able to reconstruct the discussions and the thinking that led to a particular course of treatment in the event of a challenge at a later stage – possibly years later.

The patient's open agreement to proceed with the investigation or treatment proposed after full discussion and the patient's receipt of sufficient information is sometimes called 'informed consent'.

When obtaining consent, patients should be informed of:

- details of the diagnosis and prognosis with and without treatment
- uncertainties about the diagnosis
- options available for treatment
- the purpose of all aspects of a proposed investigation or treatment
- the likely benefits and probability of success
- any possible adverse effects and the risks of the procedure proposed
- the likelihood of one or more of the risks coming to pass
- likely outcomes if a procedure is not carried out
- the need for drains, catheters, tracheostomy, etc.
- their right to change their mind at any stage
- their right to a second opinion.

Other issues that should be discussed at this stage include:

- time of appointment or admission
- eating/starving instructions
- management of usual daily medications
- specific preoperative preparation that may be required
- transport to where the procedure will be performed
- specific anaesthetic issues
- anticipated duration of procedure
- likely recovery period
- likely discharge date
- specific postoperative care
- follow-up requirements
- anticipated date of return to full activity.

'Informed' consent means that the patient must be fully aware of the procedure, its intended benefits and its possible risks, and the level of these benefits and risks. In particular, patients must be warned about:

- preoperative preparation
- possible adverse effects
- postoperative sequelae (e.g. pain)
- where they will be during their recovery
- the possibility of intravenous infusions, catheters, nasogastric tubes, any deformity, swelling, bruising, pain, etc.

All questions should be answered honestly. Information should not be withheld that might influence the decision-making process. Patients should never be coerced. Finally, for consent to be valid, the person who obtains it must have sufficient knowledge of the proposed treatment and its risks, and should be the person who is undertaking the procedure.

At any time, the information on the form can be augmented by an additional record made in the patient's notes covering conversations, discussions or warnings.

Consent may be:

- implied (a patient lying in the dental chair with an open mouth is consenting to a dental examination).
- expressed in writing.

Although rarely a legal requirement (but frequently a contractual obligation), it is good practice to seek written consent on most occasions and this is essential where the treatment is complex or involves significant risks or adverse effects. Written consent must always be obtained from all patients having an operation. The possible benefits of the treatment must be weighed against the risks and always discussed by the person carrying out the procedure; if, for some reason, this is not possible, it must be done by a delegated person with the appropriate expertise to do so (i.e. a person who is competent to carry out the proposed surgery themselves as an independent practitioner in their own right). Written consent is also essential when provision of clinical care is not the primary purpose, the treatment is part of a project or research, or there are significant consequences for personal or social life. Your organization may have a policy setting out when you need to obtain written consent. A signature on a consent form does not itself prove the consent is valid; the point of the form is to record the patient's decision and also, increasingly, the content of the discussions that have taken place. A signed consent form is not a legal waiver; if, for example, patients do not receive enough information on which to base their decision, then the consent may not be valid, even though the form has been signed. A signed consent form will not protect the clinician if there is doubt as to whether consent was actually 'informed'. Ideally, the form should be designed to serve as an *aide-mémoire* to health professionals and patients, by providing a checklist of the kind of information patients should be offered, and by enabling the patient to have a written record of the main points discussed. However, the written information provided for the patient in no way should be regarded as a substitute for face-to-face discussions with the individual. Patients are also entitled to change their mind after signing the consent form, if they retain capacity to do so.

Although the law in relation to consent continues to evolve (as does most legislation) and there are significant variations between countries, the principles are as follows:

- Before examining, treating or caring for competent adults, consent must be obtained.
- Adults are assumed to be competent unless demonstrated otherwise.
- Patients may be competent to make some health-care decisions, even if they are not competent to make others.
- Giving and obtaining consent is usually a process, not a one-off event. *Patients can change their minds and withdraw consent at any time.*

For consent to be valid, patients must receive sufficient information about their condition and proposed treatment. It is the HCP's responsibility to explain all the relevant facts to the patient and to ascertain that they are understood. If there are doubts about their competence, the question to ask is: 'Can this patient understand, retain and then weigh up the information needed to make this decision?' If patients are not offered as much information as they reasonably need to make their decision, and in a form they can understand, their consent may not be valid. For example, information for those with visual impairment should be provided in the form of audio tapes, Braille or large print.

Patients whose first language is not English may need the help of an interpreter. Most organizations have access to experienced interpreters. It is preferable to rely on a neutral interpreter (i.e. *not* a family member) when examining and seeking consent from a patient for surgery or treatment.

Ensure the patient, staff and, where appropriate and in accordance with the patient's wishes, the patient's relatives and/or partner are kept fully informed. Maintain good, clear, contemporaneous records of the nature of all discussions that take place, including the names of those involved. Good communication and documentation can prevent future dispute and litigation. If there is any reason to believe that consent may be disputed later, or if there are concerns about an individual's attitude or behaviour, meticulous documentation in the case notes is essential. The UK Department of Health's *Reference guide to consent for examination or treatment* (available at www.gov.uk/government/publications; accessed 30 September 2013) offers a comprehensive summary of the law on consent.

SPECIFIC CONSENT ISSUES

- No one else can make a decision on behalf of a competent adult.
- In an emergency, a life-saving procedure can be performed without consent.
- All actions must, however, be justifiable to one's peers.
- No one can give or withhold consent on behalf of a mentally incapacitated patient; decisions lie primarily with the clinicians, who should act in the patient's best interest. Where there is doubt, ultimately a court will decide on the best course of action, having taken expert advice. The Mental Capacity Act 2005 provides guidance for HCPs in England and Wales (see also The Adults with Incapacity (Scotland) Act 2000) who treat this group of patients. Guidance has been published by the UK Department of Health (Mental Capacity Act 2005 Code of Practice) and is available at http://www.dca.gov.uk/legal-policy/mental-capacity/mca-cp.pdf (accessed 30 September 2013).

Essentially, everyone aged 16 or more is presumed to be competent to give consent for themselves, unless the opposite is demonstrated.

Competent adults – namely, persons aged 16 and over who have the capacity to make their own decisions about treatment – can consent to dental treatment and they are also entitled to refuse treatment, even where it would clearly benefit their health. If a patient is mentally competent to give consent but is physically unable to sign a form, you should complete this form as usual and ask an independent witness to confirm that the patient has given consent orally or non-verbally.

If the patient is 18 or over and is not legally competent to give consent, you should use a form for adults who are unable to consent to investigation or treatment. Patients will not be legally competent to give consent if:

- they are unable to comprehend and retain information material to the decision; and/or
- they are unable to weigh and use this information in coming to a decision.

You should always take all reasonable steps (e.g. involving more specialist colleagues) to support patients in making their own decision before concluding that they are unable to do so.

Relatives *cannot* be asked to sign this form on behalf of an adult who is not legally competent to consent for him or herself, unless the patient has appointed a friend or relative to act for them, creating a lasting power of attorney (LPA). This LPA must have been created when the patient was competent and the LPA must be lodged with the Court of Protection. An LPA may allow the relative or friend to take decisions about the health of the patient, should the patient be found to be lacking capacity.

Children under the age of 16 years may also have capacity to consent if they have the ability to understand the nature, purpose and possible consequences of the proposed investigation or treatment, as well as the consequences of non-treatment. Children below 16 who have *Gillick* competence (i.e. they understand fully what is involved in the

proposed procedure) may therefore consent to treatment without their parents' authority or knowledge, although their parents will ideally be involved. 'Gillick competence' is a term used in medical law to decide whether a child (16 years or younger) is able to consent to medical treatment, without the need for parental permission or knowledge:

> *As a matter of Law the parental right to determine whether or not their minor child below the age of sixteen will have medical treatment terminates if and when the child achieves sufficient understanding and intelligence to understand fully what is proposed.*

The standard is based on a House of Lords' decision in the case *Gillick v West Norfolk and Wisbech Area Health Authority* [1985] 3 All ER 402 (HL). The case is binding in England, and has been approved in Australia, Canada and New Zealand. Similar provision is made in Scotland by the Age of Legal Capacity (Scotland) Act 1991. In Northern Ireland, although separate legislation applies, the then Department of Health and Social Services Northern Ireland stated that there was no reason to suppose that the House of Lords' decision would not be followed by the Northern Ireland Courts.

Where a child under 16 years old is not deemed competent to consent, a person with parental responsibility (e.g. their legal parent or guardian, or a person appointed by the courts) has authority to consent for investigations or treatment that are in the child's best interests.

There are several legal tests that have been described in relation to consent. The *Bolam* test states that a doctor who:

> *acted in accordance with a practice accepted as proper by a responsible body of medical men skilled in that particular art is not negligent if he is acting in accordance with such a practice, merely because there is a body of opinion which takes a contrary view.*

However, a judge may, on certain rare occasions, choose between two bodies of expert medical opinion, if one is to be regarded as 'logically indefensible' (*Bolitho* principle). The main alternative to the Bolam test is the *'prudent-patient test'* widely used in North America. According to this test, doctors should provide the amount of information that a 'prudent patient' would want.

Obtaining consent from adult patients without capacity

The more elective the procedure, the more care should be taken in ensuring that the patient, parent, guardian or carer has been consulted. In true emergency situations, a dentist may rely on the best-intent principle in relation to the overall well-being of the patient, although, where there is any doubt, advice should be taken. Involve the patient as far as possible; some incapacitated patients may be quite capable of giving partial consent. Decide who else should be involved in any decision to proceed with the patient's treatment. The current position (in the UK) is that no adult can consent to the treatment of another adult (with the exception of cases that fall under the Mental Capacity Act 2005). Before anyone can give valid consent to treatment, she or he must possess the requisite capacity. The law presumes that, in the absence of evidence to the contrary, patients over the age of 16 years are capable of giving (or withholding) consent to treatment. The broad test of capacity is that the person concerned should be able to understand the nature and purpose of the treatment and must be able to weigh the risks and benefits. They should be able to retain and weigh this information, as well as communicate their decision.

Where there is doubt, a decision has to be made as to the capacity of the patient. This presents a problem for dentists providing care for patients with learning impairment. Where the patient lacks the capacity to consent, then the dentist would normally act in the patient's best interests and treatment should not be withheld simply because consent has not been obtained, or a charge of failure in duty of care could be made. If a person is incapable of giving or refusing consent, and has not validly refused such care in advance, treatment may still be given lawfully if it is deemed to be in the patient's best interests. However, this should happen only after full consideration of its potential benefits and unwanted effects, and in consultation with the carer(s), relatives and other people close to the patient. Where treatment involves taking irreversible decisions or carrying greater risks, then the agreement of another dentist or doctor is appropriate. For those with learning difficulties, it is important to have a discussion with the parent, carer or, in their absence, two professionals who should sign their approval in the best interests of the patient. The discussions and agreement should be documented in the patient's record and, whilst this does not constitute consent, it represents good practice.

The Mental Health Act 1983 is primarily concerned with the care and treatment of people who are diagnosed as having a mental health problem which requires that they be detained or treated in the interests of their own health and safety or with a view to protecting other people.

The Mental Capacity Act 2005 applies to everyone involved in the care, treatment or support of people aged 16 years and over in England and Wales who lack capacity to make all or some decisions for themselves. This Act also applies to situations where a person may lack capacity to make a decision at a particular time due to illness, drugs or alcohol. Assessments of capacity should be time- and decision-specific. The Act clarifies the terms 'mental capacity' and 'lack of mental capacity', and says that a person is unable to make a particular decision if they cannot do one or more of the following:

- Understand information given to them
- Retain that information long enough to be able to make the decision
- Weigh up the information available to make the decision
- Communicate their decision; this could be done, for example, by talking, using sign language, or even making simple muscle movements such as blinking an eye or squeezing a hand.

A new criminal offence of ill-treatment or wilful neglect of people who lack capacity also came into force in 2007. Within the law, 'helping with personal hygiene' (that would include tooth-brushing) attracts protection from liability, as long as the individual has complied with the Act by assessing a person's capacity and acting in their best interests. 'Best-interest' decisions made on behalf of people who lack capacity should be the least restrictive of their basic rights and freedoms.

Further changes within the Act include the introduction of LPAs that extend to health and welfare decisions. When a health professional has a significant concern relating to decisions taken under the authority of an LPA that relate to serious medical treatment, the case can be referred for adjudication to the *Court of Protection*, which is ultimately responsible for the proper functioning of the legislation. The Act also created a new *Public Guardian* with responsibility for the registration and supervision of both LPAs and court-appointed deputies. Furthermore, *Independent Mental Capacity Advocates* (IMCAs) have been introduced to support particularly vulnerable incapacitated adults – most often those who lack any other forms of external support – in making certain decisions.

In Scotland, the position is complicated by the fact that the dentist has to comply with the Adults with Incapacity Act 2000. This requires the patient's doctor to issue a certificate before treatment. The document is procedure-specific and a new one is required for each treatment plan or in the event of a change to the plan. Episodes requiring GA or sedation not included in the original treatment plan will need further certification. The interesting nuance is that the dentist can assess capacity but it is the doctor who has to assess incapacity. This has created significant practical difficulties for many health-care providers.

Obtaining consent for child patients

Changing social patterns have meant that the position relating to who is able to consent to treatment for a child is no longer the same. Parental responsibility lies with the natural mother, natural father (if married to the mother at birth), adoptive parents or those who have temporary residence orders (where the child lives with them). The local authority may acquire responsibility. The natural father not married to the natural mother does *not* have parental responsibility. Parental responsibility can be granted by court order, by agreement with the mother or on her death, if stated in her will. Step-parents can be granted parental responsibility by court order.

It is important to remember that the legal situation with regard to consent varies around the world and is subject to continued debate and development.

THE USE OF RESTRAINT

Occasionally, patients may need some assistance in order to be able to undergo or cooperate with investigations or treatment. The dividing line between assistance and trespass to the person can be fine. Three forms of trespass to the person exist:

- Assault – the fear or threat of impending harm
- Battery – the unlawful application of force or unwanted touching
- False imprisonment – the infliction of restraint.

These issues must be considered carefully when the patient lacks the necessary capacity to understand the procedure being carried out. Any physical intervention is subject to the rule of 'reasonableness'. Sometimes it is necessary to control movements during operative procedures or to support an arm, for example, for the injection of intravenous drugs in order to prevent patients injuring themselves. It is wise to seek the assistance of a carer or relative at such times and to ensure that this is documented. Learning disabilities teams may be able to assist and are likely to have developed protocols and procedures to deal with such problems.

MEDICAL HISTORY

The history (or anamnesis) is the information gained by an HCP with the aim of formulating a diagnosis, providing medical care and identifying medical problems relevant to health care. The history is obtained from either the patient or people who know the patient and can provide the necessary information. History-taking also allows the HCP to develop rapport with the patient, place the diagnosis in the context of the patient's life, identify relevant physical signs, and assess mental state and attitude towards health care. Age and cultural factors may also be important (Appendices 2.1 and 2.2). Due cognisance must be taken of a person's "protected characteristics", of which there are nine (Table 2.9).

Table 2.9 *Protected characteristics*

Age	Where this is referred to, it refers to a person belonging to a particular age (e.g. 32 year olds) or range of ages (e.g. 18–30 year olds).
Disability	A person has a disability if s/he has a physical or mental impairment which has a substantial and long-term adverse effect on that person's ability to carry out normal day-to-day activities.
Gender reassignment	The process of transitioning from one gender to another.
Marriage and civil partnership	Marriage is defined as a 'union between a man and a woman'. Same-sex couples can have their relationships legally recognised as 'civil partnerships'. Civil partners must be treated the same as married couples on a wide range of legal matters.
Pregnancy and maternity	Pregnancy is the condition of being pregnant or expecting a baby. Maternity refers to the period after the birth, and is linked to maternity leave in the employment context. In the non-work context, protection against maternity discrimination is for 26 weeks after giving birth, and this includes treating a woman unfavourably because she is breastfeeding.
Race	Refers to the protected characteristic of Race. It refers to a group of people defined by their race, colour, and nationality (including citizenship), ethnic or national origins.
Religion and belief	Religion has the meaning usually given to it but belief includes religious and philosophical beliefs including lack of belief (e.g. Atheism). Generally, a belief should affect your life choices or the way you live for it to be included in the definition.
Sex	A man or a woman.
Sexual orientation	Whether a person's sexual attraction is towards their own sex, the opposite sex or to both sexes. http://www.equalityhumanrights.com/advice-and-guidance/new-equality-act-guidance/protected-characteristics-definitions/

Box 2.2 *Corah dental anxiety scale*

If you had to go to the dentist tomorrow, how would you feel about it?
- I would look forward to it as a reasonably enjoyable experience
- I wouldn't care one way or the other
- I would be a little uneasy about it
- I would be afraid that it would be unpleasant and painful
- I would be so anxious that I might break out in a sweat or almost feel physically sick

When you are waiting in the dental surgery for your turn in the chair, how do you feel?
- Relaxed
- A little uneasy
- Tense
- Anxious
- So anxious that I sometimes break out in a sweat or almost feel physically sick

When you are in the dentist's chair waiting while the drill is prepared to begin work on your teeth, how do you feel?
- Relaxed
- A little uneasy
- Tense
- Anxious
- So anxious that I sometimes break out in a sweat or almost feel physically sick

You are in the dentist's chair to have your teeth cleaned. While you are waiting and the dentist is getting out the instruments for scraping your teeth around the gums, how do you feel?
- Relaxed
- A little uneasy
- Tense
- Anxious
- So anxious that I sometimes break out in a sweat or almost feel physically sick

It may occasionally be helpful to carry out a formal assessment of the patient's feelings about health care, and tools such as the Corah anxiety scale are available for this (Box 2.2; Ch. 10).

When taking a history, a structured guide such as that shown in Box 2.3 should be followed. Patients should also be given a form on which to supply all the information they can about their health and any medication they are receiving. Medical and drug history should be regularly updated at subsequent dental visits. *Remember that all such information is confidential.*

Box 2.3 *Essentials of history-taking*

- Personal details
- Presenting complaint (PC)
- History of presenting complaint (HPC)
- Relevant medical history (RMH)
- Drug history
- Social history
- Family history

PERSONAL DETAILS

The patient's personal details include age, sex, educational status, religion or faith, occupation, relationship status, address and contact details. This information is necessary for administrative purposes and, since the questions are largely non-threatening, this stage provides a gentle introduction into the meeting of patient and clinician, in a format that can be individualized to suit a particular culture.

PRESENTING COMPLAINT

This should be recorded in the patient's own words (e.g. 'pain in my face').

HISTORY OF PRESENTING COMPLAINT

The timing of the complaint and its evolution should be elicited. If the patient has pain, a useful mnemonic is 'SOCRATES': S – site, O – onset (gradual/sudden), C – character, R – radiation, A – associations (other symptoms), T – timing/duration, E – exacerbating and alleviating factors, S – severity (pain rated on a visual analogue scale of 1 [minimal] to 10 [unbearable]).

RELEVANT MEDICAL HISTORY

This includes any past medical and surgical problems. Patients should be asked if they carry a medical warning card or device and careful note should be taken of it, particularly in respect of allergies, a bleeding disorder, cardiac disease or diabetes (see, for example, Medic-Alert and Talisman; Figs 2.1–2.3). Patients increasingly wear wristbands and bracelets that show the major medical issues they face. These may be seen clearly in writing; available electronically with bar codes or QR codes; supplied on a USB stick; or provided on a chip that is available for electronic scanning with a sensor (Fig. 2.4).

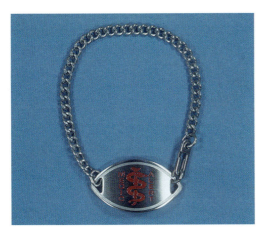

Fig. 2.1 Medic-Alert bracelet. The patient's main diagnosis or drug treatment is engraved on the reverse, together with the telephone number of the company that holds details of the medical history.

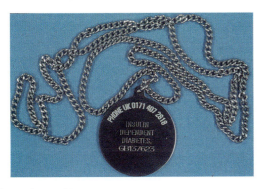

Fig. 2.2 Diabetes alert necklace.

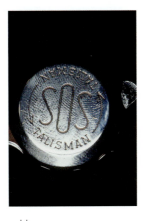

Fig. 2.3 Talisman warning emblem.

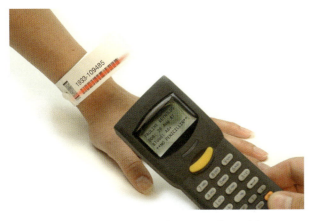

Fig. 2.4 Electronic reading of medical data. (Courtesy of Google).

> **Box 2.4** *Review of systems (see Table 2.10)*
>
> - Allergies
> - Bleeding disorders
> - Cardiorespiratory disorders
> - Drug treatment
> - Endocrine disorders
> - Fits or faints
> - Gastrointestinal disorders
> - Hospital admissions and attendances
> - Infections
> - Jaundice and liver disease
> - Kidney and genitourinary disorders
> - Likelihood of pregnancy
> - Mental state
> - Neurological problems

The completion of a medical history form provides a useful basis for the dental professional to enquire further, and the following chapters describe in more detail the nature and relevance of any diseases that are mentioned. The completion of such a form and appropriate response to its contents also constitute useful evidence when the clinician is faced with any medico-legal claims. The medical history is crucial but has limitations, not least because patients may be confused or ill informed. *The history may also change radically with time, so it is essential for it to be updated before each new course of treatment and every sedation session, and especially before surgery or GA.* For example, patients not pregnant at one course of treatment could well be by the next. One study followed a small group of middle-aged and older dental patients, and found that nearly 20% developed significant medical disorders (mostly cardiovascular) over a period of 5 years.

Functional enquiry or review of systems (ROS) helps disclose undeclared medical problems. Patients should be asked specifically about their conditions; Box 2.4 offers an alphabetical list that is easy to recall.

The relevance of the main points from the history is shown in Table 2.10. It may also be necessary to enquire about constitutional symptoms (e.g. fever, weight loss, night sweats, fatigue/malaise/lethargy, sleeping pattern, appetite, fever), musculoskeletal conditions (pain, stiffness, swelling of the joints), and rash, blistering or lumps (Figs 2.5–2.8).

DRUG (MEDICATION) HISTORY

Enquire whether the patient has any allergies, and ask for a description of any reactions that have occurred.

Often, a medical problem is revealed only after a drug history has been elicited, but some patients may be unaware of the name of, or reason for taking, their medication. Multiple drug use is common in older people with complex medical histories (Figs 2.9–2.11). Sometimes, the nature of the drug used may be suggested by the name (Table 2.11). Ask the patient if they are taking any prescription-only medication (POM; this may be tablets, injections, patches or inhalers) and also any over-the-counter (OTC) medications, including herbal preparations. Some of these can influence health care.

SOCIAL HISTORY

Enquire tactfully about occupation, marital status, partner's job and health, housing, dependants, mobility, lifestyle habits (alcohol,

Table 2.10 *Relevance of medical history to dentistry*

Condition	Main features	Other comments	Relevance in dentistry
Allergies	Range from urticaria to anaphylaxis	Rashes? Racial origins may be important, especially in the case of drug reactions. Carbamazepine-induced Stevens–Johnson syndrome is strongly associated with HLA-B1502 in Han Chinese, Hong Kong Chinese, Thais and Indians, and HLA-A3101 in Northern Europeans	Common allergies relate to latex, iodine, Elastoplast® and drugs (hence acronym 'LIED'). Anaesthetics, analgesics (e.g. aspirin or codeine) and antibiotics (e.g. penicillin) are main offending drugs
Bleeding disorders	Bleeding and/or bruising	Haematological/lymphatic: lymph node swelling? Bleeding or bruising? History of involvement of other family members or of admission to hospital for control of bleeding is particularly important	Significant hazard to surgery
Cardiorespiratory disorders	Wheezing, cough, dyspnoea, chest pain, swelling of ankles, palpitations, hypertension	Chest pain? Shortness of breath? Exercise tolerance? Orthopnoea? Oedema? Palpitations? Cough? Sputum? Wheeze? Haemoptysis? Patient's ability to climb 15–20 stairs without pain, dyspnoea or tiredness may indicate degree of fitness of cardiorespiratory system	Often a contraindication to GA or CS
Drug treatment	Obtaining useful answers about drug treatment, including over-the-counter medications, will necessitate asking: 'Do you ever have any injections or take drugs, pills, tablets, medicines or herbal preparations of *any* kind?'	Drug use may be only indication of serious underlying disease. Corticosteroids, antihypertensives, anticonvulsants, anticoagulants, antibiotics, insulin and oral hypoglycaemics are all important in this respect	Most serious drug interactions are with GA agents (intravenous or inhalational), monoamine oxidase inhibitors and antihypertensive drugs. Aspirin and other non-steroidal anti-inflammatory drugs (NSAIDs) may be a hazard in anticoagulated, asthmatic, diabetic or pregnant patients, those with peptic ulcer, or children under 16 y. If patient does not know name of medicines, defer treatment until drug is identified by patient's doctor, Drugs Information Unit or pharmacy, or by checking *Monthly Index of Medical Specialties* (MIMS), *Physicians' Desk Reference* (PDR) or *British National Formulary* (BNF)
Endocrine disorders	Diabetes mellitus may lead to collapse	Diabetes: irritability, aggression, lassitude, anorexia, weight loss Hyperthyroidism: heat intolerance, emotional lability, sweating, diarrhoea, oligomenorrhoea, weight loss despite increased appetite, tremor, palpitations, visual disturbances Hypothyroidism: dislike of cold weather, lethargy, tiredness, depression, dry skin and hair, hoarseness, menorrhagia, constipation Hyperadrenocorticism: weight gain and redistribution, moon face, hirsutism, skin striae, purpura Hypoadrenalism: weakness, weight loss, hypotension, pigmentation	Hypoglycaemia is main problem
Fits or faints	History of fits or faints	Type? Frequency? Precipitating factors? Awareness may allow preventive measures to be instituted	Fainting, epilepsy and other causes of loss of consciousness can disrupt dental treatment and may result in injury to patient
Gastrointestinal disorders	Abdominal pain, frequency and type of stool, bleeding and weight loss	Difficulty swallowing? Indigestion? Nausea/vomiting/haematemesis? Bowel habit? Faecal colour, consistency, blood (or melaena), smell, difficulty flushing away, tenesmus (feeling of incomplete evacuation) or urgency?	Crohn disease or coeliac disease may lead to oral complications, and gastric disorders may increase risk of vomiting during GA
Hospital admissions and attendances	Hospital admissions may also indicate underlying disease, and past operations may suggest possibility of future complications that can influence dental treatment		A history of operations may provide knowledge of possible reactions to GA and surgery. A patient who has had a tonsillectomy, for example, without complications is most unlikely to have a congenital bleeding disorder. Retinal operations, since they may use intraocular gases, may be a contraindication to GA or relative analgesia, which may cause rapid expansion of ocular gas and lead to blindness

(Continued)

Table 2.10 (Continued)

Condition	Main features	Other comments	Relevance in dentistry
Infections	Various, possibly rashes and/or fever	Ever attended a clinic for sexually shared infections (SSIs), or been admitted to hospital for an infection, or been accepted or refused for blood donation? Men who have sex with men, abusers of intravenous drugs and patients who have attended SSI clinics are more likely to have a history of infection with human immunodeficiency virus (HIV), hepatitis viruses, herpes simplex, syphilis, gonorrhoea and many other infections (Ch. 21)	The possibility of transmission of infections and their sequelae must be considered. Carriers of meticillin-resistant *Staphylococcus aureus* (MRSA) may be a hazard to others; carriers of *Neisseria meningitides* may be sources of meningitis outbreaks
Jaundice and liver disorders	A history of jaundice may imply carriage of hepatitis viruses, although jaundice is a clinical sign of other underlying liver diseases		Liver disease can lead to prolonged bleeding and impaired drug metabolism can result (Ch. 9). Jaundice after an operation may have resulted from halothane hepatitis and, if this is suspected, a different general anaesthetic, such as isoflurane, desflurane or sevoflurane, should be given
Kidney and genitourinary disorders	Manifestations of chronic kidney disease may include hypertension, pallor and bruising	Incontinence (stress or urge), dysuria (pain), haematuria, nocturia, frequency, polyuria, hesitancy, terminal dribbling? Vaginal discharge?	Can affect dental management, as excretion of some drugs is impaired. Tetracyclines should be given in lower doses. Complications of renal failure or transplants can produce oral signs
Likelihood of pregnancy		Menses (periods) – frequency, regularity, heaviness, duration, painfulness? First day of last menstrual period (LMP)? Number of pregnancies and births? Menarche? Menopause? Any chance of pregnancy now? Which trimester?	Any essential procedures involving drugs (even aspirin), radiography or GA should be arranged during middle trimester
Mental state	Behavioural changes	Appearance and behaviour; thought (speech) form, rate, quantity, pattern, flight of ideas, loosening of associations; mood (subjective); affect (observed); thought content, preoccupations, obsessions, overvalued ideas, ideas of reference, delusions; suicidality; abnormal experiences, hallucinations, passivity, thought interference; cognition; consciousness; attention/concentration; memory; orientation; intelligence; executive function; insight. It may sometimes be useful to assess degree of patients' anxiety in a relatively objective way by using Corah dental anxiety scale (see Box 2.2)	Anxiety is inexorably associated with attending for dental treatment. Anxious patients may sometimes react aggressively and anxiety may limit extent of dental treatment that can be provided under LA
Neurological problems		Special senses – any changes in sight, smell, hearing and/or taste? Seizures, faints, fits, funny turns? Headache? Pins and needles (paraesthesiae) or numbness? Limb weakness, poor balance? Speech problems? Sphincter disturbance?	Movement disorders can significantly disrupt operative procedures. Access can be a barrier to care

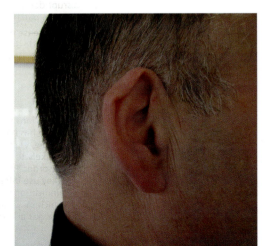

Fig. 2.5 'Boxer's ear', showing distortion.

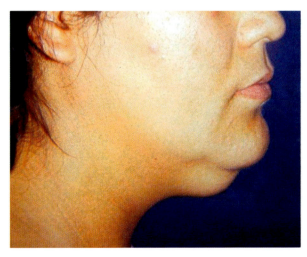

Fig. 2.6 Cyst in submental region.

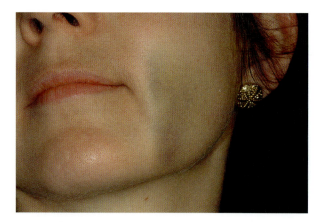

Fig. 2.7 Facial bruising.

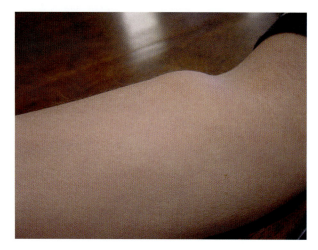

Fig. 2.8 Lipoma.

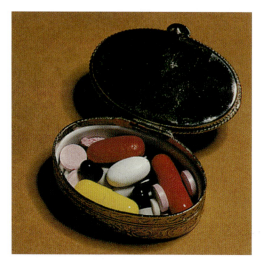

Fig. 2.9 Pill box presented by an outpatient who proved to be taking eight different medications daily, including a corticosteroid.

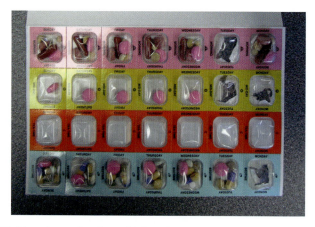

Fig. 2.10 Manual organizer for multi-drug therapy.

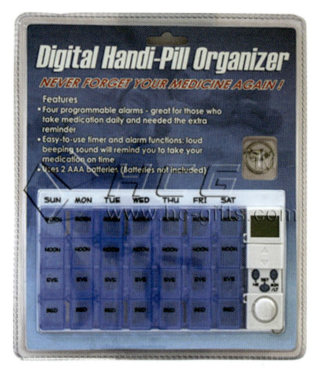

Fig. 2.11 Digital organizer for multi-drug therapy. (Courtesy of Google).

tobacco, betel, etc., and recreational drugs), culture and faith. Any social or religious engagements that are dependent on the patient being unimpeded following an elective treatment (wedding, examination, job interview) need discussion and possibly the treatment should be rescheduled; see also Chapters 25, 28 and 30.

FAMILY HISTORY

The medical history of blood relatives may be very informative.

CLINICAL EXAMINATION

It is important for dental professionals not merely to inspect and examine the mouth and neck, but also to inspect the exposed areas of the patient (the face, neck, arms and hands). The patient's appearance, behaviour, speech and body language can reveal many significant conditions (Fig. 2.12). However, it must be stressed that even very ill patients can look remarkably well. A search should be made for such readily visible signs as anxiety, movements, tremors, dyspnoea, wheezing and tiredness, and also for changes in the face (e.g. expression, pallor, cyanosis or jaundice), neck (e.g. lumps) or hands (e.g. finger clubbing, Raynaud phenomenon, rashes).

Facial movement and sensation should be assessed in the course of testing the cranial nerves (Ch. 13). Eyes and ears should be observed and examined (Fig. 2.13). Maxillary, mandibular or zygomatic deformities or swellings may be more reliably confirmed by inspection from above (maxillae, zygomas) or behind (mandible). The degree and direction of opening of the mandible should be assessed; this can be disturbed in temporomandibular joint (TMJ) disease and

Table 2.11 *Drug names and possible identification*

Drugs ending in …	Possible type of drug[a]
-am	Benzodiazepines
-ase	Fibrinolytics
-apine	Antipsychotics
-asone/one	Corticosteroids
-azine	Antipsychotics
-azole	Azole antifungals
-azosin	α-adrenoreceptor blockers
-cillin	Penicillins
-cin	Some antimicrobials
-coxib	Newer non-steroidal anti-inflammatory drugs (NSAIDs)
-cycline	Tetracyclines
-dopa	Antiparkinsonian agents
-dronate/dronic	Bisphosphonates
-erol	β_2 agonists (used for asthma)
-fibrate	Fibrates
-gatran	Newer oral anticoagulants (NOACs)
-imab/umab	Monoclonal antibodies (MoAbs)
-ipine	Calcium-channel blockers
-lukast	Leukotriene-receptor antagonists
-navir	Protease inhibitors (PIs)
-nitrate	Nitrates
-olol	Beta-blockers
-ovir	Antivirals
-parin	Heparins
-prazole	Proton-pump inhibitors (PPIs)
-pril	Angiotensin-converting enzyme inhibitors (ACEIs)
-relin	Gonadorelin analogues
-salazine	Salicylate derivatives
-sartan	Angiotensin-receptor antagonist
-setron	$5HT_3$ antagonists
-statin	Statins
-terol	β_2-adrenergic agonist
-tidine	H_2-receptor antagonists
-triptan	$5HT_1$ agonists
-tropium	Antimuscarinic bronchodilators
-vudine	Nucleoside reverse transcriptase inhibitors (NRTIs)

[a]Always check in *British National Formulary* (BNF).

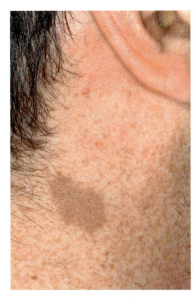

Fig. 2.12 Café-au-lait patch indicative of neurofibromatosis.

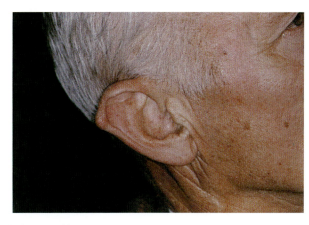

Fig. 2.13 Gouty tophi.

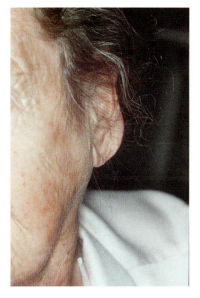

Fig. 2.14 Salivary gland swelling.

other conditions causing restricted mouth-opening (trismus) discussed in Chapter 4.

Inspection of the major salivary glands may reveal swelling of the parotid gland, which causes outward deflection of the lower part of the ear lobe, best observed by looking at the patient from behind (Fig. 2.14).

Examination of the neck is crucial. The patient should be observed from the front but also the neck should be palpated, as swollen lymph nodes are sometimes a sign of disease (Fig. 2.15). One-third of the body's lymph nodes are in the neck.

Hands can show a number of features. Deformities can be seen in arthritis (Fig. 2.16). Palmar erythema may occur in liver disease and rheumatoid arthritis. Finger-clubbing may be congenital or is seen in cardiorespiratory disease and liver cirrhosis. Koilonychia (spoon-shaped nails) is seen in iron deficiency; leukonychia (white nails) in liver cirrhosis; nail defects in lichen planus (Fig. 2.17), chronic candidosis and psoriasis; nail haemorrhages in infective endocarditis; and pigmentation in drug use (e.g. zidovudine; Fig. 2.18). Raynaud phenomenon can be a feature of connective tissue disorders. Finger-joint deformities can occur in rheumatoid arthritis. Dupuytren contracture (Ch. 4) may be seen in alcoholic cirrhosis and muscle contractures in cerebral palsy.

Hair can show features in several conditions. Alopecia may be autoimmune, may be seen in lichen planus, or may occur after radiation.

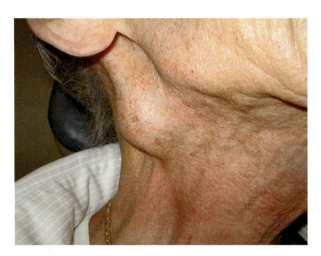

Fig. 2.15 Cervical lymphadenopathy.

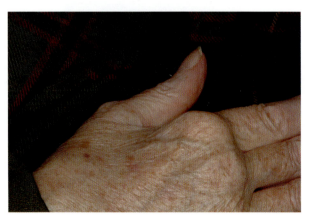

Fig. 2.16 Arthritis.

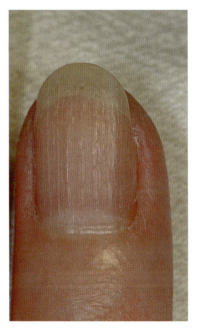

Fig. 2.17 Lichen planus nail deformity.

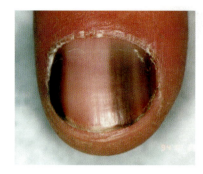

Fig. 2.18 Nail discolouration may be seen after trauma or in local disease, such as fungal infections, in drug use (as here) or in systemic disease.

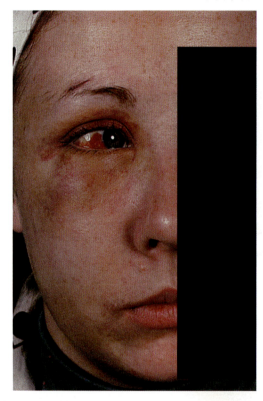

Fig. 2.19 Subconjunctival haemorrhage associated with zygomatic fracture.

Hirsutism is a feature of adrenogenital syndrome or Cushing disease, or may be caused by ciclosporin, corticosteroids, minoxidil, phenytoin or androgenic steroids.

The face may be unusual in many syndromes, such as Down syndrome or mucopolysaccharidoses. It may exhibit bruising from trauma (Fig. 2.19) or purpura; cushingoid facies due to Cushing disease or corticosteroid treatment; and a mask-like facies in scleroderma. Facial telangiectasia is seen in hereditary haemorrhagic telangiectasia, cirrhosis and CREST (*c*alcinosis, *R*aynaud, *o*esophageal dysfunction, *s*cleroderma, *t*elangiectasia) syndrome. Facial palsy may indicate stroke or Bell palsy. Neurofibromatosis (Fig. 2.20), tumours (Fig. 2.21) and cysts (Fig. 2.22) may present as lumps. Infection may cause swelling (Fig. 2.23). Myxoedema may indicate hypothyroidism. 'Butterfly rash' over the face may indicate systemic lupus erythematosus, while angiofibromas may underlie tuberous sclerosis (epiloia; Fig. 2.24). A malar flush can be seen in mitral valve stenosis, xanthelasmas in hyperlipidaemia, and cyanosis in hypoxia – cardiac or respiratory disease. Pallor is seen in anaemia or before an imminent faint; purpura may occur in thrombocytopenia or trauma; hyperpigmentation can be racial, or due to suntan, Addison disease or chronic drug (e.g. phenothiazine) use; and hypopigmentation can be caused by vitiligo (Fig. 2.25).

Eyes may show features of disease. Exophthalmos can be seen in hyperthyroidism, and ptosis in myopathy and Horner syndrome. Blue sclerae can be features of infancy and osteogenesis imperfecta.

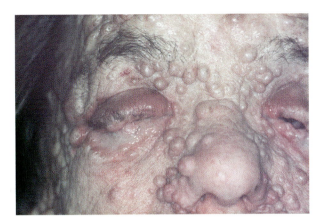

Fig. 2.20 Neurofibromatosis.

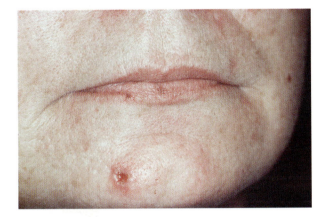

Fig. 2.21 Basal cell carcinoma.

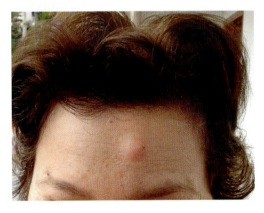

Fig. 2.22 Sebaceous cyst.

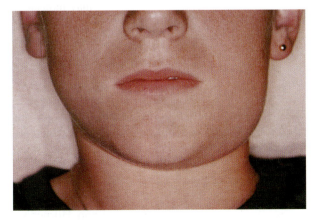

Fig. 2.23 Cat scratch disease.

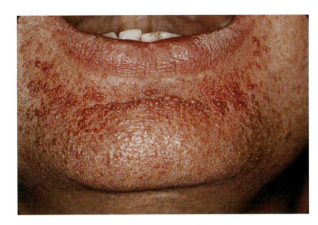

Fig. 2.24 Tuberous sclerosis showing adenoma sebaceum.

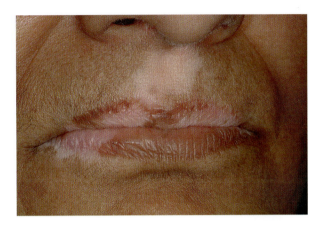

Fig. 2.25 Vitiligo.

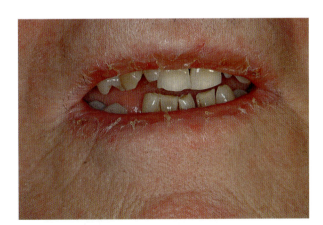

Fig. 2.26 Exfoliative cheilitis.

Conjunctival haemorrhage can indicate trauma, fractured zygoma or purpura. Jaundice can imply liver disease.

The lips can show cheilitis (e.g. factitious; Fig. 2.26), lichen planus (Fig. 2.27) or erythema multiforme. Angular stomatitis can be associated with denture-related stomatitis, anaemia, haematinic deficiency, diabetes, human immunodeficiency virus (HIV) and other diseases (Fig. 2.28). Lip swelling may be seen after trauma and in infections, neoplasms, allergies, Crohn disease, sarcoidosis or angioedema. Lip pigmentation may underlie Peutz–Jeghers syndrome. 'Hanging jaw' is a feature of myasthenia gravis.

Lumps may indicate neoplasms (Fig. 2.29). *Salivary gland* swellings can represent mumps, Sjögren syndrome, sialosis or tumour (Ch. 4).

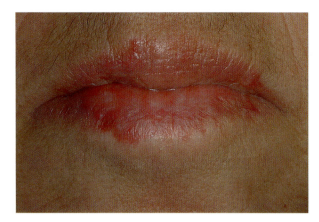

Fig. 2.27 Lichen planus on lips.

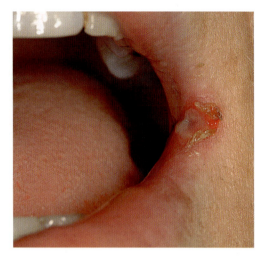

Fig. 2.28 Angular stomatitis.

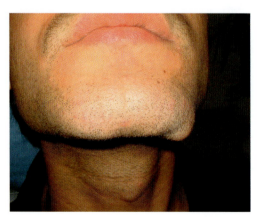

Fig. 2.29 Osteoma.

Jaw prognathism and thickened facies can be features of acromegaly. *Cervical lymph node* enlargement is seen in HIV and other infections, malignancy and leukaemia.

Loss of weight or emaciation can be features of anorexia, malignant disease, tuberculosis or HIV infection.

Speech disturbances may suggest drug intoxication, hyposalivation, learning disorder, and neurological or muscle diseases.

Inpatients must always have a full physical examination before an operation, which may include inspection, palpation, percussion and auscultation, and covers examination of at least the following systems:

- Lymph nodes
- Cardiovascular – pulse, blood pressure, heart sounds
- Respiratory – respiratory rate, lung expansion, tracheal position, lung sounds
- Gastrointestinal – any swelling or restriction of movement or tenderness, together with palpation for masses and tenderness
- Neurological – especially the cranial nerves.

Most evidence shows that the history and physical examination often reveal most, if not all, of the clinically useful data. Before any investigations are initiated, the patient's consent must be obtained. Confidentiality must be respected; the history, examination and investigation findings should not be divulged except when there is expressed consent.

INVESTIGATIONS

Investigations are useful only when the appropriate tests are requested, and interpreted in the light of the history, clinical findings, knowledge and experience. It is useless and potentially dangerous to request investigations, the results of which will have no influence on the diagnosis or management.

Screening for latent medical problems is *sometimes* appropriate, mainly when effective action can be taken on the basis of the results. Several relevant treatable conditions, particularly hypertension and diabetes, are frequently unsuspected. For example, blood and urine glucose levels may be abnormal in 5% or more of dental patients. However, it is important not to undertake testing that may cause unnecessary anxiety, trauma, delay or expense.

Many studies have shown the *disadvantages* of 'routine' and 'screening' tests, even preoperatively, carried out with little focus; too often, trivial or inexplicable findings are revealed and unnecessary anxiety and stress caused.

PREOPERATIVE TESTS

Preoperative tests may provide information to reduce possible harm or increase benefit to the patient by altering surgical or sedation/anaesthetic management, and may help risk assessment and guide discussion with the patient that is relevant to informed consent. They may predict postoperative complications and establish a baseline measurement for later reference. Before any investigation is requested, however, it is important for there to be a high enough likelihood of finding an abnormal result and for an abnormal result genuinely to change the patient's management. Most preoperative tests (typically, a full blood count, prothrombin time [PT] or international normalized ratio [INR], activated partial thromboplastin time [APTT], basic metabolic panel and urinalysis) performed on elective surgical patients prove to be normal: findings influence management in under 3% of patients tested. In almost all cases, no adverse outcomes are observed when clinically stable patients undergo elective surgery, irrespective of whether an abnormal test is identified. Preoperative testing is appropriate in symptomatic patients and those with risks factors for which diagnostic testing can provide clarification of a patient's surgical risk. The National Institute for Health and Care Excellence (NICE; formerly the National Institute for Health and Clinical Excellence) guidelines are generic and lack consensus (http://publications.nice.org.uk/preoperative-tests-cg3; accessed 25 May 2013); hospitals may have their own guidelines and individual clinicians remain ultimately responsible.

Table 2.12 *Grades of surgery*

Grade	Examples of procedures
1	Excision of lumps and bumps, incision of abscesses, tooth removal
2	Arthroscopy, herniorrhaphy, tonsillectomy, varicose veins
3	Hysterectomy, thyroidectomy, endoscopic prostatectomy
4	Major bowel, head and neck, lung and joint surgery, and joint replacement
	Neurosurgery
	Cardiovascular surgery

(adapted from NICE).

For the purpose of preoperative tests, NICE categorizes surgical procedures into four grades on the basis of complexity and physiological insult (Table 2.12).

The NICE recommendations are in the form of 'look-up' tables set out by surgery grade and ASA grade (http://www.nice.org.uk/nicemedia/live/10920/29090/29090.pdf; accessed 30 September 2013):

- Plain chest X-ray (radiograph)
- Resting electrocardiogram (ECG)
- Full blood count
- Haemostasis – including PT, APTT and INR
- Renal function – including tests for potassium, sodium, creatinine and/or urea levels
- Random blood glucose
- Urine analysis (urine dipstick tests – test for pH, protein, glucose, ketones, blood/haemoglobin).

There are also recommendations for sickle cell test and pregnancy tests, and:

- blood gases – for ASA grades II and III only
- lung function (peak expiratory flow rate, forced vital capacity and forced expiratory volume) – for ASA grades II and III only.

Chest radiograph (X-ray)

The likelihood of identifying undiagnosed cardiorespiratory disease and the desirability of re-evaluating patients with known conditions need to be balanced against the radiation exposure. In general, ASA I patients do not require preoperative chest X-rays (CXRs), with the *possible* exception of smokers over the age of 60 who are undergoing grade 3 or 4 surgery. Certain types of surgery *may* warrant a CXR at some point in the patient's work-up (e.g. cardiothoracic, oesophageal, and major head and neck surgery). ASA III patients with cardiovascular disease undergoing anything more than grade 1 surgery should probably have a CXR. This should not be repeated if one has been done within 6 months unless the patient's symptoms or signs have changed; in many cases, it could be argued that echocardiography provides more useful information and avoids radiation exposure. Respiratory disease that has changed in its nature or severity with time is a probable indication for CXR, with the exception of patients between the ages of 16 and 40 undergoing grade 1 surgery.

Electrocardiogram

An electrocardiogram (ECG) may on occasion provide evidence of asymptomatic cardiovascular disease and, in those with known cardiac disease, is useful in estimating risks of GA and surgery. An ECG should be obtained for smokers, for patients with a history or symptoms of cardiac, respiratory or renal disease undergoing grade 4 surgery, and for all patients over the age of 60, regardless of the grade of surgery.

Full blood count (full blood picture)

Full blood count (FBC) may identify and quantify pre-existing anaemia and help assessment of the patient's likely tolerance of any blood loss. FBC is probably indicated in all patients undergoing grade 3 or 4 surgery, particularly in patients with cardiovascular or respiratory disease, for all patients with renal disease, and for all patients over 60 undergoing grade 2 surgery. The white cell count (WCC) may be useful if infection is suspected, and the platelet count where there is suspicion or a history of bleeding tendency.

Haemostasis tests

Haemostatic tests include the platelet count, PT, INR and APTT (Ch. 8). Indications for such tests preoperatively are patients taking anticoagulants; those on haemodialysis; those with a past history or family history of abnormal bleeding, bruising, or liver, kidney or vascular disease; before surgery with the potential to cause a large blood loss so that the need for transfusion is likely; before surgery for cancer, especially where liver metastases may have resulted in a bleeding tendency; and before arterial reconstructive surgery. Investigations should also be considered when regional anaesthesia is planned, particularly using spinal and epidural techniques.

Renal function tests (urea and electrolytes)

Renal function should be assessed in all patients with known renal disease, diabetes, liver dysfunction, and those with an ileus, who are parenterally fed or who are likely to have intravenous fluid administration and perioperative fluid loss.

All adults and children should have urea and electrolyte tests (U&Es) before grade 4 surgery (U&Es are otherwise not generally required in children). These tests are needed in all adults of ASA III or those undergoing grade 3 surgery. Older patients may have asymptomatic deteriorating renal function, so U&Es should be obtained for those aged 60 and over, and before grade 3 surgery. In patients with cardiovascular disease, U&Es are needed in those aged 60 and over undergoing grade 2 surgery.

Sickle test

A sickle test should be requested for all patients of African and West Indian origin, and probably also for those of Mediterranean and Indian origin.

IMAGING

X-RAYS (RADIOGRAPHY)

Radiography, fully discussed elsewhere (see https://www.gov.uk/government/publications/the-ionising-radiation-medical-exposure-regulations-2000), is particularly helpful diagnostically since it is inexpensive, rapidly achieved and widely available. Conventional radiography is useful for imaging: bone and joint disease, fractures and dislocations, antral and dental disease (Table 2.13). Plain X-rays have a relatively low radiation dose and special procedures can achieve soft-tissue imaging, albeit with a higher radiation dose.

Table 2.13 *Radiographs recommended for demonstrating various head and neck sites*

Region required	Standard views	Additional views
Skull[a]	Postero-anterior (PA) 20	Submento-vertex (SMV)
	Lateral	Tangential
	Townes (1/2 axial view)	
Facial bones	Occipito-mental (OM)	Zygoma
	OM 30	Reduced exposure SMV
	Lateral	
Paranasal sinuses	OM for maxillary antra	Upper occlusal or lateral SMV
		Dental panoramic tomography (DPT), tomography
Orthodontics	DPT	
	Cephalometric lateral skull	
Pre- and post-osteotomy	DPT	
	Cephalometric lateral skull	
	Cephalometric PA skull	
Nasal bones	OM 30	
	Lateral	
	Soft tissue lateral	
Mandible	DPT	Lateral obliques
		PA mandible
		Mandibular occlusal
Temporomandibular joints	Transcranial lateral obliques or DPT (mouth open and closed)	Transpharyngeal Arthrography Reverse Townes Reverse DPT Consider CT scan/ MRI

[a] CT scanning is valuable in craniofacial injuries.

Radiography requests are essential to enable the radiographic staff to provide the best or most appropriate radiographs for the region under investigation:

1. Fill in the request form as fully as possible with full, relevant, clinical findings.
2. Request the region required rather than specific views, except for dental panoramic tomography, when the term 'DPT' will suffice.

COMPUTED (AXIAL) TOMOGRAPHY

A computed tomography (CT) or computed axial tomography (CAT) scan is a type of repeated special radiograph taken across 'slices' of the body to build up a complex image, using several beams simultaneously from a number of different angles (Fig. 2.30). Cone beam CT (CBCT) is a variant, increasingly used in dentistry for implant work especially (see below).

Advantages

- CT provides good anatomical representation of hard tissues (bone and cartilage).
- It is generally better than magnetic resonance imaging (MRI) for examining lymph nodes.
- It provides good cross-sectional representation.

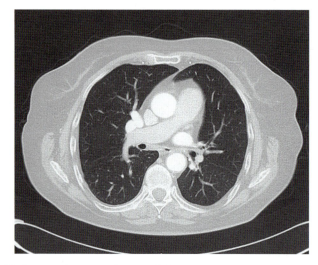

Fig. 2.30 Computed tomography scan of chest.

- Multiplanar reconstruction is possible from the raw data of the initial examination.
- Three-dimensional reconstruction is possible.
- It provides guidance for biopsies.
- Compared with MRI:
  imaging is more rapid (in seconds – compared with MRI, which takes minutes)
  it is less affected by motion artefact, since it is quicker
  it can be used on patients for whom MRI is inappropriate (e.g. claustrophobics, or people with pacemakers or ferrous or paramagnetic aneurysm clips).

Disadvantages

- CT gives a significant radiation dose.
- It provides phasic imaging of vascular structures and tumours.
- It is an expensive procedure.
- The whole CT procedure may take up to 1 hour, but often takes less than 30 minutes.
- Some patients experience claustrophobia in the CT scanner.

Indications

CT allows visualization of 3–10-mm sections of the body in two dimensions with enough clear distinction between black, grey and white areas of the image to allow pathological diagnosis in many cases.

It is particularly useful in examining the chest or abdomen. CT using contrast media makes it possible to visualize abnormalities more clearly.

Contraindications

Contraindications include pregnancy and history of severe allergies; this may preclude the use of a contrast agent.

Procedure

1. Patients may be asked not to eat beforehand.
2. Patients may have to swallow or be injected intravenously with contrast material that will show up against the tissue on the final pictures.

3. Patients must lie on a couch, which will move through the scanner.
4. The radiographer can see, hear and communicate with the patient (by means of a two-way microphone and speaker system) at all times.
5. The scanner will take a series of pictures.
6. Patients must lie still while images are being taken in order to ensure that they are in focus, and may be asked to hold their breath so the scan is not blurred.

CONE BEAM CT (CBCT)

This is CT in which the X-rays are divergent, forming a cone. CBCT is useful in implantology, endodontics and orthodontics, for accurate visualization of the jaws, teeth and roots (erupted and non-erupted) and of anomalous structures that conventional 2D radiography cannot capture.

SCINTIGRAPHY/NUCLEAR MEDICINE

Radionuclide (radioisotope) scans can be particularly useful for detecting abnormalities in bone, salivary glands, thyroid gland and lymph nodes. The common radionuclide agents used include technetium-99^{m} (Tc-99m) – labelled diphosphonates for bone scans, and gallium for imaging lymph nodes.

Radionuclide scanning involves administration of a radionuclide with an affinity for the organ or tissue of interest, and recording of the distribution of radioactivity. A very small amount of a mildly radioactive liquid is injected into a vein, usually in the arm; after the injection, the patient will have to wait up to 3 hours before the scan can be taken. The distribution of the radionuclide is detected in the tissue/organ under examination where the isotope is concentrated, by a gamma camera, which produces the images or scans after processing by a computer. Detectors record activity in retaining organs at the time of acquisition. Time/activity curves can be plotted to provide functional analysis. The images can then be produced on film or coloured paper, or as graphs or numerical data. The amount of radioactivity given to a patient is small, not dangerous either to the patient or to anyone nearby, and usually clears from the body within 24 hours.

POSITRON EMISSION TOMOGRAPHY

Radioactive molecules made from radionuclides (radioactive isotopes) with short half-lives, such as ^{11}C, ^{15}O or ^{13}N, are injected intravenously. Depending on the type of molecule injected, positron emission tomography (PET) can provide information on different biochemical functions. For example, if glucose is used, the PET scan will show an image of glucose metabolism, or how much energy the body is using in a specific area (such as the brain or a tumour).

MAGNETIC RESONANCE IMAGING (NUCLEAR MAGNETIC RESONANCE)

Magnetic resonance imaging (MRI) is a safe, non-invasive procedure that allows three-dimensional images of internal organs to be created with radio waves and large powerful electromagnets to align hydrogen atoms (protons) within the body (Fig. 2.31).

Advantages

■ There is no ionizing radiation.
■ MRI provides new, rapidly developing, good multiplanar imaging.

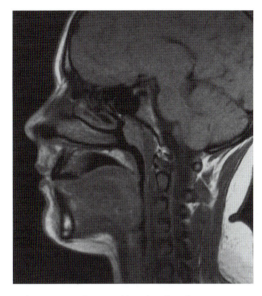

Fig. 2.31 Magnetic resonance image of head and neck.

■ It provides good soft-tissue differentiation, which is better than that with CT.
■ It provides good imaging of bone marrow.
■ It provides good imaging of perineural infiltration.
■ Pictures can be taken from multiple angles.
■ It can be performed through clothing and through dense tissue such as bone.
■ There is less distortion from dental restorations than with CT.

Disadvantages

MRI is dangerous for people with pacemakers or defibrillators and inappropriate for those with ferrous or paramagnetic aneurysm clips (Ch. 5). Currently, MRI is relatively expensive and time-consuming (it can take anything from 30 minutes to 1 hour and 30 minutes, or even 2 hours), and is rather noisy; some ———patients experience claustrophobia. It can also be affected by motion artefact, since it is slow. Gadolinium contrast medium is injected intravenously in up to 30% of MRI scans to improve the clarity.

Indications

MRI, like CT, can be used to produce cross-sectional views of the body or a body part, but can also obtain other views such as sagittal. It allows a clear distinction between black, grey and white areas of the image to aid pathological diagnosis in many cases.

Again like CT, MRI can be used on any part of the body but is frequently employed to examine the head and brain, since it is in this region that it produces clearer results than CT. MRI is also useful for detecting abnormalities in soft tissues and in chest or abdominal examination.

Contraindications

These include:

■ presence of a cardiac pacemaker, defibrillator or monitor
■ presence of vascular or surgical clips
■ presence of any type of orthopaedic prosthesis, rods or pins
■ presence of dentures or appliances of any type in the mouth, which must be removed before the scan (implants, fixed crowns or restorations are not contraindications; see below)

- presence of an intrauterine contraceptive device (IUD)
- pregnancy – any effects of MRI on pregnancy are unclear
- history of allergies – may preclude the use of contrast agent.

Procedure

1. Patients may be asked not to eat for 1 hour before the scan; not to smoke for 2 hours before; and not to drink tea, coffee, alcohol or soft drinks containing caffeine (cola, etc.) for 2 hours before. These can influence blood flow and so affect the scan. Iron interferes with MRI and thus iron-containing medications should not be taken.
2. As the MRI scan uses magnetism, metals may affect it. Persons with certain types of metal surgical clips, metal pins or plates, cardiac monitors, defibrillators or pacemakers cannot, therefore, have an MRI scan. The patient must remove everything metal, including watches, any jewellery including piercings, metal clothes closures, belts, metal-containing prostheses, hair clips, shoes, mobile phones, personal organizers, keys, purses and wallets containing magnetic strip credit cards. These must all be left outside the room.
3. MRI scans are noisy, so the patient wears ear plugs.
4. The patient must lie on a couch that can move backwards and forwards through the cylinder.
5. Patients must lie still while images are being taken in order to ensure that they are in focus, and may be asked to hold their breath so the scan is not blurred.
6. The radiographer can see, hear and communicate with the patient (by means of a two-way microphone and speaker system) at all times.
7. The MRI is in a special room that excludes radio waves, as these interfere with the scan.

ULTRASOUND (ULTRASONOGRAPHY)

Ultrasound is the use of high-frequency sound waves (at a frequency of over 20000 Hz [20 kHz]), which are reflected at interfaces between tissues. An ultrasound scan uses very high-frequency sound waves not audible to the human ear, which are passed through the body using a transmitter or scanner that is normally placed on the skin surface. The pattern of the reflected sound waves or 'echoes' is used to create an outline of the organ in question, so ultrasonography is used for soft tissues rather than bony structures. It can measure size, detect structural abnormalities, determine whether a lump is solid or fluid-filled, and monitor growth of the fetus during pregnancy.

Advantages

- Ultrasound examination is completely painless and safe.
- It produces no ionizing radiation.
- It is inexpensive and provides a good screening test.
- The equipment is mobile.
- It provides good differentiation between cystic and solid soft-tissue masses.
- Advanced technique (Doppler) assesses flow characteristics in vessels.

Indications

- To diagnose disease in liver, gallbladder, pancreas, urinary bladder, prostate, kidney, thyroid gland, lymph nodes, salivary glands, ovaries or testicles, and breast
- In obstetrics, to check that there are no fetal abnormalities, and to monitor fetal growth
- For ophthalmic imaging

- To examine blood flow
- To diagnose aneurysms
- For echocardiography.

Contraindications

None known.

Procedure

1. Ultrasound examination takes between 15 minutes and 1 hour.
2. Usually, a lubricating silicone gel applied to the skin is used to help conduct the sound waves into the body.
3. Patients must lie still during the examination.
4. For some more specialized kinds of ultrasound examination, the probe is inserted into the body.
5. In abdominal ultrasound scanning, large amounts of gas in the intestine can interfere with the images. Therefore, in these instances, low-fibre foods should be taken for 24–36 hours before the examination. Some examinations of the intestines, for example, require a preparatory enema and fasting for several hours before the appointment. Others, as used in obstetrics, may require a full bladder.

LABORATORY INVESTIGATIONS

HISTOPATHOLOGY

A biopsy that is of adequate size and representative of the lesion should be taken, placed in a fixative and sent to the pathology laboratory carefully labelled and with the appropriate form of request for histopathological examination.

- Specimens for *routine histological examination* should be fixed in 10% formol saline; at least ten times the volume of the specimen is needed for adequate fixation.
- Specimens for *immunofluorescent investigations* are not usually carried out on formol saline-fixed tissue, but should be sent in a suitable transport medium for immediate freezing at −70°C and direct immunofluorescence. Serum should also be sent for indirect immunofluorescence.

If tuberculosis or a systemic mycosis is suspected, a fresh tissue specimen should be sent for culture.

MICROBIOLOGY

Specimens should be collected before antimicrobials are started. If pus is present, a sample should be sent in a sterile container, in preference to a swab. Requests for culture and antibiotic sensitivity should indicate possible aetiology, present antimicrobial therapy and any drug allergies. If tuberculosis is suspected, this must be clearly indicated on the request form.

If the microbiological specimen cannot be dealt with within 2 hours, the swab should be placed in transport medium and kept in the refrigerator at 4°C (not a freezer) until dealt with by the microbiology department.

Actinomycosis

It is preferable to send pus for culture but, in the absence of adequate pus, send a dressing that has been in contact with the wound for several hours.

Candidosis

Swabs from the lesions and from the fitting surface of the denture may be sent for Gram stain or culture.

Viral hepatitis or HIV infection

Many centres have defined protocols for the collection of specimens from patients with suspected hepatitis or HIV infection. Particular care must be taken to avoid needlestick injuries and contamination of the outside of the containers, and to indicate that hazard may be posed by the infection. Special coloured plastic bags (usually red) to indicate this hazard can be used for transporting the specimen. Consent is required when testing.

Other viral infections

Swabs must be sent in viral transport medium; dry swabs are no use. Nucleic acid testing is increasingly common. Acute and convalescent serum samples (10 mL blood in a plain container) may be taken; convalescent serum is collected 2–3 weeks after the acute illness.

Syphilis

Oral lesions should be cleaned with saline to remove oral treponemes before a smear is made for dark-ground examination; 10 mL of serum should be sent for Venereal Disease Research Laboratory (VDRL) testing (Ch. 21).

HAEMATOLOGY

Blood for film and red cell indices must be collected in a tube containing potassium ethylenediamine tetra-acetic acid (EDTA; 4 mL into an EDTA tube). EDTA inhibits clotting through its action on cation-dependent proteolytic enzymes critical to the clotting cascade. The blood must be gently mixed to ensure that the anticoagulant is well distributed; clotted samples are useless. Blood for assay of corrected whole blood folate levels is also collected in an EDTA tube. Most other necessary investigations are performed on serum (Appendix 2.3). Any venepuncture episode requires consent, both for the insertion of the needle and for the investigations being carried out on the blood sample. See Table 2.14 for potential complications.

BIOCHEMISTRY

There is currently some variation as to whether serum or plasma is needed for certain biochemical tests, depending on the laboratory involved. Special containers may be required for automated multi-channel analysers, which give a full biochemical profile on a single blood specimen. However, most biochemical estimations can be carried out on serum (collect blood in a plain container), although plasma (collect in a lithium heparin tube) may be needed for estimation of electrolytes, cortisol and proteins. Blood glucose assays are carried out on a sample in a fluoride bottle. Urinalysis is also available (Appendices 2.4 and 2.5).

IMMUNOLOGY

Most tests of humoral immunity and complement components are carried out on serum (plain tube). Autoantibodies are detected in serum. In order to prevent the rapid decay of complement components, the

Table 2.14 *Complications of venepuncture*

Complication	Remarks
Failure in a young normal adult	Relax. Correct application of tourniquet. Warm arm/hand. Check syringe and needle will aspirate
	Try other arm; use sphygmomanometer cuff at just below diastolic pressure; make sure you can palpate vein before trying again
Difficult patients	
Fat arm: veins difficult to locate	Remember that veins are there. Palpate antecubital fossa over usual vein site (see text)
	If unsuccessful, try veins on radial side of wrist or on back of hand (painful)
Thin arm: veins move away from the needle	Most annoying! Insert needle deliberately alongside vein, preferably at a Y-junction, and immobilize vein with your other hand before penetrating vein from side
Haematoma formation	Most annoying to patient! Caused by poor technique, inadequate pressure to puncture site or removal of needle before removal of tourniquet. May cause venous thrombosis. Try not to penetrate through other side of vein. Keep firm pressure with swab on vein after venepuncture until haemostasis secured. In the elderly, maintain this pressure for several minutes

serum should be separated as soon as possible and frozen at −20°C at least and preferably at −70°C. Serum for immune complexes and cryoglobulins may need special handling, details of which can be obtained from the relevant laboratory.

Tests of cell-mediated immunity are expensive and often can be carried out only once special preparations have been made (consult the laboratory; Appendix 2.6).

See above for direct immunofluorescence specimens.

The presence of autoantibodies does not always indicate disease and absence does not necessarily exclude it. The type of autoimmune disorder or disease that occurs and the amount of destruction depend on which systems or organs are targeted by the autoantibodies, and how strongly. Disorders caused by organ-specific autoantibodies, those that primarily target a single organ, such as the thyroid in Graves disease and Hashimoto thyroiditis, are often the easiest to diagnose as they frequently present with organ-related disease.

Once a diagnosis has been made and a treatment plan has been decided on, it must be explained to the patient and informed consent must be obtained.

KEY WEBSITES

(Accessed 8 July 2013)
Dental Protection. Exercise in risk management: the medical history. <http://www.dentalprotection.org/uk/risk_management/>.
General Dental Council. Maintaining standards: guidance to dentists on professional and personal conduct. <http://www.gdc-uk.org/Newsandpublications/Publications/Publications/MaintainingStandards[1].pdf>.
General Medical Council. Consent to investigation and treatment. www.gmc-uk.org.
National Institute for Health and Care Excellence. Preoperative tests: the use of routine preoperative tests for elective surgery. <http://www.nice.org.uk/nicemedia/pdf/Preop_Fullguideline.pdf>.
National Institute for Health and Care Excellence. Preoperative tests: the use of routine preoperative tests for elective surgery. Clinical Guideline 3, June 2003. <http://www.nice.org.uk/nicemedia/pdf/CG3NICEguideline.pdf>.
NHS Choices. Blood tests – what they are used for. <http://www.nhs.uk/Conditions/Blood-tests/Pages/What-it-is-used-for.aspx>.
NHS National Patient Safety Agency. 'How to guide': five steps to safer surgery. December 2010. <http://www.patientsafetyfirst.nhs.uk/Content.aspx?path=/interventions/Perioperativecare/>.

Patient Safety First! The 'how to' guide for reducing harm in perioperative care. <http://www.patientsafetyfirst.nhs.uk/Content.aspx?path=/interventions/Perioperativecare/>.

World Health Organization. Patient safety. WHO surgical safety checklist and implementation manual. <http://www.who.int/patientsafety/safesurgery/ss_checklist/en/>.

FURTHER READING

Abraham-Inpijn, L., et al. 2008. A patient-administered medical risk related history questionnaire (EMRRH) for use in 10 European countries (multicenter trial). Oral Surg. Oral Med. Oral Pathol. Oral Radiol. Endod. 105, 597.

Brown, J., Scully, C., 2004a Advances in oral health care imaging. Part two: Private dentistry. 9 (2), 67.

Brown, J., Scully, C., 2004b. Advances in oral health care imaging. Part three: Private dentistry. 9 (3), 78.

Eijkman, M.A., et al. 2011. Oral surgery as the patient's immediate cause of death. Ned. Tijdschr. Tandheelkd. 118 (7–8), 378.

Geist, S.M., Geist, J.R., 2008. Improvement in medical consultation responses with a structured request form. J. Dent. Educ. 72, 553.

Goodchild, J.H., Glick, M., 2003. A different approach to medical risk assessment. Endodont. Topics 4, 1.

Hainsworth, J.M., et al. 2008. Psychosocial characteristics of adults who experience difficulties with retching. J. Dent. 36, 494.

Henwood, S., et al. 2006. The role of competence and capacity in relation to consent for treatment in adult patients. Br. Dent. J. 200, 18.

Leslie, D., et al. 2001. Autoantibodies as predictors of disease. J. Clin. Invest. 108, 1417.

Lockwood, A.J., Yang, Y.F., 2008. Nitrous oxide inhalation anaesthesia in the presence of intraocular gas can cause irreversible blindness. Br. Dent. J. 204, 247.

Longmore, M., et al. 2007. Oxford Handbook of Clinical Medicine, seventh ed. Oxford University Press, Oxford.

Pyle, M.A., et al. 2000. Prevalence of elevated blood pressure in students attending a college oral health program. Spec. Care Dentist. 20, 234.

Resuscitation Council. Medical emergencies and resuscitation: standards for clinical practice and training for dental practitioners and dental care professionals in general dental practice. London, July 2006 revised 2012, with updated Appendix (viii), Resuscitation Council (UK).

Royal College of Surgeons of England, 2002. Code of Practice for the Surgical Management of Jehovah's Witnesses. Royal College of Surgeons of England, London.

Spivakovsky, S., 2012. Myocardial infarction and tooth extraction associated. Evid. Based Dent. 13 (4), 110.10.1038/sj.ebd.6400894.

Thikkurissy, S., et al. 2008. Concordance and contrast between community-based physicians' and dentist anesthesiologists' history and physicals in outpatient pediatric dental surgery. Anesth. Prog. 55, 35.

APPENDIX 2.1 SUGGESTED MEDICAL QUESTIONNAIRE FOR PATIENTS TO COMPLETE[a]

	Question	Yes	No	Details
1	Have you had an operation or general anaesthetic before?			
2	Have you had any problems with anaesthetics?			
3	Have any of your relatives had any problems with anaesthetics?			
4	Are you taking any drugs or other medications (inhalers, Pill)?			
5	If female, are you or could you be pregnant?			
6	Have you had any corticosteroid drugs in the past? If yes, when?			
7	Do you have any allergies (drugs, plasters, latex, antiseptics, foodstuffs)?			
8	Do you have heart disease or have you had a heart attack?			
9	Do you ever have to take antibiotics routinely prior to dental surgery?			
10	Do you get chest pains, indigestion or tummy acid in the throat?			
11	Do you have a hiatus hernia?			
12	Do you have high blood pressure?			
13	Do you get breathless walking, climbing stairs or lying flat?			
14	Do you have asthma, bronchitis or chest disease?			
15	Have you ever had a convulsion or fit?			
16	Do you have arthritis or muscle disease?			
17	Do you have anaemia or any other blood disorder?			
18	Do you know your sickle status (if relevant)?			
19	Have you ever had liver disease or been jaundiced?			
20	Have you ever had kidney disease?			
21	Do you have diabetes (sugar in your urine)?			
22	Do you smoke? If yes, how many cigarettes a day (also last 6 months)?			
23	Do you take recreational drugs or drink alcohol? If yes, how many units per week?			
24	Do you have any crowns, loose teeth or artificial teeth? Indicate:			
25	Do you wear contact lenses?			
26	Is there anything else you think the surgeon or anaesthetist should know?			

[a]Other useful formats are available, such as that referenced in the Resuscitation Council UK document 2006 on *Medical emergencies for dental practitioners*.

APPENDIX 2.2 COMPLEX MEDICAL HISTORY AS PROVIDED BY A DENTAL PATIENT

Medical Information Sheet

Name: **Blood Group:** A +   **Situation:** Lives alone

Address:	
Phone:	
Only in real emergency:	1st contact: 2nd contact: 3rd contact:
Allergies:	To medication – Trimethoprim, preservatives and lanolin in eye ointments/drops. Airborne – Pollens, moulds. Photosensitivity reactions (Polymorphic light eruption). Oral allergy syndrome, sticky dressings, dogs, cats
Vaccinations:	Tetanus 1994, BCG 1986, Hep B booster 1997, Polio booster 1999, Hep A booster 2001, H1N1 swine flu vaccinations 2009, annual influenza vaccination, pneumococcal vaccine Nov 2010
Conditions:	<u>Current:</u> **Systemic autoimmune disease (atypical primary Sjögren syndrome) with associated complications:** Ophthalmological (Keratoconjunctivitis sicca (KCS)), CNS (Autoimmune myelitis: inflammatory non-compressive cervical cord myelopathy/Sjögren myelopathy), Renal (Chronic kidney disease (CKD) Stage 3 (lowest eGFR 49)), Urological (Interstitial cystitis (IC)/Painful bladder syndrome), Dermatological (Intermittent 'sterile neutrophilic folliculitis' rash poss associated with autoimmune disease, generalized mucosal and skin dryness), generalized (Periodic lymphadenopathy/'flu-like symptoms, severe fatigue), Gynaecological (vestibulodynia). **Other conditions:** Pineal region brain tumour (histological type not known), GI: Severe idiopathic slow-transit constipation, Psychiatric: Major depressive disorder, severe generalized anxiety, Urological: Urethral stenosis, Dermatological: Polymorphic light eruption, seborrhoeic dermatitis, intermittent acne, intermittent mild eczema, Gynaecological: Bartholin cyst (recurrence). **Resolved:** Healed pyoderma gangrenosum (PG) R. leg, costochondritis, **Recently:** Unexplained severely painful, possibly reactive, condition of tongue (instrinsic and ulcerative, desquamating) for 2 weeks between multiple infections requiring 3 antibiotics (URTIs and acute labyrinthitis and streptococcal tonsillitis). **Ongoing investigation/monitoring:** Brain tumour, myelitis, renal function.
Prescribed Drugs:	**Long-term: For autoimmune disease:** Salagen (oral pilocarpine) 5 mg every 3 h (max 6 daily) **(always kept with <u>me</u> for quick self-administration as wears off fast),** Plaquenil (hydroxychloroquine) 200 mg every other morning with food, Viscotears preservative-free single-dose vials of carbomer 974P artificial tears at least 4 times a day, more freq as needed, diazepam (and for neuro motor symptoms) 5 mg p.r.n. **For depression:** Seroquel (quetiapine) 100 mg night, Stilnoct (zolpidem) 10 mg night, trazadone 150 mg night. **For seborrhoeic dermatitis:** ketoconazole shampoo daily, aqueous cream, E45 bath oil, Lotriderm p.r.n. **For neutrophilic rash:** Dermovate p.r.n. **For IC and myelopathic paraesthesia:** imipramine 25 mg night. **For chronic idiopathic constipation:** Resolor 2 mg daily, docusate sodium 3 times a day. **For acne when returns:** Tetralysal 300 (lymecycline) 1–2 tabs. **Periodically: For pain:** Arcoxia sparingly (as contraindicated with CKD), co-codamol. **For vestibulodynia:** 5% lidocaine ointment p.r.n. **Discontinued: For KCS:** Restasis (ciclosporin 0.05% emulsion single-unit eye drops) every 12 h (on named-patient basis) for appx 4 y, Circadin (melatonin) 1 tab nocte. **For depression:** lithium, Cipralex. **Steroids previously received: For myelitis:** 3 pulsed steroid IV infusions in Feb '06 (1000 mg methylprednisolone each time), **For PG:** oral EC prednisolone (3 mths in '06), **For Sjögren lymphadenopathy/'flu-like syndrome:** IM DepoMedrone steroid injection 120 mg Nov '09, **For neutrophilic rash and lymphadenopathy:** oral EC prednisolone (4 days 30 mg Aug '10, 8 days 15 mg and 6 days 20 mg Sep '10), **For neutrophilic rash:** IM DepoMedrone steroid injection 120 mg Sep '10. **For costochondritis:** local cortisone injection into chest Sep '10. **(General note about prescribing** – consider potential of medications to exacerbate symptoms of Sjögren syndrome – e.g. caution with anticholinergics, etc.).
In case of General Anaesthetic:	*<u>To avoid exacerbation</u> of Sjögren syndrome symptoms: <u>AVOID</u> prolonged NPO, allow clear liquids till 2 h prior, omit drying agents, add humidifier to rebreathing system, lubricate ETTs/LMAs well, place w caution, use humidified O$_2$, lubricate eyes with preservative-free carbomer artificial tears, i.e. Viscotears, maintain warmth*
General Practitioner:	
Consultants: Neurologist:	Current:
Neurosurgeon:	
Ophthalmologist:	
Rheumatologist:	
Nephrologist:	
Urologist:	
Dermatologist:	
Gastroenterologist:	
Medical Insurance UK:	BUPA 'Heartbeat' Number
Travel Insurance:	'Flysure':

If in contact with BUPA or Flysure: please <u>do not disclose confidential medical history, only current reason for assistance!)</u>

Fig. 2.32 eGFR = estimated glomerular filtration rate; URTI = upper respiratory tract infection.

APPENDIX 2.3 INTERPRETATION OF HAEMATOLOGICAL RESULTS

Blood	Normal range[a]	Level ↑	Level ↓
Haemoglobin (Hb)	Male 13.0–18.0 g/dL Female 11.5–16.5 g/dL	Polycythaemia (rubra vera or physiological); myeloproliferative disease; dehydration	Anaemia
Haematocrit (packed cell volume [PCV])	Male 40–54% Female 37–47%	Polycythaemia; dehydration	Anaemia
Mean cell volume (MCV) MCV = PCV/RBC	78–99 fl	Macrocytosis in vitamin B_{12} or folate deficiency; liver disease; alcoholism; hypothyroidism; myelodysplasia; myeloproliferative disorders; aplastic anaemia; cytotoxic agent	Microcytosis in iron deficiency, thalassaemia, chronic disease
Mean cell haemoglobin (MCH) MCH = Hb/RBC	27–31 pg/cell	Pernicious anaemia	Iron deficiency; thalassaemia; sideroblastic anaemia
Mean cell haemoglobin concentration (MCHC) MCHC = Hb/PCV	32–36 g/dL		Iron deficiency; thalassaemia; sideroblastic anaemia; anaemia in chronic disease
Red cell count (RBC)	Male 4.2–6.1 × 10^{12}/L Female 4.2–5.4 × 10^{12}/L	Polycythaemia	Anaemia; fluid overload
White cell count (WCC; total)	4–10 × 10^9/L	Infection; inflammation; leukaemia; intense exercise; trauma; stress; pregnancy	Early leukaemia; some infections; bone marrow disease; drugs, including corticosteroids and chemotherapy; idiopathic
Neutrophils	Average 3.3 × 10^9/L	Pregnancy; exercise; infection; bleeding; trauma; malignancy; leukaemia; corticosteroids	Some infections; drugs; endocrinopathies; bone marrow disease; idiopathic
Lymphocytes	Average 2.5 × 10^9/L	Physiological; some infections; leukaemia; lymphoma	Some infections; some immune defects (e.g. HIV, AIDS); lymphoma; corticosteroids; systemic lupus erythematosus (SLE)
Eosinophils	Average 0.15 × 10^9/L	Allergic disease; parasitic infestations; skin disease; malignancy, including lymphoma	Some immune defects
Platelets	150–400 × 10^9/L	Thrombocytosis in bleeding; myeloproliferative disease; chronic inflammatory states	Thrombocytopenia related to leukaemia; drugs; HIV; other infections; idiopathic; autoimmune; disseminated intravascular coagulopathy (DIC)
Reticulocytes	0.5–1.5% of RBC	Haemolytic states; during treatment of anaemia	Chemotherapy; bone marrow disease
Erythrocyte sedimentation rate (ESR)	0–15 mm/h	Pregnancy; infections; anaemia; inflammation; connective tissue disease; temporal arteritis; trauma; infarction; tumours	–
Plasma viscosity	1.4–1.8 cp	As ESR	

[a]Adults unless otherwise stated. Check values with your laboratory.

APPENDIX 2.4 INTERPRETATION OF BIOCHEMICAL RESULTS[a]

Biochemistry[b]	Level[c] ↑	Level[c] ↓
Acid phosphatase	Prostatic malignancy; renal disease; acute myeloid leukaemia	–
Alanine transaminase (ALT)[d]	Liver disease; infectious mononucleosis	Hypothyroidism; hypophosphatasia; malnutrition
Alkaline phosphatase	Puberty; pregnancy; Paget disease; osteomalacia; fibrous dysplasia; malignancy in bone; liver disease; hyperparathyroidism (some); hyperphosphatasia	–
Alpha$_1$-antitrypsin	Liver cirrhosis	Congenital emphysema
Alpha-fetoprotein (AFP)	Pregnancy; gonadal tumour; liver disease	Fall in level in pregnancy indicates fetal distress
Amylase	Pancreatic disease; mumps; some other salivary diseases	–
Angiotensin-converting enzyme (ACE)	Sarcoidosis	–
Antistreptolysin O titre (ASOT)	Streptococcal infections; rheumatic fever; drugs[f]	–
Aspartate transaminase (AST)[e]	Liver disease; biliary disease; myocardial infarct; trauma; drugs[f]	–
Bilirubin (total)	Liver or biliary disease; haemolysis	–
Brain natriuretic peptide (BNP)	Cardiac failure	–
Caeruloplasmin	Pregnancy; cirrhosis; hyperthyroidism; leukaemia	Wilson disease
Calcium	Primary hyperparathyroidism; malignancy in bone; renal tubular acidosis; sarcoidosis; thiazides; calcium supplements; excess vitamin D	Hypoparathyroidism; renal failure; rickets; nephrotic syndrome; chronic renal failure; lack of vitamin D; low magnesium levels; acute pancreatitis
Cholesterol	Hypercholesterolaemia; pregnancy; hypothyroidism; diabetes; nephrotic syndrome; liver or biliary disease	Malnutrition; hyperthyroidism
Complement (C3)	Trauma; surgery; infection	Liver disease; immune complex diseases (e.g. systemic lupus erythematosus [SLE])
Complement (C4)	–	Liver disease; immune complex diseases; hereditary angioneurotic oedema (HANE)
Cortisol (see Steroids)	–	–
Creatine kinase (CK)	Myocardial infarct; trauma; muscle disease; rhabdomyolysis; statins	–
Creatinine	Renal failure; urinary obstruction	Pregnancy
C-reactive protein (CRP)	Inflammation; trauma; myocardial infarct; malignant disease	–
C1 esterase inhibitor	–	Hereditary angiodema
Cyclic citrullinated peptide (CCP)	Rheumatoid arthritis	–
Erythrocyte sedimentation rate (ESR)	Inflammation; trauma; myocardial infarct; malignant disease	–
Ferritin	Liver disease; haemochromatosis; leukaemia; lymphoma; other malignancies; thalassaemia	Iron deficiency
Fibrinogen	Pregnancy; pulmonary embolism; nephritic syndrome; lymphoma	Disseminated intravascular coagulopathy (DIC)
Folic acid	Folic acid therapy	Alcoholism; dietary deficiency; haemolytic anaemias; malabsorption; myelodysplasia; phenytoin; methotrexate; trimethoprim; pyrimethamine; sulfasalazine; cycloserine; oral contraceptives; pregnancy
Free thyroxine index (FTI; serum T4 and T3 uptake)	Hyperthyroidism	Hypothyroidism
Gamma-glutamyl transpeptidase (GGT)	Alcoholism; obesity; liver disease; myocardial infarct; pancreatitis; diabetes; renal diseases; tricyclics	–
Globulins (total; see also Protein)	Liver disease; multiple myeloma; autoimmune disease; chronic infections	Chronic lymphatic leukaemia; malnutrition; protein-losing states
Glucose	Diabetes mellitus; pancreatitis; hyperthyroidism; hyperpituitarism; Cushing disease; liver disease; post head injury	Hypoglycaemic drugs; Addison disease; hypopituitarism; hyperinsulinism; severe liver disease
Hydroxybutyrate dehydrogenase (HBD) immunoglobulins	Myocardial infarct	–
Total immunoglobulins	Liver disease; infection; sarcoidosis; connective tissue disease	Immunodeficiency; nephrotic syndrome; enteropathy
IgG	Myelomatosis; connective tissue disorders	Immunodeficiency; nephrotic syndrome
IgA	Alcoholic cirrhosis; Berger disease	Immunodeficiency

(Continued)

Biochemistry[b]	Level[c] ↑	Level[c] ↓
IgM	Primary biliary cirrhosis; nephrotic syndrome; parasites; infections	Immunodeficiency
IgE	Allergies; parasites	–
Lactate dehydrogenase (LDH)	Myocardial infarct; trauma; liver disease; haemolytic anaemias; lymphoproliferative diseases	Radiotherapy
Lipase	Pancreatic disease	–
Lipids (triglycerides)	Hyperlipidaemia; diabetes mellitus; hypothyroidism; hyper-vitaminosis D	–
Magnesium	Renal failure	Cirrhosis; malabsorption; diuretics; Conn syndrome; renal tubular defects
Nucleotidase	Liver disease	–
Percent carbohydrate-deficient transferrin	Alcoholism	–
Phosphate	Renal failure; bone disease; hypoparathyroidism; hyper-vitaminosis D	Hyperparathyroidism; rickets; malabsorption syndrome; insulin
Potassium	Renal failure; Addison disease; ACE inhibitors; potassium supplements	Vomiting; diabetes; Conn syndrome; diuretics; Cushing disease; malabsorption; corticosteroids; salbutamol
Protein (total)	Liver disease; multiple myeloma; sarcoid; connective tissue diseases	Pregnancy; nephrotic syndrome; malnutrition; enteropathy; renal failure; lymphomas
Albumin	Dehydration	Liver disease; malnutrition; malabsorption; nephrotic syndrome; multiple myeloma; connective tissue disorders
Alpha$_1$-globulin	Oestrogens	Nephrotic syndrome
Alpha$_2$-globulin	Infections; trauma	Nephrotic syndrome
Beta-globulin	Hypercholesterolaemia; liver disease; pregnancy	Chronic disease
Gamma-globulin	(see Immunoglobulins)	Nephrotic syndrome; immunodeficiency
Serum GGT (SGGT; see GGT)	–	–
Serum glutamic oxaloacetic transaminase (SGOT; see AST)	–	–
Serum glutamic pyruvic transaminase (SGPT; see ALT)	–	–
Sodium	Dehydration; Cushing disease	Cardiac failure; renal failure; syndrome of inappropriate antidiuretic hormone (SIADH); Addison disease; diuretics
Steroids (corticosteroids)	Cushing disease; some tumours	Addison disease; hypopituitarism
Thyroxine (T4)	Hyperthyroidism; pregnancy; oral contraceptive	Hypothyroidism; nephrotic syndrome; phenytoin
Troponin	Myocardial infarct	–
Urea	Renal failure; dehydration; gastrointestinal bleed	Liver disease; nephrotic syndrome; pregnancy; malnutrition
Uric acid	Gout; leukaemia; renal failure; multiple myeloma	Liver disease; probenecid; allopurinol; salicylates; other drugs
Vitamin B$_{12}$	Liver disease; leukaemia; polycythaemia rubra vera	Pernicious anaemia; gastrectomy; Crohn disease; ileal resection; veganism; metformin

[a]Absolute value ranges may differ from laboratory to laboratory. There are also many more causes of abnormal results than are outlined here. SI values: 10^{-1}, deci (d); 10^{-2}, centi (c); 10^{-3}, milli (m); 10^{-6}, micro (μ); 10^{-9}, nano (n); 10^{-12}, pico (p); 10^{15}, femto (f).
[b]Serum or plasma.
[c]Adult levels; always consult your own laboratory.
[d]ALT = SGPT (serum glutamate–pyruvate transaminase).
[e]AST = SGOT (serum glutamate–oxaloacetic transaminase).
[f]Ampicillin, cefalotin, cloxacillin, erythromycin, indometacin, methotrexate, opioids.

APPENDIX 2.5 URINALYSIS: INTERPRETATION OF RESULTS[a]

Colour	Protein	Glucose[b]	Ketones	Bilirubin[c]	Urobilinogen[c]	Blood[d]
Comment						
–	Tetrabromphenol blue dye binds to some proteins in urine – mainly albumin. Not all proteins are detected and the sensitivity is not high	–	–	–	–	Tests for intact red cells and free haemoglobin (Hb)
Health						
Yellow	Usually no protein, but a trace can be normal in young people	Usually no glucose, but a trace can be normal in 'renal glycosuria' and pregnancy	Usually no ketones but ketonuria may occur in vomiting, fasting or starvation	Usually no bilirubin	Usually present in normal healthy patients, particularly in concentrated urine	Usually no blood
False positives						
Red: beet	Alkaline urine. Container contaminated with disinfectant (e.g. chlorhexidine). Blood or pus in urine. Polyvinyl pyrrolidone infusions	Cefamandole. Container contaminated with hypochlorite	Patients on L-dopa or any phthalein compound	Chlorpromazine and other phenothiazines	Infected urine. Patients taking ascorbic acid, sulphonamides or paraminosalicylate	Menstruation. Container contaminated with some detergents
Disease						
Brown: homogentisic acid, bilirubin, urobilin, porphyrins	Renal diseases. Also cardiac failure, diabetes, endocarditis, myeloma, amyloid, some drugs, some chemicals	Diabetes mellitus. Also in pancreatitis, hyperthyroidism, Fanconi syndrome, sometimes after a head injury, other endocrinopathies	Diabetes mellitus. Also in febrile or traumatized or starved patients on low-carbohydrate diets	Only where conjugated bilirubin is increased – hepatocellular and obstructive liver disease	Haemolytic or hepatic, hepatocellular or obstructive disease. Prolonged antibiotic therapy	Genitourinary diseases. Also in bleeding tendency, haemolysis, rhabdomyolysis, some infections where bacteria contain hydroperoxidase, some drugs, endocarditis
Red: Hb						
Milky: chyluria						

[a]Using test strips (e.g. Ames reagent strips, BM-Test-5L, Diastix or Diabur strips). Normal or non-fresh urine may be alkaline; normal urine may be acid. Nitrites and leukocyte esterase positivity suggests a urinary tract infection.
[b]Dopa, ascorbate or salicylates may give false negatives.
[c]May be false negative if urine not fresh.
[d]Ascorbic acid may give false negative.

APPENDIX 2.6 SOME IMPORTANT AUTOANTIBODIES[a]

Autoantibodies	Main associations
Anti-actin	Autoimmune hepatitis, coeliac disease
Anti-epithelial	
Anti-basement membrane zone	Pemphigoid
Intercellular cement (desmoglein)	Pemphigus
Anti-ganglioside antibodies	
Anti-GD3	Guillain–Barré syndrome
Anti-GM1	Travellers' diarrhoea
Anti-GQ1b	Miller–Fisher syndrome (see Guillain–Barré syndrome)
Anti-gastric parietal cell	Pernicious anaemia
Anti-glomerular basement membrane (anti-GBM) antibody	Goodpasture syndrome
Anti-Hu	Neuroblastoma
Anti-intrinsic factor	Pernicious anaemia
Anti-islet cell	Diabetes type 1
Anti-Jo 1 (GAD65)	Polymyositis, dermatomyositis
Anti-liver/kidney microsomal 1 (anti-LKM 1 antibodies)	Chronic hepatitis C
Anti-Ku	Polymyositis/scleroderma (PM/Scl) overlap syndrome
Anti-mitochondrial	Primary biliary cirrhosis
Anti-neutrophil cytoplasmic (ANCA)	
pANCA (perinuclear; anti-myeloperoxidase)	Ulcerative colitis, polyarteritis nodosa
cANCA (cytoplasmic proteinase 3; anti-PR3)	Wegener granulomatosis
Antinuclear (ANA) anti-extractable nuclear antigen (anti-ENA)	
Anti-p62	Primary biliary cirrhosis
Anti-sp100	Primary biliary cirrhosis
Anti-glycoprotein210	Primary biliary cirrhosis
Anti-double-stranded (ds) DNA	Antibody with the highest specificity for systemic lupus erythematosus (SLE) and found in most patients
Anti-Ro (Robair)	Sjögren syndrome
Anti-La (Lattimer)	Sjögren syndrome
Anti-RNP	Mixed connective tissue disease (MCTD)
Anti-Sm	SLE
Anti-PM/Scl (anti-exosome)	PM/Scl overlap syndrome
Anti-Scl 70	
Anti-topoisomerase	Scleroderma
Anti-centromere	CREST (calcinosis, Raynaud, oesophageal dysfunction, scleroderma, telangiectasia) syndrome
Anti-smooth muscle	Autoimmune hepatitis
Anti-steroid 21-hydroxylase (21-OH)	Addison disease
Anti-thyroid	
Thyroid peroxidase (TPOAb)	Hashimoto thyroiditis, Graves disease
TSH receptor (TRAb)	Graves disease
Thyroglobulin antibodies	Autoimmune thyroid disease
Anti-transglutaminase	
Anti-tTG (tissue transglutaminase)	Coeliac disease
Anti-eTG (epidermal transglutaminase)	Dermatitis herpetiformis
Rheumatoid factor (RF)	Rheumatoid arthritis (high rate of false positives in SLE and other conditions)
Lupus anticoagulant	
Anti-thrombin antibodies	SLE

[a]See also Table 18.3.

Assessment of the patient, consent and the question of preoperative screening are discussed in Chapter 2 and much of that discussion is relevant to this chapter. Integrated care pathways are increasingly used in many countries. In the UK, the National Patient Safety Agency (NPSA) and NHS Quality Improvement Scotland (NHS QIS) are responsible for overseeing this area.

TREATMENT COMPLICATIONS

Any form of surgery or invasion of bone or soft tissues causes inflammation, with variable pain and swelling and sometimes other sequelae; therefore it is crucial that benefits outweigh the risks and that the patient has given valid consent. Even a local anaesthetic (LA) injection can be followed by complications. LA complications and medico-legal complaints arising from them are rare but include persisting anaesthesia or paraesthesia. Most cases involve lingual and/or inferior alveolar nerve sensory loss. In one study of over 12000 inferior alveolar nerve block injections, 0.15% resulted in some lingual sensory disturbance and 7% caused patients to experience an 'electric shock'-type feeling in the tongue at the time of LA injection –almost certainly indicating needle nerve damage. However, all but 1 patient regained normal sensation within 6 months. Most LAs, in particular articaine and prilocaine, are also potentially neurotoxic, and a Danish study suggested that the main cause of injury was neurotoxicity resulting from administration of the LA rather than from needle penetration. Clinicians should consider avoiding high-concentration (4%) LA for block anaesthesia and avoiding articaine for block anaesthesia. Complications from conscious sedation (CS) and general anaesthesia (GA) are considered below.

Drug use can cause adverse reactions; some of the main adverse reactions, interactions and contraindications to drugs used in dentistry are shown in Chapter 29, Tables 3.1 and 3.2, and Appendices 3.1–3.3. It is important for clinicians only to undertake a procedure or use a drug when they are aware of the attendant interactions and adverse effects (as discussed in Ch. 29), and to be able to manage any emergency (Ch. 1) or other complications. Clinicians should work only within their field of competence.

Finally, never alter a patient's medication personally, even aspirin given by another health-care professional (HCP), as this is considered, at the least, discourteous and, at worst, to be practising medicine without a licence. Always consult the patient's HCP.

PAIN MANAGEMENT

Pain is an unpleasant sensory and/or emotional experience associated with actual or potential tissue damage. Pain is a complicated process that involves an intricate interplay between chemicals (neurotransmitters), which bind to neurotransmitter receptors (nociceptors) on cell surfaces. These function as gates or ports, enabling pain messages to pass through to cells. Normally, nociceptors only respond to strong, potentially harmful stimuli; however, chemicals from injured or inflamed tissues (Box 3.1) sensitize nociceptors, causing them to transmit pain signals in response to lesser stimuli. This is referred to as allodynia, a state in which pain is produced by innocuous stimuli such as light touch.

Pain is initiated with the activation of nociceptors at the free nerve endings of A-delta and C fibres, followed by transduction, whereby one form of energy (mechanical, thermal, chemical) is converted into another (electrical – nerve impulse). Lightly myelinated A-delta nerve fibres are responsible for sharp stabbing pain usually resulting from stimulation of mechanoreceptors (e.g. primary pain following acute injury). Stimulation of unmyelinated C-polymodal nerve fibres gives rise to pain described as dull, aching and poorly localized (e.g. infection, secondary pain following acute injury, visceral pain). Pain may be superficial or deep, and somatic, visceral or neuropathic, based on the site of action of the noxious stimulus.

Following transduction, neural impulses are carried along peripheral nerves to spinal cord and brainstem, which act as relay centres (where the pain signal can potentially be blocked, enhanced or otherwise modified). They continue through the thalamus (which also serves as the storage area for body images and plays a key role in relaying messages between the brain and various parts of the body) to the cerebral cortex, where pain perception occurs.

The main excitatory neurotransmitters for pain are substance P and glutamate. Inhibitory neurotransmitters include gamma-aminobutyric acid (GABA), serotonin, noradrenaline (norepinephrine) and opioid-like chemicals such as endorphins and enkephalins (which block pain by locking on to opioid receptors and switching on pain-inhibiting pathways or circuits). Endorphins (mu-opioids) may also be responsible for the 'feel-good' effects experienced after vigorous exercise.

It must be borne in mind that pain has emotional, sensory, behavioural and cognitive components, and can be influenced by temperament, context, experience, pain sensitivity, coping skills and cognitive development, and also by biological, psychological and cultural factors.

Prevention and treatment of pain and suffering are essential. Furthermore, adequate pain control during a clinical procedure may also make management and pain control far easier for future health-care procedures. Pre-emptive analgesia is the clinical concept of introducing analgesic management before the onset of noxious stimuli, which helps to prevent pain potentiation. Reassurance, explanation, a calm environment and gentle handling will help but frequently need to be supplemented with analgesics, hypnosis, LA, CS (oral, inhalational or intravenous) or GA.

ANALGESICS

Analgesics may act at different levels of the pain transmission pathway. Aspirin and other non-steroidal anti-inflammatory agents (NSAIDs), paracetamol (acetaminophen), corticosteroids and LA act peripherally, while some other agents, such as opioids, act on the central nervous system (CNS). Neurogenic pain, originating in damaged C fibres, may also respond to membrane-stabilizing drugs, such

Table 3.1 *More common drug interactions with analgesics and local anaesthetics of significance in oral health care*[a]

Specific drugs used in dentistry	Interacting drug	Main uses of interacting drug	Possible outcomes (check text and Ch. 29)
Acetaminophen (paracetamol)	Alcohol (ethanol)	Abuse	Liver toxicity
Adrenaline (epinephrine)-containing LA	Beta-blockers (non-selective)	Hypertension	Hypertension and bradycardia
	Cocaine	Abuse	Arrhythmias
	Catechol-O-methyl transferase (COMT) inhibitors (tolcapone, entacapone)	Parkinsonism	Hypertension, tachycardias, arrhythmias
	Halothane	GA	Arrhythmias
	Tricyclics	Depression	Hypertension, tachycardias, arrhythmias
Aspirin	Alcohol	Alcoholism	Risk of gastrointestinal bleeding
	Corticosteroids	Immune suppression	Risk of gastrointestinal ulceration
	Hypoglycaemics	Diabetes	Enhanced hypoglycaemia
	Warfarin	Cardiac disease	Risk of gastrointestinal bleeding
Articaine (N.B. adrenaline [epinephrine] is included in some preparations, so care with drugs that increase QT)	Antidepressants (monoamine oxidase inhibitors [MAOIs])	Depression	Hypertension
	Antihypertensives	Hypertension	Reduced antihypertensive effect
Non-steroidal anti-inflammatory drugs (NSAIDs)	Antihypertensives	Hypertension	Reduced antihypertensive effect
	Corticosteroids	Immune suppression	Risk of gastrointestinal ulceration
	Lithium	Manic depression	Lithium toxicity
	Methotrexate	Rheumatoid disease	Methotrexate toxicity
	Warfarin	Cardiac disease	Risk of gastrointestinal bleeding
Benzocaine	Sulphonamides	Antibacterials	Methaemoglobinaemia
Benzodiazepines	Alcohol (ethanol)	Abuse	Benzodiazepine toxicity
	Cimetidine	Gastric disorders	Benzodiazepine toxicity
	Digoxin	Cardiac disease	Digitalis toxicity
	Fluoxetine	Depression	Benzodiazepine toxicity
	Isoniazid	Tuberculosis	Benzodiazepine toxicity
	Oral contraceptives	Contraception	Benzodiazepine toxicity
	Phenytoin	Epilepsy	Phenytoin toxicity
	Protease inhibitors	HIV/AIDS	Benzodiazepine toxicity
Bupivacaine	Antiarrhythmics	Arrhythmias	Cardiac depression
	Propranolol	Hypertension	Bupivacaine toxicity
Lidocaine	Acetazolamide	Diuretics	Lidocaine antagonized
	Antiarrhythmics	Arrhythmias	Cardiac depression
	Atazanavir	Antiviral	Lidocaine enhanced
	Cimetidine	Ulcer-healing agent	Lidocaine enhanced
	Fosamprenavir	Antiviral	Arrhythmias
	Loop diuretics	Diuretics	Lidocaine antagonized
	Lopinavir	Antiviral	Lidocaine enhanced
	Olanzapine or other antipsychotics	Antipsychotics	Arrhythmias
	Propranolol or other beta-blockers	Beta-blockers	Cardiac depression
	Saquinavir	Antiviral	Lidocaine enhanced
	Suxamethonium	Muscle relaxant	Neuromuscular blockade enhanced
	Thiazides	Diuretics	Lidocaine antagonized
Prilocaine	Antiarrhythmics	Arrhythmias	Cardiac depression
	Sulphonamides	Antibacterial	Methaemoglobinaemias

[a]N.B. *There are many others; check text and appendices on drugs.* ALWAYS check the *British National Formulary* or an equivalent source, as these lists cannot be complete; nor can their accuracy be guaranteed.

Table 3.2 *Main contraindications and cautions for dental analgesic agents*

Dental drugs	Avoid (as well as allergy)	Cautions apart from allergy or pregnancy/lactation
LA	Benzocaine and methaemoglobinaemia Bupivacaine in cardiacs Prilocaine in methaemoglobinaemia	Adrenaline (epinephrine) in people with cardiac disease
Anxiolytics/sedatives	Benzodiazepines with glaucoma or respiratory depressants	Children, older patients Liver or kidney disease Drug or alcohol abuse Head injury
Analgesics	Aspirin in bleeding tendency, young children or peptic ulcer	Non-steroidal anti-inflammatory drugs (NSAIDs) in bleeding tendency, cardiac failure, chronic kidney disease, children, diabetes, gastrointestinal ulcer, hypertension
	Codeine in children	Paracetamol (acetaminophen) with alcohol

as anticonvulsants (e.g. carbamazepine). Tricyclic antidepressants (e.g. amitriptyline) also have a role in the modulation of pain pathways. Muscle relaxants, such as benzodiazepines and hypnosis, may be indicated for pain related to muscle spasm. Analgesic drug use, contraindications and potential adverse reactions and interactions are fully discussed in Chapter 29 (see also Appendices 3.1, 3.2 and 3.3) but Table 3.1 summarizes the main problems relevant to dentistry. Box 27.9 shows drugs whose action may be affected by grapefruit, and Box 27.10 drugs enhanced by pomegranate.

Adjuncts to analgesia include transcutaneous electrical nerve stimulation (TENS), dorsal column stimulation (DCS), acupuncture, rubbing the skin locally (counter-irritation), psychological techniques and neurosurgical procedures.

Box 3.1 *Chemical mediators of pain*

- Bradykinin
- Hydrogen ions
- Leukotrienes
- Potassium ions
- Prostaglandins
- Serotonin
- Substance P
- Thromboxane

CONTROL OF MILD PAIN

Non-opioid analgesics are commonly used (Tables 3.3 and 3.6). NSAIDs act peripherally and are equi-analgesic with centrally acting weak opioids such as codeine. NSAIDs act by blocking cyclo-oxygenase (COX), which converts arachidonic acid to prostaglandins (PGs) that are involved in inflammation and pain. Other PGs stimulate protective gastric mucus secretion, blood platelet formation and renal excretion – and thus there can be dysfunction in these. A wide range of NSAIDs is available (Table 3.4). Most block COX-1 in particular, which is responsible for the PGs affecting stomach, platelets and kidneys – and they can thus also damage the stomach and interfere with haemostasis and renal function (Fig. 3.1 and Box 3.2). All NSAIDs can cause serious gastrointestinal effects; azapropozone confers the highest risk and ibuprofen the lowest. NSAIDs cause gastric irritation, ulceration and bleeding, especially in older individuals and patients taking corticosteroids. Piroxicam use is thus now limited to treatment by specialists – of osteoarthritis, rheumatoid arthritis and ankylosing spondylitis. Ketoprofen and ketorolac also have significant gastrointestinal adverse effects. NSAIDs should not be used in patients with current or past peptic ulcers, and not given in combinations. They can also worsen asthma and are contraindicated in pregnancy and in older patients. They inhibit platelet function, but most do so reversibly and therefore prolong the bleeding time only for the life of the drug (typically 48–72 hours). NSAIDs can interact with lithium to cause lithium toxicity. They also block renal PG synthesis and may

---

Table 3.3 *Non-opioid analgesics*

Analgesic	Tablet contains	Route	Adult dose	Comments
Non-NSAIDs				
Acetaminophen (paracetamol)	500 mg	Oral or injection	500–1000 mg up to six times a day (max. 4 mg daily)	Mild analgesic. Not anti-inflammatory. Hepatotoxic in overdose or prolonged use. Contraindicated in liver or renal disease, anorexia, or those on zidovudine. Available with methionine to prevent liver damage in overdose, as co-methiamol
Nefopam	30 mg	Oral or i.m.	30–60 mg up to three times daily	Moderate analgesic. Contraindicated in convulsive disorders. Caution in pregnancy, older patients, renal or liver disease. May cause nausea, dry mouth, sweating
NSAIDs[a]				
Aspirin	300 or 325 mg	Oral	300-600 mg up to six times a day after meals (use soluble or dispersible or enteric-coated aspirin) (max. 4 g daily)	Mild anti-inflammatory analgesic. Causes gastric irritation. Interferes with haemostasis. Contraindicated in bleeding disorders, children, asthma, late pregnancy, peptic ulcers, renal disease, aspirin allergy
Diflunisal	250 or 500 mg	Oral	250–500 mg twice a day	Anti-inflammatory analgesic for mild to moderate pain. Long action: twice-daily dose only. Effective against pain from bone and joint. Contraindicated in pregnancy, peptic ulcer, allergies, renal and liver disease
Ibuprofen	200 mg	Oral	200–400 mg up to four times a day	Mild analgesic. Fewer adverse effects than other NSAIDs. Causes gastric irritation. Interferes with haemostasis. Contraindicated in bleeding disorders, children, older people, asthma, cardiac failure, diabetes, hypertension, late pregnancy, peptic ulcers, renal disease, aspirin allergy
Ketorolac	10 mg	Injection or oral	10 mg up to three times a day	Mild anti-inflammatory analgesic. Adverse effects as other NSAIDs. May affect platelets. Allergic reactions (anaphylactoid reactions, asthma, bronchospasm, Stevens–Johnson syndrome, toxic epidermal necrolysis).Fluid retention and oedema - therefore use with caution in cardiac failure or hypertension.
Mefenamic acid	250–500 mg	Oral	250—500 mg up to three times a day	Mild anti-inflammatory analgesic. May be contraindicated in asthma, gastrointestinal, renal and liver disease, and pregnancy. May cause diarrhoea or haemolytic anaemia
Parecoxib	40 mg	Injection	40 mg prn	Mild anti-inflammatory analgesic. Adverse effects as other NSAIDs. May be contraindicated in sulphonamide sensitivity, liver or inflammatory bowel disorders. Non-approval from FDA as with other COX-2 selective inhibitors

[a]There are many other NSAIDs (see Table 3.4).

Table 3.4 *Non-steroidal anti-inflammatory drugs (NSAIDs)*

Group	Subgroup	Examples
Carboxylic acids	Carbo- and heterocyclic acids	Etodolac
		Indometacin
		Ketorolac
		Sulindac
		Tolmetin
	Fenamic acids	Flufenamic acid
		Meclofenamic acid
		Mefenamic acid
	Phenylacetic acids	Alcofenac
		Diclofenac
		Fenclofenac
	Proprionic acids	Fenbufen
		Fenoprofen
		Flurbiprofen
		Ibuprofen
		Ketoprofen
		Naproxen
		Oxaprozin
		Tiaprofenic acid
	Salicylic acids	Aspirin (acetyl salicylic acid)
		Diflunisal
Selective cyclooxygenase-2 inhibitors	Cox inhibitor	Paricoxib
		Valdecoxib
Enolic acids	Oxicams	Isoxicam
		Piroxicam (restricted use because of gastrointestinal effects and rashes)
		Tenoxicam
	Pyrazolones	Butazones
		Propazones
Non-acidic compounds		Nabumetone

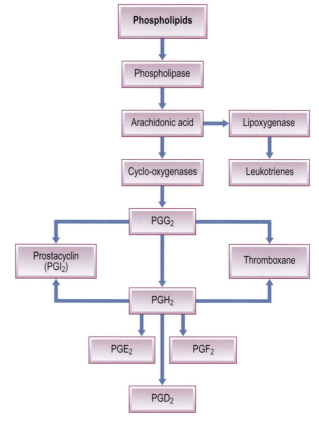

Fig. 3.1 Cyclo-oxygenase pathway. PG = prostaglandin.

Box 3.2 *Non-steroidal anti-inflammatory drugs: contraindications*

- Allergy
- Asthma
- Bleeding tendency
- Cardiac failure
- Drug interactions (e.g. lithium)
- Peptic ulceration
- Pregnancy
- Hypertension
- Renal disease
- Transplant patients

lead to acute renal failure, particularly in older patients with cardiac failure and those with renal damage, such as diabetic nephropathy. In these groups, renal function should be monitored. Aspirin is a typical NSAID, which has the effects described above but also irreversibly inhibits platelet function and therefore causes a prolonged bleeding time for the life of the platelets (about 7–8 days minimum).

Misoprostol, H2 antagonists or proton pump inhibitors can help protect the stomach in NSAID use. However, NSAIDs that act as COX-2 inhibitors, such as celecoxib and rofecoxib, spare the COX-1 enzyme and thus cause less gastric damage; they do not affect platelets and are preferred for patients with peptic ulceration, but are contraindicated in cardiac disease and should not be used together with aspirin. COX-2 inhibitors have much less effect on the stomach, platelets and kidneys but, unfortunately, are also associated with a thrombotic risk (e.g. myocardial infarction and stroke), as are non-selective NSAIDs such as diclofenac and ibuprofen, especially when used at high doses and for long periods. Rofecoxib increases the risk of myocardial infarction and has thus been withdrawn.

Paracetamol (*acetaminophen*; *N*-acetyl-para-aminophenol; APAP) has approximately the same analgesic activity as aspirin; it is a useful analgesic and antipyretic (reduces fever) but has no anti-inflammatory activity. Paracetamol appears to act by reducing the oxidized form of the COX enzyme, preventing it from forming pro-inflammatory cytokines, and it also modulates the endogenous cannabinoid system. Paracetamol is metabolized by the liver and by P450 enzymes, responsible for its toxic effects due to a minor alkylating metabolite (*N*-acetyl-*p*-benzoquinone imine, abbreviated as NAPQ1). Paracetamol causes no gastric irritation and is remarkably safe but, in overdose, it can cause liver damage. It accounts for most drug overdoses in the resource-rich world. Up to 4 g daily is the maximum dose for an adult, but toxicity is increased by starvation and by alcohol, anticonvulsants, barbiturates and possibly zidovudine. *Co-methiamol* is a combination tablet of paracetamol with methionine included to ensure that sufficient levels of glutathione in the liver are maintained in order to minimize the liver damage if an overdose is taken.

CONTROL OF MODERATE PAIN

If an NSAID or paracetamol (acetaminophen) fails to control pain, an opioid may be indicated (Tables 3.5 and 3.6). Opioids activate the mu1 receptor in the CNS that is responsible for analgesia. Weak oral opioids, such as codeine (methylmorphine), act centrally to provide useful analgesia. The analgesic efficacy of codeine is partly dependent on its O-demethylation to morphine via cytochrome P450, which exhibits genetic polymorphism, and therefore the degree of pain relief

Table 3.5 Opioids[a]

Analgesic	Tablet contains	Route	Adult dose (always check with BNF)	Comments (avoid all in known hypersensitivity to the drug or known intolerance to other opioid agonists)
Codeine phosphate	15 mg	Oral	10–60 mg up to six times a day (or 30 mg i.m.)	Analgesic for moderate pain. Contraindicated in late pregnancy, children and liver disease. Avoid alcohol. May cause sedation and constipation. Weakens cough reflex
Dextropropoxyphene	65 mg	Oral	65 mg up to four times a day	Analgesic for moderate pain. Risk of respiratory depression in overdose, especially if taken with alcohol. Can cause dependence. Occasional hepatotoxicity. No more effective as an analgesic than paracetamol/ acetaminophen or aspirin alone. Available with acetaminophen as co-proxamol
Dihydrocodeine tartrate	30 mg	Oral	30 mg up to four times a day (or 50 mg i.m.)	Analgesic for moderate pain. May cause nausea, drowsiness or constipation. Contraindicated in children, hypothyroidism, asthma and renal disease. Interacts with MAOI. May increase post-operative dental pain. Reduce dose for elderly. Available with paracetamol as co-drydamol
Fentanyl	50 micrograms	Injection. Patch and buccal tablet, lozenge and spray available	50 micrograms as required	Analgesic for moderate to severe pain. 100 times more potent than morphine. Danger of respiratory depression/ death. Contraindicated in hypovolaemia, hypotension, raised intracranial pressure, respiratory insufficiency.
Alfentanil	50 micrograms	Injection	50 micrograms as required	Analgesic for moderate to severe pain. Can cause muscle rigidity. Contraindications liver disease, bradycardia, phaeochromocytoma and as for fentanyl
Remifentanil	0.1 micrograms/kg	Injection	0.1 micrograms/kg	Analgesic for moderate to severe pain but not in conscious patients. Contraindications as for alifentanil
Pentazocine	25 mg	Oral	50 mg up to four times a day (or 30 mg i.m. or i.v.)	Analgesic for moderate pain. May produce dependence. May produce hallucinations. May provoke withdrawal symptoms in narcotic addicts. Contraindicated in pregnancy, children, hypertension, respiratory depression, head injuries or raised intracranial pressure. There is a low risk of dependence
Buprenorphine	0.2 mg	Sublingual	0.2–0.4 mg up to four times a day (or 0.3 mg i.m.)	Potent analgesic. More potent analgesic than pentazocine, longer action than morphine, no hallucinations, may cause salivation, sweating, dizziness and vomiting. Respiratory depression in overdose. Can cause dependence. Contraindicated in children, pregnancy, MAOI, liver disease and respiratory disease
Meptazinol	No tablet available	i.m. or i.v.	75–100 mg up to six times a day	Potent analgesic. Claimed to have a low incidence of respiratory depression. Side-effects as buprenorphine
Phenazocine	5 mg	Oral or sublingual	5 mg up to four times a day	Potent analgesic for severe pain. May causes nausea
Pethidine	No tablet available	s.c. or i.m.	25–100 mg up to four times a day	Potent analgesic. Less potent than morphine. Contraindicated with MAOI. Risk of dependence
Morphine	As required	s.c., i.m., oral or suppository	5–10 mg	Potent analgesic. Often causes nausea and vomiting. Reduces cough reflex, causes pupil constriction, risk of dependence
Diamorphine	10 mg	s.c., i.m. or oral	2–5 mg by injection, 5–10 mg orally	Potent analgesic. More potent than pethidine and morphine. Euphoria and dependence

[a]Not usually appropriate for dental pain.

Table 3.6 The analgesic ladder

Mild pain	Moderate pain	Severe pain
Paracetamol (acetaminophen)	Paracetamol (acetaminophen) ± oral opioid (codeine, dihydrocodeine or non-steroidal anti-inflammatory drug [NSAID])	Paracetamol (acetaminophen) + injected opioid (morphine)

and the adverse effects may vary significantly between individuals. It is thus contraindicated in children (http://www.fda.gov/Safety/MedWatch/default.htm; accessed 30 September 2013). Despite this, codeine is widely used for postoperative pain relief in adults, at a dose of 30–60 mg, often in combination with paracetamol.

Activation of the mu2 receptor by opioids can lead to the undesired effects of respiratory depression, sedation, constipation, nausea and vomiting. Opioids also depress ventilation by muting the brain response to carbon dioxide. They may therefore be contraindicated in patients who have acute or chronic respiratory disease and seizures.

Tramadol is another mild opioid that acts as an opioid receptor agonist; it also inhibits spinal monoamine reuptake and is an effective analgesic. It causes less sedation and respiratory depression than other opioids, though nausea and vomiting can be troublesome. Use of 5-hydroxytryptamine 3 ($5HT_3$) antagonists to prevent the nausea and vomiting associated with tramadol may reduce its analgesic efficacy. Tramadol is contraindicated in epilepsy and porphyria, and in patients on antidepressants or antipsychotics. It may precipitate the serotoninergic syndrome – a potentially life-threatening drug reaction that may arise mainly in combination with recreational drugs and antidepressants (monoamine oxidase inhibitors [MAOIs], selective serotonin reuptake inhibitors [SSRIs] and selective serotonin–noradrenaline reuptake inhibitors [SSNRIs]).

Table 3.7 *Hypnotics*

Hypnotic	Duration of action	Examples	Comments
Benzodiazepines	Long	Diazepam, flunitrazepam, flurazepam, nitrazepam	Residual effects on following day (hangover effect). Dependence can result
	Shorter	Loprazolam, lormetazepam, temazepam	–
Pyrazolopyrimidine	Very short	Zaleplon	–
Cyclopyrrolone	Short	Zopiclone	Dependence is possible
Imidazopyridine	Short	Zolpidem	Dependence is possible
Clomethiazole	Medium	Clomethiazole	Pronounced hangover. Anticholinergic effects such as dry mouth
Antihistamines	Medium	Diphenhydramine, promethazine	–

CONTROL OF SEVERE PAIN

Severe pain requires treatment with potent opioids (e.g. morphine, pethidine, oxycodone, fentanyl, alfentanil or remifentanil; Tables 3.4, 3.5 and 3.6). Opioids control pain, and reward addictive behaviours, exerting their actions through opioid receptors whose genes have been cloned (Oprm, Oprd1 and Oprk1, respectively). Opioid receptors are activated by a family of endogenous peptides (enkephalins, dynorphins and endorphin), or exogenously by alkaloid opiates, the prototype of which is morphine. Mu receptors mediate both the therapeutic and the adverse activities of morphine; mu-opioid receptors are a key molecular switch triggering brain reward systems and potentially initiating addictive behaviours. Delta-receptors regulate emotional responses.

Oxycodone and fentanyl are no more effective than morphine but may have fewer adverse effects. Opioids can be addictive and can cause respiratory depression, which can be reversed with naloxone; supplemental oxygen may be indicated. Other effects include pinpoint pupils, sedation, nausea, constipation and pruritus. The benefits of opioids must be weighed against their adverse effects. Choice of drug and route of administration depends on the particular clinical situation and care must be taken when converting from one form of drug or administration route to another, as doses will vary.

Postoperatively, morphine may be administered orally but, as some patients may need to be kept nil by mouth, or gastrointestinal absorption may be reduced or unpredictable, intramuscular or subcutaneous administration may be needed. Nevertheless, intramuscular injections are painful, absorption is unpredictable and dangerous, and analgesia cannot be accurately titrated to clinical need. Intravenous morphine is the only way to establish a suitable degree of analgesia reliably, but issues about the timing of administration and who may safely administer it have led to the development of more demand-dependent systems of analgesic delivery.

Patient-controlled analgesia

The disadvantages of giving morphine as required (p.r.n.) are due to the peak effects, which may oversedate and cause nausea and vomiting while, during the trough, the patient may have inadequate analgesia. Patient-controlled analgesia (PCA), which consists of an infusion pump which delivers a small bolus whenever a demand button is pressed within the confines of a set 'lock-out' time, solves some of these problems.

CONTROL OF CHRONIC AND NEUROPATHIC PAIN

Sustained-release oral formulations of morphine or oxycodone or transdermal administration of fentanyl may help some patients with chronic pain. Antidepressants and anticonvulsants can also be useful.

Psychological therapies, as well as alternative techniques such as TENS, may also help, as may one of several neurosurgical procedures.

CHOICE OF ANAESTHETIC TECHNIQUE FOR DENTAL PROCEDURES

Dental professionals should ensure that due regard is given to all aspects of behavioural management and anxiety control before deciding to treat under LA, CS or GA. The choice of an appropriate method for a particular patient undergoing a specific procedure depends on several factors, including the type of procedure or operation indicated, the physical and mental health of the patient (Appendix 3.4), the effects of the agents used and the patient's wishes. Attempts have been made to grade patients as regards physical fitness for operation (Ch. 2) and these may help in decision-making (Appendix 3.5). The degree of cooperation must be taken into account; this may be lacking in some children and other people. Other factors that may influence the decision include social circumstances (e.g. is the patient able to be accompanied, and cared for at home?), urgency and facilities available at the time.

Hypnotics can be useful preoperatively, to help the patient relax and sleep (Table 3.7); most, apart from antihistamines and clomethiazole, act on receptors for GABA. However, all can impair decision-making and driving.

LA should be used wherever possible for outpatient dentistry (Table 3.8), with CS if necessary. GA and so-called 'sedation with intravenous barbiturates' are significant causes of morbidity or even mortality, and should be given only in a hospital with critical care facilities.

LOCAL ANAESTHESIA (LOCAL ANALGESIA)

The first use of cocaine as LA in surgery is credited to an Austrian ophthalmologist, Koller, who, in 1884, used cocaine at the suggestion of Freud. Subsequently, dozens of LA compounds have been developed and used in solution to block nerve conduction temporarily. LA molecules bind specifically to sodium channel proteins in axonal membranes of neurons near the injection site, with essentially no effects centrally unless given in overdose. LAs used in dentistry are mostly amides (Box 3.3) (e.g. articaine, bupivacaine, lidocaine, mepivacaine, prilocaine, ropivacaine). Earlier ester-type agents (e.g. procaine, benzocaine) are only rarely used. A vasoconstrictor is usually included to maintain the duration of anaesthesia. Adrenaline (epinephrine) is the most commonly used vasoconstrictor; felypressin (Octapressin®) is an alternative and is used with prilocaine.

Adverse reactions to LAs may also include dose-related toxic responses (cardiovascular and CNS) in normal individuals (especially

Table 3.8 *Possible indications for and contraindications to local anaesthesia (LA)*

May be contraindicated	May be indicated
Patients on beta-blockers if very large doses are given	After a recent meal
Patients with sensory loss in the trigeminal region	Inadequate facilities for general anaesthesia (GA)
Local infection	No GA available
LA 'allergy'	Poor-risk patients for GA
Liver disease: doses should be reduced	Minor surgery or procedure
Very young children	
Needle-phobics	
Haemangioma in field	
Pseudocholinesterase deficiency	
Bleeding tendency	
Major surgery	
Uncooperative patients	
Sepsis in field	

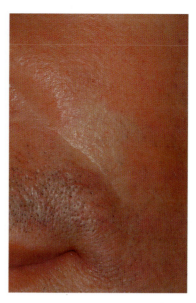

Fig. 3.2 Skin vasoconstriction after dental local anaesthetic injection.

Box 3.3 *Amide local anaesthetic agents*

- Articaine (carticaine)
- Bupivacaine and etidocaine (sometimes used for their prolonged action)
- Lidocaine
- Mepivacaine
- Prilocaine
- Ropivacaine

---

if the agents enters the vasculature), and idiosyncratic or allergic responses. Most adverse reactions to LA administration are unrelated to the drug and are caused by fainting or by inadvertent entry of the drug into the circulation. One study showed blood aspiration into the LA cartridge in nearly 3% of injections. LA injections should be given with an aspirating syringe to avoid intravascular injection of adrenaline (epinephrine) in particular. It is also wise to use a safety syringe in order to reduce the risk of needlestick (sharps) injury. The LA should then be injected slowly. Reactions unrelated to LA agents include psychomotor responses and sympathetic or other nerve stimulation. The common adverse reactions of inadvertent intravenous administration of LA should be appropriately recognized and explained to the patient. Arrhythmias and electrocardiogram (ECG) changes, such as ST-segment depression, may be detectable during dental extractions or operations under LA, presumably due to trigeminal stimulation. Patients being treated with digoxin for atrial fibrillation or congestive heart failure are more prone to these arrhythmias.

Overdosage has caused deaths associated with LA but otherwise mortality is very rare indeed. Over a 10-year period, there were only three deaths in persons receiving dental care under LA in Britain when last recorded (1980–1989). *All* were related to the use of prilocaine. This fact does not suggest that prilocaine is dangerous but serves to emphasize that it is not necessarily safer than lidocaine. *Amide LAs have been given to millions of patients, many of whom must have been medically compromised, for nearly half a century, with few serious untoward reactions.* It is difficult, therefore, to believe that, in moderated doses, they can cause significant toxic or allergic reactions.

It is questionable whether there have been many genuine (immunoglobulin E [IgE]-mediated) allergic reactions to lidocaine. However, there have been occasional reactions to other components, such as the preservative, since vasoconstrictor solutions may also contain antioxidants such as bisulphites (Ch. 17).

The overall incidence of complications of all types from LA is reportedly around 4.5% but most of these are of a trifling nature. Local adverse effects may include blanching of the facial skin (Fig. 3.2), transient facial palsy (LA misplaced and entering the parotid gland, where it affects the facial nerve), visual disturbance (misplaced posterior superior alveolar nerve LA can produce diplopia, mydriasis, palpebral ptosis and abduction difficulties of the affected eye), persistent anaesthesia (prilocaine and articaine in particular are mildly neurotoxic, and any LA injection can physically damage nerves), trismus (damage to nerve supply or medial pterygoid muscle, or bleeding into the area) or lip trauma (due to the patient biting an anaesthetized lip). None of these is common or permanent.

Drug interactions with LA solutions are rare, if at least theoretically possible (see Table 3.1 and Ch. 29). Adrenaline (epinephrine) was alleged to be potentiated in patients taking tricyclic antidepressants but this has been disproved. In patients on beta-blockers, interactions may be possible because of the unopposed beta-sympathomimetic activity of adrenaline, but this only happens when excessively large doses of an adrenaline-containing LA are given. Other interactions are exceedingly rare (see below) and contraindications may include some cardiac disorders (especially heart block or other conduction disturbances), porphyria and myasthenia gravis (see individual LA agents below).

Local anaesthetic creams (e.g. Ametop; tetracaine [amethocaine] or Emla; lidocaine plus prilocaine) effectively reduce the pain of needle pricks and are thus useful for skin injections in children.

LOCAL ANAESTHETIC AGENTS

Most LAs are metabolized in the liver.

Articaine (carticaine)

Articaine is an amide-type LA that has an onset and duration of anaesthesia similar to those of other intermediate-acting amide LAs. The most significant benefit of articaine over lidocaine is that it may have somewhat faster onset and greater depth of action. Articaine is 1.5 times as potent and only 0.6 times as toxic as lidocaine and has

Table 3.9 *Indications for and contraindications to LA with articaine**

May be contraindicated	May be indicated
Porphyria	Patients on beta-blockers
Heart block	
Cholinesterase deficiency	
Narrow-angle glaucoma	

*Some advise against use in block anaesthesia.

Table 3.10 *Indications for and contraindications to LA with bupivacaine*

May be contraindicated	May be indicated
Pregnancy: may cause maternal cardiac effects and fetal hypoxia	When unusually prolonged analgesia is required
Cardiac disease	

Table 3.11 *Indications for and contraindications to LA with lidocaine*

May be contraindicated	May be indicated
Porphyria	Pregnancy: lidocaine is the LA of choice
Patients on suxamethonium, since apnoea is prolonged	

been shown to be superior in achieving successful anaesthesia following infiltration. It is not for injection in children under 4 years of age. However, the use of inferior alveolar nerve blocks can be almost eliminated in children by using articaine due to its ability to anaesthetize teeth effectively by infiltration up to the first permanent molar region. In addition, diffusion of articaine on to the palatal surface may also eliminate the discomfort of palatal infiltration. It can also be used in patients taking beta-blockers.

Articaine may be mildly neurotoxic and can cause prolonged anaesthesia, but its other adverse effects, toxic reactions and drug interactions (solutions containing a vasoconstrictor) are the same as those of other amide LAs (Table 3.9). The maximum recommended adult dose for articaine is 7 mg/kg. It should possibly not be given in porphyria.

Bupivacaine

Bupivacaine is an amide-type LA with a slow onset but long duration of action. It is therefore useful intraoperatively for patients under GA, to reduce the trigeminal nerve stimulation that can cause arrhythmias, and to give prolonged pain control postoperatively. It binds to plasma proteins and has a plasma half-life of 1.5–5.5 hours. Bupivacaine is largely metabolized in the liver. Maximum dose is 2.5 mg/kg.

Bupivacaine is the most cardiotoxic of the LAs (Table 3.10), the cardiotoxic effects being enhanced by hypoxia, hypercapnia, acidosis and hyperkalaemia. It inhibits cardiac conductivity and contractility, and may induce ventricular fibrillation. Bupivacaine therefore should not be used for patients with cardiac disease. Levobupivacaine, the L-isomer of bupivacaine, is of similar potency to bupivacaine but has the advantage of being significantly less cardiotoxic and neurotoxic than racemic bupivacaine.

Lidocaine

Lidocaine is the most widely used LA in many countries. Because of its effectiveness and the paucity of significant adverse reactions to it after half a century of use, lidocaine with adrenaline (epinephrine) is the standard against which other LAs are judged. It is an amide type with a rapid onset of action, providing LA of intermediate to long duration. Less than 10% of lidocaine is excreted unchanged in the urine. Lidocaine is metabolized mainly by the liver with an elimination half-life of 1–2 hours, and rapidly undergoes first-pass metabolism. The main metabolites also have LA activity and contribute to the effects of lidocaine as they have longer half-lives. Lidocaine can cross the placenta and may enter breast milk.

Serious adverse effects of lidocaine are exceedingly rare and most adverse reactions are due to misplacement of the needle, incompetent administration or overdose. There may not, however, be a linear relationship between the dose of lidocaine and the resultant blood level. In general, toxicity is more likely in children, older people and some acutely ill patients. Early features of overdose include tinnitus,

circumoral paraesthesia, metallic taste, light-headedness, nausea, vomiting and double vision. At higher levels, nystagmus, slurred speech, auditory and visual hallucinations, localized muscle twitching and tremors of the hands and feet are possible. Convulsions followed by loss of consciousness, respiratory arrest and eventual cardiovascular collapse may also occur. Lidocaine may cause some degree of depression of atrial and atrioventricular nodal activity, intraventricular conductivity and ventricular contraction. *Excessive* doses of lidocaine have been followed by death.

Lidocaine should not be given in a dose exceeding 4.4 mg/kg body weight. The maximum dose of lidocaine for the average adult is therefore 300 mg. If lidocaine is used in combination with adrenaline (epinephrine), the safe dose is up to 7 mg/kg, increasing the maximum dose of lidocaine to 500 mg for an average adult. A dental LA cartridge of 2.2 mL containing lidocaine 2% with adrenaline contains 44 mg of lidocaine, and thus the maximum safe number of cartridges for a normal adult would be 11 cartridges (7 cartridges if used without adrenaline). Lidocaine solution with adrenaline contains sodium metabisulphite to prevent oxidation of adrenaline; it should not be given to patients allergic to sulphites. Lidocaine may be contraindicated (Table 3.11) in patients with some cardiac disorders (especially hypovolaemia, heart block or other conduction disturbances), porphyria and myasthenia gravis. Lidocaine should be used in lower doses in children and older patients, and in cardiac, hepatic or renal disease. Impaired lidocaine metabolism may be found in severe cardiac failure and liver disease. Factors that affect hepatic blood supply and/or enzyme function can also significantly influence lidocaine metabolism.

Adrenaline can cause unopposed alpha-adrenergic activity in patients taking beta-blockers but only if LAs are given in far larger doses than appropriate for dentistry. Beta-blockers may also reduce hepatic blood flow and inhibit hepatic microsomal enzymes. By contrast, phenytoin, benzodiazepines and barbiturates may induce hepatic enzymes, lowering levels of free lidocaine.

Mepivacaine

Mepivacaine is an amide-type LA with a more rapid onset and shorter duration of action than lidocaine, and is rapidly metabolized in the liver. It binds to plasma proteins and has a plasma half-life of 2–3 hours. About 50% of the metabolites of mepivacaine are excreted in urine. Mepivacaine can cross the placenta.

Prilocaine

Prilocaine is an amide-type LA of fast onset and intermediate duration of action. Prilocaine metabolism is similar to that of lidocaine,

Table 3.12 *Indications for and contraindications to LA with prilocaine*

May be contraindicated	May be indicated
Glucose-6-phosphatase deficiency: greater risk of methaemoglobinaemia	In some patients with cardiovascular disease
Porphyria	
In patients on antimalarials: greater risk of methaemoglobinaemia	
In patients on sulphonamides: greater risk of methaemoglobinaemia	

Table 3.13 *Indications for and contraindications to LA containing adrenaline*

May be contraindicated	May be indicated
After radiotherapy to the area	For maximally effective anaesthesia
Liability to dry socket	
Asthma: patients can be sensitive to sulphites	
In patients on digoxin: may precipitate arrhythmias	
Cardiac bypass grafts: may precipitate arrhythmias	
In patients on beta-blockers: hypertensive crises may result but only in overdose	
In patients on norepinephrine-uptake blockers, St John's wort, atomoxetine, antipsychotic drugs or other psychoactive agents	
In patients who have used drugs of abuse, especially cannabis, ephedrine, clenbuterol or cocaine, in the previous 24 h: additive sympathomimetic effects may develop	
In patients on antiemetics	
Untreated hyperthyroidism	
Phaeochromocytoma	

being rapidly metabolized by the liver and excreted in the urine as *o*-toluidine. The main adverse effect of prilocaine is a dose-dependent production of methaemoglobinaemia resulting in impaired oxygen-carrying capacity. Cyanosis may occur 2–3 hours following administration. The local and systemic adverse effects of prilocaine on the CNS and heart are similar to those of lidocaine. Prilocaine may occasionally cause local neurotoxicity. The maximum adult dose is 400 mg. Prilocaine is contraindicated in methaemoglobinaemia and possibly in porphyria or children (Table 3.12).

Ropivacaine

Ropivacaine is an amide LA that may have a faster onset of action and longer duration of action than lidocaine but lesser pulpal anaesthesia; it can increase blood pressure (BP) and heart rate. It was found to be less cardiotoxic than bupivacaine in animal models. The local and systemic adverse effects of ropivacaine on the CNS and heart are similar to those of lidocaine. Use is prohibited in children of less than 12 years of age, the elderly, people with severe liver disease, and those with hypersensitivity.

VASOCONSTRICTORS

Adrenaline (epinephrine)

The addition of adrenaline to an LA improves haemostasis and anaesthesia; 1 in 80 000 to 1 in 100 000 adrenaline enhances pulpal anaesthesia ninefold and soft-tissue anaesthesia fourfold. It also increases the duration of action of lidocaine and enhances its safety margin. There is controversy about the possible systemic effects of adrenaline in an LA solution (Table 3.13). Adrenaline is a potent sympathomimetic, having significant beta-adrenergic activity (β_1 action raises cardiac rate and contraction force while β_2 activity causes bronchodilatation); it can thus cause a rise in BP, and some alpha activity, which causes vasoconstriction of vessels of the skin and mucosae.

The cardiac effects of adrenaline-containing LA solutions are usually slight but can be significant. Even with the use of aspirating techniques, up to 20% of all LA injections made into the highly vascular head and neck region may result in a significant rapid, albeit transient, rise of peripheral blood levels of adrenaline. There is also a slow rise in peripheral blood levels of adrenaline as a consequence of the gradual release of LA solution from the site of injection into local blood vessels. Adrenaline in LAs can raise cardiac output or BP. This is seen in healthy persons and others with cardiovascular disease. This does not happen when adrenaline is omitted. There is a very small rise in systolic BP (up to 8 mmHg) and a slight fall in diastolic pressure when lidocaine with 1:100 000 adrenaline is used, and up to a 14-mmHg rise with 1:25 000 adrenaline. By virtue of the enhanced anaesthesia, adrenaline may reduce the release of endogenous catecholamines. This is shown by data using tritiated adrenaline, where the rise in peripheral blood

catecholamine levels associated with intraoral injection of adrenaline-containing LA was mainly due to endogenous adrenaline. Patients with hypertension have greater elevation of systolic pressures after administration of LAs, but patients with ischaemic heart disease or prosthetic cardiac valves have changes similar to those of healthy people. However, systolic and diastolic pressures and cardiac rate can be raised even before the patient attends for dental treatment. The mere sight of a clinician can cause a slight rise in BP ('white-coat hypertension'). Immediately before the injection of LA, there can be significant rises in cardiac rate, systolic pressure and, to a lesser extent, diastolic pressure. Cardiac rate may fall but systolic pressure may rise slightly during administration of the LA. Similar cardiovascular changes may be seen when saline is injected or even if a syringe is placed in the mouth but the needle does not touch the mucosa. Anxiety clearly underlies these changes.

The clinical significance, if any, of the above remains unclear, but some argue that adrenaline is best avoided in cardiac patients or those on beta-blockers. However, this remains debatable. If a less effective LA is used, pain may not be completely abolished and this can have significant adverse effects on the heart. Also, in the case of patients on beta-blockers, interactions have only resulted when excessively large doses of an adrenaline-containing LA have been given.

Adrenaline-containing LAs may cause a significant but transient fall in plasma potassium, an effect particularly noticeable in patients on non-potassium-sparing diuretics (e.g. thiazide and loop diuretics). This hypokalaemic action appears due to a β_2-adrenergic action on membrane-bound adenosine triphosphase (ATPase). Adrenaline-containing LAs may also cause a transient rise in plasma glucose levels, due to α_2-adrenergic inhibition of insulin release, but these changes appear to have no clinical significance.

In the case of cocaine intoxication, adrenaline-containing LAs and other adrenergic vasoconstrictors are completely contraindicated. Adrenaline-containing LAs may also slightly delay wound healing after dental surgery and may increase the frequency of post-extraction alveolar osteitis ('dry socket').

Adrenaline is rapidly inactivated by the liver via both catechol-*O*-methyl transferases (COMTs) and monoamine oxidases (MAOs). The metabolites are excreted in urine, mainly as glucuronides or ethereal sulphate conjugates.

Table 3.14 *Possible indications for and contraindications to prilocaine with felypressin*

May be contraindicated	May be indicated
In cardiac patients	For better anaesthesia than with prilocaine alone
In patients with a liability to dry socket	
Theoretically, in pregnant patients	

Table 3.15 *Indications and contraindications for LA by intraligamentary injection*

May be contraindicated	May be indicated
Possibly in patients predisposed to infective endocarditis	Bleeding tendencies

Table 3.16 *Indications for and contraindications to electronic dental analgesia*

May be contraindicated	May be indicated
Demand-type pacemakers	–
Cerebrovascular disease	
Epilepsy	

Felypressin

Felypressin is a synthetic analogue of vasopressin with little of its anti-diuretic or oxytocin-like actions. Theoretically, it can cause coronary artery vasoconstriction and might affect the uterus in pregnancy, but these effects are unlikely with dental LA preparations. The administration of large amounts of felypressin to patients receiving GA with halothane may result in cyanosis and a slight rise in BP, but these changes are not serious. Felypressin has little toxicity, even if given intravenously in amounts far in excess of those used for LA (Table 3.14).

Over the years however, prilocaine with felypressin has not been shown to be safer than lidocaine with adrenaline (epinephrine), which generally provides deeper and more effective pain control.

OTHER METHODS OF LOCAL ANALGESIA

Intraligamentary (intraligamental) injections

Intraligamentary injections given after topical anaesthesia are recommended for restorative procedures in mandibular teeth in haemophiliac patients. The intraligamentary injection administered with a computer-controlled local anaesthetic delivery system (wand) is successful, particularly in palatal injections and when an inferior alveolar nerve block fails to provide profound pulpal anaesthesia in mandibular posterior teeth of patients presenting with irreversible pulpitis. Indications and contraindications are shown in Table 3.15.

Electronic dental analgesia

A number of dedicated electronic dental analgesia (EDA) systems are available. Some studies found that many patients (60%) preferred EDA to LA for restorative dentistry; however, others found that the levels of effectiveness of EDA were similar to those of topical anaesthesia, reducing the discomfort of LA injections in only 26% of cases. Indications and contraindications are shown in Table 3.16.

CONSCIOUS SEDATION

Changes in the provision of GA for UK dental services, and recommendations by repeated working groups that GA for dental treatment should only be used when there is no other method of pain and anxiety management appropriate for that patient, have led to the growing use of conscious sedation (CS). This is defined as:

> *a technique in which the use of a drug or drugs produces a state of depression of the central nervous system enabling treatment to be carried out, but during which verbal contact with the patient is maintained throughout. No interventions are required to maintain a patent airway, spontaneous ventilation is adequate and cardiovascular function is maintained. The drugs and techniques used to provide conscious sedation for dental treatment should carry a margin of safety wide enough to render loss of consciousness unlikely. (Department of Health. Conscious sedation in the provision of dental care: report of an expert group on sedation for dentistry – see Useful websites.)*

The Indicator of Sedation Need (IOSN) is increasingly used to assess needs.

PROCEDURAL SEDATION

Procedural sedation is 'a technique of administering sedatives or dissociative agents with or without analgesics to induce a state that allows the patient to tolerate unpleasant procedures while maintaining cardiorespiratory function'. Procedural sedation and analgesia (PSA) is intended to depress conscious level but to allow the patient to maintain oxygenation and airway control independently.

Degree of conscious level loss

ASA has defined the various sedation depths:

Minimal sedation (anxiolysis)

- Response to verbal stimulation is normal
- Cognitive function and coordination may be impaired
- Ventilatory and cardiovascular functions are unaffected.

Moderate sedation/analgesia (also called conscious sedation)

- Depression of consciousness is drug-induced
- Patient responds purposefully to verbal commands
- Airway is patent and spontaneous ventilation is adequate
- Cardiovascular function is usually unaffected.

Deep sedation/analgesia

- Depression of consciousness is drug-induced
- Patient is not easily aroused but responds purposefully following repeated or painful stimulation
- Independent maintenance of ventilatory function may be impaired
- Patient may require assistance in maintaining a patent airway
- Spontaneous ventilation may be inadequate
- Cardiovascular function is usually maintained.

General anesthesia

- Loss of consciousness is drug-induced, where the patient cannot be aroused, even by painful stimulation
- Patient's ability to maintain ventilatory function independently is impaired
- Patient requires assistance to maintain patent airway, and positive pressure ventilation may be required because of depressed spontaneous ventilation or drug-induced depression of neuromuscular function
- Cardiovascular function may be impaired.

Monitoring sedation

- Monitor vital signs before, during and after the procedure
- Monitor the ECG continuously in high-risk patients, during prolonged procedures or during deep sedation
- Consider continuous pulse oximetry for patients with co-morbidities (e.g. chronic obstructive pulmonary disease [COPD], asthma, congestive heart failure) or when high doses of sedatives or multiple drugs that may depress respirations are used
- Monitor the patient's appearance
- Monitor airway patency
- Monitor response to physical stimuli and verbal command
- Remember that measurement of blood gas level may be required
- Consider capnography for high-risk patients.

Suitability for CS

Only patients who are in ASA categories I and II are suitable for treatment under CS outside a hospital department. CS can be helpful for treating patients with needle phobia or other fears, pronounced gag reflex or anxiety, and for complex procedure such as endodontic and surgical work. It is normally used in conjunction with appropriate LA.

Most anxious patients can be treated with oral sedation (with benzodiazepines such as temazepam) or intravenous techniques with benzodiazepines (e.g. midazolam), or transmucosal sedation with benzodiazepines (usually nasal or sublingual midazolam) or inhalational sedation (with nitrous oxide and oxygen). Others may respond to a combination of alternative techniques, such as intravenous sedation with propofol or more than one drug.

Particular care is necessary in patients who are old, pregnant or very young, or who have cardiovascular, respiratory, liver, kidney or psychiatric disorders (Table 3.17). All patients should have thorough medical, dental and social histories taken and their dental examinations should be recorded for each course of treatment. BP measurement (Fig. 3.3), colour, pulse and respiration are important, as they determine patient selection and monitoring of the procedure. The ASA status should be determined.

Written informed consent must be obtained before each operation. Suitable consent forms are supplied by the medical defence societies. It is desirable, and there is increasing pressure, to provide patients with written information relevant to their treatment. Due consideration should be given to the patient's regular medication, if any (Table 3.18).

Sedated and anaesthetized patients may lose their cough reflex and the ability to protect their airway adequately. Material from the mouth or elsewhere can thus be aspirated into the larynx or lungs. Thus the airway must be protected by the anaesthetist/sedationist.

Table 3.17 *Indications for and contraindications to conscious sedation*

May be contraindicated	May be indicated
Intravenous sedation	
Psychotic personalities	Involuntary movements (e.g. chorea, parkinsonism)
Severe (disabling) heart disease	Uncooperative patients (e.g. learning impairment)
Respiratory infections	
Airways obstruction	Patients who faint with local anaesthesia
Fascial space infections	Patients with a tendency to retch
Chronic obstructive pulmonary disease	Where stress may induce attacks of angina
	Where stress may induce attacks of epilepsy
Unescorted patients	Where stress may induce attacks of asthma
Pregnancy	Where stress may induce attacks of hypertension
Children	
Needle-phobics	Patients too anxious to accept treatment under LA
Liver disease	
Myasthenia gravis	Many prolonged operations, such as removal of third molars or preparation for multiple implants for which GA would otherwise be needed
Glaucoma	
	Upper airways obstruction
	Claustrophobic patients
Inhalational sedation	
Psychoses	Children
Pregnancy during the first trimester	Drug users
	Myasthenia gravis
Claustrophobic patients (mask phobia)	Asthma
Respiratory infections	Needle-phobics
After some eye surgery	Patients with tendency to retch
In patients with vitamin B_{12} deficiency or on methotrexate	Epilepsy
Where access to the nose is required	

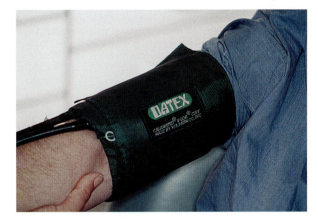

Fig. 3.3 Blood pressure measurement using sphygmomanometry.

PRE-MEDICATION

Pre-medication may still be administered for the purposes of diminishing anxiety, decreasing secretions, and reducing pain and vomiting (Table 3.19).

CONDUCTING CONSCIOUS SEDATION

In conducting sedation in the UK, the requirements of the Code of Practice issued by the General Dental Council must be fulfilled (Box 3.4;

Table 3.18 *Preoperative modification of regularly used medications before operation under conscious sedation or general anaesthesia*

Medication	Action (always discuss with the physician responsible for the patient)
Alpha-blockers	Continue
Analgesics	Continue
Angiotensin-converting enzyme inhibitors (ACEIs)	Continue
Antiarrhythmics	Continue
Anticholinesterase eye drops	May theoretically prolong the effect of suxamethonium and mivacurium; usually continue
Anticoagulants	Continue or consult haematologist
Anticonvulsants	Continue
Antimicrobial	Continue
Aspirin	Continue except for some surgery (e.g. urological and neurosurgery)
Beta-blockers	Continue
Calcium-channel blockers	Continue
Contraceptive pill	Continue
Corticosteroids	Continue, and raise dose (Ch. 6)
Digoxin	Continue
Diuretics (potassium-sparing)	Omit on morning of operation
Diuretics (thiazides or loop)	Continue
Heparin	Last prophylactic dose must be 6h before operation
Insulin or antidiabetics	Consult diabetologist; usually change to a sliding scale (Ch. 6)
Lithium	Stop 1 day before major surgery
Monoamine oxidase inhibitors (MAOIs)	Dangerous hypertensive interaction with certain opioid drugs. Preferably stop a few weeks before surgery if opioids are to be used
Non-steroidal anti-inflammatory drugs (NSAIDs)	Continue
Oral hypoglycaemics	Last dose is administered the night before a morning operating list, or the morning of an afternoon list
Selective serotonin reuptake inhibitors (SSRIs)	May interact with other drugs that facilitate serotonin (e.g. tramadol and other antidepressants): possibility of serotonin syndrome (dangerous neuromuscular and autonomic overactivity); consult anaesthetist
Statins	Continue
Tricyclic antidepressants	Exaggerate the effects of catecholamines; consult anaesthetist
Warfarin	Continue usually; consult haematologist

Table 3.19 *Pre-medication*

Aim	Drugs used
Reduction of anxiety	Temazepam 10–30mg p.o. (adults); oral midazolam 0.5mg/kg or alimemazine (trimeprazine) 2mg/kg p.o. (children)
Decrease in secretions	Glycopyrrolate
Analgesia	NSAIDs are commonly administered in adults; paracetamol in children
Antiemetic	Promethazine or alimemazine

Box 3.4 *Requirements before using conscious sedation*

- Written medical history
- Previous dental history
- Written instructions have been provided pre- and postoperatively
- The presence of an accompanying adult
- The patient has complied with pre-treatment instructions
- The medical history has been checked and acted on
- Records of drugs employed, dosages and times given, including site and method of administration
- Previous conscious sedation/general anaesthesia history
- Pre-sedation assessment
- Any individual specific patient requirements
- Suitable supervision has been arranged
- Written documentation of consent for sedation (consent form)
- Records of monitoring techniques
- Full details of dental treatment provided
- Post-sedation assessment

designed relative analgesia (inhalational sedation; IS) machines for dentistry should be used. Such machines should be maintained according to manufacturers' guidance with regular documented servicing. Gas supply lines for IS machines must be connected by non-interchangeable colour-coded pipelines to the medical gas supply or a mobile four-cylinder stand. On installed pipelines there must be a low-pressure warning device and an audible alarm. Nitrous oxide and oxygen cylinders must be stored safely with regard to current regulations. Cylinders must be secured safely to prevent injury. There should be adequate scavenging of waste gases. Inadequate scavenging may result in unacceptable risks to the health of the dental team. Scavenging of gases should not rely on window-opening or air-conditioning alone, and in the UK should conform to current Control of Substances Hazardous to Health (COSHH) Regulations (2002; http://www.hse.gov.uk/coshh/, accessed 30 September 2013). The long-term exposure limit (LTEL) represents a time-weighted average (TWA) over an 8-hour reference period defined in COSHH Regulation EH40 as the procedure whereby the occupational exposures in any 24-hour period are treated as equivalent to a single uniform exposure for 8 hours – the TWA exposure; recommended LTELs range from 25 to 100ppm. Breathing systems should have separate inspiratory and expiratory limbs to allow proper scavenging. Active and passive systems are available for scavenging. Nasal masks should be close-fitting to provide a good seal without air entrainment valves. All the appropriate equipment for the administration of sedation must be available in the surgery. This includes syringes, needles, cannulae, surgical wipes/tapes/dressings, tourniquets and labels. Purpose-designed, calibrated and appropriately maintained equipment is essential for all infusion techniques. It is mandatory to be able to administer supplementary oxygen or oxygen under intermittent positive pressure ventilation (IPPV) to the patient, should the need arise.

There must be at least one other person present at all times, who is suitably qualified and experienced enough to monitor the level of sedation and well-being of the patient. The levels of theoretical and practical training required by team members, regulations regarding standard and emergency equipment, monitoring, recovery facilities, consent, and instructions to patients and carers have been described in two UK Department of Health reports (see Further reading). An overview of the practical techniques only is provided here.

The clinical record for CS should include the reason for it and evidence of the consent process (Box 3.5). Instructions should be given in

see Appendix 3.4). Suitable resuscitative equipment, including a defibrillator, must always be available.

The dental surgery should be large enough to allow adequate access for the dental team all around the patient. The dental chair must be capable of being placed in the horizontal position. Dedicated purpose-

Box 3.5 *Inhalation sedation (IS) technique*

1. Check that the IS (relative analgesia) machine and scavenging are functioning properly and that an alternative supply of oxygen (O_2) is available

2. Recline the patient with legs uncrossed and position the mask over the patient's nose

3. Close the air entrainment valve on the mask (if present) and start administering 100% O_2 at a flow rate to approximate the patient's minute volume. This has been achieved when the reservoir bag moves with each breath without collapsing or overinflating and the patient does not have to mouth-breathe. (Correct flow rates are typically 5–8 L/min for an adult. Paediatric minute volumes vary with age)

4. Turn the nitrous oxide (N_2O) inspired concentration to 10% and advise the patient that they may start to feel warm or light-headed, or experience tingling of the extremities

5. After ensuring that the patient's speech (which may be slurred) is maintained for 1 min, increase the N_2O in increments of 5–10% at 1-min intervals until a relaxed state is reached. Inspired N_2O concentrations of 25–35% are typically used; concentrations exceeding 50% should be avoided

6. Supplement the inhalational sedation throughout with positive comments of reassurance and instructions

7. Delayed verbal or motor responses, visual or auditory changes, warmth and paraesthesia are all signs of an adequately sedated patient. Inability to maintain mouth-opening, snoring (indicating some degree of airway compromise) or moving into a state of restlessness are signs of oversedation and the concentration of N_2O should thus be decreased

8. Protect the airway with a rubber dam or butterfly sponge in the sedated patient

9. Monitor clinical signs (e.g. pulse and respiratory rate, unobstructed breathing and lack of cyanosis) throughout the surgery. Pulse oximetry may help

10. Turn the O_2 concentration to 100% at the end of the procedure

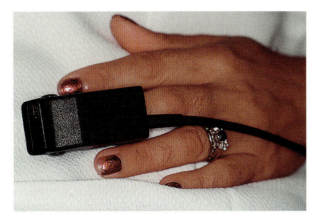

Fig. 3.4 Pulse oximetry to monitor blood oxygen saturation (nail varnish should be removed!).

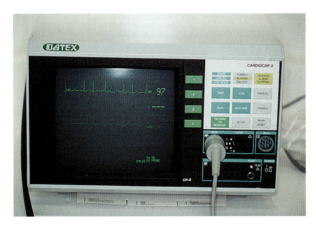

Fig. 3.5 Cardiac monitor.

written form when sedation is proposed. Patients often fail to take in what they are told or quickly forget. The patient's name and the reason for having sedation must be confirmed. This apparently obvious precaution avoids embarrassing confusion between patients coming from a crowded waiting room. The operation site should be confirmed and, if appropriate, marked in ink by the operator. This must be done while the patient is conscious, and checked with the patient. One of the most effective methods of lessening anxiety is by reassurance and brief discussion of a patient's particular anxieties.

Appliances such as orthodontic removable appliances or dentures should be removed preoperatively. The sedationist must be aware of the presence of crowned, fragile or loose teeth, bridges that could be damaged, contact lenses, hearing aids or colostomy bags. The bladder should be emptied preoperatively.

It is essential that a dental professional does not administer sedation in the absence of a second trained person. The latter is required not merely to assist and help deal with any mishaps, but also to act as a chaperone. Fantasies of sexual assault may arise during benzodiazepine sedation. Further, the patient may become disinhibited and make advances to the dentist.

Monitoring for intravenous sedation must include constant monitoring of conscious state, colour, BP, respiration and pulse. Use should be made of a BP monitor and pulse oximeter (Fig. 3.4); this provides a measure of the degree of haemoglobin oxygen saturation by means of spectrophotometry. Pulse oximeters are usually accurate and are a valuable safety measure. They pass red light at 660 nm (absorbed by oxygenated haemoglobin) and infrared light at 920 nm (absorbed by deoxygenated haemoglobin) across the vascular bed (usually of a finger or ear lobe), which permits display of the percentage of haemoglobin saturated with oxygen. This is safe when above 90%. A stethoscope and, ideally, an ECG monitor too (Fig. 3.5) should be used. However,

this is rarely practicable in the absence of expert interpretation of the tracing, such as in a hospital, unless an automatic read-out of possible diagnoses is available. Disadvantages of using ECG are that it can generate anxiety in the patient and is disturbed by movements, so its use is often restricted to patients with serious cardiac disease being treated in a hospital.

CHECKS AND INSTRUCTIONS FOR PATIENTS

Routine checks before conscious sedation for dental treatment

Always check the following:

1. Patient's name (and hospital number)
2. Nature, side and site of operation
3. Medical history, particularly of cardiorespiratory disease or bleeding tendency
4. Consent has been obtained in writing from the patient or, in a person under 16 years of age, from parent or guardian, and that the patient adequately understands the nature of the operation and sequelae
5. Necessary oral investigations (e.g. radiographs) are available
6. What the patient has had by mouth, including drugs, over the previous 4 hours
7. Patient has emptied the bladder
8. Patient's dentures have been removed and bridges, crowns and loose teeth have been noted by the anaesthetist

9. Pre-medication (and, where indicated, regular medication such as the contraceptive pill, anticonvulsants or antidepressants) has been given but not usually within the previous 4 hours
10. Anaesthetic and suction apparatus are working satisfactorily and that emergency drugs are available and not date-expired
11. Patient is escorted by a responsible adult
12. Patient has been warned not to drive, operate unguarded machinery, drink alcohol or make important decisions for 24 hours postoperatively.

Instructions to patients before conscious sedation

These instructions should preferably be given in writing:

1. You must be accompanied by a responsible adult, over the age of 18 years, who will undertake to escort you home and remain with you for 24 hours after treatment. You must not be accompanied by children under 14 years of age.
2. Do not wear nail varnish or make-up.
3. After sedation, you must not on the same day:
   A. drive a motor vehicle
   B. ride a bicycle or motorcycle, even as a passenger
   C. cook or use unguarded machinery
   D. take alcohol
   E. take sedative drugs without medical advice
   F. make important decisions or sign any documents.
4. If you develop a cold before your appointment, please telephone the hospital or dental surgery for advice.

Patients who fail to comply with these simple safety precautions will not be given sedation.

STANDING DENTAL ADVISORY COMMITTEE: REPORT OF AN EXPERT GROUP ON SEDATION FOR DENTISTRY

Conscious sedation in the provision of dental care: executive summary

- *Despite the publication of a number of authoritative documents on pain and anxiety control for dentistry, it has become evident that there remain areas of confusion and lack of consensus.*
- *This document is designed to lay down specific recommendations to all practitioners providing conscious sedation for the provision of dental care in general dental practice, community and hospital settings.*
- *The effective management of pain and anxiety is of paramount importance for patients requiring dental care and conscious sedation is a fundamental component of this.*
- *Competently provided conscious sedation is safe, valuable and effective.*
- *It is absolutely essential that a wide margin of safety be maintained between conscious sedation and the unconscious state of general anaesthesia. Conscious sedation must under no circumstances be interpreted as light general anaesthesia.*
- *A high level of competence based on a solid foundation of theoretical and practical supervised training, progressive updating of skills and continuing experience is the key to safe practice.*

- *Education and training must ensure that all members of the dental team providing treatment under conscious sedation have received appropriate supervised theoretical, practical and clinical training.*
- *Training in the management of complications, in addition to regularly rehearsed proficiency in life-support techniques, is essential for all clinical staff. Retention and improvement of knowledge and skills rely upon regular updating.*
- *Operating chairs and patient trolleys must be capable of being placed in the head-down tilt position and equipment for resuscitation from respiratory and cardiac arrest must be readily available.*
- *Dedicated purpose-designed machines for inhalational sedation should be used.*
- *It is essential to ensure that hypoxic mixtures cannot be delivered.*
- *There should be adequate active scavenging of waste gases.*
- *All equipment for the administration of intravenous sedation, including appropriate antagonist drugs, must be available in the treatment area and appropriately maintained.*
- *Supplemental oxygen delivered under intermittent positive pressure, together with back-up, must be immediately available.*
- *It is important to ensure that each exposure to conscious sedation is justified. Careful and thorough assessment of the patient ensures that correct decisions are made regarding the planning of treatment.*
- *A thorough medical, dental and social history should be taken and recorded prior to each course of treatment for every patient.*
- *There are few absolute contraindications for conscious sedation, though special care is required in the assessment and treatment of children and elderly patients.*
- *Patients must receive careful instructions and written valid consent must be obtained.*
- *Fasting for conscious sedation is not normally required but some authorities recommend the same fasting requirements as for general anaesthesia.*
- *Recovery from sedation is a progressive step down from completion of treatment through to discharge. A member of the dental team must supervise and monitor the patient throughout this period.*
- *The decision to discharge a patient into the care of the escort following any type of sedation must be the responsibility of the sedationist.*
- *The patient and escort should be provided with details of potential complications, aftercare and adequate information regarding emergency contact.*
- *The three standard techniques of inhalation and oral and intravenous sedation employed in dentistry are effective and adequate for the vast majority of patients. The simplest technique to match the requirements should be used.*
- *The only currently recommended technique for inhalation sedation is a titrated dose of nitrous oxide with oxygen and it is absolutely essential to ensure that a hypoxic mixture cannot be administered.*
- *The standard technique for intravenous sedation is the use of a titrated dose of a single drug: for example, the current use of a benzodiazepine. This can be given into a vein on the dorsum of hand or elsewhere in the arm (Fig. 3.6)*

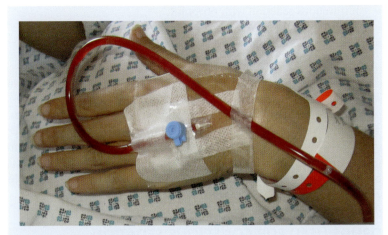

Fig. 3.6 Intravenous line.

- *Oral pre-medication with an effective low dose of a sedative agent may be prescribed.*
- *No single technique will be successful for all patients.*
- *All drugs and all syringes in use in the treatment area must be clearly labelled and each drug should be given according to accepted recommendations.*
- *Stringent clinical monitoring during the procedure is of particular importance and all members of the clinical team must be capable of undertaking this.*
- *Conscious sedation for children must only be undertaken by teams which have adequate training and experience.*
- *Nitrous oxide/oxygen should be the first choice for paediatric dental patients.*
- *Intravenous sedation for children is only appropriate in a minority of cases.*
- *The management of any complication, including loss of consciousness, requires the whole dental team to be aware of the risks, appropriately trained and fully equipped. It is vitally important for the whole team to be prepared and regularly rehearsed.*
- *Attention must be given to risk awareness, risk control and risk containment.*
- *Evidence of active participation in continuing professional development (CPD) and personal clinic audit is an essential feature of clinical governance.*

PREPARATION AND CHOICE OF TECHNIQUE

Only patients of ASA classes I and II are suitable for sedation as outpatients. ASA III patients should be referred to at least an appropriate secondary care unit and ASA IV patients to the hospital service, ideally with an anaesthetist present. Unlike sedation in the hospital operating-theatre setting, fasting is not required for CS in the dental practice when resorting to GA in the event of failure is not an option. There are few absolute contraindications but special care should be taken with children and the elderly. Treatment during pregnancy should be avoided where possible, certainly as regards the use of nitrous oxide and probably benzodiazepines in the first trimester.

'Standard' sedation techniques involve the use of *one only* of the options outlined below.

Oral sedative drug alone

This method is ideal where it is not possible to use one of the titratable techniques (e.g. needle-phobic patients for whom nitrous oxide is unlikely to provide sufficient relaxation). Oral sedation should only be used by those capable of intravenous cannulation. Benzodiazepines may cause paradoxical hyperexcitability in some children or oversedation in older people, and the level of sedation cannot be altered.

Pre-medication before conscious sedation

Pre-medication may be desirable to lessen anxiety. However, this is not usually feasible in general dental practice as it delays recovery. Any pre-medication is typically given 30–35 minutes preoperatively. If pre-medication has to be given, benzodiazepines are useful because of their anxiolytic and amnesic actions, their relative freedom from side-effects and their wide safety margin. Diazepam, lorazepam and temazepam are used more and more widely for pre-medication. Beta-blockers may also be employed and may help to prevent arrhythmias induced by surgery. Opioids such as pethidine are traditional pre-medicants because of their sedative action. However, they frequently cause nausea, vomiting and respiratory depression. Promethazine or alimemazine (trimeprazine) may be used for its sedative and antiemetic effect, for pre-medication of children, but these drugs have a prolonged action and are often ineffective. They also raise blood sugar levels – a consideration when treating diabetics. Patients vary widely in their requirements for pre-medication and this may be discussed with the anaesthetist/sedationist.

Inhalational sedation with nitrous oxide and oxygen

This technique does not cause significant cardiorespiratory or respiratory depression in patients who are well enough to have outpatient treatment. Nitrous oxide diffuses into body cavities and thus is contraindicated after recent eye retinal surgery where parfluoropropane sulphur hexafluoride has been used, and where there is bowel obstruction or cysts on pathological cavities. The gases persist in the eye for up to 3 months after surgery. Chronic exposure may interfere with vitamin B_{12}. An 'IS machine' with built-in safety features is used to titrate nitrous oxide and non-hypoxic (30%+) flows of oxygen (see Box 3.5). The oxygen concentration is set to 100% at the end of surgery to minimize diffusion hypoxia. Patients are monitored using clinical signs (i.e. responsiveness, adequate breathing, pulse and colour). Before being allowed to leave professional supervision, the patient should be able to walk unaided without stumbling or feeling unstable. Adults who have received inhalation sedation may leave unaccompanied.

Intravenous sedation with midazolam alone

Midazolam is currently the accepted benzodiazepine of 'standard' intravenous sedation and has displaced diazepam (Box 3.6). Benzodiazepines may cause disinhibition in children, and intravenous sedation for children under 12 is only appropriate for a minority of cases. Outpatient sedation is contraindicated for patients with cardiorespiratory disease of ASA grade IV and in those with significant renal or hepatic dysfunction.

Patients must be accompanied postoperatively and receive advice similar to that issued after GA. Flumazenil is a specific antagonist at the benzodiazepine binding site on the GABA receptor and will reverse sedation in emergencies.

Advanced techniques

More experienced and suitably trained teams working in tightly controlled clinical settings with additional facilities as outlined by the UK Department of Health may use 'alternative techniques' such as:

- sedation for children under 12 other than with nitrous oxide
- inhalational sedation using anything other than nitrous oxide (e.g. sevoflurane)

Box 3.6 *Intravenous sedation (IS) technique*

1. Establish reliable intravenous access
2. Inject 2–3 mg of midazolam over 30 s and assess the patient's response over the next 2–3 min
3. Administer further 0.5–1 mg increments of midazolam at 2-min intervals until adequate sedation is achieved, as indicated by a relaxed but cooperative patient with slight speech slurring (eyelid signs, as formerly used in diazepam sedation, are not reliable)
4. Careful titration is necessary because some patients may require more and some may require a lot less than the average dose requirement of 0.07 mg/kg (i.e. 5 mg for a 70 kg person)
5. Protect the airway with the use of a rubber dam or butterfly sponge; this is particularly important in the patient sedated with midazolam
6. Note that sedation will realistically be maintained for about 30 min of operating time. Monitor the patient clinically as for inhalational sedation (see earlier) and also with pulse oximetry
7. Remember that signs of oversedation are as for inhalation sedation (see earlier). In addition, if oxygen (O_2) saturation is seen to fall, reassess the patient's airway and respiratory effort. Simply instructing the patient to take deeper breaths and administering supplemental nasal or face-mask O_2 may be all that is necessary for surgery to continue, provided verbal contact is also still maintained. However, in the presence of other signs of oversedation (see earlier), it may be advisable not to start surgery
8. Use flumazenil (200 mcg bolus then 100-mcg increments at 1-min intervals until improvement) only if this fails; flumazenil should never be used solely to hasten postoperative recovery
9. Continue direct postoperative observation for 15 min and discharge with an escort after 1 h

---

- intravenous sedation with propofol
- the use of additional intravenous drugs, an opioid or ketamine
- combined inhalational and intravenous sedation (except use of nitrous oxide to site a cannula).

Where techniques involve the continuous intravenous administration of a drug, or where three or more drugs are used together regardless of their routes, a dedicated non-operator sedationist must be present. This may be a dentist or doctor, registered for 4 years with experience of at least 100 procedures, who has undergone recognized training in conscious sedation in the context of the dental environment. It has been suggested that an anaesthetist with 2 years' experience would comply with *most* of these requirements.

DRUGS USED FOR CONSCIOUS SEDATION

Sedative agents for sedation include mainly the benzodiazepines (midazolam and diazepam), propofol and nitrous oxide. Before their use, the administrator's experience, the facilities and the relative safety of the different agents must be taken into consideration (see also Table 3.20).

Benzodiazepines

- Benzodiazepines are potent sedative drugs, acting on the limbic system to block reuptake of GABA.
- They have been widely used for conscious sedation.
- They are usually given intravenously, but some can be given orally, rectally or intranasally.
- Their effects include amnesia, anticonvulsant activity, anxiolysis, muscle relaxation and sedation but they can also cause respiratory depression.
- Benzodiazepines do not affect the cardiovascular system.
- Achievement of the depth of sedation necessary is established when the patient shows Eve's sign (the inability to touch the end of the nose accurately).

Table 3.20 *Agents for conscious intravenous sedation[a]*

Drug	Proprietary names (UK)	Adult dose	Comments
Diazepam	Valium	Up to 20 mg	Benzodiazepine: gives sedation with amnesia but no analgesia. Give slowly intravenously in 2.5-mg increments until ptosis begins (i.e. eyelids begin to droop; Verrill's sign) – rapid injection may cause respiratory depression. Then give local analgesia. Disadvantages: • May cause pain or thrombophlebitis • Drowsiness returns transiently 4–6 h postoperatively due to metabolites desmethyl diazepam, triazolam and oxazepam, and enterohepatic recirculation • May cause mild hypotension and respiratory depression.
	Diazemuls	Up to 20 mg	Preferred to Valium. Has most of the actions above but causes less thrombophlebitis and therefore can be given into veins on dorsum of hand. Expensive. Do not give intramuscularly.
Midazolam	Hypnovel	0.07 mg/kg (up to 7.5 mg total dose)	Benzodiazepine. Compared to diazepam: • onset of action is quicker (30 s) • amnesia is more profound, starting 2–5 min after administration and lasting up to 40 min (with no retrograde amnesia) • recovery is more rapid; midazolam is virtually completely eliminated within 5 h without the recurrence of drowsiness that may follow the use of diazepam • incidence of venous thrombosis is lower than with diazepam • at least twice as potent • signs of sedation are less predictable – very slow injection required. Occasional deaths in elderly.
Propofol	Propofol, Diprivan	2 mg/kg	Contraindicated in children under 18 years. May cause pain on injection. Contraindicated in patients taking anticonvulsants. Occasional fits or anaphylaxis.

[a]Midazolam is the main agent used.

- The effect of benzodiazepines is reversed by flumazenil.
- Benzodiazepines may be ineffective in children, in whom they may paradoxically cause hyperactivity, and in persons on long-term medication with psychoactive drugs. Be very careful about prescribing benzodiazepines in combination with an opioid, as both are respiratory depressants.
- Diazepam has a long half-life (0.8–2.25 days) that is markedly increased in obese or elderly patients (3.9 days and 3.29 days, respectively), and its active metabolites have long half-lives (i.e. *N*-desmethyldiazepam [1.6–4.2 days]; nordiazepam [about 8 days]).
- Diazepam is a mild respiratory depressant with minimal risk to healthy persons, but is potentially dangerous to those with cardiorespiratory disease, particularly COPD. Diazepam is metabolized to products that have sedative actions (desmethyldiazepam, temazepam and oxazepam) and thus effects can persist, with a half-life of 20–72 hours.
- Midazolam is now the most commonly used agent for procedural sedation. It is considerably (two or three times) more potent than diazepam, amnesia is more profound and recovery more rapid (Tables 3.21 and 3.22). The maximal effect of midazolam on the brain appears to be about 10–15 minutes after intravenous administration. Intranasal midazolam has a faster onset of sedation than oral diazepam, with better sedation and faster recovery.
- Intravenous midazolam produces a faster onset of sedation, less pain on injection, and improved awakening when compared with diazepam. Midazolam is cleared by hepatic hydroxylation to 1-hydroxymidazolam (which has only 10% of the pharmacological activity of midazolam).

- Lorazepam has a peak onset of action 15–20 minutes after administration and the duration of action is longer (i.e. 6–8 hours) than that of midazolam (30–60 minutes). In addition, lorazepam has roughly double the potency of midazolam. Because of this, lorazepam is more typically used for long-term sedation, such as in the intensive care unit.
- A short-acting benzodiazepine (e.g. midazolam), usually alone or in combination with an opioid analgesic (e.g. fentanyl, morphine), is commonly selected but the combination increases risks of oxygen desaturation and cardiorespiratory complications. Specific reversal agents for benzodiazepines (flumazenil) and opiates (naloxone) must be readily available throughout the procedure. The sedative and respiratory-depressant effects and the risk of cardiovascular depression conferred by all benzodiazepines are

Table 3.22 *Midazolam: possible adverse reactions and contraindications*

Adverse reactions	Contraindications
Hiccough	Hypersensitivity to midazolam
Cough	Erythromycin use (potentiates midazolam)
Oversedation	Concomitant use of barbiturates, alcohol, narcotics or other CNS depressants, cimetidine, omeprazole, kava or valerian
Pain at the injection site	
Nausea and vomiting	
Headache	Glaucoma
Blurred vision	Depressed vital signs, shock or coma
Fluctuations in vital signs	
Hypotension	
Respiratory depression	
Respiratory arrest	

Table 3.21 *Procedural sedation*[a]

Drug	Dose (adult)	Onset of action (min)	Duration (min)	Comments
Midazolam (Versed)	0.02–0.1 mg/kg i.v. initially; if further sedation is required, may repeat with 25% of initial dose after 3–5 min; do not exceed 2.5 mg/dose (1.5 mg for elderly persons) and 5 mg cumulative dose (3.5 mg for elderly persons)	1–2	30–60	Respiratory depression or hypotension possible, particularly when rapidly administered or given with fentanyl; does not provide analgesia. Flumazenil can reverse
Fentanyl	1–2 mcg/kg slow i.v. push over 1–2 min; may repeat dose after 30 min	1–2	30–60	May cause chest wall rigidity, apnoea, respiratory depression or hypotension; elicits minimal cardiovascular depression; may cause dysphoria, nausea, vomiting or EEG changes. Naloxone can reverse
Etomidate (Amidate)	0.1–0.2 mg/kg slow i.v. push over 30–60 s	<1	3–5	Often causes pain on injection, myoclonus or adrenal suppression (typically no clinical significance unless repeated doses are used within a limited time span). May cause nausea and vomiting, and lowers seizure threshold; causes a slight-to-moderate decrease in intracranial pressure lasting for several minutes; does not cause histamine release; useful for patients with trauma and hypotension
Ketamine	1–4.5 mg/kg i.v. over 60 s; total dose 0.5–2 mg/kg	1	10–15	Emergence delirium in approximately 12% of patients, which may last from 1–3 h but not usual in children <15 y or in older patients (i.e. >65 y)
Dexmedetomidine	0.7 mcg/kg/h; if further sedation is required, may repeat	5–30	60–120	Slow onset. Produces a sedation level similar to the other agents noted here but no respiratory depression and no major cardiac depression; patients are able to follow commands and respond to verbal and tactile stimulus
Propofol (Diprivan)	0.5–1 mg/kg i.v. loading dose; may repeat by 0.5-mg increments every 3–5 min	<1	3–10	Provides rapid onset, brief duration of action and quick recovery; has anticonvulsant properties; can rapidly cause deepening sedation; causes cardiovascular depression and hypotension

[a]Medscape Reference. Dosage guidelines for adults. http://emedicine.medscape.com/article/109695-overview#aw2aab6b8 (accessed 27 May 2013).

greatly increased if these drugs are combined with alcohol or opioids (opiates). Opiates may be used to provide analgesia and sedation during painful procedures. Fentanyl is favoured because of its prompt onset and short duration of action, with minimal cardiovascular depressive effects and hypotension. Fentanyl binds with stereospecific receptors at many sites within the CNS and increases pain threshold, alters pain reception and inhibits ascending pain pathways. In addition to analgesia, opioid agonists suppress the cough reflex and cause respiratory depression, drowsiness and sedation. The half-life is 2–4 hours.

Propofol

- Propofol provides potent, ultra-short-acting sedation or anaesthesia but has no analgesic properties. It is associated with a deep sedation level approaching that of GA. Because of this, an anaesthetist or sedation team often administers it and monitors its use outside the operating room.
- It appears to have the advantages of a rapid sedative response, with a quicker recovery and better effects on mood compared with midazolam. Propofol's onset of action is rapid at 90–100 seconds. Duration of action is dose-dependent and ranges from 5 to 10 minutes after bolus administration.
- Propofol is rapidly metabolized by the liver.
- It leads to a dose-dependent decrease in arterial BP and cardiac output.
- It has a relatively high rate of discomfort, including severe pain, with injection in up to 28–90% of patients. Transient local pain can be minimized if the larger veins of the forearm or antecubital fossa are used.
- Propofol is slightly more cost-effective than midazolam because of its shorter recovery times, and is safer than benzodiazepines and opiates. There are no antagonists.
- Long-term treatment with high doses can cause a propofol infusion syndrome (PRIS) – a rare but often lethal reaction characterized by rhabdomyolysis, acidosis, and renal and cardiac failure.
- It is therefore contraindicated for children under the age of 18 years, either during surgical or diagnostic procedures or in the ICU.
- It is sometimes used with remifentanil (short-acting and not affected by obesity or liver or kidney disease) for maintenance of total intravenous anaesthesia.

Nitrous oxide

- Nitrous oxide (NO) produces analgesia and sedation with a far quicker recovery than most sedatives/analgesics. Nitrous oxide with oxygen is overall the safest agent for CS because of its rapid reversibility and lack of respiratory or cardiodepressant effects.
- For needle-phobics, children, epileptics, some drug users or those with asthma and myasthenia gravis, inhalational sedation is preferable to intravenous sedation because it provides better control of the patient. For inhalation sedation, clinical monitoring of the patient is adequate.
- For claustrophobic patients or those with upper airways obstruction, inhalation sedation may be contraindicated.

Other agents

Other agents may occasionally include etomidate, ketamine and dexmedetomidine.

Etomidate

- Etomidate produces minimal haemodynamic effects and has a reliable onset of action.
- It is an ultra-short-acting, non-barbiturate hypnotic used mainly for GA. It produces rapid induction without histamine release and with minimal cardiovascular and respiratory effects. Etomidate transiently lowers cerebral blood flow by 20–30% and slightly reduces intracranial and intraocular pressure. It has no analgesic properties. Onset of action is 5–30 seconds with peak action at 1 minute. Etomidate has a duration of 2–10 minutes, depending on the dose.
- The major adverse effect is transient adrenal suppression secondary to inhibition of 11-β-hydroxylase and 17-α-hydroxylase enzymes, which are important in cortisol synthesis. There is also a high incidence of pain on injection, and nausea and vomiting associated with bolus administration.

Ketamine

- Ketamine produces a dissociative state and patients may not be able to speak or respond purposefully to verbal commands. Onset of action for intravenous administration is within 1 minute, and duration of action about 10–15 minutes.
- It is usually not recommended for adults because it often causes emergence delirium (i.e. vivid imagery, hallucinations, confusion, excitement, irrational behaviour). Emergence delirium is not typical in children younger than 15 years or in older patients (i.e. over 65 years).
- Emergence reactions are estimated to occur in approximately 12% of patients and can be expected to last from 1–3 hours. The incidence may be reduced by decreasing the recommended dose of ketamine and using it in conjunction with a benzodiazepine. A small hypnotic dose of a short-acting barbiturate or benzodiazepine is recommended to terminate severe emergence reactions.
- In doses typically used for procedural sedation, ketamine does not affect pharyngeal–laryngeal reflexes and thus allows a patent airway as well as maintaining spontaneous respiration. Therefore it is useful for emergency procedures when fasting cannot be assured. The unique dissociative action and partial agonism at opiate mu receptors permit painful procedures to be performed in a consistent state of sedation and patient comfort. Ketamine is contraindicated when an increased BP would pose a risk of complications. An increase in oropharyngeal secretions is often triggered and laryngospasms are possible.
- At a 1:1 mixture with propofol, ketamine can be used in adults for procedural sedation and analgesia. This mixture has been associated with a reduced incidence of emergence delirium and may negate the need for concomitant benzodiazepine use.

Dexmedetomidine (DEX)

- Dexmedetomidine produces a level of sedation similar to the other agents mentioned but no respiratory depression and no major cardiac depression. Patients are able to follow commands and respond to verbal and tactile stimulus but fall quickly asleep when not stimulated. It does provide some pain relief. Minimal cardiovascular effects are seen and include mild bradycardia and a decrease in systemic vascular resistance.
- It is an α_2-adrenergic agonist that provides sedation, anxiolysis, hypnosis, analgesia and sympatholysis. Onset of action is

relatively slow and the context-sensitive half-life is approximately 4 minutes after a 10-minute infusion. It is 1600 times more selective for α_2 than α_1 receptors and therefore has very few adverse effects and provides predictable results.

■ Dexmedetomidine has a minimal respiratory depressive effect, which is beneficial for dentistry; however, it has the disadvantage of permitting an intraoperative arousal response such that the patient suddenly appears to be no longer sedated, and it has a variable amnestic effect.

POSTOPERATIVE CARE

The immediate postoperative period is a particularly dangerous time and the patient must be closely supervised with pulse oximetry, until completely conscious, by the dental surgeon; supervision by the nurse or other responsible adult should continue until the patient is alert and able to stand without dizziness or ataxia. A member of the dental team should supervise the patient during recovery. The first stage of recovery is normally in the dental chair. Once patients have recovered sufficiently to move to a resting area, they should be carefully guided and supported. During recovery, patients should be laid on their side in the semi-prone (tonsillar) position and the airway must be protected. Up to 20% of patients may become hypoxic after intravenous sedation and therefore supplemental oxygen should be given during recovery. Equipment and drugs for dealing with medical emergencies must be on hand. The sedationist must be constantly available to see the patient for any emergency.

Monitoring discharge

Patients cannot be considered fully recovered until they have returned to their preoperative physiological state. Early recovery (phase I) lasts from discontinuation of the procedure until patients have recovered protective reflexes and motor function. This requires close monitoring and supervision, normally in a high-dependency atmosphere with suitably trained nursing staff. In deciding when patients have recovered enough to allow their safe transfer to phase II recovery, the Aldrete scoring system may be used (Table 3.23). This assigns a score of 0, 1 or 2 to activity, respiration, circulation, consciousness and colour, giving a maximal score of 10. A score of 9 indicates recovery sufficient for the patient to be transferred from high dependency. However, with the advent of pulse oximetry, a more reliable indicator of oxygenation than clinical observation, the ability to maintain O_2 saturation >92% on room air is regarded as a satisfactory end-point. After patients are discharged, they can then undergo full recovery at home (phase III recovery).

The decision to discharge a patient into the care of the responsible adult escort after any type of sedation must be the responsibility of the dentist or anaesthetist/sedationist (see also Appendices to this chapter). The patient must be accompanied home by a responsible adult. If this is not possible, sedation is contraindicated. Exceptions may be made occasionally in the case of inhalation sedation with nitrous oxide and oxygen when, at the discretion of the sedationist, the patient may leave unaccompanied if medically fit and responsible. Arrangements should be made for the patient to travel home by private car driven by the escort or by taxi rather than on public transport. When this is not possible, the escort must be made aware of the added responsibilities of caring for the patient during the journey home. If either the patient or the escort appears to be unwilling or unable to comply with these requirements, sedation should not be given. It is desirable that the escort should look after the patient for the rest of the day.

Table 3.23 *Aldrete score*

	2	1	0
Respiration	Able to take deep breath and cough	Dyspnoea/shallow breathing	Apnoea
O_2 saturation	Maintains >92% on room air	Needs O_2 inhalation to maintain O_2 saturation >90%	Saturation <90% even with supplemental oxygen
Consciousness	Fully awake	Arousable on calling	Not responding
Circulation	BP ± 20 mmHg preoperatively	BP ± 20–50 mmHg preoperatively	BP ± 50 mmHg preoperatively
Activity	Able to move 4 extremities	Able to move 2 extremities	Able to move 0 extremities

Table 3.24 *Indications for and contraindications to general anaesthesia*

May be contraindicated	May be indicated
Pregnancy	Refusal of or allergy to local anaesthesia
Unescorted patients	
Severe infections in the floor of the mouth	Acute local infections (but not Ludwig angina)
Severe anaemia (especially sickle cell anaemia)	
Severe renal disease	Injection phobia
Severe hepatic disease	Learning impairment
Severe respiratory disease	Major surgery
Severe cardiac disease	Multiple extractions

Alternatively, arrangements should be made for a reliable adult to undertake that care.

GENERAL ANAESTHESIA

It is inappropriate in this book to discuss general anaesthetic agents or intraoperative care in detail, since GA is the remit of specialist anaesthetists and, in the UK, must be given only in a hospital (see *A conscious decision: a review of the use of general anaesthesia and conscious sedation in primary dental care*, Department of Health, 2003).

However, dental surgeons working in hospital may have to care for such patients perioperatively. Indications for GA are shown in Table 3.24. Due consideration should be given to the patient's medication, if any (see Table 3.7), which should be discussed with the anaesthetist.

PREOPERATIVE PREPARATION

It is the anaesthetist's responsibility to assess suitability for, and the best approach to, GA but a thorough clerking by the surgical team makes this process more efficient. Information about previous GA (tolerance and associated problems), induction or airway management (e.g. starvation, mouth-opening, dentition, heartburn and reflux), and history or family history of conditions relevant to GA (e.g. cholinesterase deficiency, malignant hyperpyrexia) are important.

Preoperative starvation guidelines

If gastric contents are regurgitated, they risk being aspirated into the lungs and causing asphyxiation or Mendelsohn syndrome. This risk has traditionally been reduced, whenever possible, by minimizing intake of food and drink before GA. In reality, however, many patients are starved for excessive times. Prolonged fast of fluid is illogical since, in fasting patients, the stomach can secrete up to 50 mL of gastric juice an hour. Further, ingested clear fluids rapidly leave the stomach of healthy people, with about half the volume disappearing in 10–20 minutes. Prolonged fluid deprivation has also been shown to raise the volume and decrease the pH of gastric juice, which increases the likelihood and consequences of gastric acid aspiration. Although patients who are likely to have delayed gastric emptying through underlying disease or drug treatment should not drink before GA, there is now overwhelming evidence in favour of allowing other patients with ASA grades I or II to drink clear fluids up to 2 hours before the procedure. If medication needs to be administered preoperatively, tablets and capsules can be swallowed with a small quantity of water at any time before GA.

The risks apply mainly (and rarely) to GA. Protective reflexes should remain largely intact in CS, and so the risks of aspiration should be lower. The available guidelines are somewhat equivocal but there are no hard data to support starvation before CS.

If aspiration is likely, metoclopramide hastens gastric emptying and may contribute to risk reduction. Ranitidine or sodium citrate can neutralize the acidity of gastric secretions in those at risk of aspiration.

Rapid sequence induction

It may not be appropriate to wait for adequate starvation when emergency surgery is required. In such circumstances, a rapid sequence induction of GA is required. In addition, certain conditions may render starvation times less effective (Box 3.7).

Patients with significant reflux or gastro-oesophageal incompetence are also at risk of aspirating the contents of their stomach, whether filled with food or not; in general, they should also be considered for a rapid sequence induction. The patient breathes 100% oxygen for at least 3 minutes to extend the time during which they may remain well saturated while apnoeic if there are difficulties intubating (pre-oxygenation). A predetermined dose of induction agent is delivered as a bolus while an assistant applies backward pressure to the cricoid cartilage. The latter manœuvre occludes the oesophagus and further reduces the likelihood of regurgitation. A fast-acting muscle relaxant (suxamethonium or rocuronium) is given, the patient intubated, and cricoid pressure only released when endotracheal tube position is confirmed and its cuff inflated.

INTRAVENOUS ANAESTHETICS

Most intravenous sedative and GA agents are modulators of the $GABA_A$ receptor, facilitating inhibitory neurotransmission at a site on the receptor away from that of GABA itself. Ketamine, however, is an *N*-methyl-D-aspartate (NMDA) receptor blocker and clonidine-like agents are α_2-receptor agonists (Table 3.25).

Etomidate

Etomidate, an imidazole derivative, causes less cardiovascular depression than either propofol or thiopental, although its use, even in hypotensive patients, has declined owing to other undesirable effects such as nausea and vomiting, pain on injection and excitatory movements. It inhibits the enzymes 11-β-hydroxylase and 17-α-hydroxylase, suppressing adrenal function, an effect which may occur even after a single dose.

Box 3.7 *Conditions rendering preoperative starvation ineffective*

- Trauma at less than the usual starvation time after eating
- Use of potent opioids preoperatively
- Acute abdominal condition (particularly bowel obstruction)
- Active labour

Table 3.25 *Drugs for intravenous anaesthesia*

Drug	Proprietary names (UK)	Adult dose	Comments
Etomidate	Hypnomidate	0.2 mg/kg	Good for outpatient anaesthesia. Pain on injection: use large vein and give fentanyl 200 mcg first. After operation give naloxone 0.1–0.2 mg and oxygen. Little cardiovascular effect. Often involuntary movements, cough and hiccough. Hepatic metabolism. Avoid in repeated doses in traumatized patient – may suppress adrenal steroid production
Ketamine	Ketalar	0.5–2 mg/kg	Rise in BP, cardiac rate and intraocular pressure. Little respiratory depression. Often hallucinations. Contraindicated in hypertension, psychiatric, cerebrovascular or ocular disorders. Rarely used in dentistry
Propofol	Diprivan	2 mg/kg	May cause pain on injection. Occasional fits or anaphylaxis. Contraindicated in children under 18
Thiopental	Intraval	2.5 mg/kg (2.5% solution)	Ultra-short-acting barbiturate. No analgesia. Danger of laryngospasm. Rapid injection may cause apnoea. Irritant if injected into artery or extravascularly

Ketamine

Ketamine anaesthesia is dissociative, separating the electrical activity of the thalamocortical system from that of the limbic system. There is a delay preceding the onset of anaesthesia. Unlike other induction agents, ketamine stimulates the sympathetic nervous system, increasing heart rate and BP (but also cerebral blood flow, intracranial pressure, and both myocardial and cerebral oxygen demand). Ketamine should be avoided in patients with raised intracranial pressure and open eye injuries, and used with caution in hypertension. It is a bronchodilator and useful in patients with severe bronchospasm refractory to other bronchodilators. Vivid and unpleasant dreams may follow its use.

Propofol

Propofol is the most commonly used intravenous induction agent (see above). It is a highly lipid-soluble, weak organic acid, formulated as a 1% or 2% lipid emulsion with soya bean oil and egg phosphatide. Patients with egg allergy are usually sensitive to egg *albumin* and therefore may still be given propofol.

Propofol suppresses upper airway reflexes, making coughing and laryngospasm rare, and it is therefore particularly suited to the use of the laryngeal mask airway (LMA). Propofol causes systemic vascular resistance to fall and is associated with less reflex tachycardia than other induction agents. BP invariably falls and propofol should be administered slowly and cautiously to older or haemodynamically compromised patients. Awakening is due largely to redistribution rather than metabolism. Pain on injection may be decreased by the addition of lidocaine or formulation in an alternative base.

Thiopental

Thiopental is a barbiturate that leaves airway reflexes relatively preserved, but airway manipulation without a muscle relaxant (i.e. the LMA) can cause laryngospasm. Thiopental was the agent originally described for rapid sequence induction and is often (by convention only) the agent of choice in these circumstances. Thiopental is contraindicated in patients with porphyria. Accidental extravascular injection causes pain and necrosis, and intra-arterial injection may result in gangrene.

Total intravenous anaesthesia

Anaesthesia may be maintained by repeated boluses or an infusion of intravenous agents – total intravenous anaesthesia (TIVA). Infusion pumps can deliver propofol by a continuous infusion that maintains a constant level in the plasma – target-controlled infusion (TCI).

AIRWAY MANAGEMENT

Effective GA abolishes pain and awareness during surgery, and also the tone of head and neck muscles that normally maintain the airway patency and the cough and gag reflexes crucial to protecting the airway from aspiratable material. Some form of airway-opening technique is thus always required, with an additional need to protect the patient's respiratory tract from aspiratable material.

Airway manœuvres with or without a face mask

The patency of the airway of an unconscious patient may be maintained using a head-tilt and chin-lift or jaw-thrust technique. Where GA is being administered, a face mask is usually necessary to deliver both oxygen and GA to keep the patient alive and asleep, respectively. An oropharyngeal and/or nasopharyngeal airway may be used to aid manual airway maintenance. Although a head-down lateral position with vigilant observation and suction may help minimize the risk of airway soiling from aspiratable material, more reliable means of airway protection are generally needed. Furthermore, the insertion of a more substantial airway-opening device means the anaesthetist is free to deliver an appropriate GA at the same time.

Laryngeal mask

The laryngeal mask airway is an inflatable 'mask' that acts as a face mask but is connected to a tube or stem so that it may be inserted into the oropharynx just at the laryngeal entrance. An airway seal is achieved by inflation of the 'mask' cuff, which also provides some degree of isolation from the oesophagus. The LMA requires less skill to insert than an endotracheal tube and usually presents a smaller risk of trauma to tissues and teeth. Once inserted, it does not need to be held in place and it is possible to maintain an airway probably for as long as necessary. Although the classic LMA (cLMA) offers

---

Box 3.8 *Indications for intubation*

- Restricted access to airway or whole patient (ear, nose and throat; neurosurgery; prone patient)
- Protection against contamination of airway from above
- Protection against contamination of airway from below
- Requirement for muscle relaxation where resulting airway pressure may exceed that suitable for a laryngeal mask airway

---

Box 3.9 *Intubation technique*

1. Check equipment and monitoring
2. Induce anaesthesia and manually ventilate the patient before a muscle relaxant is administered
3. Flex the patient's neck with the atlanto-occipital joint extended ('sniffing the morning air'), allowing direct visual alignment of the larynx with the open mouth at laryngoscopy
4. Hold the laryngoscope blade (in the left hand) and pass along the right side of the floor of the mouth, displacing the tongue to the right
5. When the epiglottis is seen, advance the tip of the blade into the space between it and the base of tongue
6. Lift the laryngoscope up and away, bringing the vocal cords into view and allowing the introduction of the endotracheal tube, either directly or after first inserting a bougie and 'rail-roading' the endotracheal tube over it
7. Commence ventilation and inflate the tube cuff until the leak disappears. Confirm the tube position by auscultating both lung bases and apices, looking for chest movement and preferably demonstration of carbon dioxide in the exhaled gases with a capnograph. An endotracheal tube inserted too far will tend to go down the right bronchus, in which case partially deflate the cuff and withdraw the tube slightly. If in doubt, remove the tube, ensure the patient is well oxygenated and anaesthetized, and start again

---

reasonable protection from material coming from the airway above, it does not guarantee airway protection from gastric material; therefore, where there is a risk of regurgitation, endotracheal intubation is usually required. The ProSeal LMA™ has a second lumen that 'sits' at the opening of the oesophagus, creating a channel through which gastric contents may be vented away from the trachea or through which a nasogastric tube may be inserted; it may thus reduce the risk of inadvertent aspiration. The intubating LMA (ILMA) is another variation of the cLMA that may be used to aid the intubation of the trachea, either when this has proved difficult or where there is a need to avoid positioning the head and neck for intubation in the usual manner (e.g. cervical spine injury or rheumatoid arthritis). The cLMA, though a bulky device that limits surgical access to the mouth, has become an acceptable alternative to intubation for many dental, oral, maxillofacial and ear, nose and throat procedures.

Intubation

Use of a tracheal tube with an inflated cuff is the only way to *guarantee* protection of the respiratory tract from soiling. Indications for intubation are shown in Box 3.8.

A cuffed tracheal tube may be inserted orally, nasally or as a surgical airway (trachcostomy or cricothyroidotomy). A muscle relaxant is usually used for intubation (see Box 3.9 for intubation technique).

Endotracheal intubation may be difficult in some instances; this difficulty may be suggested by a high Mallampati score (Table 3.26) and a number of other factors (Box 3.10).

Table 3.26 *Mallampati scoring*

Class	Definition
1	Full visibility of tonsils, uvula and soft palate
2	Visibility of hard and soft palate, upper portion of tonsils and uvula
3	Visibility of soft and hard palate and base of the uvula
4	Visibility of hard palate only

Box 3.10 *Observations that suggest difficulty in intubation*

- Neck – reduced distance from thyroid cartilage to mandibular symphysis, short and/or fat, thyroid goitre, neck masses
- Mandible – retrognathic with class II malocclusion, particularly class II division 1
- Ankylosing spondylitis
- Rheumatoid arthritis
- Trismus

Fibreoptic intubation

For patients at known or high risk of difficult intubation, an awake fibreoptic procedure allows intubation without loss of the protective airway reflexes and ability to breathe. Anaesthesia of the entire upper airway from nasopharynx to glottis is established using topical LA in a variety of concentrations with or without some carefully titrated sedation. A short narrow endoscope with endotracheal tube mounted is introduced via the nose or mouth into the trachea by direct visualization and the tube is rail-roaded over it. GA is subsequently induced in the normal way and the cuff inflated. Fibreoptic intubation is often performed in patients who are asleep (not at risk of aspiration and unlikely to be difficult to ventilate), for the purpose of avoiding a traumatic direct laryngoscopy where a nasal tube is required, to avoid neck manipulation in those with cervical spine pathology, and to teach and develop the skill of fibreoptic intubation.

MUSCLE RELAXANTS

With the exception of the rapid sequence induction situation, an ability to ventilate the patient manually with a bag and face mask should always be verified prior to the administration of a muscle relaxant. These are neuromuscular-blocking drugs. There are two main categories – non-depolarizing and depolarizing. Non-depolarizing agents (mivacurium, rocuronium, vecuronium and atracurium) act by blocking acetylcholine (ACh) receptors at the motor endplate. Depolarizing agents (suxamethonium) are ACh agonists that, after an initial stimulation, desensitize muscle fibres to further ACh stimulation, preventing nearby Na^+ channels from repolarizing and producing a neuromuscular block.

Suxamethonium

Suxamethonium is the only depolarizing muscle relaxant in use. Its usefulness lies in its rapid action and very brief effects. The rapid onset and short duration of action make it useful for induction of GA. Suxamethonium may stimulate muscarinic receptors in the sinoatrial node, causing bradycardia (atropine should be given before a repeat dose and considered in all infants). Because of the initial muscle spasm, this can result in hyperkalaemia postoperatively. The small rise in K^+ is usually of little significance but may be dangerous in patients with pre-existing electrolyte abnormalities, renal failure, burns, spinal injuries and progressive neuromuscular disorders. Muscle pains also occur postoperatively and intraocular pressure rises. Prolonged neuromuscular block (suxamethonium apnoea) occurs in 4% of patients owing to inherited deficiency in the enzyme plasma cholinesterase, apnoea ranging from 10 minutes to several hours. Suxamethonium may also precipitate malignant hyperpyrexia.

Atracurium

Atracurium is an antagonist at the nicotinic ACh receptor of the neuromuscular junction. Histamine release can occasionally cause hypotension or bronchospasm. Atracurium is eliminated completely, independently of hepatic and renal metabolism, by ester hydrolysis and spontaneous breakdown. *Cis*-atracurium causes less histamine release but has a slower onset time.

Vecuronium

Vecuronium is an aminosteroidal muscle relaxant, which does not affect the cardiovascular system or release histamine. It is metabolized by hepatic de-acetylation and renal excretion.

Rocuronium

Rocuronium is an aminosteroidal muscle relaxant used as an alternative to suxamethonium for rapid sequence intubation.

Mivacurium

Mivacurium is a benzylisoquinolinium muscle relaxant, which has a shorter duration of action than the other non-depolarizing relaxants. It is metabolized by plasma cholinesterase and therefore patients prone to suxamethonium apnoea should also not receive mivacurium.

Reversal of neuromuscular blockade

Neostigmine is an anticholinesterase that reverses the competitive effects of non-depolarizing muscle relaxants. It also acts at autonomic ganglia and is therefore given with either atropine or glycopyrrolate to prevent bradycardia.

Sugammadex is used for the reversal of rocuronium and vecuronium neuromuscular blockade.

ANAESTHETIC GASES

General anaesthesia acts via effects on proteins in cell membranes, probably ion channels. Several inhalational and intravenous anaesthetic agents appear to facilitate the function of inhibitory ion channels similarly while attenuating the function of excitatory ion channels, to produce a state of anaesthesia. Nitrous oxide has been used for many years for GA. Halothane was the main drug used for inhalational anaesthesia until the 1980s but the rare severe liver injury following repeated exposures to halothane in some patients (Ch. 9) led to the development of other volatile agents such as enflurane, isoflurane, desflurane and sevoflurane. Arrhythmias may accompany halothane use, especially if adrenaline (epinephrine) is given. Cardiac rhythm is also more stable with the other agents, though they cause greater respiratory depression than halothane and induction is less pleasant. Enflurane causes cardiorespiratory depression and can be

Table 3.27 *Inhalational agents*

Drug	Proprietary names (UK)	Comments
Desflurane	Suprane	Less potent than isoflurane. May cause apnoea or coughing and is contraindicated in children
Enflurane	Ethrane/ Alyrane	Less potent anaesthetic than halothane. Non-explosive. Less likely to induce arrhythmias or affect liver than halothane. Induction and recovery are slower than with halothane
Halothane	Fluothane	Non-explosive. Anaesthetic but weak analgesic. Causes fall in blood pressure, cardiac arrhythmias and bradycardia. Hepatotoxic on repeated administration. Post-anaesthetic shivering is common, vomiting rare. Contraindicated for dental procedures in patients younger than 18 years unless treated in hospital
Isoflurane	Forane/ Aerrane	Isomer of enflurane. Causes less cardiac but more respiratory depression than halothane. Induction and recovery are slower than with halothane
Nitrous oxide	–	Analgesic but weak anaesthetic. Non-explosive. No cardiorespiratory effects. May cause eye damage from expansion of intravitreal gases
Sevoflurane	Sevoflurane	Rapid action and recovery. May cause agitation in children

epileptogenic. Immediate recovery is slower after isoflurane than after halothane and there may be some coughing. Recovery after sevoflurane is rapid but it may agitate children. Desflurane may cause apnoea or breath-holding, and increased secretions, and is not for use in children (Table 3.27).

Following induction of GA and the establishment of airway control, anaesthesia is maintained by the continuous administration of either a volatile anaesthetic or intravenous agent, with or without nitrous oxide or another means of analgesia.

The potency of an inhalational agent is determined by its lipid solubility or oil:gas partition coefficient, whereas its speed of action is determined by its blood:gas partition coefficient. Historically, some volatile anaesthetic agents were inflammable or even explosive, but modern agents are not inflammable. The commonly used volatile agents are all bronchodilators but depress ventilation.

Nitrous oxide

Nitrous oxide has a very low blood:gas partition coefficient and thus a very rapid onset and offset, but it approaches anaesthetic potency only in a grossly hypoxic mixture. It has good analgesic properties (useful for inhalational pain relief with oxygen as Entonox). Nitrous oxide with its analgesic properties may also be used as a 'carrier' gas to complement the sleep-inducing properties of a volatile agent. In addition, nitrous oxide, which moves into blood faster than nitrogen moves out, has the ability to increase the alveolar concentration of a volatile agent and speed up its effects. Conversely, at the end of GA, nitrous oxide rapidly leaves the blood, reducing the concentration of available oxygen in the alveoli (diffusion hypoxia). Additional oxygen is thus usually administered to a patient recovering from nitrous oxide anaesthesia to counteract this. Nitrous oxide has additional undesirable properties in some circumstances. It contributes to postoperative nausea and vomiting, and expands enclosed gas spaces and may thus be detrimental to certain bowel, ocular and middle ear procedures.

Prolonged exposure to nitrous oxide affects vitamin B_{12} metabolism and can result in megaloblastic and neurological syndromes.

Isoflurane

Isoflurane is the longest established and cheapest of the three commonly used volatile anaesthetics (isoflurane, sevoflurane, desflurane). It is irritant and unpleasant to inhale, and is therefore rarely used for induction of anaesthesia, but otherwise has properties that make it a good maintenance agent. It may reduce systemic vascular resistance and cause a reflex tachycardia.

Sevoflurane

Sevoflurane has a faster onset than isoflurane and is more pleasant to inhale. Like halothane, it also causes a fall in systemic vascular resistance but, because it attenuates reflex changes in heart rate, the BP tends to fall further. Compared to isoflurane, a greater proportion of sevoflurane is metabolized to potentially toxic by-products and there are theoretical if controversial concerns regarding its suitability in renal failure. It is considerably more expensive than isoflurane.

Desflurane

Desflurane has a blood:gas partition coefficient lower than that of nitrous oxide, and thus the onset and offset of its effects are rapid. Like isoflurane, it is unsuitable for inhalation induction but its effects wear off rapidly, even after prolonged anaesthesia, and this can be an advantage for long surgical cases where prolonged administration of other agents may be associated with prolonged recovery. Desflurane's unusual physical properties necessitate an electrically heated vaporizer.

Halothane

The risk of cardiac arrhythmias and hepatotoxicity means halothane has been superseded by other volatile agents in most situations. Because of a relatively high blood:gas coefficient, halothane does not wear off as quickly as sevoflurane. Thus induction is slower but also anaesthesia will be deeper for longer when the mask is removed; this may be an advantage where airway manipulation with minimal risk of laryngospasm is necessary.

Enflurane

Enflurane is an isomer of isoflurane. Its cardiovascular side-effects fall between those of halothane and isoflurane, and it has been associated with epileptiform electroencephalogram (EEG) changes. Its use has therefore declined.

ANALGESIA

Opioids are commonly used at induction and act rapidly so that effective analgesia is established before surgery. Alfentanil, fentanyl, morphine and remifentanil are opioids that are frequently used.

COMPLICATIONS OF GENERAL ANAESTHESIA

Many patients have a relatively smooth postoperative recovery, especially after short procedures. Superficial vein thrombosis may follow intravenous injections that are irritant or entry of cannulae into the tissues. Analgesics usually suffice, though antibiotics are occasionally indicated.

Medical emergencies, such as anaphylaxis, Addisonian crisis and acute severe asthma, among others, may occur perioperatively, as they may at any time.

Local complications after GA

Operative care carried out expeditiously, with careful handling of tissues, asepsis, wound toilet and careful wound closure, will minimize local complications, as will the appropriate use of analgesics and antimicrobials. Nevertheless, some pain is to be expected after surgical procedures, and bleeding or wound infection is not always totally avoidable.

Pain

Pain after surgery usually starts after anaesthetic drugs have worn off and may result from unavoidable operative trauma. Alternatively, it may stem from a complication such as infection. Postoperatively, analgesics should be given as necessary, but if a GA has been given, the anaesthetist should be consulted first. Immediately after oral surgery, it may be necessary to use a long-acting local analgesic or a strong analgesic such as morphine. In some cases, this is best controlled by the patient (PCA). However, after most dental procedures, a combination of ibuprofen and paracetamol (acetaminophen; see Tables 3.3 and 3.4) should be effective.

Wound infection

Wound infection is uncommon after oral and maxillofacial procedures unless there has been significant contamination, such as in a road traffic accident, or if foreign bodies are present, local vascularity is poor or the patient is immunocompromised. Infection may cause pain, discharge or sepsis and is best managed by drainage, wound toilet, antimicrobials and analgesics as indicated. The diagnosis must first be made, and treatment guided by the likely pathogen (Ch. 21). If streptococci are implicated, the first-choice therapy in the absence of allergy is amoxicillin ± clavulanic acid. If staphylococci are involved, flucloxacillin is appropriate. For anaerobic infections, metronidazole is the first choice. For Gram-negative infections (e.g. contamination of wound with bowel organisms, urinary tract infection (UTI), hospital-acquired and aspiration pneumonia), it is best to take advice from the microbiologist; useful antibiotics include amoxicillin, piperacillin plus tazobactam, and gentamicin.

Bleeding

Postoperative haemorrhage usually has a local cause (i.e. damaged soft tissues; Ch. 8). It responds to local pressure, insertion of haemostatic agents or suturing of the soft tissues. Patients should be given written as well as verbal guidance on how to care for their wounds (Appendix 3.6). If there is a contributing systemic cause (e.g. anticoagulated patients), appropriate pre- and postoperative measures must be taken.

Systemic complications after GA

Drowsiness, headache, sore throat, muscle pains and vomiting are seen in over 60% of patients after outpatient GA. Headache seems more common in women, especially if halothane has been used. Sore throat is common if the patient was intubated, as are muscle pains if suxamethonium has been given. More important complications are shown in Box 3.11 and discussed below.

> **Box 3.11** *Postoperative complications*
> * Collapse
> * Nausea and vomiting
> * Fever
> * Jaundice
> * Behavioural problems
> * Low urine output
> * Thrombosis
> * Awareness
> * Delayed recovery of consciousness
> * Cardiac complications
> * Laryngospasm
> * Respiratory complications
> * Malignant hyperpyrexia
> * Death

Collapse

There may be signs of weakness, sweating, rapid pulse, pallor, hypotension, shock or loss of consciousness. The causes can be difficult to find but may include haemorrhage, pulmonary embolism, cardiac arrest (usually myocardial infarction), sepsis, anaphylaxis, adrenal insufficiency and adverse reactions to GA agents. These are outlined in Chapters 1 and 5.

Postoperative nausea and vomiting (PONV)

Postoperative vomiting is both unpleasant for the patient and dangerous if protective laryngeal reflexes have not returned after GA or sedation; it may have serious sequelae (risk of aspiration with intermaxillary fixation, wound dehiscence, etc.). Risk factors include female sex, being a non-smoker, a previous history of PONV or travel sickness, and use of postoperative morphine. Volatile agents are thought to be responsible for most vomiting immediately after waking from GA. One possible explanation is that these agents potentiate the function of $5HT_3$ receptors in addition to their effect on the $GABA_A$ receptor. Optimum prevention or treatment is by combining drugs with different modes of action. In many cases, the cause of postoperative nausea is unclear, but some patients seem to be particularly susceptible. An antiemetic is usually effective (Tables 3.19 and 3.28). Metoclopramide and domperidone, however, are best avoided in the young and in older people, as they can induce dystonic reactions. Parenteral administration may be needed if vomiting is severe.

Fever

A transient rise in temperature postoperatively is common within a few hours of GA and major operations, and is regarded as 'physiological'. Persistent fever shortly after an operation may indicate malignant hyperthermia (Ch. 23). Persistent fever for several days postoperatively, especially if spiking, may indicate haematoma, wound infection, deep vein thrombosis (DVT), UTI, infection of an intravenous line or more serious pulmonary infection. Persistent mild fever continuing or appearing several weeks postoperatively may indicate infective endocarditis (Ch. 5).

Jaundice

Postoperative jaundice after GA can result from many causes, including viral and drug-induced hepatitis. Halothane should be avoided if the

Table 3.28 *Antiemetics*

Class	Used mainly for nausea and vomiting related to	Main possible adverse effects
Antihistamines (e.g. cyclizine)	Many causes, including postoperative	May cause sedation
Dexamethasone	Postoperative nausea and vomiting or that associated with cancer chemotherapy	
Domperidone	Cancer chemotherapy	Few problems with sedation or dystonic reactions
Metoclopramide	Gastrointestinal disorders, including postoperative	May cause dystonic reactions
Nabilone	Cancer chemotherapy	A cannabinoid that may cause drowsiness
Phenothiazines	Neoplastic disease, radiation, general anaesthesia or drug use, including postoperative	May cause dystonic reactions
5HT₃ antagonists (granisetron, ondansetron, tropisetron)	Postoperative nausea and vomiting or that associated with cancer chemotherapy	May cause headaches or hypersensitivity reactions

Box 3.12 *Causes of delayed recovery from GA*

- Residual intravenous or gaseous agents, sedatives, opioids
- Residual muscle relaxation (use a nerve stimulator)
- Anticholinergic drugs
- Hypoxia, hypercapnia
- Hypothermia
- Hypothyroidism
- Electrolytes (Na⁺, Ca²⁺ particularly)
- Cerebrovascular accident or other pathology

patient has been exposed to it within the previous 6 months or has had a previous episode of halothane hepatitis. In a series of 300 patients who had been given halothane on more than one occasion within a month and who subsequently developed hepatitis, no fewer than 46% died.

Alcoholic hepatitis can be a problem. GA for high-risk patients cannot be avoided for emergencies, such as maxillofacial injuries, and this group of patients includes an unduly high proportion of alcoholics.

Aggravation of pre-existing liver disease (including gallstones), hepatic necrosis secondary to circulatory failure, transfusion reactions and Gilbert syndrome are other causes.

Behavioural complications

Causes of confusion after GA or sedation may include: drugs (anaesthetic, analgesic, others), hypoglycaemia, alcohol or other drug withdrawal, pre-existing psychiatric states, hypoxia, infection (wound, lungs, urinary tract, abscess, septicaemia), urine retention or disturbed urea and electrolytes. Amnesia that persists for at least 5 hours is common after sedation with diazepam or midazolam. As a result, patients are likely to forget post-sedation instructions, or worse, have an accident as a result of forgetting to take normal precautions when using power tools or other dangerous equipment. Bizarre behaviour has also been described even 24 hours after sedation. It is also important to make sure that the patient is not anticipating going abroad immediately after the GA or sedation. Airports are difficult to navigate even by the fully alert, and complications might develop on board an aircraft or at a destination where medical care is limited.

Low urine output

Absolute anuria is usually caused by urine retention – a common postoperative complication, especially in the older male. The patient should be catheterized unless urine can be passed after a warm bath. If the patient is already catheterized, make sure the catheter is not blocked. Low urine output is a cardinal sign of dehydration, hypovolaemia and shock. The patient should be given fluids orally or intravenously. Start with a fluid challenge and continue according to the response. Care must be taken with patients in heart failure.

Deep vein thrombosis

DVT is mainly seen after prolonged major operations under GA and affects the leg veins. It may lead to pulmonary embolism (Ch. 5). Always suspect this in a patient whose haemoglobin saturation falls several days after major surgery or who develops hypotension, tachycardia, chest pain, etc. (Ch. 5). Factor V Leiden deficiency and other causes of thrombophilia should be considered (Ch. 8).

Awareness

For patients, the possibility of being awake during GA is a cause of worry. Unfortunately, it is not unheard of; it is an established cause of complaints against anaesthetists and is a precipitant of post-traumatic stress disorder. Awareness most often manifests as recollection of an auditory perception; sensations of pain are less likely. These experiences are more likely to occur when GA may become light, such as during airway manipulation and transfer of the patient into the operating room. Significant awareness is generally felt to be unlikely during surgery where a muscle relaxant has not been used, because movement in response to a noxious stimulus precedes awareness – and depth of anaesthesia may be adjusted accordingly. There is currently much interest in depth of anaesthesia monitoring, which utilizes various calculations from a simplified EEG recording (e.g. bispectral index [BIS]), but whether or not these technologies are likely to reduce the incidence of awareness is unknown.

Delayed recovery of consciousness after GA

Important causes are overdose of GA agents or the use of long-acting opioids for pre-medication, suxamethonium sensitivity, diabetic coma or hypoglycaemia, cardiac complications as mentioned earlier, or cerebrovascular accidents. The latter may occur either in susceptible patients (elderly hypertensives) or as a result of emboli. Occasionally, neurotic patients may feign persistent unconsciousness.

Patients should not be discharged from recovery if they are at risk of laryngospasm or not fully conscious. Certain conditions resulting in an abnormally prolonged time to recovery of either consciousness or ventilation may, however, cause more subtle respiratory problems or postoperative confusion, as shown in Box 3.12.

Cardiac complications

Myocardial infarction, cardiac failure or severe arrhythmias can follow GA and are the main risks in those with pre-existing cardiac disease (Ch. 5). Pre-existing cardiac disease may be aggravated or myocardial infarction can follow at an unpredictable interval after the anaesthetic, especially in those with ischaemic heart disease (Ch. 5). Myocardial infarction is one of the chief causes of deaths associated with anaesthesia. There is no logical reason why GA *per se* should be expected to cause myocardial infarction or arrhythmias, and evidence is emerging that certain GA agents may have myocardial *protective* properties. Nevertheless, perioperative cardiac complications account for many of the deaths 'under GA', although these can probably be explained by gross haemodynamic abnormalities (blood loss, hypotension, hypertension, bradycardia, tachycardia) and/or metabolic abnormalities (hypoxia, hypercapnia, electrolyte problems) in patients who cannot compensate for them. Cardiac risk factors are notoriously difficult to apply generally, though there have been many scoring systems over the years. Shock (circulatory failure leading to tissue and organ hypoperfusion) is more likely to be a complication of major surgery; contributory factors include pre-existing heart disease, dehydration, haemorrhage, sepsis or anaphylactic reactions.

Laryngospasm

Upper airway stimulation causes coughing in a fully awake patient and no reaction in one who is deeply anaesthetized. Instead of a coordinated cough, the patient in between these states is at risk of their vocal cords closing and failing to open again (laryngospasm). This results in stridor when mild to moderate, but complete airway obstruction when severe. The cords often relax with positive airway pressure (and increasing the inspired volatile concentration when inducing anaesthesia) but occasionally it is necessary to re-administer a muscle relaxant.

Other respiratory complications

Airway obstruction is particularly important in dental surgery because of operating around the airway and the risk of foreign material being inhaled. Facilities such as suction must always be immediately available for locating and clearing any blockage. *The recovery period is the most dangerous time and great care must be taken to keep the airway clear.*

Lung alveoli begin to collapse within minutes of GA, as respiratory muscle tone is lost (atelectasis). This occurs particularly in lower zones and with higher inspired oxygen concentrations when there is less nitrogen to 'splint' open the alveoli. If excessive, it may cause shunting to occur with a tendency to impaired postoperative gas exchange. This is extremely common but quickly compensated for in the healthy patient. At the other end of the spectrum, patients with poor preoperative respiratory function or inadequate pain relief preventing coughing and clearance of secretions may develop pneumonia and respiratory failure. Immobility for any reason leaves patients at risk of thromboembolism and thus GA is a contributory factor. This is reflected in the markedly different risks associated with different types of surgery. After prolonged GA, especially in older people, there is high risk of atelectasis (Ch. 15); therefore, the patient should be strongly encouraged to undertake breathing exercises and to cough up any sputum. Accumulation of secretions is a frequent cause of lower airway obstruction and subsequent chest infection. This can be particularly severe in patients with chronic bronchitis (Ch. 15). A transient rise in temperature is common and is usually caused by atelectasis or localized pulmonary infection that may not be clinically detectable. Physiotherapy may be helpful. In dentistry, inhalation of a tooth or fragments of materials is another possible cause of atelectasis and subsequent lung abscess. Also, if an emergency operation has had to be carried out despite an acute upper respiratory tract infection, lower respiratory tract infection is more likely. Occasionally, bronchospasm can result from a hypersensitivity reaction to an intravenous anaesthetic or other drug used during the operation.

Respiratory weakness may be due to the action of muscle relaxants. Reversal of the action of neuromuscular blocking drugs depends on many factors but, if delayed, results in weak respiratory movements that cannot be made stronger by the patient's conscious efforts. Suxamethonium apnoea is discussed in Chapter 23. Impaired chest movements may be caused by damage to the chest, a common accompaniment of maxillofacial injuries, particularly when they result from road traffic accidents (Ch. 24). This may inhibit respiration and coughing.

Respiratory depression can result from the effects of the anaesthetic and ancillary drugs. Midazolam and pentazocine, for example, form a potent combination of respiratory depressants, which can be aggravated by hypoxia, often from a similar cause, and have caused occasional deaths.

Malignant hyperpyrexia

See Chapter 23.

PARTICULAR CONSIDERATIONS IN OUTPATIENT SEDATION OR GA IN DENTISTRY

Since the operation site is close to the airway, any inflammatory oedema, haemorrhage or foreign bodies can endanger respiration. Appropriate instruction must be given preoperatively, recorded in the case notes and re-emphasized before discharge. Patients must be made aware that, after a GA, it is dangerous to drive a vehicle, ride a bicycle, ride pillion on a motorcycle, work with unguarded machinery or make important decisions. They should also be warned not to drink alcohol or take certain drugs, particularly sleeping tablets. Obviously, it is impossible to control the behaviour of irresponsible patients, but it is essential to point out the dangers in the clearest possible terms. Patients may also fail to take in or forget verbal instructions, particularly after benzodiazepine use. To protect both patient and operator, the patient and escort should be given written instructions (Fig. 3.7). In the case of sedation given in the dental surgery, it is important to use a questionnaire to make sure that nothing has been forgotten and, in the event of any mishap, to provide documentary evidence that this assessment has been carried out.

DEATHS IN PATIENTS RECEIVING GA FOR DENTAL TREATMENT

Although deaths are now uncommon during or immediately after GA for dental treatment, they are more frequent than with other pain and anxiety control methods. Every death is a tragedy for the individual and family. Investigation of deaths has too often highlighted factors that seemed potentially avoidable. In the UK, there has been a fall in the number of deaths associated with GA for dental treatment outside hospital since the 1960s, in line with the decline in the use of GA in dental practice. Tragically, though, there were a number of deaths in children associated with GA for dental treatment outside hospital in the late 1990s. Investigations and inquiries into these deaths have been critical of the standard of care provided in fundamental areas such as preoperative assessment, monitoring of electrical heart activity, BP, oxygen and carbon dioxide levels, start of resuscitation and transfer to specialist critical care. GA for dental treatment is not permitted in the UK outside a hospital with critical care facilities (amendment in 'Maintaining standards' published by the British General Dental Council, 2001). Dentists arranging or providing dental treatment under GA should also make sure they have explored and discussed with the patient all possible alternatives and enquired about possible contraindications. They must also take measures to avoid the need for GA in the future.

Mark each item with a tick or N/A for *every* sedation given   Patient label

STAFF CHECK DATE:						
Experienced qualified DN present ?						
Another dentist/doctor/nurse/DN is within easy call?						
Operator and assistants know emergency procedures?						
EQUIPMENT CHECK Site of emergency equipment known?						
Have the following been checked by the operator? Oxygen						
Suction — dental unit						
Suction — mobile/back-up						
Positive pressure ventilating bag						
Sphygmomanometer						
Pulse oximeter						
Other automatic monitor (BP/ECG)						
Emergency drugs (Flumazenil)						
Sedation equipment						
Have the following been checked? Dental equipment						
Dental unit						
PATIENT CHECK Patient, parent or guardian know what is planned?						
Written consent has been obtained?						
Written pre- + post-operative instruction issued?						
Medical and dental history checked?						
Routine medication taken?						
Last meal or drink checked?						
Fasting patient?						
If Yes — has glucose been given?						
Patient has consumed alcohol today?						
If Yes — advise to postpone session?						
Responsible escort present?						
Weight recorded?						
BP recorded?						
OPERATOR'S NAME IN CAPITALS:						

Fig. 3.7 Checklist for operators before giving sedation. DN = dental nurse. (Courtesy of Miss AM Skelly)

CENTRAL LINES (CATHETERS)

Attempting to give infusions of antimicrobials, antiemetics, blood and blood products, chemotherapeutic drugs, nutrients and other fluids into a small vein may cause pain. Most such infusions should therefore be delivered into a larger vein (Fig. 3.8). This is achieved with a central line – a central venous catheter (e.g. Hickman® or Groshong® line) – which can also be used to take blood samples (Table 3.29). A central line is a long, hollow, silicone rubber tube inserted into a large vein, leaving the limb free to move. The catheter tube tip is positioned in the vein just above the heart; the other end of the line is usually sealed with a cap or bung that can be attached to an intravenous drip (Fig. 3.9) or syringe. Sometimes the tube has more than a solitary lumen, to permit different infusions or

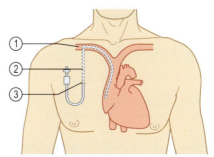

1 Central line is inserted into chest
2 Line is tunnelled under skin
3 Line emerges here

Fig. 3.8 Central catheter.

Table 3.29 *Catheters for venous and arterial access*

Catheter type	Entry site	Length	Comments
Peripheral venous catheters	Veins of forearm or hand	<7 cm	Phlebitis with prolonged use; rarely associated with bloodstream infection
Peripheral arterial catheters	Usually radial artery; sometimes femoral, axillary, brachial, posterior tibial arteries	<7 cm	Low infection risk; rarely associated with bloodstream infection
Midline catheters	Via antecubital fossa into proximal basilic or cephalic veins; do not enter central veins	7–230 cm	Anaphylactoid reactions reported with catheters made of elastomeric hydrogel; lower rates of phlebitis than short peripheral catheters
Non-tunnelled central venous catheters	Percutaneously into central (subclavian, internal jugular or femoral) veins	≥8 cm	Account for majority of catheter-related bloodstream infections
Pulmonary artery catheters	Inserted through a Teflon® introducer in a central (subclavian, internal jugular or femoral) vein	≥30 cm	Usually heparin-bonded; similar rates of bloodstream infection as central catheters; subclavian site preferred to reduce infection risk
Peripherally inserted central venous catheters (PICC)	Inserted into basilic, cephalic or brachial veins and enter superior vena cava	≥20 cm	Lower rate of infection than non-tunnelled central catheters
Tunnelled central venous catheters	Implanted into subclavian, internal jugular or femoral veins	≥8 cm	Lower rate of infection than non-tunnelled central catheters
Totally implantable	Tunnelled beneath skin; implanted in subclavian or internal jugular vein; have subcutaneous port accessed with needle	≥8 cm	Lowest risk for infection; improved patient self-image; no local catheter-site care required; surgery required for removal
Umbilical catheters	Inserted into either umbilical vein or artery	≤6 cm	Risk of infection similar with catheters placed in umbilical vein or artery

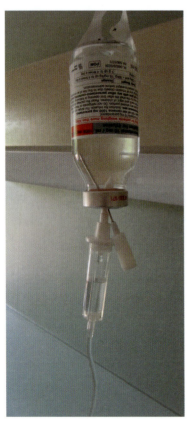

Fig. 3.9 Intravenous fluid delivery ('drip').

injections to be given simultaneously. Such a vascular catheter can be designated by:

- the type of vessel it occupies (e.g. peripheral venous, central venous, or arterial)
- the intended life span (e.g. temporary or short-term versus permanent or long term)
- the site of insertion (e.g. subclavian, axillary, innominate, femoral, internal jugular veins, or peripherally inserted central catheter [PICC])
- the pathway from skin to blood vessel (e.g. tunnelled versus non-tunnelled)

- the physical length (e.g. long versus short)
- some special characteristic (e.g. presence or absence of a cuff, impregnation with heparin, antibiotics or antiseptics, and the number of lumens).

The more common central lines are:

- *subclavian line* – the simplest central line and a *triple-lumen catheter*. It is easy to place, but is not well protected from infection and therefore should typically be replaced every 5–7 days. Attempts have been made to prolong catheter longevity by coating subclavian lines with chlorhexidine or antibiotics.
- *Hickman® catheter* – also placed in the subclavian vein. This type is softer and the distal end is tunnelled under the skin for 13–25 cm for protection against infection, to appear on the chest close to the nipple. These catheters can stay in place for weeks to months. *Groshong®* and *Broviac® catheters* are similar.
- *pheresis* catheters – larger and sturdier than Hickman® catheters. These are often called 'dialysis catheters', as they can be used for haemodialysis. They can be inserted either with (e.g. *PermCath®*) or without a tunnel (e.g. *Arrow Catheter®*).
- *implantable ports* –inserted in the subclavian vein but completely under the skin, with the distal end formed by a small metal 'drum' or reservoir, which has a membrane on one side for needle access. This drum is surgically placed under the skin, just below the clavicle, with the membrane immediately beneath the skin. Since the entire catheter is under the skin, there is minimal infection risk. Access is with a special needle that is pushed through the skin and the membrane into the reservoir.
- *peripherally inserted central catheter* (PICC line) – inserted into one of the antecubital fossa veins. PICCs can stay in place for several weeks, but typically need replacement earlier than a Hickman® or implantable port.

A central line is usually inserted under LA. A suitable vein is identified with ultrasound, a skin incision made near the clavicle and the tip of the line threaded into a large vein. A chest X-ray confirms that the line is correctly located. Once every week:

- heparin is 'flushed' into the line to prevent it clotting
- caps or bungs are changed

■ the exit site is cleaned to reduce the risk of infection and an antibiotic patch is placed around the exit site.

Complications related to central line insertion may include:

■ accidental arterial puncture
■ air in the line; clamps should always be closed when the line is not in use
■ dislodgement
■ infection – should be suspected if:
  ◆ the exit site becomes red, swollen or painful
  ◆ discoloured fluid discharges
  ◆ fever develops
■ pneumothorax
■ thrombosis – should be suspected if there is swelling, redness, tenderness in the ipsilateral arm, chest area or up into the neck, or if there is:
  ◆ shortness of breath
  ◆ chest tightness.

ANTIMICROBIAL PROPHYLAXIS

Antimicrobials are used in dentistry to treat an existing infection therapeutically or to prevent an infection prophylactically. To prevent a perioperative infection (primary prophylaxis), prophylactic antibiotics may be administered when a surgical device, such as a prosthetic cardiac valve, is placed. They also may be administered to patients who have an existing medical condition or have received a previously placed device to reduce the risk of infection from a bacteraemia (secondary prophylaxis). Although it is common to prescribe secondary prophylaxis for many dental conditions, there is a general lack of scientific evidence of its effectiveness and accumulating evidence suggests that such prescriptions may be unnecessary. In the past, antibiotic prophylaxis has been used for conditions with no proven benefit. Risks associated with antibiotics include allergic reactions (e.g. anaphylaxis), development of antibiotic-resistant bacteria, development of superinfections, pseudomembranous colitis, cross-reactions with other drugs, and death. The costs involved with the use of antibiotics can be significant as well. This is discussed above and in chapters covering the various organ systems, while Appendix 3.7 summarizes situations where antibiotic prophylaxis has been considered or used in some cases.

KEY WEBSITES

(Accessed 25 May 2013)
Dental Protection. Exercise in risk management: the medical history. <http://www.dentalprotection.org/uk/risk_management/>.
General Dental Council. Maintaining standards: guidance to dentists on professional and personal conduct. <http://www.gdc-uk.org/Newsandpublications/Publications/Publications/MaintainingStandards[1].pdf>.
National Institute for Health and Care Excellence. Evidence search. Perioperative care: guidance. <http://www.evidence.nhs.uk/topic/perioperative-care>.
National Institute for Health and Care Excellence. Preoperative tests: the use of routine preoperative tests for elective surgery. <http://www.nice.org.uk/nicemedia/pdf/Preop_Fullguideline.pdf>.
National Institute for Health and Care Excellence. Preoperative tests: the use of routine preoperative tests for elective surgery. Clinical guideline 3, June 2003. <http://www.nice.org.uk/nicemedia/pdf/CG3NICEguideline.pdf>.
NHS Choices. Blood tests – what they are used for. <http://www.nhs.uk/Conditions/Blood-tests/Pages/What-it-is-used-for.aspx>.
NHS National Patient Safety Agency. 'How to guide': five steps to safer surgery, December 2010. <http://www.patientsafetyfirst.nhs.uk/Content.aspx?path=/interventions/Perioperativecare/>.
NHS Patient Safety. Practical information, tools and support to improve patient safety in the NHS. <http://www.nrls.npsa.nhs.uk/>.
Patient Safety First! The 'how to' guide for reducing harm in perioperative care. <http://www.patientsafetyfirst.nhs.uk/Content.aspx?path=/interventions/Perioperativecare/>.

Scottish Dental Clinical Effectiveness Programme (SDCEP). <http://www.sdcep.org.uk/>.
Society for the Advancement of Anaesthesia in Dentistry (SAAD). <http://www.saad.org.uk/documents/conscious-sedation>.
World Health Organization. Patient safety. WHO surgical safety checklist and implementation manual. <http://www.who.int/patientsafety/safesurgery/ss_checklist/en/>.

USEFUL WEBSITES

(Accessed 25 May 2013)
Association of Anaesthetists of Great Britain and Ireland. <http://www.aagbi.org>.
British Medical Association. <http://www.bma.org.uk>.
European Society for Clinical Nutrition and Metabolism (ESPEN). <http://www.espen.org/>.
General Dental Council. Standards for the dental team. <http://www.gdc-uk.org/dentalprofessionals/standards/Pages/default.aspx>.
Medscape Reference. Drug interactions checker. <http://reference.medscape.com/>.
Medscape Reference. Perioperative care articles. <http://emedicine.medscape.com>.
Mental Capacity Act 2005. Guidance for health professionals 2007. <http://bma.org.uk/practical-support-at-work/ethics/mental-capacity>.
National Institute for Health and Care Excellence. Nutrition support in adults (CG32). February 2006. <http://www.nice.org.uk/CG032>.
Royal College of Nursing. Perioperative fasting. <http://www.rcn.org.uk/development/practice/perioperative_fasting>.
Royal College of Surgeons of England Faculty of Dental Surgery. <http://www.rcseng.ac.uk/fds>.
Scottish Intercollegiate Guidelines Network. Postoperative management in adults: a practical guide to postoperative care for clinical staff, August 2004. <http://www.sign.ac.uk/pdf/sign77.pdf>.
Surgical-tutor.org.uk. Perioperative care. <http://www.surgical-tutor.org.uk/default-home.htm?principles/perioperative.htm~right>.

Conscious sedation and general anaesthesia

The statement by the General Dental Council (GDC) on both conscious sedation and general anaesthesia is found in the GDC's *Standards for the dental team*. It supports the recommendations and guidance of the Department of Health. Full details are available at <http://www.gdc-uk.org/dentalprofessionals/standards/Pages/default.aspx>.
Department of Health. *A conscious decision: a review of the use of general anaesthesia and conscious sedation in primary dental care.* <http://www.dh.gov.uk/en/Publicationsandstatistics/Publications/PublicationsPolicyAndGuidance/DH_4074702>.
Department of Health, Standing Dental Advisory Committee. *Conscious sedation in the provision of dental care: report of an expert group on sedation for dentistry.* <http://www.dh.gov.uk/en/Publicationsandstatistics/Publications/PublicationsPolicyAndGuidance/DH_4069257>.

Consent

The GDC has produced supporting guidance to its standards specifically on consent – *Principles of patient consent*. <http://www.gdc-uk.org/Newsandpublications/Publications/Publications/PatientConsent[1].pdf>.

FURTHER READING

Arrow, P., 2012. A comparison of articaine 4% and lignocaine 2% in block and infiltration analgesia in children. Aust. Dent. J. 57 (3), 325.10.1111/j.1834-7819.2012.01699.x Epub. 2012 May 28. PubMed PMID: 22924356.
Ashford, R.U., et al. 2002. Obtaining informed consent. Hosp. Med. 62, 374.
Axelsson, S., Isacsson, G., 2004. The efficacy of ropivacaine as a dental local anaesthetic. Swed. Dent. J. 28 (2), 85. PubMed PMID: 15272513.
Becker, D.E., Reed, K.L., 2012. Local anesthetics: review of pharmacological considerations. Anesth. Prog. 59 (2), 90. quiz 102. doi: 10.2344/0003-3006-59.2.90. Review. PubMed PMID: 22822998. PubMed Central PMCID: PMC3403589.
Bishop, L., et al. 2007. Guidelines on the insertion and management of central venous access devices in adults. Int. J. Lab. Hematol. 29 (4), 261. Review. PubMed PMID: 17617077.
Boyle, C.A., 2012. Summary of: compliance with pre-operative instructions for procedures with conscious sedation: a complete audit cycle. Br. Dent. J. 212 (3), 132.10.1038/sj.bdj.2012.118 PubMed PMID: 22322766.
British Medical Association and Law Society, 2004. Assessment of Mental Capacity: Guidance for Doctors and Lawyers. BMJ, London.
Bryant, C., Boyle, C., 2011. Sickle cell disease, dentistry and conscious sedation. Dent. Update 38 (7) 486, 491. PubMed PMID: 22046909.
Cohn, S.L., Goldman, L., 2003. Preoperative risk evaluation and perioperative management of patients with coronary artery disease. Med. Clin. North Am. 87, 111.
Crowe, S., 2002. Obtaining consent in the elderly patient. Hosp. Med. 63, 61.

Curl, C., Boyle, C., 2012. Sedation for patients with movement disorders. Dent. Update 39 (1), 45. PubMed PMID: 22720380.

Department of Health, 2000. A Conscious Decision: Report of an Expert Group Chaired by the Chief Medical and Dental Officer. Department of Health, London.

Department of Health, 2002. Guidelines for Conscious Sedation in the Provision of Dental Care. Standing Dental Advisory Committee, London.

Flynn, P.J., Strunin, L., 2005. General anaesthesia for dentistry. Anaesth. Intensive Care Med. 6, 263.

Furness, P.M., 2003. Obtaining and using human tissues for research: ethical and practical dilemmas. Hosp. Med. 64, 198.

Goodwin, M., et al. 2012. Estimating the need for dental sedation: 4. Using IOSN as a referral tool. Br. Dent. J. 212 (5), E9. doi:10.1038/sj.bdj.2012.183. PubMed PMID: 22402564.

Haas, D.A., 2002. An update on analgesics for the management of acute postoperative dental pain. J. Can. Dent. Assoc. 68, 476.

Hillerup, S., et al. 2011. Trigeminal nerve injury associated with injection of local anesthetics: needle lesion or neurotoxicity? J. Am. Dent. Assoc. 142 (5), 531. PubMed PMID: 21531935.

Jones, R., 2012. Weak evidence that oral midazolam is an effective sedative agent for children undergoing dental treatment. Evid. Based Dent. 13 (3), 76. http://dx.doi.org/10.1038/sj.ebd.6400873. PubMed PMID: 23059919.

Krzemiński, T.F., et al. 2011. Comparison of ropivacaine and lidocaine with epinephrine for infiltration anesthesia in dentistry: a randomized study. Am. J. Dent. 24 (5), 305. PubMed PMID: 22165459.

LaPointe, L., et al. 2012. State regulations governing oral sedation in dental practice. Pediatr. Dent. 34 (7), 489. PubMed PMID: 23265167.

Leith, R., et al. 2012. Articaine use in children: a review. Eur. Arch. Paediatr. Dent. 13 (6), 293. Review. PubMed PMID: 23235128

Little, J.W., et al. 2008. Antibiotic prophylaxis in dentistry: an update. Gen. Dent. 56 (1), 20.

Lourenço-Matharu, L., et al. 2012. Sedation of children undergoing dental treatment. Cochrane Database Syst. Rev. CD003877, doi: 10.1002/14651858. CD003877.pub4. Review. PubMed PMID: 22419289.

McKenna, G., Manton, S., 2008. Pre-operative fasting for intravenous conscious sedation used in dental treatment: are conclusions based on relative risk management or evidence? Br. Dent. J. 205, 173.

Meechan, J.G., 2002. A comparison of ropivacaine and lidocaine with epinephrine for intraligamentary anesthesia. Oral Surg. Oral Med. Oral Pathol. Oral Radiol. Endod. 93 (4), 469. PubMed PMID: 12029287.

Miller, C.S., et al. 2001. Supplemental corticosteroids for dental patients with adrenal insufficiency: reconsideration of the problem. J. Am. Dent. Assoc. 132 (11), 1570. quiz 1596.

Newton, T., 2011a. Summary of: estimating the need for dental sedation: 1. The Indicator of Sedation Need (IOSN) – a novel assessment tool. Br. Dent. J. 211 (5), 218. http://dx.doi.org/10.1038/sj.bdj.2011.745 PubMed PMID: 21904357.

Newton, T., 2011b. Summary of: estimating the need for dental sedation: 2. Using IOSN as a health needs assessment tool. Br. Dent. J. 211 (5), 220. http://dx.doi.org/10.1038/sj.bdj.2011.746 PubMed PMID: 21904358.

Ogle, O.E., Hertz, M.B., 2012. Anxiety control in the dental patient. Dent. Clin. North Am. 56 (1) 1, vii. doi: 10.1016/j.cden.2011.06.001. Epub. 2011 Jul 28. PubMed PMID: 22117939.

Padfield, A., 2007. 'Just a little whiff of gas': a partial history of UK dental chair anaesthesia. Anaesth. News 243, 27.

Powell, C.A., Caplan, C.E., 2001. Pulmonary function tests in the preoperative pulmonary evaluation. Clin. Chest Med. 22, 703.

Pretty, I.A., et al. 2011. Estimating the need for dental sedation: 2. Using IOSN as a health needs assessment tool. Br. Dent. J. 211 (5), E11.http://dx.doi.org/10.1038/sj.bdj.2011.726. PubMed PMID: 21904335.

Reference guide to consent for examination or treatment. 2001, Department of Health, London.

Schwamburger, N.T., et al. 2012. The rate of adverse events during IV conscious sedation. Gen. Dent. 60 (5), e341. PubMed PMID: 23032244.

Smetana, G.W., 2003. Preoperative pulmonary assessment of the older patient. Clin. Geriatr. Med. 19, 35.

Smith, A.F., Pittaway, A.J., 2003. Premedication for anxiety in adult day surgery. Cochrane Database Syst. Rev. CD002192.

Snoeck, M., 2012. Articaine: a review of its use for local and regional anesthesia. Local Reg. Anesth. 5, 23. http://dx.doi.org/10.2147/LRA.S16682. Epub. 2012 Jun 5. PubMed PMID: 22915899; PubMed Central PMCID: PMC3417979.

Standing Dental Advisory Committee, 2007. Standards for Conscious Sedation in Dentistry: Alternative Techniques. Report of an Expert Group on Sedation for Dentistry. Standing Dental Advisory Committee, London.

Wakita, R., et al. 2012. A comparison of dexmedetomidine sedation with and without midazolam for dental implant surgery. Anesth. Prog. 59 (2), 62. doi: 10.2344/11-11.1. PubMed PMID: 22822992. PubMed Central PMCID: PMC3403583

Wheeler, R., 2006. Consent in surgery. Ann. R. Coll. Surg. Engl. 88, 261.

Wilson, K.E., et al. 2011. Complications associated with intravenous midazolam sedation in anxious dental patients. Prim. Dent. Care 18 (4), 161. http://dx.doi.org/10.1308/135576111797512801. PubMed PMID: 21968043.

APPENDIX 3.1 DRUGS TO BE AVOIDED OR ONLY USED IN LOW DOSAGE IN SPECIFIC CONDITIONS[a]

Condition	Drugs that may be contraindicated[b]
Addison disease (hypoadrenocorticism)	Any general anaesthetic
Alcoholism	Antidepressants
	Any general anaesthetic
	Aspirin
	Baclofen
	Carbamazepine
	Cefamandole
	Chlorpropamide
	Metronidazole
	Paracetamol (acetaminophen)
	Salicylate
	Tinidazole
Allergies	Aspirin
	Penicillin
Anorexia	Paracetamol (acetaminophen)
Asthma	Aspirin
	Beta-blockers
	Non-steroidal anti-inflammatory drugs (NSAIDs)
	Opioids
	Radiocontrast media
Bleeding disorders	Aspirin
	Corticosteroids
	NSAIDs
Breast-feeding	Aciclovir
	Alcohol
	Antidepressants
	Aspirin
	Azithromycin
	Benzodiazepines
	Buspirone
	Clarithromycin
	Corticosteroids
	Co-trimoxazole
	Dapsone
	Dihydrocodeine
	Famciclovir
	Indometacin
	Iodides
	Itraconazole
	Ketoconazole
	Oxcarbazepine
	Pentazocine
	Phenytoin
	Povidone-iodine
	Sulphonamides
	Sumatriptan
	Tetracyclines
	Voriconazole
	Warfarin
Burns	Suxamethonium
Carcinoid syndrome	Opioids
Cardiovascular diseases	Adrenaline (epinephrine)
	Aspirin
	Chloral hydrate
	Halothane

(Continued)

Condition	Drugs that may be contraindicated[b]
	Itraconazole
	NSAIDs
	Pentazocine
	Rofecoxib
	Thiopental
	Tricyclics
Cerebrovascular disease	Diazepam[c]
Children under 16 years	Aspirin
	NSAIDs
	Codeine
	Tetracyclines
Chronic lymphocytic leukaemia	Amoxicillin
	Ampicillin
Constipation	Codeine
Diabetes mellitus	Aspirin
	Corticosteroids
	NSAIDs
	Quinolones
Diarrhoea	Clindamycin
	Mefenamic acid
Drug addiction	Pentazocine
Dystrophia myotonica (myotonic dystrophy)	Suxamethonium
	Thiopental
Elderly	Atropinics
	Diazepam
	Dihydrocodeine
	Ketamine
	Midazolam
	NSAIDs
	Tricyclics
Epilepsy	Enflurane
	Flumazenil
	Fluoxetine
	Ketamine
	Phenothiazines
	Quinolones
	Tricyclics
Glaucoma	Atropinics
	Carbamazepine
	Corticosteroids
	Diazepam[c]
	Imipramine
	Midazolam
	Selective serotonin reuptake inhibitors (SSRIs)
	Topiramate
	Tricyclics
Glucose-6-phosphate dehydrogenase deficiency	Aspirin
	Co-trimoxazole
	Sulphonamides
Gout	Amoxicillin
	Ampicillin
	Aspirin
Head injury	Ketamine
	Opioids
Hypertension	Adrenaline (epinephrine)
	Aspirin

Condition	Drugs that may be contraindicated[b]
	Corticosteroids
	Ketamine
	NSAIDs
	Pentazocine
Hyperthyroidism	Adrenaline (epinephrine)
	Atropinics
Hypothyroidism	Any general anaesthetic
	Codeine
	Diazepam
	Dihydrocodeine
	Midazolam
	Opioids
	Pethidine
	Thiopental
Infectious mononucleosis	Amoxicillin
	Ampicillin
Liver disease	Antidepressants
	Aspirin
	Azithromycin
	Carbamazepine
	Carbenoxolone
	Chloral hydrate
	Clarithromycin
	Co-amoxiclav
	Corticosteroids
	Co-trimoxazole
	Dextropropoxyphene
	Diazepam
	Erythromycin estolate
	Etretinate
	Flucloxacillin
	Flumazenil
	General anaesthetics
	Halothane
	Itraconazole
	Ketoconazole
	Lamotrigine
	Metronidazole
	Miconazole
	Midazolam
	Moxifloxacin
	NSAIDs
	Opioids or codeine
	Paracetamol (acetaminophen)
	Pentazocine
	Phenothiazines
	Phenytoin
	Pilocarpine
	Prednisolone (prednisone)
	Promethazine
	Propofol
	Rifampicin
	Sumatriptan
	Suxamethonium
	Tetracyclines
	Thiopental
	Tricyclics
	Warfarin

(Continued)

Condition	Drugs that may be contraindicated[b]	Condition	Drugs that may be contraindicated[b]
Malignant hyperpyrexia	Desflurane		NSAIDs
	Enflurane		Opioids
	Halothane		Oxcarbazepine
	Ketamine		Phenytoin
	Sevoflurane		Prilocaine
	Suxamethonium		Sulphonamides
Myasthenia gravis	Aminoglycosides		Teicoplanin
	Clindamycin		Tetracyclines
	General anaesthetics		Tranexamic acid
	Lincomycin		Vancomycin
	Quinolones		Voriconazole
	Sulphonamides	Psychiatric disease	Ketamine
	Tetracyclines	Raised intracranial pressure	Ketamine
Neuromuscular diseases	Diazepam		Opioids
	Midazolam	Renal disease (systemic)	Aciclovir
	Suxamethonium		Aminoglycosides
	Tetracyclines		Amoxicillin
	Thiopental		Any general anaesthetic or CNS depressant or NSAID
Parkinsonism	Benzodiazepines		
Peptic ulcer	Aspirin		Aspirin
	Chloral hydrate		Azathioprine
	Corticosteroids		Baclofen
	Mefenamic acid		Bupivacaine
	NSAIDs		Carbamazepine
Phaeochromocytoma	Adrenaline (epinephrine)		Cefadroxil
	Barbiturates		Cefalexin
	Enflurane		Cefixime
Porphyria	Carbamazepine		Chloral hydrate
	Co-trimoxazole		Ciprofloxacin
	Dextropropoxyphene		Co-amoxiclav
	Diazepam		Co-trimoxazole
	Erythromycin		Diazepam
	MAOIs		Dihydrocodeine
	Metronidazole		Ephedrine
	Midazolam		Erythromycin
	Phenytoin		Famciclovir
	Sulphonamides		Flucloxacillin
	Thiopental		Fluconazole
Pregnancy[d]	Care with all drugs		Gabapentin
	Alcohol		Itraconazole
	Aminoglycosides		Lamotrigine
	Aspirin		Mefenamic acid
	Carbamazepine		Metronidazole
	Corticosteroids		Midazolam
	Co-trimoxazole		NSAIDs
	Dapsone		Opioids
	Diazepam		Paracetamol (acetaminophen)
	Ephedrine		Pentazocine
	Epsilon aminocaproic acid (EACA)		Pilocarpine
	Erythromycin		Prilocaine
	Etretinate		Sulphonamides
	Fluconazole		Suxamethonium
	Flumazenil		Tetracyclines
	Gabapentin		Valaciclovir
	Itraconazole		Vancomycin
	Ketoconazole		Voriconazole
	Mefenamic acid[d]		Warfarin
	Methotrexate	Respiratory disease	Any general anaesthetic
	Metronidazole		Dextropropoxyphene
	Midazolam		Diazepam

(Continued)

Condition	Drugs that may be contraindicated[b]
	Dihydrocodeine
	Midazolam
	Opioids
	Thiopental
Sjögren syndrome	Co-trimoxazole
Suxamethonium sensitivity	Local anaesthetics
	Suxamethonium
Systemic lupus erythematosus	Tetracyclines
Teenagers	Metoclopramide
Thrombotic disease	Epsilon aminocaproic acid (EACA)
	Tranexamic acid
Thyroid disease	Povidone–iodine

Condition	Drugs that may be contraindicated[b]
Tuberculosis	Corticosteroids
Urinary retention (prostatic disease)	Atropinics
	Opioids

[a]ALWAYS check the *British National Formulary* or an equivalent source, as these lists cannot be complete; nor can their accuracy be guaranteed. Box 27.9 shows drugs whose action may be affected by grapefruit; Box 27.10 shows drugs enhanced by pomegranate. See also Appendices 3.2 and 3.3.
[b]Contraindications are often relative or of theoretical interest only; other drugs may also be contraindicated.
[c]Midazolam may be safer but should still be used with caution.
[d]And breast-feeding.

APPENDIX 3.2 POSSIBLE CONTRAINDICATIONS TO DRUGS USED IN DENTISTRY[a]

Drug	Possible contraindications	Possible reaction
Aciclovir (systemic)	Renal disease	Rise in urea
Adrenaline (epinephrine)	Hypertension (theoretically)	Rise in BP
	Hyperthyroidism (theoretically)	Arrhythmias
	Ischaemic heart disease	Arrhythmias
	Phaeochromocytoma	Hypertension
Ampicillin (or amoxicillin)	Allergy to penicillin	Anaphylaxis
	Chronic lymphocytic leukaemia	Rash
	Gout	Rash
	Infectious mononucleosis	Rash
Antidepressants	Alcoholism	Potentiated
Aspirin	Alcoholism	Gastric bleeding
	Allergy to aspirin including aspirin-induced asthma	Anaphylaxis or asthma
	Bleeding disorders	Gastric bleeding
	Breast-feeding	Reye syndrome
	Cardiac failure	Fluid retention
	Children under 16 years	Reye syndrome
	Diabetes mellitus	Interferes with control
	Glucose-6-phosphate dehydrogenase deficiency	Haemolysis
	Gout	Exacerbation of gout
	Hypertension	Fluid retention
	Liver disease	Bleeding tendency
	Peptic ulcer	Gastric bleeding
	Pregnancy	Haemorrhage
	Renal disease	Fluid retention and gastric bleeding
Atropinics	Elderly	Confusion
	Glaucoma	Exacerbation of glaucoma
	Hyperthyroidism	Tachycardias
	Urinary retention or prostatic hypertrophy	Urine retention
Benzodiazepines (see Midazolam)		
Carbamazepine	Alcoholism	Sedation
	Blood disorders	Dyscrasia
	Elderly	Agitation or confusion
	Glaucoma	Raised intraocular pressure
	Liver disease	Hepatotoxicity
	Porphyria	Acute porphyria
	Pregnancy	Teratogenicity
Carbenoxolone	Liver disease	Toxicity
Cephalosporins	Allergy to cephalosporins	Anaphylaxis
	Allergy to penicillins	Allergy
	Renal disease	Nephrotoxicity

(Continued)

Drug	Possible contraindications	Possible reaction
Chloral hydrate	Cardiovascular disease	Fluid retention
	Gastritis	Gastric irritation
	Liver disease	Coma
	Renal disease	CNS depression
Clindamycin	Diarrhoea	Aggravation of diarrhoea
	Liver disease	Increased toxicity
	Renal disease	Increased toxicity
Codeine	Children	Potential toxicity
	Colonic disease	Constipation
	Hypothyroidism	Coma
	Liver disease	Respiratory depression
Corticosteroids	Diabetes mellitus	Exacerbation of diabetes
	Glaucoma	Exacerbation of glaucoma
	Hypertension	Increased hypertension
	Liver disease	Increased side-effects
	Peptic ulcer	Perforation
	Tuberculosis	Possible dissemination
Co-trimoxazole	Elderly	Agranulocytosis
	Glucose-6-phosphate-dehydrogenase deficiency	Haemolysis
	Liver disease	Enhanced toxicity
	Porphyria	Acute porphyria
	Pregnancy	Folate deficiency
	Renal disease	Increased toxicity
	Sjögren syndrome	Aseptic meningitis
Dextropropoxyphene	Liver disease	Potentiated paralysis
	Porphyria	Hypertension
	Pregnancy	Fetal depression
	Respiratory disease	Respiratory depression
Desflurane	Malignant hyperpyrexia	Pyrexia
Diazepam (see Midazolam)		
Dihydrocodeine	Elderly	Increased toxicity
	Hypothyroidism	Coma
	Renal disease	Increased toxicity
	Respiratory disease	Respiratory depression
Enflurane	Epilepsy	Epileptogenic
	Halothane hepatitis	Hepatitis
	Malignant hyperpyrexia	Pyrexia
	Phaeochromocytoma	Hypertension
Epsilon aminocaproic acid (EACA)	Haematuria	Renal tract obstruction
	Pregnancy	Thrombosis
	Thrombotic disease	Thrombosis
Erythromycin	Breast-feeding	Entry of milk
	Liver disease	Hepatotoxicity
	Porphyria	Paralysis
	Pregnancy	?Teratogenicity
	Renal disease	Toxicity
Etomidate	Adrenal disease	Adrenal suppression
Etretinate	Liver disease	Hepatotoxicity
	Pregnancy	Teratogenicity
Flucloxacillin	Liver disease	Hepatotoxicity
Fluconazole	Cardiac failure	Cardiac failure
	Liver disease	Hepatotoxicity
	Porphyria	Crisis
	Pregnancy	Teratogenicity
	Renal disease	Toxicity
Flumazenil	Allergy	Allergy
	Epilepsy	Epileptogenicity
	Liver disease	Delayed excretion
	Pregnancy	Teratogenicity

(Continued)

Drug	Possible contraindications	Possible reaction
Fluoxetine	Epilepsy	Epileptogenicity
Halothane	Cardiac arrhythmias	Increased arrhythmias
	Halothane hepatitis	Hepatitis
	Malignant hyperpyrexia	Pyrexia
	Recent anaesthesia with halothane	Hepatitis
Isoflurane	Malignant hyperpyrexia	Pyrexia
Itraconazole (see also Fluconazole)	Heart failure	Heart failure
Ketamine	Elderly	Hallucinations
	Epilepsy	Fits
	Hallucinations	Hallucinations
	Hypertension	Hypertension
	Malignant hyperpyrexia	Pyrexia
	Psychiatric disease	Psychotic reactions
	Raised intracranial pressure	Increased intracranial pressure
Ketoconazole (see also Fluconazole)	Liver disease	Hepatotoxicity
Lincomycin (as for Clindamycin)		
Local anaesthetics	Suxamethonium sensitivity	Respiratory depression
Mefenamic acid	Asthma	Bronchospasm
	Diarrhoea	Exacerbation of diarrhoea
	Peptic ulcer	Bleeding
	Pregnancy and lactation	?Teratogenicity
	Renal disease	Renal damage
Metoclopramide	Teenagers	Dystonic reactions
Metronidazole	Alcoholism	Headache
	Blood dyscrasias	Leucopenia
	Breast-feeding	Entry into milk
	CNS disease	Neuropathy
	Epilepsy	Epileptogenicity
	Liver disease	Toxicity
	Porphyria	Acute porphyria
	Pregnancy	?Teratogenicity
	Renal disease	Increased drug effect
Miconazole (see Fluconazole)		
Midazolam	Cerebrovascular disease	Cerebral ischaemia
	Children	Anomalous effects
	Chronic obstructive airways disease	Respiratory depression
	Elderly	Cerebral ischaemia
	Glaucoma	Increased intraocular pressure
	Head injury	Disturbed signs
	Hypothyroidism	Coma
	Neuromuscular disorders	Deterioration of condition
	Porphyria	Acute porphyria
	Pregnancy	Fetal hypoxia/dependence
	Severe kidney disease	Increased midazolam effect
	Severe liver disease	Increased midazolam effect
NSAIDs	Asthma	Bronchospasm
	Bleeding tendency	Bleeding
	Cardiac failure	Cardiac failure
	Children	Toxicity
	Diabetes	Disturbed control
	Elderly	Toxicity
	Hypertension	Disturbed control
	Liver disease	Hepatotoxicity
	Peptic ulcer	Gastric bleeding
	Pregnancy	Patent ductus arteriosus
	Renal disease	Nephrotoxicity

(Continued)

Drug	Possible contraindications	Possible reaction
Opioids	Asthma	Bronchospasm
	Carcinoid syndrome	Increased toxicity
	Chronic obstructive airways disease	Respiratory depression
	Head injury	Confusion of 'eye signs'
	Hypothyroidism	Coma
	Liver disease	Increased respiratory depression
	Pregnancy	Fetal depression
	Renal disease	Increased respiratory depression
	Urinary retention or prostatic enlargement	Urinary retention
Paracetamol (acetaminophen)	Alcoholism	Hepatotoxicity
	Anorexia	Hepatotoxicity
	Liver disease	Hepatotoxicity
	Renal disease	Nephrotoxicity
Penicillins	Allergy to penicillin	Anaphylaxis
	Renal disease	Hyperkalaemia with i.m. benzyl penicillin
Pentazocine	Hypertension	Hypertension
	Liver disease	Enhanced activity
	Myocardial infarct (recent)	Cardiac arrest
	Narcotic addiction	Withdrawal syndrome
	Pregnancy	Fetal depression
Pethidine	Hypothyroidism	Coma
Povidone–iodine	Lactation	Toxicity
	Pregnancy	Toxicity
	Thyroid disease	Toxicity
Promethazine	Liver disease	Coma
Propofol	Children under 17 y	May cause convulsions
Quinolones	Diabetes	Hypoglycaemia
	Epilepsy	Epileptogenicity
	Myasthenia gravis	Muscle weakness
Rifampicin	Liver disease	Hepatotoxicity
Rofecoxib	Cardiac disease	Risk of infarction
Sevoflurane	Malignant hyperpyrexia	Pyrexia
Sulphonamides	Glucose-6-phosphate dehydrogenase deficiency	Haemolysis
	Liver disease	Toxicity
	Porphyria	Acute porphyria
	Pregnancy	Fetal haemolysis
	Renal disease	Crystalluria
Suxamethonium	Burns	Arrhythmias
	Dystrophia myotonica	Increased muscle weakness
	Liver disease	Apnoea
	Malignant hyperpyrexia	Pyrexia
	Myasthenia gravis	Increased muscle weakness
	Renal disease	Apnoea
	Suxamethonium sensitivity	Apnoea
Tetracyclines	After gastrointestinal surgery	Enterocolitis
	Children	Tooth staining
	Myasthenia gravis	Increased muscle weakness
	Pregnancy	Tooth staining (fetus)
	Renal disease	Nephrotoxicity
	Systemic lupus erythematosus	Photosensitivity
Thiopental	Addison disease	Coma
	Barbiturate sensitivity	Anaphylaxis
	Cardiovascular disease	Cardiovascular depression
	Dystrophia myotonica	Increased weakness
	Hypothyroidism	Coma
	Liver disease	Increased anaesthesia
	Myasthenia gravis	Increased weakness
	Porphyria	Acute porphyria
	Postnasal drip	Laryngeal spasm
	Respiratory disease	Respiratory depression

(Continued)

Drug	Possible contraindications	Possible reaction
Tranexamic acid	Haematuria	Renal tract obstruction
	Pregnancy	Thromboses
Triclofos	Thromboembolic disease	Thromboses
Tricyclics	Cardiovascular disease	Postural hypotension, arrhythmias
	Elderly	Hypotension
	Epilepsy	Increased fits
	Glaucoma	Exacerbation of glaucoma
	Liver disease	Increased drug effect
Trimethoprim	Sjögren syndrome	Trimethoprim-induced aseptic meningitis
Voriconazole (see Fluconazole)		

[a]ALWAYS check the *British National Formulary* or an equivalent source, as these lists cannot be complete; nor can their accuracy be guaranteed. Many of these reactions are likely to be of more theoretical interest than clinical significance, so that reference should also be made to the appropriate chapters for particular diseases. Box 27.9 shows drugs whose action may be affected by grapefruit; Box 27.10 shows drugs enhanced by pomegranate. See also Appendices 3.1 and 3.3.

APPENDIX 3.3 POSSIBLE DRUG INTERACTIONS IN DENTISTRY[a]

Drug used in dentistry	Interaction with	Possible effects
Aciclovir	Ciclosporin	Nephrotoxicity
	Tacrolimus	Nephrotoxicity
	Zidovudine	Lethargy
Adrenaline (epinephrine)	Halothane	Arrhythmias
	Propranolol	Hypertension
	Tricyclics	Pressor response in overdose
Amphotericin (i.v.)	Aminoglycosides	Enhanced nephrotoxicity
	Ciclosporin	Enhanced nephrotoxicity
	Corticosteroids	Hypokalaemia
	Diuretics	Hypokalaemia
	Tacrolimus	Nephrotoxicity
Anaesthetics (general)	Antihypertensives	Hypotension
	Monoamine oxidase inhibitors (MAOIs)	Enhanced hypotension; anaesthetics potentiated
Antibiotics	Anticoagulants	Enhanced anticoagulant effect
	Oral contraceptives	Reduced contraceptive effect
	Retinoids	Intracranial hypertension
Aspirin (doses >4 g/day)	Angiotensin-converting enzyme inhibitors (ACEIs)	ACEI impaired?
	Alcohol	Increased risk of gastric bleeding
	Antacids	Reduced aspirin absorption
	Anticoagulants	Enhanced anticoagulant effect
	Cilostazol	Toxicity
	Clopidogrel	Increased bleeding
	Corticosteroids	Peptic ulceration
	Digoxin	Digoxin increased
	Iloprost	Increased bleeding
	Lithium	Lithium toxicity
	Methotrexate	Enhanced methotrexate activity
	Metoclopramide	Potentiation of aspirin absorption
	Mifepristone	Toxicity
	Non-steroidal anti-inflammatory drugs (NSAIDs)	Peptic ulceration
	Oral hypoglycaemics	Enhanced hypoglycaemic effect
	Paracetamol (acetaminophen)	Enhanced hepatotoxicity
	Phenylbutazone	Increased liability of peptic ulceration
	Phenytoin	Phenytoin toxicity
	Probenecid	Uricosuric action reduced
	Sodium valproate	Bleeding tendency
	Selective serotonin reuptake inhibitors (SSRIs)	Bleeding tendency
	Spironolactone	Spironolactone impaired
	Subitramine	Bleeding tendency
	Sulfinpyrazone	Uricosuric action reduced
	Venlafaxine	Bleeding tendency
	Varicella zoster virus (VZV) vaccine	Reye syndrome
	Zafirlukast	Enhanced leukotrienes

(Continued)

Drug used in dentistry	Interaction with	Possible effects
Atropine	Metoclopramide	Antagonism
Azathioprine	Allopurinol	Toxicity
	Clozapine	Blood dycrasia
	Co-trimoxazole	Blood dyscrasia
	Rifampicin	Transplant rejection
	Trimethoprim	Blood dyscrasia
	Warfarin	Reduced warfarin effect
Azithromycin (see Erythromycin and Clarithromycin)	Antipsychotics	Long QT syndrome (LQTS; Ch. 5)
	Ciclosporin	Increased ciclosporin effect
	Pimozide	Arrhythmias
	Terfenadine	Arrhythmias
	Theophylline	Increased theophylline
Baclofen	ACEIs	Enhanced hypotension
	Alcohol	Sedation
	NSAIDs	Toxicity
Barbiturates	Alcohol	May be increased sedation or resistance
	Anticoagulants	Reduced anticoagulant activity
	Antihistamines	Enhanced sedation
	Antihypertensives	Hypotension
	Corticosteroids	May precipitate hypotensive crises
	Ciclosporin	Reduced effect of ciclosporin
	MAOIs	Enhanced sedation
	Phenothiazines	Tremor
	Phenytoin	Reduced phenytoin effect
	Tricyclics	Cardiac arrest
Carbamazepine	Alcohol	Toxicity
	Antidepressants	Effect increased
	Calcium channel blockers	Carbamazepine toxicity
	Ciclosporin	Reduced effect of ciclosporin
	Cimetidine	Carbamazepine toxicity
	Clarithromycin	Carbamazepine toxicity
	Danazol	Carbamazepine toxicity
	Dextropropoxyphene	Carbamazepine enhanced
	Doxycycline	Reduced doxycycline effect
	Erythromycin	Carbamazepine toxicity
	Fluoxetine	Confusion
	Irinotecan	Irinotecan effect reduced
	Lithium	Lithium toxicity
	MAOIs	Hypertension
	Oral anticoagulants	Reduced anticoagulant effect
	Oral contraceptive	Reduced contraceptive effect
	Paracetamol (acetaminophen)	Liver damage
	Phenytoin	Reduced phenytoin effect
	Protease inhibitors	Interference
	Sodium valproate	Reduced effect of valproate
Cefamandole	Alcohol	Disulfiram-type reaction
	Anticoagulants	Increased anticoagulant activity
Cephalosporins	Antacids	Reduced absorption
	Anticoagulants	Increased anticoagulant activity
	Diuretics	Increased nephrotoxicity
Ciclosporin	ACEIs	Hyperkalaemia
	Aciclovir	Nephrotoxicity
	Allopurinol	Nephrotoxicity
	Aminoglycosides	Nephrotoxicity
	Azoles	Ciclosporin toxicity
	Carbamazepine	Ciclosporin reduced
	Clarithromycin	Ciclosporin toxicity
	Colchicine	Nephrotoxicity and myotoxicity
	Corticosteroids	Both drugs increased
	Diclofenac	Diclofenac enhanced
	Erythromycin	Ciclosporin toxicity
	NSAIDs	Nephrotoxicity

(Continued)

Drug used in dentistry	Interaction with	Possible effects
Clarithromycin	Pimozide	Arrhythmias
	Terfenadine	Arrhythmias
Codeine	MAOIs	Coma
Colchicine	Ciclosporin	Nephrotoxicity and myotoxicity
Corticosteroids	ACEIs	Reduced hypotensive effect
	Aminoglycosides	Reduced steroid effects
	Anticoagulants	Gastric bleeding
	Aspirin/NSAIDs	Increased liability of peptic ulceration
	Oral antidiabetics	Reduced effect
Danazol	Anticoagulants	Potentiated anticoagulation
	Carbamazepine	Carbamazepine toxicity
Dextropropoxyphene	Alcohol	CNS depression
	Anticoagulants	Enhanced anticoagulant effect
	Carbamazepine	Serotonin syndrome
	Orphenadrine	Tremor, anxiety and confusion
	MAOIs	Serotonin syndrome
Doxycycline (see Tetracyclines)		
Ephedrine	MAOIs	Hypertension
	Tricyclics	Hypertension
Erythromycin	Alfentanil	Increased alfentanil effect
	Amiodarone	Arrhythmias
	Amprenavir	Erythromycin toxicity
	Anticoagulants	Increased bleeding
	Antipsychotics	LQTS
	Artemether	Erythromycin toxicity
	Atazanavir	Erythromycin toxicity
	Atomoxetine	Arrhythmias
	Bromocriptine	Erythromycin toxicity
	Buspirone	Buspirone toxicity
	Cabergoline	Erythromycin toxicity
	Carbamazepine	Carbamazepine toxicity
	Ciclosporin	Ciclosporin toxicity
	Cimetidine	Erythromycin toxicity
	Clozapine	Convulsions
	Colchicine	Colchicine toxicity
	Corticosteroids	Metabolism reduced
	Darifenacin	Increased darifenacin level
	Digoxin	Digoxin toxicity
	Efavirenz	Erythromycin toxicity
	Eletriptan	Eletriptan toxicity
	Eplerenone	Increased eplerenone level
	Ergotamine	Ergotism
	Felodipine	Increased felodipine level
	Fluoxetine	LQTS
	Galantamine	Increased galantamine level
	Ivabradine	Arrhythmias
	Loratidine	Loratidine toxicity
	Methysergide	Ergotism
	Midazolam	Midazolam enhanced
	Mizolastine	Mizolastine toxicity
	Moxifloxacin	Arrhythmias
	Oral contraceptive	Reduced effect
	Pentamidine	Arrhythmias
	Phenytoin	Phenytoin toxicity
	Pimozide	Arrhythmias
	Rifabutin	Uveitis
	Ritonavir	Erythromycin toxicity
	Sertindole	Arrhythmias
	Sildenafil	Sildenafil level increased
	Sirolimus	Enhanced drug level
	Statins	Myopathy increased
	Tacrolimus	Tacrolimus toxicity
	Tadalafil	Tadalafil increased

(Continued)

Drug used in dentistry	Interaction with	Possible effects
	Terfenadine	Arrhythmias
	Theophyllines	Toxicity
	Tolterodine	Increased tolterodine level
	Tricyclics	LQTS
	Valproate	Toxicity
	Vardenafil	Increased toxicity
	Venlafaxine	LQTS
	Verapamil	Toxicity
	Zopiclone	Increased zopiclone level
Fluconazole	Anticoagulants	Enhanced anticoagulant effect
	Anticonvulsants	Anticonvulsant enhanced
	Antipsychotics	Antipsychotics enhanced
	Calcium-channel blockers	Cardiac failure
	Carbamazepine	Carbamazepine enhanced
	Celecoxib	Celecoxib enhanced
	Ciclosporin	Ciclosporin enhanced
	Digoxin	Digoxin enhanced
	Midazolam	Midazolam enhanced
	Mizolastine	Mizolastine enhanced
	Oral antidiabetics	Enhanced antidiabetic effect
	Oral contraceptive	May impair contraception
	Parecoxib	Parecoxib enhanced
	Phenytoin	Phenytoin enhanced
	Pimozide	Arrhythmias
	Protease inhibitors (PIs)	PIs enhanced
	Quinidine	Arrhythmias
	Rifampicin	Fluconazole effect reduced
	Sirolimus	Sirolimus enhanced
	Statins	Increased myopathy
	Tacrolimus	Tacrolimus enhanced
	Terfenadine	Arrhythmias
	Vincristine	Vincristine enhanced
	Zidovudine	Myelotoxicity
Flumazenil	Tricyclics	Sedation
Fluoxetine	Alcohol	Enhanced alcohol effect
	Antiepileptics	Antagonism
	Carbamazepine	Confusion
	MAOIs	CNS effects
	Warfarin	Enhanced anticoagulant effect
Ganciclovir	Zidovudine	Marrow suppression
Gentamicin	Furosemide	Toxicity and nephrotoxicity
Halothane	Aminophylline	Arrhythmias
	Anticonvulsants	Phenytoin toxicity
	Antihypertensives	Hypotension
	Diazepam	Enhanced activity of halothane
	Fenfluramine	Arrhythmias
	Isoprenaline	Arrhythmias
	L-dopa	Arrhythmias
	Lithium	Arrhythmias
	Opioids	Respiratory depression
	Phenothiazines	Respiratory depression; hypotension
Indometacin	Haloperidol	Drowsiness
Itraconazole (as for Fluconazole)		
Ketamine	CNS depressants	Increased sedation
Ketoconazole (see Fluconazole)	Ciclosporin	Nephrotoxicity
	Simvastatin	Risk of myopathy
	Terfenadine	Cardiotoxicity
Mefenamic acid	Anticoagulants	Enhanced anticoagulant effect
	Oral hypoglycaemics	Enhanced hypoglycaemia

(Continued)

Drug used in dentistry	Interaction with	Possible effects
Metronidazole	Alcohol	Headache and hypotension
	Anticoagulants	Increased bleeding tendency
	Anticonvulsants	Phenytoin toxicity
	BCNU (bis-chloroethylnitrosourea)	BCNU toxicity
	Busulfan	Busulfan toxicity
	Ciclosporin	Ciclosporin toxicity
	Cimetidine	Metronidazole toxicity
	Cyclophosphamide	Cyclophosphamide toxicity
	Fluorouracil	Fluorouracil toxicity
	Lithium	Lithium toxicity
Miconazole (as for Fluconazole)		
Midazolam and other sedatives	Alcohol	Enhanced sedation
	Anticoagulants	Increased bleeding
	Anticonvulsants	Midazolam potentiated
	Antidepressants	Enhanced sedation
	Antihistamines	Enhanced sedation
	Antipsychotics	Enhanced sedation
	Azoles	Midazolam potentiated
	Baclofen	Midazolam potentiated
	Benzodiazepines	Enhanced sedation
	Calcium-channel blockers	Midazolam potentiated
	Cimetidine	Enhanced sedation
	Clarithromycin	Midazolam potentiated
	Disulfiram	Midazolam potentiated?
	Esomeprazole	Midazolam potentiated?
	Erythromycin	Midazolam potentiated
	Fluvoxamine	Midazolam potentiated
	General anaesthetics	Anaesthesia enhanced
	L-dopa	Antagonism
	Lithium	Hypothermia
	Macrolides	Midazolam potentiated
	Omeprazole	Midazolam potentiated?
	Opioids	Respiratory depression
	Pentazocine	Respiratory depression
	Phenytoin	Phenytoin toxicity
	PIs	Midazolam potentiated
	Quinupristin	Midazolam potentiated
	Rifampicin	Midazolam effect reduced
	Suxamethonium	Activity of suxamethonium reduced
	Telithromycin	Midazolam potentiated
	Tizanidine	Enhanced sedation
	Tricyclics	Enhanced sedation
Monoamine oxidase inhibitors (MAOIs)	Anticoagulants	Enhanced anticoagulant effect
	Antihypertensives	Reduced or increased hypotensive effect
	Codeine	Hypertension
	General anaesthetics	Hypertension
	L-dopa	Hypertensive crisis
	Opioids	Respiratory depression
	Oral hypoglycaemics	Enhanced hypoglycaemia
	Pethidine	Hypertensive crisis
	Propranolol	Hypertensive crisis
	Tricyclics	Excitation and other interactions
	Tyramine-containing foods	Hypertensive crisis
Non-steroidal anti-inflammatory drugs (NSAIDs; >4 g/day)	Alcohol	Gastric irritation
	Anticoagulants	Increased bleeding tendency
	Anticonvulsants	Phenytoin toxicity
	Antihypertensives	Hypotension, hyperkalaemia
	Baclofen	Toxicity
	Ciclosporin	Nephrotoxicity
	Corticosteroids	Gastric irrritation
	Cytotoxics	Toxicity

(Continued)

Drug used in dentistry	Interaction with	Possible effects
	Diuretics	Nephrotoxicity
	Lithium	Lithium toxicity
	Moclobemide	NSAID enhanced
	Oral antidiabetics	Enhanced antidiabetic activity
	Paracetamol (acetaminophen)	Hepatotoxicity
	Pentoxifylline	Increased bleeding
	Quinolones	Convulsions
	SSRIs	Bleeding
	Tacrolimus	Nephrotoxicity
	Warfarin	Increased bleeding
	Zidovudine	Blood dyscrasia
Noradrenaline (norepinephrine)	Tricyclics	Hypertension
Opioids	Diazepam	Respiratory depression
	Halothane	Respiratory depression
	MAOIs	Respiratory depression or coma
	Thiopental	Respiratory depression
Paracetamol (acetaminophen)	Alcohol	Hepatotoxicity
	Anticoagulants	Increased bleeding tendency
	Anticonvulsants	Hepatotoxicity
	Busulfan	Toxicity
	Carbamazepine	Hepatotoxicity
	Colestyramine	Reduced absorption of paracetamol (acetaminophen)
	Domperidone	Increased absorption of paracetamol (acetaminophen)
	Isonicotinic acid hydrazide (INAH)	Enhanced INAH hepatotoxicity
	Metoclopramide	Increased absorption of paracetamol (acetaminophen)
	Zidovudine	Increased myelosuppression
Pentazocine	Diazepam	Respiratory depression
Pethidine	Antidepressants	Serotonin syndrome
	MAOIs	Hypertensive crisis
	Phenothiazines	Respiratory depression
Phenothiazines	Alcohol	May be increased sedation
	Anticoagulants	Enhanced anticoagulant effect
	Antihistamines	Enhanced sedation
	Antihypertensives	Hypotension
	Barbiturates	Tremor
	Diazepam	Respiratory depression
	Opioids	Respiratory depression
	Pethidine	Respiratory depression
	Tricyclics	Convulsions
Phenylbutazone	Aspirin	Increased liability to peptic ulceration
Phenytoin	Aspirin	Phenytoin toxicity
	Azoles	Phenytoin toxicity
	Baclofen	Phenytoin toxicity
	Carbamazepine	Reduced carbamazepine effect
	Cimetidine	Phenytoin toxicity
	Clarithromycin	Phenytoin toxicity
	Disulfiram	Disulfiram potentiated
	INAH	INAH potentiated
	Midazolam	Phenytoin toxicity
	NSAIDs	Phenytoin toxicity
	Phenylbutazone	Phenylbutazone potentiated
Promethazine	Thiopental	Respiratory depression
Quinolones	Antacids	Reduced absorption
	Anticoagulants	Bleeding increased
	Antidiabetics	Antidiabetic enhanced
	Anticonvulsants	Phenytoin enhanced
	Artemether	Toxicity
	Ciclosporin	Nephrotoxicity
	Iron	Reduced absoprtion
	Theophylline	Convulsions
	Zolmitriptan	Increased effect of zolmitriptan

(Continued)

Drug used in dentistry	Interaction with	Possible effects
Rifampicin	Antacids	Reduced rifampicin absorption
	Anticoagulants	Reduced bleeding tendency
	Antifungals	Increased metabolism of antifungals
	Ciclosporin	Reduced effect of ciclosporin
	Oral contraceptive	Reduced contraceptive effect
Selective serotonin reuptake inhibitors (SSRIs)	Anticoagulants	Bleeding
	Lithium	Serotonin syndrome
	NSAIDs	Bleeding
	Tramadol	Serotonin syndrome
Sulphonamides	Anticoagulants	Enhanced anticoagulant effect
	Methotrexate	Increased methotrexate toxicity
	Oral hypoglycaemics	Enhanced hypoglycaemia
	Phenytoin	Phenytoin toxicity
Suxamethonium	Cytotoxic drugs	Prolonged muscle paralysis
	Diazepam	Activity of suxamethonium reduced
	Diethylstilbestrol	Prolonged muscle paralysis
	Digitalis	Digitalis toxicity enhanced
	Ecothiopate	Prolonged muscle paralysis
	Lithium	Onset of suxamethonium delayed; action prolonged
	Spironolactone	Plasma potassium rises; potential arrhythmias
Tetracyclines	ACEIs	Reduced serum levels of tetracyclines
	Antacids	Lower serum levels of tetracyclines
	Anticoagulants	Bleeding tendency
	Barbiturates	Reduced doxycycline blood levels
	Cimetidine	Reduced serum tetracycline levels
	Iron	Reduced serum tetracycline levels
	Lithium	Lithium toxicity
	Methoxyflurane	Renal damage
	Milk	Reduced tetracycline absorption
	Oral contraceptive	Reduced contraceptive effect
	Retinoids	Benign intracranial hypertension
Thiopental	Alcohol	Increased sedation
	Antihypertensives	Hypotension
	MAOIs	Coma
	Opioids	Respiratory depression
	Phenothiazines	Respiratory depression
	Sulphonamides	Barbiturate potentiated
Tramadol	Antidepressants	Serotonin syndrome
Tricyclics	Adrenaline (epinephrine)	Hypertensive response in overdose
	Alcohol	Enhanced CNS effects
	Anticoagulants	Enhanced anticoagulant effect
	Antihypertensives	Impaired blood pressure control
	Atropinics	Enhanced atropinic effect
	Carbamazepine	Confusion
	Cimetidine	Tricyclic enhanced
	Contraceptive pill	Tricyclic effect reduced
	Diazepam	Enhanced sedation
	General anaesthetics	Cardiac arrest
	MAOIs	Excitation and other interactions
	Phenothiazines	Convulsions
Valproate	Anticoagulants	Bleeding
	Erythromycin	Valproate enhanced
Voriconazole (see Fluconazole)		

^aALWAYS check the *British National Formulary* or an equivalent source, as these lists cannot be complete; nor can their accuracy be guaranteed. Many of these drug interactions are of little more than theoretical importance in dentistry, or are the result of overdose of one or both agents. However, there can be a wide range of individual variations in response to drugs, especially sedating agents. Box 27.9 shows drugs whose action may be affected by grapefruit; Box 27.10 shows drugs enhanced by pomegranate. See also Appendices 3.1 and 3.2.

APPENDIX 3.4 GENERAL ANAESTHESIA, SEDATION AND RESUSCITATION

RECOMMENDATIONS FROM THE POSWILLO REPORT (DEPARTMENT OF HEALTH)

- The use of general anaesthesia should be avoided wherever possible.
- The same general standards in respect of personnel, premises and equipment must apply irrespective of where the general anaesthetic is administered. (Para 3.8)
- Dental anaesthesia must be regarded as a postgraduate subject. (Para 3.11)
- All anaesthetics should be administered by accredited anaesthetists who must recognize their responsibility for providing dental anaesthetic services. (Para 3.13)
- Anaesthetic training should include specific experience in dental anaesthesia. (Para 3.14)
- Health authorities should review the provision of consultant dental anaesthetic sessions to ensure that they are sufficient to meet local needs. (Para 3.14)
- Doctors and dentists with knowledge, experience and competence sufficient to satisfy the College of Anaesthetists and the Faculty of Dental Surgery are to be under no detriment. (Para 3.16)
- The no detriment arrangements must have been implemented within 2 years of the publication of this report. (Para 3.17)
- The administration of general anaesthesia in dental surgeries and clinics equipped to the recommended standards of monitoring necessary for patient safety shall continue. (Para 3.17)
- An electrocardiogram, a pulse oximeter and a non-invasive blood pressure device are essential for the non-invasive monitoring of a patient under general anaesthesia. (Paras 3.16 and 3.19)
- A capnograph is to be used where tracheal anaesthesia is practised. (Para 3.20)
- A defibrillator must be available. (Para 3.21)
- Equipment conforming to recognized standards should be purchased and installed, regularly serviced and maintained in accordance with the manufacturer's instructions. (Para 3.21)
- Intravenous agents should be administered via an indwelling needle or cannula, which should not be moved until the patient has fully recovered. (Para 3.22)
- Appropriate training must be provided for those assisting the anaesthetist and dentist. (Paras 3.25 and 4.15)
- At no time should the recovering patient be left unattended. (Para 3.26)
- Adequate recovery facilities should be available. (Para 3.26)
- Good contemporaneous records of all treatments and procedures should be kept. (Para 3.26)
- Written consent should be obtained on each occasion prior to the administration of a general anaesthetic. (Para 3.30)
- Consideration should be given to developing a national general anaesthetic/sedation consent form for general dental practitioners. (Para 3.31)
- Patients should be provided with comprehensive pre- and post-treatment instructions and advice. (Para 3.31)

APPENDIX 3.5 CLASSIFICATION OF OPERATIONS AND ADMISSIONS

CLASSIFICATION OF OPERATIONS

Emergency

Immediate life-saving operation, resuscitation simultaneous with surgical treatment (e.g. trauma, ruptured aortic aneurysm). Operation usually within 1 h.

Urgent

Operation as soon as possible after resuscitation (e.g. irreducible hernia, intussusception, oesophageal atresia, intestinal obstruction, major fractures). Operation within 24 h.

Scheduled

An early operation but not immediately life-saving (e.g. malignancy). Operation usually within 3 weeks.

Elective

Operation at a time to suit both patient and surgeon (e.g. cholecystectomy, joint replacement).

Day case

A patient who is admitted for investigation or operation on a planned non-resident basis (i.e. no overnight stay).

CLASSIFICATION OF ADMISSIONS

Elective

At a time agreed between the patient and the surgical service.

Urgent

Within 48 h of referral/consultation.

Emergency

Immediately following referral/consultation, when admission is unpredictable and at short notice because of the clinical need.

APPENDIX 3.6 INSTRUCTIONS TO PATIENTS AFTER TOOTH EXTRACTION

These should preferably be given to the patient in writing.

After a tooth has been extracted, the socket will usually bleed for a short time. This bleeding stops because a healthy blood clot forms in the tooth socket. These clots are easily disturbed, and if this happens, bleeding will recur. To avoid disturbance of the clot, please follow these instructions:

1. After leaving the hospital or dental surgery, do not rinse out your mouth for 24 h, unless you have been told otherwise by the dentist.

2. Do not disturb the clot in the socket with your tongue or fingers.
3. For the rest of the day, take only soft foods.
4. Try not to chew on the affected side for at least 3 days.
5. Avoid unnecessary talking, excitement or exercise for the rest of the day.
6. Do not take alcoholic or very hot drinks for the rest of the day.
7. If the tooth socket continues to bleed after you have left the surgery, do not be alarmed – much of the liquid that appears to be blood is actually saliva. If bleeding persists, make a small pad from a clean handkerchief or cotton wool, place over the socket and close the teeth firmly on it. Keep up the pressure for 15–30 min. If the bleeding still does not stop, seek dental or medical advice.

APPENDIX 3.7 ANTIMICROBIAL PROPHYLAXIS

ANTIBIOTIC PROPHYLAXIS CONSIDERED IN SOME CASES

- Prosthetic heart valves
- Heart murmurs, e.g. mitral valve prolapse (with incompetence) and history of rheumatic fever, rheumatic heart disease
- Patients with congenital heart disease
- Dialysis patients – those with arteriovenous shunts and those on continuous ambulatory peritoneal dialysis (CAPD)
- Organ transplant patients, pre- and post-transplant – depends on 'counts'
- Chemotherapy patients, including bone marrow transplant – depends on 'counts'
- Artificial joint patients
- Poorly controlled diabetic patients
- Radiation therapy patients, depending on procedure
- Down syndrome patients (many have cardiac defects)
- Immunosuppressed patients, depending on treatment).

ENDOCARDITIS PROPHYLAXIS RECOMMENDED

High-risk category

- Prosthetic cardiac valves, including bioprosthetic and homograft valves
- Previous bacterial endocarditis
- Complex cyanotic congenital heart disease (e.g. single ventricle states, transposition of the great arteries, tetralogy of Fallot)
- Surgically constructed systemic–pulmonary shunts or conduits.

Moderate-risk category

- Most other congenital cardiac malformations (other than above and below)
- Acquired valvular dysfunction (e.g. rheumatic heart disease)
- Hypertrophic cardiomyopathy
- Mitral valve prolapse with valvular regurgitation and/or thickened leaflets.

ENDOCARDITIS PROPHYLAXIS NOT RECOMMENDED

Negligible-risk category (no greater risk than general population)

- Isolated secundum atrial septal defect
- Surgical repair of atrial septal defect, ventricular septal defect or patent ductus arteriosus (without residual beyond 6 months)
- Previous coronary artery bypass graft surgery
- Mitral valve prolapse without valvular regurgitation
- Physiological, functional or innocent heart murmurs
- Previous Kawasaki disease without valvular dysfunction
- Previous rheumatic fever without valvular dysfunction
- Cardiac pacemakers (intravascular and epicardial) and implanted defibrillators.

Prophylaxis is recommended for high-risk patients and optional for medium-risk patients.

Prophylaxis is optional for high-risk patients.

PROPHYLAXIS MAY BE CONSIDERED

- Immunocompromised/immunosuppressed patients
- Inflammatory arthropathies: rheumatoid arthritis, systemic lupus erythematosus
- Disease-, drug- or radiation-induced immunosuppression
- Other patients:
  - Type 1 (insulin-dependent) diabetes
  - First 2 years following joint placement
  - Previous prosthetic joint infections
  - Malnourishment
  - Haemophilia.

HIGHER-INCIDENCE BACTERAEMIC DENTAL PROCEDURES

- Dental extractions
- Periodontal procedures, including surgery, subgingival placement of antibiotic fibres/strips, scaling and root planing, probing, recall maintenance
- Dental implant placement and reimplantation of avulsed teeth
- Endodontic (root canal) instrumentation or surgery only beyond the apex
- Initial placement of orthodontic bands but not brackets
- Intraligamentary LA injections
- Prophylactic cleaning of teeth or implants where bleeding is anticipated.

LOWER-INCIDENCE BACTERAEMIC DENTAL PROCEDURES

- Restorative dentistry (operative and prosthodontic) with/without retraction cord
- LA injections (non-intraligamentary)
- Intracanal endodontic treatment; post-placement and build-up
- Placement of rubber dam
- Postoperative suture removal
- Placement of removable prosthodontic/orthodontic appliances
- Taking of oral impressions

- Fluoride treatments
- Taking of oral radiographs
- Orthodontic appliance adjustment.

Adapted from:

Dajani, A.S., et al. 1997. Prevention of bacterial endocarditis: recommendations by the American Heart Association. J. Am. Dent. Assoc. 128(8):1142. PubMed PMID: 9260427.

Dajani, A.S., et al. 1997. Prevention of bacterial endocarditis: recommendations by the American Heart Association. Circulation 96(1):358. Review. PubMed PMID: 9236458.

Dajani, A.S., et al. 1997. Prevention of bacterial endocarditis: recommendations by the American Heart Association. JAMA 277(22):1794. Review. PubMed PMID: 9178793.

Signs and symptoms 4

This chapter alphabetically summarizes a range of the more important medical conditions.

ABDOMINAL PAIN

Abdominal pain is common and often due to gastroenteritis. Acute and severe pain may be a symptom of more serious intra-abdominal disease, from inflammatory bowel disease to various 'surgical emergencies' ('acute abdomen'); this includes appendicitis, intestinal obstruction, perforated peptic ulcer, perforated diverticulitis, ectopic pregnancy, twisted ovarian cyst, dissecting abdominal aneurysm, mesenteric embolism or thrombosis, biliary tract disease, pancreatitis and renal stone. A leaking abdominal aneurysm is an emergency.

Gangrene and intestinal perforation can follow as little as 6 hours after interruption of the intestinal blood supply from appendicitis, a strangulating obstruction or arterial embolism – and can lead to potentially fatal peritonitis.

ALOPECIA

Alopecia (hair loss) may be temporary and caused, for example, by radiotherapy, cytotoxic chemotherapy, other drugs (e.g. anticoagulants, retinoids, beta-blockers and oral contraceptives) or tinea capitis (ringworm). More permanent alopecia may be:

- *involutional alopecia* – the gradual progressive normal thinning of the hair seen in ageing in both sexes
- *androgenic alopecia* – a genetically predisposed condition that affects both sexes, earlier in men than women, with the hairline receding and hair from the crown gradually and permanently disappearing (male-pattern baldness)
- *alopecia areata* – patchy hair loss in children and young adults of uncertain cause, often sudden in onset and sometimes causing complete baldness, though the hair regrows within a few years in 90%
- *alopecia universalis* – loss of all body hair of uncertain cause, with a low chance of regrowth, especially when in children.

Autoimmune diseases, particularly lupus erythematosus, may also cause hair loss, as may factitious (self-induced) hair-pulling.

AMENORRHOEA

Amenorrhoea – absence of menstruation (menses) – is pathological, except before puberty, during pregnancy or early lactation, and after the menopause. Amenorrhoea may be caused by anatomical abnormalities, endocrine dysfunction (hypothalamic, pituitary, adrenal, thyroid, anorexia nervosa or other), cirrhosis, chemo- or radio-therapy, ovarian failure or genetic defects.

Amenorrhoea is either primary (menarche has not occurred by age 16) or secondary (menses have not occurred for 3 or more months in women who have had menses).

ANAEMIA

Anaemia is a reduction in the haemoglobin level for an individual's age and sex. Anaemia may be normocytic, microcytic or macrocytic, according to the cause (Ch. 8).

ANGINA PECTORIS

See 'Chest pain' and Chapter 5.

ANOREXIA

Anorexia, or loss of appetite, is a non-specific symptom seen in many conditions, but notably in malignant disease (Ch. 22), chronic infections and eating disorders (Ch. 27).

ANOSMIA

Anosmia (loss of the sense of smell) is usually due to nasal occlusion from the common cold, rhinitis, hay fever or nasal polyps. Some loss of smell may be normal with ageing but medications may change or impair the ability to detect odours. Anosmia can also arise from damage to olfactory nerves after head injury, radiotherapy or viral infections. Systemic causes include cerebrovascular events, Alzheimer dementia, tabes (syphilis), brain tumours, and many endocrine, nutritional and nervous disorders.

ANXIETY

Anxiety is common, and may be normal or part of a psychiatric disorder (Ch. 10), but it may also be caused by stimulant drugs such as amphetamines, caffeine, cocaine, ecstasy and many others – or by their withdrawal; neurological disorders (brain trauma, infections, inner ear disorders); cardiovascular disorders (cardiac failure, arrhythmias); endocrine diseases (adrenal or thyroid hyperfunction, hypoglycaemia, phaeochromocytoma); or respiratory diseases (asthma, chronic obstructive pulmonary disease).

APHASIA

Aphasia is a language disorder that impairs both expression and understanding of language, as well as reading and writing. Aphasia results from damage to the left cerebral hemisphere, often as the result

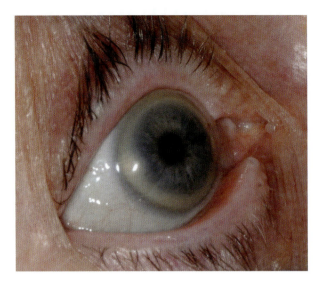

Fig. 4.1 Corneal arcus.

of a stroke, injury or tumour. Speech disorders such as dysarthria or apraxia of speech, which also result from brain damage, may be associated.

ARCUS (CORNEAL ARCUS)

Corneal arcus (arcus senilis) is a white or grey ring in the eyes due to cholesterol deposits in the cornea (Fig. 4.1); it is seen mainly in older age groups. These rings cause no visual problems but can indicate a problem with cholesterol metabolism – and an increased risk of ischaemic heart disease. Corneal arcus not only is associated with high cholesterol levels, but also can be seen in people with diabetes or hypertension, or those who smoke tobacco.

ARRHYTHMIAS

See Chapter 5.

ASCITES

Ascites is the accumulation of fluid in the peritoneal cavity, either from peritoneal sources (bacterial, fungal or parasitic disease; cancer [malignant ascites]; endometriosis or starch peritonitis) or from extraperitoneal sources (cirrhosis, congestive heart failure, hypoalbuminaemia, myxoedema or ovarian disease, e.g. Meig syndrome).

ATAXIA

Ataxia is incoordination or clumsiness of movement that has a cerebellar, vestibular or sensory (proprioceptive) origin rather than being the result of muscle weakness. In ataxia, movement is uncoordinated – defined as an inability to coordinate movements finely. Causes include: drugs (e.g. alcohol, aminoglutethimide, anticholinergics, phenytoin, carbamazepine, phenobarbital and tricyclic antidepressants); stroke or transient ischaemic attack (TIA); multiple sclerosis; head trauma; poisoning; and hereditary conditions (congenital cerebellar ataxia, Friedreich ataxia, ataxia telangiectasia). Ataxia may also follow infection (typically chickenpox or encephalitis).

Cerebellar ataxia is produced by lesions of the cerebellum or its afferent or efferent connections in cerebellar peduncles, pons or red nucleus.

Vestibular ataxia is produced by lesions anywhere along the eighth nerve pathway from labyrinth to brainstem or in the vestibular nuclei. Viral labyrinthitis is a typical cause. Nystagmus is frequently present, typically unilateral, and most pronounced on gaze away from the side of vestibular involvement. Vestibular ataxia is also gravity-dependent – incoordination of limb movements cannot be demonstrated when the patient is examined lying down but only when the patient attempts to stand or walk.

Sensory ataxia can result from abnormalities anywhere along the afferent pathway from peripheral nerve to the parietal cortex. Clinical findings include defective joint position and vibration sense in the leg and sometimes the arms, unstable stance with Romberg sign (sways with eyes shut), and a gait of slapping quality.

BACK PAIN

Back pain is a very common complaint; nearly four out of five people experience it at some time. Most cases do not have a definable cause but sedentary jobs and lifestyles predispose, as can obesity, or strenuous sports such as football and gymnastics. Women who have been pregnant, smokers, and workers who repetitively lift heavy objects are all at greater risk of back pain.

Back pain can develop from:

■ spinal causes – muscular disorders or strain, back overuse or injury, pressure on a nerve root or ruptured intervertebral/vertebral disc ('slipped disc'), spinal arthritis, fractures or metastases
■ non-spinal causes – menstruation or premenstrual syndrome (PMS), endometriosis or ovarian cysts.

BLEEDING TENDENCIES

Prolonged bleeding usually has a local cause such as excessive operative trauma (Ch. 5). Other causes include: haemorrhagic disease; anticoagulants; uncontrolled hypertension; and aspirin or other drugs that interfere with platelet function.

BLINDNESS

See 'Visual impairment'.

BRADYCARDIA

Bradycardia (slow pulse rate) may have intrinsic or extrinsic causes (Ch. 5).

Intrinsic causes include: myocardial infarction, ischaemia or idiopathic degeneration; infiltrative diseases (sarcoidosis, amyloidosis or haemochromatosis); collagen diseases; myotonic muscular dystrophy; surgical trauma; and endocarditis.

Extrinsic causes include: autonomically mediated syndromes (vomiting, coughing, micturition, defecation, etc.); carotid-sinus hypersensitivity from vagal hypertonicity; drugs (beta-adrenergic blockers, calcium-channel blockers, clonidine, digoxin, antiarrhythmic agents); hypothyroidism; hypothermia; neurological disorders (affecting the autonomic nervous system); and electrolyte imbalances (hypokalaemia, hyperkalaemia).

Table 4.1 *Main causes of acute chest pain*

Cause of pain	Features	Predisposing factors
Myocardial infarction	Severe persistent crushing retrosternal pain, possibly radiating to left arm. Unrelieved by glyceryl trinitrate. May be accompanied by nausea or vomiting	Coronary heart disease Hypertension
Angina pectoris	Retrosternal pain, possibly radiating to left arm. Often previously experienced. Relieved in 3 min by glyceryl trinitrate	Coronary heart disease Hypertension
Acute abdominal pain	Pain location is of particular importance. Depending on cause, there may be concomitant symptoms such as gastro-oesophageal reflux, nausea, vomiting, diarrhoea, constipation, jaundice, melaena, haematuria, haematemesis, weight loss, and mucus or blood in stool	Serious causes: ruptured abdominal aortic aneurysm, perforated viscus, mesenteric ischaemia, ruptured ectopic pregnancy, intestinal obstruction, appendicitis, pancreatitis
Dissecting aneurysm	Sudden severe chest or upper back pain, often described as tearing, ripping or shearing sensation that radiates down back, loss of consciousness, shortness of breath	Men between 40 and 70 y
Oesophagitis	Low retrosternal pain on lying down or stooping. Improved by antacids	Hiatus hernia
Anxiety (hyperventilation)	Anxious patients with precordial pain. Overbreathing, panic and precordial pain	Stress
Trauma	Obvious history	–
Lung infection or tumour	Pain on inspiration. May be accompanied by dyspnoea or cough	Pneumonia Pleurisy Bronchogenic carcinoma

Table 4.2 *Causes of finger clubbing*

Hereditary	Respiratory	Cardiovascular	Gastrointestinal	Metabolic
	Lung cancer	Endocarditis	Ulcerative colitis	Thyrotoxicosis
	Bronchiolitis	Cyanotic congenital heart disease	Crohn disease	Acromegaly
	Fibrosing alveolitis		Coeliac disease	
	Asbestosis		Liver disease	
	HIV, fungal and mycoplasmal infections			
	Mesothelioma			

CERVICAL LYMPH NODE ENLARGEMENT

See 'Lymphadenopathy'.

CHEST PAIN

Angina and myocardial infarction (acute coronary syndromes) are the main causes of acute chest pain (Table 4.1; Ch. 5).

CLUBBING OF FINGERS

Finger-clubbing is enlargement of the end of the digits. The cause is uncertain but might be hypoxia and circulating hormones such as erythropoietin. Clubbing can be hereditary but is usually acquired (Table 4.2).

COMA

A coma is profound unconsciousness in which the person is alive but unable to react or respond to stimuli. Coma results from central nervous system (CNS) diseases and conditions that affect CNS function, especially brain trauma, stroke, tumour, epilepsy, infection (e.g. meningitis), metabolic abnormalities (diabetic coma, ketoacidosis or electrolyte abnormality – hypernatraemia, hypercalcaemia), intoxication (e.g. alcohol, drugs of abuse, analgesics, anticonvulsants, antihistamines,

benzodiazepines, digoxin, heavy metals, hydrocarbons, barbiturates, insulin, lithium, organophosphates, phencyclidine, phenothiazines, salicylates or tricyclic antidepressants), shock, hypoxia or hypotension (arrhythmia, heart failure).

Persistent coma is termed the vegetative state. Level of consciousness is assessed by the Glasgow Coma Scale (Ch. 24).

CONFUSION

The confused patient has fluctuating consciousness and impaired orientation and short-term memory, and is usually more confused at night. Causes are multiple and include old age, dementia and most of the causes of coma. See also "delirium". Delusions or hallucinations can cause severe agitation. The confused patient should receive immediate medical attention since brain damage may result from many of the causes (see 'Coma'). Confusional states need to be differentiated from dementia, in which there are similar disturbances of orientation and memory, with unimpaired consciousness.

CONSTIPATION

Constipation is the passage of small amounts of hard, dry faeces, usually fewer than three times a week. If they do not have a bowel movement every day, some people believe they are constipated or irregular – but there are no criteria for 'normal'. Constipation is the most common gastrointestinal complaint.

Common causes include: lifestyle habits; inadequate dietary fibre, liquids or exercise; changes in life or routine, such as pregnancy, older age and travel; abuse of laxatives; or ignoring the urge to have a bowel movement. Codeine, opioids, antacids that contain aluminium, antispasmodics, antidepressants, iron supplements, diuretics and anticonvulsants may be implicated. More important but less common causes include colorectal disease (obstruction, scar tissue [adhesions]), diverticulosis, tumours, strictures, irritable bowel syndrome and Hirschsprung disease. Constipation may also be caused by systemic disease, such as neurological disorders (multiple sclerosis, Parkinson disease, chronic idiopathic intestinal pseudo-obstruction, stroke, spinal cord injuries), metabolic and endocrine conditions (diabetes, thyroid dysfunction, uraemia), or immunological disorders (amyloidosis, lupus, scleroderma).

COUGH

A cough is a sudden, voluntary or involuntary, explosive expiratory manœuvre that intends to clear material (sputum) from the airways. Transient cough may simply be a mechanism to expel mucus or an inhaled foreign body. Cough is typical of respiratory, and sometimes of cardiac, disorders. Angiotensin-converting enzyme inhibitors (ACEIs) may also produce a cough.

A morning cough persisting until sputum is expectorated typifies chronic bronchitis. A cough that is provoked by exposure to cold air or during exercise may suggest asthma. Cough associated with rhinitis or wheezing or that is seasonal may be allergic. Cough induced by postural change may suggest chronic lung abscess, tuberculosis, bronchiectasis or a tumour. Cough associated with eating suggests a swallowing disturbance, or possibly pharyngeal pouch or tracheo-oesophageal fistula. A persistent cough should be taken seriously and tumours and infections excluded. See also "haemoptysis"

CYANOSIS

Cyanosis is a bluish or purplish tinge to the skin due to very low oxygen saturation (SaO_2) and thus excess reduced (deoxygenated) haemoglobin. Approximately 5 g/dL of reduced haemoglobin has to be present in the capillaries to generate the dark blue colour of cyanosis. For this reason, patients who are anaemic may be hypoxaemic without showing any cyanosis.

Peripheral cyanosis is a dusky or bluish tinge to the fingers and toes. When unaccompanied by hypoxaemia, it is caused by peripheral vasoconstriction as in the cold, especially in Raynaud disease.

Central cyanosis (where the colour is also seen in the lips or the mouth) is more serious and is usually an indication of hypoxaemia because of cardiac failure or respiratory disease, or both in cor pulmonale. Many factors, from natural skin pigment to room lighting, can affect detection of cyanosis and, if hypoxaemia is suspected, measurement of the oxygen level is necessary (arterial blood gas determination, pulse oximetry). Central cyanosis is an indication of gross hypoxia; such patients needing conscious sedation must be dealt with in hospital.

DELIRIUM

Delirium is a state of mental confusion, caused by a disturbance in normal brain functioning, which develops quickly and usually fluctuates in intensity. More frequent in older people, delirium affects 1 in 10 hospitalized patients and is common in many terminal illnesses.

In contrast to dementia, delirium appears quickly, in hours or days, with a fluctuating level of consciousness. There may be limited awareness of the environment; confusion or disorientation (especially of time); memory impairment, especially of recent events; hallucinations, illusions and misinterpreted stimuli; mood disturbance, possibly including anxiety, euphoria or depression; and language or speech impairment. There are many possible causes of delirium, including:

- metabolic encephalopathy – hepatic or renal failure, diabetes, hyperthyroidism or hypothyroidism, vitamin deficiencies, fluid and electrolytes imbalance or severe dehydration
- drug intoxication – alcohol, anticholinergics (including atropine, hyoscine [scopolamine], chlorpromazine and diphenhydramine), sedatives (including barbiturates and benzodiazepines), antidepressants (including lithium, anticonvulsant drugs, corticosteroids), anticancer drugs (including methotrexate, procarbazine, cimetidine) and street drugs (e.g. marijuana, lysergic acid diethylamide [LSD], amphetamines, cocaine, opioids, phenylcyclidine, inhalants, legal highs)
- poisons – e.g. carbon monoxide, heavy metals, insecticides (e.g. parathion and carbaryl), mushrooms (such as *Amanita* spp.) and plants (jimsonweed [*Datura*] and morning glory [*Ipomoea* spp.])
- fever, cerebral disorders (infection, head trauma, epilepsy, cerebrovascular events, brain tumour), blood gas changes (hypoxaemia, hypercapnia) or following surgery.

DEMENTIA

Dementia is a progressive loss of mental ability, including the ability to remember, think and reason (Ch. 10). The most common features include changes in memory, behaviour, mood and personality, and difficulty in communicating or understanding. Alzheimer disease is the most common form and responsible for about 50% of cases. Vascular dementia is the second leading cause and is a result of several TIAs. Other causes include parkinsonism, Huntington disease, human immunodeficiency virus (HIV) infection and Creutzfeldt–Jakob disease. Dementia may be reversible if caused by brain diseases or conditions such as tumours, depression or alcoholism.

DIARRHOEA

Diarrhoea is defined as loose, watery stools passed more than three times in a day. Diarrhoea may be temporary, such as from an infection; this is common, usually lasts a day or two and resolves spontaneously. Prolonged diarrhoea can be a sign of other disorders, particularly intestinal disease such as infections: bacterial infections or toxins, such as preformed staphylococcal enterotoxin (from *S. aureus*) in contaminated food or water; viral infections; parasites; food intolerances (e.g. to lactose); drug reactions (such as to antibiotics like clindamycin, and antacids containing magnesium); intestinal diseases (inflammatory bowel disease, coeliac disease or irritable bowel syndrome); or after surgery (e.g. gastric surgery or cholecystectomy).

Where food hygiene is poor, diarrhoea can be life-threatening, especially if due to infections such as shigellosis (bacillary dysentery), *Escherichia coli* or cholera. The passing of blood in the stools is typical of severe diarrhoea – termed dysentery.

DIPLOPIA

Double vision (diplopia) is the simultaneous perception of two images of a single object displaced horizontally, vertically or diagonally (i.e. both

Table 4.3 *Causes of diplopia*

Structure involved	Site	Causes	Features that may be associated
Extraocular muscles	Orbit	Trauma	Middle-third facial fracture
		Exophthalmos	Thyrotoxicosis
		Myasthenia gravis	Myopathy
Cranial nerves III, IV and VI	Orbit	Trauma, tumour, sarcoid	Middle-third facial fracture
	Superior orbital fissure	Trauma, tumour, sarcoid	Often several muscles paralysed. Involvement of ophthalmic division of trigeminal. Pupil often normal
	Cavernous sinus	Aneurysms, infection, fistula, trauma	Similar to superior orbital fissure syndrome
	Skull base	Aneurysms, tumours, meningitis, fractures	May be involvement of single nerves; may be pupil dilatation
Cranial nerve nuclei	Brainstem	Vascular lesions, tumours, multiple sclerosis	May be involvement of trigeminal or facial nerves or complex neurological disorders

vertically and horizontally) in relation to each other. Diplopia is caused by misalignment of the eyes due to visual functional defects, mainly stemming from eye muscle or neurological disorders; by a structural defect in the eye's optical system; or by drugs (e.g. alcohol, phenytoin, carbamazepine or lamotrigine). Diplopia may be an occasional transient complication of dental LA injections, presumably because anaesthetic tracks to the inferior orbital fissure, where it can block orbital nerves. Diplopia is not uncommon after maxillofacial or head trauma (from assault, accident and/or alcohol or drugs) but usually resolves spontaneously within a few days or weeks. Persistent diplopia after trauma can be caused by blow-out fractures of the floor of the orbit, entrapment of (or damage to) the orbital muscles or damage to the suspensory ligament to the frontal process or the zygomatic bone. Later fibrous adhesions between the orbital periosteum and coverings of the eye may cause permanent limitation of movement, as may injury to cranial nerves III, IV and VI (Table 4.3). Paralytic strabismus is characterized by variable deviation of the ocular axes according to the position of gaze and is the usual type of strabismus that follows maxillofacial injuries.

DIZZINESS

Dizziness (vertigo) is a sensation of feeling unsteady or giddy, sometimes with a sensation of movement, spinning or floating. It is often due to disorders of the labyrinth. Movement of fluid in the semicircular canals signals the direction and speed of rotation of the head. Dizziness can also be due to central vestibular disorders (a problem in the brain or its connecting nerves); Ménière disease – an inner-ear fluid balance disorder that also causes fluctuating hearing loss and tinnitus (ringing in the ears); or perilymph fistula – a leakage of inner ear fluid to the middle ear. Dizziness can follow head injury or physical exertion; rarely, it has no known cause. Benign paroxysmal positional vertigo (a brief intense sensation of vertigo caused by a specific positional change of the head), labyrinthitis (inner ear infection) and vestibular neuronitis (a viral infection of the vestibular nerve) are other causes. Systemic disorders (vascular disorders) may occasionally be implicated.

DROOLING

See 'Sialorrhoea'.

DRY MOUTH

Important causes of dry mouth (hyposalivation) are drugs, irradiation of major salivary glands, Sjögren syndrome and infections (Box 4.1).

Box 4.1 *Causes of dry mouth*

Iatrogenic
- Drugs (antimuscarinics, sympathomimetics)
- Cancer therapy (irradiation of salivary glands, radioactive iodine, cytotoxic drugs)
- Graft-versus-host disease

Salivary gland disease
- Aplasia
- Sjögren syndrome
- Sarcoidosis
- Infection with HIV, human T-lymphotropic virus 1 (HTLV-1), hepatitis C or other viruses
- Infiltrates (amyloidosis; haemochromatosis)
- Cystic fibrosis
- Others

Dehydration
- Diabetes mellitus
- Diabetes insipidus
- Renal failure
- Haemorrhage
- Other causes of fluid loss or deprivation

If dry mouth occurs when salivary flow is normal, it may be psychogenic. Smoking and alcohol use aggravate the complaint of dry mouth – xerostomia.

DUPUYTREN CONTRACTURE

Dupuytren contracture affects the hands and fingers, cause one or more finger, on one or both hands, to bend into the palm (Fig. 4.2). Apart from familial cases, diabetes, epilepsy, heavy smoking and heavy alcohol consumption have also been linked to the contracture.

DYSPHAGIA

Swallowing is a process by which food and liquid move from the mouth, through the pharynx and then the oesophagus, and into the stomach. Each individual swallows 500–2000 times per day and swallowing also occurs during sleep. It is divided into three phases:

- Oral – food is reduced to a bolus, chewed, mixed with saliva and then transported from the anterior to the posterior oral cavity.

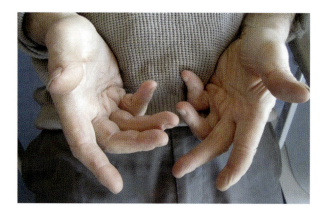

Fig. 4.2 Dupuytren contracture affecting both hands.

- Pharyngeal – the velopharyngeal opening completely closes, the hyoid and larynx ascend and the epiglottis folds down. The tongue base makes contact with the pharyngeal wall to form a seal and the pharyngeal muscles start to contract. The laryngeal inlet closes and the vocal cords adduct. The cricopharyngeus then relaxes, the upper oesophageal inlet opens and apnoea prevents food from entering the airway.
- Oesophageal – the upper oesophageal sphincter opens and peristalsis carries the bolus through the oesophagus to the stomach. This phase may take 10–12 seconds.

Cranial nerves IX to XII, and the pharyngeal muscles in particular, are essential to swallowing (Box 4.2). Dysphagia is 'difficulty in swallowing' (from the Greek *dys* meaning difficulty or disordered, and *phagia* 'to eat') and has many causes; older people in particular may develop swallowing dysfunction. This is due mainly to conditions such as cerebrovascular events or Parkinson's disease. People with mental impairment often have cognitive and physiological impairments that may result in dysphagia.

Dysphagia may be secondary to defects in any stage of the swallowing process:

- *Neurological causes* – may be fixed or progressive (Table 4.4)
- *Mechanical and obstructive causes*:
  - Infections, e.g. tonsillitis, dental abscess, tuberculosis
  - Traumatic injuries to the face/neck
  - Reduced muscle compliance
  - Zenker diverticulum (pharyngeal pouch)
  - Thyromegaly
  - Oesophageal strictures
  - Oesophageal malignancies
  - Lung malignancies/lymphomas
  - Head/neck malignancies
  - Cervical osteophytes.
- *Drug-induced, caused by*:
  - medications affecting the oesophageal muscles, e.g. oxybutynin, tolterodine
  - combinations of medications that produce a dry mouth, e.g. diuretics, calcium-channel blockers, antihistamines; antipsychotic/neuroleptic drugs may cause a dry mouth and, additionally, some can cause movement disorders that may affect the muscles of the face and tongue used in swallowing (e.g. haloperidol, risperidone, clozapine)
  - local anaesthetics used for dental treatment, which may cause a temporary loss of sensation and ability to swallow

  - drugs affecting the CNS and swallowing (antiepileptic medication, benzodiazepines, narcotics and smooth muscle relaxants).

Swallowing may be assessed by watching for signs of leakage from the mouth, facial weakness, poor muscular coordination, delayed pharyngeal/laryngeal elevation, choking, breathlessness and changes in voice quality after swallowing. The 'gold standard' is videofluoroscopy

---

Box 4.2 *Causes of dysphagia*

Psychogenic
- Globus hystericus

Organic
Mouth
- Dry mouth
- Inflammatory or neoplastic lesions

Pharynx
- Inflammatory or neoplastic lesions
- Foreign bodies
- Sideropenic dysphagia (Paterson–Brown-Kelly syndrome)
- Pouch

Oesophagus
- Benign stricture
- Inflammatory or neoplastic lesions
- Scleroderma
- External pressure from mediastinal lymph nodes

Neurological and neuromuscular causes
- Achalasia
- Cerebellar disease
- Cerebral palsy
- Cerebrovascular accidents
- Cerebrovascular disease (pseudobulbar palsy)
- Dermatomyositis
- Diphtheria
- Guillain–Barré syndrome
- Motor neuron disease
- Muscular dystrophies
- Myasthenia gravis
- Myopathies
- Parkinsonism
- Poliomyelitis
- Syringobulbia

Table 4.4 *Neurological causes of dysphagia*

Non-progressive	Progressive
Cerebral palsy	Amyotrophic lateral sclerosis
Cerebrovascular events	Cerebrovascular events
Post-surgery	Dementia
Traumatic brain injury	Head and neck malignancies
	Huntington disease
	Multiple sclerosis
	Muscular/myotonic dystrophy
	Myasthenia gravis
	Parkinson disease
	Supranuclear palsy

(VFS; modified barium swallow), in which radio-opaque barium liquid is swallowed by the patient and moving images of swallowing are captured. Fibreoptic endoscopic evaluation of swallowing (FEES) with nasoendoscopy has an advantage over VFS in that it is a bedside procedure with no radiation exposure.

Swallowing problems may lead to inhalation of either oropharyngeal or gastric contents into the airway. Aspiration may lead to chest infections, which are the leading cause of death in such people. The main risk of dysphagia is choking if the passage of air to the lungs is blocked by a foreign body; this is a precursor to asphyxiation. Signs of choking include coughing, gagging, inability to speak, breathe or cry, loss of consciousness and cyanosis. If the obstruction is not successfully removed, the patient is at risk from asphyxiation and ultimately death.

The major dental concern when treating patients with dysphagia is the risk of aspiration during treatment, which may lead to choking or aspiration pneumonia.

DYSPNOEA

Dyspnoea is difficulty in breathing. Functional causes include anxiety, panic disorders and hyperventilation. Organic causes include cardiac and respiratory disorders and anaemia. Dyspnoea is typically exacerbated by exercise, but may occur at rest and persist or worsen when lying down (orthopnoea). Paroxysmal nocturnal dyspnoea (cardiac asthma) is a sudden attack of severe dyspnoea due to pulmonary oedema that wakes the patient from sleep with a terrifying sensation of suffocation.

DYSRHYTHMIAS

See Chapter 5.

DYSURIA

Dysuria is the sensation of pain or burning on urination. It is more common in women than in men, and then bacterial cystitis (usually after intercourse) is the commonest cause. In men too, dysuria is usually a result of urinary tract infection – in younger patients most often caused by a sexually transmitted organism such as *Chlamydia trachomatis*. In those over 35 years, coliform bacteria predominate and infection typically results from urinary stasis secondary to prostatic hyperplasia.

Dysuria in either sex may occasionally be caused by renal calculus, genitourinary malignancy, spondyloarthropathy and medications.

EARACHE

As aircraft descend, pressure rises even in the normal middle ear, and this can cause excruciating pain. Earache (otalgia) is commonly due to middle ear infection (otitis media) and is especially common in children, often following a sore throat or cold. There is severe pain and often a temporary loss of hearing; with severe infections, the ear drum may perforate, causing a leakage of pus from the ear. Tumours in the middle ear are uncommon but include cholesteatoma. Pain may be referred to the ear from elsewhere, such as tongue cancer, the antra, dental abscesses and temporomandibular disorders.

ENCOPRESIS

Encopresis is the soiling of underwear with stool by children who are past the age of toilet training, but it is not considered a medical condition unless the child is at least 4 years old. A large amount of hard stool is in the intestine, and stool leaks around this mass and out through the anus. The best way to prevent encopresis is to avoid constipation by eating a varied diet with plenty of fruits and vegetables and wholegrain bread and cereals.

EPILEPSY

See Chapter 13.

EPISTAXIS (NOSEBLEEDS)

Most nosebleeds are caused by nose-picking, minor nose injuries, the common cold, or vigorous nose-blowing or sneezing. Rarely, they may be caused by a foreign body lodged in the nose, barotrauma, chemical irritants, drugs (e.g. anticoagulants, anti-platelet agents, non-steroidal anti-inflammatory drugs [NSAIDs] or vitamin E), maxillofacial or nasal surgery, hereditary telangiectasia or thrombocytopenia.

EROSION OF TEETH

Tooth erosion can result from exposure to dietary acidic sources (carbonated drinks, citrus fruits and juices, pickles, vinegar, wine) or some drugs (e.g. chewable vitamin C); regurgitated gastric contents (anorexia nervosa, bulimia, gastro-oesophageal reflux or alcoholism); industrial sources (various acids); or, rarely, other sources (e.g. swimming-pool water).

EXOPHTHALMOS

See 'Proptosis'.

FAINTING (VASOVAGAL SYNCOPE)

Syncope, commonly called fainting or 'passing out', is a temporary loss of consciousness due to a sudden decline of brain blood flow. Syncope can occur in otherwise healthy people and affects all age groups, but does so more often in older people. Vasovagal syncope is a reflex mediated by autonomic nerves in which there is splanchnic and skeletal muscle vasodilatation, bradycardia and thus diminished cerebral blood flow, leading to loss of consciousness. Fainting can be precipitated by psychological factors (e.g. pain, or fear at the sight of a needle or blood); postural changes; hypoxia; or carotid sinus syndrome. The latter is usually seen in older patients in whom mild pressure on the neck causes a vagal reaction, leading to syncope with bradycardia or cardiac arrest. Vasovagal syncope is treated by having the patient lie down with their legs raised (Ch. 1).

Recurrent syncope with complex associated symptoms in so-called neurally mediated syncope (NMS) is associated with any of the following: preceding or succeeding sleepiness, preceding visual disturbance ('spots before the eyes'), sweating and light-headedness. Other types of syncope include:

■ *carotid sinus* – happens because of carotid artery constriction after turning the head, while shaving, or when wearing a tight collar

- *vertebrobasilar* – occurs when arterial disease in the upper spinal cord or lower brain causes syncope if there is a reduction in blood supply, which may occur with extending the neck
- *cardiogenic* – is more common in older patients, and includes arrhythmic, obstructive, ischaemic, drug or cardiomyopathic causes
- *orthostatic (postural)* – is as common as vasovagal syncope but caused by a change in body posture, most often associated with movement from lying or sitting to a standing position; it does not necessarily signal any serious underlying disease. The most susceptible individuals are older frail people, or persons dehydrated from hot environments or inadequate fluid intake
- *neuropathic* – may be seen in neurological disorders such as parkinsonism, postural orthostatic tachycardia syndrome (POTS), and diabetic or other types of neuropathy
- *drug-related* – is caused by diuretics, beta-blockers, calcium antagonists, ACEI, nitrates, antipsychotics, antihistamines, L-dopa, narcotics and alcohol.

FACIAL PARALYSIS

See Chapter 13.

FACIAL SENSORY LOSS

See Chapter 13.

FEVER (PYREXIA)

Normal body temperature (37°C) has a diurnal rhythm, lower in the morning before dawn and higher in the afternoon. Temperature control activities balance heat loss and production. An abnormal rise in body temperature is caused by either hyperthermia or fever. In fever, the body temperature controls are functioning correctly, but the hypothalamic set point is raised by exogenous or endogenous pyrogens; temperature rises as the body responds to cytokines such as interleukin-1, produced by microorganisms or immunocytes.

The main causes of fever include: infections, tumours, drugs (e.g. chemotherapy drugs, biological response modifiers, and antibiotics such as vancomycin and amphotericin), neuroleptic malignant syndrome, blood transfusion reactions, connective tissue disorders, cerebrovascular events and or graft-versus-host disease.

Fever may, in children under 6 years, be complicated by seizures (febrile convulsions) and, in older persons when the hypothalamus temperature-regulating centres may function poorly, by arrhythmias, heart failure, cerebral hypoxia and confusion.

GASTROINTESTINAL BLEEDING

Bleeding in the digestive tract can be the result of many different conditions, some of which are life-threatening. Bleeding can sometimes be unnoticed (occult or hidden bleeding), but the faecal occult blood test (FOBT) checks stool samples for traces of blood, detecting bleeding from almost anywhere in the digestive tract. Causes of gastrointestinal bleeding, apart from drugs such as NSAIDs, include lesions in: the oesophagus (oesophagitis [hiatus hernia], varices, tears [Mallory–Weiss syndrome, after severe vomiting], cancer); the stomach (ulcers,

gastritis, cancer); the small intestine (duodenal ulcer, inflammatory bowel disease); and the large intestine and rectum (haemorrhoids, infections, ulcerative colitis, diverticular disease, polyps or cancer).

The appearance of blood in the faeces depends upon the site and severity of bleeding. Bleeding from the oesophagus, stomach or duodenum can cause black or tarry stools (melaena). The stool may be mixed with darker blood if the bleeding is higher in the colon. Blood originating from the rectum or lower colon is bright red.

Vomited blood may be bright red or have the appearance of coffee grounds.

Endoscopy permits examination of the oesophagus, stomach, duodenum (oesophagoduodenoscopy), colon (colonoscopy) and rectum (sigmoidoscopy), and facilitates biopsies. Magnetic resonance imaging (MRI), computed tomography (CT), barium radiography, angiography, radionuclide scans and ultrasound can also be used to locate sources of chronic occult gastrointestinal bleeding.

GINGIVAL SWELLING

Gingival swelling may be localized or generalized. It is usually drug-induced gingival overgrowth (DIGO), but occasionally is due to a systemic disease (Box 4.3).

HAEMATEMESIS

Haematemesis (blood in the vomit) typically results from blood regurgitation from the gastrointestinal tract (mouth, pharynx, oesophagus, stomach and small intestine). Conditions that cause haematemesis include bleeding ulcer(s), neoplasms, angiomas or varices in the stomach, duodenum or oesophagus; prolonged and vigorous retching, which may tear small blood vessels of the throat or oesophagus; drugs; and ingested blood (e.g. swallowed after a nosebleed) or gastroenteritis. It may be difficult to distinguish haematemesis from coughing up blood from the lung (haemoptysis) or a nosebleed (bloody postnasal drainage), but it can also cause blood in the stool.

HAEMATURIA

Haematuria, blood in the urine, typically originates in the urinary tract (urethra, bladder or ureter) but, in women, vaginal/uterine blood may appear in the urine and, in men, a bloody ejaculate is usually due to a prostate disorder. Causes of haematuria include: haematological disorders (e.g. coagulopathies, sickle cell disease, renal vein thrombosis or thrombocytopenias); renal and urinary tract diseases (calculi, benign familial haematuria, infection, tumours, renal vein thrombosis, systemic lupus erythematosus, haemolytic–uraemic syndrome, anaphylactoid (Henoch–Schönlein) purpura, polycystic kidney disease, glomerulonephritis, congenital anomalies); prostatitis; hypercalciuria (increased calcium in urine); urethral ulceration or meatal stenosis; trauma (fractured pelvis, renal trauma, urethral trauma, surgical procedures, including catheterization, circumcision, surgery and biopsy); or drugs (anticoagulants, cyclophosphamide, metirosine, oxyphenbutazone, phenylbutazone or tiabendazole).

HAEMOPTYSIS

Haemoptysis is the coughing or expectoration or spitting up of blood or bloody mucus from the lungs. It may be confused with bleeding

Box 4.3 *Causes of gingival enlargement*

Generalized
Congenital
- Aspartylglycosaminuria
- Fucosidosis
- Hereditary gingival fibromatosis and related disorders
- Hypoplasminogenaemia
- Infantile systemic hyalinosis
- Leprechaunism (Donohue syndrome)
- Mucopolysaccharidosis I–H
- Pfeiffer syndrome
- Primary amyloidosis

Acquired
Haematological
- Acute myeloid leukaemia
- Pre-leukaemic leukaemia(s)
- Aplastic anaemia
- Vitamin C deficiency

Drugs
- Phenytoin
- Ciclosporin
- Calcium-channel blockers

Localized
Congenital
- Fabry syndrome (angiokeratoma corporis diffusum universale)
- Cowden syndrome (multiple hamartoma and neoplasia syndrome)
- Tuberous sclerosis
- Sturge–Weber angiomatosis
- Congenital gingival granular cell tumour

Acquired
Epulides
- Pregnancy epulis
- Fibrous epulis
- Giant-cell epulis (e.g. secondary to primary hyperparathyroidism)

Granulomatous conditions
- Pyogenic granuloma
- Sarcoidosis
- Crohn disease
- Orofacial granulomatosis
- Wegener granulomatosis

Infections with human papillomavirus (HPV)
- Papilloma
- Condyloma
- Warts
- Heck disease

Tumours
- Squamous cell carcinoma
- Lymphomas
- Langerhans cell tumours
- Multiple myeloma
- Kaposi sarcoma
- Plasmacytomas
- Other primary and secondary neoplasms

from the mouth, nose, throat or gastrointestinal tract. Apart from a simple recent nosebleed and irritation of the throat from violent coughing, causes may include diagnostic tests (bronchoscopy, laryngoscopy, biopsy, mediastinoscopy or spirometry), pulmonary infection, bronchitis, bronchiectasis, cancer, embolus, oedema, cystic fibrosis and systemic lupus erythematosus.

HALITOSIS (ORAL MALODOUR)

Volatile sulphur compounds (VSC) of microbial origin are at least partly responsible for oral malodour (bad breath). Oral malodour is common on awakening (morning breath), and then transient and rarely of any special significance, probably resulting from increased microbial metabolic activity during sleep, aggravated by a physiological reduction in salivary flow, lack of nocturnal physiological oral cleansing (e.g. movement of the facial and oral muscles) and variable oral hygiene procedures prior to sleep. Starvation can lead to a similar malodour.

Malodour at other times may be due to ingestion of certain food and drinks, such as spices, garlic, onion, durian, cabbage, cauliflower and radish, or of habits such as smoking tobacco or drinking alcohol, and is usually transient. It is considered to arise from both intraoral (food debris) and extraoral (respiratory) origins. Halitosis is most frequently due to oral infection (such as the tongue flora or periodontal disease), and rarely stems from systemic causes (Table 4.5).

HEADACHE

See Chapter 13.

HEARING IMPAIRMENT

Hearing loss is categorized on which part of the auditory system is damaged. There are three basic types of hearing loss: conductive, sensorineural and mixed.

Conductive hearing loss is due to middle or external ear disorders – when sounds that should be carried from the tympanic membrane to the inner ear are blocked by, for example, foreign bodies, wax, fluid, infection or abnormal bone growth.

Sensorineural hearing loss is due to defects of the cochlear nerve or its central connections – as in damage to the inner ear or auditory nerve (e.g. in birth defects, head injury, surgery, tumours, certain drugs, hypertension or stroke). Hearing can be lost by exposure to very loud noises, (pop music, explosions, loud machinery, etc.), particularly for long periods.

Deafness is common and, in 30% of cases, is hereditary. It may occasionally be associated with congenital malformations, such as first arch syndromes. Age-related changes include especially *presbycusis* – the most common hearing problem in older people and linked to inner ear changes.

Hearing aids are available to help. Differing in design, size, amount of amplification, ease of handling, volume control and special features, all have similar components that include a microphone to detect sound, an amplifier to make the sound louder, and a receiver (miniature loudspeaker) to deliver the sound into the ear. Bone-anchored hearing aids are implantable devices that act by directly stimulating the inner ear through the bone. Hearing assistive devices are available for use with or without hearing aids. Electromagnetic interference can be an issue with these aids (Ch. 5).

People with a severe-to-profound hearing loss who cannot be helped with hearing aids may find cochlear implants of benefit. Cochlear implants stimulate the auditory nerve directly, helping sensorineural

Table 4.5 *Main causes of halitosis*

Causes	Examples
Plaque-related gingival and periodontal disease	Gingivitis
	Periodontitis
	Necrotizing ulcerative gingivitis
	Pericoronitis
	Abscesses
Oral ulceration	Systemic disease (inflammatory/infectious disorders, cutaneous, gastrointestinal and haematological disease)
	Malignancy
	Local causes
	Aphthae
	Drugs
Hyposalivation	Drugs
	Sjögren syndrome
	Radiotherapy
	Chemotherapy
Tongue coating	Poor hygiene
Wearing dental appliances	Poor hygiene
Dental conditions	Food packing
Bone diseases	Jaw dry sockets
	Osteomyelitis
	Osteonecrosis
	Malignancy
Respiratory system	Sinusitis
	Antral malignancy
	Cleft palate
	Foreign bodies in the nose
	Nasal malignancy
	Tonsilloliths
	Tonsillitis
	Pharyngeal malignancy
	Lung infections
	Bronchitis
	Bronchiectasis
	Lung malignancy
Gastrointestinal tract	Oesophageal diverticulum
	Gastro-oesophageal reflux disease
	Malignancy
Metabolic disorders (blood-borne)	Acetone-like smell in uncontrolled diabetes
	Uraemic breath in renal failure
	Foetor hepaticus in liver disease
	Trimethylaminuria (fish odour syndrome)
	Hypermethioninaemia
	Cystinosis
Drugs (blood-borne)	Amphetamines
	Chloral hydrate
	Cytotoxic agents
	Dimethyl sulfoxide (DMSO)
	Disulfiram
	Nitrates and nitrites
	Phenothiazines
	Solvent abuse
Psychogenic causes	

hearing loss. They have external parts behind the ear (receiver) and internal (surgically implanted) electrodes. People with cochlear implants are more likely to contract bacterial meningitis than those without. In addition, some children who are candidates for cochlear implants have inner ear anatomical abnormalities that may increase their risk for meningitis. The Centers for Disease Control (CDC) recommend that these children receive pneumococcal vaccination.

Precautions are needed for electrosurgery in patients with cochlear implants; use bipolar where possible. If monopolar diathermy is necessary, ensure that the distance between the active electrode and the return electrode is as short as possible by using a return electrode mat. It is always important when communicating with people with hearing impairment to face them, without a face mask, and to speak clearly, in the absence of extraneous noise. The sign language ('deaf') alphabet helps (Fig. 4.3).

HEART FAILURE

Heart failure is usually the result of cardiac disease, but an otherwise normal heart can fail as a consequence of overload (e.g. severe anaemia). The common causes are ischaemic heart disease, hypertension, valve disease and chronic obstructive pulmonary disease. Failure can affect either the left or the right side of the heart predominantly, but left-sided heart failure is more common. Failure of one side of the heart usually leads to failure of the other. Right-sided failure often follows left-sided failure, particularly when there is mitral stenosis, and causes congestive cardiac failure (CCF). See also Chapter 5.

HEPATOMEGALY

Hepatomegaly is enlargement of the liver beyond its normal size. The lower edge of the liver normally comes just to the lower edge of the ribs (costal margin) on the right side and it cannot be palpated. The diagnosis must be confirmed by imaging.

Causes include infections (viral, bacterial or parasitic, e.g. viral hepatitis, infectious mononucleosis); malignancy (leukaemias, tumour metastases, neuroblastoma, hepatocellular carcinoma); anaemias; storage diseases (Niemann–Pick disease, hereditary fructose intolerance, glycogen storage disease); heart failure; congenital heart disease; toxins (e.g. alcohol); primary biliary cirrhosis; sarcoidosis; sclerosing cholangitis; haemolytic–uraemic syndrome; or Reye syndrome.

HIRSUTISM (HYPERTRICHOSIS)

Hirsutism is the excessive growth of dark, coarse body hair in women (and children), and typically appears in a male distribution pattern. Excessive facial hair is usually the most troublesome aspect. Signs of masculinization, such as voice deepening, increased muscle mass, decreased breast size, increased genital size and menstrual irregularities, may be associated.

Common causes of hirsutism include: genetic factors, endocrine abnormalities (polycystic ovarian syndrome, Cushing syndrome, adrenocortical carcinoma, congenital adrenal hyperplasia, precocious puberty, pregnancy, menopause, ovarian tumour or cancer, ovarian overproduction of androgens) or drugs (androgens, aminoglutethimide, calcium-channel blockers, ciclosporin, finasteride, phenytoin, glucocorticoids, metoclopramide and minoxidil).

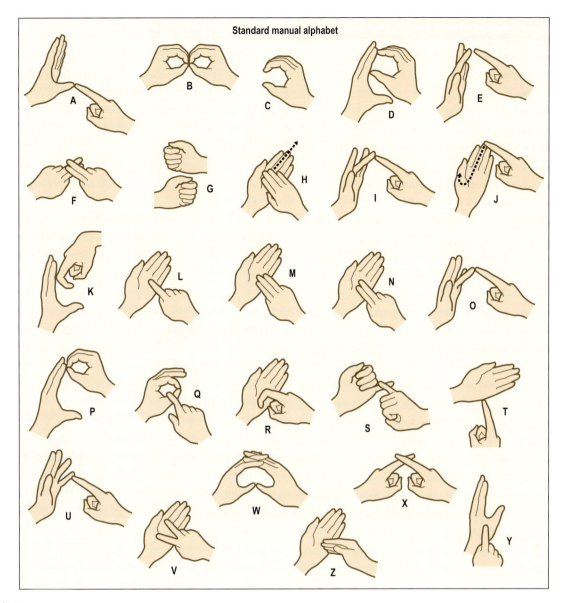

Fig. 4.3 Manual alphabet.

HOARSENESS

Hoarseness is usually due to acute laryngitis, secondary to excessive talking/singing/shouting, or caused by a viral upper respiratory infection such as a cold, and is self-limiting. Chronic laryngitis is the commonest cause of persistent hoarseness; predisposing factors are usually smoking and voice abuse. However, any patient with hoarseness persisting for over 1 month should be investigated for trauma to the vocal cords (from persistent shouting or singing – singer's nodules); thyroid cancer; laryngeal cancer; surgical damage to the vagus or recurrent laryngeal nerve during thyroid or cardiovascular surgery; and psychological problems.

HOSTILITY

Hostile (acutely disturbed) patients can totally disrupt their environment and harm those with whom they come into contact. Frequently, the cause is drug/alcohol intoxication or an acute psychosis. Otherwise, the disorder may be due to infection or withdrawal of drugs (alcohol or other drugs of abuse). If the patient appears unresponsive to

reason, no treatment should be attempted, but the physician or psychiatrist should be contacted. No attempt should be made to sedate the patient; benzodiazepines usually worsen violently psychotic behaviour and adequate doses of phenothiazines, such as chlorpromazine, can cause severe hypotension. If the patient becomes violent, the police have to be called to restrain them; ambulance personnel cannot usually manage such cases. The usual treatment, once the patient has been forcibly restrained, is to give haloperidol by injection.

HYPERPIGMENTATION

Most pigmentation is racial in origin. Local pigmentations, such as a tattoo, are common. Systemic causes of hyperpigmentation, apart from suntan, are rare (Box 4.4).

HYPERTHERMIA

Hyperthermia is an unusual rise in body temperature above normal, caused by disordered body temperature control. A group of inherited

Box 4.4 *Causes of hyperpigmentation*

Congenital
- Racial (even in some Caucasians)
- Naevi
- Syndromes

  Peutz–Jeghers syndrome: oral and perioral hyperpigmentation with small intestine polyps

  Carney complex: lentiginosis due to adrenal disease, and multiple neoplasia such as myxomas of skin, heart and breast, schwannomas, pituitary adenomas, testicular and thyroid tumours

  Laugier–Hunziker syndrome: oral and perioral hyperpigmentation with nail pigmentation

  NAME syndrome (naevi, atrial myxoma, myxoid neurofibromas and ephelides)

  LAMB syndrome (lentigines, atrial myxoma, mucocutaneous myxoma, blue naevi)

  LEOPARD syndrome: lentigines with hypertrophic cardiomyopathy, or arterial dissections

Acquired
Endocrine or metabolic
- Addison disease
- Adrenocorticotropic hormone (ACTH) therapy
- ACTH-producing tumours (lung cancer)
- Haemochromatosis
- Nelson syndrome

Neoplastic
- Melanoma
- Kaposi sarcoma

Foreign bodies
Drugs
- Smoking
- Antimalarials
- Cytotoxics (particularly busulfan)
- Oral contraceptives
- Phenothiazines
- Minocycline
- Zidovudine
- Clofazimine

Others
- Human immunodeficiency syndrome (HIV) infection and acquired immunodeficiency syndrome (AIDS)

muscle problems, characterized by muscle breakdown following certain stimuli, is termed malignant hyperthermia. Attacks can be precipitated by anaesthesia, extreme exercise, fever or certain drugs (Ch. 23).

HYPERVENTILATION

See 'Tachypnoea'.

HYPODONTIA

Most missing teeth are caused by tooth extraction. Hypodontia is the developmental absence of teeth and affects about 5% of the population. The teeth most commonly missing, apart from third molars, are the mandibular second premolars, maxillary lateral incisors and maxillary second premolars. Severe hypodontia is the absence of six or more teeth and can be a feature of ectodermal dysplasia, Down syndrome, hemifacial microsomia and van der Woude syndrome.

HYPOGLYCAEMIA

Hypoglycaemia (low blood sugar) is when blood glucose levels drop, causing the patient to feel weak, drowsy, confused, hungry, aggressive and dizzy. Pallor, headache, irritability, trembling, sweating, rapid pulse and a cold, clammy feeling are other signs and, in severe cases, unconsciousness or coma can result.

Hypoglycaemia is caused by diabetes (insulin or drug overdose, missing or delaying a meal, eating too little food for the amount of insulin taken); exercising too strenuously, particularly when associated with beta-blocker medication; prolonged fasting; certain foods and drinks (alcohol, aspirin [in some children], unripe Jamaican ackee fruit); liver disease; hormonal states (early pregnancy, insulinomas, growth hormone deficiency, breast cancer and adrenal cancer); or hereditary enzyme deficiencies (hereditary fructose intolerance [attacks of hypoglycaemia, marked by seizures, vomiting and unconsciousness] or galactosaemia [also causes vomiting, weight loss and cataracts]).

HYPOTENSION

See 'Low blood pressure'.

HYPOTHERMIA

Cold exposure is the main cause of hypothermia (low body temperature). Conditions that may predispose include drugs (alcohol, anxiolytics, antidepressants, antiemetics and some over-the-counter cold remedies); illnesses that restrict activity (stroke or other causes of paralysis, severe arthritis, Parkinson disease, Alzheimer disease); or hypothyroidism.

IMPOTENCE

Impotence is the term used particularly for erectile dysfunction (ED), lack of sexual desire and ejaculation or orgasm problems. ED is the repeated inability to achieve or maintain an erection adequate for intercourse. Causes of impotence are psychological factors, including stress, anxiety, guilt, depression, low self-esteem and fear of sexual failure; smoking; drugs (antihypertensives, antihistamines, antidepressants, finasteride, tranquillizers, appetite suppressants and cimetidine); various diseases (diabetes, renal disease, alcoholism, multiple sclerosis, atherosclerosis, neurological disease); hormonal abnormalities (inadequate testosterone); and injuries to the nerves or conditions that impair penile blood flow. These include trauma in particular (to penis, spinal cord, prostate, bladder or pelvis), including that from surgery (especially radical prostate surgery). Sildenafil citrate (Viagra) is effective treatment.

INSOMNIA

See Chapter 13.

JAUNDICE

Jaundice (icterus) is the accumulation of, and colouring of the skin and mucous membranes by, bilirubin, if it appears in excessive amounts or is not conjugated or excreted. Jaundice can be a manifestation of haemolytic anaemias, liver disease, biliary disease or pancreatic disorders (Ch. 9).

LOW BLOOD PRESSURE (HYPOTENSION)

The main causes of hypotension are described here.
Drugs causes include:

- alcohol
- analgesics
- antidepressants
- anxiolytics
- diuretics.

Orthostatic hypotension, including postprandial orthostatic hypotension, is brought on by a sudden change in body position, most often when shifting from lying down to standing. This type of hypotension usually lasts only a few seconds or minutes. It most commonly affects older adults, those with high blood pressure, and persons with parkinsonism, excessive use of diuretics, vasodilators or other drugs, dehydration, Addison disease, atherosclerosis or dysautonomias, such as in diabetes.
Neurally mediated hypotension (NMH) occurs when a person has been standing for a long time and most often affects young adults and children.
Disease causes of low blood pressure include:

- anaphylaxis
- arrhythmias
- dehydration
- diabetes
- fainting
- heart failure
- infection
- myocardial infarction
- sudden blood loss.

Symptoms of hypotension may include:

- blurred vision
- confusion
- dizziness
- fainting
- light-headedness
- sleepiness
- weakness.

LYMPHADENOPATHY

Many diseases can cause lesions in the neck, but most commonly they involve swellings and/or pain in the cervical lymph nodes. About one-third of all lymph nodes are in the neck and the dental surgeon can often detect serious disease by examination of the neck.
A limited number of lymph nodes swell, usually because of infection in the area of drainage. The nodes are then often firm, discrete and tender but mobile (lymphadenitis), and the focus of inflammation can usually be found in the drainage area, which is anywhere on the face, scalp, nasal cavity, sinuses, ears, pharynx and oral cavity.
Lymphadenopathy in the anterior triangle of the neck alone is often due to local disease, especially if the nodes are enlarged on one side only. Infection and malignancy in the drainage area are important

causes. Metastatic infiltration causes the node to feel distinctly hard, and it may become bound down to adjacent tissues ('fixed') and, in advanced cases, may ulcerate through the skin.
Lymph nodes may also swell in systemic infections or disorders involving the immune system, and then there is usually involvement of more than one node, and often several in different sites. Most children or young people may have small palpable cervical, axillary and/or inguinal nodes. Most of these are caused by viral infections.
Lymph node enlargement may have several disparate causes including infections; lymphadenitis (inflammation of lymph nodes) is the most common cause of lymphadenopathy. The location of the affected nodes is usually related to the site of the underlying infection (Box 4.5).

MALABSORPTION

Malabsorption is difficulty with the digestion or absorption of nutrients from food, such as failure to absorb specific sugars, fats, proteins or other nutrients (such as vitamins). Diarrhoea, bloating or cramping, weakness, failure to thrive, frequent bulky stools that are difficult to flush, muscle-wasting and a distended abdomen may result; in children, malabsorption can affect growth and development.
Causes of malabsorption include: intestinal, biliary or pancreatic disease (cystic fibrosis, biliary atresia, Whipple disease, Shwachman–Bodian-Diamond syndrome); food allergies or intolerances (coeliac disease, lactose intolerance, bovine lactalbumin intolerance [cow's milk protein], soy milk protein intolerance); vitamin B_{12} malabsorption (pernicious anaemia, ileal disease, *Diphyllobothrium latum* [fish tapeworm] infestation); other parasites (*Giardia lamblia*, *Strongyloides stercoralis* [threadworm], *Necator americanus* [hookworm]); or, rarely, acrodermatitis enteropathica or abetalipoproteinaemia.

MALAISE

Malaise is a generalized feeling of discomfort, illness, uneasiness, fatigue or lack of well-being, often associated with a disease state. However, it is a very non-specific symptom and can be due to almost any infection, cancer and metabolic, endocrine, psychiatric or neurological disorders, and may develop slowly or rapidly, depending on the nature of the disease.

MELAENA

Melaena is the passage of black, tarry and foul-smelling stools, and usually indicates bleeding from the upper gastrointestinal tract. Other substances, such as blackberries, iron or liquorice, can cause black stools (false melaena), so that black stools should be formally tested for blood. Table 4.6 shows the causes of stools of various colours.

MENORRHAGIA

Menorrhagia is heavy regular bleeding over consecutive menstrual cycles ('periods'). The definition of heavy periods is the loss of 80 mL or more of blood, but passage of clots and overuse of sanitary towels or tampons may be suggestive. It may cause anaemia.
Common causes of menorrhagia are dysfunctional uterine bleeding (DUB) and uterine fibroids. Other causes are endometriosis, clotting disorders and anticoagulants.

Box 4.5 *Causes of cervical lymphadenopathy*

Bacterial
- Dental, face or scalp infections
- Tuberculosis
- Syphilis
- Cat scratch disease
- Brucellosis

Viral
- Herpetic stomatitis
- Infectious mononucleosis
- Adenovirus infections
- HIV
- Cytomegalovirus

Parasitic
- Toxoplasmosis

Connective tissue disorders
- Rheumatoid arthritis
- Systemic lupus erythematosus

Lymphoid or reticuloendothelial disease
- Leukaemias
- Hodgkin disease
- Non-Hodgkin lymphomas

Neoplasms
- Metastases from any tumour in the drainage area
- Nasopharyngeal carcinoma
- Neuroblastoma
- Thyroid carcinoma, chronic lymphocytic thyroiditis
- Kaposi sarcoma
- Langerhans histiocytosis

Immunodeficiency syndromes and phagocytic dysfunction
- Chronic granulomatous disease
- Hyperimmunoglobulin E (Job) syndrome
- HIV/AIDS

Metabolic and storage diseases
- Gaucher disease
- Niemann–Pick disease
- Cystinosis

Haemopoietic diseases
- Sickle cell anaemia
- Thalassaemia
- Congenital haemolytic anaemia
- Autoimmune haemolytic anaemia

Drug-induced hypersensitivity syndrome
- Phenytoin
- Others (such as cephalosporins, penicillins or sulphonamides)

Immunological disorders
- Serum sickness
- Chronic graft-versus-host disease
- Benign sinus histiocytosis
- Angioimmunoblastic or immunoblastic lymphadenopathy
- Chronic pseudolymphomatous lymphadenopathy (chronic benign lymphadenopathy)
- Sarcoidosis, Crohn disease and orofacial granulomatosis
- Kawasaki disease (mucocutaneous lymph node syndrome)
- Angiolymphoid hyperplasia with eosinophilia, haemangioma, with eosinophilic infiltration and lymphoid hyperplasia
- Castleman disease (angiofollicular lymphoid hyperplasia or benign giant lymph node hyperplasia).
- Kikuchi syndrome (Ch. 37)

Table 4.6 *Causes of coloured stools (apart from foods/drinks/drugs)*

Black	Maroon	Red
Bleeding gastric ulcer	All the causes of black-coloured stool	All the causes of black- or maroon-coloured stool
Gastritis	Bleeding diverticula	Haemorrhoids
Oesophageal varices	Bleeding vascular malformation	Anal fissures
Mallory–Weiss tear	Intestinal infection (e.g. bacterial enterocolitis)	
Bleeding disorder	Inflammatory bowel disease	
	Colonic polyps	
	Colonic cancer	

MOUTH ULCERS

Oral ulcers are common; most are traumatic or recurrent aphthae, but more serious causes must always be excluded. Particular care must be taken to exclude drugs, cancer, blood dyscrasias, infections, and gastrointestinal or mucocutaneous disease (Box 4.6 and Ch. 11).

MURMURS

Heart murmurs are caused by turbulence of blood flow through valves or ventricular outflow tracts. The prevalence of cardiac murmurs in the general population is very high, and some indicate cardiac disease. Functional (high-flow – also called physiological) murmurs are innocent murmurs that are heard in the absence of cardiac valvular disease. An example is an aortic systolic ejection murmur caused by a high cardiac output state, as in athletes and anaemia. Another example is pregnancy, where the rise in cardiac output, especially when coupled with anaemia, can result in physiological ejection murmurs.

NAUSEA AND VOMITING

Nausea is the sensation leading to the urge to vomit; vomiting is the forced ejection of stomach contents through the oesophagus and out of the mouth. Causes of nausea and vomiting are varied, but may include unusual motion (e.g. travel/motion sickness); gastroenterological causes (infections, food poisoning, food allergies, gastroenteritis, pyloric stenosis); neuropsychiatric factors (bulimia, cyclic vomiting syndrome, emotional stress, labyrinthitis, migraine); morning sickness during pregnancy; and many drugs (especially alcohol, chemotherapy, erythromycin, general anaesthetics). Complications of vomiting include dehydration, loss of electrolytes, peptic oesophagitis, haematemesis, aspiration, Mallory–Weiss tear, and tooth erosion if vomiting is chronic. Apart from treating underlying causes, antiemetic drugs may help.

NECK LUMPS

The lumps in the neck of most significance are enlarged cervical lymph nodes, but lumps may also be due to other pathology (Box 4.7).

Box 4.6 *Causes of oral ulceration*

Systemic causes

Blood diseases (Ch. 8)
- Leukopenias, including HIV disease
- Leukaemias and myelodysplastic syndrome
- Deficiency states or anaemia
- Hypereosinophilic syndrome

Infections

Viral, mainly (Ch. 21)
- Herpes viruses
- Coxsackie viruses
- ECHO viruses

Bacterial
- Acute necrotizing gingivitis
- Syphilis
- Tuberculosis

Fungal
- Cryptococcosis
- Histoplasmosis
- Paracoccidioidomycosis
- Blastomycosis
- Zygomycosis
- Aspergillosis

Protozoal
- Leishmaniasis

Gastrointestinal disease (Ch. 7)
- Coeliac disease
- Crohn disease
- Ulcerative colitis

Mucocutaneous diseases (Ch. 11)
- Lichen planus
- Chronic ulcerative stomatitis
- Pemphigus
- Pemphigoid
- Localized oral purpura
- Erythema multiforme
- Epidermolysis bullosa
- Dermatitis herpetiformis
- Linear immunoglobulin A (IgA) disease
- Behçet and Sweet syndromes

Connective tissue and other diseases (Ch. 16)
- Lupus erythematosus
- Reiter syndrome
- Vasculitides
- Giant cell arteritis
- Wegener granulomatosis
- Periarteritis nodosa

Malignant neoplasms (Ch. 22)
- Squamous cell carcinoma
- Others

Local causes
- Trauma
- Chemical irritation
- Burns
- Irradiation

Aphthae and aphthous-like ulcers

Drugs (Ch. 29)

Box 4.7 *Causes of neck lumps other than lymphadenopathy*

Infections
- Abscess
- Actinomycosis

Cysts
- Thyroglossal
- Branchial
- Cystic hygroma
- Sebaceous cyst
- Dermoid cyst

Hamartomas
- Haemangioma/lymphangioma

Thyroid
- Goitre
- Nodules (and carcinoma)

Carotid
- Aneurysm
- Body tumour

Skin
- Lipoma
- Seroma
- Carcinoma
- Pharyngeal pouch

NECK STIFFNESS

Neck pain and stiffness may originate from any neck structure or from the shoulders and arms, ranging from the cervical vertebrae to blood vessels, muscles and lymphatic tissue. Causes mainly include strain and spasm of neck muscles; trauma (road traffic accidents); or arthritis. Neck stiffness can have serious significance since it can also originate from meningeal irritation in meningitis (there may also be fever, an aversion to light, vomiting, and severe headache) and meningism – a non-infective syndrome with similar features, caused by meningeal irritation by, for example, an intracranial haemorrhage or tumour.

NOCTURIA

Nocturia is the passing of too much urine at night. Young people tend to excrete their daily urine output mostly in the day; older people commonly also pass urine once or twice at night. Causes of nocturia include, in particular, drinks such as coffee or tea too close to bedtime; insomnia or other sleep-related difficulties; urinary or prostatic disorders (e.g. benign prostate disease or cystitis); chronic kidney disease; diabetes; or cardiac failure.

NYSTAGMUS

A few irregular eye jerks are normal in some individuals when the eyes are deviated far to one side. Nystagmus is involuntary rapid, back-and-forth, repetitive eye movements, caused by abnormalities of function in the areas of the brain that control eye movements. It may be congenital (the most common cause), when it is usually mild, unchanging in severity, and not associated with any other disorder. Causes include cataract, glaucoma, retinal disease, Down syndrome and albinism.

Nystagmus may be acquired and caused by disease or injury later in life, most commonly by head injury or, in older people, by stroke, but any brain diseases, such as multiple sclerosis or tumours, inner ear problems or drugs, can be responsible.

The most common form of nystagmus is rhythmic (jerk), which is usually horizontal but can be vertical or rotary. It results from drug intoxication (barbiturates, phenytoin toxicity and alcohol intoxication); inner ear disease (Ménière disease); cerebellar disease; or brainstem disease.

OBESITY

See Chapter 27.

OEDEMA

Oedema is the accumulation of fluid in the tissues. Slight oedema of the legs is common in healthy persons, especially in the warm summer months, after prolonged standing and/or on long flights or car journeys. Injury or trauma, insect bite or sting, burns, allergic reactions or angioedema can cause oedema. It may also stem from more serious conditions. When venous pressure rises in cardiac failure, subcutaneous oedema gravitates to dependent parts; ankle oedema is seen in ambulant patients and sacral oedema in those in bed. Oedema may be pitting (when a finger is pressed against a swollen area for 10 seconds and then quickly removed, an indentation is left that fills slowly) or non-pitting (no indentation is left). In pregnancy (pre-eclampsia – hypertension with albuminuria), oedema can appear between the 20th week of pregnancy and the end of the first week postpartum. Other causes include loss of plasma proteins from renal factors or malnutrition (causing the nephrotic syndrome) and medical treatments (body fluid overload, infiltration of an intravenous site, diagnostic tests, e.g. venogram), including drugs (corticosteroids, androgenic and anabolic steroids, oestrogens, antihypertensives, NSAIDs).

PALMAR ERYTHEMA

Redness of the palms of the hands may be seen in cirrhosis, pregnancy, rheumatoid arthritis, systemic lupus erythematosus and hyperthyroidism.

PALPITATIONS

Palpitations are the consciousness of rapid heart action (Ch. 5). Cardiac activity is controlled by the autonomic nervous system and is commonly sensed only by persons with abnormally heightened awareness of their body functions, as in anxiety states, or following exercise – when heart stroke volume or rate rises. Palpitations are most commonly caused by arrhythmias but may also stem from disorders such as anaemia, aortic regurgitation or thyrotoxicosis. Palpitations accompanied by myocardial ischaemia-type chest pain probably indicate coronary artery disease. Enquiry into the rate and the rhythm of palpitations helps differentiate pathological from physiological, since palpitations due to an arrhythmia may be accompanied by weakness, dyspnoea or light-headedness.

Atrial or ventricular extrasystoles are often described as skipped beats, and atrial fibrillation as total irregularity, while supraventricular or ventricular tachycardia is most often perceived as being rapid and regular, and of sudden onset and termination.

PAPILLOEDEMA

Papilloedema is a swelling of the optic nerve seen on ophthalmoscopy. The optic nerve anatomy makes it sensitive to slight rises in cerebrospinal fluid (CSF) pressure, and when the optic nerve is exposed to such pressure or when it becomes inflamed, it can bulge (papilloedema). Causes of raised CSF pressure and papilloedema are brain disease, raised intracranial pressure (e.g. haemorrhage, tumours, infections – brain abscess, meningitis or encephalitis) and pseudotumour cerebri or benign intracranial hypertension (results from CSF overproduction). This is more common in women who are obese and of childbearing age, and seems to be triggered at times of hormone change, such as pregnancy, the start of contraceptive pill use, tetracycline use, the first menstrual period or menopause. Papilloedema can also arise from local inflammation (optic neuritis); multiple sclerosis is the most common cause.

Symptoms related to papilloedema are mainly caused by raised intracranial pressure and include headache and nausea with vomiting. About 25% of patients with advanced papilloedema also develop some visual symptoms, such as recurring brief episodes in which the vision turns grey or 'blacks out', as if a veil has fallen over the eyes. Ophthalmoscopy shows an elevated optic disc with a blurred margin, and there is a wider blind spot and narrowing of peripheral vision.

PARAESTHESIA

Paraesthesia is a burning or prickling sensation, most common when there is sustained pressure on a nerve and experienced as temporary paraesthesia – 'pins and needles' – when individuals have sat with their legs crossed for too long or fallen asleep with an arm crooked under their head; the feeling abates once the pressure is relieved. Nerve entrapment syndromes, such as carpal tunnel syndrome, can cause paraesthesia sometimes accompanied by pain but are usually very peripheral and obvious. Chronic paraesthesia may be a feature of traumatic nerve damage or an underlying neurological disease, such as cerebrovascular issues (stroke and TIAs), multiple sclerosis, connective tissue diseases, sarcoidosis, transverse myelitis, brain or spinal cord tumour or vascular lesion, encephalitis and some drugs. Some LA agents can be neurotoxic (Ch. 3).

POLYDIPSIA

Polydipsia is an abnormal feeling of constant thirst. The most common cause is the excessive intake of salty foods but the desire to drink excessively beyond a certain limit may reflect underlying disease, either physical or emotional. Causes include excessive loss of water and salt (as with water deprivation, profuse sweating, diarrhoea or vomiting, severe infections or widespread burns); fluid loss during exercise; bleeding sufficient to cause a significant fall in blood volume; drugs (including anticholinergics, demeclocycline, diuretics, lithium, phenothiazines); endocrine disorders (diabetes mellitus, Conn disease, Cushing disease, hyperthyroidism, diabetes insipidus); and cardiac, hepatic or renal failure. Psychogenic causes are most commonly seen in women over age 30.

POLYURIA

Polyuria – the passing of abnormally large amounts of urine (for an adult, at least 2.5 L per day) – is fairly common and often first noticed at night. Polyuria is to be expected with excessive intake of fluids, particularly ones containing caffeine or alcohol, or too much salt or glucose (especially if diabetic); the use of diuretics can also lead to polyuria. Other causes include diabetes mellitus or insipidus; psychogenic polydipsia; renal failure; sickle cell anaemia; and radiography using contrast media.

PRESSURE ULCERS (BED SORES)

Pressure sores or ulcers are injuries to skin and underlying tissues from prolonged pressure on skin that covers bony areas of the body, such as the heel, ankles, hips or buttocks. People most at risk are those with medical conditions that limit their ability to change position, requires them to use a wheelchair or confines them to bed for long periods. Sores develop through a series of stages:

- Stage I
  The skin is intact and red in people with lighter skin colour, failing to blanch when touched.
  The site may be painful, firm, soft, warmer or cooler compared with surrounding skin.
- Stage II
  A pressure ulcer may appear – as a shallow, pinkish-red ulcer.
  It may also appear as an intact or ruptured fluid-filled blister.
- Stage III
  There is a deep wound, usually with fat exposed.
  The bottom of the wound may have some slough.
  Damage may extend beyond the primary wound below layers of healthy skin.
- Stage IV
  The wound may expose muscle, bone and tendons.
  The wound base contains slough or eschar.
  Damage often extends beyond the primary wound below layers of healthy skin.

Risk factors, apart from continued pressure, include:

- age
- lack of sensory perception; spinal cord injuries, neurological disorders and other conditions can result in a loss of sensation
- weight loss
- poor nutrition and hydration
- urinary or faecal incontinence
- excess moisture or dryness
- diabetes and vascular disease, affecting the circulation
- smoking
- decreased mental awareness
- muscle spasms.

Complications of pressure ulcers include:

- sepsis
- cellulitis
- bone and joint infections
- cancer (Marjolin ulcer).

Treatment consists of the following measures:

- Relief of pressure by repositioning. Special cushions, pads, mattresses and beds may be used.
- Removal of damaged tissue by surgical mechanical, enzymatic or autolytic debridement.
- Cleaning and dressing of wounds.

- Pain management. Interventions may include the use of NSAIDs, such as ibuprofen and naproxen, particularly before and after repositioning, debridement procedures and dressing changes. Topical pain medications, such as a combination of lidocaine and prilocaine, also may be used during debridement and dressing changes.
- Antibiotics.
- Healthy diet.
- Muscle spasm relief. Relaxants such as diazepam, tizanidine, dantrolene and baclofen may inhibit spasms.
- Surgical repair.

PROPTOSIS

Proptosis is the anterior displacement of one or both eye globes within the bony orbit. The term exophthalmos is sometimes used, particularly when the proptosis is related to thyroid dysfunction. The normal amount of ocular protrusion as measured (with an exophthalmometer) from the lateral orbital rim to the corneal apex is 14–21 mm in adults; protrusion greater than 21 mm or a 2-mm change is abnormal. On scans, proptosis is defined as globe protrusion greater than 21 mm anterior to the interzygomatic line on axial scans at the level of the lens.

Proptosis without displacement (axial) is due to intraconal, most commonly dysthyroid, eye disease. In this case, the protrusion is caused by inflammatory swelling of the small eye-moving muscles behind the globe. Thyroid exophthalmos may appear months or years after the onset of a thyroid disorder but may occasionally precede it. Tumours (such as glioma and meningioma of the optic nerve and cavernous haemangioma) may also be responsible.

Proptosis with displacement (non-axial) is due to extraconal disease, most commonly lacrimal tumours or a mucocoele.

Pseudoproptosis is either the simulation of abnormal eye prominence, or a true asymmetry that is not the result of increased orbital contents. Causes include enlarged eye globe (high myopia, buphthalmos); extraocular muscle weakness or paralysis; contralateral enophthalmos; asymmetrical orbital size (congenital, post-irradiation, post-surgical); and asymmetrical palpebral fissures (e.g. caused by ipsilateral eyelid retraction, scarring, facial nerve paralysis or contralateral ptosis).

PRURITUS (ITCHING)

Pruritus is a peculiar tingling or uneasy irritation of the skin, which leads to a desire to scratch the affected area. Causes include skin irritation from insect bites, stings and chemicals; environmental causes (drying, sunburn); or urticaria. Parasites (e.g. lice) or skin conditions (e.g. lichen planus, dermatitis herpetiformis) are other causes. Less commonly, pruritus is due to infectious diseases (chickenpox), pregnancy, allergic reactions, biliary obstruction, chronic kidney disease, lymphomas, drugs (penicillin, sulphonamides, gold, griseofulvin, isoniazid, opiates, phenothiazines or vitamin A) or contact irritants (such as soaps, chemicals or wool).

Pruritus ani is a common and troublesome complaint that can result from such causes as haemorrhoids or irritable bowel syndrome; fistulas or fissures; mucocutaneous diseases such as lichen planus; or infections such as candidosis or worms.

PTOSIS

Ptosis is drooping eyelids, caused by weakness of the muscle responsible for raising the eyelid (levator palpebrae superioris), as in

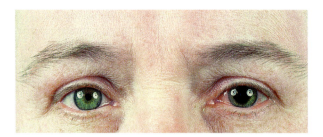

Fig. 4.4 Mydriasis.

myasthenia gravis, damage to the extraocular nerves, or skin laxity in the upper eyelids.

Congenital ptosis is most commonly due to a defect in the levator palpebrae superioris or rare myopathies (e.g. myotonica congenita). Marcus Gunn 'jaw-winking' syndrome is ptosis usually in one eye only; it is due to the lid partially opening as the jaw opens because of an abnormal nerve connection.

Acquired ptosis can be through age-related defects of the eyelid muscles and nerves, or by damage to the sympathetic nerve supply or the oculomotor nerve. A mechanical defect caused by anything that increases the weight of the eyelid, such as a cyst, may also cause ptosis.

PUPIL ANOMALIES

The pupils normally are equal in size, and they constrict on exposure to bright light and on accommodation for near objects. Light shone in one eye causes pupillary constriction in that eye (direct light reflex) and also in the unexposed eye (indirect or consensual reflex).

Pupil size is determined by dilator fibres (the sympathetic nerve supply from the superior cervical ganglion runs along the internal carotid artery and joins the ophthalmic division of the trigeminal nerve and the long ciliary nerves) and the sympathetic nerve supply is also partially responsible for contraction of the levator palpebrae superioris muscle (raising the upper eyelid). Pupil size is also determined by constrictor fibres (the parasympathetic supply runs with the oculomotor nerve). Pupil constriction (miosis) can be caused by a lesion of the sympathetic supply, and dilatation (mydriasis) by a third nerve lesion (Fig. 4.4). The most important cause of an abnormally dilated pupil is a rise in intracranial pressure, when the pupil also becomes non-reactive owing to pressure on the oculomotor nerve (Table 4.7).

PURPURA

Purpura is abnormal bruising (Fig. 4.5) with small bleeds into the skin (petechiae) or larger bleeds (ecchymoses), and bleeding from mucosae (epistaxes – nosebleeds – and gingival bleeding).

Causes of purpura include:

- *purpura simplex* (easy bruising) – the most common vascular bleeding disorder, due to excessive vascular fragility and usually seen in women in whom the platelet count and tests of platelet function, blood coagulation and fibrinolysis are normal. Bruises develop without known trauma on the thighs, buttocks and upper arms, and are typically small.
- *senile purpura* – a common disorder affecting older patients, mainly on the extensor surfaces of the hands and forearms, particularly in those who have had excessive sun exposure. Lesions appear often without known trauma as dark purple

Table 4.7 *Causes of pupillary abnormalities*

Pupils	Other signs	Significance
Constricted bilaterally	±Signs of drug abuse	Opiate use
Constricted bilaterally, unequal, react to accommodation but not light	–	Argyll Robertson pupils – neurosyphilis, multiple sclerosis, diabetes mellitus, sarcoid, brain tumour, amyloid, trauma, Lyme disease
Constricted unilaterally	Ptosis, absence of facial sweating, enophthalmos sometimes	Horner syndrome – damage to sympathetic fibres, usually in neck (e.g. by trauma or bronchial carcinoma)
Dilated unilaterally	Ptosis	Third nerve lesion
Dilated unilaterally and react slowly to light or convergence	Possible absence of ankle or knee jerks	Usually benign Adie (Holmes–Adie) pupil
Dilated bilaterally and reactive	±Signs of drug abuse	Cocaine or other drug use
Dilated bilaterally and unreactive	±Headaches	Raised intracranial pressure

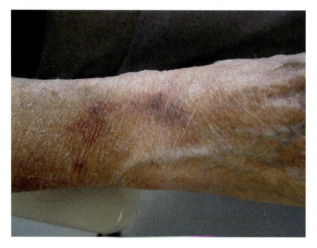

Fig. 4.5 Purpura.

ecchymoses and slowly resolve over several days, leaving a brownish discolouration caused by deposits of haemosiderin. The condition has no serious consequences. Angina bullosa haemorrhagica may be a localized form of purpura seen in the mouth or throat.

- *thrombocytopenia* – the most important systemic cause of purpura (Ch. 8).

RAISED INTRACRANIAL PRESSURE

Normal intracranial pressure (ICP) for an adult at rest is 7–15 mmHg supine, becoming negative (−10 mmHg) in the vertical position. Changes in ICP are attributed to volume changes in one or more of the constituents contained in the cranium; any expansion of cranial contents causes a rise of ICP, which tends to impede the venous return from the brain and to increase the pressure further. Cerebral blood flow is thus diminished, even though the raised CSF pressure causes a reflex rise in systemic blood pressure in an attempt to improve cerebral blood flow.

Table 4.8 *Types of glaucoma*

Type	Features	Treatment
Open-angle	Most common. The angle that allows fluid to drain out of the anterior chamber is *open*. However, the fluid passes too slowly through the meshwork drain. Optic nerve damage and narrowed side vision develop. Risk groups include people of African heritage over the age of 40, anyone over age 60 and a family history of glaucoma	Drugs or laser trabeculoplasty
Low-tension or normal-tension	Optic nerve damage and narrowed side vision develop unexpectedly in people with normal eye pressure	Drugs or laser trabeculoplasty
Closed-angle	The fluid at the front of the eye cannot reach the angle and leave it because the angle is blocked by part of the iris. Without treatment, the eye can become blind within 48 h	A medical emergency. Immediate laser treatment
Congenital	Involves defects in the angle of the eye that slow the normal drainage of fluid	Surgery
Secondary	Develops as a complication of other medical conditions, cataracts, uveitis, eye surgery, injuries or tumours	Various

Causes of raised ICP include hydrocephalus, intracranial haemorrhage (after head injury), space-occupying lesions (abscess, tumour or haematoma), oedema (trauma, malignant hypertension, vascular lesions or tumours of the brain), or obstruction to the flow of CSF (blockage of the aqueduct of Sylvius, or subarachnoid adhesions due to meningitis).

Idiopathic intracranial hypertension, sometimes called benign intracranial hypertension or pseudotumour cerebri, occurs in the absence of a tumour or other disease affecting the brain or meninges.

Characteristic symptoms of raised ICP are headache, transient visual changes or loss in one or both eyes usually lasting seconds, pulse-synchronous tinnitus (a 'whooshing noise'), diplopia (double vision) and visual loss. Signs of raised ICP include papilloedema (bulging of the optic disc with engorgement of its vessels seen by ophthalmoscopy); restlessness (in the unconscious patient); vomiting; decreasing consciousness; rising blood pressure and slowing of the pulse; dilatation of the pupil on the side of the lesion with diminished reaction to light, and loss of visual acuity and fields. Diplopia, if present, may be due to abducens palsy.

Raised ICP can be fatal, as the pressure can cause herniation of the brain (displacement of part of the brain from one dural compartment to another) and pressure is exerted on the brainstem and medullary respiratory and cardiac control centres (this is called 'coning'). *Lumbar puncture is contraindicated*, as it can precipitate brain herniation and death by coning. The possibility of herniation is suggested by signs of raised ICP, particularly pupil dilatation and reduced reactivity to light caused by stretching of the oculomotor nerves.

RAISED INTRAOCULAR PRESSURE

Normal intraocular pressure is between 12 and 21 mmHg. Glaucoma is a group of diseases of raised intraocular pressure that can lead to damage to the eye's optic nerve and result in impaired vision (Table 4.8). Glaucoma often affects both eyes, usually in varying degrees but one eye may develop glaucoma quicker than the other. Glaucoma occurs when the eye drainage tubes (trabecular meshwork) become slightly blocked, impeding eye fluid (aqueous humour) drainage. When the fluid cannot drain properly, intraocular pressure (IOP) increases and can damage the optic nerve and the retina. The main types of glaucoma are:

- *chronic open-angle glaucoma* – the most common type; develops slowly
- *primary angle-closure glaucoma* – rare; can develop slowly, or rapidly with a sudden, painful build-up of pressure

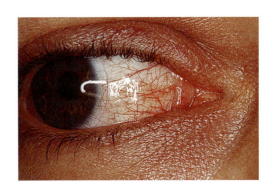

Fig. 4.6 Red eye.

- *secondary glaucoma* – the result of an eye injury or another eye condition, such as uveitis
- *developmental (congenital) glaucoma* – rare but serious; usually presents at birth or develops shortly after.

Early diagnosis is important because any damage cannot be reversed. Treatment aims to control the condition and minimize future damage with eye medication drops (prostaglandin inhibitors, sympathomimetics, beta-blockers or carbonic anhydrase inhibitors), laser trabeculoplasty, cyclodiode therapy or surgery (trabeculectomy).

Drug-induced elevation of intraocular pressure is more common by an open-angle mechanism; some antidepressants, atropine, corticosteroids, diazepam, glycopyrrolate, hyoscine (scopolamine) and topiramate are implicated and therefore contraindicated. Most drugs that have glaucoma as a contraindication or adverse effect, however, are concerned with inducing acute angle-closure glaucoma and include topical anticholinergic or sympathomimetic dilating drops; antidepressants (tricyclic antidepressants, monoamine oxidase inhibitors [MAOIs]); antihistamines; antiparkinsonians; antipsychotics; antispasmolytics; and benzodiazepines.

Overviews of drug-induced glaucoma can be found at http://emedicine.medscape.com/article/1205298-overview and http://www.fmshk.org/database/articles/03mb6_5.pdf (accessed 25 May 2013).

RED EYE

There are many causes of red eye (Fig. 4.6), ranging from trauma or simple superficial inflammation (conjunctivitis) to more serious corneal ulceration, uveitis (inflammation of iris, ciliary body and choroids) and acute glaucoma – a medical emergency.

Box 4.8 *Causes of salivary gland swelling*

Inflammatory
- Mumps
- Bacterial ascending sialadenitis
- Obstructive sialadenitis
- Allergic sialadenitis (e.g. to iodides or chlorhexidine)
- Sjögren syndrome and IgG4 syndrome
- Sarcoidosis
- HIV infection
- Tuberculosis and non-tuberculous mycobacteriosis
- Actinomycosis
- Toxoplasmosis

Neoplastic
- Pleomorphic adenoma and many others

Endocrine and metabolic
- Alcoholic and other types of cirrhosis
- Diabetes mellitus
- Acromegaly
- Malnutrition or bulimia
- Cystic fibrosis
- Chronic renal failure
- Amyloidosis
- Haemochromatosis

Drugs (rarely)
- Antiretroviral drugs (lipomatosis)
- Chlorhexidine
- Iodides
- Isoprenaline
- Phenylbutazone

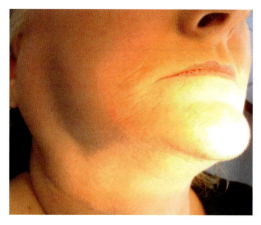

Fig. 4.7 Unilateral parotid swelling.

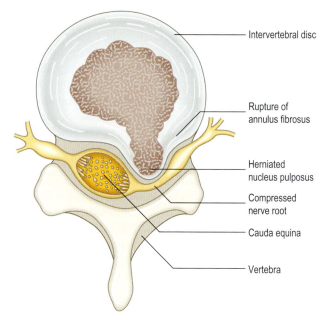

Intervertebral disc

Rupture of annulus fibrosus

Herniated nucleus pulposus

Compressed nerve root

Cauda equina

Vertebra

Fig. 4.8 Prolapsed intervertebral disc ('slipped disc').

RED LESIONS IN THE MOUTH

Many oral mucosal red lesions are due to infections or are inflammatory with no identified infectious agent (sarcoidosis, Crohn disease); vascular anomalies (e.g. telangiectasias); or mucosal atrophy (erythema migrans [geographic tongue], desquamative gingivitis, erythroplasia or deficiency state). Lichen planus, lupus erythematosus and candidosis may cause red or white lesions (Ch. 11). Red lesions are sometimes due to Kaposi sarcoma or Wegener granulomatosis.

SALIVARY SWELLING

The most common cause of salivary swelling is mumps (Ch. 21), which usually affects children and typically causes bilateral painful swellings, but there are many other causes (Box 4.8). Salivary obstruction, as by a calculus (stone), is the common cause of a unilateral swelling. Neoplasms (usually pleomorphic adenoma) must be considered, particularly when there is a persistent unilateral swelling in older patients (Fig. 4.7). Painless bilateral salivary swelling in an adult is usually due to sialadenosis (sialosis) and to autonomic dysfunction; it is thus a rare feature of alcoholic cirrhosis, diabetes mellitus, acromegaly, starvation or bulimia, or may be idiopathic. Sjögren syndrome and immunoglobulin G4 (IgG4) disease may also cause salivary gland swelling (see Box 4.8).

SCIATICA

Sciatica is pain down the leg, caused by irritation of the sciatic nerve, the main nerve to the leg. The pain travels below the knee and may involve the foot, and there may be numbness and weakness of the lower leg muscles. The most common cause is a 'slipped disc' (a prolapsed intervertebral disc or herniated nucleus pulposus). Pressures within intervertebral discs can be high on bending or twisting, even without carrying a load. If part of the fibrous outer ring of the disc is weak, the softer nucleus pulposus centre may push its way through, and if it presses against a nerve it causes symptoms. Sciatica occurs when the herniated disc presses against the sciatic nerve (Fig. 4.8).

CT or MRI scans determine whether an operation will help cure the sciatica. Simple analgesics, such as paracetamol or ibuprofen, help. Activities likely to put unnecessary strain on the back should be avoided. In the minority of cases in which sciatica does not settle or complications arise, surgery is needed.

SELF-HARM

See Chapter 10.

SIALORRHOEA (HYPERSALIVATION)

Normally, any excess of saliva is swallowed and causes no symptoms. However, in normal infants, and in patients who have learning impairment, poor neuromuscular coordination or pharyngeal or oesophageal obstruction, drooling is common without any true overproduction of saliva (hypersalivation).

Causes of decreased saliva clearance include:

- infections such as tonsillitis, retropharyngeal and peritonsillar abscesses, epiglottitis and mumps
- jaw problems, e.g. fracture or dislocation
- neurological disorders such as myasthenia gravis, Parkinson disease, rabies, bulbar paralysis, bilateral facial nerve palsy and hypoglossal nerve palsy
- radiation therapy.

Causes of saliva overproduction include:

- excessive starch intake
- foreign bodies (e.g. new mouth appliances)
- gastro-oesophageal reflux disease, in such cases specifically called water brash, and characterized by a sour fluid or almost tasteless saliva
- liver disease
- oral infections or ulcers
- pancreatitis
- pregnancy
- rabies
- serotonin syndrome.

Drugs that can cause saliva overproduction include:

- clozapine
- ketamine
- pilocarpine
- potassium chlorate
- rabeprazole sodium
- risperidone.

Toxins that can cause hypersalivation include:

- arsenic
- copper
- mercury
- organophosphates (insecticide).

However, there is often no objective evidence for hypersalivation – when it may have a psychogenic basis.

Hypersalivation or drooling may be controllable with anticholinergic drugs (benzatropine, glycopyrronium and trihexyphenidyl hydrochloride) or antimuscarinic agents such as sublingual atropine or propantheline bromide. Botulinum toxin injections can be effective in certain circumstances. If hypersalivation is very severe, surgical relocation of the parotid duct, such that it discharges into the pharynx, may be effective, and the submandibular duct can also be moved.

SNEEZING (STERNUTATION)

Sneezing is a sudden, forceful, involuntary burst of air through the nose and mouth, almost invariably caused by irritation to the mucous membranes of the nose or throat. Rarely a sign of serious disease, sneezing typically is caused by allergy or hay fever, upper respiratory tract infections, opioid withdrawal or corticosteroid inhalation.

SNORING

Snoring is caused by obstructed breathing; the sound is usually made by the palate vibrating when the muscles relax, narrowing the airway. Snoring is usually normal, of unknown cause and not an indication of any underlying disorder. Excess alcohol or sedation can contribute. However, snoring can also be a sign of the *sleep apnoea syndrome*, with chronic nasal congestion or obstruction by enlarged tonsils and adenoids – or more serious pathology. It often causes nocturnal xerostomia. Snoring may often be reduced by not taking too much alcohol or sedation at bedtime, by avoiding sleeping flat on the back, and by weight loss (Ch. 14).

SORE THROAT

A sore throat is discomfort, pain or scratchiness in the throat, often associated with pain on swallowing. Sore throats are common, especially in children between the ages of 5 and 10, most often caused by upper respiratory viruses (Ch. 14). Streptococcal throat is the most common bacterial cause and can occasionally lead to rheumatic fever, so antibiotics are indicated. Other causes of sore throat include trauma (a fish or chicken bone or other foreign substance stuck in the throat, endotracheal intubation, or local surgery, such as tonsillectomy and adenoidectomy). Occasionally, more serious pathology underlies the complaint.

SPLENOMEGALY

Splenomegaly is enlargement of the spleen beyond its normal size. The spleen is involved in the production and maintenance of erythrocytes and the production of certain immunocytes; it may be affected and enlarged by many conditions involving the blood or lymph system, and by infection, liver disease, haemolytic anaemias, malignancies and parasites. Causes of splenomegaly can include those listed in Box 4.9.

Rupture of the enlarged spleen is possible and usually due to trauma.

STROKE (CEREBROVASCULAR EVENT OR ACCIDENT; CVA)

See Chapter 13.

STUTTERING

Stuttering (stammering) is a speech disorder in which the normal flow of speech is disrupted by frequent repetitions or prolongations of speech sounds, syllables or words, or by an individual's inability to start a word. Stuttering usually has a genetic basis but other causes can be neurogenic – following a stroke or other brain injury, or psychogenic – particularly anxiety. Stuttering may be accompanied by rapid eye blinks, lip and/or jaw tremors or other movements. Certain situations, such as lecturing, talking on the telephone or being interviewed, tend to aggravate stuttering, whereas others, such as singing or speaking alone, often improve it.

SWEATING

Sweating is a heat-regulatory mechanism, mediated by the hypothalamus, when in a warm environment or exercising. The evaporation of

Box 4.9 *Causes of splenomegaly*

Infections
- Malaria (worldwide the most common cause)
- Infectious mononucleosis
- Cytomegalovirus infection
- Other viral infections
- Parasitic infections
- Cat scratch disease
- Bacterial infections

Liver diseases
- Cirrhosis (portal vein obstruction, portal hypertension)
- Sclerosing cholangitis
- Wilson disease
- Biliary atresia
- Cystic fibrosis

Haemolytic anaemias
- Thalassaemia
- Haemoglobinopathies
- Glucose-6-phosphate dehydrogenase (G6PD) deficiency
- Idiopathic autoimmune haemolytic anaemia
- Immune haemolytic anaemia

Malignant disease
- Leukaemia
- Lymphoma
- Hodgkin disease

Other causes
- Sarcoidosis
- Sickle cell splenic crisis
- Banti syndrome
- Felty syndrome

Box 4.10 *Causes of sweating*

- Exercise
- Infections
- Menopause
- Malignant disease
  Breast cancer
  Prostate cancer
  Hodgkin disease
  Phaeochromocytoma
  CNS tumours
  Endocrine tumours
- Drugs
  Tamoxifen
  Opioids
  Antidepressants
  Steroids
  Recreational drugs
- Hypothalamic disease
- Sweating disorders (hyperhidrosis)

Box 4.11 *Causes of tachypnoea*

- Psychological states
  Anxiety
  Stress
  Situations in which there is a psychological advantage in having a sudden dramatic illness
- Drug use
  Stimulant use
  Drugs (e.g. aspirin overdose)
- Respiratory disorders
  Asthma
  Chronic obstructive pulmonary disease
  Pneumonia
  Pulmonary fibrosis
  Pleurisy
  Pulmonary embolism
- Cardiac disease
  Congestive heart failure
  Coronary artery disease
  Valvular disease
- Severe pain
- Ketoacidosis and similar medical conditions

sweat, produced by sweat glands in the skin, leads to heat loss. Other causes of sweating are shown in Box 4.10.

SYNCOPE

Syncope is a feeling of faintness, dizziness or light-headedness (presyncope), or loss of consciousness (syncope), due to a sudden decline in blood flow to the brain. Syncope can affect otherwise healthy people but may also be caused by an irregular cardiac rate or rhythm, or by changes of blood volume or distribution. The main causes include: vasovagal attack (fainting, Ch. 1); respiratory factors (severe coughing causing vagal stimulation); cardiac disease (arrhythmias, heart block, aortic stenosis); paralytic factors – in the elderly, especially those taking drugs such as phenothiazines, L-dopa, hypotensive agents, tricyclics or benzodiazepines; brainstem factors – owing to migraine or vertebrobasilar disease, usually in the elderly; and carotid sinus syndrome – an exaggerated baroreceptor response resulting in periods of inappropriately high vagal tone and sympathetic suppression. The diagnosis is frequently made in men over 50 and in patients with atherosclerosis and hypertension. Syncope may also be caused by turning or pressing on the neck.

TACHYCARDIA

See Chapter 5.

TACHYPNOEA

Tachypnoea or hyperventilation is excessive, rapid and deep breathing, resulting in a fall in the carbon dioxide level in the blood. Hyperventilation is not uncommon in young adults, especially in women, usually when they are nervous and tense. It can also be a symptom of other disorders. Causes of tachypnoea include those shown in Box 4.11.

TASTE DISORDERS

See Chapter 13.

Box 4.12 *Causes of tiredness*

- Excessive physical exertion
- Poor nutrition
- Infections (e.g. tuberculosis, bacterial endocarditis, HIV, hepatitis, influenza and mononucleosis)
- Chronic fatigue syndrome
- Psychological disorders
  Anxiety and depression
  Chronic boredom
  Grief
  Sleep disorders, such as insomnia
  Stress
- Anaemia
- Endocrinopathies (e.g. diabetes, hypothyroidism, Addison disease, acromegaly)
- Drugs (e.g. antihistamines, antihypertensives, sedatives or diuretics)
- Chronic disease (e.g. cancer, rheumatoid arthritis, systemic lupus erythematosus)
- Most types of surgery
- Cardiac failure

Table 4.9 *Causes of discolouration of teeth*

Extrinsic	Intrinsic
Most teeth affected	
Smoking, beverages, e.g. tea Drugs, e.g. Iron, chlorhexidine, minocycline Poor oral hygiene, betel chewing	Tetracycline, fluorosis, amelogenesis imperfecta, dentinogenesis imperfecta, kernicterus, biliary atresia, porphyria
One or a few teeth affected	
As above	Trauma, caries, resorption

Table 4.10 *Different types of tremor*

Type	Causes
Contraction tremors (e.g. making a tight fist while the arm is resting and supported)	Essential tremor, cerebellar disease, hyperthyroidism, drugs such as caffeine and anticholinergic agents
Intention (action or kinetic) tremors (e.g. finger-to-nose test)	Cerebellar disorders and alcohol
Posture tremors (e.g. with the arms raised against gravity)	Essential tremor, physiological tremor, tremor with basal ganglia disease (as in parkinsonism), cerebellar disease, peripheral neuropathy, post-traumatic and alcoholic
Resting tremors (e.g. when the hands are lying on the lap)	Parkinsonism, antipsychotic drugs, essential tremor

TEETHING

Restlessness, irritability, finger-sucking, gum-rubbing and drooling may be associated with the eruption of deciduous teeth. Teething is traditionally blamed for a variety of other signs and symptoms in infancy, but is not responsible for diarrhoea, fever, convulsions or other systemic disorders. These have systemic causes, usually infections – often herpetic stomatitis.

TINNITUS

Tinnitus is a ringing, roaring or other sound inside the ears. It may be caused by ear problems (wax, infection, Ménière disease); neurological causes; or aspirin or certain antibiotics (aminoglycosides mainly). However, the reason for the tinnitus often cannot be found. Tinnitus can fluctuate or can resolve spontaneously, but is frequently untreatable.

TIREDNESS

Tiredness is a feeling of lack of energy, fatigue or weariness. Fatigue represents a normal response to physical exertion, emotional stress or lack of sleep, but can also be a non-specific symptom of a psychological or physiological disorder. In many cases, fatigue is related to boredom, unhappiness, disappointment, lack of sleep or hard work. Because it is such a common complaint and is often caused by psychological problems, its potential seriousness is often overlooked.

Pathological (illness-related) fatigue is not relieved by rest, adequate sleep or removal of stressful factors. An example is the so-called *chronic fatigue syndrome*.

The pattern of fatigue may help delineate its underlying cause: individuals who arise in the morning rested but, with activity, rapidly fatigue may have a disease, while individuals who awaken fatigued and the level of fatigue remains constant throughout the day may be suffering from depression. Other causes are shown in Box 4.12.

TOOTH DISCOLOURATION

Most causes of discolouration of several teeth are extrinsic stains. Discolouration of isolated teeth is commonly related to caries or trauma. Fluorosis, tetracyclines or congenital defects of enamel or dentine may cause brown or white intrinsic discolouration of most or all teeth; biliary atresia may cause green teeth, and erythropoietic porphyria may cause red teeth (Table 4.9).

TREMOR

Tremor is an unintentional, somewhat rhythmic, involuntary muscle movement involving to-and-fro movements (oscillations) of one or more parts of the body, most commonly affecting the hands. Tremor may also affect the arms, head, face, vocal cords, trunk and legs (Table 4.10). Caffeine (e.g. in coffee and carbonated beverages) and other stimulants should be avoided because they commonly worsen a tremor, as may emotion, stress, fever or physical exercise.

The most common form of tremor occurs in otherwise healthy people; this is essential tremor (no known cause). Tremor may also be caused by drugs (e.g. alcohol, amphetamines, caffeine, corticosteroids, ciclosporin, lithium, major tranquillizers and valproate); poisoning (e.g. mercury); neurological disorders (e.g. parkinsonism, multiple sclerosis, cerebellar disease); psychogenic reactions; or metabolic disorders (hypoglycaemia, hyperthyroidism, liver failure).

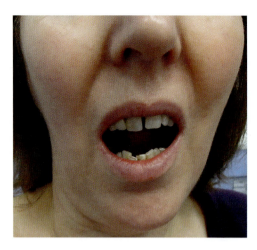

Fig. 4.9 Trismus.

TRISMUS

40–50 mm from incisal edge to incisal edge is considered normal mouth opening but 3 fingers is usually a rough guide. Limited oral opening (Fig. 4.9) can arise from temporomandibular joint disorders or from extra-articular causes such as infection, submucous fibrosis or scarring, or even tetanus.

Intra-articular causes may include:

- ankylosis
  - bony ankylosis: after trauma, infections and prolonged immobilization
  - fibrous ankylosis: due to trauma and infection
- arthitis
- synovitis.

Extra-articular causes may include:

- infection
  - odontogenic
  - non-odontogenic: peritonsillar abscess, tetanus, meningitis, brain abscess, parotid abscess.

URINARY INCONTINENCE

Urinary incontinence is an inability to hold urine until a lavatory is reached. It results from an underlying medical condition and is often only temporary. Women, particularly older women, experience incontinence twice as often as men because of problems associated with pregnancy and childbirth, and the menopause. Both women and men can become incontinent from neurological injury, birth defects, strokes, multiple sclerosis and physical problems associated with ageing.

Stress incontinence results from physical changes from pregnancy, childbirth and the menopause, and causes incontinence when coughing, laughing, sneezing or other movements that put pressure on the bladder.

Urge incontinence is caused by inappropriate bladder contractions, which result from overactive nervous control of the bladder. Urine is lost for no apparent reason while suddenly feeling the need or urge to urinate. Urge incontinence can mean that the bladder empties during sleep, after drinking a small amount of water, or when touching water or hearing it running (as when washing dishes or hearing someone else taking a shower). Involuntary actions of bladder muscles can occur due to damage to the nerves of the bladder, to the nervous system (spinal cord and brain), or to the muscles themselves as in multiple sclerosis, Parkinson disease, Alzheimer disease, stroke and injury.

Functional incontinence appears in people who have problems thinking, moving or communicating that prevent them from reaching a lavatory fast enough, as in Alzheimer disease. A person in a wheelchair may be blocked from getting to a lavatory in time.

Overflow incontinence is seen when the bladder is always full because of weak bladder muscles or a blocked urethra (e.g. prostatic disease), so that it leaks urine frequently. Nerve damage from diabetes or other diseases can lead to weak bladder muscles; tumours and urinary stones can block the urethra.

VERTIGO

See 'Dizziness'.

VISUAL IMPAIRMENT

Visual impairment may be suspected if a patient has overcautious driving habits; finds lighting either too bright or too dim; has frequent spectacle prescription changes; holds books or reading material close to the face or at arm's length; squints or tilts the head to see; has difficulty in recognizing people; changes leisure-time activities, personal appearance or table etiquette; moves about cautiously or bumps into objects; or acts confusedly or is disoriented.

Visual impairment can have a range of causes, from disease of the lens such as cataract, to albinism, glaucoma, retinitis pigmentosa, retinal detachment or nerve lesions. Blindness or defects of visual fields can be caused by ocular, optic nerve or cortical damage, but the type of defect varies according to the site and extent of the lesion. A complete lesion of one optic nerve causes that eye to be totally blind. There is no direct reaction of the pupil to light (loss of constriction) and, if a light is shone into the affected eye, the pupil of the unaffected eye also fails to respond (loss of the consensual reflex). However, the nerves to the affected eye that are responsible for pupil constriction run in the third cranial nerve and should be intact. If, therefore, a light is shone into the *unaffected eye*, the pupil of the affected eye also constricts, even though that eye is sightless.

Lesions of the optic tract, chiasma, radiation or optic cortex cause various visual field defects involving both visual fields but without total field loss on either side.

Visual field examination (perimetry) tests the total area where objects can be seen in the peripheral vision while the eye is focused on a central point. Confrontation visual field examination is a quick and basic evaluation of the visual field done by an examiner sitting directly in front of the patient, who is asked to look at the examiner's eye and say when they can see the examiner's hand. Tangent screen examination involves the patient looking at a central target and telling the examiner when an object brought into the peripheral vision can be seen.

Automated perimetry is when the patient sits in front of a computer-driven program that flashes small lights at different locations, and presses a button whenever the lights in the peripheral vision are seen. An ophthalmological opinion should always be obtained if there is any suggestion of a visual field defect.

Vision is tested by visual acuity testing using the Snellen eye chart or another standard eye chart. This displays a series of letters or letters and numbers, with the largest at the top. As the person being tested reads down the chart, the letters gradually become smaller. When visual acuity is being checked, one eye is covered at a time and the vision of each eye is recorded separately, as well as both eyes together. Normal vision is 20/20, which means that the eye being tested can read

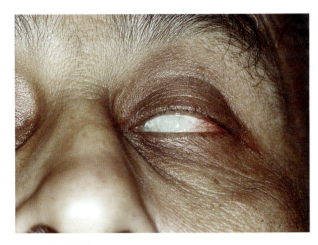

Fig. 4.10 Complete blindness: an opaque eye.

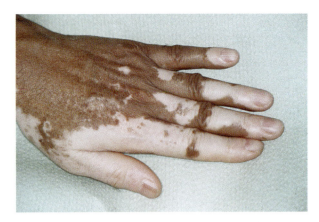

Fig. 4.11 Vitiligo (see also Fig. 2.25).

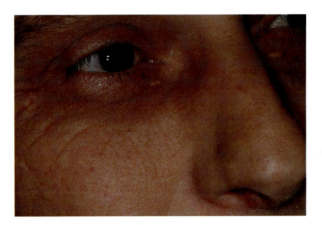

Fig. 4.12 Xanthelasma.

a letter of a certain size when it is 20 feet away. If a person sees 20/40, then at 20 feet from the chart that person can read letters that a person with 20/20 vision could read from 40 feet away. The 20/40 letters are twice the size of 20/20 letters; however, if 20/20 is considered 100% visual efficiency, 20/40 visual acuity is 85% efficient. For people who have worse than 20/400 vision, a different eye chart can be used. It is common to record vision worse than 20/400 as count fingers (CF at a certain number of feet), hand motion (HM at a certain number of feet), light perception (LP) or no light perception (NLP). As for legal blindness, in the UK the statutory definition of 'blind' is 'so blind as to be unable to perform any work for which eyesight is essential' (the Blind Persons Act 1920). There is no statutory definition of 'partial sight', although the guideline is 'substantially and permanently handicapped by defective vision caused by congenital defect, illness, or injury' (the National Assistance Act 1948).

After the pupils have been dilated, direct *ophthalmoscopy/ fundoscopy* provides a wider magnified view of the retina. *Tonometry* measures pressure inside the eye and is one of several tests necessary to detect glaucoma. *Slit-lamp examination* allows examination of the front of the eye. *Phoroptery* detects refractive errors.

Visual impairment can vary from limitations in sight for distance, colour, size or shape to full blindness (Fig. 4.10). It is an important disability that invariably restricts activity to some degree. Most visual impairment is caused by disease or malnutrition. The main causes include:

- cataracts
- glaucoma
- uveitis
- age-related macular degeneration (ARMD)
- trachoma
- corneal opacity
- diabetic retinopathy.

Cataracts, the most common cause of visual impairment in older people, are lens opacities that are more common in diabetes or after excess exposure to sunlight, ionizing irradiation or corticosteroids.

Visual defects are also among the most common genetic disorders, and congenital blindness may be associated with other handicaps such as epilepsy.

Clearly, communication is best verbally, though, for the partially sighted, writing matter can sometimes be used but must be in large, bold, black type on a white background.

Adaptive technology that may help includes adaptations around the home, as well as large-print books, books on tape and in Braille, and low-vision and blindness-related products.

VITILIGO

Vitiligo is loss of skin pigmentation (Fig. 4.11), which can be dramatically unaesthetic. It is usually an autoimmune disorder.

WEIGHT LOSS

Involuntary weight loss is a non-specific finding but is of concern. Causes, apart from malnutrition, are diabetes, hyperthyroidism, eating disorders, cancer (e.g. lung, gastrointestinal), infections (e.g. HIV disease, tuberculosis), depression and drugs.

WHITE LESIONS IN THE MOUTH

Most white oral lesions are due to local causes, such as keratoses caused by irritation, or idiopathic leukoplakia. Rare congenital causes include white sponge naevus (can involve the vagina and anus), dyskeratosis congenita and pachyonychia congenita.

Candidosis may cause white or red lesions (Ch. 21). Lichen planus and lupus erythematosus are discussed in Chapter 11. Cancer may present as a white lesion.

XANTHELASMA

These are flat yellow plaques over the upper or lower eyelids, most often near the inner canthus (Fig. 4.12). They are areas of lipid-containing macrophages; the presence of xanthelasma and corneal arcus indicates a higher risk of developing ischaemic heart disease and, though xanthelasma also have other causes, patients should have fasting lipid levels checked and those with hyperlipidaemia should have a formal cardiac assessment.

KEY WEBSITES

(Accessed 25 May 2013)

AIDS.gov. <http://aids.gov/hiv-aids-basics/hiv-aids-101/signs-and-symptoms/>.

American Cancer Society. <http://www.cancer.org/cancer/cancerbasics/signs-and-symptoms-of-cancer>.

WebMD symptom checker. <http://www.medicinenet.com/symptoms_and_signs/article.htm>.

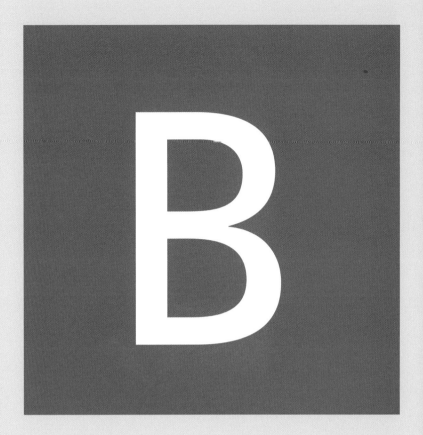

Organ systems medicine

The heart is vital to life, as its essential function is pumping oxygenated blood to the brain and vital organs. Blood is oxygenated in the lungs and travels in the pulmonary vein to the heart at the left atrium, from where it flows to the left ventricle through the mitral valve. Blood leaves the left ventricle through the aortic valve to the aorta (the body's main artery) and is distributed via arteries throughout the body. Thus the left ventricle is the most powerful chamber, as it has to move blood all around the body. Oxygen is transported on the red bloodcell (erythrocyte) pigment haemoglobin, which colours the blood red. Arteries branch to arterioles and then to capillaries to transport oxygen to the tissues (Fig. 5.1) and collect waste carbon dioxide. A vast venous network collects deoxygenated blood from all the tissues and returns it to the superior vena cava and inferior vena cava and thence to the right atrium of the heart (Fig. 5.2). This blood flows through the tricuspid valve to the right ventricle and then leaves the right ventricle through the pulmonary valve to the pulmonary artery and thence to the lungs, where it takes up oxygen. The heart thus consists of four chambers: two ventricles and two atria. It is centrally located in the chest (thorax) but, because the left ventricle is larger, the heart beat (apex beat) is found to the left side (Fig. 5.3).

The heart rate and force of contraction are controlled by nerves (mainly vagus and sympathetic) and hormones (especially adrenaline [epinephrine], which increases both rate and force). Anxiety and exercise can increase the pulse rate and force of the heart beat.

Heart disease is a major killer; in the USA, possibly one person dies from heart disease every 30 seconds. It also causes significant morbidity and disability in many aspects of life, including effects on entitlement to drive a motor vehicle. There is a wide range of disorders that can affect the heart (Box 5.1).

CONGENITAL HEART DISEASE (CHD)

General aspects

Congenital heart defects are the most common type of heart problem in children, present in about 1% of live births. Lesions may involve the

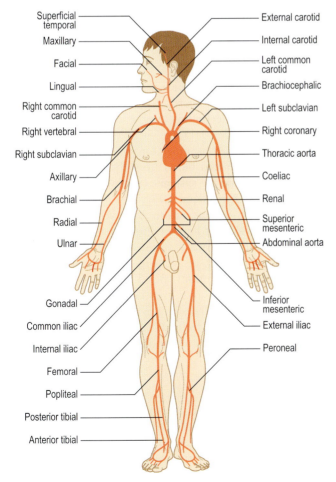

Fig. 5.1 Major arteries.

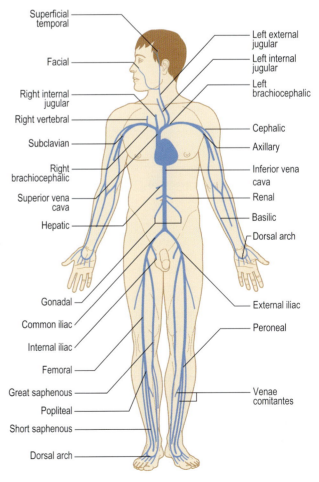

Fig. 5.2 Major veins.

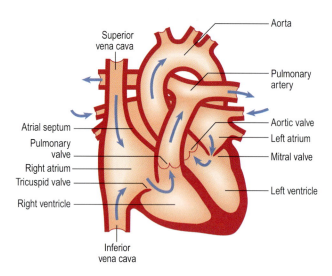

Superior vena cava
Aorta
Pulmonary artery
Atrial septum
Pulmonary valve
Aortic valve
Left atrium
Right atrium
Mitral valve
Tricuspid valve
Left ventricle
Right ventricle
Inferior vena cava

Fig. 5.3 Cardiac anatomy.

Table 5.1 *Types of congenital heart disease*[a]

| | | Acyanotic | |
Cyanotic	With no shunt	With left-to-right shunt
Eisenmenger syndrome	Aortic stenosis (AS)	Atrial septal defect (ASD)
Fallot tetralogy	Bicuspid aortic valve	Patent ductus arteriosus (PDA)
Pulmonary atresia (PA)	Coarctation of the aorta	Ventricular septal defect (VSD)
Pulmonary valve stenosis	Dextrocardia	
Total anomalous venous drainage (TAVD)	Mitral valve prolapse	
Transposition of the great vessels		
Tricuspid atresia (TA)		

[a]See also Table 5.2.

Box 5.1 *Causes of cardiovascular disease*

Organic heart disease
- Myocardial
  Overload secondary to hypertension or valve disease[a]
  Coronary (ischaemic) heart disease[a]
  Cardiomyopathies
- Endocardial
  Rheumatic heart disease
  Congenital anomalies[a]
  Infective endocarditis
- Pericardial
  Pericarditis
  Pericardial effusion

Functional disorders
- Due to hypertension[a]
- Due to abnormalities in heart rate
  Tachycardias
  Bradycardias
  Other arrhythmias
- Changes in circulatory volume
  Hypervolaemia (shock syndrome)
  Hypervolaemia (circulatory overload)
  Others

[a]Common causes of heart failure.

---

heart or adjacent great vessels, in isolation or in a variety of combinations, and include a wide variety of structural defects that can lead to malfunction such as arrhythmias or flow problems. Vessel or valve stenosis or obstruction and septal defects strain the myocardium.

The types of CHD are summarized in Table 5.1. CHD may be: cyanotic ('blue babies'), where there is right-to-left shunting – in general these are more severe defects; or acyanotic. Cyanosis and hypoxia can lead to neurological deficits, polycythaemia (with hypercoagulability and thromboses) and systemic infections (e.g. brain abscess). Approximately 20% of patients with CHD also have other congenital anomalies.

The cause of CHD is often unidentified but some causes are genetic (e.g. Down syndrome; see Ch. 28). There are many other causes (Table 5.2;

Appendices 5.1 and 5.2) and syndromes (e.g. oesophageal atresia and heart disease, and forearm/digit abnormalities and atrial septal defect [ASD]). The main acquired causes of CHD are maternal infections such as TORCH – congenital *to*xoplasmosis, *r*ubella, *c*ytomegalovirus or *h*erpes infection – which can lead to patent ductus arteriosus (PDA), pulmonary stenosis, ventricular septal defect (VSD) and coarctation of the aorta; maternal drug use (e.g. alcohol, anticonvulsants, lithium, recreational drugs, thalidomide and warfarin); or maternal systemic disease (systemic lupus erythematosus and Sjögren syndrome [both can cause heart block], and diabetes [which is associated with an increased incidence of VSD, coarctation and transposition of the great arteries and/or a characteristic hypertrophic cardiomyopathy]); and, rarely, maternal irradiation.

Clinical features

Cyanotic CHD is, in general, a much more severe defect than acyanotic (Fig. 5.4), which can lead to cardiac failure or be life-threatening or fatal without surgical intervention. In the absence of treatment, 40% of children with cyanotic CHD die within the first 5 years. Cyanosis (caused by >5 g of reduced haemoglobin per decilitre of blood) results from shunting deoxygenated blood from the right ventricle into the left side of the heart and the systemic circulation (*right-to-left shunt*), and leads to chronic hypoxaemia (Fig. 5.5). Patients may crouch in an effort to improve venous return but eventually polycythaemia develops – with consequent haemorrhagic or thrombotic tendencies. Finger- and toe-clubbing are associated with cyanotic CHD, but appear after about 3 months of age (Fig. 5.6). Patients with CHD are liable to a range of complications (Box 5.2).

Pulmonary hypertension and, eventually, right ventricular hypertrophy may be seen where the shunt is *left-to-right* and some of the output of the left ventricle is recirculated through the lungs. The shunt may eventually reverse and then cyanosis develops.

General management

An obstetric ultrasound scan is often used to screen pregnant women at around 20 weeks for signs of CHD in their unborn babies. Most defects, however, are well tolerated *in utero* and it is only after birth that the impact of the anatomical and subsequently haemodynamic abnormality becomes evident. In young children, chest radiography may show cardiomegaly. Electrocardiography (ECG) may

Table 5.2 *Main features of congenital heart disease (CHD)*

CHD	Main pathology/location	Main features
Aortic stenosis	Narrowing of the aortic valve	Angina, dyspnoea and syncope. Balloon valvuloplasty or surgery may be indicated
Atrial septal defect (ASD)	Usually near foramen ovale and termed a secundum defect. Associated in 10–20% with mitral valve prolapse	Initially acyanotic, with survival into middle age in most cases, and therefore is the most common CHD presenting in adults. In the absence of surgical correction, right ventricular failure eventually develops. Usually repaired by primary closure or by pericardial or Dacron patch
Bicuspid aortic valve	Valve is bicuspid instead of tricuspid. Often associated with other left-sided lesions (e.g. coarctation of the aorta or interrupted aortic arch)	Usually asymptomatic, even in athletes, but there is a high risk of infective endocarditis
Coarctation of the aorta	In the aorta beyond the origin of the subclavian arteries	Normal blood supply to the head, neck and upper body but restricted to the lower body. Surgery is indicated
Dextrocardia	Right-sided heart	Usually asymptomatic but may be part of situs inversus (all organs transposed) with bronchiectasis and sinusitis (Kartagener syndrome)
Ebstein anomaly	Congenital abnormality of the tricuspid valve, usually associated with ASD	Ebstein anomaly is mild in most and surgery is needed only if the tricuspid valve leaks severely enough to result in heart failure or cyanosis
Eisenmenger syndrome or reaction	The process in which a left-to-right shunt in the heart causes increased flow through the pulmonary vasculature (and pulmonary hypertension) which, in turn, causes increased pressures in the right heart and reversal into a right-to-left shunt	Ventricular or atrial septal defects, patent ductus arteriosus and more complex types of acyanotic heart disease can underlie this. Initially there is pulmonary hypertension, polycythaemia and a hyperviscosity syndrome with haemorrhagic and thrombotic tendencies. Later there is right ventricular hypertrophy and cyanosis. Anticoagulants and pulmonary vasodilators (e.g. bosentan) may be indicated
Fallot tetralogy	Ventricular septal defect, pulmonary stenosis, right ventricular hypertrophy and an aorta that overrides both ventricles. Fluconazole use in pregnancy may predispose	Cyanosis progressive from birth. Chronic hypoxia causes decreased neurological function. Episodes of acute hypoxia from infundibular spasm are life-threatening. Polycythaemia causes hypercoagulability and thrombosis. Right-to-left shunting is associated with a higher incidence of systemic infection such as a brain abscess. Surgery is indicated
Mitral valve prolapse (floppy mitral valve; Barlow syndrome)	The most common CHD, affecting 5–10% of the population. Seen mainly in women. Strong hereditary tendency. Seen especially in Marfan, Ehlers–Danlos and Down syndromes. May be associated with polycystic kidney disease and panic disorder	May cause no symptoms but, if there is mitral regurgitation, some patients develop pain, irregular or racing pulse, or fatigue and heart failure
Patent ductus arteriosus (PDA)	A persistent opening (normally closed by the third month of life) between aorta and pulmonary artery, common in prematurity and maternal rubella	Shunt is left to right, initially acyanotic, and a typical complication is right ventricular failure. Closure can be promoted in early infancy by giving intravenous indometacin, a prostaglandin inhibitor
Patent foramen ovale	Communication between atria	Often symptomless
Pulmonary atresia	No pulmonary valve exists, so blood cannot flow from the right ventricle into the pulmonary artery and to the lungs. The right ventricle is not well developed. The tricuspid valve is often poorly developed. An ASD allows blood to exit the right atrium, so the baby is cyanotic. The only source of lung blood flow is the PDA	Early treatment often includes using a drug to keep the PDA from closing, and surgery to create a shunt between the aorta and the pulmonary artery
Pulmonary stenosis	Narrowing of the pulmonary valve	Symptoms are breathlessness and right ventricular failure. Balloon valvuloplasty or surgery may be indicated
Total anomalous pulmonary venous return (TAPVR)	Blood returns from the lungs to the right rather than left atrium	Survivors also have ASD or patent foramen ovale
Transposition of the great vessels	Reversal of pulmonary artery and aorta origins	Cyanosis and breathlessness from birth, with early congestive cardiac failure and death in infancy unless there are associated defects providing sufficient collateral circulation (such as a patent interventricular septum or PDA)
Tricuspid atresia	Absence of the tricuspid valve means no blood can flow from the right atrium to the right ventricle. Thus the right ventricle is small. Survival depends on there being an ASD and usually a ventricular septal defect	A surgical shunting procedure is often needed to increase the lung blood flow and reduce cyanosis. Some children may need pulmonary artery banding to *reduce* blood flow to the lungs. Others may need a more functional repair (Fontan procedure)
Ventricular septal defect (VSD)	One of the most common CHDs. Ranges from a pinhole compatible with survival at least into middle age, to a large defect causing death in infancy if untreated. Some 90% of children with VSD have an additional cardiac defect	Initially left-to-right shunt but, with right ventricular hypertrophy, shunt may eventually reverse with late-onset cyanosis. Right ventricular failure may develop. Usually repaired by primary closure or by a pericardial or Dacron patch

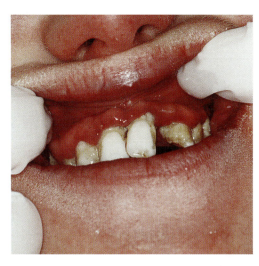

Fig. 5.4 Central cyanosis in a child with a congenital heart defect, showing purple lips and gingivae.

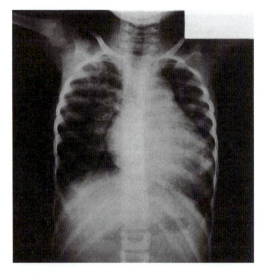

Fig. 5.5 Chest radiograph of a child with congenital heart disease showing gross cardiac enlargement. (The heart normally occupies less than half the width of the chest).

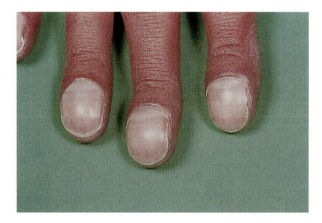

Fig. 5.6 Finger-clubbing in a patient with Fallot tetralogy. Finger-clubbing can be found in several different disorders, particularly cyanotic heart disease, chronic respiratory disease, lung cancer, Crohn disease, etc., but is sometimes benign and hereditary.

Box 5.2 *Possible complications in congenital heart disease*

- Bleeding tendency
- Cardiac failure
- Cyanosis
- Fatigue
- Growth retardation
- Infections (e.g. brain abscess, endocarditis)
- Polycythaemia
- Pulmonary oedema

demonstrate an abnormal cardiac axis, ventricular hypertrophy and strain, depending on the lesion present. CHD is more commonly diagnosed through echocardiography, which has superseded intracardiac catheter studies, and confirmed by cardiac magnetic resonance imaging (MRI).

Early correction of the congenital defect, often by transvenous catheter techniques, is the treatment of choice. More complex defects may require an operation. Medical treatment may be needed for the management of pulmonary oedema, heart failure, polycythaemia, infection or emotional disturbances. Modern surgical and medical care helps children survive into adult life and patients are then often said to have adult or 'grown-up' CHD. Nevertheless, complications observed in adults who were previously thought to have had successful repair of CHD include arrhythmias, valve disorders and cardiac failure, and residual defects can still predispose to complications such as infective endocarditis.

Dental aspects

All dental health-care professionals (HCPs) should be certified in basic cardiopulmonary resuscitation (CPR), and the entire team should rehearse emergency protocol procedures regularly (Ch. 1).

Patients with heart disease should take their medications as usual on the day of the dental procedure, and should bring all their medications to the dental surgery for review at the time of the first appointment. The most important aspect for dentists to consider is how well the patient's heart condition is compensated. Patients with stable heart disease receiving atraumatic treatment under local anaesthesia (LA) can receive treatment in the dental surgery. Since cardiac events are most likely to occur in the early morning, patients with cardiac disease should be treated in the late morning or early afternoon. The dental team should provide dental care with a stress-reduction protocol and with good analgesia, limiting the dosage of adrenaline (epinephrine). An aspirating syringe should be used to give an LA, since adrenaline in the anaesthetic entering a vessel may theoretically raise the BP or precipitate arrhythmias. Gingival retraction cords containing adrenaline should be avoided. Conscious sedation, preferably with nitrous oxide, can be given with the approval of the physician. General anaesthesia (GA) is a matter for expert anaesthetists in hospital.

Congestive cardiac failure may complicate management. In cyanotic CHD there may also be polycythaemia-related bleeding tendencies caused by thrombocytopenia, platelet dysfunction, coagulation defects (from liver hypoxia – causing reduced vitamin K-dependent factors) and excessive fibrinolytic activity. Thus platelets may be reduced, and the haematocrit, prothrombin time (PT [and International Normal Ratio, INR]; Ch. 8) and activated partial thromboplastin time (APTT) increased. Occasionally, there is a thrombotic tendency. A special hazard in some CHD is the development of cerebral abscess, sometimes due to oral bacteria. Leukopenia may be a factor in some right-to-left shunts. There may be susceptibility to infective endocarditis. Oral abnormalities can be associated with cyanotic CHD and may include:

- delayed eruption of both dentitions
- positional anomalies
- enamel hypoplasia – the teeth often have a bluish-white, 'skimmed milk' appearance and there is gross vasodilatation in the pulps
- greater caries and periodontal disease activity, probably because of poor oral hygiene and lack of dental attention
- after cardiotomy, the possible appearance of transient small, white, non-ulcerated mucosal lesions of unknown aetiology.

CONGENITAL HEART DISEASE IN OTHER SYNDROMES

Down syndrome

See Chapter 28.

Noonan syndrome

Noonan syndrome, usually an autosomal dominant trait, is characterized by CHD (the commonest cardiac lesions are pulmonary stenosis, septal defects and hypertrophic cardiomyopathy), short stature, unusual facies, chest deformity, learning disability, and cryptorchidism in males. Facial features may include an elongated mid-face, hypertelorism, retrognathia, a lower nasal bridge and nasal root, a wider mouth, a more prominent upper lip and low-set ears. Abnormal vision and hearing are common. Other associations include hepatosplenomegaly and an abnormal bleeding tendency associated with low levels of clotting factors (particularly XI and XII), and with cherubism, jaw giant-cell lesions and neurofibromatosis.

Hypercalcaemia–supravalvular aortic stenosis syndrome (Williams syndrome)

Williams syndrome comprises, in its rare complete form, infantile hypercalcaemia, elfin facies, learning disability and CHD. Most cases appear to be sporadic. These children may be sociable and talkative ('cocktail party manner'). Hypercalcaemia typically remits in infancy but leaves growth deficiency, osteosclerosis and craniostenosis. Cardiovascular lesions include supravalvular subaortic stenosis or other abnormalities, and may contraindicate GA. Also, masseter spasm has been reported during GA with halothane and suxamethonium, but it is not malignant hyperthermia. Dental defects may include hypodontia, microdontia and hypoplastic, bud-shaped teeth. The upper dental arch may be disproportionately wide and overlap the lower.

ACQUIRED HEART DISEASE

General aspects

Most acquired heart disease is ischaemic heart disease (IHD; coronary artery disease, CAD) – the most important cardiac disease, which can lead to heart failure and is the major killer in the high-income world. Functional disorders, where there is no organic disease of the heart itself, can also cause circulatory failure, as in shock. A variety of common extracardiac diseases can aggravate heart disease, particularly if there is impaired oxygenation, as in severe anaemia.

Clinical features

Serious heart disease is not always symptomatic and patients can die suddenly from myocardial infarction (MI), despite having experienced neither chest pain nor any other symptom ("silent infarction"). Also, many patients with manifest cardiac disease can have signs and symptoms effectively controlled so that they may superficially appear well and, often, only the drug history gives a clue to the nature of any cardiac illness. Common clinical features of cardiac disease include breathlessness, chest pain, palpitations and cyanosis, while signs may be seen on the hands (clubbing, cyanosis) or deduced from measuring the BP, palpating the pulse or listening to the heart (auscultation).

General management

The heart rate, force of contraction and rhythm can be assessed from palpation of the pulse; disturbances of rhythm may signify cardiac disease.

The BP is measured by sphygmomanometry. The finding of either normal levels (pressures of 120 mmHg systolic and 80 mmHg diastolic) or grossly raised levels (>160/90 mmHg for a male of 45 years or over) is informative. However, these must be checked on further occasions, as the BP frequently increases in anxiety. In an injured patient, a falling BP is also a danger sign that must not be ignored, since it implies a serious complication such as haemorrhage or shock.

Experienced cardiologists can identify by auscultation the vast majority of innocent functional murmurs and can differentiate these from the serious murmurs of aortic stenosis, mitral regurgitation, tricuspid regurgitation, pulmonary stenosis, VSD and hypertrophic cardiomyopathy.

Other investigations include blood assays of cardiac enzymes (troponin, troponin T (cTnT), creatine kinase), which are raised after cardiac damage such as an MI. Chest radiography (CXR) helps detect heart enlargement (e.g. in cardiac failure or hypertension). ECG, invaluable for the diagnosis of arrhythmias and of IHD, is a graphic tracing of the variations in electrical potential caused by the excitation of the atria (Fig. 5.7). The QRS deflections are due to excitation (depolarization) of the ventricles. The T wave is due to recovery of the ventricles (repolarization). Doppler echocardiography (cardiac ultrasonography done trans-thoracically or trans-oesophageally) is a valuable non-invasive imaging tool for the heart; it is helpful in establishing a specific diagnosis and estimating the severity of various diseases by evaluating cardiac chamber size, wall thickness, wall motion, valve configuration

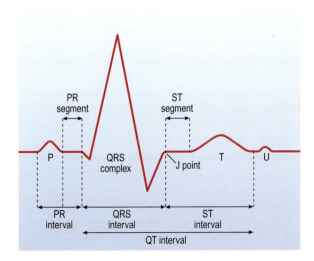

Fig. 5.7 Normal ECG tracing.

Table 5.3 *Predictors of high cardiovascular risk*

Very high risk	Medium risk	Low risk
MI in previous month	Mild angina	Old age
Unstable or severe angina	Myocardial infarction (MI) more than 1 month previously	ECG abnormalities only
Atrioventricular block		Atrial fibrillation
		Stroke
Ventricular arrhythmias	Compensated heart failure	Uncontrolled hypertension
Severe cardiac valvular disease		Mild heart failure
Advanced heart failure		

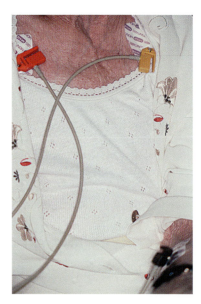

Fig. 5.8 Cardiac monitoring – chest leads.

and motion, and the proximal great vessels. This technique also provides a sensitive method for detecting pericardial and pleural fluid accumulation, and can allow identification of mass lesions within and adjacent to the heart. Cardiac MRI, scans using gadolinium, thallium-201 or technetium-99, and positron emission tomography (PET) using 18F-deoxyglucose (FDG) are also extremely useful.

Medical treatments are available to control many cardiac disorders, but surgery may be required, especially for IHD.

Dental aspects

Management implications in oral health care depend mainly on the type of intervention and the degree of cardiovascular risk (Table 5.3 and see below). Both the anxiety and the pain that may be associated with dental care can cause enhanced sympathetic activity and adrenaline (epinephrine) release, which increases the load on the heart and the risk of angina or arrhythmias. Therefore, patients with unstable angina (pain pattern changing in occurrence, frequency, intensity or duration; pain at rest) and those with MI <3 months previously should have dental treatment in a hospital environment. Patients with stable angina and those who are at least 3 months post-MI may be treated in primary care. However, appointments should be made for the late morning, with the patient's glyceryl trinitrate (GTN) available and used preoperatively, and the use of pulse oximetry and prophylactic sedatives considered. Nitrate drugs, which include glyceryl trinitrate (GTN), isosorbide dinitrate and isosorbide mononitrate are vasodilators and act by reducing load on the heart. GTN is available for sublingual use as a tablet or a spray, or as a skin patch. Tables have a limited shelf life of about 8 weeks. Oral use works within a minute or so and lasts 30 mins but the patch takes about an hour to work and is often left on for 12 hours. The most common adverse effects of nitrates are a throbbing headache, flushing, and dizziness, and they interfere with sildenafil. Pain control is crucial to minimize endogenous adrenaline release. LA must be given with aspiration and it may be prudent to avoid adrenaline-containing LA. If a patient is taking a non-selective beta-blocker (e.g. propanolol), no more than two carpules of LA with adrenaline 1:80 000 should be administered. The combination of aspirin with other antiplatelet drugs increases the chances of significant postoperative bleeding. Furthermore, drugs such as erythromycin and clarithromycin should be avoided in long QT syndrome and in patients also taking statins (antihyperlipidaemics). In the case of intraoperative chest pain, medical assistance should be summoned and emergency management commenced, including the use of GTN aspirin and oxygen. Cardiac monitoring is desirable in many instances (Figs 5.8 and 5.9).

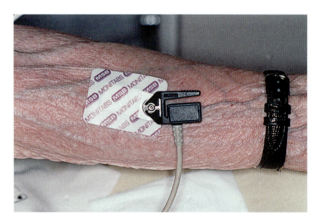

Fig. 5.9 Cardiac monitoring – arm lead.

Effective painless LA is essential. An aspirating syringe should be used since adrenaline in the anaesthetic may get into the blood and may (theoretically) raise the BP and precipitate arrhythmias. BP tends to rise during oral surgery under LA, and adrenaline theoretically can contribute, but this is usually of little practical importance. However, adrenaline-containing LA should not be given in excessive doses to patients taking beta-blockers, as this may induce hypertension and cardiovascular complications. *Note*: A woman on beta-blockers, who was (inexcusably) given 16 dental cartridges of LA, died from lidocaine overdosage, *not* from accelerated hypertension. Gingival retraction cords containing adrenaline should be avoided wherever possible. General anaesthesia for dental care in cardiac patients should be avoided unless essential.

A range of cardiovascular drugs can influence oral health care (Table 5.4), while drugs used in dentistry can interact with cardiac drugs. Aspirin may cause sodium and fluid retention, which may be contraindicated in severe hypertension or cardiac failure. Indometacin may interfere with antihypertensive agents. Macrolides and azoles may cause statins to produce increased muscle damage.

An association between periodontal disease and cardiovascular disease has been suggested but several evidence-based reviews question this association.

Table 5.4 *Cardiovascular drugs: potential effects on oral health care*

Group	Oral adverse effects	Possible interaction or reaction
Alpha-blockers	Dry mouth	Orthostatic hypotension
Alpha-/beta-blockers	–	Enhanced pressor response to adrenaline (epinephrine)
Angiotensin-converting enzyme inhibitors (ACEIs)	Burning sensation Ulceration Taste changes Dry mouth Angioedema Lichenoid reactions	Impairment by indometacin
Angiotensin II receptor blockers (ARBs)	Facial flushing Taste disturbance Dry mouth Increased gag reflex Lupoid reactions	Good toleration
Antihypertensives (see Table 5.8)	Predisposition to lip cancer (hydrochlorothiazide, nifedipine, triamterene, lisinopril, atenolol)	Photosensitivity
Antiplatelets	Purpura Bleeding	Bleeding tendency enhanced by erythromycin
Beta-blockers (non-cardioselective)	Dry mouth Paraesthesia Lichenoid lesions	Enhanced pressor response to adrenaline (epinephrine)
Calcium-channel blockers (CCBs)	Gingival swelling: 30% using nifedipine develop this Angioedema	–
Digitalis glycosides	Dry mouth	Possible induction of arrhythmias by LA vasoconstrictor Gag reflex increased
Diuretics	Dry mouth	–
Potassium-channel blockers	Ulceration	–
Statins	–	Muscle damage increased by macrolides (erythromycin, clarithromycin, telithromycin) and azoles (fluconazole, itraconazole, ketoconazole, miconazole) but rosuvastatin, pravastatin and fluvastatin do not appear to have this problem

Box 5.3 *Manual technique for recording blood pressure*

1. Ask patient to avoid alcohol and smoking for 30 min before measurement
2. Allow patient to sit at rest for as long as possible
3. Place sphygmomanometer cuff on right upper arm with about 3 cm of skin visible at antecubital fossa; bladder should encircle at least two-thirds of arm
4. Palpate right brachial pulse
5. After 5 min, inflate cuff slowly to about 200–250 mmHg, or until pulse is no longer palpable
6. Deflate cuff slowly while listening with stethoscope over brachial artery over skin on inside of arm below cuff
7. Record systolic pressure as pressure when first tapping sounds appear (Korotkoff sounds)
8. Deflate cuff further until tapping sounds become muffled (diastolic pressure) and then disappear
9. Repeat; record BP as systolic/diastolic pressures

a progressive rise in BP. Untreated hypertension is one of the most important preventable causes of morbidity and mortality, since it is a major risk factor for ischaemic and haemorrhagic strokes (cerebro-vascular events), myocardial infarction, heart failure, chronic kidney disease, cognitive decline and premature death. The risk associated with increasing BP is continuous, with each 2 mmHg rise in systolic BP linked with a 7% rise in risk of mortality from ischaemic heart disease and a 10% increased risk of mortality from stroke. The vascular and renal damage that hypertension may cause can culminate in a treatment-resistant state. The BP is the product of cardiac output and peripheral resistance, and is dependent on the heart and vasculature, autonomic nervous system, endocrine system and kidneys. Regulatory mechanisms, though unclear, involve baroreceptors in various organs that detect changes in BP, and adjust it by altering both the heart rate and the force of contractions, as well as the peripheral resistance. Other factors are the kidney renin–angiotensin system, which responds to a fall in BP by activating a vasoconstrictor (angiotensin II), and the adrenocortical release of aldosterone in response to angiotensin II, causing fluid retention via the kidney – increasing sodium retention and potassium excretion. The most potent vasoconstrictor is endothelin-1, released by vascular endothelium in response to expansion of plasma volume, hypoxia or growth factors, and which regulates vascular tone. Nitric oxide (NO) also modulates vasodilator tone in the control of BP.

The BP will vary, depending on age, gender, ethnicity, environment, emotional state and activity. Since it rises with anxiety, measurements should be made with the patient relaxed and fully at rest. The BP is lowest at night and highest first thing in the morning. It tends to increase with age.

If the clinic BP is 140/90 mmHg or higher, ambulatory blood pressure monitoring (ABPM) is needed to confirm the diagnosis of hypertension (average value of at least 14 measurements taken during the person's usual waking hours). Home BP monitoring (HBPM) can be used to confirm a diagnosis of hypertension, provided that:

- for each BP recording, two consecutive measurements are taken, at least 1 minute apart and with the person seated
- BP is recorded twice daily, ideally in the morning and evening
- BP recording continues for at least 4 days, and ideally for 7 days.

Hypertension is a persistently raised BP. There is no agreed BP cut-off point above which 'hypertension' exists and below which it does not. At least one-quarter of adults (and more than half of those older

HYPERTENSION

General aspects

Hypertension (high blood pressure) is common, often unrecognised and potentially lethal. The blood pressure is measured with a sphygmomanometer (Box 5.3), in units of millimetres of mercury (mmHg). A 'normal' adult blood pressure (BP) is 120/80 (systolic/diastolic) mmHg. High blood pressure (hypertension) is usually associated with

Table 5.5 *Blood pressure levels*

Stage	Designation	Level
Normal		Systolic: less than 120 mmHg
		Diastolic: less than 80 mmHg
At risk	Pre-hypertension	Systolic: 120–139 mmHg
		Diastolic: 80–89 mmHg
Stage 1	Hypertension	Systolic: 140/90 mmHg or higher and subsequent ambulatory monitoring (ABPM) daytime average or home monitoring (HBPM) average is 135/85 mmHg or higher
Stage 2	Hypertension	Systolic: 160/100 mmHg or higher and subsequent ABPM daytime average or HBPM average is 150/95 mmHg or higher
Severe	Hypertension	Systolic: 180 mmHg or higher
		Diastolic: 110 mmHg or higher

Table 5.6 *American Society of Anesthesiologists (ASA) grading of hypertension and dental management considerations*

Blood pressure (mmHg; systolic, diastolic)	ASA grade	Hypertension stage	Dental aspects
<140, <90	I	–	Routine dental care
140–159, 90–99	II	1	Recheck BP before starting routine dental care
160–179, 95–109	III	2	Recheck BP and seek medical advice before routine dental care
			Restrict use of adrenaline (epinephrine)
			Conscious sedation may help
>180, >110	IV	3	Recheck BP after 5 min quiet rest
			Medical advice before dental care
			Only emergency care until BP controlled
			Avoid vasoconstrictors

Table 5.7 *Causes of hypertension*

Secondary hypertension	Idiopathic (essential) hypertension
Renal disease (80% of cases) – renal artery disease, pyelonephritis, glomerulonephritis, polycystic disease, post-transplant	Genetic predisposition
	High alcohol intake
	High salt intake (possibly)
Endocrine conditions – pregnancy, Cushing syndrome and corticosteroid therapy, hyperaldosteronism, phaeochromocytoma, acromegaly	High basal metabolic index (BMI)
	Insulin resistance
	Sympathetic overactivity: 40% of hypertensive patients have raised catecholamines (adrenaline [epinephrine] and noradrenaline [norepinephrine])
Cerebral disease – cerebral oedema (mainly strokes, head injuries or tumours)	
Coarctation of aorta – hypertension in upper half of body only	
Drugs – oral contraceptive pill, corticosteroids, non-steroidal anti-inflammatory drugs (NSAIDs), liquorice	
Sleep apnoea	

Table 5.8 *Lifestyle risk factors modifying hypertension*

Factors raising blood pressure	Factors lowering blood pressure
Obesity	No obesity
High dietary salt intake	Low salt intake
Excess alcohol	Low alcohol intake
Smoking	Stopping smoking
Excessive physical inactivity	Physical activity
Stress/anxiety	Relaxation
	High-fibre diet
	Omega-3 fatty acids possibly
	Fruit and vegetables
	Supplemental potassium

than 60) have high BP. Hypertension is thus common, especially with advancing age, when systolic hypertension becomes a more significant problem, as a result of the progressive stiffening and loss of compliance of larger arteries. Diastolic pressure is more commonly raised in people younger than 50 years (Table 5.5). Hypertension nevertheless is generally defined as a BP of at least 140/90 mmHg, based on at least two readings on separate occasions. Indeed, the Seventh Report of the Joint National Committee on Prevention, Detection, Evaluation, and Treatment of High Blood Pressure defined a BP of 120/80–139/89 mmHg as pre-hypertension – a designation chosen to identify individuals at high risk of developing hypertension. The National Heart, Lung and Blood Institute (NHLBI) has even recommended that 'pre-hypertension' should be considered as beginning when BP is 115/75 mmHg. Hypertension may be staged as shown in Tables 5.5 and 5.6.

Some 40% of adults in the developed world have hypertension but in more than 90% the cause is unknown; this is termed 'primary', 'idiopathic' or 'essential' hypertension. In 1–2% of hypertensive patients, an identifiable cause is present and this is termed 'secondary' hypertension. Aetiological factors are shown in Table 5.7. Lifestyle factors that can raise the BP include stress, obesity, salt intake, smoking,

alcohol, illicit drugs (cocaine, amphetamines) or prescribed drugs (e.g. immunosuppressives, glucocorticoids, mineralocorticoids, anabolic steroids), but other factors can lower the BP (Table 5.8).

Clinical features

At least one-third of people with hypertension are asymptomatic or have only trivial complications, such as epistaxes. Hypertension can affect many tissues, however, and especially the brain, heart, eyes and kidneys, with complications that include coronary artery disease, myocardial infarction, heart failure and cerebrovascular events in particular (Table 5.9). Long-standing hypertension accelerates atheroma and predisposes to: coronary artery disease; cerebrovascular disease; chronic kidney disease (hypertensive nephrosclerosis is the term given to long-term essential hypertension, hypertensive retinopathy, left ventricular hypertrophy, minimal proteinuria and progressive renal insufficiency); peripheral vascular disease; and hypertensive retinopathy leading to retinal haemorrhages, retinopathy or optic neuropathy and blindness. Hypertension shortens life by 10–20 years. The risk of these sequelae is greater in people who also have diabetes and cardiac or renal disease.

General management

The National Institute for Health and Care Excellence (NICE)'s clinical guideline 127, *Hypertension: clinical management of primary*

Table 5.9 *Features of advanced hypertension*

Symptoms	Signs
Headaches	Hypertension on testing
Visual disorders	Retinal changes
Tinnitus	Left ventricular hypertrophy
Dizziness	Proteinuria
Angina	Haematuria

Table 5.10 *Antihypertensive drugs*

Antihypertensive agents	Examples
Alpha-adrenergic blockers	Doxazosin, indoramin, prazosin, terazosin
Angiotensin-converting enzyme inhibitors (ACEIs)	Captopril, cilazapril, enalapril, fosinopril, imidapril, lisinopril, moexipril, perindopril, quinapril, ramipril, trandolapril
Angiotensinogen II receptor blockers (ARBs)	Azilsartan, candesartan, eprosartan, losartan, olmesartan, temisartan, valsartan
Beta-adrenergic blockers	Acebutolol, atenolol, bisoprolol, carvedilol, celiprolol, esmolol, labetalol, metoprolol, nadolol, nebivolol, oxprenolol, pindolol, propranolol, timolol
Calcium-channel blockers (CCBs)	Amlodipine, diltiazem, felodipine, isradipine, lacidipine, lercanidipine, nicardipine, nifedipine, verapamil
Diuretics	Amiloride, bendroflumethiazide, bumetanide, chlortalidone, furosemide, indapamide, metolazone, spironolactone, torasemide, triamterene, xipamide
Sympatholytics	Clonidine, methyldopa
Vasodilators	Hydralazine, minoxidil

hypertension in adults, is available at http://publications.nice.org.uk/hypertension-cg127 (accessed 25 May 2013).

Hypertension is diagnosed by standardized serial BP measurements, as above. Investigations to identify a 'secondary' cause and assess end-organ damage include: chest radiography (cardiomegaly is suggestive of hypertensive heart disease); ECG (may indicate ischaemic heart disease); serum urea and electrolytes (deranged in hypertensive renal disease and endocrine causes of secondary hypertension); and urine Stix testing (blood and protein suggest renal disease).

Treatment of hypertension reduces the risk of stroke, heart failure and renal failure but has less effect on ischaemic cardiac events. Hypertension and its complications can be modulated by changing lifestyle (see Table 5.8) through: relaxation, weight loss, a high-fibre diet, reduction in salt intake, restriction of alcohol consumption, restriction of caffeine intake, smoking cessation and greater amounts of exercise. Acute emotion, particularly anger, fear and anxiety, can cause great rises in catecholamine output and transient rises in BP and should, therefore, be avoided or controlled.

Antihypertensive therapy is given with the goal of using the minimum dose of drugs commensurate with achieving the desired BP, and with minimal adverse effects. Therapy is urgently indicated where the systolic pressure exceeds 200 mmHg, or the diastolic 110 mmHg, and is indicated at lower levels particularly if there are vascular complications, diabetes or end-organ damage such as renal impairment. Current guidelines are to offer antihypertensive drug treatment to:

- people below 80 years of age with stage 1 hypertension (see Tables 5.5 and 5.6), who have one or more of the following:
  - Target organ damage
  - Established cardiovascular disease
  - Renal disease
  - Diabetes
  - A 10-year cardiovascular risk equivalent to 20% or greater
- people of any age with stage 2 hypertension.

A large number of antihypertensive drugs are available (Table 5.10); beta-blockers are not now a preferred initial antihypertensive therapy. Treatment is stepwise:

A BP of less than 140/90 mmHg is generally the aim. There is strong evidence to support treating hypertensive persons aged 60 years or older to a BP goal of less than 150/90 mmHg and hypertensive persons 30 through 59 years of age to a diastolic goal of less than 90 mmHg. There is moderate evidence to support starting treatment with an angiotensin-converting enzyme inhibitor, angiotensin receptor blocker, calcium channel blocker, or thiazide-type diuretic in the nonblack hypertensive population and in the black hypertensive population, initial therapy is a calcium channel blocker or thiazide-type diuretic. There is moderate evidence to support initial or add-on antihypertensive therapy with an angiotensin-converting enzyme inhibitor or angiotensin receptor blocker in persons with CKD to improve renal outcomes.

Step 1

- Offer people *<55 years* an angiotensin-converting enzyme inhibitor (ACEI) or angiotensin II receptor blocker (ARB).
- Offer a calcium-channel blocker (CCB) to people aged *>55 years and to people of African or Caribbean family origin* of any age. If a CCB is unsuitable, or if there is evidence or a high risk of heart failure, offer a thiazide-like diuretic. If a diuretic is to be initiated or changed, offer a thiazide-like diuretic (e.g. chlortalidone or indapamide) rather than a conventional thiazide diuretic (bendroflumethiazide or hydrochlorothiazide).

Step 2

If BP is not controlled by step 1 treatment:

- offer a CCB with either an ACEI or an ARB, *but*
- if a CCB is unsuitable, or if there is evidence or a high risk of heart failure, offer a thiazide-like diuretic. For black people of African or Caribbean family origin, consider an ARB in preference to an ACEI, in combination with a CCB.

Step 3

If step 2 treatment is not effective:

- use the combination of ACEI or ARB, CCB and thiazide-like diuretic.

Step 4

If BP remains >140/90 mmHg after treatment with ACEI or ARB plus CCB plus a diuretic, this may be resistant hypertension. In this case:

- treat with spironolactone or a higher-dose thiazide-like diuretic (specialist advice is indicated).

Adverse effects of antihypertensive treatment can sometimes be troublesome and treatment has to be tailored to each patient's response (Table 5.11).

Accelerated (malignant) hypertension

This typically affects young adults, especially those of African or Afro-Caribbean black heritage and, like essential hypertension, often causes no symptoms until complications develop. It may present with headaches, visual impairment, nausea, vomiting, fits (seizures) or

Table 5.11 *Adverse effects from antihypertensive and other cardioactive drugs*

Group	Comments and adverse effects
Alpha-adrenergic blockers	Thrombocytopenia
Angiotensin-converting enzyme inhibitors (ACEIs)	First dose may cause sudden fall in BP May impede renal function, especially if NSAIDs also given Cough, angioedema
Angiotensin II receptor blockers (ARBs)	Generally well tolerated but olmesartan can cause a sprue-like disease
Beta-blockers	Bronchospasm
	Contraindicated in asthma, heart failure or heart block
	Muscle weakness
	Lassitude
	Disturbed sleep
Calcium-channel blockers (CCBs)	Headache and flushing
	Swollen legs
Centrally acting antihypertensives (largely obsolete)	Haemolysis Hepatitis
Diuretics	Hypovolaemia
	Electrolyte changes
Potassium-channel blockers	Headache
	May cause flushing
Vasodilators	Lupoid reactions

Table 5.12 *Causes of orthostatic hypotension*

Primary autonomic causes	Secondary autonomic causes	Non-autonomic causes
Familial dysautonomia (Riley–Day syndrome)	B vitamin deficiency	Hypovolaemia
	Alcoholism	Ageing
Pure autonomic failure (idiopathic orthostatic hypotension)	Diabetes	Prolonged bed rest
	Parkinsonism	Pregnancy
	Porphyria	Drugs (e.g. antihypertensives)
Shy–Drager syndrome		
Dopamine		
Beta-hydroxylase deficiency		

acute cardiac failure. The chief complication is severe ischaemic damage to the kidneys and renal failure, which can be fatal within 1 year of diagnosis. Other causes of death are cardiac failure or cerebrovascular accidents. Life-threatening accelerated hypertension requires urgent hospital admission with the aim of reducing the BP slowly with oral antihypertensives. Rarely, intravenous antihypertensives (sodium nitroprusside) are used but a sudden drop in BP may result in a stroke (cerebral infarction). Vigorous treatment, if started before renal damage is too far advanced, can greatly improve the life expectancy; about 50% of patients can now expect to live for at least 5 years. Renal sympathetic denervation is a promising recent therapy for resistant hypertension.

Dental aspects of hypertension

There are no recognized orofacial manifestations of hypertension but facial palsy is an occasional complication of malignant hypertension. Antihypertensive drugs can sometimes cause orofacial side-effects, such as hyposalivation (clonidine in particular), salivary gland swelling or pain, lichenoid reactions, erythema multiforme, angioedema, gingival swelling, sore mouth or paraesthesiae (see Table 5.10).

BP should be controlled before elective dental treatment or the opinion of a physician should be sought, since the BP often rises even before a visit for dental care; preoperative reassurance is important and sedation using temazepam may be helpful. Endogenous adrenaline (epinephrine) levels peak during the morning hours and adverse cardiac events are most likely in the early morning, so patients are best treated in the late morning. Those with stable hypertension may receive dental care, in short, minimally stressful appointments. It is essential to avoid anxiety and pain, since endogenous adrenaline released in response to pain or fear may induce arrhythmias. Adequate analgesia must be provided. Both the pain threshold and tolerance are higher in hypertensive than normotensive subjects; the mechanism is

unclear but drug treatment of the hypertension normalizes the pain perception. An aspirating syringe should be used to give an LA, since adrenaline given intravenously may (theoretically) increase hypertension and precipitate arrhythmias. BP tends to rise during oral surgery under LA, and adrenaline theoretically can contribute to this, but this is usually of little practical importance. Under most circumstances, the use of adrenaline in combination with LA is not contraindicated in the hypertensive patient unless the systolic pressure is >200 mmHg and/or the diastolic is >115 mmHg. Adrenaline-containing LA should not be given in large doses to patients taking beta-blockers, since interactions between adrenaline and the beta-blocker may induce hypertension and cardiovascular complications. Lidocaine should be used with caution in patients taking beta-blockers. Adrenaline effects may be reversed in patients taking alpha-blockers causing vasodilatation. Gingival retraction cords containing adrenaline should be avoided.

Conscious sedation may be advisable to control anxiety. Continuous BP monitoring is indicated. Raising the patient suddenly from the supine position may cause postural hypotension and loss of consciousness if the patient is using antihypertensive drugs such as thiazides, furosemide or a CCB.

GA agents potentiate antihypertensive drugs, which can induce dangerous hypotension. Intravenous barbiturates in particular can be dangerous, but halothane, enflurane and isoflurane may also cause hypotension in patients on beta-blockers. However, antihypertensive drugs should not be stopped, since rebound hypertension can result, and the risks of cerebrovascular accidents and cardiovascular instability that stem from withdrawal of antihypertensive medication and rebound hypertension outweigh the dangers of drug interactions, which to some extent are predictable and manageable by an expert anaesthetist. Therefore, antihypertensive treatment is usually continued, the management of such patients being a matter for the specialist anaesthetist in hospital. A severely reduced blood supply to vital organs can be dangerous, even in a normal person. In the chronically hypertensive patient, tissues have become adapted to the raised BP, which becomes essential (hence the term 'essential hypertension') to overcome the resistance of the vessels and maintain adequate perfusion. A fall in BP below the critical level needed for adequate perfusion of vital organs, particularly the kidneys, can therefore be fatal. Hypertension may be a contraindication to GA if complicated by cardiac failure, coronary or cerebral artery insufficiency, or renal insufficiency. Chronic administration of some diuretics such as furosemide may lead to potassium deficiency, which should, therefore, be checked preoperatively in order to avoid arrhythmias and increased sensitivity to muscle relaxants such as curare, gallamine and pancuronium.

The management of hypertensive patients may also be complicated by diseases such as cardiac or renal failure. Systemic corticosteroids may raise the BP and antihypertensive treatment may have to be

Table 5.13 *Risk and protective factors for atheroma*

Primary risk factors	Secondary risk factors	Unclear factors	Protective factors
High low-density lipoprotein (LDL)	Low LDL	Low dietary fibre	Raising HDL to LDL ratio
Hypertension	Diabetes	Soft water	More exercise
Smoking	Obesity	High plasma fibrinogen	Moderate red wine or other alcohol
	Family history of coronary heart disease (CAD)	Raised blood factor VII Raised lipoprotein levels	
	Physical inactivity	Homocysteine levels	
	Type A personality	Folate levels	
	Gout	C-reactive protein levels	
	Ethnicity (Asians)		
	Male gender		
	Increasing age		
	Low social class		
	Chronic renal failure		

Table 5.14 *Main sites and results of atheroma*

Site	Consequence	Possible clinical syndromes
Coronary arteries	Coronary artery disease	Impairs oxygenation and can lead to chest pain (angina), arrhythmias or myocardial infarction
Carotid and other cerebral arteries	Cerebrovascular disease	Stroke or transient ischaemic attacks
Peripheral arteries	Peripheral vascular disease	Impaired oxygenation, pain (intermittent claudication) and sometimes gangrene

Table 5.15 *Blood lipids*

	Total cholesterol	LDL ('bad') cholesterol	Lipid HDL ('good') cholesterol	Triglycerides
Significance of high level	May indicate atheroma	Main source of atheroma	Inhibits atheroma <40 mg/dL is a major risk factor for coronary artery disease	May indicate atheroma
Target blood levels for health	<200 mg/dL	<100 mg/dL	≥60 mg/dL	<150–199 mg/dL

adjusted accordingly. Some non-steroidal anti-inflammatory drugs (NSAIDs; indometacin, ibuprofen and naproxen) can reduce the efficacy of antihypertensive agents.

HYPOTENSION

Hypotension is uncommon but can have many causes (Table 5.12). Raising the patient suddenly from the supine position may cause postural (orthostatic) hypotension and loss of consciousness.

ATHEROMA AND ISCHAEMIC HEART DISEASE/ CORONARY ARTERY DISEASE

General aspects

Atheroma (atherosclerosis; arteriosclerosis) is the accumulation of cholesterol and lipids in the intima of arterial walls; it can lead to thromboses (clots), which sometimes break off and move within the vessels to lodge in and occlude small vessels (embolism). Atheroma can thus lead to CAD/IHD with angina, MI, cerebrovascular disease and stroke (Table 5.13). It also affects other arteries and can cause, for example, ischaemic

pain in the calves whilst walking – intermittent claudication – seen especially in young smokers, when it is termed Buerger disease.

In Western populations, atheroma may affect up to 45% of young adult males, and IHD affects at least 20% and increasingly thereafter, and accounts for about 35% of total mortality in Britain and the USA (Table 5.14). Atheroma results from a combination of genetic and lifestyle factors. Irreversible (fixed) risk factors include increasing age, male gender and family history of atheroma. Potentially reversible (modifiable) risk factors for atheroma include:

- cigarette smoking
- blood lipids
- hypertension
- diabetes mellitus
- obesity and lack of exercise
- the metabolic syndrome (Ch. 23).

High blood cholesterol is one of the major risk factors for IHD. Low-density lipoproteins (LDLs) are associated with a high risk of atheroma, whilst high-density lipoproteins (HDLs) appear to be anti-atherogenic (Table 5.15).

Atheroma is predominantly a disease of males, particularly in affluent societies, and is linked to smoking, lack of exercise, hypertension

Table 5.16 *Risk factors for ischaemic heart disease[a]*

H	Heredity
A	Age (older age)
S	Sex (male)
L	Lipidaemia
I	Increased weight (obesity)
P	Pressure (arterial hypertension)
I	Inactivity (sedentary lifestyle)
D	Diabetes
S	Smoking tobacco

[a]Adapted from Damjanov I. *Pathology secrets*, 2nd edn. New York, 2004, Mosby.

Table 5.17 *Main consequences of ischaemic heart disease*

Site	Consequence	Possible clinical syndromes
Coronary arteries	Coronary occlusion	Arrhythmias or acute coronary syndrome (angina, myocardial infarction)
Carotid and other cerebral arteries	Cerebrovascular occlusion	Stroke or transient ischaemic attacks, dementia
Peripheral arteries	Peripheral vascular disease	Pain (intermittent claudication) and gangrene

and hyperlipidaemia. Dietary fat is processed by the liver to form four main lipoproteins – chylomicrons, very-low-density lipoproteins (VLDLs), LDLs and HDLs. VLDL reforms to LDL, and it is these fats that are incorporated into atherosclerotic plaque and associated with a high risk of IHD/CAD. By contrast, HDLs clear cholesterol from the blood via the liver, appear to be anti-atherogenic, and are associated with a lower risk of IHD/CAD (Table 5.16). Cholesterol may be raised genetically and with increasing age in both sexes. Before the menopause, women have lower total cholesterol levels than men of the same age but, after the menopause, women's LDL levels tend to rise with inactivity and excess weight, a diet low in fruit and vegetables, smoking and other diseases such as hypertension and diabetes.

There is a higher incidence of IHD/CAD in patients with diabetes, hyperlipidaemia, the metabolic syndrome and hypothyroidism. Hyperlipidaemia and hypertension seem to be linked, and immigrants from the Indian subcontinent have a higher than average morbidity and mortality from IHD/CAD. Apolipoprotein E genotyping may help confirm a diagnosis of type III hyperlipoproteinaemia (also known as dysbetalipoproteinaemia), to evaluate a possible genetic cause of atheroma.

Periodontal disease could be an independent risk factor for IHD/CAD because oral bacteria, inflammatory mediators and endotoxaemia might contribute. Other infectious agents implicated have included *Chlamydia pneumoniae*, *Helicobacter pylori* and *cytomegalovirus*, but none of these associations has been proven.

Clinical features

Atheroma has a patchy distribution and, depending on the site and extent of disease, can give rise to a variety of clinical presentations. Atheromatous plaques may rupture and 'heal' spontaneously. Alternatively, a platelet–fibrin thrombus (clot) may form, then break up and travel in the bloodstream (thromboembolism), with potentially life-threatening consequences.

IHD/CAD is due to occlusion of the coronary arteries and leads to angina pectoris (pain arising when the myocardial oxygen demand exceeds the supply). Rare causes of IHD/CAD include embolism and coronary artery spasm. Patients with IHD/CAD are at greatest risk from MI, which, if severe, causes cardiac arrest with acute failure of the whole circulation, loss of cerebral blood supply and often death within a few minutes. MI differs from angina in that it causes more severe and persistent chest pain that is not controlled by rest; it leads to irreversible cardiac damage or sudden death. A chronically reduced blood supply to the myocardium progressively damages the heart and may lead to cardiac arrhythmias and cardiac failure (Table 5.17).

Box 5.4 *Lifestyle recommendations for lowering ischaemic heart disease risk*

- Healthy weight
- Smoking cessation
- Moderate alcohol consumption
- Regular exercise (e.g. brisk walking for at least 30 min daily)
- Fresh fruit and vegetable intake of at least five servings a day
- Grain intake of at least six servings a day with at least one-third wholegrain

Prevention

The primary aim is to prevent or reduce progression of atheroma by lifestyle changes, as shown in Box 5.4. IHD/CAD prophylaxis is by lowering cholesterol levels that are too high. If the total cholesterol is 200 mg/dL or more, or if HDL is less than 40 mg/dL, a lipoprotein profile should be done after a 9–12-hour fast. Abnormal cholesterol levels can be altered by:

- improving diet (reducing saturated fat and cholesterol)
- losing weight, which can help lower LDL and total cholesterol levels, as well as raise HDL and lower triglyceride levels
- increasing physical activity, which can help lower LDL and raise HDL levels, and also helps weight loss
- stopping cigarette smoking
- controlling hypertension
- taking drugs to lower LDL cholesterol if it is 130 mg/dL or more – statins (simvastatin, pravastatin, etc.), which inhibit the *de novo* production of cholesterol via hydroxymethylglutaryl coenzyme A (HMG-CoA) reductase
- taking bile acid sequestrants (colesevelam), resins (colestyramine, colestipol), nicotinic acid-related drugs (nicotinic acid and acipimox) or fibrates (clofibrate, fenofibrate, gemfibrozil) as alternatives to statins.

A diet high in marine triglycerides (and omega-3 fatty acids – though this is contentious) and high in fruit and vegetables may be cardioprotective. Fish such as salmon, tuna and mackerel containing omega-3 fatty acids may offer protection against CAD by reducing inflammation. Polyunsaturated fatty acids of the omega-3 type are present as alpha-linolenic acid, mainly in certain vegetable sources such as soybean, canola oil and English walnuts, and in fish oils such as eicosapentaenoic acid (EPA) and docosahexaenoic acid (DHA). Fruits and vegetables, and other foods high in antioxidants, are associated with a lower risk of IHD/CAD. Moderate red wine consumption is also associated with lower mortality (possibly because of the contained antioxidant resveratrol), and eating less salt may reduce the chances of developing high BP.

General management

The diagnosis of IHD/CAD may be suggested by the history. Resting ECG may help but, if normal, exercise ECG is indicated. Coronary arteriography (angiography; CAG) demonstrates the anatomy and patency of the arteries and also allows for intervention if necessary (percutaneous coronary intervention [PCI]). Use of a radionuclide such as thallium-201 or MIBI (2-methoxy isobutyl isonitrile; sestamibi) can enhance the sensitivity. Myocardial perfusion scans (thallium-201) may reveal ischaemic areas, which show as 'cold spots' during exercise. Often an exercise stress test (EST) is the first-choice investigation but this and other non-invasive techniques, such as myocardial perfusion single photon emission computed tomography (SPECT), can only identify patients with advanced CAD. Electron-beam computed tomography (EBCT) can detect and quantify coronary artery calcification (CAC) and there is a strong independent association between CAC and CAD detected with CAG, and also with cerebrovascular disease.

The most effective ways to treat patients with IHD/CAD include the lifestyle changes described above, particularly stopping smoking. Drugs that may help include antiplatelet drugs (aspirin or clopidogrel) to prevent thrombosis; beta-blockers (atenolol, metoprolol, etc.) to lower the BP; ACEIs (enalapril, fosinopril, etc.) to lower peripheral resistance and cardiac workload, and hence BP; and statins to lower blood cholesterol. Statins may cause muscle damage, sleep disturbances, memory loss, depression, sexual dysfunction or interstitial lung disease. Other measures include good control of blood glucose levels in diabetics.

Pain relief and prophylaxis of angina is with GTN 0.3–0.6 mg sublingually during attacks or before anticipated physical activity or stress. Long-acting nitrates (e.g. isosorbide dinitrate) may help prevent attacks. When IHD/CAD is extensive and symptoms are worsening despite general measures and optimal medical management, cardiac revascularization techniques should be considered. These include: *coronary angioplasty* – stents may be placed percutaneously (by PCI) to re-establish coronary blood flow and improve myocardial perfusion; or *coronary artery bypass graft* (CABG) – to bridge severe obstructions in the coronary blood vessels.

Dental aspects of ischaemic heart disease

Stress, anxiety, exertion or pain can provoke angina and, therefore, patients should receive dental care, in short, minimally stressful appointments in the late morning. Effective painless LA is essential. An aspirating syringe should be used since adrenaline (epinephrine) in the LA may enter the blood and may (theoretically) raise the BP and precipitate arrhythmias. Adrenaline-containing LA should not be given in excessive doses to patients taking beta-blockers, since the interaction may induce hypertension and cardiovascular complications if excessively large doses are given. Gingival retraction cords containing adrenaline should be avoided.

Conscious sedation should be deferred for at least 3 months after MI, recent-onset angina, unstable angina or recent development of bundle branch block and, in any case, should be given in hospital. GA should be avoided wherever possible and at the least deferred for 3 months after MI.

Drugs and other therapies may affect dental care. Angina can rarely cause pain in the mandible, teeth or other oral tissues. Patients with IHD/CAD appear to have more severe dental caries and periodontal disease than the general population. Whether these infections bear any causative relationship to heart disease remains controversial but periodontal disease could be an independent risk factor because oral bacteria, inflammatory mediators and endotoxaemia might contribute.

Coronary artery stenosis and dental pulp calcification are significantly associated. Dental radiography has the potential to be used as a rapid screening method for the early detection of coronary artery stenosis.

ACUTE CORONARY SYNDROMES (ACS)

General aspects

Acute coronary syndrome is the term used to refer to clinical features attributed to coronary artery obstruction. They are typically due to IHD/CAD but are occasionally caused by cocaine, anaemias or arrhythmias. The most common feature is acute chest pain, often radiating to the left arm or jaw, and sometimes associated with nausea and sweating.

ACS is usually the result of unstable angina (38%) or MI; the latter can be ST-elevation MI (STEMI: 30%) or non–ST-elevation MI (NSTEMI, also known as non–Q-wave MI: 25%). Unstable angina occurs suddenly, often at rest or with minimal exertion, or at lesser degrees of exertion than precipitated previous angina attacks ('crescendo angina'). New-onset angina is also considered as unstable angina.

General management

If a 12-lead ECG suggests STEMI (ST elevations in specific leads, a new left bundle branch block or a true posterior MI pattern), then urgent triage, transfer and treatment with thrombolytics or angioplasty are essential. Troponin I or troponin T is a useful cardiac damage marker. Give pain relief as soon as possible, using GTN, and offer intravenous opioids such as morphine, if an acute MI is suspected. Offer a single loading dose of 300 mg aspirin as soon as possible, unless there is clear evidence that the patient is allergic to aspirin. Do not routinely administer oxygen but undertake early coronary angiography with a view to revascularization either by PCI, usually with stent implantation, or CABG.

However, at least 50% of survivors of attacks of sudden cardiac death have no evidence of myocardial damage from the ECG or serum enzyme levels; the pathogenesis appears not to be the same as in typical MI, and therefore the term NSTEMI is used. If the ECG suggests NSTEMI, treatment is with glycoprotein IIb/IIIa inhibitors (eptifibatide or tirofiban), plus aspirin, low-molecular-weight heparin (LMWH) and clopidogrel, with intravenous GTN and opioids if the pain persists; where appropriate, early coronary angiography is undertaken with a view to revascularization either by PCI, usually with stent implantation, or CABG. Abciximab is a monoclonal antibody that targets the glycoprotein IIb/IIIa receptor on platelets. If, 12 hours after onset of the pain, cardiac troponins (cTnT) are positive, urgent coronary angiography is typically indicated, as this is highly predictive of an impending MI. If the troponin is negative, a treadmill exercise test or a thallium scintigram may be indicated.

The NICE guidelines on MI are available at http://guidance.nice.org.uk and NICE technology appraisal guidance on the use of glycoprotein IIb/IIIa inhibitors in the treatment of ACS (TA47) at http://publications.nice.org.uk (both accessed 25 May 2013).

ANGINA PECTORIS

General aspects

Angina pectoris is the name given to episodes of chest pain caused by myocardial ischaemia secondary to IHD/CAD. It affects around 1% of adults and its prevalence rises with increasing age. The usual underlying causes are atherosclerotic plaques that rupture with resulting platelet activation, adhesion and aggregation, and thrombosis impeding coronary artery blood flow (or, if this is complete occlusion, MI). Arterial spasm alone may, rarely, be responsible. The mortality rate in angina is about 4% per year, the prognosis depending on the degree of coronary artery narrowing.

Clinical features

Angina is often an unmistakable pain described as a sense of strangling or choking, or tightness, heaviness, compression or constriction of the chest, sometimes radiating to the left arm or jaw *but relieved by rest* (Box 5.5). The most common precipitating causes of angina pain are physical exertion (particularly in cold weather); emotion (especially anger or anxiety); and stress caused by fear or pain, leading to adrenal release of catecholamines (adrenaline [epinephrine] and noradrenaline [norepinephrine]) and consequent tachycardia, vasoconstriction and raised BP. Consequently, an increased cardiac workload is accompanied by a paradoxical drop in blood flow and myocardial ischaemia occurs, resulting in angina.

The severity and prognosis of angina depend upon the degree of coronary artery narrowing and there is a varied clinical presentation (Box 5.6). Unstable angina is the term given to a pain pattern changing in occurrence, frequency, intensity, duration or pain at rest, and these patients are at high risk of progression to MI or death. The British Cardiac Society guidelines state the circumstances associated with an increased risk of early adverse outcome, which include:

- age above 65 years
- co-morbidity, especially diabetes
- prolonged (>15 min) cardiac pain at rest
- ischaemic ECG ST-segment depression on admission or during symptoms
- ECG T-wave inversion (associated with an intermediate risk, lying between that associated with ST-segment depression and normal ECG)
- evidence of impairment of left ventricular function (either pre-existing or during MI)
- elevated C-reactive protein (CRP)
- raised levels of cardiac troponin.

Patients may have repeated attacks of angina over a long period, or have an MI soon after the first one or two attacks. Many patients have *painless* myocardial ischaemia, as shown by arteriography (angiography) and exercise ECG changes. Some even have hyposensitivity to pain.

General management

The diagnosis is primarily clinical. Occasionally, gastro-oesophageal reflux disease (GORD) or chest wall diseases mimic angina, and neither the results of physical examination nor investigations are necessarily abnormal. The latter may especially include resting ECG, which typically shows ST-segment depression with a flat or inverted T wave, but is usually normal between episodes of angina. Exercise ECG testing is positive in approximately 75% of people with severe CAD. Myocardial perfusion scans (thallium-201) highlight ischaemic myocardium. Coronary angiography can assess coronary blood flow in diagnostically challenging cases.

Risk factors for IHD/CAD (cigarette smoking, physical inactivity, obesity, hypertension, diabetes, hypercholesterolaemia) should be identified and corrected. During acute episodes of angina, pain is relieved by oxygen, GTN and reduction of anxiety. The pain, though relieved by rest, is ameliorated more quickly by nitrates – usually GTN – which act by lowering the peripheral vascular resistance and reducing the oxygen demands of the heart. Most patients use GTN in the buccal sulcus or sublingually, as a spray or tablet. Other nitrates, CCBs and occasionally potassium-channel activators such as nicorandil may also be prescribed. Nitrates are not used to relieve an angina attack if the patient has recently taken sildenafil, as there may be a precipitous fall in BP; analgesics should be used.

When angina is frequent, long-acting nitrates (isosorbide mononitrate), beta-adrenergic–blocking drugs (e.g. atenolol) and calcium antagonists (e.g. amlodipine) are used. Many patients with stable angina are given a beta-blocker or a CCB but, if this fails to control symptoms adequately, a combination of a beta-blocker and a dihydropyridine CCB (e.g. amlodipine, felodipine, modified-release nifedipine) may be used. If this combination is inappropriate because of intolerance of, or contraindication to, *either* beta-blockers *or* CCBs *or* both, a long-acting nitrate, ivabradine, nicorandil or ranolazine can be considered (Box 5.7). Ivabradine, a cardiotonic agent, helps to lower the heart rate, which can be helpful in angina (and heart failure). It can be used when beta-blockers fail or can be used in combination with a beta-blocker for people whose symptoms are not adequately controlled with a beta-blocker, providing their heart rate is greater than 60 beats/min). Grapefruit can affect the metabolism of ivabradine. Adverse effects of ivabradine include luminous visual phenomena and there are multiple contraindications to its use. Drugs used to prevent thrombosis in unstable angina in particular include:

- aspirin, which acetylates platelet cyclo-oxygenase (COX) and thereby inhibits platelet function for about 7 days, and also inhibits platelet aggregation by preventing the synthesis of thromboxane A2; it is more effective when used with clopidogrel
- glycoprotein IIb and IIIa inhibitors, such as abciximab, to prevent adherence of fibrinogen to receptors on platelets and to block their aggregation
- lipid-lowering drugs
- LMWH.

In angina that does not respond to drugs, PCI procedures or CABG may be indicated.

Dental aspects

Preoperative GTN and sometimes oral sedation (e.g. temazepam) are advised. Dental care should be carried out in such a way as to cause minimal anxiety, and with oxygen saturation, BP and pulse monitoring. Effective LA is essential. Ready access to medical help, oxygen and GTN is crucial.

If a patient with a history of angina experiences chest pain in the dental surgery, dental treatment must be stopped and the patient should be given GTN sublingually and oxygen; the patient should be kept sitting upright. Vital signs should be monitored. The pain should be relieved in 2–3 minutes; the patient should then rest and be accompanied home.

If chest pain is not relieved within about 3 minutes, MI is a possible cause (see below) and medical help should be summoned. Pain that persists after three doses of GTN given every 5 minutes, lasts more than 15–20 minutes, or is associated with nausea, vomiting, syncope or hypertension is highly suggestive of MI. If pain persists, the patient should continue on oxygen and *chew* 300 mg of aspirin (Ch. 1).

Tricyclic antidepressants are best avoided, as they can disturb cardiac rhythm. Sumatriptan is contraindicated, as it may cause coronary artery vasoconstriction.

Angina is a rare cause of pain in the mandible, teeth or other oral tissues, or pharynx. Drugs used in the care of patients with angina may cause oral adverse effects, such as lichenoid lesions (CCBs), gingival swelling (CCBs) or ulcers (nicorandil).

Conscious sedation should be deferred for at least 3 months in patients with recent-onset angina, unstable angina or recent development of bundle branch block; in any case, it should be given in hospital.

GA should be deferred for at least 3 months in patients with recent-onset angina, unstable angina or recent development of bundle branch block; in any case, it must be given in hospital. Intravenous barbiturates are particularly dangerous.

Stable angina

For anything but minor treatment under LA, the physician should be consulted and consideration should be given to any other complicating factors, such as beta-blocker therapy, hypertension or cardiac failure. Other medication should not be interfered with. Before dental treatment, patients with stable angina should be reassured and possibly sedated with oral diazepam. Prophylactic administration of GTN may be indicated if the patient has angina more than once a week.

Unstable angina

Elective dental care should be deferred until a physician has agreed to it, because of the risk of infarction. Preoperative GTN should be given, together with relative analgesia monitored by pulse oximetry, and LA; however, such patients are best cared for in hospital, as intravenous nitrates may be indicated.

Emergency dental care should be the least invasive possible, using preoperative GTN, together with relative analgesia monitored by pulse oximetry and LA; however, such patients are best cared for in a hospital environment, as coronary vasodilators may be indicated intravenously. Other medication should not be interfered with.

MYOCARDIAL INFARCTION

General aspects

Myocardial infarction (coronary thrombosis or heart attack) results from the complete occlusion (blockage) of one or more coronary arteries. It arises when atherosclerotic plaques rupture, causing platelet activation, adhesion and aggregation with subsequent thrombus formation within the coronary circulation. Angina may progress to MI but fewer than 50% of patients with MI have any preceding symptoms.

Clinical features

MI most commonly presents with central chest pain similar to that of angina *but is not relieved by rest or with sublingual nitrates*. MI may appear without warning or is sometimes precipitated by exercise or stress. The pain is often unmistakable and described as an unbearably severe sense of strangling or choking, or tightness, heaviness, compression or constriction of the chest. It sometimes radiates to the left arm or jaw. Sometimes MI is preceded by angina, often felt as indigestion-like pain (Box 5.8). It can persist for hours, if death does not supervene.

The pain of MI may sometimes start at rest, and is not relieved by nitrates. Vomiting, facial pallor, sweating, restlessness, shortness of breath and apprehension are common. Other features may include cough and loss of consciousness, but the clinical picture is variable and fewer than 50% of patients with an MI have any premonitory symptoms. Approximately 10–20% of individuals have silent (painless) infarctions and the first sign may be the catastrophic onset of left ventricular failure, shock, loss of consciousness and death.

Death soon after the onset of the chest pain is common, often from ventricular fibrillation or cardiac arrest. Less often, there is sudden cardiac death characterized by immediate collapse without premonitory symptoms, and loss of pulses. In such cases, the precipitating event is a severe arrhythmia such as ventricular fibrillation. Up to 50% of patients die within the first hour of MI and a further 10–20% within the next few days. The prognosis of MI may be judged from the Killip classification (Table 5.18).

Cardiac failure and arrhythmias may develop in MI survivors and the chances of reinfarction are high in the immediate post-infarction

Table 5.18 *Killip classification of acute myocardial infarction*

Killip class	Defining features	Mortality rate (%)
I	No clinical signs of heart failure	6
II	Rales or crackles in the lungs, an S3 gallop and elevated jugular venous pressure	17
II	Frank acute pulmonary oedema	38
IV	Cardiogenic shock or hypotension (systolic BP < 90 mmHg), and evidence of peripheral vasoconstriction (oliguria, cyanosis or sweating)	81

Table 5.19 *Serum enzyme level changes after myocardial infarction*

Enzyme	Abbreviation	Number of days after MI that maximum rise is seen
Troponin T (troponin 1)	TT	0.5–1.0
Creatine kinase-MB	CK-MB	1.5
Aspartate transaminase	AST	2.0
Lactic dehydrogenase	LDH	3.0

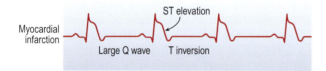

Fig. 5.10 Electrocardiogram tracings in myocardial infarction: large Q wave, ST elevation, inverted T wave.

weeks. Dressler syndrome, also known as post-myocardial infarction syndrome or post-cardiotomy pericarditis, is a form of pericarditis complicating MI. Valvular dysfunction and myocardial rupture may also complicate an MI.

General management

MI is diagnosed mainly from clinical features supported by ECG (Fig. 5.10) and changes in serum levels of enzymes termed 'cardiac enzymes' (Box 5.9). In the first few hours, T waves become abnormally tall (hyperacute with the loss of their normal concavity) and ST segments begin to rise. Pathological Q waves may appear within hours or up to more than 24 hours. Thus the characteristic pattern of MI is a normal or raised ST segment, with hyperacute T and acute Q waves (see Fig. 5.10). By 24 hours, the T wave becomes inverted as the ST elevation begins to resolve. Long-term ECG changes include persistent Q and T waves.

Damaged (infarcted) cardiac muscle releases several enzymes into the blood, including troponin T (TT), cardiac-specific creatine kinase (CK-MB), aspartate transaminase (AST) and lactic dehydrogenase (LDH). The earliest changes are in cardiac TT, an enzyme expressed only in the myocardium and not in other muscles, and which can be detected in the blood 3–6 hours after onset of the chest pain of MI, reaching peak levels within 16–25 hours. TT is also useful for the late diagnosis of MI because raised blood concentrations can be seen even 5–8 days after MI onset (Table 5.19).

MI requires immediate hospital admission and treatment (which halves the mortality rate). Management aims to relieve pain, limit myocardial damage (infarct size) and prevent/treat complications (Box 5.10; see also Ch. 1). Ventricular fibrillation is the most common cause of death and nearly 50% of deaths are in the first hour, so immediate defibrillation and CPR can be life-saving (Ch. 1).

In the convalescent stage, ACEIs or beta-blockers can reduce mortality and the risk of recurrence. Early mobilization, a cardiac

Table 5.20 *Oral health-care effects on automatic implantable cardiac defibrillators (AICDs)*

Procedures that are safe from interference with AICD	Procedures in which interference with AICD can be reduced by safety measures	Procedures in which interference with an AICD is likely
Diagnostic radiography and CT: if the AICD is placed in the upper chest area, the radiography equipment may be adjusted to lessen pressure on the defibrillator	Transcutaneous electrical nerve stimulation (TENS) Ultrasound for diagnostic or therapeutic purposes: keep the transducer head 25 cm from the defibrillator	Cardioversion Diathermy, electrocautery, lithotripsy, radiation therapy
Dental procedures; use of equipment such as dental drills, ultrasonic scalers or endosonic instruments; dental radiography		Electrocoagulation Electrocutting Electrosurgery
ECG Microwave Peripheral nerve stimulators Radiography		External defibrillation: if this is needed, the health-care professional should not place the paddles directly over the defibrillator
Ultrasonography Use of laser scalpels		MRI: *contraindicated* for a person with a defibrillator. Even if the MRI scanner is off, there is a strong magnetic field that may affect the defibrillator
		Radiofrequency ablation
		TENS (with AICD or pacemaker)

rehabili-tation programme and correction of risk factors for IHD/CAD (as in angina management) are indicated. Mechanical circulatory support (MCS) may be used for treatment of patients with severe cardiogenic shock, over a period of several days up to months before heart transplantation. A multicentre automatic defibrillator implantation trial showed a 30% relative risk reduction in all-cause mortality from the prophylactic use of an automatic implantable cardiac defibrillator (AICD) in patients after MI. NICE also recommends the use of an AICD in people who have survived a cardiac arrest that was due to either ventricular tachycardia or ventricular fibrillation.

Dental aspects

Dental intervention after MI can precipitate arrhythmias or aggravate cardiac ischaemia. This is more likely in severe MI, when the actual infarct is close in time and in the presence of cardiac complications. The severity of an MI can be assessed from the resulting disability, the length of the acute illness and whether or not the patient was hospitalized; nevertheless, it is important to consult the patient's physician before undertaking operative treatment.

In general, patients within 6 months of an MI (recent MI) are at greatest risk of further MI, chest pain, arrhythmias or other complications, and have generally been classed as ASA class IV. A level of reinfarction of 50% has been reported in major surgery done during this period; therefore, higher-risk procedures such as elective and major surgery should be deferred. Simple emergency dental treatment under LA may be given during the first 6 months after MI but the opinion of a physician should be sought first.

In symptomatic patients with previous older MI (between 6 and 12 months), elective simple dental care can normally be carried out safely but it is wise to minimize pain and anxiety. Higher-risk procedures such as elective surgery may need to be deferred since a level of reinfarction of 20% has been reported in major surgery and about 5% in minor surgery done during this period.

In asymptomatic patients with previous but older MI (more than 12 months), elective dental care can normally be carried out safely but it is always wise to minimize pain and anxiety. A level of reinfarction of 5% has been reported in major surgery done during this period.

At any time, the level of risk will depend on the type of intervention; surgery is a higher risk, for example, than conservative dentistry. There must be ready access to oxygen and medical help. Anxiety and pain must be minimized, and the physician may advocate preoperative use of GTN. Effective LA, possibly supplemented with relative analgesia, and monitoring of BP, ECG, pulse and oxygen saturation are indicated. Dental procedures should be stopped if there is chest pain, dyspnoea, a rise in heart rate of 40 beats/min or more, a rise in the ST-segment displacement of above 0.2 mV on ECG, arrhythmias, or a rise in systolic BP of more than 20 mmHg.

The incidence of MI after GA in patients with a documented preoperative MI is up to eight times that of patients with no previous history. Nearly 30% of patients having a GA within 3 months of an infarct have another MI in the first postoperative week and at least 50% die. Elective surgery under GA should therefore be postponed for at least 3 months and preferably a year, since the prognosis of recurrent MI is also influenced by the time after the first attack.

After mechanical circulatory support, management is complicated by a combination of anticoagulant and antiplatelet medication, and sometimes by an increased risk of thromboembolic events and infections. Elective interventions should be postponed.

Adrenaline (epinephrine) or other vasoconstrictors should be used with caution (lower dose and careful monitoring) in patients with AICDs and there are certain procedures where interference with an AICD is possible (especially MRI) (Table 5.20). Patients with AICDs do not need antibiotic cover to prevent endocarditis.

CARDIOMYOPATHIES

General aspects

Cardiomyopathy (from the Latin) means a heart muscle disease. Extrinsic or specific cardiomyopathies include those associated with IHD/CAD; nutritional diseases; hypertension; cardiac valvular disease; inflammatory diseases; or systemic metabolic disease. Intrinsic cardiomyopathy has a number of causes, including drug and alcohol toxicity, certain infections (including hepatitis C), and various genetic and idiopathic causes. Alcohol is a major cause. Four separate and distinct types of intrinsic cardiomyopathy are recognized (Box 5.11).

Clinical features

Frequently, there are no symptoms until complications develop. Most affected individuals have a normal quality and duration of life. Congestive

Table 5.21 *Arrhythmia-inducing drugs and foods*

Tachycardias	Bradycardias	Other arrhythmias
Adrenaline (epinephrine)	Beta-blockers	Adrenaline (epinephrine)
Alcohol	Calcium-channel blockers	Alcohol
Atropine		Amphetamines
Caffeine	Digitalis	Cocaine
Nicotine	Morphine	Digitalis
		Procainamide
		Quinidine
		Tricyclics

cardiac failure (CCF) with atrial fibrillation or other serious complications (mitral regurgitation, angina, sudden death or infective endocarditis) can, however, result. Exercise-induced sudden death is a constant risk.

General management

Medical care prolongs life to a variable degree and aims to ameliorate symptoms. Medication, ablation, an implanted pacemaker, defibrillator or ventricular assist device (VAD), or cardiac transplantation often becomes necessary.

Dental aspects

Adrenaline (epinephrine) should be used in limited amounts, and GTN or similar drugs are contraindicated. Conscious sedation with nitrous oxide and oxygen may be used if necessary, with the approval of the physician. Patients with cardiomyopathy are a poor risk for GA because of alcoholism, arrhythmias, cardiac failure or myocardial ischaemia.

If angina pectoris, MI or fibrillation occurs, oxygen should be given and preparations made to perform CPR and to activate the emergency response system.

ARRHYTHMIAS (DYSRHYTHMIAS)

Normally, the heart chambers (atria and ventricles) contract in a co-ordinated manner initiated by an electrical signal in the sinoatrial node (sinus node or SA node), a small mass of heart tissue with characteristics of both muscle and nerve, located in the right atrial wall. The electrical signal is conducted through the atria, stimulating them to contract, and then passes through the atrioventricular node (AV node), where the impulse transmission to the ventricles is delayed transiently while the atria complete their contraction (consistent with the P wave on the ECG) and empty their blood into the ventricles. (These are already partially filled with blood that has drained passively from the large veins – vena cava on the right side and the pulmonary veins on the left side – into the atria during diastole.) Once the impulse leaves the AV node, it descends in the interventricular septum via the bundle of His and reaches the Purkinje fibres of the ventricle walls, causing them to contract (i.e. the ventricular component of systole), as noted on the ECG by the QRS complex. Following excitation and depolarization, the conductive tissue repolarizes to be ready for the next pulse.

In adults, the heart beats regularly, the resting rate ranging from 60 to 100 beats/min. In children the rate is much faster.

General and clinical aspects

Arrhythmia is any disorder of heart rate or rhythm; the heart beats too quickly (tachycardia), too slowly (bradycardia) or irregularly. Some arrhythmias are so brief (e.g. a temporary pause or premature beat) that the overall heart rate or rhythm is not greatly affected. However, if, for any period of time, the heart fails to beat properly (too fast or too slow, regular or irregular) and pumps ineffectively, the lungs, brain and all other organs may malfunction.

Most arrhythmias arise from problems in the cardiac electrical system but some may be provoked by stress, catecholamines or drugs (illegal, prescription or over-the-counter), as well as alcohol, tobacco, foods and other substances (Table 5.21). Arrhythmias may further arise from cardiac, respiratory, autonomic or endocrine disease, fever, hypoxia or electrolyte disturbances. Surgery is sometimes implicated; the trigeminocardiac reflex (TCR), which may be associated with surgery, consists of bradycardia, hypotension, apnoea and gastric hypermotility. The parasympathetic nerve supply to the face is carried in the trigeminal nerve; alternative afferent pathways must exist via the maxillary and/or mandibular divisions, in addition to the commonly reported pathway via the ophthalmic division of the trigeminal in the classic oculocardiac reflex. The efferent arc involves the vagus. Central stimulation of the trigeminal nerve can cause reflex bradycardic responses during maxillofacial or ocular surgical procedures or neurosurgery, but some have followed oral or perioral procedures. Cardiac surgery may also be followed by arrhythmias; junctional ectopic tachycardia is then the most common arrhythmia, presumed to be initiated from a small focus of abnormal automaticity somewhere in the AV node or bundle of His.

The significance of arrhythmias varies from the fatal to the inconsequential (Table 5.22), some being regarded as normal variants, others merely annoying – such as an abnormal awareness of heartbeat (palpitations) – but some reducing cardiac efficiency and output and causing palpitations with dyspnoea, angina or syncope. Some can be life-threatening and lead to cardiac arrest. Others cause no symptoms but still predispose to potentially life-threatening complications such as cerebrovascular events (stroke and transient ischaemic attacks).

Types of arrhythmia

Up to 15% of the population have arrhythmias. There is a wide range of arrhythmias, which may be classified by rate (tachycardia, bradycardia), mechanism (automaticity, re-entry, fibrillation) or origin (Table 5.23). Extrasystoles are the most common true arrhythmia. *Sinus arrhythmia* is not a true arrhythmia but a normal phenomenon of mild acceleration and slowing of the heart rate that occurs with breathing in and out; it is usually quite pronounced in children and lessens with age.

Table 5.24 shows agents used to treat arrhythmias.

Information about arrhythmias is available from the American Heart Association (AHA) at http://www.heart.org/, under the 'Conditions' tab (accessed 30 September 2013).

Table 5.22 *Arrhythmias posing different levels of risk to the patient (usual level of risk)*

High	Medium	Low	None
Atrial fibrillation	Atrial arrhythmias which are symptomatic or under treatment	Atrial arrhythmias which are asymptomatic and not under treatment	Bradycardia in athletes
Bradycardia plus other arrhythmia			Extrasystoles (atrial)
Bradycardia plus pacemaker	Drug-induced arrhythmias	Premature ventricular beats	
Irregular pulse ventricular extrasystoles	Pacemaker		
Irregular pulse plus bradycardia	Paroxysmal supraventricular tachycardia		
Tachycardia plus other arrhythmia	Ventricular arrhythmias which are symptomatic or under treatment		
Ventricular fibrillation			
Ventricular tachycardia			
Wolff–Parkinson–White syndrome			

Table 5.23 *Significance of arrhythmias*

Arrhythmia	Description	Significance
Atrial fibrillation	Quivering	Dangerous because of thromboses
Bradycardia	Too slow	Occasionally dangerous
Premature contraction	Early beat	May be insignificant
Tachycardia	Too fast	Can be dangerous
Ventricular fibrillation	Fluttering	Emergency; cardiac arrest

Table 5.24 *Antiarrhythmic agents*

Type of arrhythmia	Examples of drugs used	
	Main	Others
Supraventricular	Verapamil	Adenosine, digoxin, beta-blockers
Supraventricular and ventricular	Disopyramide	Amiodarone, beta-blockers, flecainide, procainamide, propafenone
Ventricular	Lidocaine	Mexiletine, moracizine

EXTRASYSTOLES (ECTOPICS)

Extrasystoles are essentially extra beats, or contractions, which occur when there is electrical discharge from somewhere in the heart other than the SA node. Extrasystoles can sometimes be a feature of cardiac disease, and even *in people with otherwise apparently normal hearts*, extrasystoles occurring during exercise and in the recovery period after exercise can have increased mortality risk.

Premature beats are common in normal children and teenagers. An extra beat comes sooner than normal; then there is a pause that causes the next beat to be more forceful. Most people have them at some time and usually no cause can be found. Those without identifiable cause usually disappear on their own. Only occasionally are premature beats caused by cardiac disease or injury.

Atrial extrasystoles (premature atrial contractions; PACs) are common in healthy people with normal hearts, especially with advancing age, but can also occur when there is increased pressure on the atria, such as in cardiac failure or mitral valve disease; in such cases, they may arise prior to the development of atrial fibrillation. Atrial extrasystoles may also be of little consequence but are exacerbated by alcohol and caffeine (as a former UK Prime Minister found!) (see Table 5.22).

The 'sick sinus syndrome' is when the SA node fires irregularly, the heart rate sometimes changing back and forth between a bradycardia and a tachycardia.

Ventricular extrasystoles occur when the abnormal discharge arises from the ventricles; though they can occur in people with normal hearts, they are more commonly found in heart disease. Ventricular extrasystoles (ectopics) are the commonest type of arrhythmia arising after MI and may also occur in severe left ventricular hyper-trophy, hypertrophic cardiomyopathy and congestive cardiac failure. The British Heart Foundation has stated that ventricular ectopics, in the absence of structural heart disease or a family history of sudden death, are benign and do not require specialist intervention or specific drug therapy.

TACHYCARDIAS

A tachycardia is a resting heart rate of more than 100 beats/min in an adult. It may result in palpitations but is not *necessarily* an arrhythmia.

Sinus tachycardia is an increased heart rate that is a normal response to exercise or emotional stress, mediated by the effects of the sympathetic nervous system and catecholamines on the SA node. Hyperthyroidism and ingested or injected substances, such as cocaine, ecstasy, amphetamines or caffeine, can produce or exaggerate this effect. In sinus tachycardia, the heart beats regularly. It may also be a response to conditions such as:

- anxiety
- emotional distress
- fever
- fright
- strenuous exercise.

Less commonly, it may indicate:

- anaemia
- haemorrhage
- heart muscle damage
- hyperthyroidism.

Treatments address the cause of the sinus tachycardia rather than the condition itself.

Supraventricular tachycardias

Supraventricular tachycardia (SVT or atrial tachycardia) is a fast heart rate that starts in the cardiac upper chambers (Table 5.25). Some forms are called paroxysmal atrial tachycardia (PAT) or paroxysmal supraventricular tachycardia (PSVT). The rapid heart beat does not allow enough time for the heart to fill before it contracts, so blood flow to the rest of the body is compromised. SVT is most commonly seen in:

- children
- females

Table 5.25 *Supraventricular tachycardias*

Tachycardia	Heart rate	Frequency	Precipitants
Irregular heart rhythm			
Atrial fibrillation	Often rapid onset, rate 60–220 beats/min	Most common pathological tachycardia	Older age, male sex, hypertension, cardiac disease, pulmonary embolism, hyperthyroidism, surgery
Multifocal atrial tachycardia	Gradual onset, rate 100–150 beats/min		Pulmonary disease, theophylline
Atrial premature contractions	Gradual onset, rate 100–150 beats/min		Caffeine or other stimulants
Regular heart rhythm			
Sinus tachycardia	<220 beats/min	Most common supraventricular tachycardia	Physiological; sepsis, hypovolaemia, pain, fear, hyperthyroidism
Atrial flutter	Rapid onset, rate 140–150 beats/min	Common tachycardia	Cardiac disease (congenital heart disease, myocardial infarction, atrial fibrillation); chronic obstructive pulmonary disease, cardiac surgery
Group consisting of atrioventricular nodal re-entrant tachycardia, atrioventricular reciprocating (re-entrant) tachycardia, and atrial tachycardia	Rapid onset, rate 150–250 beats/min	Common tachycardias Atrioventricular nodal re-entrant tachycardia most common among persons >20 y of age, atrioventricular reciprocating tachycardia more frequent in children. Atrial tachycardia is least common of these. Occasionally Ebstein anomaly	

- anxious young people
- people who are fatigued
- people who drink large amounts of coffee
- people who drink alcohol heavily
- people who smoke heavily.

Some people with SVT have no symptoms, while others may experience:

- angina
- dizziness
- dyspnoea
- light-headedness
- palpitations.

In extreme cases, SVT may cause:

- unconsciousness
- cardiac arrest.

Treatment of SVT, considered if episodes are prolonged or frequent, may include:

- vagal stimulation by:
  - carotid sinus massage – gentle pressure on the neck
  - gentle pressure on the eyeballs with eyes closed
  - Valsalva manœuvre – holding the patient's nostrils closed while blowing air through the nose
- reduction of coffee, alcohol and tobacco use
- sedation
- antiarrhythmic drugs (Table 5.26 and Appendix 5.3)
- cardiac ablation, defibrillation or cardioversion; these may be needed if the measures above do not work (see later; Table 5.27), while anticoagulants and antiplatelet drugs are often also used to reduce the risk of clotting.

Table 5.26 *Treatment of arrhythmias*

Heart rhythm changes	Usual treatments
Atrial fibrillation (AF)	Cardioversion
	Digoxin
	Anticoagulants advocated
Atrial tachycardia	–
Bradycardia (pathological)	Atropine may be indicated
	May need a pacemaker
Extrasystoles	–
Long QT syndrome	Avoidance of precipitants
	Beta-blockers
Paroxysmal supraventricular tachycardia (SVT)	Vagal pressure or intravenous adenosine
	Cardiac glycosides or verapamil may be needed
Sinus tachycardia	–
Ventricular fibrillation (VF)	Defibrillation
	For acute VF, flecainide and disopyramide are indicated. Lidocaine is the usual treatment but bretylium or mexiletine may be required
	Implantable cardiac defibrillators may be used
Ventricular tachycardia	Cardioversion
	Lidocaine
Wolff–Parkinson–White syndrome	Medications, or catheter ablation to destroy the abnormal pathway

Wolff–Parkinson–White (WPW) syndrome

This is a syndrome of ventricular pre-excitation due to an accessory conduction pathway (the bundle of Kent) conducting anterogradely. Many people with WPW syndrome have a tachycardia, and may have dizziness, palpitations or faints. It is associated with atrial fibrillation

Table 5.27 *Relevant treatments in certain arrhythmias*

Simple	Medical	Drugs	Surgery
Vagal manœuvres – can stop or slow some supraventricular arrhythmias:	Catheter ablation	Drugs used to slow a fast heart rate – beta-blockers (metoprolol, atenolol)	Coronary artery bypass grafting (CABG)
• Gagging • Holding breath and bearing down (Valsalva manœuvre)	Cardioversion	Calcium-channel blockers (e.g. diltiazem and verapamil) and digoxin (digitalis) – often used to treat atrial fibrillation	Maze surgery (small cuts or burns in the atria) – can help atrial fibrillation
• Immersing face in ice-cold water • Coughing • Gently pressing fingers on eyelids	Implantable cardiac defibrillator	Amiodarone, sotalol, flecainide, propafenone, dofetilide, ibutilide, quinidine, procainamide and disopyramide – used to restore normal heart rhythm	
	Pacemaker	Anticoagulants	

and, in rare instances, results in ventricular fibrillation. Some people with WPW syndrome have no symptoms but still have an increased risk for sudden death.

Treatment depends on symptom severity and frequency, risk for future arrhythmias and patient preference. If medication fails to work, cardioversion (shock) may be used to correct the heart rate. Radiofrequency ablation is the usual therapy to block the unwanted conduction shortcut.

Paroxysmal supraventricular tachycardia (PSVT)

This is an atrioventricular nodal re-entrant tachycardia that occurs most often in young people and infants. Excessive smoking, caffeine and alcohol use, and digitalis toxicity also predispose to it. PSVT may remit spontaneously but can recur. Electrical cardioversion (shock) is successful in conversion of PSVT to a normal sinus rhythm in many other cases. Another way to convert a PSVT rapidly is to administer adenosine or verapamil.

Atrial fibrillation (AF)

Atrial fibrillation is the most common arrhythmia, with a prevalence of 1.0 % in the general population. The risk is fivefold greater in those over 65 years. AF is a common end-point for many cardiac diseases that cause atrial myocyte damage and fibrosis. People with AF do not necessarily have symptoms but others may experience one or more of:

- chest pain or pressure
- dizziness
- dyspnoea
- fainting or confusion
- fatigue
- rapid and irregular heart beat
- sweating
- weakness.

There are 3 types of AF; Paroxysmal AF (last 2-7 days); Persistent AF (longer than 7 days and needs medication or cardioversion) or Permanent AF. AF is associated with thrombus formation, particularly in the left atrial appendage. Both aspirin, clopidogrel and anticoagulants (warfarin or NOACs) have been shown to reduce this and the consequent stroke risk but a patient's absolute risk depends on other risk factors like age, left ventricular function, hypertension and previous thromboembolic events. After stroke risk has been managed, the basis of treatment is either to control the ventricular rate with drugs that block the AV node or to try to maintain sinus rhythm, and restore the heart to a normal rate and rhythm.

Atrial flutter

Rapidly fired signals cause the muscles in the atria to contract quickly, leading to a very fast, steady heart beat. Features may include:

- angina
- dizziness
- dyspnoea
- fainting
- light-headedness
- palpitations.

Ventricular tachycardias

Ventricular tachycardia is usually the result of heart disease, most commonly a previous MI, and is dangerous as it can result in chest pain, cardiac failure, syncope or ventricular fibrillation. In ventricular tachycardia, the rapid heart beat does not allow enough time for the heart to fill before it contracts, so blood flow to the rest of the body is compromised. Causes include:

- cardiac problems, including:
  - coronary heart disease
  - cardiomyopathy
  - mitral valve prolapse
  - valvular heart disease
- other causes, such as:
  - sarcoidosis
  - drugs (e.g. digitalis and antiarrhythmics)
  - change in posture
  - exercise
  - emotional excitement
  - vagal stimulation.

Ventricular fibrillation is effectively a type of cardiac arrest and is imminently life-threatening. It is typically a consequence of MI or structural heart disease, occasionally of idiopathic fibrosis affecting the conduction mechanism, thyrotoxicosis, halothane anaesthesia, or adrenaline (epinephrine), cocaine or digitalis overdosage.

Clinical features

These are dizziness, light-headedness, collapse or cardiac arrest.

General management

Treatment may include:

- cardioversion
- drugs

Table 5.28 *Conduction disorders*

Type of block	Comments	Management
Bundle branch	One ventricle contracts a fraction of a second slower than the other; often symptomless; may show on ECG	Usually no treatment is required
First-degree heart	The electrical impulse moves through the atrioventricular node more slowly than normal. The heart beat usually has a slower rate and may cause light-headedness and dizziness, or no noticeable symptoms. Can be caused by certain drugs (digitalis, beta-blockers and calcium-channel blockers)	May not require specific treatment
Second-degree heart	Some electrical signals from the atria do not reach the ventricles, resulting in 'dropped beats'. Can be classified as Mobitz type 1 (Wenckebach) and may not cause noticeable symptoms; or Mobitz type 2, typified by symptoms such as chest pain, syncope, faintness and palpitations, breathing difficulties (e.g. shortness of breath with exertion), rapid breathing, nausea and fatigue	Second-degree type 1 may not require treatment but can be a forerunner for type 2 and needs to be monitored regularly Pacemaker may be indicated
Third-degree or complete heart	The electrical impulse does not pass from the atria to the ventricles. Complete heart block in adults is caused by heart conditions, heart surgery or drug toxicity. People with third-degree heart block experience irregular and unreliable heart beats	Because of the potential for cardiac arrest, a permanent pacemaker is often indicated to treat complete heart block

- radiofrequency ablation
- surgery.

BRADYCARDIAS

Bradycardia is a slow cardiac rhythm (<60 beats/min). This may be caused by a slowed electrical signal from the SA node (sinus bradycardia), a pause in the normal activity of the SA node (sinus arrest), or blocking of the impulse between the atria and ventricles (atrioventricular block or heart block). Bradycardia may be unimportant in a young person and is often found in athletes. Physically active adults frequently have a resting heart rate slower than 60 beats/min but it causes no problems. The heart rate may fall below 60 beats/min during deep sleep.

Bradycardia in an older person, however, especially when associated with heart disease, can cause sudden loss of consciousness (syncope). Among the more common causes are IHD, drugs (especially digitalis), surgery, connective tissue disorders, including Sjögren syndrome, and, in the past, rheumatic fever.

First-degree heart block (mild heart block) may only be detectable as PR prolongation on an EGG.

Second-degree heart block (type 1 second-degree heart block [Mobitz I or Wenckebach] or type 2 second-degree heart block [Mobitz II]) may be symptomatic.

Third-degree heart block (complete heart block), when the ventricle contracts at its intrinsic rate of about 30–40 beats/min, causes severely reduced cardiac output with pallor or cyanosis, dyspnoea and syncopal (Stokes–Adams) attacks. Such patients may also have convulsions.

Causes of bradycardia include:

- conduction pathway problems (Table 5.28)
- heart disease
- hypothermia
- SA node problems.

Clinical features

The main features arise from cerebral hypoxia and include:

- dizziness
- fatigue
- fainting or near-fainting spells
- light-headedness
- cardiac arrest, in extreme cases.

Severe, prolonged, untreated bradycardia can cause:

- angina
- cardiac failure
- hypertension
- syncope.

General management

Treatment is not usually needed, except with prolonged or repeated symptoms, when bradycardia can normally be corrected with a pacemaker. Medication may need to be adjusted.

LONG QT SYNDROME

Patients with long QT syndrome (LQTS) are liable to sudden death. They have lengthening of the cardiac cycle repolarization phase, which shows on ECG. The typical changes can include a long QT interval (the time between the start of the Q wave and the end of the T wave) with delayed ventricular repolarisation; T wave abnormalities; and progression to torsades de pointes (TdP; a French term meaning 'twisting of the spikes') and ventricular fibrillation, especially in females, and sometimes to sudden cardiac death. LQTS affects about 1–2% of the population and is probably the second most common cause of sudden cardiac arrest in children and young adults, next to hypertrophic cardiomyopathy. More than half of individuals with inherited LQTS die within 10 years. A history of unexplained syncope in a young person (age 10-25 years usually), or a family history of sudden death, should raise suspicions.

LQTS often is inherited, and there are several known types:

- LQTS 1, with arrhythmias triggered by emotional stress or exercise (especially swimming)
- LQTS 2, with arrhythmias triggered by extreme emotions, such as surprise, or by noise, exercise or rest
- LQTS 3, with arrhythmias triggered by a slow heart rate during sleep.

LQTS 4, 5 and 6 are rare, as is the Jervell and Lange-Nielsen syndrome (LQTS and deafness). The term Romano-Ward syndrome is sometimes used when there is LQTS without deafness. LQTS can also be acquired, in which case it is mainly caused by a number of factors (Appendix 5.4). Adrenaline (epinephrine), stress, drugs such as olanzapine, erythromycin or azithromycin, and use of more than one psychotropic, such as a selective serotonin reuptake inhibitor (SSRI), increase the QT interval and pose a hazard of TdP, especially in:

- cardiac disease
- female patients
- older patients (>65 years)
- hypokalaemia.

Clinical features

The clinical presentations of LQTS range from dizziness to syncope and sudden death. Sometimes families are mistakenly diagnosed with 'seizure disorders' when the cause of their 'seizures' is brain hypoxia caused by a cardiac problem. Some children with LQTS are misdiagnosed as having 'exercise-induced' asthma.

General management

The diagnosis of LQTS is based on the clinical features, family history and ECG. However, for about 10% of people with LQTS, the condition is not apparent on an ECG until it is triggered by drugs such as those mentioned above.

Lifestyle changes and treatments that may prevent complications include:

- avoidance of competitive physical activity
- avoidance of startling noises
- increase in dietary potassium
- beta-blockers for LQTS 1 and 2 (mexiletine for some types)
- implantable cardiac devices
- left stellectomy.

Dental aspects

Evaluation by a cardiac specialist is advisable before any dental intervention. Stress and GA must be avoided. Beta-blockers are often used. Use of anxiolytic protocols, avoidance of adrenaline (epinephrine) and other drugs that might prolong the QT interval (see Appendix 5.4 and http://crediblemeds.org/everyone/drugs-avoid-congenital-lqts/?rf=All), and provision of treatment in a setting in which emergencies can be managed expeditiously are appropriate. LA containing adrenaline or bupivacaine, antimicrobials such as erythromycin, azole antifungals and GA-associated agents, including ketamine, succinylcholine and atropine, are contraindicated, particularly if there is any other factor predisposing to TdP.

Lidocaine and mepivacaine, which have a lesser cardiac effect than some other local anaesthetics, may be preferred for analgesia. Midazolam or propofol may be used. Isoflurane is the GA agent of choice.

If an LQTS arrhythmia progresses to sudden cardiac arrest, the only known treatment is prompt shock from an automated external defibrillator (AED).

SUDDEN ARRHYTHMIA DEATH SYNDROME (SADS)

This term refers to the sudden death of an apparently fit and healthy young person. The conditions responsible for SADS precipitate ventricular arrhythmia, the main causes being the uncommon ion channelopathies, including:

- long QT syndrome (LQTS)
- Brugada syndrome (an inherited disorder characterized by one of several ECG patterns with incomplete right bundle

branch block and ST elevations in the anterior precordial leads predisposing to ventricular tachycardia, with syncopal episodes usually in sleep, that can be misinterpreted as epilepsy. An ICD may be considered. Drugs to be avoided include bupivacaine, carbamazepine, ketamine and propofol (see http://www.brugadadrugs.org))
- catecholaminergic polymorphic ventricular tachycardia (PVT)
- progressive cardiac conduction defect (PCCD)
- short QT syndrome
- early repolarization syndrome
- sodium channel disease
- familial atrial fibrillation.

Less frequently, SADS can be caused by extra electrical pathways or cardiomyopathies. In about 1 in every 20 cases of all-age sudden cardiac arrest, and up to 1 in 5 of young cases, no definite cause can be found.

GENERAL MANAGEMENT OF ARRHYTHMIAS

An ECG is needed to diagnose and assess the risk of an arrhythmia. Management includes:

- *Radiofrequency ablation (catheter ablation)*. This is used for most simple arrhythmias and many more complex rhythm disorders (e.g. atrial fibrillation and ventricular tachycardia). Catheter ablation uses a flexible catheter with an electrode at its tip, which is introduced under radiographic guidance (fluoroscopy) via the blood vessels. A burst of radiofrequency energy or cautery with heat, cold, or electrical or laser probes allows abnormal areas of conduction to be located and destroyed.
- *Cardiovascular implantable electronic devices (CIEDs)*. If the arrhythmia is serious, the patient may need to have one of two devices implanted under the skin: a cardiac pacemaker (CP) or an automatic implantable cardioverter defibrillator (AICD). Pacemakers and AICDs (also called cardiovascular implantable electronic devices [CIEDs] or implantable rhythm devices [IRDs]) work by sensing intrinsic cardiac electrical activity. The number of patients with CIEDs is rising dramatically due to an ageing population, and clinical trials show benefits in reducing both mortality and morbidity (http://www.ncbi.nlm.nih.gov/pmc/articles/PMC2001150/; accessed 30 September 2013).

Pacemakers

A pacemaker monitors the cardiac electrical impulses and, by delivering low-energy electrical pulses, helps overcome the faulty electrical signalling. Pacemakers may be needed for people with:

- Heart block or sick sinus syndrome
- Atrial fibrillation
- Cardiac syncope
- Cardiac failure.

Pacemakers can create a more normal rhythm by:

- speeding up a bradycardia
- controlling tachyarrhythmias
- coordinating electrical signalling between the atria and ventricles
- coordinating electrical signalling between ventricles (cardiac resynchronization therapy [CRT])
- ensuring that the ventricles contract normally if there is atrial fibrillation

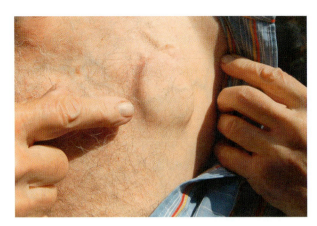

Fig. 5.11 Pacemaker. (Courtesy of Google).

- preventing dangerous arrhythmias caused by the long QT syndrome.

Some modern pacemakers can also monitor blood temperature, breathing rate and other factors.
Pacemakers can be:

- *temporary* – used to treat short-term heart problems, such as bradycardia caused by an MI, cardiac surgery or a drug overdose
- *permanent* – used to control long-term arrhythmias

and

- *single-chamber* – use one lead in the right atrium or right ventricle to pace the heart; often employed for patients whose SA node signals too slowly
- *dual-chamber* – use two leads, one in the right atrium and one in the right ventricle; the electrical pulses are timed to ensure that the beats in the atria and ventricles are synchronized.

Modern pacemakers have non-rechargeable lithium batteries that can last up to 10 years, are bipolar and are implanted transvenously via the subclavian or cephalic vein. They are typically sited in the right ventricle; on the chest wall, either within the pectoral muscle or beneath the skin (Fig. 5.11); or in the abdominal wall. Most work mainly on demand, are rate-adaptive and can be programmed to adjust the heart rate by tracking sinus node activity or by responding to sensors that monitor body motion and depth or rate of respiration. Adjustments to the pacemaker can be made non-invasively, using a specially designed radiofrequency programmer, with a wand placed on the skin over the device. Patients should carry a pacemaker registration card bearing details of the make and model.

Automatic implantable cardioverter defibrillators (AICDs)

Electric shock across the heart (defibrillation or cardioversion), either externally to the chest or internally to the heart via implanted electrodes, may be needed, via:

- *defibrillation* – the application of a shock that is *not synchronized*; this is needed for the chaotic rhythm of ventricular fibrillation and for pulseless ventricular tachycardia
- *cardioversion* – the application of a shock *synchronized* to the underlying heart beat; this is used for the treatment of supraventricular tachycardias, such as atrial tachycardia, including atrial fibrillation.

Defibrillation or cardioversion accomplished by an AICD is the most successful treatment to prevent ventricular fibrillation and is 99% effective in stopping life-threatening arrhythmias. An AICD is similar to a pacemaker and most newer models can act as both pacemakers and defibrillators. If the AICD detects an irregular ventricular rhythm, it will use low-energy electrical pulses to restore normal rhythm; if the low-energy pulses fail to restore normal rhythm, the AICD will switch to high-energy pulses for defibrillation. An AICD also can use high-energy pulses to treat life-threatening arrhythmias, especially those that can cause sudden cardiac arrest. Though the high-energy pulses last only a fraction of a second, they can be painful. An AICD continuously monitors the heart rhythm, automatically functions as a pacemaker for heart rates that are too slow, and delivers life-saving shocks if a dangerous rhythm is detected. Because AICDs must be built both to pace and to deliver shocks, they are larger than pacemakers and their batteries do not last as long.

Interference with pacemakers/defibrillators

Soon after the introduction of non-competitive, 'demand' pacemakers, examples of extraneous signals causing undesired triggering or inhibition of pacemaker output were identified; this was termed electromagnetic interference (EMI). Coupled with the increase in the number of patients with CIEDs is the proliferation of technology that emits electromagnetic signals, which can potentially interfere with it. EMI has two components: an electric and a magnetic field. EMI can come from radiofrequency (RF) waves (e.g. radio and television transmitters, electrical power and electrosurgery); microwaves (e.g. radar transmitters, mobile phones and microwave ovens); ionizing radiation; acoustic radiation; static and pulsed magnetic fields; and electrical currents.

High-frequency external electromagnetic radiation, ionizing radiation, ultrasonic and EMI from a wide range of sources can interfere with the sensing function of both pacemakers and AICDs (Table 5.29). The most frequent responses of CIEDs to EMI are inappropriate inhibition or triggering of pacemaker stimuli, reversion to asynchronous pacing, and spurious AICD tachyarrhythmia detection.

Device interactions have occurred in hospitals, where EMI sources are ubiquitous, especially from exposures to:

- radiation
- electrocautery
- MRI (Appendix 5.5).

MRI is the main EMI contraindication for patients with pacemakers or AICDs. EMI sources should be avoided where possible. Guidelines generally suggest that all handheld electronic devices be kept 15 cm away from an IRD. However, hermetic shielding in metal cases, filtering and interference rejection circuits, together with bipolar sensing, have made contemporary pacemakers and AICDs relatively immune to most EMI in household and workplace environments.

Sources of EMI

Many sources of EMI are predictable and avoidable. EMI can be conducted by direct contact (e.g. electrosurgery) or by contact with inadequately grounded equipment, or can radiate from a distance. The degree of EMI depends on the external source of power, distance from the device, signal duration, and its frequency, orientation and modulation. New technologies that use more of the electromagnetic spectrum (i.e. wireless telephones, electronic article surveillance [EAS] devices)

Table 5.29 *Sources of possible interference with cardiac pacemaker function*

Electrically coupled	Magnetic	Galvanic	Ultrasonic	Ionizing radiation
Medical sources				
Electrical appliances – particularly those with large motors and/or large power supplies. Problems more likely if appliance is in poor working condition, with motors or relays that are arcing or sparking	Magnetic resonance imaging (MRI)	Defibrillation/cardioversion Electrocautery Diathermy Transcutaneous electrical nerve stimulation (TENS)	Ultrasound equipment (see text) Lithotripsy	Radiotherapy
Non-medical sources				
Petrol-powered lawn mowers Petrol-powered saws High-voltage power lines Ham radios Arc welders Mobile phones High-power car ignition systems Metal detectors	Close proximity to powerful and large loudspeakers Induction furnaces, e.g. those used in steel industry Large generators, e.g. those used in power industry Electromagnets, e.g. those used in car-wrecking yards	Workplace situations (e.g. in electrical/computer manufacturing industry) Domestic situations (e.g. current leakage due to defective or poorly maintained house or appliance wiring)	Ultrasound equipment	Ionizing radiation sources
Comments				
Interference requires no direct contact with patient[a]	Interference requires no direct contact with patient[a]	Interference requires pacemaker patient to be in direct contact with electrical current[a] Disengaging contact from source of interference will usually return pacemaker to normal behaviour		

[a]The likelihood of interference from these sources of interference increases with the strength of the source and with the proximity of the pacemaker to the source.

have, however, reignited interest in EMI risks. Radiated EMI can arise from energy emitted for communication purposes or as an unintended effect of other electrical activity (e.g. motor operation in an electric razor). EMI from electric power can occur if patients are in proximity to high-voltage overhead power lines (accidentally or by occupation) or it may be caused by electrical appliances held close to or in direct contact with the chest. EMI from household appliances is more likely with improper grounding (Appendix 5.6).

Interference with pacemakers

The responses of pacemakers to interference are varied, usually transient and only seen while the patient remains in range of the source of interference; moving away from the source will usually return the device to its normal behaviour. The response largely depends on the interference signal characteristics and includes a single-beat inhibition (where the pacemaker may not pace the heart for a single cardiac cycle); total inhibition (where the pacemaker ceases to pace the heart); asynchronous pacing (where the pacemaker paces the heart at a fixed rate); and rate rise or erratic pacing rate. The most common pacemaker response to EMI is oversensing, which may cause transient or, rarely, permanent damage to the pacemaker. In extreme cases, where the interference is of a sufficiently high magnitude, the circuitry may be damaged, leading to persistently abnormal pacing. Modern bipolar pacemakers have improved titanium-insulated, interference-resistant circuitry and the risk of EMI is thus very small; the main and real hazard is with MRI because of the static magnetic, alternating magnetic and RF fields (Table 5.30). The pacemaker's stainless steel metal casing, and some of its components, can also trigger security devices, typically found in airports, shops and libraries, but the pacemaker function is *not* significantly affected by them. Brief exposure of a pacemaker to electromagnetic antitheft or surveillance devices causes no significant disruption of

Table 5.30 *Oral health-care equipment effects on cardiac pacemakers*

Equipment unlikely to cause interference	Equipment likely to cause interference
Amalgamator	Diathermy units
Composite curing lights	Electronic dental analgesia units
Dental chair or light	Electrosurgical units
Dental handpieces Dental radiography unit	Ferromagnetic (magnetostrictive) ultrasonic scalers
Electric toothbrushes	Lithotripsy units
Electronic apex locators	Magnetic resonance imaging (MRI)
Electronic pulp testers Microwave ovens	Transcutaneous electrical nerve stimulation (TENS) units
Piezoelectric ultrasonic scalers	Ultrasonic instrument baths
Sonic scalers	

function. Digital mobile phones, and even television transmitters and faulty or badly earthed equipment, may also cause EMI, but the risk is very small and only present when they are used close to the pacemaker. With most digital phones, EMI has no effect on most pacemakers now in use unless the phone is closer than about 15cm to the implanted pacemaker. Domestic electrical appliances – even remote controls, CB radios, electric blankets, heating pads, shavers, sewing machines, kitchen appliances and microwave ovens – are safe, but some old microwave ovens (20 years or older) may leak and cause a pacemaker temporary confusion.

If a pacemaker does shut off, all possible sources of interference should be switched off and the patient given CPR in the supine position. Artificial respiration should force the heart to resume its rhythm and the pacemaker to restart.

Patients with pacemakers do not need antibiotic cover to prevent endocarditis.

Interference with AICDs

If the AICD's magnetic switch is affected by an external magnetic field, erroneous detection and shocks may occur. AICDs are also subject to noise that can be misinterpreted as ventricular tachycardia or ventricular fibrillation, with consequent inappropriate delivery of shocks. Not only will an AICD trigger airport security alarms but also the use of strong magnets over the device may adversely affect its function and even render it non-operational. It is sensible to alert security staff to the presence of an AICD.

Patients with AICDs do not need antibiotic cover to prevent endocarditis.

DENTAL ASPECTS OF ARRHYTHMIAS

Most sudden cardiac arrests arise during endogenous adrenaline (epinephrine) peak levels (8–11 a.m.) and appointments therefore are best made for late morning or early afternoon. Arrhythmias can be induced, particularly in older patients and those with IHD or aortic stenosis, by:

- manipulation of the neck, carotid sinus or eyes (vagal reflex)
- LA (rarely)
- supraventricular or ventricular ectopics, which may develop during dental extractions or dentoalveolar surgery (these are rarely significant)
- drugs – GA agents, especially halothane (isoflurane is safer), digitalis, erythromycin or azole antifungal drugs, especially in patients taking terfenadine, cisapride or astemizole.

Ventricular fibrillation is clinically indistinguishable from asystole and is one of the most serious emergencies that may have to be managed in the dental surgery (Ch. 1). Syncope can also result from bradycardia, heart block or atrial tachycardia, and may need to be distinguished from a simple fainting attack by the slowness or irregularity of the pulse. Patients with atrial fibrillation may be treated with anticoagulants, which influence operative care (Ch. 8). As far as conscious sedation is concerned, a physician should decide whether this is acceptable for any given patient. GA is generally to be avoided. If unavoidable, it is a matter for an expert anaesthetist in hospital.

Dental aspects of CEIDs

Patients with CEIDs are usually advised to avoid elective dental care for the first few weeks after receiving the device. An aspirating syringe is recommended, as always for LA. Adequate analgesia is essential since pain can cause an outpouring of endogenous adrenaline (epinephrine). Vasoconstrictors such as adrenaline or levonordefrin in LA may raise BP or lead to atrial or ventricular arrhythmias, including fibrillation or even asystole. Intraosseous or intraligamental injections with LA agents containing vasoconstrictor should usually be avoided to prevent excessive systemic absorption. Gingival retraction cords containing adrenaline should be avoided. Adrenaline accidentally entering a blood vessel may (theoretically) increase hypertension and precipitate arrhythmias. BP tends to rise during oral surgery under LA, and adrenaline theoretically can contribute to this – though this is usually of little practical importance.

In large doses, LA may adversely interact with digoxin, non-selective beta-adrenergic-blocking drugs, antidepressants or cocaine. Adrenaline-containing LA should not be given in large doses to patients on these agents; interaction may induce hypertension and cardiovascular complications. Mepivacaine 3% is thought to be preferable to lidocaine.

Dental aspects of pacemakers

Some dental electrical devices capable of generating electromagnetic radiation may pose a threat to dental patients with a pacemaker *but this is usually low-grade and only present if the devices are placed very close to the pacemaker* (see Table 5.30). Cardiac pacemakers usually now have two (bipolar) electrode leads and present few problems for dental treatment. In patients with pacemakers, MRI, electrosurgery, diathermy and transcutaneous nerve stimulation are contraindicated. Pacemaker single-beat inhibition of little consequence may occasionally be caused by dental equipment, such as piezoelectric ultrasonic scalers and ultrasonic baths, older ferromagnetic ultrasonic scalers, pulp testers, electronic apex locators, dental induction casting machines, belt-driven motors in dental chairs, and older radiography machines. Modern piezoelectric scalers have no significant effect, but activity rate-responsive devices may exhibit faster pacing rates. The only safe procedure under such circumstances is to avoid the use of all such equipment whenever a patient with a pacemaker is being treated, as it is difficult to assess the level of risk in any individual patient. Patients with pacemakers should be treated supine; electrical equipment kept over 30 cm away; and rapid, repetitive switching of electrical instruments avoided. Diagnostic radiation and ultrasonography have no effect on pacemakers, even with cumulative doses, but faulty equipment may cause problems. After experiencing EMI, the IRD will usually revert to normal functioning as soon as the patient moves away from the EMI source. If procedures associated with increased EMI risk are indicated, the dependency status should be verified and the device temporarily reprogrammed to the optimal setting. Post-procedure device verification is recommended if there is any evidence of or any doubt about EMI.

Patients with permanent pacemakers do not need antibiotic cover to prevent endocarditis. If a temporary transvenous pacemaker is present, however, the physician should be consulted first.

Dental aspects of AICDs

Adrenaline (epinephrine) or other vasoconstrictors should be used with caution (lower dose and careful monitoring) in patients with AICDs.

AICDs may activate without significant warning, possibly causing the patient to flinch, bite down or perform other sudden movements that may result in injury to the patient or clinician. Some patients with AICDs may lose consciousness when the device is activated. This is less likely with newer devices, which initially emit low-level electrical bursts followed by stronger shocks if cardioversion does not follow immediately. After experiencing EMI, the AICD will usually revert to normal functioning as soon as the patient moves away from the EMI source. If procedures associated with increased EMI risk are indicated, the dependency status should be verified and the device temporarily reprogrammed to the optimal setting. Post-procedure device verification is recommended if there is any evidence of or any doubt about EMI.

Patients with AICDs do not need antibiotic cover to prevent endocarditis.

Several antiarrhythmic drugs can cause oral lesions. Verapamil, enalapril and diltiazem can cause gingival swelling; some beta-blockers may rarely cause lichenoid ulceration; and procainamide can cause a lupus-like reaction.

THYROID-RELATED HEART DISEASE

See also Chapter 6.

General aspects

Hyperthyroidism raises the metabolic rate and activity of the heart, and sensitizes the myocardium to sympathetic activity. The heart may be unable to meet the greater demands resulting from the raised metabolic activity of the rest of the body, particularly in the elderly.

Hypothyroidism slows the metabolic rate and activity of the heart and other tissues.

Clinical features

Untreated thyrotoxicosis causes tachycardia and a tendency to arrhythmias, which can lead to cardiac failure or MI, especially in the elderly.

Hypothyroidism slows the heart rate and myxoedema patients may have hypercholesterolaemia associated with atheroma. IHD often develops but is unusual in that it predominantly affects women.

General management

Beta-blockers are useful to control hyperthyroid heart disease.

Dental aspects

Patients with uncontrolled hyperthyroidism can sometimes be difficult to manage, as a result of heightened anxiety, hyperexcitability and excessive sympathetic activity.

Effective analgesia must be provided. An aspirating syringe should be used to give an LA, and LA containing adrenaline (epinephrine) should, in theory, be avoided because of the possible risk of dangerous arrhythmias. However, there seems little clinical evidence for this and the risk is probably real only if an overdose is given. There is no evidence that prilocaine with felypressin is any safer.

Gingival retraction cords containing adrenaline should be avoided.

Conscious sedation, preferably with nitrous oxide and oxygen, may be beneficial in that it calms the patient. The same reservations about GA apply to patients with uncontrolled thyroid heart disease as to those with other dangerous heart diseases.

Hypothyroid patients may be at risk in the dental surgery if they have CAD. Sjögren syndrome is occasionally associated. In severe myxoedema, diazepam and other CNS depressants can precipitate coma.

PULMONARY HEART DISEASE (COR PULMONALE)

General aspects

Cor pulmonale is heart disease resulting from the excessive load imposed on the right ventricle by diseases of the lungs or pulmonary circulation, especially chronic obstructive pulmonary (airways) disease (COPD, COAD; Ch. 15).

Clinical features

Right ventricular hypertrophy may lead to right-sided failure with systemic venous congestion and persistent hypoxia. In the early stages, there is dyspnoea, a chronic cough, wheezing and often cyanosis. Later, there is also ankle oedema and ascites.

General management

Oxygen, diuretics, vasodilators, salbutamol and ipratropium are among the measures that may be needed.

Dental aspects

Ipratropium can cause a dry mouth.

Local analgesia is the main means of pain control. Conscious sedation with diazepam or midazolam is contraindicated because of the respiratory depressant action in a hypoxic patient. Nitrous oxide and oxygen may be acceptable. Intravenous barbiturates are also contraindicated because of their respiratory depressant effect.

KAWASAKI DISEASE (MUCOCUTANEOUS LYMPH NODE SYNDROME)

General aspects

Kawasaki disease is an acute febrile illness with lymphadenopathy and desquamation of lips, fingers and toes, simulating scarlet fever and erythema multiforme. It is now a considerably more common cause of severe childhood heart disease than rheumatic fever in many countries. It is significantly more prevalent in Japanese and Korean people.

Although an infection is probably causal, presumably in persons of certain genetic backgrounds, no agent has yet been consistently isolated. Superantigens (bacterial toxins that stimulate T lymphocytes) are another possible cause. The main pathological process is a widespread vasculitis, which can, in approximately 25%, affect the coronary arteries – with aneurysm formation.

Clinical features

Eighty per cent of affected children are aged less than 5 years, with a male preponderance in a ratio of more than 2 to 1.

Fever lasting at least 5 days, erythema and oedema of the extremities, followed by desquamation, a polymorphous rash, labial and oral mucosal erythema, cervical lymphadenopathy, conjunctival injection and mood changes (extreme misery) are seen. The mortality is 5–10%, death mainly stemming from MI secondary to aneurysmal thrombus formation.

General management

Erythrocyte sedimentation rate (ESR) and CRP are raised; liver function is abnormal; there may be pyuria and normocytic anaemia. Ultrasonography may show an enlarged gallbladder; ECG and echocardiography may demonstrate abnormalities; and lumbar puncture may provide evidence of aseptic meningitis. Patients should be admitted to hospital for intravenous gammaglobulin treatment. Aspirin or a systemic steroid is usually also given.

Dental aspects

Characteristic oral changes include a strawberry tongue, labial oedema, crusting or cracking of the lips, pharyngitis, oropharyngeal erythema and cervical lymphadenopathy – usually unilateral but occasionally massive. Facial palsy is sometimes seen, but is self-limiting and usually associated with cardiovascular disease. Treatment is unlikely to be given to a young child in the acute phase but, for a dental emergency, LA may be given. Conscious sedation is inappropriate and GA is contraindicated.

VALVULAR HEART DISEASE

RHEUMATIC FEVER

General aspects

Rheumatic fever sometimes follows a sore throat caused by certain strains of beta-haemolytic streptococci (*Streptococcus pyogenes*). Rheumatic fever is now a very rare disease in the Western world but is common in countries such as the Indian subcontinent, the Middle East and some of the Caribbean islands. Children between 5 and 15 years are predominantly affected.

Rheumatic fever may occasionally be followed by chronic rheumatic carditis with permanent cardiac valvular damage. The inflammatory reaction of rheumatic carditis appears to result from immunological cross-reactivity with streptococcal antigens and immunologically mediated tissue damage, which may lead, after the lapse of years, to fibrosis and distortion of the cardiac valves (chronic rheumatic heart disease).

Clinical features

A sore throat may be followed after about 3 weeks (2–26 weeks) by an acute febrile illness with pain flitting from one joint to another (migratory arthralgia). Usually there is resolution within 6–12 weeks without apparent after-effects. Pain in the large joints (which gives rheumatic fever its name) is conspicuous but heals without permanent damage in about 3 weeks.

Other effects may include: cerebral involvement – causing spasmodic involuntary movements (Sydenham chorea, St Vitus dance); a characteristic rash (erythema marginatum); lung involvement; and subcutaneous nodules (usually around the elbows).

The most serious cardiac complication is subendocardial inflammation, particularly along the lines of closure of the mitral and aortic valve cusps, resulting in the formation of minute fibrinous vegetations and later scarring. There is usually little detectable effect on cardiac function in the acute phase but, in unusually severe cases, myocarditis can cause death from cardiac failure. The essential features of chronic rheumatic heart disease are fibrotic stiffening and distortion of the heart valves, often causing mitral stenosis. This is essentially a mechanical, haemodynamic disorder, in which the defective valves may become infected at any time, leading to infective endocarditis. Cardiac failure can develop, often after many years.

General management

The clinical manifestations of acute rheumatic fever are so variable that the diagnosis is made only if at least two of the major criteria are fulfilled (Table 5.31).

Preceding streptococcal infection is confirmed by a high or rising titre of antistreptolysin O antibodies (ASOT), which is suggestive, but not diagnostic, of rheumatic fever; a low ASOT virtually excludes the diagnosis.

Streptococcal sore throat is an indication for treatment with antibiotics, usually penicillin. Prompt antimicrobial treatment (within 24 hours of onset) prevents the development of rheumatic fever in most cases. Complications such as cardiac failure are treated along conventional lines. Chorea may recur during pregnancy or in patients taking the contraceptive pill, but does not indicate recurrent carditis.

After an attack of rheumatic carditis, there is a risk of recurrence, and continuous antibiotic prophylaxis becomes necessary to lessen the risk of permanent cardiac damage. The drug of choice is usually

Table 5.31 *Rheumatic fever: diagnostic criteria*

Major	Minor
Carditis	Pyrexia
Polyarthritis	Arthralgia
Chorea	Previous rheumatic fever
Erythema marginatum	Raised ESR and CRP
Subcutaneous nodules	Characteristic ECG changes

oral phenoxymethylpenicillin until the age of 20. For those allergic to penicillin, sulfadimidine should be given.

In the past, approximately 60% of children who survived acute rheumatic fever developed a cardiac lesion detectable after 10 years, but heart failure frequently took 10 or more years to emerge. However, such complications have become increasingly rare in the high-income world and chronic rheumatic heart disease is only likely to be seen now in the middle-aged and some immigrants. The mitral valve is usually affected, either alone in 60–70% or with the aortic valve in a further 20%. The aortic valve alone is affected in only 10%. Valve narrowing (stenosis) and regurgitation (incompetence) are associated in varying degrees. The earliest sign of valve damage is a murmur. Later effects, particularly enlargement of the heart, may be detected clinically, radiographically and by ECG and echocardiography changes. Treatment is by mitral balloon valvuloplasty, using an Inoue balloon.

Dental aspects

Acute rheumatic fever patients are exceedingly unlikely to be seen during an attack but emergency dental treatment may be necessary. Most patients with chronic rheumatic fever are anticoagulated; treatment can be done under LA in consultation with the physician. Conscious sedation with nitrous oxide may be given if cardiac function is good and with the approval of the physician.

DRUG-INDUCED CARDIAC VALVULAR LESIONS

Use of a combination of the appetite suppressants fenfluramine and phentermine has been associated with a risk of cardiac valve regurgitation, particularly aortic regurgitation. All patients who have taken these drugs for longer than 3 months should have a clinical examination and, if any abnormality is detected, should be referred to a cardiologist for echocardiography.

INFECTIVE (BACTERIAL) ENDOCARDITIS

Infectious endocarditis (IE) results from bacterial or fungal infection of the endocardium, and is associated with significant morbidity and mortality. It is rare but potentially life-threatening, predominantly affecting damaged heart valves. Risk factors include the presence of a prosthetic heart valve, structural or congenital heart disease, intravenous drug use and a recent history of invasive procedures. IE has changed in profile, moving from being a streptococcal disease in patients with previously known heart disease to a staphylococcal health-care-associated disease in older patients suffering from many co-morbidities or having intracardiac devices.

Individuals who have had uncomplicated myocardial infarcts, coronary angioplasty or CABG, or who have had cardiac pacemakers inserted, do not have an increased risk of developing IE. Natural heart valves (native valve endocarditis), sometimes damaged by disease

Table 5.32 *Main groups affected by infective endocarditis*

Aetiology	Approximate % of all cases of infective endocarditis
No obvious cardiac valve disease	40
Chronic rheumatic heart disease	30
Congenital heart disease	10
Prosthetic cardiac valves	10
Intravenous drug abuse	10

Box 5.12 *Patients at highest risk from infective endocarditis*

- Prosthetic valves
- Previous infective endocarditis
- Complex cyanotic congenital heart defect, e.g. tetralogy of Fallot, transposition of the great arteries or Gerbode defect
- Surgically constructed systemic–pulmonary shunts or conduits
- Mitral valve prolapse with regurgitation or thickened leaflets

(e.g. rheumatic carditis), are usually affected by IE, but it can also affect people with CHD or patients who have undergone valve surgery (Table 5.32). Cardiac valves already damaged by infective endocarditis, or prosthetic cardiac valves (prosthetic valve endocarditis), are particularly at risk of infection (Box 5.12).

Platelet–fibrin deposits may accumulate along the free margins of valves, where there is turbulent blood flow; here they form sterile vegetations (aseptic thrombotic endocarditis) that may become infected with microorganisms, resulting in large friable vegetations (IE). Most bacteraemias are transient, self-limiting and not associated with any systemic complications. The factors that determine the development of IE are complex, but a susceptible surface (damaged endocardium) and high bacterial loads in the circulation appear to be important. Oral viridans streptococci (*Streptococcus mutans* and *sanguis*) from plaque enter the bloodstream (bacteraemia) during chewing, oral hygiene, tooth extractions and other oral procedures. They have complex attachment mechanisms, which enable them to adhere to damaged endocardium. Other microorganisms are also implicated, particularly *Staphylococcus aureus* and enterococci. Very few healthy ambulant patients, probably less than 5%, acquire IE as a result of dental treatment, and it is also clear that bacteria enter the blood from the mouth (and other sites) on innumerable occasions unrelated to operative intervention but usually cause no harm. In statistical terms, the chance of dental extractions causing IE, even in a patient with valvular disease, may possibly be as low as 1 in 3000.

Intravascular access devices, such as central intravenous lines, Hickman lines or Uldall catheters, often become infected but there is no evidence for a dental focus for such infections. An uncommon but dangerous type of right-sided IE in a previously healthy heart results from intravenous drug abuse, when highly virulent bacteria such as staphylococci can be introduced from the skin into the bloodstream with the addict's needle.

Guidelines from the AHA on the prevention of endocarditis can be found by searching on 'infective endocarditis' at http://circ.ahajournals.org or http://www.americanheart.org (accessed 30 September 2013).

Clinical features

The clinical features of IE are highly variable. It often has an insidious onset but should be considered in any individual presenting with fever and a new or changing heart murmur. IE cases range from fulminatingly acute to chronic.

Pallor (anaemia) or light (café-au-lait) pigmentation of the skin, joint pains and hepatosplenomegaly are typical, but the main effect of endocarditis is progressive heart damage (valve destruction and heart failure). Increasing disability is associated with changing cardiac murmurs indicative of progressive heart damage, infection or embolic damage of many organs, especially the kidneys (fever, malaise, night sweats and weight loss). Release of emboli can have widespread effects (on brain, lungs, spleen and kidneys), ranging from loss of a peripheral pulse to (rarely) sudden death from a stroke. Embolic phenomena include haematuria, cerebrovascular occlusion, petechiae or purpura of skin and mucous membranes, and splinter haemorrhages under the fingernails. Roth spots are small retinal haemorrhages. Immune complex formation from the antigens and resultant antibodies can lead to vasculitis, arthritis, and retinal and renal damage. Osler's nodes are small, tender, vasculitic lesions in the skin.

Endocarditis should be suspected in patients with unexplained fevers, night sweats or signs of systemic illness.

General management

Diagnosis is made using the Duke criteria, which include clinical, laboratory and echocardiographic findings, and is based on changing murmurs, ECG (may show conduction abnormalities), echocardiography (may identify vegetations and enables assessment of valvular and cardiac function) and blood culture. The latter is essential when IE is suspected and must be carried out before antimicrobial treatment is started; at least three samples of blood should be taken aseptically, at half-hourly intervals, to increase the chances of obtaining a positive culture. Urine Stix may detect microscopic haematuria. Serological testing helps identify atypical organisms (e.g. *Legionella*).

Common blood culture isolates include *Staphylococcus aureus*, viridans streptococci, enterococci and coagulase-negative staphylococci. Antibiotic treatment of IE depends on whether the involved valve is native or prosthetic, as well as the causative microorganism and its antibiotic susceptibilities. Without treatment, IE is fatal in approximately 30% of cases, so the patient should be admitted to hospital for intravenous antibiotic therapy, usually benzylpenicillin and gentamicin. If staphylococcal endocarditis is suspected, vancomycin should be substituted in place of penicillin. In severe cases, such as prosthetic valve endocarditis, early removal of the infected valve and insertion of a sterile replacement may be needed.

After completion of antibiotic therapy, patients should be educated about the importance of daily dental hygiene and regular visits for oral health care.

According to 2007 AHA guidelines, the only individuals who will need antibiotic pre-medication are those who:

- have a prosthetic cardiac valve
- have a history of previous IE
- have a history of CHD:
  - an unrepaired cyanotic congenital heart defect, including palliative shunts and conduits
  - a completely repaired congenital heart defect with prosthetic material or prosthetic device, whether placed by surgery or by catheter intervention, during the first 6 months after the procedure
  - a repaired congenital heart defect with residual defects at the site or adjacent to the site of a prosthetic patch or prosthetic device (which inhibit endothelialization)

■ are cardiac transplantation recipients who develop cardiac valvulopathy.

The AHA and American Dental Association (ADA) recommend the following 'talking points' to assuage the concerns of patients and colleagues:

■ IE is much more likely to result from frequent exposure to random bacteraemias associated with daily activities than from bacteraemia caused by a dental, gastrointestinal tract or genitourinary tract procedure.
■ Prophylaxis may prevent an exceedingly small number of cases of IE, if any, in individuals who undergo a dental, gastrointestinal tract or genitourinary tract procedure.
■ The risk of antibiotic-associated adverse events exceeds the benefit, if any, from prophylactic antibiotic therapy.
■ Maintenance of optimal oral health and hygiene may reduce the incidence of bacteraemia from daily activities and is more important than prophylactic antibiotics for a dental procedure to reduce the risk of IE.

Dental aspects

The main points are as follows:

■ The cardiac endocarditis risk is now stratified into high, moderate and low. The low-risk categories do not require antibiotic prophylaxis for dental procedures.
■ Dental procedures associated with bleeding are no longer exclusively indicated for antibiotic prophylaxis:
  ◆ Only procedures with a statistically significant difference in bacteraemia between a pre- and a post-procedure blood sample are recommended for prophylaxis. This provides a logical and easily identifiable way of identifying procedures requiring antibiotic prophylaxis.
  ◆ The use of azithromycin syrup for children who refuse tablets or capsules and for patients with dysphagia, already advocated by the *British National Formulary* (BNF), has now been formally recommended but this can affect cardiac QT (see 'Long QT syndrome' above).

Patients at risk of endocarditis should receive intensive preventive dental care to minimize the need for dental intervention. However, this aspect of care is frequently neglected; a very high proportion of patients attending cardiology clinics have periodontal disease. There is no reliable evidence to suggest that oral hygiene aids, such as electric toothbrushes, water-piks or similar devices, pose a risk.

In many countries, there are national guidelines on the use of antimicrobial prophylaxis against IE, if dental interventions are needed. However, the efficacy of such antimicrobial prophylaxis has been questionable and antibiotic prophylaxis is no longer mandatory for IE-susceptible patients who are to undergo dental care (Box 5.13).

There is always a risk of adverse reactions to the antimicrobial (such as anaphylaxis), which can approach 5% and can be as high from the oral administration of amoxicillin as from intramuscular administration of the same. Estimates suggest that deaths from an anaphylactic reaction to antibiotics are possibly 5–6 times more likely than deaths from IE.

Medico-legal and other considerations suggest that one should err on the side of caution in relation to antibiotic prophylaxis of IE by following these guidelines:

■ Fully inform the patient about antimicrobial prophylaxis against IE and discuss it with them.
■ Take medical advice in any case of doubt.

Box 5.13 *Reasons for abandoning use of antibiotic prophylaxis for endocarditis*

• Dental treatment is a proven cause of few cases of IE. One US study showed that in the 3 months before IE diagnosis, dental treatment was no more frequent than in controls, concluding that few cases would be prevented even if antibiotic prophylaxis were provided and were 100% effective. Another study concluded that, if antibiotic prophylaxis were 100% effective and provided for all at-risk patients receiving dental treatment, only a fraction of cases (5.3%) would be potentially prevented
• Prophylactic antibiotic regimens fail in some instances
• Adverse reactions to antimicrobials are possible, including anaphylaxis
• The cost-effectiveness of antimicrobial prophylaxis is questionable
• There is an increased risk of resistant bacteria

■ Remember that, in countries where there are national guidelines, it is mandatory, for medico-legal reasons, to give such prophylaxis to patients at risk. For example, in 2007, the ADA, endorsed by the Infectious Diseases Society of America and the Pediatric Infectious Diseases Society, recommended prophylaxis, but only in the high-risk circumstances described above.

In the UK, over the years, a number of regimens have been suggested for endocarditis cover. In 1992, the British Society for Antimicrobial Chemotherapy (BSAC) recommended cover for all procedures associated with bleeding. The British Cardiac Society/Royal College of Physicians (BCS/RCP) suggested in 2004 that antibiotic prophylaxis be given for all bacteraemic dental procedures and for a large range of cardiac defects and/or surgery. However, in 2006, the BSAC recommended antibiotic prophylaxis in only three (high-risk) circumstances:

■ Previous IE
■ Prosthetic valves
■ Surgically constructed pulmonary shunts or conduits.

NICE then issued recommendations in 2008, completely removing the need for antibiotic prophylaxis in relation to dentistry. *Antibiotic prophylaxis is now not recommended for patients at risk of endocarditis undergoing dental procedures.* Patients at risk of endocarditis should achieve and maintain high standards of oral health. NICE recommended that patients at risk for endocarditis should receive intensive preventive oral health care, to try to minimize the need for dental intervention. See also Appendix 5.7.

CARDIAC FAILURE

General aspects

Not to be confused with cardiac *arrest*, cardiac or heart failure is when any structural or functional impairment of the pumping action of the heart leads to blood output insufficient to meet the body's demands. Lack of tissue and organ perfusion with congestion results, and thus the term 'congestive cardiac failure' is often used. Heart failure (HF; or congestive heart or cardiac failure [CHF, CCF]) is common and the prevalence is rising. It is associated with considerable morbidity and mortality (Table 5.33), being the leading cause of hospitalization in people over 65 and having an annual mortality rate of 10%.

The most common cause of cardiac failure is IHD but there are many others (Table 5.34), and cardiac failure may arise as a consequence of myocardial, valvular, pericardial, endocardial or electrical problems (or some combination). The remainder have a non-ischaemic

Table 5.33 *New York Heart Association (NYHA) heart failure classification and treatment*

NYHA class	Features	Therapy
I	No limitation: ordinary physical exercise does not cause undue fatigue, dyspnoea or palpitations	ACE inhibitor (ACEI) Beta-blocker
II	Slight limitation of physical activity: comfortable at rest but ordinary activity results in fatigue, palpitations or dyspnoea	ACEI Beta-blocker Candesartan (initiation requires specialist advice)
III	Marked limitation of physical activity: comfortable at rest but less than ordinary activity results in symptoms	ACEI Beta-blocker
IV	Unable to carry out any physical activity without discomfort: symptoms of heart failure are present even at rest with increased discomfort with any physical activity	Spironolactone (initiation requires specialist advice) For patients in sinus rhythm with drug-refractory symptoms of heart failure due to left ventricular systolic dysfunction and who have a QRS duration of >120 ms, cardiac resynchronization should be considered

Table 5.34 *Main causes of heart failure*

Left-sided mainly	Right-sided mainly	Biventricular
Ischaemic heart disease	Chronic obstructive pulmonary disease	Ischaemic heart disease
Aortic valve disease	Pulmonary embolism	Aortic valve disease
Mitral valve disease		Mitral valve disease
Hypertension		Hypertension
		Cardiomyopathies
		Hyperthyroidism
		Chronic anaemias
		Arrhythmias

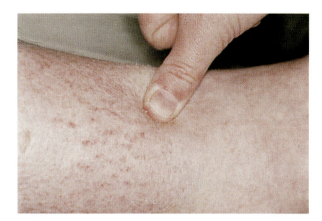

Fig 5.12 Pressure on ankle in a person with suspected ankle oedema.

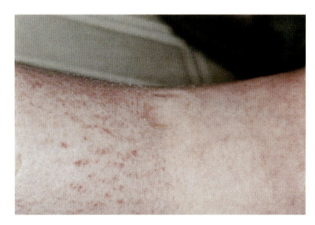

Fig. 5.13 Pitting oedema, indicating oedema and probable cardiac failure.

cardiomyo-pathy, with either an identifiable cause (e.g. hypertension, thyroid disease, valvular disease, alcohol excess or myocarditis) or an unknown cause (e.g. idiopathic dilated cardiomyopathy). The term 'acute heart failure' is used to mean acute (cardiogenic) dyspnoea characterized by signs of pulmonary congestion, including pulmonary oedema. Chronic HF is a complex syndrome that can result from any structural or functional cardiac or non-cardiac disorder that impairs the ability of the heart to respond to physiological demands for increased cardiac output.

Clinical features

HF is characterized by fatigue, exertional breathlessness and signs of fluid retention. CHF can be associated with left ventricular systolic dysfunction (LVSD) and/or left ventricular diastolic dysfunction (LVDD). It can progress to involve right ventricular dysfunction (RVD). The result is an inadequate supply of oxygenated blood to the circulation. Features depend on which side of the heart – left or right – is predominantly involved and on the type of failure, either diastolic or systolic. The following signs are specific for heart failure:

- Raised jugular venous pressure (JVP)
- Lateral displacement of the apex beat
- Presence of a third heart sound (S3)
- Basal lung crepitations
- Peripheral oedema.

Symptoms can be few until activity becomes limited by breathlessness (dyspnoea), cyanosis and dependent oedema (usually swollen ankles or sacral oedema; Figs 5.12 and 5.13). CHF is often undiagnosed, owing to lack of a universally agreed definition and difficulties in diagnosis, particularly when the condition is considered 'mild'.

Left-sided heart failure results in damming of blood back from the left ventricle to the pulmonary circulation with pulmonary hypertension, pulmonary oedema and dyspnoea. Lying down worsens pulmonary congestion, oedema and dyspnoea (orthopnoea). It also makes respiration less efficient, and cyanosis likely, because the abdominal viscera move the diaphragm higher and reduce the vital capacity of the lungs. Coughing is another typical consequence; the sputum is frothy and, in severe cases, pink with blood. In the more advanced stages of left-sided heart failure, there is inadequate cerebral oxygenation leading to symptoms such as loss of concentration, restlessness and irritability or, in older people, disorientation.

Right-sided heart failure causes congestion of the main venous systems and thus affects the liver, gastrointestinal tract, kidneys and subcutaneous tissues primarily. It presents with peripheral (dependent) oedema, fatigue and hepatomegaly due to passive congestion, causing abdominal discomfort and, in severe cardiac failure, raised portal venous pressure, which also leads to the escape of large amounts of fluid into the peritoneal cavity (ascites).

Failure of one side of the heart usually leads to failure of the other – biventricular failure. The pulse may then become rapid and irregular, particularly if there is atrial fibrillation; in extreme cases, patients are cyanotic, polycythaemic, dyspnoeic at rest and oedematous with pulmonary oedema and distension of the neck veins (raised JVP). Arrhythmias and sudden death may result. The American College of Cardiology/AHA/New York Heart Association (NYHA) has defined four stages in the progression of cardiac failure (see Table 5.33).

General management

Heart failure is diagnosed clinically and by chest radiography (cardiomegaly), echocardiography, ECG and biochemistry (*B-type natriuretic peptide* [BNP]). Echocardiography determines the *stroke volume* (SV; the amount of blood that exits the ventricles with each heart beat), the *end-diastolic volume* (EDV; the amount of blood at the end of diastole), and the SV in proportion to the EDV (the *ejection fraction*; EF). Normally, the EF should lie between 50 and 70% but, in cardiac failure, it is less than 40%. A raised BNP is a specific test result indicative of cardiac failure. There may also be abnormal liver and renal function tests, hyponatraemia and alkalosis.

Heart failure is managed by treating the symptoms and signs via reduction of the heart workload and correction of precipitating factors (e.g. hypertension, anaemia, valvular disease and thyrotoxicosis). General measures may include rest, stress reduction, control of hypertension, weight loss, smoking cessation and salt restriction. Treatment aims to prevent HF progressing, thereby reducing symptoms, hospital admissions and mortality. Many treatments reduce either one or more (often all) of these but each can produce adverse effects. Careful monitoring is essential to maximize benefit and minimize adverse effects.

First-line therapies

These are ACEIs (e.g. enalapril, ramipril, quinapril, perindopril, lisinopril and benazepril) or angiotensin II receptor blockers (ARBs) or sartans (e.g. valsartan, telmisartan, losartan, irbesartan and olmesartan). These delay progression and reduce mortality, improving myocardial contractility, tissue and organ perfusion, and oxygenation. ACEIs reduce the relative risk of mortality by 25% and should be considered in patients with all NYHA functional classes of heart failure due to LVSD. Adverse effects include cough, hypotension, renal impairment, a sprue-like syndrome, and hyperkalaemia. Angioedema is rare but can be life-threatening (due to laryngeal involvement). ACEI-induced renal dysfunction is likely to occur in those with unsuspected renovascular disease. Concomitant ACEI and aspirin use is safe and effective in reducing cardiovascular events in patients with HF.

Beta-blockers

Beta-blockers may be indicated for patients with systolic heart failure due to LVSD after stabilization with ACEIs and diuretics. Beta-blockers are needed in all patients with HF due to LVSD of all NYHA classes. Beta-blocker therapy is needed as soon as their condition is stable (unless contraindicated by a history of asthma, heart block or symptomatic hypotension). Beta$_1$-selective (bisoprolol, metoprolol, nebivolol) or non-selective (carvedilol) blockers produce a consistent reduction in mortality of approximately one-third.

Angiotensin receptor blockers (ARBs)

ARBs block the biological effect of angiotensin II, mimicking the effect of ACEIs without cough as an adverse effect. Patients with chronic heart failure due to LVSD alone, or HF, LVSD or both following MI who are intolerant of ACEIs should be considered for an ARB. Patients with heart failure due to LVSD who are still symptomatic despite therapy with an ACEI and a beta-blocker may benefit from the addition of candesartan, following specialist advice.

Aldosterone antagonists

Aldosterone antagonists, such as spironolactone, added to an ACEI reduce mortality by 30%. Spironolactone can produce gynaecomastia, hyperkalaemia and renal dysfunction. Following specialist advice, patients with moderate to severe HF due to LVSD should be considered for spironolactone, unless this is contraindicated by renal impairment or a high potassium concentration. Eplerenone is an alternative aldosterone receptor antagonist that is less likely to produce sexual adverse effects such as gynaecomastia, breast pain or menstrual irregularities. Patients who have suffered an MI, and who have a left ventricular EF of 40% or less and either diabetes or clinical signs of HF, should be considered for eplerenone unless this is contra-indicated by the presence of renal impairment or a high potassium concentration. Even when added to maximum medication therapy in patients with mild to moderate heart failure, eplerenone reduces the risk of both death and hospitalization.

Diuretics

Diuretics (mainly loop diuretics such as furosemide or bumetanide) increase sodium and water excretion. Diuretics/loop diuretics/metolazone should be considered for HF patients with dyspnoea or oedema (ankle or pulmonary). The dose should eliminate ankle or pulmonary oedema without dehydrating the patient and placing them at risk of renal dysfunction or hypotension.

Digoxin

Digoxin may help when failure is associated with atrial fibrillation and should be considered as an add-on therapy for HF patients in sinus rhythm who are still symptomatic after optimum therapy. Digoxin improves symptoms but not survival, and benefit must be weighed against the possibility of an increase in sudden deaths associated with digoxin. The risk of digoxin toxicity is increased by hypokalaemia. In patients with HF and atrial fibrillation, a beta-blocker is preferred for control of the ventricular rate, though digoxin may be used initially while the beta-blocker is being introduced. If excessive bradycardia occurs with both drugs, digoxin should be stopped.

Vasodilators

Vasodilators, particularly isosorbide dinitrate plus hydralazine, may be valuable for people who fail to respond to ACEIs. Recombinant BNP (nesiritide) is indicated for patients with acute HF who have dyspnoea at rest. Antagonists of vasopressin (tolvaptan and conivaptan) and aldosterone (spironolactone and eplerenone) receptors are newer therapies. Phosphodiesterase inhibitors (enoximone or milrinone) may help to support cardiac function. Drug treatment is shown in Box 5.14.

Other therapies

Nesiritide, the recombinant form of B-type natriuretic peptide despite earlier promise, appears of little benefit. The *BNF* advises that, due to interactions with prescribed medications, certain supplements and fruit juices should be avoided:

■ Patients with CHF who are taking warfarin should be advised to avoid cranberry juice (which may increase drug potency).

Box 5.14 *Treatment of heart failure*

Medical
- Diuretic
- Angiotensin-converting enzyme inhibitor (ACEI)
- Beta-blocker
- Aldosterone antagonist

Devices
- Pacemaker
- Cardiac resynchronization device
- Implantable cardiac defibrillator

Surgical
- Valve surgery
- Coronary artery bypass graft
- Transplant

- Patients with CHF who are taking simvastatin should be advised to avoid grapefruit juice (which may interfere with liver metabolism of statins).
- Patients with CHF should not take St John's wort due to the interaction with warfarin, digoxin, eplerenone and SSRIs.

Supplemental oxygen may be required and surgery (heart transplantation) is occasionally used to treat severe cardiac failure. New technologies include:

- *Heart pump* – this involves a left ventricular assist device (VAD) implanted into the abdomen and attached to the heart. A mechanical pump supports heart function and blood flow by taking blood from the ventricle and helping pump it to the body and vital organs. For patients with severe decompensated HF, ventricular mechanical support can be considered as a bridge to transplantation. VADs or total artificial hearts (TAHs) are used for HF, as bridges to transplantation or cardiotomy. VADs are used during or after heart surgery, or whilst a patient is awaiting a heart transplant. A small tube carries blood out of the heart into a pump and another carries it back to the blood vessels, to deliver the blood to the body. A control unit monitors the VAD functions. Some VADs work with a pumping action, while others keep up a continuous blood flow. The most common type is a left ventricular assist device, which conveys blood back to the aorta. A right ventricular assist device is used only for short-term support of the right ventricle after heart surgery; it helps the right ventricle pump blood to the pulmonary artery. If both ventricles are failing, both types of VAD are used simultaneously as a biventricular assist device. An alternative treatment option for this is a TAH. A transcutaneous VAD has its pump and power source located outside of the body. Tubes connect the pump to the heart through small holes in the abdomen. This type of VAD might be used for short-term support during or after surgery.
- *Biventricular cardiac pacemaker* – this sends specifically timed electrical impulses to the ventricles for cardiac resynchronization therapy.
- *Xenotransplantation* – a genetically manipulated pig's heart is transplanted into a human.
- *Artificial heart* – all-mechanical artificial hearts have already been implanted in humans.

- *Cardiac resynchronization therapy* – this is considered for patients in sinus rhythm with drug-refractory symptoms of HF due to LVSD (left ventricular ejection fraction $\leq 35\%$) and who are in NYHA class III or IV and have a QRS duration of >120 ms.
- *Implantable cardiac defibrillator* – this is an important part of management of CHF.

The Scottish Intercollegiate Guidelines Network (SIGN) national clinical guideline 95 on the management of chronic heart failure is available at http://www.sign.ac.uk/pdf/sign95.pdf (accessed 25 May 2013).

Dental aspects

For patients with poorly controlled or uncontrolled cardiac failure (worsening dyspnoea with minimal exertion, dyspnoea at rest or nocturnal angina), medical attention should be obtained before any dental treatment. Elective dental treatment should be delayed until the condition has been stabilized medically. Emergency dental care should be conservative, principally with analgesics and antibiotics.

Routine dental care can usually be provided with little modification for patients with mild controlled cardiac failure. Appointments for patients with cardiac failure should be short and in the late morning. Endogenous adrenaline (epinephrine) levels peak during the morning hours and cardiac complications are most likely in the early morning.

The dental chair should be kept in a partially reclining or erect position. It is dangerous to lay any patient with left-sided heart failure supine, as this may severely worsen dyspnoea.

Pain and anxiety may precipitate arrhythmias, angina or heart failure, and thus effective analgesia must be provided. Lidocaine or prilocaine can be used but bupivacaine should be avoided, as it is cardiotoxic. An aspirating syringe should be used to give the LA. Adrenaline (epinephrine) may theoretically increase hypertension and precipitate arrhythmias. BP tends to rise during oral surgery under LA, and adrenaline can theoretically contribute, but this is usually of little practical importance. Adrenaline-containing LA should not be given in large doses to patients taking beta-blockers. Interactions between adrenaline and the beta-blocker may induce hypertension if excessive doses of the LA are given. Gingival retraction cords containing adrenaline should be avoided. Cardiac monitoring is desirable and supplemental oxygen should be readily available.

Conscious sedation can usually be used safely. However, consideration must be given to the underlying cause of the cardiac failure (see Table 5.34). GA is contraindicated in cardiac failure until it is under control. Care should be taken after GA since there is a predisposition to venous thrombosis and pulmonary embolism.

Some drugs used in HF may complicate dental treatment (Table 5.35).

ARTERIAL DISSECTION

General aspects

Arterial dissection is an abnormal, usually abrupt, formation of a tear along the inside wall of an artery. Aortic aneurysm (AA) is a ballooning or dilatation of the aorta; in the chest, it is called a thoracic AA, in the abdomen an abdominal AA (AAA), and across both areas a thoracoabdominal AA.

Risk factors for aortic aneurysm include:

- male gender
- advancing age
- smoking
- family history of aortic aneurysm

Table 5.35 *Cardiac failure treatment drugs in oral health care*

Medical drugs	Oral complications/complications that may disturb dental care	Dentistry drugs to be used with caution	Possible complications
ACE inhibitors (ACEIs)	Coughing	Itraconazole	Can aggravate cardiac failure
	Erythema multiforme, angioedema, burning mouth	NSAIDs other than aspirin	Increases the risk of renal damage from ACEI
Digitalis	ECG changes (e.g. ST-segment depression during dental extractions)	Erythromycin Tetracycline	May induce digitalis toxicity by impairing its gut flora metabolism
	Vomiting		
Diuretics	Orthostatic hypotension	Carbamazepine	Hyponatraemia

- hypertension
- high cholesterol
- atherosclerosis
- Marfan syndrome and similar inherited conditions
- infection
- trauma.

Clinical features

Aortic dissection occurs when the lining of the aorta tears and this can lead to aneurysm formation. The most common symptom is pain; thoracic AA causes chest or upper back pain, while AAA results in pain in the abdomen or lower back that may radiate to buttocks, groin or legs.

General management

AA can be diagnosed by ultrasound and CT. When it reaches a certain size or interferes with surrounding blood vessels or organs, surgical repair or placement of an aortic stent may be necessary. AA prevention is by smoking cessation and control of BP and cholesterol.

Carotid or vertebral artery dissection is uncommon but the arteries can be damaged by neck injuries or forceful neck movements. Spontaneous dissection of the carotid and vertebral arteries may arise in Marfan or Ehlers–Danlos syndromes, osteogenesis imperfecta or polycystic kidney disease, and is an uncommon cause of stroke. Features may include:

- pain on one or both sides of the face, head or neck
- eye pain or one unusually small pupil (unilateral Horner syndrome)
- ptosis or diplopia
- vertigo, tinnitus
- facial paralysis.

Dental aspects may also include changes in or loss of taste.

SURGERY

VASCULAR SURGERY

Bypass grafts to the aorta and lower limb vasculature (femoropopliteal bypass) are often made of synthetic materials. They remain non-endothelialized and are liable to infection, typically with *Staphylococcus epidermidis*. There is no evidence for odontogenic infection of such grafts, nor any good evidence that antimicrobial prophylaxis should be given for dental procedures.

MRI is contraindicated where ferromagnetic vascular clips have been placed.

Patients undergoing vascular surgery have a high incidence of periodontal disease.

CARDIAC SURGERY

Cardiac (heart) surgery can:

- replace occluded coronary arteries
- repair or replace heart valves
- repair abnormal or damaged structures
- use implant devices to help control the heart beat or support function and blood flow
- replace a damaged heart.

The most common cardiac surgery for adults is coronary artery bypass grafting (CABG), in which a healthy artery or vein from outside the heart is grafted to a blocked coronary artery.

Car drivers should avoid driving for 1 week after PTCA or pacemaker insertion, and for 1 month after MI or CABG, or when they have unstable angina. Patients with implantable defibrillators usually lose their driving licence but may regain it if they are shock-free for at least 6 months.

OPEN HEART SURGERY

Traditional heart surgery, called *open-heart surgery*, is done by splitting the sternum to open the chest wall for access to the heart. Often, the patient is connected to a heart–lung bypass machine to allow the surgeon to operate on a non-beating heart that has no blood flowing through it. In *off-pump, or beating heart, surgery* such as is carried out in CABG, however, a heart–lung bypass machine is not used.

PERCUTANEOUS TRANSLUMINAL CORONARY ANGIOPLASTY (PTCA)

This aims to open up the coronary blood flow by inserting a balloon-tipped catheter through the groin and up via the femoral artery and aorta into the area of arterial blockage. However, 40–50% of coronary arteries block again within 6 months, though this may be partially prevented with clopidogrel, aspirin or other antiplatelet drugs. PTCA has a lower morbidity than coronary bypass. Stents (miniature wire coils) may be inserted at the time of angioplasty to keep the arteries open, but renarrowing (restenosis) follows in about 25% of patients. Stents coated with the immunosuppressive drug sirolimus reduce this restenosis. Minute amounts of beta-radiation in vascular brachytherapy (intravascular brachytherapy or endovascular brachytherapy) can inhibit or reduce restenosis.

CORONARY ARTERY BYPASS GRAFTING (CABG)

Coronary artery bypass grafts are vascular grafts made to bridge the obstructions in the coronary blood vessels. Saphenous veins (from the leg) are placed, accessing the heart by full sternotomy. Minimally invasive CABG uses arteries such as the internal mammary artery without the need for full sternotomy. CABG results in a 5-year survival of over 85% and a 10-year survival of around 70%. Goals may include:

- improving quality of life and reducing angina and other CHD symptoms
- allowing a more active lifestyle
- improving the heart pumping action
- lowering the risk of a heart attack
- improving survival.

CABG usually improves or completely relieves angina for as long as 10–15 years and may also reduce the risk of having a heart attack.

MINIMALLY INVASIVE HEART SURGERY

Minimally invasive heart surgery is also known as limited access coronary artery surgery and includes port-access coronary artery bypass (PACAB or PortCAB) and minimally invasive coronary artery bypass graft (MIDCAB). It is an alternative to standard bypass surgery (CABG). Access to the heart is gained via small incisions ('ports') between the ribs; the sternum is not opened. The surgeon views these operations on video monitors rather than directly. In PACAB, the heart is stopped and blood is pumped through an oxygenator or heart–lung machine; MIDCAB is used to avoid the use of a heart–lung machine.

CARDIAC CATHETERIZATION

In this procedure, radio-opaque dye is injected into blood vessels via a catheter; angiography is then used to examine the inside of the cardiac blood vessels.

ANGIOPLASTY

Angioplasty is done because it can:

- increase blood flow through the blocked artery
- decrease angina
- increase ability for physical activity
- reduce the risk of a heart attack
- open neck arteries to help prevent stroke (carotid endarterectomy).

Also known as percutaneous coronary intervention (PCI), balloon angioplasty and coronary artery balloon dilation, angioplasty involves threading special tubing with an attached deflated balloon up from the groin to the coronary arteries. The balloon is inflated to widen blocked areas, where blood flow to the heart muscle has been reduced. This procedure is often followed by insertion of a small wire mesh tube (a stent) in the coronary artery to keep it open and to decrease the chance of another blockage.

A coronary artery stent physically opens the lumen of an artery during and after angioplasty. The stent is collapsed to a small diameter and placed over a balloon catheter for insertion. The stent is then moved into the area of blockage through the artery. When the balloon is inflated, the stent expands and locks into place, forming a scaffold that endothelializes and holds the newly dilated artery open. The stent stays in the artery permanently and improves blood flow. However, stent-mediated arterial injury causes neointimal hyperplasia, leading to restenosis and the need for repeat revascularization in up to one-third of patients. Therefore, drug-eluting stents with controlled local release of antiproliferative agents were developed; they have reduced the risk of repeat revascularization, although their long-term safety has been questioned. Current recommendations are to extend dual antiplatelet therapy (see below) for at least 12 months after stent implantation. Stents are made of stainless steel, cobalt–chrome or platinum–chrome, and coated with a polymer; they are able to release sirolimus, everolimus or zotarolimus. Restenosis is now very uncommon.

Patients with stents in place receive dual antiplatelet/antithrombotic medications consisting of aspirin and a platelet receptor (P2Y12) inhibitor to reduce the risk of ischaemic events and to decrease the chances of restenosis. When these patients are being treated for other medical or dental problems, concerns include the effects of possible bacteraemia on recently stented vessels, the risk of post-treatment bleeding and the possibility of interactions with drugs.

Considered less invasive than some other techniques because the body is not cut open, angioplasty takes 30 minutes to several hours to perform. Laser angioplasty catheter has a laser tip that opens the blocked artery; pulsating beams of light vaporize the plaque build-up. In atherectomy, the catheter has a rotating shaver on its tip to cut away plaque from the artery. After angioplasty, patients are usually given aspirin on a permanent basis, as well as clopidogrel, prasugrel or ticagrelor for 1–12 months.

Perioperative antithrombotic management is based on risk assessment for thromboembolism and bleeding. Dental anaesthetics with standard concentrations of adrenaline (epinephrine) seem to alter heart rate and BP, although no cardiac ischaemic alterations or any other cardiovascular complications are observed.

The AHA provides an educational module on stent insertion at http://watchlearnlive.heart.org/CVML_Player.php?moduleSelect=cstent (accessed 25 May 2013).

TRANSMYOCARDIAL REVASCULARIZATION (TMR)

This procedure may be used to relieve severe angina in very ill patients who are not candidates for bypass surgery or angioplasty. TMR involves an incision on the left breast to expose the heart. A laser is then used to drill a series of holes from the outside of the heart into the interior. In some patients, TMR is combined with bypass surgery, in which case an incision through the breastbone is used for the bypass.

CARDIAC VALVE SURGERY

Heart valve defects may be corrected by valvotomy, grafts or prosthetic valves.

Dental aspects of cardiac surgery

Dental management of patients on anticoagulants or antiplatelets is summarized in Table 5.36.

Post-angioplasty

Elective dental care should be deferred for 6 months; emergency dental care should be given in a hospital setting.

Table 5.36 *Dental management of patients on anticoagulants or antiplatelets*

Patient status	Antithrombotic management
At low risk for thromboembolism	Do not give bridging anticoagulation
Requiring vitamin K antagonist (VKA) interruption before surgery	Stop VKA 5 days before surgery
At high risk for thromboembolism and having a mechanical heart valve, atrial fibrillation or venous thromboembolism	Give bridging anticoagulation
At moderate to high risk for thromboembolism and receiving acetylsalicylic acid (ASA)	Continue ASA perioperatively
Requiring a dental procedure	Continue VKA with an oral prohaemostatic agent
Requiring surgery and having a coronary stent	Defer surgery for >6 weeks after bare-metal stent placement and >6 months after drug-eluting stent placement
Requiring surgery within 6 weeks of bare-metal stent placement or within 6 months of drug-eluting stent placement	Continue antiplatelet therapy perioperatively

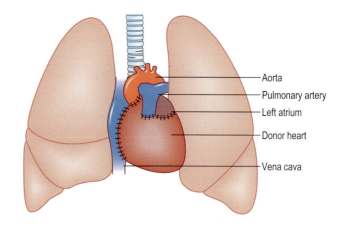

Fig. 5.14 Heart transplantation.

Table 5.37 *Average survival of patients after cardiac transplant*

At year	1	3	5
% survival	>80	>75	>70

Patients with coronary artery bypass graft

These patients should not receive an adrenaline (epinephrine)-containing LA, since it may possibly precipitate arrhythmias. For the first couple of weeks after surgery, the patient may feel severe pain when reclining in the dental chair as a side-effect of the surgery.

Patients with vascular stents that are successfully engrafted

The main points have been discussed earlier. It may be prudent to provide antibiotic coverage if emergency dental treatment is required during the first 6 weeks after the operation. Elective dental care should be deferred. Patients may require long-term anticoagulant medication. Appropriate action is required to deal with any bleeding tendencies (Ch. 8), but most patients are on aspirin or clopidogrel rather than warfarin.

Cardiac valve surgery

Patients scheduled for cardiac surgery should ideally have excellent oral health established before operation. Generally speaking, teeth with a poor pulpal or periodontal prognosis are best removed, particularly before a valve replacement, major surgery for congenital anomalies or a heart transplant. Teeth with no more than shallow caries and periodontal pocketing should be conserved.

Elective dental care should be avoided for the first 6 months after cardiac surgery. Some patients are on anticoagulant treatment, immunosuppressives or other drugs, or may also have a residual lesion. Prosthetic valves are particularly susceptible to IE and in that case there is a high mortality rate. Endocarditis within the first 6 months is usually caused by *Staphylococcus aureus*, is rarely of dental origin and has a mortality rate of around 60%.

CARDIAC (HEART) TRANSPLANTATION

General aspects

Heart transplantation is increasingly used to treat patients with otherwise uncontrollable cardiac failure, especially cardiomyopathy, CHD, CAD, heart valve disease and life-threatening arrhythmias.

The procedure uses a heart that has usually come from a brain-dead organ donor (*allograft*). The recipient patient's own heart may be either removed (*orthotopic procedure*) or, less commonly, left *in situ* to support the donor heart (*heterotopic procedure*; Fig. 5.14). Survival after cardiac transplantation is improving (Table 5.37) and some patients have lived for around 30 years. Heart–lung transplantation is also increasingly performed. Outcomes using a heart from another species (*xenograft*) or an *artificial heart* have been less successful.

All transplant recipients require lifelong immunosuppression to prevent a T-cell, alloimmune rejection response, usually with ciclosporin, mycophenolate or azathioprine, corticosteroids and antithymocyte globulin, or tacrolimus.

Patients may be anticoagulated or taking aspirin and dipyridamole to reduce platelet adhesion and prolong the bleeding time. They are often given a statin to minimize the risk of atheroma in the transplanted heart.

Since the vagus nerve is severed during the transplant operation, the donated heart will beat at around 100 beats/min until nerve regrowth occurs. There is evidence of increased cardiac sensitivity to catecholamines such as adrenaline (epinephrine). Owing to the absence of innervation, angina is rare and patients may experience 'silent' MI or sudden death.

Dental aspects

The following points should be noted, in addition to those discussed in Chapter 35. Immunosuppressive therapy can lead to liability to infections and to a bleeding tendency.

A meticulous pre-surgery oral assessment is required and dental treatment should be undertaken with particular attention to establishing optimal oral hygiene and eradicating sources of potential infection. Dental treatment should be completed before surgery.

For 6 months after surgery, elective dental care is best deferred. If dental surgical treatment is needed during the 6 months that follow the heart surgery, or until the ECG is normal, antibiotic prophylaxis against endocarditis (see 'Infective endocarditis' above) may be requested by the surgeons.

It has been suggested that heart transplant patients cannot show any vasovagal reaction because the donor heart is completely deprived of any vagal or sympathetic innervation. However, episodes of vasovagal syncope in heart transplant patients undergoing periodontal surgery have been reported.

LA without adrenaline (epinephrine) is indicated.

KEY WEBSITES

(Accessed 25 May 2013)

BMJ. <http://www.bmj.com/specialties/cardiovascular-medicine>.
British Heart Foundation. <http://www.bhf.org.uk/heart-health/conditions/cardiovascular-disease.aspx>.
Centers for Disease Control and Prevention. <http://www.cdc.gov/heartdisease/>.
National Institutes of Health. <http://health.nih.gov/topic/HeartDiseasesGeneral/>.

USEFUL WEBSITES

(Accessed 25 May 2013)

American Heart Association. <http://www.heart.org/HEARTORG/>.
American Society of Hypertension. <http://www.ash-us.org>.
Heart Health Center. <http://heartdisease.about.com/cs/valvulardisease/>.
Medscape Reference. Infective endocarditis. <http://emedicine.medscape.com/article/216650-overview>.
National Institute for Health and Care Excellence. Prophylaxis against infective endocarditis (CG64). <http://www.nice.org.uk/CG064>.

REFERENCES AND FURTHER READING

Academy report. Periodontal management of patients with cardiovascular diseases. J Periodontol 2002; 73:954.

Ahmed, M.F., Elseed, A.I., 2005. The medical management and dental implications of long QT syndrome. Dent. Update 32 (8), 472.

Auluck, A., Manohar, C., 2006. Haematological considerations in patients with cyanotic congenital heart disease. Dent. Update 33, 617.

Bader, J.D., et al., 2002. Cardiovascular effects of epinephrine on hypertensive dental patients. Agency for Healthcare Research and Quality Evidence Report 48.

Baddour, L.M., et al., 2011. A summary of the update on cardiovascular implantable electronic device infections and their management: a scientific statement from the American Heart Association. J. Am. Dent. Assoc. 142 (2), 159.

Bajorek, B.V., et al., 2005. Optimizing the use of antithrombic therapy for atrial fibrillation in older people: a pharmacist-led multidisciplinary intervention. J. Am. Geriatr. Soc. 53, 1912.

Becker, R.C., et al., 2008. The primary and secondary prevention of coronary artery disease: American College of Chest Physicians evidence-based clinical practice guidelines, 8th edn. Chest 133 (Suppl. 6), 776S.

Beirne, O.R., 2005. Evidence to continue oral anticoagulant therapy for ambulatory oral surgery. J. Oral Maxillofac. Surg. 63, 540.

Carmona, I.T., et al., 2002. An update on the controversies in bacterial endocarditis of oral origin. Oral Surg. Oral Med. Oral Pathol. Oral Radiol. Endod. 93, 660.

Carmona, I.T., et al., 2007. Efficacy of antibiotic prophylactic regimens for the prevention of bacterial endocarditis of oral origin. J. Dent. Res. 86, 1142.

D'Aiuto, F., et al., 2007. Acute effects of periodontal therapy on bio-markers of vascular health. J. Clin. Periodontol. 34, 124.

Douketis, J.D., et al., 2012. Perioperative management of antithrombotic therapy: antithrombotic therapy and prevention of thrombosis, 9th edn: American College of Chest Physicians Evidence-based clinical practice guidelines. Chest 141 (Suppl. 2), e326S.

Friedlander, A.H., et al., 2009. Atrial fibrillation: pathogenesis, medical–surgical management and dental implications. J. Am. Dent. Assoc. 140, 167.

Fuster, V., et al., 2006. Guidelines for the management of patients with atrial fibrillation: a report of the American College of Cardiology/American Heart Association Task Force on Practice Guidelines and the European Society of Cardiology Committee for Practice Guidelines (Writing Committee to Revise the 2001 Guidelines for the Management of Patients With Atrial Fibrillation): developed in collaboration with the European Heart Rhythm Association and the Heart Rhythm Society. Circulation 114, e257.

Gibson, R.M., Meechan, J.G., 2007. The effects of antihypertensive medication on dental treatment. Dent. Update 34, 70.

Goldstein, L.B., et al., 2006. Primary prevention of ischemic stroke: a guideline from the American Heart Association/American Stroke Association Stroke Council: cosponsored by the Atherosclerotic Peripheral Vascular Disease Interdisciplinary Working Group; Cardiovascular Nursing Council; Clinical Cardiology Council; Nutrition, Physical Activity, and Metabolism Council; and the Quality of Care and Outcomes Research Interdisciplinary Working Group. Circulation 113, e873. [erratum in Circulation 2006; 114:e617]

Gould, F.K., et al., 2006. Guidelines for the prevention of endocarditis: report of the Working Party of the British Society for Antimicrobial Chemotherapy. J. Antimicrob. Chemother. 58, 896.

Holmstrup, P., et al., 2003. Oral infections and systemic diseases. Dent. Clin. North Am. 47, 575.

James, P.A., et al., 2013. 2014 Evidence-Based Guideline for the Management of High Blood Pressure in Adults: Report from the Panel Members Appointed to the Eighth Joint National Committee (JNC 8). JAMA doi: 10.1001/jama.2013.284427 [Epub ahead of print] PubMed PMID: 24352797.

Karp, J.M., Moss, A.J., 2006. Dental treatment of patients with long QT syndrome. J. Am. Dent. Assoc. 137 (5), 630.

Kistler, P.M., 2007. Management of atrial fibrillation. Aust. Fam. Physician 36, 506.

Lessard, E., et al., 2005. The patient with a heart murmur: evaluation, assessment and dental considerations. J. Am. Dent. Assoc. 136, 347.

Lip, G.Y., Tse, H.F., 2007. Management of atrial fibrillation. Lancet 370, 604.

Lund, J.P., et al., 2002. Oral surgical management of patients with mechanical circulatory support. Int. J. Oral Maxillofac. Surg. 31, 629.

Mahmood, M., et al., 2007. Potential drug–drug interactions within Veterans Affairs medical centers. Am. J. Health Syst. Pharm. 64, 1500.

McDonagh, T.A., et al., 2011. European Society of Cardiology Heart Failure Association Standards for delivering heart failure care. Eur. J. Heart Fail 13 (3), 235. doi: 10.1093/eurjhf/hfq221. Epub 2010 Dec 15. PubMed PMID: 21159794

Mead, G.E., et al., 2005. Electrical cardioversion for atrial fibrillation and flutter. Cochrane Database Syst. Rev. 3 CD002903.

National Collaborating Centre for Chronic Conditions, 2006. Atrial Fibrillation: National Clinical Guideline for Management in Primary and Secondary Care. Royal College of Physicians, London.

Oliver, R., et al., 2004. Penicillins for the prophylaxis of bacterial endocarditis in dentistry. Cochrane Database Syst. Rev. 2 CD003813.

Pérez-Gómez, F., et al., 2007. Antithrombotic therapy in elderly patients with atrial fibrillation: effects and bleeding complications: a stratified analysis of the NASPEAF randomized trial. Eur. Heart J. 28, 996.

Pinski, S.L., Trohman, R.G., 2002. Interference in implanted cardiac devices. J. Pacing Clin. Electrophysiol. 25 (9) 1367, 1496.

Rhodus, N.L., Falace, D.A., 2002. Management of the dental patient with congestive heart failure. Gen. Dent. 50 (3), 260. quiz 266.

Roberts, G.J., 2004. New recommendations on antibiotic prophylaxis of infective endocarditis. Ann. R. Coll. Surg. Engl. (Suppl.) 86, 163.

Roberts, H.W., Mitnisky, E.F., 2001. Cardiac risk stratification for postmyocardial infarction in dental patients. Oral Surg. 91, 676.

Rochford, C., Seldin, R.D., 2009. Review and management of the dental patient with long QT syndrome (LQTS). Anesth. Prog. 56, 42.

Rustemeyer, J., Bremerich, A., 2007. Necessity of surgical dental foci treatment prior to organ transplantation and heart valve replacement. Clin. Oral Invest. 11, 171.

Saffitz, J.E., 2006. Connexins, conduction, and atrial fibrillation. N. Engl. J. Med. 354, 2712.

Saxena, R., Koudstaal, P.J., 2004. Anticoagulants versus antiplatelet therapy for preventing stroke in patients with nonrheumatic atrial fibrillation and a history of stroke or transient ischemic attack. Cochrane Database Syst. Rev. 4 CD000187

Schauer, D.P., et al., 2005. Psychosocial risk factors for adverse outcomes in patients with nonvalvular atrial fibrillation receiving warfarin. J. Gen. Intern. Med. 20, 1114.

Scully, C., Chaudhry, S., 2006a. Aspects of human disease 1. Atheroma and coronary artery (ischaemic heart) disease. Dent. Update 33, 251.

Scully, C., Chaudhry, S., 2006b. Aspects of human disease 2. Angina pectoris. Dent. Update 33, 317.

Scully, C., Chaudhry, S., 2006c. Aspects of human disease 3. Myocardial infarction. Dent. Update 33, 381.

Scully, C., Chaudhry, S., 2006d. Aspects of human disease 4. Hypertension. Dent. Update 33, 443.

Scully, C., Chaudhry, S., 2006e. Aspects of human disease 5. Infective endocarditis. Dent. Update 33, 509.

Scully, C., Chaudhry, S., 2006f. Aspects of human disease 6. Congenital heart disease. Dent. Update 33, 573.

Scully, C., Ettinger, R., 2007. The influence of systemic diseases on oral health care in older adults. JADA 138 (Suppl.), 7S.

Scully, C., Wolff, A., 2002. Oral surgery in patients on anticoagulant therapy. Oral Surg. Oral Med. Oral Pathol. Oral Radiol. Endod. 94, 57.

Scully, C., et al., 2001. The mouth in heart disease. Practitioner 245, 432.

Scully, C., et al., 2007. Special Care in Dentistry: Handbook of Oral Healthcare. Churchill Livingstone, Edinburgh.

Seymour, R.A., Whitworth, J.M., 2002. Antibiotic prophylaxis for endocarditis, prosthetic joints, and surgery. Dent. Clin. North Am. 46, 635.

Snow, V., et al., 2003. Management of newly detected atrial fibrillation: a clinical practice guideline from the American Academy of Family Physicians and the American College of Physicians. Ann. Intern. Med. 139, 1009.

Stecksén-Blicks, C., et al., 2004. Dental caries experience in children with congenital heart disease: a case-control study. Int. J. Paediatr. Dent. 14, 94.

Stefanini, G.G., Holmes, D.R., 2013. Drug-eluting coronary-artery stents. N. Engl. J. Med. 368, 254.10.1056/NEJMra1210816

Stevenson, H., et al., 2006. The statins: drug interactions of significance to the dental practitioner. Dent. Update 33, 14.

Stroke Risk in Atrial Fibrillation Working Group, 2007. Independent predictors of stroke in patients with atrial fibrillation: a systematic review. Neurology 69, 546.

Tempe, D.K., Virmani, S., 2002. Coagulation abnormality in patients with cyanotic congenital heart disease. J. Cardiothorac. Vasc. Anaesth. 16, 752.

Tomás Carmona, I., et al., 2007. A clorhexidine mouthwash reduces the risk of post-extraction bacteraemia. Infect. Control Hosp. Epidemiol. 28, 577.

Wilson, W., et al., 2007. Prevention of infective endocarditis: guidelines from the American Heart Association. J. Am. Dent. Assoc. 138 (739), 747.

APPENDIX 5.1 GENETIC SYNDROMES WITH ASSOCIATED CARDIAC DEFECTS

Names of disorder	Further information
Chromosomal disorders	
Down	Ch. 28
Edwards	Ch. 28
Patau	Ch. 28
Turner (XXY)	Ch. 28
XXXY	Learning disability, hypogonadism
XXXXX	Learning disability, small hands
Hereditary disorders	
Ehlers–Danlos	Ch. 16
Marfan	Ch. 16
Osteogenesis imperfecta	Ch. 16
The mucopolysaccharidoses (Hurler and related syndromes)	Ch. 23
Ellis–van Creveld	Ch. 37
TAR	Thrombocytopenia, absent radius
Holt–Oram	Hypoplastic clavicles, upper limb defect
Multiple lentigines	Basal cell naevi, rib defects
Rubenstein–Taybi	Broad thumbs and toes, hypoplastic maxilla

APPENDIX 5.2 MAIN CONGENITAL HEART DEFECTS THAT MAY BE ASSOCIATED WITH VARIOUS EPONYMOUS SYNDROMES

Syndrome	Defects
Down	Atrioventricular defect and also patent ductus arteriosus and Fallot tetralogy
Ehlers–Danlos	Mitral valve prolapse
Friedreich	Hypertrophic cardiomyopathy
Holt–Oram	Atrial septal defect, ventricular septal defect
Klinefelter	Atrial septal defect
Marfan	Mitral valve prolapse, aortic regurgitation
Noonan	Pulmonary stenosis, sometimes Fallot tetralogy
Turner	Coarctation, aortic stenosis
Williams	Supravalvular aortic stenosis

APPENDIX 5.3 VAUGHAN–WILLIAMS CLASSIFICATION OF ANTI-ARRHYTHMIC AGENTS

Mechanism	Class	Examples	Main uses
Membrane stabilizers (sodium-channel blockers)	Ia	Disopyramide	Ventricular arrhythmias
		Procainamide	Wolff–Parkinson–White syndrome
		Quinidine	
	Ib	Lidocaine	Ventricular tachycardia
		Phenytoin	Atrial fibrillation
	Ic	Flecainide	Paroxysmal atrial fibrillation
		Propafenone	
Beta-blockers	II	Atenolol	Tachyarrhythmias
		Metoprolol	
		Propranolol	
		Sotalol	
		Timolol	
Unknown	III	Amiodarone	Atrial fibrillation
		Dofetilide	Ventricular tachycardias
		Nibentan	Wolff–Parkinson–White syndrome
		Sotalol	
Calcium-channel blockers	IV	Diltiazem	Paroxysmal supraventricular tachycardia
		Verapamil	Atrial fibrillation

APPENDIX 5.4 DRUGS TO AVOID IN LONG QT SYNDROME (MAY PROLONG THE QT INTERVAL AND INDUCE TORSADES DE POINTES)

- Amiodarone
- Arsenic trioxide
- Astemizole
- Azithromycin
- Bepridil
- Chloroquine
- Chlorpromazine
- Cisapride
- Citalopram
- Clarithromycin
- Disopyramide
- Dofetilide
- Domperidone
- Droperidol
- Erythromycin
- Flecainide
- Halofantrine
- Haloperidol
- Ibutilide
- Levacetylmethadol (levomethadyl)
- Mesoridazine
- Methadone
- Moxifloxacin
- Pentamidine
- Pimozide
- Probucol
- Procainamide
- Quinidine
- Sotalol
- Sparfloxacin
- Terfenadine
- Thioridazine
- Vandetanib

Drugs that may prolong QT

- Alfuzosin
- Amantadine
- Dihydroartemisinin (artenimol) + piperaquine
- Atazanavir
- Chloral hydrate
- Clozapine
- Dolasetron
- Dronedarone
- Eribulin
- Escitalopram
- Famotidine
- Felbamate
- Fingolimod
- Foscarnet
- Fosphenytoin
- Gatifloxacin
- Gemifloxacin
- Granisetron
- Iloperidone
- Indapamide
- Isradipine
- Lapatinib
- Levofloxacin
- Lithium
- Moexipril/hydrochlorothiazide (HCTZ)
- Nicardipine
- Nilotinib
- Octreotide
- Ofloxacin
- Ondansetron
- Oxytocin

(Continued)

- Paliperidone
- Perflutren lipid microspheres
- Quetiapine
- Ranolazine
- Risperidone
- Roxithromycin
- Sertindole
- Sunitinib
- Tacrolimus
- Tamoxifen
- Telithromycin
- Tizanidine
- Vardenafil
- Venlafaxine
- Voriconazole
- Ziprasidone

Others drugs that may affect the ECG

- Amisulpride
- Amitriptyline
- Ciprofloxacin
- Clomipramine
- Desipramine
- Diphenhydramine
- Doxepin
- Fluconazole
- Fluoxetine
- Galantamine
- Imipramine
- Itraconazole
- Ketoconazole
- Nortriptyline
- Paroxetine
- Protriptyline
- Ritonavir
- Sertraline
- Solifenacin
- Trazodone
- Trimethoprim/sulfamethoxazole (co-trimoxazole)
- Trimipramine

Drugs to avoid in congenital long QT syndrome

- Adrenaline (epinephrine)
- Albuterol
- Alfuzosin
- Amantadine
- Amiodarone
- Amisulpride
- Amitriptyline
- Amphetamine
- Arsenic trioxide
- Dihydroartemisinin (artenimol) + piperaquine
- Astemizole
- Atazanavir
- Atomoxetine
- Azithromycin
- Bepridil
- Chloral hydrate
- Chloroquine
- Chlorpromazine
- Ciprofloxacin
- Cisapride

- Citalopram
- Clarithromycin
- Clomipramine
- Clozapine
- Cocaine
- Desipramine
- Dexmethylphenidate
- Diphenhydramine
- Disopyramide
- Dobutamine
- Dofetilide
- Dolasetron
- Domperidone
- Dopamine
- Doxepin
- Dronedarone
- Droperidol
- Ephedrine
- Eribulin
- Erythromycin
- Escitalopram
- Famotidine
- Felbamate
- Fenfluramine
- Fingolimod
- Flecainide
- Fluconazole
- Fluoxetine
- Foscarnet
- Fosphenytoin
- Galantamine
- Gatifloxacin
- Gemifloxacin
- Granisetron
- Halofantrine
- Haloperidol
- Ibutilide
- Iloperidone
- Imipramine
- Indapamide
- Isoproterenol
- Isradipine
- Itraconazole
- Ketoconazole
- Lapatinib
- Levofloxacin
- Levacetylmethadol (levomethadyl)
- Levosalbutamol (levalbuterol)
- Lisdexamfetamine
- Lithium
- Mesoridazine
- Methadone
- Methylphenidate
- Midodrine
- Moexipril/HCTZ
- Moxifloxacin
- Nicardipine
- Nilotinib
- Noradrenaline (norepinephrine)
- Nortriptyline
- Octreotide

(Continued)

- Ofloxacin
- Olanzapine
- Ondansetron
- Orciprenaline (metaproterenol)
- Oxytocin
- Paliperidone
- Paroxetine
- Pentamidine
- Perflutren lipid microspheres
- Phentermine
- Phenylephrine
- Phenylpropanolamine
- Pimozide
- Probucol
- Procainamide
- Protriptyline
- Pseudoephedrine
- Quetiapine
- Quinidine
- Ranolazine
- Risperidone
- Ritodrine
- Ritonavir
- Roxithromycin[*]
- Salmeterol

- Sertindole
- Sertraline
- Sibutramine
- Solifenacin
- Sotalol
- Sparfloxacin
- Sunitinib
- Tacrolimus
- Tamoxifen
- Telithromycin
- Terbutaline
- Terfenadine
- Thioridazine
- Tizanidine
- Tolterodine
- Trazodone
- Trimethoprim/sulfamethoxazole (co-trimoxazole)
- Trimipramine
- Vandetanib
- Vardenafil
- Venlafaxine
- Voriconazole
- Ziprasidone

[*]More information is available at http://www.crediblemeds.org (accessed 30 September 2013).

APPENDIX 5.5 MODIFICATION OF CLINICAL PROCEDURES IN PATIENTS WITH CEIDS

INVESTIGATIONS AND PROCEDURES

MRI

Avoid MRI scanning in patients with pacemakers. Concerns about exposure of AICDs to MRI are similar to pacemakers – with the additional risk of interpreting noise as ventricular arrhythmias and the consequent delivery of shocks and/or rapid ventricular pacing.

Radiotherapy

There is little risk as long as the irradiation field avoids pacemakers. Although the effect of radiation on the newest AICDs is variable, the AICD may inappropriately deliver anti-tachycardia therapy if tachycardia monitoring and therapies are active during irradiation:

- Avoid the CEID location.
- Avoid the betatron.
- Evaluate device and pacemaker dependency prior to therapy.
- Plan radiotherapy to minimize the total dose (including scatter) received by the generator.
- Avoid direct irradiation.
- Maximize shielding and distance of the pulse generator from the radiation beam.
- Consider moving the pulse generator away from the field if the estimated dose is over 10 Gy.
- Institute an appropriate level of monitoring:
  - If the estimated dose is less than 2 Gy and the patient is not pacemaker-dependent, clinical monitoring suffices.

  - If the estimated dose is over 2 Gy or the patient is pacemaker-dependent, high-level monitoring is necessary.
- Ensure continuous ECG monitoring during treatments.
- Have staff competent in advanced cardiac life support nearby.
- Check device function after each therapy session and regularly for several weeks thereafter.

External cardioversion and defibrillation

The newer IRDs are better protected and thus more resistant to external cardioversion and defibrillation currents, but all devices are at risk of reversion to back-up mode, transient increase in capture threshold, loss of capture, destruction of the pulse generator and circuitry, and thermal damage to myocardial tissue in contact with the lead(s).

Electrocautery/electrosurgery

Radiofrequency currents may be interpreted by an IRD as an intracardiac signal, which can inhibit pacing, trigger ventricular pacing, switch mode in a pacemaker, and spuriously detect tachyarrhythmia in an AICD. Patients with pacemakers should have continual ECG monitoring during electrosurgery. The following additional precautions should be observed for children with pacemakers:

- Ensure the distance between the active electrode and the dispersive electrode is as short as possible.
- Keep all electrosurgery cables away from the pacemaker and its leads.
- Have a defibrillator immediately available for emergencies.
- Use a bipolar pacemaker where possible.
- Have a magnet or control unit available.

All patients with AICDs should have a defibrillator immediately available and the AICD device should be deactivated before the electrosurgery is initiated.

Lithotripsy

Extracorporeal shock wave lithotripsy can theoretically damage pacemakers and AICDs by emitting a shock wave. The lithotriptor should be placed at least 5 cm away from the IRD.

Transcutaneous electrical nerve stimulation (TENS)

TENS may be sensed by unipolar IRD systems. Although TENS is relatively safe for use with pacemakers, these patients should undergo monitored assessment during first-time use, and repeatedly if therapy is applied to different locations. TENS should be discouraged in patients with AICDs since there may be inappropriate shocks, and noise reversion may inhibit appropriate AICD shocks.

OTHER EQUIPMENT

Mobile (cellular) phones

The recommended distance between the operating phone and the pacemaker is 15 cm; alternatively, the contralateral ear should be used. Modern mobile phones have little effect on AICDs, but manufacturers recommend a 15-cm distance between active telephones and AICDs.

Personal digital assistants (PDAs)

PDAs fitted with wireless local area network technology may run electromagnetic interference (EMI) risks so the advised precautionary measure is to maintain a 15-cm safety margin between PDAs and IRDs.

Portable media players (e.g. iPods)

Despite the fact that portable media players appear to have no EMI effects on IRDs, manufacturers recommend that they should not be stowed in ipsilateral pockets, shoulder bags or arm carrier straps.

Security systems

Metal detectors may cause EMI but with PMs there is no atrial oversensing, inappropriate mode switching, ventricular oversensing, atrial or ventricular loss of capture, pacing in the magnet mode or spontaneous reprogramming. In AICD patients, ventricular oversensing does not result in inappropriate detection, spontaneous reprogramming or temporary suspension of therapies. Nevertheless, IRD casings may trigger alarms, so patients should forewarn security agents. Patients should be advised to carry their device identification card, to request alternate search methods if possible, and to walk through detectors at a normal pace, avoiding leaning or lingering within the field of the detector.

EMERGENCY PROCEDURES

(After http://www.ncbi.nlm.nih.gov/pmc/articles/PMC2001150/; accessed 30 September 2013)

- Ensure that cardiopulmonary resuscitation, temporary external/transvenous pacing, and external defibrillation equipment are readily available.
- Where the presence of a device is suspected but not confirmed, use normal radiographic procedures to identify any such devices. Note that:
  - Most devices are implanted in the anterior left pectoral region.

- Older implants may be implanted abdominally.
- X-ray identification symbols can be used to identify the manufacturer (consult a cardiac pacing clinic for the manufacturer).
- Obtain pacemaker/AICD details from the patient's device registration card/'passport', which holds the pertinent details. Where possible, obtain the following key information and alert the cardiology department for assistance:
  - Device manufacturer, model number, serial number
  - Implanting hospital, follow-up hospital
  - Reason for implant.
- Where possible, contact the cardiac pacing department to determine to what extent support may be required in pacemaker/AICD reprogramming. AICDs may need to be programmed to 'monitor only' mode to prevent inappropriate sensing and shock delivery. Securing a magnet over the AICD implant site may, in many cases, inhibit the delivery of shock therapy. However, this cannot always be guaranteed. Similarly, securing a magnet over the pacemaker implant site will not necessarily guarantee asynchronous (non-sensing) pacing. Magnet response may vary between manufacturers' models and according to particular programmed settings.
- If the AICD is deactivated, consider connecting the patient to an external defibrillator using remote pads, if access to the anterior chest wall will interfere with surgery or sterile field.
- Monitor the patient's ECG before the induction of anaesthesia.
- Since some ECG monitors (having a 'paced' mode) may misinterpret pacing spikes as the patient's QRS complexes and incorrectly display a heart rate (when the patient is in asystole), an alternative method of detecting a patient's pulse, such as a pulse oximeter or an arterial line, should be used.
- Monitoring systems that use thoracic impedance measurements can cause an increase in paced rate for pacemakers that use the minute ventilation system to determine the patient's exercise level. Where interaction is suspected, consider using a patient monitoring system that does not employ thoracic impedance measurements.
- On detection of any pacemaker inhibition or rate increase, inform the surgeon immediately and use diathermy either intermittently or not at all.
- Consider using an external pacemaker to overdrive and inhibit pacing from the implanted pacemaker (when necessary).
- Use monopolar diathermy/electrocautery as a last resort and:
  - use in short bursts
  - ensure that the return electrode is anatomically positioned so the current pathway is far away from the pacemaker/defibrillator (and leads)
  - keep diathermy/electrocautery cables well away from the site of implant
  - consider alternative external/transvenous pacing where pacing from the implant is significantly affected during the use of monopolar diathermy.
- On completion of surgery, or as soon as possible, contact the cardiac pacing clinic to request a pacemaker/AICD check to ensure the correct functioning of the device.

There are no scientific data to support the use of antimicrobial prophylaxis for dental or other invasive procedures in people with CIEDs.

APPENDIX 5.6 NON-HEALTH-CARE SOURCES OF ELECTROMAGNETIC INTERFERENCE (EMI) AFFECTING MODERN DEVICES, WITH THEIR SAFETY LEVELS

Safe	Used with caution	To be avoided
Personal care		
Electric razors	Do not place directly over IRD:	Electrolysis (hair removal)
Hair dryers	Hand-held massagers	
Tanning beds	Power toothbrushes	
Thermolysis (hair removal)		
Domestic items		
Air purifiers	Keep 15 cm away or in contralateral ear/pocket:	Hand-held body fat measuring scales
Blenders	Mobile phones	Magnetic mattresses and chairs
Clothes dryers	Cordless phones	
Convection ovens	Personal digital assistants (with mobile phone features)	
Electric blankets		
Electric ovens and stoves		
Electric can openers		
Gas ovens and stoves		
Heating pads		
Microwave ovens		
Pagers		
Patient-alert devices		
Personal digital assistants (without mobile phone features)		
Portable space heaters		
Radio-controlled clocks		
Vacuum cleaners		
Washing machines		
Watches		
Radio, TV, security, etc., equipment		
AM/FM radio	Keep 60 cm away:	
CD/DVD players	CB and police radio aerials	
Remote controls (TV, stereo, garage door, video equipment, cameras)	Keep 30 cm away:	
	Slot machines	
TV/video recorder	Stereo speakers	
Video games	Keep 15 cm away:	
	Bingo games	
	Magnetic wands	
	Do not linger near:	
	Electronic antitheft systems	
	High-voltage lines	
	Radio/TV towers	
	Residential power generators	
	Transformers	
	Walk through airport security systems at normal pace, tell security and show device ID card	
	Request alternative search method with security wands: should not be held over pacemaker for >2 s every 10 s, or over AICD for >2 s every 30 s	
Workplace		
Electric invisible fences	Keep 60 cm away:	Jackhammers
Fax machines	Arc welding equipment	Neodymium–iron–boron magnets
Personal computers	Running motors or alternators	
Photocopiers	Keep 30 cm away:	
	Battery-powered power tools	
	Chainsaws	
	Cordless drills	
	Lawn mowers	
	Leaf blowers	
	Power tools such as drills and saws	
	Snow blowers	
	Soldering guns	

(Continued)

Safe	Used with caution	To be avoided
Daily life		
Electronic article surveillance (EAS) devices (also known as antitheft devices or antishoplifting gates)	EAS devices are ubiquitous in retail stores and libraries. There are several major types of system:	
Improperly grounded appliances held in close contact with body	Magnetic, also known as magnetoharmonic	
	Acoustomagnetic, also known as magnetostrictive	
	Radiofrequency	
Metal detectors	Microwave	
Mobile phones	Video surveillance (to some extent)	
Slot machines	On interacting, the tag emits a signal that is detected by the receiver. All EAS systems emit electromagnetic energy and thus can interfere with electronics; there are reported instances where magnetic or acoustomagnetic EAS systems have caused a pacemaker to fail and a defibrillator to trigger	
Some home appliances (e.g. electric razor)		
Toy remote controls		
Industrial environment		
Degaussing coils	Arc or spot welders	
Electric motors	Industrial welding machines	
High-voltage power lines	Additional general precautions include ensuring appropriate grounding of equipment and avoiding close contact with EMI source	
Induction furnaces		
Transformers		
Welders		

APPENDIX 5.7 DO PATIENTS UNDERGOING DENTAL PROCEDURES REQUIRE ENDOCARDITIS PROPHYLAXIS?

(Reproduced with permission from UK Medicines Information (UKMi) pharmacists for NHS health-care professionals)

BACKGROUND

Infective endocarditis is an inflammation of the inner lining of the heart (endocardium), particularly affecting the heart valves and caused mainly by bacterial infection. Patients with structural abnormalities of the heart, hypertrophic cardiomyopathy, replacement heart valves or with a history of infective endocarditis are considered to be at risk of developing infective endocarditis.

Traditionally, prophylactic antibiotics have been given to patients at risk of infective endocarditis before undergoing dental procedures. Typically, three grams of oral amoxicillin would be taken one hour beforehand. The rationale for using antibiotics was that dental procedures lead to increased numbers of bacteria in the blood (bacteraemia) and it was assumed that bacteraemia was a key factor in the development of infective endocarditis.

In recent years, there have been conflicting guidelines as to which patients and dental procedures warranted the use of prophylactic antibiotics.[1,2,3] This led to confusion for health professionals and patients. The National Institute for Health and Care Excellence (NICE) has now issued definitive, evidence-based guidance on the prophylaxis of infective endocarditis.[4] This guidance has been adopted nationally and is reflected in the current British National Formulary, published March 2008.[5]

ANSWER

Antibiotic prophylaxis is not recommended for the prevention of infective endocarditis in adults or children undergoing any dental procedure.[4]

The basis for this recommendation is:

- *There is no consistent association between dental procedures and an increased risk of infective endocarditis;*
- *Bacteraemia associated with dental procedures is no greater than that from toothbrushing;*
- *Regular toothbrushing almost certainly presents a greater risk of infective endocarditis than a single dental procedure because of repetitive exposure to bacteraemia;*
- *Antibiotics are not proven to reduce the risk of infective endocarditis;*
- *Antibiotics are themselves not without risk and can cause fatal anaphylaxis.*

Patients who previously received endocarditis prophylaxis for dental procedures will require a clear explanation as to why prophylaxis is no longer recommended. A summary of the NICE guideline for patients[6] and a 'quick reference leaflet'[7] are available online. Printed copies can be ordered from NICE Publications via 0845 003 7783 (quote reference numbers N1488 and N1487 when ordering the patient summary and quick reference leaflet, respectively).

(Continued)

NICE states that healthcare professionals should offer clear and consistent advice to patients on four points, details of which are on page 2 of this document.

The NICE summary for patients[6] includes a list of questions that patients might ask their healthcare team; answers are suggested on page 3 of this document.

ADVICE FOR HEALTHCARE PROFESSIONALS TO OFFER TO PATIENTS

Patients at risk of infective endocarditis should be reassured that antibiotic prophylaxis is no longer recommended and offered information regarding:

The benefits and risks of antibiotic prophylaxis, and an explanation of why antibiotic prophylaxis is no longer recommended

Patients at risk of infective endocarditis have traditionally received prophylactic antibiotics prior to dental procedures. Procedures that disturb bacteria in the mouth increase the number of bacteria in the blood (bacteraemia). High levels of bacteraemia have been shown (in animal models) to increase the risk of infective endocarditis. On this basis, it was considered prudent to provide antibiotic prophylaxis to reduce bacteraemia in patients considered to be at risk of infective endocarditis. Over recent years, there have been conflicting guidelines as to which patients required antibiotic prophylaxis and for which dental procedures.

NICE has reviewed the evidence regarding infective endocarditis and concluded that there is no clear association between dental procedures and infective endocarditis. Evidence shows that levels of bacteraemia associated with dental procedures are no greater than those associated with regular toothbrushing. The risk of infective endocarditis is almost certainly greater from toothbrushing than from a single dental procedure due to repeated exposure to bacteraemia.

Antibiotic prophylaxis given before dental procedures has not been shown to eliminate bacteraemia or to reduce the risk of infective endocarditis and is associated with risks of its own. Antibiotics can cause adverse reactions including fatal anaphylaxis. Using antibiotics when not indicated puts patients at risk from adverse effects and can increase bacterial resistance to antibiotics. For all these reasons, antibiotic prophylaxis is no longer recommended for the prevention of infective endocarditis in patients undergoing dental procedures.

The importance of maintaining good oral health

Maintaining good oral health reduces the numbers of bacteria in the mouth and helps prevent tooth decay and gum disease. Patients should be advised to keep their mouth and teeth clean with twice-daily toothbrushing, to have regular dental check-ups and not to let any dental problems such as abscess or gum disease go untreated.

Symptoms that may indicate infective endocarditis and when to seek expert advice

Infective endocarditis is rare and patients are unlikely to develop it. Early symptoms of infective endocarditis are similar to flu symptoms: fever, night sweats and chills, weakness and tiredness, and also breathlessness, weight loss and joint pain. Patients at risk of infective endocarditis should be advised to see a GP if they have such symptoms for longer than a week.[8]

The risks of undergoing invasive procedures, including non-medical procedures such as body piercing or tattooing

Bacteraemia can develop following piercing or tattooing, particularly if non-sterile equipment or techniques are involved. Patients at risk of infective endocarditis should be discouraged from having procedures such as piercing or tattooing.[8]

People with the following cardiac conditions are considered to be at risk of developing infective endocarditis and would have received antibiotics for endocarditis prophylaxis in the past:

- *Previous infective endocarditis,*
- *Replacement heart valve,*
- *Structural congenital heart disease (but not isolated atrial septal defect, fully repaired septal defect, fully repaired patent ductus arteriosus or congenital heart disease repaired with closure devices that are judged to be endothelialised)*
- *Valvular heart disease with stenosis or regurgitation,*
- *Hypertrophic cardiomyopathy.*

QUESTIONS PATIENTS MAY ASK

In the past I have been given antibiotics to prevent infective endocarditis for the same dental procedure but have not been offered them now. Why has this changed?

In the past, guidelines recommended that people at risk of infective endocarditis were given prophylactic (preventative) antibiotics before certain procedures. The National Institute for Health and Care Excellence (NICE) has reviewed the evidence regarding infective endocarditis and concluded that prophylactic antibiotics are not required for dental procedures.

To understand why the guidelines have changed, it is helpful to know why antibiotics were recommended in the first place: Dental procedures (such as scaling or tooth extraction) disturb bacteria in the mouth and these bacteria can then enter the bloodstream. It was thought that the rise in the number of bacteria in the bloodstream (bacteraemia) that occurred following dental procedures increased the risk of getting endocarditis, and antibiotics were given to combat this rise.

NICE has found that the levels of bacteria in the bloodstream associated with dental procedures are no higher than those associated with toothbrushing. So, patients undergoing dental procedures are not at any greater risk of getting endocarditis than they are from brushing their teeth. The bacteria that enter the bloodstream are killed by the body's immune system.

Antibiotics can cause side effects, some of which can be very serious, or even fatal. Taking antibiotics when they are not needed puts patients at unnecessary risk. Because antibiotics have not been shown to reduce the chance of getting endocarditis, and because dental procedures are no longer thought to be a cause of endocarditis, taking antibiotics before dental procedures is no longer recommended.

I've used a chlorhexidine mouthwash when I have had dental treatment in the past. Is this helpful?

Chlorhexidine mouthwash is not recommended to prevent infective endocarditis. It has not been shown to reduce the chance of getting endocarditis and, as explained above, dental procedures are no longer thought to be a cause of endocarditis.

Is there some written material (like a leaflet) about infective endocarditis that I can have?

The British Heart Foundation has information about infective endocarditis on its website. Go to the home page and type 'endocarditis' in the search box at the top of the screen.

What can I do to improve my oral health?

Keep your teeth and mouth clean with twice-daily toothbrushing. Visit your dentist for regular check-ups and don't let any dental problems such as a dental abscess or gum disease go untreated.

(Continued)

What are the symptoms of infective endocarditis? What should I do if I think I have it?

Infective endocarditis is very rare. Symptoms are flu-like, and include fever, night sweats and chills, weakness and tiredness as well as breathlessness, weight loss and joint pain. It is very unlikely that you will ever suffer from endocarditis but if you are at risk (e.g. if you have a replacement heart valve, valvular heart disease or hypertrophic cardiomyopathy) and have flu-like symptoms for longer than a week you should see a GP.

What do I do if I think I have an infection?

Guidelines for the treatment of infections have not changed. If you think you have an infection, contact a healthcare professional (e.g. pharmacist, GP, dentist or optician) as you would normally.

NICE provides guidance for the NHS in England and Wales. Further information about NICE, its work and how it reaches decisions is available online.

SUMMARY

Antibiotic prophylaxis is not recommended for the prevention of infective endocarditis in patients undergoing dental procedures.

LIMITATIONS

This document does not relate to the use of pre-procedural antibiotics to prevent infections other than infective endocarditis.

DISCLAIMER

- *Medicines Q&As are intended for healthcare professionals and reflect UK practice.*
- *Each Medicines Q&A relates only to the clinical scenario described.*
- *Medicines Q&As are believed to accurately reflect the medical literature at the time of writing.*

REFERENCES

1. *Joint Formulary Committee. British National Formulary, 54th edition. London: British Medical Association and Royal Pharmaceutical Society of Great Britain; 2007. Chapter 5.1, Table 2: Summary of antibacterial prophylaxis (page 279).*
2. *Ramsdale DR, Turner-Stokes L, Advisory Group of the British Cardiac Society Clinical Practice Committee, et al. Prophylaxis and treatment of infective endocarditis in adults: a concise guide. Clin Med 2004;4:545–550.*
3. *Gould FK, Elliott TSJ, Foweraker J et al. Guidelines for prevention of endocarditis: report of the Working Party of the British Society for Antimicrobial Chemotherapy. J Antimicrob Chemother 2006;57:1035–1042. Accessed on 25/5/2013 at: http://jac.oxfordjournals.org/cgi/reprint/dkl121v1.*
4. *NICE. Prophylaxis against infective endocarditis. March 2008 (NICE Clinical Guideline No.64). Accessed on 8/4/2008 at: NICE full guideline (107 pages) and NICE appendices to the full guideline (270 pages).*
5. *Joint Formulary Committee. British National Formulary, 55th edition. London: British Medical Association and Royal Pharmaceutical Society of Great Britain; 2007. Chapter 5.1, Table 2: Summary of antibacterial prophylaxis (page 283).*
6. *NICE. Understanding NICE guidance: information for people who use NHS services. Preventing infective endocarditis. Reference N1488. Accessed on 8/4/2008.*
7. *NICE. Prophylaxis against infective endocarditis. Quick reference guide. Reference N1487. Accessed on 8/4/2008.*
8. *British Heart Foundation. Infective endocarditis: the facts. Accessed on 8/4/2008.*

QUALITY ASSURANCE
Prepared by
Karoline Brennan, North West Medicines Information Centre
Date prepared
April 2008
Checked by
Christine Randall, North West Medicines Information Centre
Date of check
April 2008.

Endocrinology 6

The endocrine system is widespread and consists of glands that exert their effects by means of chemicals (hormones) secreted into the blood circulation (Fig. 6.1). Hormones are chemical messengers of various types, which usually act at some distance from their source, and can be classified according to their main function.

Nervous and endocrine control mechanisms normally maintain body homeostasis, coordinated via the neuroendocrine system and most apparent in the hypothalamus. The hypothalamus, along with the pituitary gland, controls many other endocrine functions.

Pregnancy and the menopause cause important endocrine changes (Ch. 25). It is also common to see endocrine disorders in people who overexercise or who are anorectic, starving, stressed or ill (Table 6.1). Obesity may be due to endocrine disease (e.g. hypothyroidism, insulinoma, Cushing syndrome, polycystic ovary disease).

Endocrine glands can underproduce (hypofunction) or overproduce (hyperfunction) their hormones. Endocrine disorders (endocrinopathies) may be caused by diminished hormone release (e.g. hypothyroidism), by hormone resistance (e.g. type 2 diabetes) or by excess (e.g. primary hyperparathyroidism). Endocrinopathies can cause a range of symptoms and signs but fatigue is common to many (e.g. thyroid dysfunction, hyper- or hypoglycaemia, dyslipidaemia and gonadal dysfunction).

Endocrine function can be assessed by measuring the hormone in the blood plasma (many have a circadian rhythm – the level varies over 24 hours), or the hormone or its metabolite in the urine; alternatively, dynamic tests of hormone secretion or regulation may be performed – by suppressing (tests hormone excess) or stimulating (tests hormone deficiency) hormone release; or by assessing levels of hormone receptors or effects on the target tissues.

The most common and important specific endocrine disorder is diabetes mellitus, but the hypothalamus is the conductor of the endocrine 'orchestra' (Table 6.2).

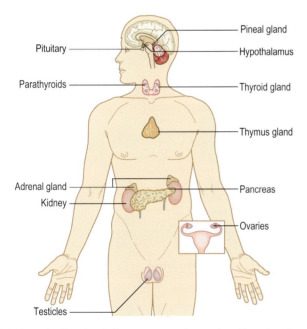

Pituitary — Pineal gland
Hypothalamus
Parathyroids — Thyroid gland
Thymus gland
Adrenal gland — Pancreas
Kidney
Ovaries
Testicles

Fig. 6.1 Main endocrine glands (hormones are also produced by other tissues).

Table 6.1 *Endocrine responses to severe stress or illness*

Plasma levels of hormone rise	Plasma levels of hormone fall	Resistance of hormone increases
Adrenaline (epinephrine)	Luteinizing hormone and follicle-stimulating hormone	Insulin
Glucagon	Sex steroids	
Glucocorticoids and adrenocorticotropic hormone	Thyroid hormones and thyroid-stimulating hormone	
Growth hormone		
Prolactin		

Table 6.2 *Hormones – classified by function*

Electrolyte/fluid/vascular	Metabolic	Liver and digestive	Reproductive	Stress
Aldosterone	Adrenaline (epinephrine) and noradrenaline (norepinephrine)	Cholecystokinin	Aetiocholanolone	Adrenaline (epinephrine) and noradrenaline (norepinephrine)
Androstenedione		Gastrin	Chorionic gonadotropin	
Bradykinin	Cortisol	Vasoactive intestinal peptide	Oestradiol	Adrenocorticotropic hormone
Calcitonin	Growth hormone		Oestriol	Corticosterone
Erythropoietin	Glucagon		Oestrone	Growth hormone
Neurotensin	Insulin		Progesterone	Hydrocortisone (cortisol)
Vasopressin (antidiuretic hormone)	Parathyroid hormone		Prolactin	
	Thyroid hormone		Testosterone	
	Vitamin D			

HYPOTHALAMUS AND PITUITARY GLAND

The hypothalamus is the part of the brain that controls many other endocrine glands, via pituitary function and hypophysiotropic hormones sometimes termed 'releasing factors'.

The anterior pituitary (adenohypophysis) originates as an outgrowth from the stomatodeum (Rathke pouch) and, although anatomically distinct from the hypothalamus, falls under its influence by factors passing through a portal venous system (Fig. 6.2). Hypothalamic hormones that act on the anterior pituitary gland include *thyrotropin-releasing hormone* (TRH), *gonadotropin-releasing hormone* (GnRH), *growth hormone-releasing hormone* (GHRH), *corticotropin-releasing hormone* (CRH) and *somatostatin* (Table 6.3).

The posterior pituitary (neurohypophysis) is a downgrowth from the base of the brain and is connected with the hypothalamus by neurons. Two hypothalamic hormones act on the posterior pituitary gland – *antidiuretic hormone* (ADH) and *oxytocin*.

The hypothalamus is under the control of higher centres in the brain and inhibited by the hormone somatostatin (octreotide). Feedback control influences the amount of hypothalamic hypophysiotropic hormone secreted. *Dopamine* inhibits pituitary release of *prolactin* (PRL).

Pituitary hyperfunction is sometimes caused by pituitary tumours, usually microadenomas (smaller than 1 cm), which can have pressure effects on adjacent structures such as the rest of the anterior pituitary gland and the optic chiasm (Fig. 6.3), causing headaches and visual defects as well as effects on hormone release. Around 50% of pituitary adenomas are hormone-secreting – half producing prolactin, the rest producing growth hormone, adrenocorticotropic hormone (ACTH) or thyroid-stimulating hormone (TSH).

Pituitary hormones, used to stimulate growth, have been implicated in the transmission of some cases of iatrogenic Creutzfeldt–Jakob disease (Ch. 13).

POSTERIOR PITUITARY HYPOFUNCTION

Diabetes insipidus

General aspects

Diabetes insipidus is a rare disease caused by lack of ADH effect. Rarely, this is because of renal insensitivity to ADH (nephrogenic diabetes insipidus – a rare X-linked disorder affecting renal tubular ADH

Table 6.3 *Hypothalamic hormones*

Hypothalamic hormone	Primary activities	Effects
Thyrotropin-releasing hormone (TRH)	Stimulates pituitary release of thyroid-stimulating hormone (TSH) and prolactin (PRL)	Stimulates thyroid hormone synthesis and release
Gonadotropin-releasing hormone (GnRH)	Stimulates pituitary release of luteinizing hormone (LH) and follicle-stimulating hormone (FSH)	LH stimulates follicle to secrete oestrogen in first half of menstrual cycle, triggers completion of meiosis and egg release (ovulation) in mid-cycle, and stimulates empty follicle to develop into corpus luteum, which secretes progesterone during latter half of cycle
		LH acts on interstitial cells of testes, stimulating them to synthesize and secrete testosterone. FSH acts on follicle to stimulate it to release oestrogens and on spermatogonia, stimulating (with aid of testosterone) sperm production
Growth hormone-releasing hormone (GHRH)	Stimulates pituitary release of growth hormone (GH)	Growth (also diabetogenic)
Corticotropin-releasing hormone (CRH)	Stimulates pituitary release of adrenocorticotropic hormone (ACTH)	Stimulates glucocorticoid synthesis and release
Somatostatin	Inhibits pituitary release of TSH and GH	Pituitary control
Antidiuretic hormone (ADH)	Promotes water absorption in renal tubules	Water control
Oxytocin	Stimulates uterine contraction and breast-milk ejection	Lactation

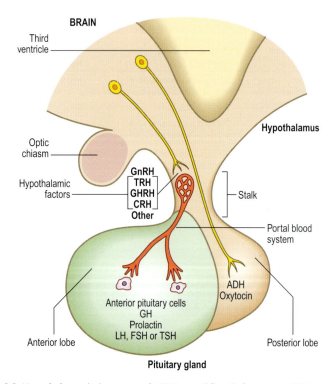

Fig. 6.2 Hypothalamopituitary control. ADH = antidiuretic hormone; CRH = corticotropin-releasing hormone; FSH = follicle stimulating hormone; GH = growth hormone; GHRH = growth hormone-releasing hormone; GnRH = gonadotropin-releasing hormone; LH = luteinizing hormone; TRH = thyrotropin-releasing hormone; TSH = thyroid-stimulating hormone.

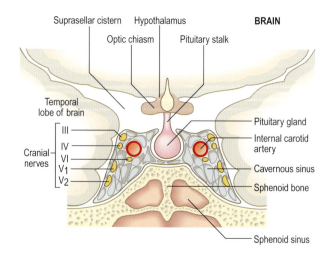

Fig. 6.3 Anatomical relations of the pituitary gland.

receptors, or due to hypercalcaemia, hypokalaemia, renal disease or drugs such as lithium). More commonly, it is because of reduced ADH secretion – cranial diabetes insipidus, which is caused by head injuries (when it may be temporary), a tumour (usually craniopharyngioma), infiltration or vascular disease in the region of the hypothalamus or pituitary, or it may be idiopathic.

Clinical features

Diabetes insipidus is characterized by an excessive volume of dilute urine (polyuria) and by persistent thirst and drinking (polydipsia). *Cranial* diabetes insipidus may also cause pressure on the optic chiasm, leading to visual or cranial nerve defects, or raised intracranial pressure and headaches.

General management

The diagnosis is established by assessing the relation of plasma to urine osmolality and by demonstrating an inability to concentrate the urine during a water-deprivation test. The local extent of disease is assessed by imaging (skull radiography and magnetic resonance imaging [MRI]), visual field charting and tests of anterior pituitary function.

Diabetes insipidus is treated with the ADH-like peptide desmopressin or antidiuretic drugs such as chlorpropamide or carbamazepine.

Dental aspects

Local anaesthesia (LA) is the most satisfactory means of pain control. Conscious sedation (CS) may be needed to control anxiety. Dentistry is usually uncomplicated by this disorder except for dryness of the mouth.

Carbamazepine used in the treatment of trigeminal neuralgia may have an additive effect with other drugs used to treat diabetes insipidus. Transient diabetes insipidus can be a complication of head injury, but head injury can also cause the opposite effect – excessive ADH levels.

Syndrome of inappropriate antidiuretic hormone secretion (SIADH)

Excessive ADH levels may be caused by: maxillofacial injury or even elective maxillofacial surgery, head injury or intracranial lesions; general anaesthesia (GA); pain; fits; smoking; tumours (especially some lung cancers); or drugs (carbamazepine, chlorpropamide, vinca alkaloids).

Inappropriate ADH secretion causes water retention, overhydration, confusion, behavioural disturbances, ataxia and dysphagia. Diagnosis is by finding hyponatraemia with concentrated urine and high plasma and urinary ADH, and an abnormal water-excretion test.

Patients with SIADH are treated with fluid restriction, corticosteroids or demeclocycline.

ANTERIOR PITUITARY HYPOFUNCTION

General aspects

The usual causes of hypopituitarism are local hypothalamic or pituitary lesions, such as tumours, or irradiation (similar factors to those causing cranial diabetes insipidus) or infarction of the pituitary following postpartum haemorrhage (Sheehan syndrome).

Clinical features

The results of hypopituitarism (Table 6.4) are essentially hypofunction of the target glands (the gonads, thyroid and/or adrenal cortex) with soft skin, hypotension, hypoadrenalism and hypothyroidism.

Multiple (panhypopituitarism) hormone deficiencies can result (Fig. 6.4).

General management

Hormone substitution therapy (corticosteroids and thyroxine) is needed. Surgery may be required if there are tumours, cranial nerve defects or hydrocephalus.

Dental aspects

Patients are at risk from adrenal crisis (Ch. 1) and from hypopituitary coma, which is precipitated by stress (trauma, surgery, GA, sedatives

Table 6.4 *Hypopituitarism: clinical effects*

Sequence of hormone deficiencies		Effects
1	LH	Impotence
	FSH	Amenorrhoea
		Infertility
		Loss of pubic hair
2	GH	Impaired growth in children
3	Prolactin	Failure of lactation if postpartum (Sheehan syndrome)
4	ACTH	Hypoadrenocorticism
5	TSH	Hypothyroidism

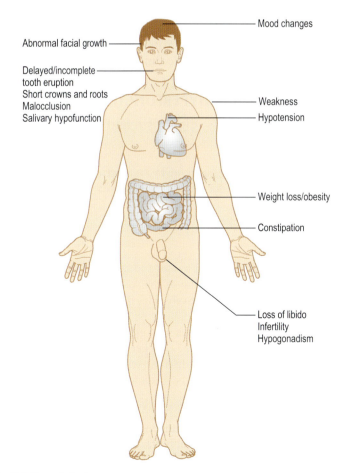

Fig. 6.4 Hypopituitarism.

Mood changes

Abnormal facial growth

Delayed/incomplete tooth eruption
Short crowns and roots
Malocclusion
Salivary hypofunction

Weakness

Hypotension

Weight loss/obesity

Constipation

Loss of libido
Infertility
Hypogonadism

or hypnotics, or infection), much in the way that an adrenal crisis may be.

Hypopituitary coma should be treated by laying the patient flat and giving an immediate intravenous injection of 200 mg hydrocortisone sodium succinate. Blood should be taken for assay of glucose, thyroid hormones and cortisol, and 25–50 g dextrose should be given intravenously if there is hypoglycaemia (defined as a blood glucose <3.0 mmol/L). Oxygen should be given by face mask, medical assistance summoned and emergency admission to hospital arranged.

Gonadotropin (GnRH) deficiency

Hyposecretion of GnRH may be seen most commonly in intense physical training or anorexia nervosa, and rarely in syndromes (Box 6.1).

Kallmann syndrome (hypogonadotropin eunuchoidism) is the most frequent form of isolated gonadotropin deficiency – a rare X-linked recessive disease caused by a defect in a cell adhesion protein that participates in the migration of the GnRH neurons. These normally originate in olfactory tissues and migrate to the hypothalamus. Impaired sense of smell is caused by the absence of the olfactory bulbs. Kallmann syndrome mainly affects males and becomes apparent when they fail to develop secondary sexual characteristics. Thus, hypogonadism and anosmia, with underdeveloped genitalia and sterile gonads, are classic presentations. Treatment involves oestrogen or testosterone replacement, and pulsatile GnRH injections.

ANTERIOR PITUITARY HYPERFUNCTION

Growth hormone excess: gigantism and acromegaly

General aspects

Overproduction of growth hormone by an anterior pituitary adenoma causes gigantism before the epiphyses have fused, and acromegaly thereafter.

Clinical features

In *gigantism*, all the organs, soft tissues and skeleton enlarge, leading to excessively tall stature, thickening of the soft tissues with prominence of the supraorbital ridge, coarse oily skin, thick spade-like fingers and deepening of the voice.

In *acromegaly*, only those bones with growth potential, particularly the mandible, can enlarge. There is thickening of the soft tissues and the hands become large and spade-like. Acromegaly is one of the few endocrine diseases that should be instantly recognized – even in a passer-by – by the gross prognathism and the thickened facial features and hands (Fig. 6.5).

In *both gigantism and acromegaly*, local pressure effects from the pituitary tumour may cause hypopituitarism plus compression of the optic chiasma, with visual field defects and raised intracranial pressure with severe headaches.

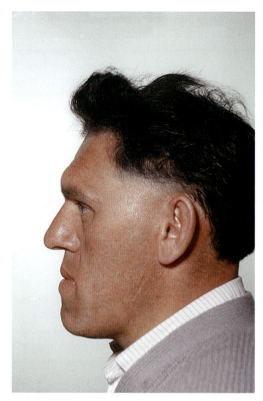

Fig. 6.5 Acromegaly showing prominent supraorbital ridges and prognathism.

Growth hormone disorders may be complicated by diabetes mellitus, hypertension, cardiomyopathy, sleep apnoea, hypercalcaemia and osteoarthritis (Fig. 6.6). Life expectancy is also shortened by diseases such as colonic carcinoma.

General management

Family photographs may clearly demonstrate the increasingly coarse features. Skull radiography, computed tomography (CT) and MRI scans (for pituitary – sella turcica – enlargement) are indicated. Sella enlargement is also sometimes due to other causes, such as hypothalamic masses or cysts or the empty sella syndrome (this is caused by herniation of a sac of leptomeninges into the sella). Rhinorrhoea may warrant surgical correction, but no other treatment is needed.

Other investigations in growth hormone excess are visual field assessment (to detect optic chiasm involvement), glucose tolerance tests (to exclude diabetes and to assess the plasma growth hormone response), levels of growth hormone and insulin-like growth factor 1 (IGF-1), and assessment of function of the remaining pituitary.

The pituitary adenoma may be resected trans-sphenoidally or the whole gland may have to be irradiated (e.g. by transnasal yttrium). Hypopituitarism or diabetes insipidus follows such treatment.

Bromocriptine or octreotide (an analogue of the hypothalamic release-inhibiting hormone somatostatin) may also help treatment.

Dental aspects

Local analgesia is suitable. CS may be given, if necessary, provided the airway is clear. GA may be hazardous because of complications (see later).

Dental management may be complicated by:

- blindness, diabetes mellitus, hypertension, cardiomyopathy, arrhythmias and hypopituitarism

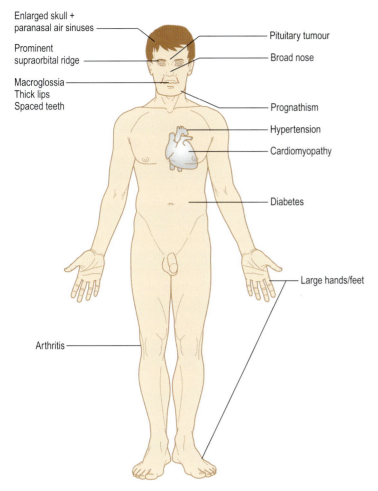

Fig. 6.6 Acromegaly.

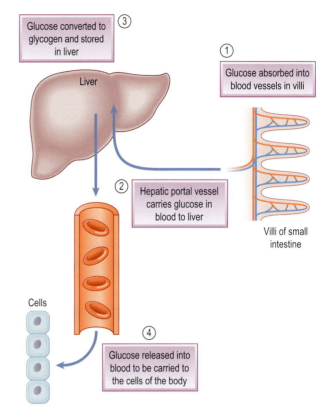

Fig. 6.7 Glucose absorption and homeostasis.

- kyphosis and other deformities affecting respiration, which may make GA hazardous. The glottic opening may be narrowed and the cords' mobility reduced. A goitre may further embarrass the airway
- rarely, the development of Cushing syndrome or hyperparathyroidism due to associated multiple endocrine adenoma syndrome.

Mandibular enlargement leads to prognathism (class III malocclusion) with spacing of the teeth and thickening of all soft tissues, but most conspicuously of the face. Orthognathic surgery may be needed and fatalities have followed such surgery in the past because of airway obstruction. The paranasal air sinuses are enlarged and the skull thickened. Sialosis may develop.

PANCREAS

All carbohydrate eaten is digested into glucose, which passes from the stomach and intestine into the blood and is the main source of energy. Glucose homeostasis depends mainly on the pancreatic hormones insulin (from the beta-cells of the islets of Langerhans) and glucagon from the alpha-cells in the islets.

Insulin facilitates glucose transport into cells and thus lowers blood sugar (glucose) levels. Glucagon stimulates the liver to convert glycogen into glucose, thus raising glucose levels and having the opposite effect to insulin (Fig. 6.7). The beta-cells also produce amylin, which modulates gastric emptying and satiety, and decreases the postprandial

rise in glucagon. Also involved in glucose homeostasis are gastric inhibitory polypeptide (GIP) and glucagon-like peptide 1 (GLP-1) – small intestine hormones (incretins) secreted when eating. GLP-1 has a glucose-lowering effect via stimulation of insulin production and inhibition of glucagon (as well as preserving pancreatic beta-cell function, slowing gastric emptying and suppressing food intake). Several other hormones that can influence glucose include catecholamines (adrenaline [epinephrine] and noradrenaline [norepinephrine]), corticosteroids, thyroid hormone and growth hormone.

DIABETES MELLITUS

General aspects

Diabetes mellitus (DM) is a disorder caused by an absolute or relative lack of insulin; there can be a low output of insulin from the pancreas, or the peripheral tissues may resist insulin. In diabetes, with insulin lacking or its action blocked, glucose cannot enter cells and, without energy, weakness results. Glucose also then accumulates in the blood (hyperglycaemia) and spills over into the urine (glucosuria), taking with it, osmotically, a large amount of water (polyuria). This leads to dehydration and thus thirst and the need to drink excessively (polydipsia). As glucose is then no longer a viable energy source, fat and protein stores are metabolized with weight loss, peripheral muscle wasting and, in type 1 diabetes, the production of ketone bodies (acetoacetate, β-hydroxybutyrate and acetone). In severe cases, ketone bodies may be detected on the breath (in particular, acetone) and accumulate in the blood (ketonaemia), as well as being excreted in the urine (ketonuria). The resultant metabolic ketoacidosis leads to a compensatory increase in respiratory rate (hyperventilation) and a secondary respiratory alkalosis.

Chronic hyperglycaemia causes microvascular complications and atherosclerosis, and is a leading cause of death and disability.

ENDOCRINOLOGY

Diabetes affects about 3–4% of the general population but may be recognized in only 75% of those individuals, yet it is a leading cause of death and disability. Worldwide, about 246 million people are affected. Risk factors for diabetes include family history (the risk of developing diabetes rises if a close relative, such as a parent or sibling, has the disease); being overweight; inactivity; age (the risk of developing type 2 diabetes rises with age, especially after age 45); and race. Genetics has a role. Type 1 diabetes is more common in Caucasians and in European countries, such as Finland and Sweden. Type 2 diabetes is especially common in people of African heritage, Asians and Hispanics, and has a stronger genetic background. Diabetes affects up to one-third of the elderly from the Asian subcontinent. Among the Pima Indians in the USA and in Nauru in the Pacific, around half of all adults have type 2 diabetes – the highest rates in the world. The prevalence of diabetes appears to be rising, mainly as more children and adolescents become overweight. In contrast, fewer diabetics remain undiagnosed, and associated ischaemic heart disease and retinal disease are falling.

Diabetes may be primary, or secondary to some other factor(s), as shown in Table 6.5. Type 2 is by far the most common type (Table 6.6).

Type 1 diabetes (T1DM)

Type 1 diabetes develops when the immune system attacks insulin-producing cells of the pancreatic islets of Langerhans. Weight reduction and exercise increase sensitivity to insulin, thus helping to control blood glucose elevations, but these patients still require insulin.

Type 1 diabetes – formerly termed insulin-dependent (IDDM) or juvenile-onset diabetes – is most commonly diagnosed at about 12 years of age and commonly presents before the third decade, but can appear at any age. Associated with other organ-specific autoimmune diseases, it is characterized by antibodies directed against insulin and the pancreatic islets of Langerhans. It may have a viral (possibly Coxsackie or rubella) aetiology. Latent autoimmune diabetes in adults (LADA) is essentially a slow presentation of type 1 diabetes, which is seen in slimmer patients who progress quickly to insulin requirement. Anti-glutamic acid decarboxylase (GAD) antibodies may be helpful in the diagnosis.

Type 2 diabetes (T2DM)

Type 2 diabetes – formerly termed non-insulin-dependent (NIDDM) or maturity-onset diabetes – accounts for at least 90% of diabetics. Generally, it occurs in genetically predisposed individuals over the age of 40, who are typically overweight. Patients are insulin-resistant and have diminished beta-cell function. Alcohol binge drinking may induce insulin resistance independent of caloric intake and increase the risk for developing metabolic syndrome and T2DM. Maturity-onset diabetes of the young (MODY) is a rare form of type 2 diabetes; it caused by autosomal dominant mutations and so there is vertical transmission of diabetes within families. The phenotype varies from mild glucose intolerance to insulin-requiring diabetes, typically diagnosed before the age of 25 years.

Type 3 diabetes (T3DM)

Gestational diabetes is basically an insulin-resistant state exposing the patient to a future risk of type 2 diabetes (see Table 6.6).

Clinical features

Patients with diabetes may be asymptomatic and detected on routine or opportunistic screening, or present in a variety of ways related to severity and degree of onset (Table 6.7).

Table 6.7 *Acute and chronic presenting features of diabetes mellitus*

Acute	Chronic
Thirst	Thirst
Polyuria and polydipsia	Polyuria and polydipsia
Weight loss and weakness	Weight loss and weakness
Lethargy	Lethargy
Confusion/aggression/behavioural changes	Irritability
	Recurrent skin, oral and genital infections
Abdominal pain	Visual deterioration
Nausea and vomiting	Paraesthesia (hands and feet)
Ketoacidosis	
Dehydration	
Renal failure	
Coma	

Table 6.5 *Classification of diabetes mellitus*

Primary	Type 1 – insulin-dependent (IDDM); juvenile onset
	Type 2 – non-insulin-dependent (NIDDM); maturity onset
Secondary	Drugs (corticosteroids, thiazide diuretics, beta-blockers)
	Endocrine disorders (phaeochromocytoma, acromegaly, Cushing syndrome)
	Pancreatic disease (pancreatitis), haemochromatosis
	Pregnancy (gestational diabetes) – usually represents type 2 diabetes exposed by the increased insulin resistance of pregnancy

Table 6.6 *Types of diabetes mellitus*

Type	Formerly called	Typical time of onset	% of all diabetes	Aetiopathogenesis	Autoantibodies	Other factors
1	Insulin-dependent (IDDM)	Juvenile onset	5–10	Insulin deficiency	Islet cell antibodies in up to 90%	Genetic: HLA-DR3/4 in 95%. Viruses (mumps or Coxsackie) affect beta-cells: implicated in autoimmune disease
2	Non-insulin-dependent (NIDDM)	Maturity onset	90–95	Insulin resistance	None	Overweight, often family history of diabetes; no HLA association. Subtypes result from mutations in glucokinase gene, changes in insulin signalling, defective phosphatidylinositol kinases or other mechanisms
3	Gestational	Appears usually in second or third trimester of pregnancy	Rare	Affects up to 5% of pregnant women. Placental hormones interfere with insulin	None	Most common in people of African heritage or with a family history of diabetes. Increased risk of type 2 diabetes later

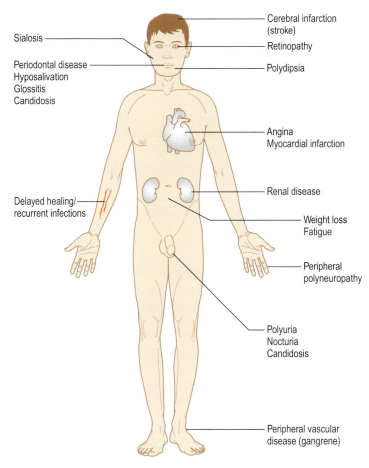

Fig. 6.8 Diabetes mellitus.

Labels on figure:
- Sialosis
- Periodontal disease / Hyposalivation / Glossitis / Candidosis
- Delayed healing/ recurrent infections
- Cerebral infarction (stroke)
- Retinopathy
- Polydipsia
- Angina / Myocardial infarction
- Renal disease
- Weight loss / Fatigue
- Peripheral polyneuropathy
- Polyuria / Nocturia / Candidosis
- Peripheral vascular disease (gangrene)

Table 6.8 *Causes of hypoglycaemia*

Common (diabetics)	Rare (non-diabetics)
Excess insulin or hypoglycaemic drug	Insulinoma
	Hepatic disease
Missed meal	Hypoadrenocorticism
Unaccustomed exercise	Hypopituitarism
Alcohol (the effect of which is delayed)	Functional hypoglycaemia
	Beta-blockers

Lethargy is the most common symptom but hyperglycaemia, polyuria and thirst (polydipsia) are prominent. Since glucose is lost as an energy source in type 1 diabetes, fats must be metabolized, leading to weight loss from fat breakdown to fatty acids and ketone bodies, which appear in the blood, causing acidosis and hyperventilation, in the urine (ketonuria) and to some extent in the breath (acetone). Overproduction of acetoacetate is converted to the other ketone bodies, hydroxybutyrate and acetone. Diabetes is also associated with immune deficiencies, particularly polymorph dysfunction, leading to susceptibility to infections (mainly skin infections and mucosal candidosis; Fig. 6.8).

Type 1 diabetes develops most often in children and young adults, generally before the age of 25. Symptoms usually develop over a short period. Excessive thirst and urination, constant hunger, weight loss, blurred vision and extreme fatigue are typical. Life-threatening diabetic coma (diabetic ketoacidosis) is a significant risk. Insulin is required daily for treatment, for life, and diet must be controlled. Hypoglycaemia is a risk.

Type 2 diabetes develops most often in overweight patients. Symptoms usually develop gradually. Fatigue, frequent urination, unusual thirst, weight loss, blurred vision, frequent infections, and slow healing of wounds or sores are seen. Most patients with type 2 diabetes can be managed on diet and oral hypoglycaemic drugs. Many will eventually need insulin but are often resistant. About 80% of people with type 2 diabetes have the *metabolic syndrome*, which includes obesity, elevated blood pressure and high levels of blood lipids (Ch. 23).

Factors that affect the blood glucose level are shown in Box 6.2.

Acute complications

Diabetes can lead to coma. Hypoglycaemic coma is the main acute complication of diabetes, is growing in frequency with the trend towards tighter metabolic control of diabetes, and is usually the result of one or more of the above factors. Less common causes are shown in Table 6.8. Many insulin-treated patients are liable to hypoglycaemia, due to an imbalance between food intake and usage, and insulin therapy. Hypoglycaemia can be of rapid onset and may resemble fainting. Adrenaline (epinephrine) is released, leading to a strong and bounding pulse, sweaty skin, and often anxiety, irritability and disorientation, before consciousness is lost. Occasionally, the patient may convulse.

The patient should be treated immediately (Table 6.9); hypoglycaemia must be quickly corrected with glucose or brain damage can result. Glucose will cause little harm in hyperglycaemic coma but will improve hypoglycaemia. Never give insulin since this can cause severe brain damage or kill a hypoglycaemic patient. Assess the glucose level with a testing strip.

If the patient is conscious, give glucose solution or gel (GlucoGel) immediately by mouth or 10 g sugar but, if the patient is comatose, give 10–20 mL of 20–50% sterile dextrose intravenously or, if a vein cannot readily be found, glucagon 1 mg intramuscularly. On arousal, the patient should also be given glucose orally, usually in the form of longer-acting carbohydrate (e.g. bread, biscuits).

Other diabetics are difficult to control (brittle diabetes – a term usually used in association with adolescent girls who may be self-harming) and more prone to ketosis, severe acidosis and hyperglycaemia (diabetic coma), the result of a relative or absolute deficiency of insulin. In patients under treatment, it may be precipitated by factors such as infections.

Hyperglycaemic coma usually has a slow onset over many hours, with deepening drowsiness (but unconsciousness is rare, so an unconscious diabetic should always be assumed to be hypoglycaemic), signs of dehydration (dry skin, weak pulse, hypotension), acidosis (deep breathing), and ketosis (acetone smell on breath and vomiting) mainly in type 1 diabetes. If it is certain that collapse is due to hyperglycaemic

Table 6.9 *Hypoglycaemic and hyperglycaemic comas and their treatment*

Hypoglycaemic coma	Hyperglycaemic coma
Diabetes usually known	Diabetes may be unrecognized
Too much insulin or too little food, or too much exercise or alcohol	Too little insulin, infection or myocardial infarct
Adrenaline (epinephrine) release causes:	Acidosis in some variants causes:
Sweaty warm skin	Vomiting
Rapid bounding pulse	Hyperventilation
Dilated (reacting) pupils	Ketonuria
Anxiety, tremor, aggression	Acetone breath
Tingling around mouth	Osmotic diuresis and polyuria cause:
Cerebral hypoglycaemia causes:	Dehydration
Confusion, disorientation, aggression	Hypotension
	Tachycardia
Headache	Dry mouth and skin
Dysarthria	Abdominal pain
Unconsciousness	
Focal neurological signs (e.g. fits)	
Management	
Take blood for baseline glucose, electrolytes, urea, Hb and packed cell volume (PCV)	
If conscious, give Hypostop (GlucoGel) or 25 g glucose orally (2 teaspoons sugar, 3 lumps sugar, 3 Dextrosol tablets, 60 mL Lucozade, 15 mL Ribena, 90 mL cola drink (*not* 'diet' variety) or 170 mL milk)	Put up infusion to rehydrate and give insulin
If comatose, give 20 mg 20% or 50% dextrose i.v. and on arousal 25 mg orally	
If i.v. injection impossible, give glucagon 1 mg i.m.	
Call ambulance (Ch. 1)	

Table 6.10 *Chronic complications of diabetes*

Cardiovascular	Atherosclerosis leading to ischaemic heart disease, cerebrovascular disease and peripheral gangrene
	Cardiorespiratory arrest
Renal	Renal damage and failure
Ocular	Retinopathy
	Cataracts
Neuropathies	Peripheral polyneuropathy
	Mononeuropathies
	Autonomic neuropathy (postural hypotension)
Infections	Candidosis
	Staphylococcal infections
	Systemic mycoses (rarely)

Table 6.11 *Glucose assays in the diagnosis of diabetes*

Test	Confirms diabetes[a]	Excludes diabetes
Fasting plasma glucose (after a person has fasted for 8 h)	>7.0 mmol/L	<6 mmol/L
Random blood glucose (taken at any time of day)	≥11.1 mmol/L	<8 mmol/L[b]
Plasma glucose taken 2 h after a person has consumed a drink containing 75 g of glucose in oral glucose tolerance test (OGTT)	>11.1 mmol/L[a]	<11.1 mmol/L

[a]If associated with symptoms, or abnormal on repeat testing.
[b]Must be checked with fasting glucose.

ketoacidotic coma, the immediate priority is to establish an intravenous infusion line. This enables rapid rehydration to correct dehydration and electrolyte (especially potassium) losses, and the administration of insulin. Blood should be taken for baseline measurements of glucose, electrolytes, pH and blood gases. Raised plasma ketone body levels can be demonstrated with a testing strip such as Ketostix (Ames). Insulin is then started, such as 20 units i.m. stat. Medical help should be obtained as soon as possible.

Coma in a diabetic patient, though usually due to hypo- or hyperglycaemia, may have other causes such as myocardial infarction (Ch. 5).

Chronic complications

Diabetes is associated with long-term microvascular and macrovascular complications that can affect almost every part of the body (Table 6.10). It is a leading cause of death and disability due to premature cardiovascular disease; the risk of myocardial infarction is at least tripled. Renal and retinal complications are also incapacitating, as is gangrene of toes.

Smoking increases the risk of many chronic complications. Phagocytic defects contribute to an immune defect and liability to infections. Babies born to women with diabetes are often large and sometimes have birth defects. Occasionally, there are associations of type 1 diabetes with autoimmune disorders, especially Addison disease. There may be a predilection to oral cancer.

General management

Glycosuria is *usually* indicative of diabetes, but absence of glycosuria does not completely exclude it and confirmation by blood glucose levels is essential. Diagnosis is from the presence of raised blood (venous plasma) glucose level (Table 6.11).

A diagnosis of diabetes is made when any one of the glycosuria, random blood glucose and fasting blood glucose tests is positive, with a second test positive on a different day (not needed if symptomatic). *Pre-diabetes* is the term applied when there is either of the following:

- An impaired glucose tolerance (IGT) test – blood glucose during the oral glucose tolerance test (OGTT) is higher than normal but not high enough for a diagnosis of diabetes (7.8–11.0 mmol/L)
- An impaired fasting glucose (IFG; impaired fasting glycaemia) test – fasting plasma glucose is higher than normal (6.1–6.9 mmol/L) but less than the level confirming the presence of diabetes.

Patients with IGT and IFG are more likely to develop type 2 diabetes, and have an increased risk of cardiovascular disease.

Prevention

- Weight should be reduced and physical activity stepped up.
- Diet may help diabetic control; recommendations are to:

Eat more starches, such as bread, cereal and starchy vegetables
Eat five portions of fruits and vegetables every day. Soluble fibres, found mainly in fruits, vegetables and some seeds, are especially useful as they help slow down or reduce intestinal absorption of glucose. Legumes, such as cooked kidney beans, are among the highest soluble-fibre foods. Other fibre-containing foods, such as carrots, also have a positive levelling effect on blood glucose.
Eat fewer sugars and sweets.

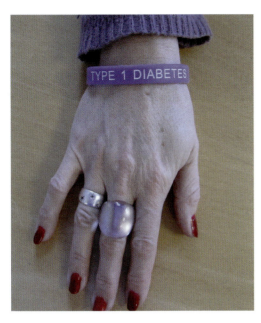

Fig. 6.9 Diabetes wristband.

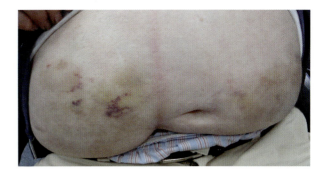

Fig. 6.10 Insulin injection sites.

Treatment

Treatment objectives are:

- reduction of hyperglycaemia – to alleviate presenting symptoms
- prevention of hypoglycaemia and other acute complications
- maintenance of near-normal blood glucose levels – to minimize microvascular complications
- reduction of other cardiovascular risk factors (smoking, exercise, hypertension and lipids).

Individuals should be educated about the importance of good long-term diabetic control; they should have a thorough knowledge of the disease and may wish to warn others that they have it (Fig. 6.9). All diabetics should carry a card indicating the diagnosis, treatment schedule and physician in charge, and should be encouraged to wear a MedicAlert-type device.

The progressive nature of diabetes, its complications and management aims should be well understood. Patients should also be aware of the range of diabetic services available and how to make appropriate use of them. A multidisciplinary team approach is required for their effective management. Meals should be taken at regular intervals, with a high fibre and relatively high carbohydrate content but avoiding sugars, and with a caloric intake strictly related to physical activity. Lifestyle changes, such as exercise, diet, fasting, travel (including changing time zones) and changes in working practices, can have an impact on diabetic control.

Urine testing has little or no place in the assessment or control of diabetes. Control is assessed by blood glucose levels and used to guide medication. A glucometer allows glucose readings to be taken easily by the patient at home. Fasting glucose <6 mmol/L is normal. Long-term assessment of glucose control is made by estimation of the blood level of glycosylated haemoglobin (HbA_{1c}). HbA_{1c} is normal adult haemoglobin that binds glucose and remains in the circulation for the life of the erythrocyte, therefore acting as a cumulative index of diabetic control over the preceding 3 months; the higher the glycosylated haemoglobin level, the greater the risk of chronic complications. Patients should have an HbA_{1c} test every 3–6 months; glycosylated haemoglobin below 4.8% of total haemoglobin is normal. Fructosamine is an alternative assay of long-term diabetic control.

Optimum control would be to aim to keep blood glucose levels at 4–7 mmol/L before meals (preprandial) and at no higher than

Table 6.12 *Different insulins*

Insulin type	Protocol	Peak activity	Approximate duration of activity
Rapid-acting analogues	Injected just before, with or after food	0–3 h	2–5 hours
Long-acting analogues	Injected once a day, not necessarily with food	–	24 h
Short-acting insulins	Injected 15–30 min before a meal to cover the rise in blood glucose levels that occurs after eating	2–6 h	8 h
Medium- and long-acting insulins	Injected once or twice a day to provide background insulin or in combination with short-acting insulins/ rapid-acting analogues	4–12 h	30 h
Mixed insulin	Combination of medium- and short-acting insulin	Varies	Varies
Mixed analogue	Medium-acting insulin and rapid-acting analogue	Varies	Varies

10 mmol/L 2 hours after meals (postprandial), and HbA_{1c} (long-term glucose level) at 7% or less.

Type 1 diabetes

Basic treatment of type 1 diabetes is subcutaneous insulin, the amount being balanced against food intake and daily activities, and monitored via home blood glucose testing. Insulin cannot be taken orally but must be given via injection, subcutaneously, either in the abdominal wall (Fig. 6.10), buttocks, thighs or upper arms, using a syringe, pen device or insulin pump. An artificial pancreas, a "closed loop" system that monitors blood glucose levels to adjust the insulin being administered by a pump is being developed. There are three groups of insulins – animal, human (actually synthetic) and analogues. There are six main types of insulin, available in various combinations and all working in different ways (Table 6.12). Most insulin regimes are based on a long-acting insulin combined with a smaller amount of faster-acting insulin, all normally taken via two or more injections each day. Insulin pump therapy (continuous subcutaneous insulin infusion [CSII]) is fast-acting insulin given continually day and night, at a rate preset according to needs. An insulin pump is not a closed loop system; rather, patients learn to set the dose according to diet, activity and blood glucose levels. Most test a minimum of four times a day, in order to obtain the information needed to set an appropriate insulin dose. An advantage of insulin pump therapy is that it can help improve control and minimize the frequency of 'hypos'. The types of insulin used include those shown in Table 6.12.

Table 6.13 *Hypoglycaemic drugs other than insulin*

Group	Principles of action	Comments
Sulphonylureas	Increase pancreatic output of insulin	Sulfa-containing drugs, which should be avoided by patients who are allergic to sulfas. Bind to insulin-producing cell receptors and lower blood glucose by increasing pancreatic release of insulin, but run the risk of hypoglycaemia. Older generations include chlorpropamide and tolbutamide; newer drugs include glibenclamide (glyburide), glipizide and glimepiride. May enhance, or be enhanced by, aspirin, anticoagulants, monoamine oxidase inhibitors (MAOIs), beta-blockers or clofibrate
Meglitinides		Meglitinides – repaglinide and nateglinide – promote pancreatic insulin secretion via a cell-surface potassium-based channel. Like sulphonylureas, they cause hypoglycaemia but are very short-acting, with peak effects within 1h. Prandial glucose regulators
Biguanides		Metformin is unique in its ability to decrease liver glucose production. It does not increase insulin levels and therefore rarely causes hypoglycaemia. In addition, it suppresses appetite, which may be beneficial in overweight diabetics. Biguanides decrease target tissue insulin resistance, affect the absorption and metabolism of glucose, and reduce appetite, but can induce lactic acidosis. Metformin may be used alone or together with other oral drugs or insulin. It should not be used in renal disease and must be used with caution in liver disease. Metformin should be discontinued for 24h before surgery or any procedure involving the intravenous injection of dyes (such as for some renal radiographic studies), as the dyes may impair kidney function and cause metformin accumulation
Thiazolidinediones (glitazones)	Help overcome insulin resistance by binding to the adipocyte receptor to increase the response of cells to insulin	Lower blood glucose by increasing cell sensitivity to insulin. Troglitazone has been withdrawn because it causes severe hepatotoxicity. Pioglitazone and rosiglitazone are safer, and effective in lowering blood glucose within 1h of administration. Rosiglitazone, however, has been associated with an increased risk of cardiovascular events and with fractures of distal long bones of limbs. Glitazones mainly used in addition to metformin/sulphonylurea. Contraindicated in heart failure, ischaemic heart disease or peripheral vascular disease
Alpha-glucosidase inhibitors	Slightly delay intestinal breakdown of oligosaccharides to glucose and monosaccharides, and decrease carbohydrate absorption from the intestine	Carbohydrates are broken down by small-intestine enzymes, such as alpha-glucosidase, into sugars, such as glucose. Acarbose is an alpha-glucosidase inhibitor, whose use results in less efficient breakdown of carbohydrates and thus delay in glucose absorption. It has significant gastrointestinal side-effects, at least for a few weeks, although some patients report persistent problems
Dipeptidyl peptidase-4 inhibitors (DPP-IV; incretins)	Impede breakdown of endogenous incretin glucagon-like peptide 1 (GLP-1), thus stimulating insulin secretion but rarely causing hypoglycaemia	Sitagliptin and saxagliptin have a similar adverse effect profile to exenatide but are in pill form. Linagliptin increases the level of hormones that stimulate the release of insulin after a meal
Exenatide		Exenatide is an incretin mimetic, similar to the gut glucagon-like peptide-1 (GLP-1) hormone, which is broken down in the body by DPP-IV. Incretins, such as GLP-1, enhance glucose-dependent insulin secretion. GLP-1, produced in the small intestine, and amylin, produced by the pancreas, also have glucose-lowering effects. GLP-1, also released in a postprandial manner, promotes insulin production and secretion, reduces glucagon secretion, delays gastric emptying and induces a feeling of fullness. GLP-1 mimetics may produce nausea but have the advantage over other drugs of not leading to weight gain. Exenatide promotes insulin release from beta-cells, mimics certain antihyperglycaemic actions of GLP-1, is not a substitute for insulin, and is used with a thiazolidinedione with or without metformin. Exenatide is injected subcutaneously, twice a day. It may interact with paracetamol (acetaminophen), antibiotics, contraceptive pills, digoxin, lovastatin, sulphonylureas and warfarin
Liraglutide		A GLP-1 receptor agonist, which helps the pancreas make more insulin after a meal. As an injectable medicine, it improves blood glucose in adults with type 2 diabetes when used with a diet and exercise programme
Pramlintide	Affects glycaemic control	The first new injectable, antihyperglycaemic, a synthetic analogue of human amylin, a naturally occurring hormone synthesized by pancreatic beta-cells. Amylin helps control glucose after meals, and is absent or deficient in patients with diabetes

Type 2 diabetes

Medications for type 2 diabetes are designed to:

- increase the pancreatic output of insulin
- increase the response of cells to insulin
- decrease carbohydrate absorption from the intestine
- affect glycaemic control.

When selecting therapy, consideration should be given to:

- the magnitude of change in blood glucose control
- co-morbidities (high cholesterol, hypertension, etc.)
- medication:
  adverse effects
  contraindications
  compliance
  cost.

Some people with type 2 diabetes find that, despite having their diabetes medication adjusted, their blood glucose levels remain too high and insulin treatment is needed. Combination drugs, such as glibenclamide (glyburide)/metformin, rosiglitazone/metformin, glipizide/metformin, pioglitazone/metformin and metformin/sitagliptin, are available (Table 6.13).

Emerging treatments

Phlorizin, a naturally occurring product found in the bark of pear (*Pyrus communis*), apple, cherry and other fruit trees, is a competitive inhibitor of sodium–glucose co-transporters SGLT1 and SGLT2; it reduces renal glucose transport and lowers blood glucose. Although it is a potential treatment for type 2 diabetes, it has been superseded by more selective and more promising synthetic analogues, dapagliflozin and canagliflozin. Dapagliflozin is a selective and reversible inhibitor of SGLT2 and has European regulatory approval for treatment of type 2 diabetes.

Combined kidney and pancreas transplantation is used for renal failure from type 1 diabetes in persons who are otherwise in acceptable health. Most people who receive a donor pancreas fall into this group. Approximately 85% of those who receive a combined kidney and pancreas transplant no longer require insulin a year after surgery. Pancreatic transplantation can be associated with all the problems that accompany immunosuppression (Ch. 35).

Islet cell transplantation offers a less invasive, expensive and risky option than a pancreas transplant. In islet cell transplantation, insulin-producing beta-cells are taken from a donor pancreas and transferred into a person with diabetes. Once transplanted, the donor islets begin to make and release insulin, actively regulating the level of blood glucose.

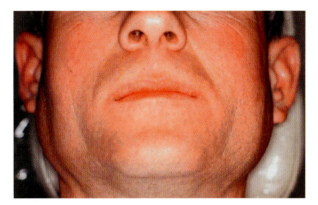

Fig. 6.11 Sialosis in diabetes.

Dental aspects

There are no specific oral manifestations of diabetes mellitus but, even if it is well controlled, diabetic patients are predisposed to infections and have more severe periodontal disease than controls. Severe periodontitis may also upset glycaemic control. If diabetic control is poor, oral candidosis can develop and cause, for example, angular stomatitis. Severe diabetes with ketoacidosis predisposes to and is the main cause of mucormycosis originating in the paranasal sinuses and nose (Ch. 21). Severe dentoalveolar abscesses with fascial space involvement in seemingly healthy individuals may indicate diabetes. Any such patients should be investigated to exclude it and other immune defects.

In patients with insulin-treated diabetes, circumoral paraesthesia is a common and important sign of impending hypoglycaemia. Neuropathy may occasionally cause cranial nerve deficits and occasionally there is swelling of the salivary glands (sialosis; Fig. 6.11) due to autonomic neuropathy. Temporary lingual and labial paraesthesia may follow the removal of mandibular third molar teeth. A burning mouth sensation in the absence of physical changes may be possible. A dry mouth may result from dehydration. The 'Grinspan syndrome' (diabetes, lichen planus and hypertension) may be the result of purely coincidental associations of common disorders probably related to drug use.

Diabetes may have significant complications, such as hypoglycaemia, visual impairment, renal failure, gangrene, stroke or myocardial infarction, which can profoundly influence oral health care. The main hazard is hypoglycaemia, as dental disease and treatment may disrupt the normal pattern of food intake. This should be prevented by planning ahead, such as by administering oral glucose just before the appointment if a patient has taken their medication but has not had the appropriate meal. Furthermore, the patient's blood glucose level may be tested using a point-of-care device prior to treatment, particularly before surgical procedures, and oral glucose given if the level is too low – less than about 5 mmol/L (180 mg/dL). If normal eating will not be resumed at lunchtime, a postoperative blood glucose level may be taken and further glucose given.

Drugs used should be sugar-free, avoiding those that can disturb diabetic control: corticosteroids, which increase blood glucose; and doxycycline, tetracyclines and ciprofloxacin, which enhance insulin hypoglycaemia. Paracetamol (acetaminophen) or codeine is the analgesic of choice. NSAIDs should be used with caution in view of renal damage and risk of gastrointestinal bleeding, especially as many diabetics are already on low-dose aspirin for prophylaxis of ischaemic heart disease. The dentist should manage infections aggressively, as people with diabetes may be immunocompromised (Ch. 20); amoxicillin is the antibiotic of choice.

LA can usually be safely used in diabetics; the dose of adrenaline (epinephrine) is unlikely to increase blood glucose levels significantly. CS with benzodiazepines can usually be safely used. Autonomic neuropathy in diabetes can cause orthostatic hypotension; therefore the supine patient should be slowly raised upright in the dental chair. Routine non-surgical procedures or short minor surgical procedures under LA can be carried out with no special precautions, apart from ensuring that treatment does not interfere with eating.

In a well-controlled diabetic patient, providing that normal diet has been, and can be, taken, it is feasible to carry out even minor surgical procedures, such as simple single extractions under LA, as long as the procedure is carried out within 2 hours of breakfast and the morning insulin injection, with no change in the insulin regimen. More protracted procedures, such as multiple extractions, must only be carried out in hospital. Poorly controlled diabetics (whether type 1 or 2) should also be referred for improved control of their blood glucose before non-emergency treatment is performed.

Diabetics on insulin

In a well-controlled insulin-dependent diabetic, providing that a normal diet can be taken and that the procedure is carried out within 2 hours of breakfast and the morning insulin injection, with no change in the insulin regimen, it is feasible to carry out minor surgical procedures (e.g. simple single extractions under LA, or minor operations under GA in hospital) by operating early in the morning and withholding both food and insulin from the previous midnight, until after the procedure.

The management of diabetes requiring GA is shown in Table 6.14.

Some medications can hide the warning symptoms of hypoglycaemia. These include:

- beta-blockers
- clonidine
- guanethidine
- reserpine.

Other drugs can cause hypoglycaemia (Box 6.3).

Perioperative management

The following section has been adapted from the UK National Health Service's guidelines on emergency and inpatient perioperative management in diabetic patients and from the *Tayside Area Formulary: Guidelines for the perioperative management of patients with diabetes* (www.nhstaysideadtc.scot.nhs.uk; accessed 30 September 2013).

Table 6.14 *Management of diabetes requiring general anaesthesia*[a]

	Type 2 diabetes[b]	Type 1 diabetes
Preoperative	Stop biguanides	Stabilize on at least twice-daily insulin for 2–3 days preoperatively. One day preoperatively, use only short-acting insulin (Actrapid soluble or neutral)
Perioperative	Omit oral hypoglycaemic. Estimate blood glucose level	Do not give sulphonylurea or subcutaneous insulin on day of operation. Estimate blood glucose level. Set up intravenous infusion of 10% glucose 500 mL containing Actrapid or Leo neutral insulin 10 units plus potassium chloride 1 g at 8.00 am. Infuse over 4 h. Estimate blood glucose and potassium levels 2-hourly. Adjust insulin and potassium to keep glucose at 5–10 mmol/L and normokalaemic
Postoperative	Estimate blood glucose 4 h postoperatively	Continue infusion 4-hourly. Estimate blood glucose 4-hourly. Estimate potassium 8-hourly
On resuming normal diet	Start sulphonylurea or other usual regimen	Stop infusion. Start Actrapid or Leo neutral insulin and continue over the next 2 days. Start sulphonylurea. Start normal insulin regimen

[a]Check for local guidance protocols, and with anaesthetist.
[b]If well controlled, otherwise treat as type 1.

Box 6.3 *Drugs that may change blood glucose*

- Adrenaline (epinephrine)
- Alcohol
- Anabolic steroids
- Angiotensin-converting enzyme inhibitors
- Antiretroviral protease inhibitors
- Appetite suppressants
- Aspirin and aspirin-like drugs
- Beta-blockers
- Certain medicines used for depression and emotional or psychotic disturbances
- Chromium
- Ciclosporin
- Cisapride
- Clonidine
- Corticosteroids
- Diazoxide
- Diuretics
- Female hormones
- Glucagon
- Growth hormone (somatotropin)
- Guanethidine
- Lithium
- Male hormones
- Medicines for allergies, asthma, cold or cough
- Metoclopramide
- Pentamidine
- Pentoxifylline
- Phenytoin
- Propoxyphene
- Quinolone antibiotics
- Some herbal dietary supplements
- Sulphonamides
- Tacrolimus
- Thyroid hormones

Careful planning is required at all stages of the patient pathway from GP referral to postoperative discharge. The patient should be involved in planning for all stages. Hospital patient administration systems should be able to identify all patients with diabetes so that they can be prioritized on the operating list. High-risk patients (poor glycaemic control/complications of diabetes) should be identified in surgical outpatients or at preoperative assessment, and plans should be put in place to manage their risk.

Early preoperative assessment should be arranged to determine a perioperative diabetes management strategy and to identify and optimize other co-morbidities.

Routine overnight admission for preoperative management of diabetes should not be necessary.

Starvation time should be minimized by prioritizing patients on the operating list.

The aim should be earlier mobilization with resumption of normal diet and return to usual diabetes management. Multimodal analgesia should be combined with appropriate antiemetics to enable an early return to normal diet and the usual diabetes regimen.

The term 'variable rate intravenous insulin infusion' (VRIII) should replace the ambiguous 'sliding scale'. Patients with a planned short starvation period (no more than one missed meal in total) should be managed by modification of their usual diabetes medication, avoiding a VRIII wherever possible. Those expected to miss more than one meal should have a VRIII. The recommended first-choice substrate solution for a VRIII is 0.45% sodium chloride with 5% glucose and either 0.15% potassium chloride (KCl) or 0.3% KCl.

Insulin should be prescribed according to National Patient Safety Agency (NPSA) recommendations for its safe use. Capillary blood glucose (CBG) levels should be monitored and recorded at least hourly during the procedure and in the immediate postoperative period.

The World Health Organization (WHO) surgical safety checklist bundle should be implemented. The target blood glucose should be 6–10 mmol/L (acceptable range 4–12 mmol/L).

The above also applies to patients presenting for emergency surgery, with the proviso that many such patients are high-risk and are likely to require an intravenous insulin infusion and level 1 care (acute ward with input from critical care team) as a minimum.

General assessment

Exclude cardiac, renal and neurological issues that may complicate perioperative management and increase patient risk. Ensure that no other diabetes-related problems (e.g. retinopathy) need attention.

Assessment of glycaemic control

HbA$_{1c}$ is an indicator of recent control (the previous 3 months). If it is above 9%, control is poor; if above 12%, control must be improved before elective surgery.

Perioperative blood glucose control

Patients on diet alone or oral hypoglycaemic agents

Minor operations (dental, body surface or endoscopic procedures).

- Omit oral hypoglycaemic therapy on the day of the operation and avoid glucose infusions.
- Check fingerprick blood glucose on the morning of the operation and regularly thereafter.
- Operate on these patients early in the morning.
- Note that there is no need to stop metformin any sooner than on the day of surgery. Oral medication, *except for metformin*, should be restarted as normally prescribed with the first meal. Lactic acidosis is more likely if renal impairment is present and so metformin should not be restarted postoperatively unless renal function is known to be satisfactory. Metformin should not be used if the estimated glomerular filtration rate (eGFR) is below 30, and doses not higher than 500 mg b.d. are advised for patients with an eGFR of 30–49. If metformin is contraindicated, then additional hypoglycaemic therapy may be required. If in doubt, contact the diabetes team for advice.

Major operations
- Patients undergoing major operations will require intravenous insulin therapy after fasting.
- Patients on oral therapy who are inadequately controlled (i.e. random venous blood glucose >15.0 mmol/L or HbA$_{1c}$ >9%) should be stabilized on insulin preoperatively and managed in the same way as insulin-treated patients (see below).

Management of patients (type 1 and type 2) on insulin
For surgical procedures, the essential requirement is to avoid hypoglycaemia but to keep hyperglycaemia below levels that may be harmful because of delayed wound healing or phagocyte dysfunction. The desired whole-blood glucose level is therefore 3–5 mmol/L. For major surgery, intermediate insulins are usually omitted and an intravenous infusion is given that contains glucose, to which, according to the level of plasma glucose, regularly measured, soluble (regular) insulin can be added as required. The effects of stress and trauma may raise insulin requirements and precipitate ketosis.

More protracted procedures, such as multiple extractions, must only be carried out in hospital, with the precautions described below.

Preoperatively
- All patients on insulin should be adequately controlled preoperatively and stabilized over 48 hours:
  For patients using twice-daily insulin, this may be possible with their usual regime but may involve switching them to a multiple injection regimen.
  For people with type 1 diabetes on multiple daily insulin regimens, it is advisable to continue their 'usual' daily long-acting analogue insulin, as this will reduce the risk of diabetic ketoacidosis if intravenous insulin is interrupted, and will facilitate a smooth transition to subcutaneous insulin at a suitable mealtime postoperatively.
- Remember that *some patients with type 2 diabetes may be treated with both insulin and metformin* – see above before restarting metformin.
- On the day prior to operation, check random venous blood glucose and urea and electrolytes.

Day-case surgery
- Aim for 'first on list'.
- For those on a multiple injection regimen, continue the usual basal (long-acting) insulin on the evening prior to the procedure.
- For patients on twice-daily insulin, continue the usual evening insulin prior to the procedure.

- Fast the patient from midnight and omit the morning insulin.
- Check a fingerprick blood glucose before and after the procedure.
- Resume the usual insulin and diet after the procedure. If a b.d. insulin regimen is restarted at lunchtime, it is recommended that half of the normal 'breakfast' insulin dose should be prescribed with lunch after the procedure.
- The above applies if rapid recovery is expected, i.e. the patient is expected to be eating within 2 hours of the procedure.
- If the patient is unable to tolerate the diet or the blood glucose is >14 mmol/L, then a glucose, potassium and insulin (GKI) infusion or alternative will be required.

Major surgery
On the morning of the operation:

- check blood glucose and commence an intravenous GKI infusion
- *ensure that the patient does not receive subcutaneous rapid-acting or premixed insulin on the day of surgery.* The last dose of either type of insulin should have been given on the previous evening
- continue checking blood glucose hourly – before, during and after the operation.

Postoperatively
- Change to subcutaneous insulin postoperatively when the patient is eating normally.
- *Continue the intravenous insulin infusion for 60 minutes after the first subcutaneous insulin injection.*
- If the patient has previously been poorly controlled (HbA$_{1c}$ >9%), refer to the diabetes team for advice before discharge.

ADRENAL CORTEX

The hypothalamus is in overall control of adrenocortical function by producing factors that stimulate the pituitary to release adrenocorticotropic hormone (Fig. 6.12). ACTH arises from a precursor, pro-opiomelanocortin, and is released in response to hypothalamic corticotropin-releasing hormone (CRH), with a diurnal rhythm (peak early morning, nadir on retiring). Circulating corticosteroids have a negative feedback control on hypothalamic activity and ACTH production. There is thus a hypothalamic–pituitary–adrenocortical (HPA) axis. Glucocorticoid production is stimulated by ACTH (corticotropin) from the anterior pituitary gland, and cortisol exerts a negative feedback on the pituitary and hypothalamus. The adrenal cortex produces a series of corticosteroids, mainly cortisol (hydrocortisone) and corticosterone (the glucocorticoids), and aldosterone (the mineralocorticoid).

Corticosteroids are an essential part of the body's response to stresses such as trauma, infection, GA or operation, pain, stress, fever, burns and hypoglycaemia. At such times, there is normally raised adrenal corticosteroid production and the size of the response is proportional to the degree of stress.

Mineralocorticoid (aldosterone) production is regulated mainly by the renin–angiotensin system, renal blood pressure, and sodium and potassium levels. Renin, an enzyme that converts angiotensinogen to angiotensin 1, is produced by the renal juxtaglomerular apparatus in response to low sodium or renal perfusion (Fig. 6.13). Angiotensin 1 is converted by angiotensin-converting enzyme in the lung parenchyma, to the active angiotensin 2, which stimulates aldosterone release. Aldosterone acts on the kidney to promote sodium retention, potassium excretion and fluid retention, and causes vasoconstriction and thirst.

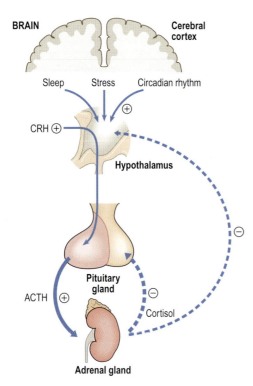

Fig. 6.12 Adrenal control homeostasis. ACTH = adrenocorticotropic hormone; CRH = corticotropin-releasing hormone.

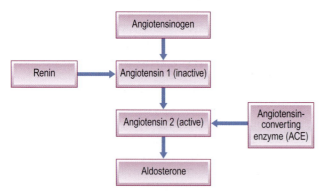

Fig. 6.13 Blood pressure regulation via aldosterone production.

Table 6.15 *Causes of adrenal insufficiency*

Patient on systemic corticosteroids	Adrenal disorders	Hypopituitarism
Trauma	Addison disease	
Operation	Post-adrenalectomy	
General anaesthesia	Waterhouse–Friderichsen syndrome (adrenal haemorrhage caused by septicaemia, anticoagulants or epilepsy)	
Infection		
	Congenital adrenal hyperplasia	

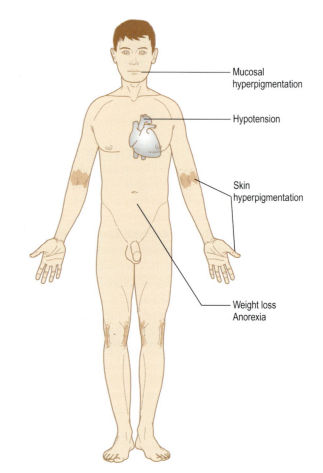

Fig. 6.14 Hypoadrenocorticism.

Atrial natriuretic peptide, synthesized by myocytes in the right atrium and ventricles, causes sodium loss and thus counters the effect of aldosterone.

ADRENOCORTICAL HYPOFUNCTION

Adrenocortical hypofunction can lead to hypotension, shock and death if the individual is stressed – for example, by operation, infection or trauma.

Adrenocortical hypofunction is due most commonly to ACTH (corticotropin) deficiency caused by the suppression of adrenocortical function following the use of systemic corticosteroids (secondary hypoadrenocorticism); occasionally by acquired adrenal disease (primary hypoadrenocorticism); and rarely, by a congenital defect in corticosteroid biosynthesis (congenital adrenal hyperplasia; Table 6.15).

Primary hypoadrenocorticism (Addison disease)

Primary hypoadrenocorticism is rare; it is caused by autoantibodies to the adrenal cortex, leading to adrenocortical atrophy and failed hormone secretion – cortisol (hydrocortisone) and aldosterone. Patients also have a higher incidence of other endocrine deficiencies (see later), vitiligo and, occasionally, chronic mucocutaneous candidosis.

Primary hypoadrenocorticism occasionally has other adrenal causes (though the term *primary* is then really a misnomer), such as tuberculosis, histoplasmosis (particularly secondary to human immunodeficiency virus [HIV] infection), malignancy, haemorrhage, sarcoidosis, amyloidosis, or adrenalectomy for metastatic breast cancer.

Clinical features

Lack of cortisol predisposes to hypotension and hypoglycaemia but stimulates the HPA, causing release of pro-opiomelanocortin, which has ACTH and melanocyte-stimulating hormone (MSH) activity and can cause hyperpigmentation. Lack of aldosterone leads to sodium depletion, reduced extracellular fluid volume and hypotension (Fig. 6.14).

The lack of adrenocortical reserve makes patients vulnerable to any stress such as infection, trauma, surgery or anaesthesia, though they may be asymptomatic otherwise. An acute adrenal crisis (Addisonian crisis or shock) is thus characterized by collapse, bradycardia, hypotension, profound weakness, hypoglycaemia, vomiting and dehydration.

Patients with hypoadrenocorticism also suffer from fatigue and weakness, lethargy, weight loss, anorexia, nausea, vomiting, diarrhoea, hyperpigmentation, dizziness and postural hypotension (Box 6.4).

General management

Diagnosis of hypoadrenocorticism is confirmed by: hypotension; sometimes, low plasma sodium and raised potassium; plasma glucose assay (hypoglycaemia is common); and low plasma cortisol levels and depressed cortisol responses to ACTH stimulation. Blood for plasma cortisol estimation (10 mL in a lithium heparin tube, or plain tube) should be taken at 8.00 or 9.00 a.m. In hypoadrenocorticism, the basal plasma cortisol level is usually lower than 6 mg/100 mL (170 nmol/L), often lower than 100 nmol/L. In early hypoadrenocorticism, the cortisol levels may still be in the low normal range and therefore a short ACTH stimulation test is indicated. Plasma is collected before and 30 min after 250 mg of tetracosactrin (synthetic ACTH; Synacthen) is injected intramuscularly or intravenously. In health, the plasma cortisol level normally doubles from at least 200 nmol/L to more than 500 nmol/L after tetracosactrin. In hypoadrenocorticism, the basal cortisol level is low and does not rise by more than 200 nmol/L after tetracosactrin is given.

Estimation of serum ACTH levels differentiates primary (ACTH raised, usually above 200 ng/L) from secondary (ACTH low or normal) hypoadrenocorticism.

Serum should be tested for autoantibodies to various tissues, especially endocrine glands, and other investigations may be needed, including radiography or CT or MRI scans of the skull (for pituitary abnormalities), chest (for tuberculosis) or abdomen (for adrenal calcification suggestive of tuberculosis or a mycosis).

A warning card should be carried (Fig. 6.15) and most patients are treated with oral hydrocortisone and fludrocortisone.

Dental aspects

Adrenal crisis is rare in dentistry; a recent publication identified only six reports in the past 65 years or so. Risks included unrecognized adrenal insufficiency, poor health status and stability at the time of treatment, pain, infection, having undergone an invasive procedure and receipt of a barbiturate GA. Drugs such as barbiturates can accelerate cortisol metabolism and can exacerbate the situation, as can aminoglutethimide, azole antifungals, etomidate, metyrapone, phenytoin and rifampicin.

Nevertheless, despite the low risk, the danger of precipitating hypotensive collapse is such that corticosteroids must be given

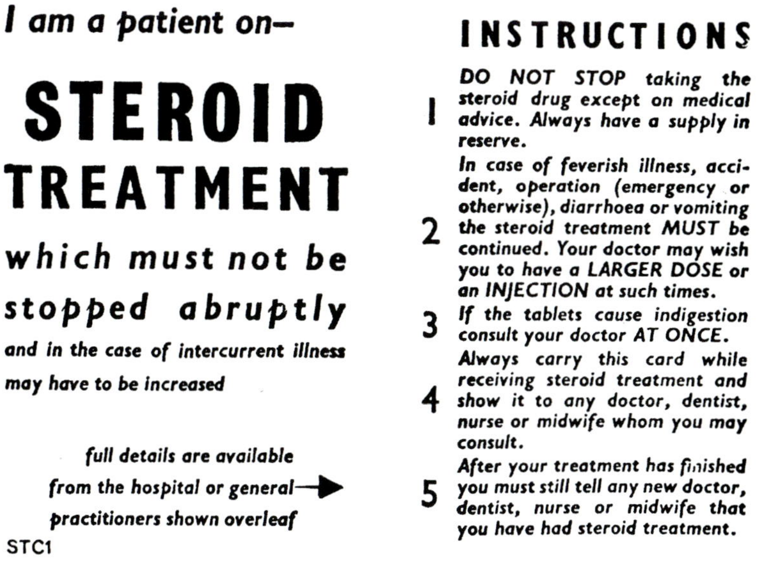

I am a patient on—

STEROID
TREATMENT

which must not be stopped abruptly and in the case of intercurrent illness may have to be increased

full details are available from the hospital or general → practitioners shown overleaf

STC1

INSTRUCTIONS

1. **DO NOT STOP** taking the steroid drug except on medical advice. Always have a supply in reserve.

2. In case of feverish illness, accident, operation (emergency or otherwise), diarrhoea or vomiting the steroid treatment MUST be continued. Your doctor may wish you to have a LARGER DOSE or an INJECTION at such times.

3. If the tablets cause indigestion consult your doctor AT ONCE.

4. Always carry this card while receiving steroid treatment and show it to any doctor, dentist, nurse or midwife whom you may consult.

5. After your treatment has finished you must still tell any new doctor, dentist, nurse or midwife that you have had steroid treatment.

Fig. 6.15 Steroid warning card. This is a blue card that should be carried at all times by patients with hypoadrenocorticism or on systemic corticosteroids in view of the danger of an adrenocortical crisis and collapse if the patient is subject to trauma, stress or anaesthesia. (By permission of the Controller of Her Majesty's Stationery Office).

preoperatively. CS should generally be avoided unless the patient has had corticosteroid cover. GA is obviously a matter for the expert anaesthetist in hospital.

For dental surgery under LA, the glucocorticoid dose should be doubled (up to 20 mg hydrocortisone) 1 hour before surgery. After the procedure, the dose of oral medication is doubled for 24 hours, and then the normal dose is reinstated (http://cks.nice.org.uk/addisons-disease; accessed 30 September 2013).

Brown or black pigmentation of the mucosa is seen in over 75% of patients with Addison disease, but is not a feature of corticosteroid-induced hypoadrenocorticism or of hypoadrenocorticism secondary to hypothalamopituitary disease. Hyperpigmentation is related to high levels of MSH and affects particularly those areas normally pigmented or exposed to trauma (e.g. in the buccal mucosa at the occlusal line, or the tongue, but also the gingivae). Other causes of oral pigmentation (Ch. 11; especially racial pigmentation) are far more common and need to be differentiated. Addison disease is a rare cause but must be considered, particularly if there is hypotension, weakness, weight loss, anorexia, nausea, vomiting or abdominal pain.

Acute adrenal insufficiency has several causes (see Table 6.15) and is managed as described in Chapter 1.

Secondary adrenocortical insufficiency

Secondary adrenocortical insufficiency can be caused by corticosteroid therapy and ACTH deficiency as a result of hypothalamic or pituitary disease. It is then associated with other endocrine defects but *no* hyperpigmentation (ACTH levels are low) and blood pressure is virtually normal (aldosterone secretion is normal).

Congenital adrenal hyperplasia

Congenital adrenal hyperplasia is the term given to a group of rare autosomal recessive inborn errors of corticosteroid metabolism characterized by defects in 21-hydroxylase or 11-hydroxylase, resulting in lack of cortisol (adrenal insufficiency) and androgen excess. Male precocious puberty or female ambiguous genitalia can result.

Box 6.5 *Hyperadrenocorticism: clinical features*

- Weakness
- Weight gain
- Truncal obesity
- Hypertension
- Hirsutism
- Amenorrhoea
- Cutaneous striae
- Personality changes

ADRENOCORTICAL HYPERFUNCTION

Adrenocortical hyperfunction may lead to release of excessive:

- glucocorticoids (Cushing disease)
- mineralocorticoids (Conn syndrome or hyperaldosteronism)
- androgens (congenital adrenal hyperplasia).

Cushing disease

General aspects

Cushing disease is caused by excess glucocorticoid production by adrenal hyperplasia secondary to excess ACTH production by pituitary basophil adenomas. It is occasionally caused by ectopic ACTH from adrenal or other tumours, such as small-cell lung carcinomas or carcinoid tumours. A similar clinical picture results where there is ectopic production by a tumour (usually a bronchial carcinoid tumour) of CRH.

Cushing syndrome is clinically similar but is caused by primary adrenal disease (adenoma or rarely carcinoma or micronodular bilateral hyperplasia). However, most cases of Cushing syndrome have been found to be due to microadenomas of the pituitary, so that the terms Cushing disease and Cushing syndrome are in effect synonymous.

A similar clinical picture is produced by corticosteroid therapy or rarely by the multiple endocrine adenoma syndromes (see later).

Clinical features

These are listed in Box 6.5. The most obvious feature is central obesity, affecting the abdomen and also the face (moon face; Fig. 6.16). Facial photographs from the past and more recently may show the development of moon face, interscapular region (buffalo hump) and trunk, but with relative sparing of the limbs. Hypertension is common. Breakdown of proteins with conversion to glucose (gluconeogenesis) leads to hyperglycaemia and possibly diabetes mellitus, osteoporosis, muscle weakness, thinning of the skin, purpura and purplish skin striae (Figs. 6.17 and 6.18). Other features may include hirsutism and acne, oligomenorrhoea, infections and psychoses (Fig. 6.19).

General management

The main differential diagnoses are severe depression and alcoholism.

The diagnosis is confirmed by a raised plasma cortisol level and absence of the normal diurnal variation in cortisol levels, normally highest in the morning around 8.00 a.m. and lowest at midnight. Another useful screening test is to measure plasma cortisol at 8.00–9.00 a.m. after giving 1 mg dexamethasone orally at midnight to suppress the adrenal glands temporarily; in health, cortisol levels fall but in Cushing syndrome there is no such fall (low-dose overnight dexamethasone suppression test).

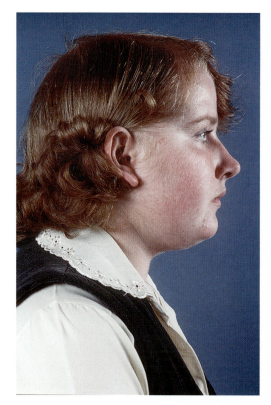

Fig. 6.16 Moon face in a patient with Cushing syndrome.

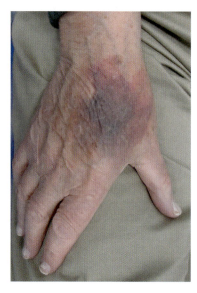

Fig. 6.17 Steroid purpura.

Localization of the cause as adrenal, pituitary or ectopic tumour relies on the CRH stimulation test, which in turn depends on the fact that the pituitary responds to CRH, whereas adrenal and other tumours producing ectopic ACTH do not. Baseline plasma ACTH and cortisol levels are first obtained, CRH is then given, and an exaggerated rise in ACTH and cortisol levels is demonstrated by patients with pituitary Cushing but not by patients with other types of Cushing syndrome. Other special dexamethasone tests or sampling from the inferior petrosal sinus are needed to distinguish pituitary from adrenal causes of Cushing syndrome. Other diagnostic aids include pituitary MRI, tomography of the sella turcica, abdominal CT and adrenal ultrasound scans.

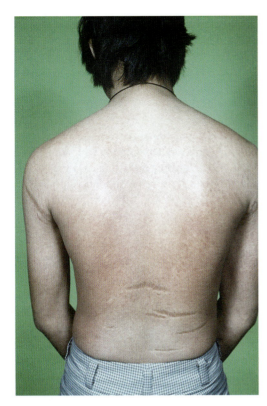

Fig. 6.18 Systemic corticosteroid therapy causes several complications, including cutaneous striae as shown here.

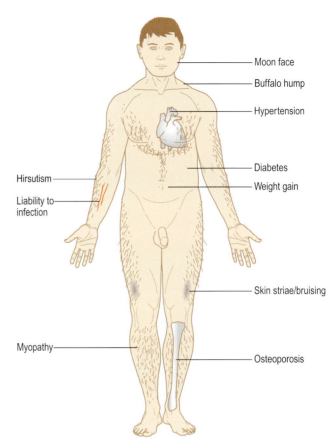

Moon face
Buffalo hump
Hypertension
Diabetes
Hirsutism
Weight gain
Liability to infection
Skin striae/bruising
Myopathy
Osteoporosis

Fig. 6.19 Cushing syndrome.

In Cushing disease, the pituitary tumour is treated by trans-sphenoidal microadenectomy and then, for those not cured, by pituitary irradiation or an yttrium implant. Cyproheptadine or sodium valproate is sometimes used where surgery is inappropriate.

In Cushing syndrome, the adrenal gland is usually irradiated or excised (adrenalectomy), though ketoconazole, mitotane, aminoglutethimide or metyrapone can also be effective. Some patients subjected to bilateral adrenalectomy develop pituitary ACTH-producing adenomas with hyperpigmentation and symptoms related to the pituitary tumour (Nelson syndrome). Cushing syndrome secondary to carcinoma of the bronchus is not controllable by surgery but metyrapone, an inhibitor of hydroxylation in the adrenal cortex, can relieve symptoms.

Steroid replacement is subsequently necessary in treated Cushing disease/syndrome. Subacute adrenal insufficiency develops if corticosteroid dosage is reduced too quickly after replacement therapy in postsurgical patients with Cushing syndrome. Features include lethargy, abdominal pain, hypotension and psychological disturbances, and a characteristic sign is scaly desquamation of the facial skin, particularly of the forehead.

Dental aspects

LA is preferred for pain control. CS can be given, preferably with nitrous oxide and oxygen. GA must be carried out in hospital.

Management complications may include:

- the need for corticosteroid cover; patients, once treated, are maintained on corticosteroid replacement therapy and then are at risk from an adrenal crisis if subjected to operation, anaesthesia or trauma
- hypertension
- cardiovascular disease
- diabetes mellitus
- psychosis

- vertebral collapse or myopathy causing limited mobility
- multiple endocrine adenomatosis (MEA I; see later).

There are no specific oral manifestations of Cushing disease, but patients have been referred for a suspected dental cause of the swollen face.

Hyperaldosteronism

General aspects

Primary hyperaldosteronism (Conn syndrome) arises from an adrenal cortex benign tumour or hyperplasia. Secondary hyperaldosteronism arises from activation of the renin–angiotensin system in cirrhosis, nephrotic syndrome, severe cardiac failure or renal artery stenosis.

Clinical features

High aldosterone secretion leads to potassium loss (hypokalaemia) – causing muscle weakness and cramps, paraesthesia, polyuria and polydipsia, and, since it is associated with a metabolic alkalosis, possibly tetany – and sodium retention (causing hypertension but rarely oedema).

General management

Amiloride, or the aldosterone antagonist spironolactone, is given until the affected adrenal gland can be excised.

Dental aspects

LA is used for pain control. CS may be helpful, especially if there is hypertension. GA must, as always, be carried out in hospital. In the

Table 6.16 *Some uses of systemic corticosteroids*

Adrenal insufficiency	Addison disease
	Adrenalectomy
	Hypopituitarism
Allergic disorders	Asthma
Blood dyscrasias	Idiopathic thrombocytopenia
	Lymphocytic leukaemia
	Lymphoma
Connective tissue disorders	Rheumatoid arthritis (rarely)
	Systemic lupus erythematosus
Gastrointestinal disorders	Ulcerative colitis
	Crohn disease
Mucocutaneous diseases	Pemphigus
Post-transplantation	Any organ transplant
Renal disorders	Nephrotic syndrome
	Renal transplants

Table 6.17 *Approximate potencies of systemic corticosteroids relative to cortisol[a]*

Short-acting		Medium-acting		Long-acting	
Cortisone	1	Triamcinolone	5	Betamethasone	25
Methylprednisolone	5			Dexamethasone	30
Prednisolone	4				
Prednisone	4				

[a]Cortisol (hydrocortisone) = 1.

untreated patient, hypertension and muscle weakness are the main complications. Competitive muscle relaxants may be dangerous, as they can cause profound paralysis.

If bilateral adrenalectomy has been carried out, the patient is at risk from collapse during dental treatment and therefore requires corticosteroid cover.

Autoimmune polyendocrinopathy syndrome

See later.

SYSTEMIC CORTICOSTEROID THERAPY

General aspects

Corticosteroids are frequently used to suppress inflammation and to suppress graft rejection, and occasionally to replace missing hormones (in Addison disease or after adrenalectomy; Table 6.16). Steroids have different potencies (Table 6.17).

Corticosteroids are an essential part of the body's response to stresses such as trauma, infection, GA or operation. At such times there is normally an enhanced adrenal corticosteroid response related to the degree of stress. In patients given exogenous steroids, the enhanced adrenal corticosteroid response may not follow.

Corticosteroids have a negative feedback control on hypothalamic activity and ACTH production; there is thus suppression of the HPA axis and the adrenals may become unable to produce a steroid response to stress. When the adrenal cortex is unable to produce the necessary steroid response to stress, acute adrenal insufficiency (adrenal crisis) can result, with rapidly developing hypotension, collapse and possibly death.

Suppression of the HPA axis becomes profound if corticosteroid treatment has been prolonged and/or the dose of steroids exceeds physiological levels (more than about 7.5 mg/day of prednisolone [prednisone]). Adrenal suppression is less when the exogenous steroid is given on alternate days or as a single morning dose (rather than as divided doses through the day). ACTH (corticotropin) has been used in the hope of reducing adrenal suppression but the response is variable and unpredictable, and wanes with time.

However, adrenal function may even be suppressed for up to a week after cessation of steroid treatment lasting only 5 days. If steroid treatment is for longer periods, adrenal function may be suppressed for at least 30 days and perhaps for 2–24 months after the cessation of treatment. Patients who are on corticosteroid therapy, or have been on it within the past 30 days, may be at risk from adrenal crisis; those who have been on corticosteroids during the previous 24 months may also be at risk, if they are not given supplementary corticosteroids before and during periods of stress such as operation, GA, infection or trauma. Patients who have used systemic corticosteroids should be warned of the danger and should carry a steroid card indicating the dosage and the responsible physician (see Fig. 6.15). Metal bracelets or necklaces with the diagnosis engraved on them are available: for example, from MedicAlert Foundation (http://www.medicalert.org.uk).

However, the frequency and extent of the adrenocortical suppression (and the need for supplementary corticosteroids before and during periods of stress) are unclear and have been questioned. Although the evidence for the need for steroid cover may be questionable, medicolegal and other considerations suggest that one should err on the side of caution and fully inform and discuss with the patient, take medical advice in any case of doubt, and give steroid cover unless confident that collapse is unlikely.

Clinical features

Long-term systemic use of corticosteroids can cause many other adverse effects, often beginning soon after the start of treatment, and can lead to significant morbidity or mortality (Table 6.18). Complications includes immediately obvious effects such as Cushingoid weight gain around the face (moon face) and upper back (buffalo hump), and hirsutism. Other possible complications are shown in Table 6.18.

General management

Complications may be reduced but not abolished if steroids are given on alternate days. In order listed above, patients on systemic steroids are usually monitored and given drugs prophylactically:

- There should be no contraindications such as hypertension (Ch. 5), diabetes or latent tuberculosis.
- The smallest effective steroid dose should be given, ideally in the morning on alternate days.
- Systemic corticosteroids cause the greatest risk of adrenocortical suppression, so topical steroids should always be used in preference, provided that the desired therapeutic effect is achievable. However, there can even be adrenocortical suppression from extensive application of steroid skin preparations, particularly if occlusive dressings are used, or from some use in the mouth if ulceration is extensive and potent steroids are used.
- The patient must be given a warning card and told about the dangers of withdrawal and about side-effects. There should never be abrupt withdrawal of the steroid. The dose should be raised if there is illness, infection, trauma or operation.

Table 6.18 *Complications of systemic corticosteroid therapy*

Cardiovascular	Cerebrovascular accidents
	Hypertension
	Myocardial infarction
Dermatological	Acne
	Bruising
	Hirsutism
	Striae
Gastrointestinal	Peptic ulcer
Immunosuppressive	Increased susceptibility to infections
	Neoplasms in the long term
Neurological	Cataracts
	Mood changes
	Psychosis
Metabolic	Fat redistribution (moon face and buffalo hump)
	Growth retardation
	Hypothalamic–pituitary–adrenal suppression
	Impaired glucose tolerance or diabetes mellitus
	Loss of sodium and potassium
	Muscle weakness
	Osteoporosis
	Weight gain

- Weight, chest radiography, bone mineral density, blood pressure and blood glucose baseline measures should be taken and these parameters monitored.
- Ranitidine and calcitriol or disodium etidronate are often given.

Dental aspects

Cortisol is the major glucocorticoid in humans and is involved in metabolic processes, vascular tonicity, inflammatory responses and the control of response to stresses such as trauma, infection, GA or surgery. Secretion from the adrenals is regulated via the HPA axis by involving ACTH. In patients given exogenous corticosteroids (steroids), this feedback response may not occur and acute adrenal insufficiency (adrenal crisis) may result, as the adrenal cortex is unable to produce the necessary steroid response to stress.

Suppression of the HPA axis becomes deeper if treatment with exogenous steroids is prolonged and the dose exceeds physiological levels (over 7.5 mg/day of prednisolone [prednisone]).

Adrenal suppression is likely if the patient is currently on daily systemic corticosteroids at doses of 10 mg prednisolone or above, or has been in the last 3 months.

Adrenocortical function may be suppressed if:

- the patient is currently on daily systemic corticosteroids at doses above 5 mg prednisolone
- corticosteroids have been taken regularly during the previous 30 days
- corticosteroids have been taken for more than 1 month during the past year.

During intercurrent illness or infection, after trauma, or before operation or anaesthesia, these patients may require a higher steroid dosage. Steroid supplementation should be considered before stressful procedures. It is recognized that dentoalveolar or maxillofacial surgery may result in stress, but most other forms of dental treatment cause little response.

Table 6.19 *Suggested management of patients with a history of systemic corticosteroid therapy*

Procedure	No steroids for previous 12 months	Steroids taken during previous 12 months	Steroids currently taken
Conservative dentistry or dentoalveolar surgery (e.g. single extraction under LA)	No cover required	Give usual oral steroid dose in morning or hydrocortisone[a] 25–50 mg i.v. preoperatively	Double oral steroid dose in morning or give hydrocortisone[a] 25–50 mg i.v. preoperatively Continue normal steroid medication postoperatively
Intermediate surgery (e.g. multiple extractions, or surgery under GA)	Consider cover if large doses of steroid were given. Test adrenocortical function (ACTH stimulation test)	Give usual oral steroid dose in morning plus hydrocortisone[a] 25–50 mg i.v. preoperatively and i.m. 6-hourly for 24 h	Double oral steroid dose in morning plus give hydrocortisone[a] 25–50 mg i.v. preoperatively and i.m. 6-hourly for 24 h. Then continue normal medication
Maxillofacial surgery or trauma	Consider cover if large doses of steroid were given. Test adrenocortical function (ACTH stimulation test)	Give usual oral steroid dose in morning plus hydrocortisone[a] 25–50 mg i.v. preoperatively and i.m. 6-hourly for 72 h	Double oral steroid dose in morning plus give hydrocortisone[a] 25–50 mg i.v. preoperatively and i.m. 6-hourly for 72 h. Then continue normal medication

[a]Hydrocortisone sodium succinate (e.g. Efcortelan soluble) or phosphate given immediately preoperatively and blood pressure monitored.

Patients on long-term systemic steroid medication have been recommended to receive supplementary glucocorticoids or 'steroid cover' when undergoing certain types of stressful treatment, including dentistry. Several studies, however, confirm the low likelihood of significant adrenal insufficiency, even following major surgical procedures.

Patients on long-term steroid medication may therefore not require supplementary 'steroid cover' for routine dentistry, including minor surgical procedures, under LA. Those with adrenal hypofunction or those undergoing GA for surgical procedures may require supplement-ary steroids, depending on the dose of steroid and duration of treatment. Individuals who have taken steroids in excess of 10 mg prednisolone, or equivalent, within the last 3 months, should be considered for supplementation. Patients who have not received steroids for more than 3 months are considered to have full recovery of the HPA axis and require no supplementation. Traditionally, minor operations under LA were covered by giving the usual oral steroid dose in the morning and oral steroids 2–4 hours pre- and postoperatively (25–50 mg hydrocortisone or 20 mg prednisolone or 4 mg dexamethasone) or by giving intravenous 25–50 mg hydrocortisone immediately before operation (Table 6.19). These Nicholson's guidelines are not universally accepted, as they require intravenous administration of steroids. For this reason, regimens such as doubling the normal daily oral steroid dose on the day of procedure (Gibson & Ferguson, 2004) are now more commonly used.

The blood pressure must be carefully watched during surgery and especially during recovery, and steroid supplementation given immediately if it starts to fall. Intravenous hydrocortisone must be immediately available for use if the blood pressure falls or the patient collapses.

Cover for major operations can be provided by giving at least 25–50 mg hydrocortisone sodium succinate intramuscularly or intravenously (with the pre-medication) and then 6-hourly for a further 24–72 hours (see Table 6.19). Corticosteroids given by intramuscular injection are more slowly absorbed and reach lower plasma levels than when given intravenously or orally.

Drugs, especially sedatives and general anaesthetics, are a hazard and it is extremely important to avoid hypoxia, hypotension or haemorrhage. Patients may also require special management as a result of diabetes, hypertension, poor wound healing or infections. Aspirin and other NSAIDs should be avoided, as they may increase the risk of peptic ulceration. Osteoporosis introduces the danger of fractures when handling the patient.

Topical corticosteroids for use in the mouth are unlikely to have any systemic effect but predispose to oral candidosis. Susceptibility to infection is increased by systemic steroid use (see later) and there is a predisposition to herpes virus infections (particularly herpes simplex). Chickenpox is an especial hazard to those who are not immune and fulminant disease can result. Passive immunization with varicella zoster immunoglobulin is indicated for non-immune patients who are on systemic corticosteroids (or who have been on them within the previous 3 months), if exposed to chickenpox or zoster. Immunization should be given within 3 days of exposure.

Wound healing is impaired and wound infections are more frequent. In addition to careful aseptic surgery, prophylactic antimicrobials may be indicated.

Long-term and profound immunosuppression may lead to the appearance of hairy leukoplakia, Kaposi sarcoma, lymphomas, lip cancer, oral keratosis or other oral complications (Ch. 20).

Corticosteroids can also mask the presence of many serious diseases that may influence dental care, as well as causing suppression of the adrenocortical response to stress (see Table 6.19 for management).

POLYCYSTIC OVARY SYNDROME (PCOS)

Polycystic ovary syndrome (PCOS) presents with hirsutism, acne, oligo-menorrhoea and subfertility. Other features include obesity, acanthosis nigricans and hypertension (and premature balding in male relatives).

ADRENAL MEDULLA

The adrenal medulla secretes the catecholamines noradrenaline (norepinephrine) and adrenaline (epinephrine) in response to hypotension, hypoglycaemia and other stress, their release being regulated by the central nervous system.

PHAEOCHROMOCYTOMA

General aspects

Phaeochromocytomas are rare, usually benign tumours; they are most commonly found in the adrenal medulla (producing adrenaline [epinephrine]) but others arise in other neuroectodermal tissues such as paraganglia or the sympathetic chain and produce noradrenaline (norepinephrine) or dopamine. Ten per cent of phaeochromocytomas are familial, 10% are bilateral, 10% are outside the adrenals and 10% are malignant. Phaeochromocytomas may occasionally be associated with other tumours – neurofibromatosis; endocrine tumours, particularly medullary carcinoma of the thyroid and hyperparathyroidism (multiple endocrine adenomatosis: MEA II or III [see later]); von Hippel–Lindau disease (cerebelloretinal haemangioblastomatosis); and

gastric leiomyosarcoma, pulmonary chondroma and testicular tumours (Carney triad).

Clinical features

Typical features are episodes of anxiety, headache, epigastric discomfort, palpitations, tachycardia, arrhythmias, hypertension, sweating, pyrexia, flushing and glycosuria.

General management

Plasma catecholamines (collected at rest in the supine position) may be raised but are less reliable than urinary assays. Diagnosis is supported by finding excessive urinary catecholamines and their metabolites, such as vanillylmandelic acid (VMA) or metanephrines. The tumour is located by CT, MRI, venous catheterization, arteriography, ultrasonography and radionuclide scanning, such as iodine-131–meta-iodobenzylguanidine (MIBG). The tumour is excised after the blood pressure has been controlled with an alpha-blocking agent (e.g. phenoxybenzamine) and a beta-blocker.

Dental aspects

Acute hypertension and arrhythmias may complicate dental treatment. Elective treatment should therefore be deferred until after surgical treatment of the phaeochromocytoma. If emergency care is required, the blood pressure should first be controlled with alpha-blockers (such as phenoxybenzamine or prazosin) and then beta-adrenergic blockers (such as propanolol).

Patients who have had adrenal surgery may suffer from hypoadreno-corticism, since the adrenal cortex is inevitably damaged at operation. These patients therefore require steroid cover at operation. Local analgesia is then generally safe and adrenaline (epinephrine) in modest amounts is unlikely to have any significant adverse effect. CS may be desirable to control anxiety and endogenous adrenaline production.

GA must only be given in hospital; neuroleptanalgesia, using a combination such as droperidol, fentanyl and midazolam, may be the most satisfactory choice.

Phaeochromocytoma is occasionally associated with oral mucosal neuromas (MEA III syndrome; see later).

THYROID GLAND

The thyroid gland is under the influence of thyroid-stimulating hormone (TSH or thyrotropin) from the pituitary gland, which is itself regulated by thyrotropin-releasing hormone (TRH) from the hypothalamus. Thyroid hormones stored as iodide-rich 'thyroid colloid' are thyroxine (T4; tetra-iodothyronine), which has a half-life of 1 week, and is converted to tri-iodothyronine (T3), the active form, which has a half-life of 1 day. Thyroid hormones feed back to the hypothalamus and pituitary to regulate TSH release.

Thyroid hormones act on metabolism by regulating protein synthesis via effects on gene transcription and messenger RNA stabilization, and have profound effects on the sensitivity of tissues to catecholamines, as well as on mitochondrial oxidative activity, synthesis and degradation of proteins, differentiation of muscle fibres, capillary growth and levels of antioxidant compounds.

Thyroid function tests (Table 6.20) include serum levels of T4 and T3. Free T4 and free T3 provide a better assessment of the thyroid status than do total T4 and T3 since about 95% of thyroid hormones is

Table 6.20 *Tests of thyroid function*

Test	Hyperthyroidism	Hypothyroidism
T4 serum level	↑	↓
T3 serum level	↑	↓
Free thyroxine index	↑	↓
T3 resin uptake	↑	↓
Serum thyroid-stimulating hormone (TSH)	↓	↑[a]
Thyroid-releasing hormone (TRH) test (release of TSH by TRH)	ND	↓
Radio-iodine uptake	↑[b]	ND
Thyroid autoantibodies	LATS	Thyroglobulin autoantibodies

LATS = long-acting thyroid stimulator; ND = not done; T3 = tri-iodothyronine; T4 = thyroxine (tetraiodothyronine).
[a]Depressed in pituitary hypofunction.
[b]Not suppressed by administration of T3.

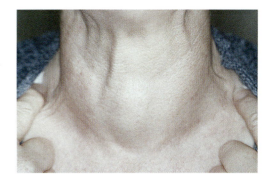

Fig. 6.20 Goitre.

Box 6.6 *Causes of goitre*

- Physiological
  - Puberty
  - Pregnancy
- Low iodine intake or natural goitrogens (endemic goitre)
- Drugs
  - Thiouracil
  - Carbimazole
  - Potassium perchlorate
  - Lithium
  - Phenylbutazone
- Thyroid disease
  - Graves disease (toxic goitre)
  - Dyshormonogenesis
  - Carcinoma
  - Hashimoto thyroiditis

bound to plasma proteins, especially thyroid-binding globulin (TBG) and thyroid-binding pre-albumin (TBPA). TSH levels can be assayed. Thyroid antibody tests, ultrasound and radio-iodine uptake using iodine-131 or 123 are the other common thyroid function tests.

LINGUAL THYROID

The thyroid normally develops as a downgrowth from the foramen caecum at the junction of the posterior third with the anterior two-thirds of the tongue. Rarely, ectopic thyroid tissue remains in this tract and may be seen as a lump in the midline between the foramen caecum and epiglottis, but has also been recorded in the oropharynx, infra-hyoid region, larynx, oesophagus, heart and mediastinum. A lingual thyroid is seen mainly in females and is often asymptomatic, but it may cause dysphagia, airway obstruction or even haemorrhage. Hypothyroidism may be associated in about one-third of cases and, occasionally, the lingual thyroid becomes malignant. There is a raised incidence of thyroid disease in relatives.

A lingual thyroid may not be suspected until the lump in the tongue has been biopsied or excised and examined histologically. The diagnosis can be confirmed by iodine-123, iodine-131 or technetium-99 uptake in the tongue, by biopsy, by CT scanning without contrast or by MRI.

Treatment depends on the size of the lingual thyroid but thyroxine may be needed and, if the lump does not regress sufficiently, the lingual thyroid can be ablated; this is best done by surgery, or, if the patient is unfit, by iodine-131, if normal functioning thyroid tissue is identified in the neck.

GOITRE

A goitre is an enlarged thyroid gland (Fig. 6.20). Most goitres are acquired and seen in Graves disease or thyroiditis (Box 6.6).

The cause of the goitre should be sought. One rare cause is a medullary carcinoma of the thyroid, which can be part of a multiple endocrine adenomatosis syndrome (MEA II and MEA III).

Thyroid function is assessed to determine whether it is normal (euthyroid), hyperactive (hyperthyroid) or hypoactive (hypothyroid).

Most goitres do not require surgery but this is indicated if there is a danger of airways obstruction (cough, voice changes, dyspnoea, tracheal deviation or dysphagia) or for cosmetic reasons.

Dental management in goitre may be influenced by abnormal thyroid function, by the underlying cause of the goitre or by complications such as respiratory obstruction.

THYROID NODULES

A nodule in the thyroid gland may represent a neoplasm (Fig. 6.21). Thyroid function tests and ultrasound-guided needle biopsy are indicated. Radio-iodine thyroid scans (nuclear medicine thyroid scanning) does not conclusively determine whether thyroid nodules are benign or malignant but are useful to evaluate the functional status of thyroid nodules in patients who are hyperthyroid. A nodule that takes up radio-iodine is termed a hot nodule and is unlikely to be malignant – more usually it is an adenoma. A nodule that fails to take up the radio-iodine is termed a cold nodule, and may be malignant – usually a papillary, follicular or medullary cell carcinoma; needle biopsy is indicated. Treatment may be surgical, irradiation or sorafenib – now approved to treat differentiated thyroid carcinoma (DTC).

HYPOTHYROIDISM

General aspects

Hypothyroidism may be primary (due to thyroid disease) or secondary (due to hypothalamic or pituitary dysfunction). The common causes are thyroid loss from surgery or destruction by irradiation of the neck or thyroid gland. Autoimmune disease (Hashimoto thyroiditis), associated with autoantibodies to thyroglobulin and thyroid microsomes, and drugs such as amiodarone, carbimazole, lithium or radio-iodine may be implicated. Rare cases in the developed world are caused by iodine deficiency.

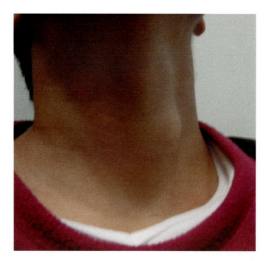

Fig. 6.21 Thyroid nodule.

Box 6.7 *Hypothyroidism: typical clinical features*

- Angina
- Bradycardia
- Cold intolerance
- Constipation
- Decreased appetite
- Decreased sweating
- Dry cold skin
- Hair loss
- Hoarseness
- Ischaemic heart disease
- Menorrhagia
- Periorbital oedema
- Psychosis
- Serous effusions
- Slow cerebration, poor memory
- Slow reactions
- Weight gain

Clinical features

Hypothyroidism is often unrecognized. Subclinical hypothyroidism, with raised TSH but normal T4 levels, may be found in up to 10% of postmenopausal females. However, hypothyroidism can cause weight gain, lassitude, dry skin, myxoedema, loss of hair, cardiac failure, ischaemic heart disease, bradycardia, anaemia, neurological or psychiatric changes, hypotonia, cerebellar signs of ataxia, tremor, dysmetria, polyneuropathy, cranial nerve deficits, entrapment neuropathy (e.g. carpal tunnel syndrome), myopathic weakness, dementia, apathy, mental dullness, irritability and sleepiness (Box 6.7; Fig. 6.22).

Hoarseness and hypothermia and may be complicated by coma. Sjögren syndrome (Ch. 16) may be associated. Congenital hypothyroidism (cretinism) has similar features, together with an enlarged tongue and learning impairment.

General management

The diagnosis is confirmed by demonstrating low serum T4 and T3 levels. TSH levels are raised in primary hypothyroidism and depressed in secondary hypothyroidism. Serum antibodies are detectable in Hashimoto thyroiditis – thyroid microsomal antibodies (TMAbs) in 95%, thyroglobulin antibodies (TGAbs) in 60%.

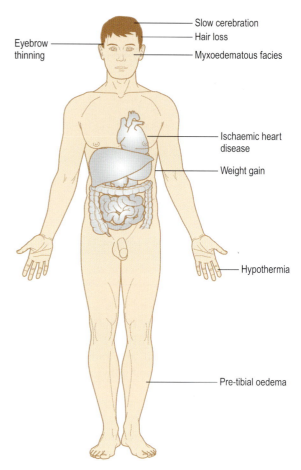

Fig. 6.22 Hypothyroidism.

Symptomatic patients are managed with daily oral thyroxine sodium. Treatment is started slowly but angina, myocardial infarction or sudden death may be precipitated, especially if there is evidence of ischaemic heart disease.

Dental aspects

The main danger is precipitation of myxoedema coma by the use of sedatives (including diazepam or midazolam), opioid analgesics (including codeine) or tranquillizers. These should therefore be either avoided or given in a low dose. LA is satisfactory for pain control. CS can be carried out with nitrous oxide and oxygen. Diazepam or midazolam may precipitate coma.

GA may be complicated because of possible ischaemic heart disease and the danger of coma, and the respiratory centre is also hypersensitive to drugs such as opioids or sedatives. GA, if unavoidable, should be delayed if possible until thyroxine has been started.

Associated problems may include hypoadrenocorticism, anaemia, hypotension, diminished cardiac output and bradycardia. Occasional associations include hypopituitarism and other autoimmune disorders such as Sjögren syndrome.

Povidone–iodine and similar compounds are best avoided.

HYPERTHYROIDISM

General aspects

Hyperthyroidism is usually associated with a diffuse goitre due to autoimmune disease (Graves disease, primary hyperthyroidism) when there are thyroid-stimulating autoantibodies against TSH receptor antibodies (TRAbs) and TMAbs. Sometimes, a hyperfunctioning

Box 6.8 *Hyperthyroidism: typical clinical features*

- Amenorrhoea
- Atrial fibrillation
- Diarrhoea
- Excess sweating
- Exophthalmos in some
- Gynaecomastia
- Heart failure
- Heat intolerance
- Increased appetite
- Irritability
- No hair loss
- No voice change
- Psychosis
- Tachycardia
- Tremor
- Warm moist skin
- Weight loss

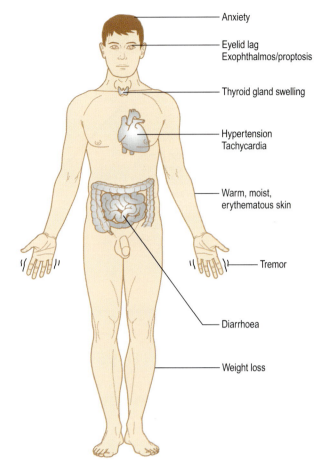

Fig. 6.23 Hyperthyroidism.

(toxic) multinodular goitre or nodule due to one or more thyroid adenomas produces excess thyroxine. Ninety per cent of the swellings are benign. Rarely, thyroiditis, thyroid hormone overdosage or ectopic thyroid tissue causes a goitre.

Clinical features

Hyperthyroidism may cause exophthalmos, eyelid lag and eyelid retraction (Box 6.8, Figs. 6.23 and 6.24); it mimics the effects of adrenaline (epinephrine), and can cause anorexia, vomiting or diarrhoea, weight loss, anxiety and tremor, sweating and heat intolerance. Cardiac disturbances, particularly in older patients, include tachycardia, arrhythmias (especially atrial fibrillation) or cardiac failure.

Thyrotoxic periodic paralysis comprises attacks of mild to severe weakness, during which serum potassium levels are generally low.

Myasthenia gravis may occasionally be associated.

General management

The diagnosis is confirmed by raised serum levels of T3 and T4. Circulating TMAbs and TRAbs are found in 55% of patients with Graves disease. A scan or radioactive iodine uptake can differentiate causes of hyperthyroidism: subacute thyroiditis (low uptake) versus Graves disease (high uptake).

Hyperthyroidism can be treated with beta-blockers (which achieve rapid control of many of the signs and symptoms by moderating sympathetic overactivity, but suddenly stopping beta-blocker treatment can precipitate a thyroid crisis within 4 hours). Carbimazole, the usual antithyroid drug, can suppress the bone marrow and cause rashes. Iodine-131 is effective but can result in hypothyroidism. There appears to be no risk of neoplastic change. Surgery is effective but leads to hypothyroidism in about 30%. Hypoparathyroidism and recurrent laryngeal nerve palsy are rare complications.

In untreated patients with hyperthyroidism, pain, anxiety, trauma, GA or premature cessation of antithyroid treatment may precipitate a thyroid (thyrotoxic) crisis, characterized by anxiety, tremor and dyspnoea, which can progress to ventricular fibrillation. Medical assistance is essential, as treatment requires the use of potassium iodide and propylthiouracil, and propranolol or chlorpromazine.

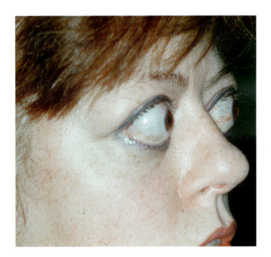

Fig. 6.24 Exophthalmos.

Dental aspects

Patients with sympathetic overactivity in untreated hyperthyroidism can be anxious and irritable, and may faint. LA is the main means of pain control; any risk of adrenaline (epinephrine) exacerbating sympathetic overactivity is only theoretical and prilocaine with felypressin is not known to be safer than lidocaine. CS is frequently desirable to control excessive anxiety. Benzodiazepines may potentiate antithyroid drugs, and therefore nitrous oxide, which is more rapidly controllable, is probably safer.

Povidone–iodine and similar compounds are best avoided. Carbimazole occasionally causes agranulocytosis, which may cause oral or oropharyngeal ulceration. Otherwise, the treated thyrotoxic

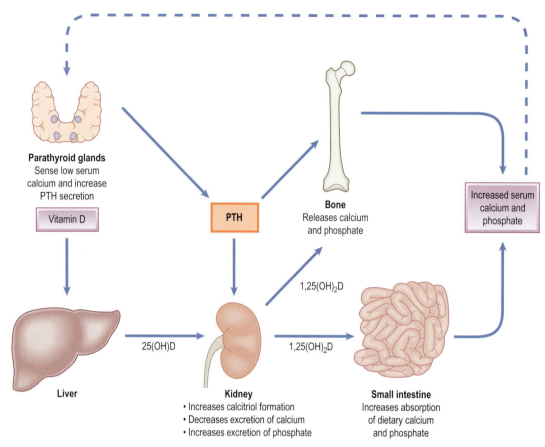

Fig. 6.25 Parathyroid vitamin D and calcium metabolism.

Table 6.21 *Parathyroid function tests*				
	Calcium[a]	Phosphate[a]	Alkaline phosphatase	Urea[a]
Primary hyperparathyroidism				
Without bone lesions	↑	↓	N	N
With bone lesions	↑	N or ↓	↑	N or ↑
Secondary hyperparathyroidism				
Due to renal failure	N or ↓	N or ↑	N or ↑	↑
Due to malabsorption	N or ↓	↓	↑	N
Tertiary hyperparathyroidism				
With bone lesions	↑	N or ↓	↑	N or ↑
Without bone lesions	↑	↓	N	N or ↑
Hypoparathyroidism	↓	↑	N	N
Pseudohypoparathyroidism	↓	↑	N	N
Pseudo-pseudohypoparathyroidism	N	N	N	N
Vitamin D deficiency	↓	N or ↓	↑	N

N = normal.
[a]Serum concentrations.

patient presents no special problems in dental treatment. However, after treatment of hyperthyroidism, the patient is at risk from hypothyroidism, which may pass unrecognized. This point must be borne in mind especially if a GA is required.

PARATHYROID GLANDS

The parathyroids are four pea-sized glands located on the back of the thyroid gland in the neck, which produce parathyroid hormone (PTH). Occasionally, congenitally ectopic parathyroid glands are embedded in the thyroid, the thymus or the chest. In most such cases, ectopic glands function normally.

PTH and vitamin D both act to control plasma calcium levels. PTH secretion is stimulated by a fall in the level of the plasma ionized calcium. PTH acts on the kidneys to increase renal reabsorption of calcium and impair phosphate reabsorption (Fig. 6.25). PTH enhances gastrointestinal absorption of calcium and promotes osteoclastic bone resorption, causing a rise in the plasma level of calcium and of the osteoblastic enzyme alkaline phosphatase (Table 6.21). Both bone mineral and matrix are degraded, and the amino acids, such as hydroxyproline, thus released are not reused but are excreted in the urine.

- Acute pancreatitis
- Candidosis[a]
- Cataracts[a]
- Constipation
- Dental defects[a]
- Epilepsy
- Hypertension
- Psychiatric disorders
- Tetany
- Weakness

[a] *Only in some types of congenital hypoparathyroidism.*

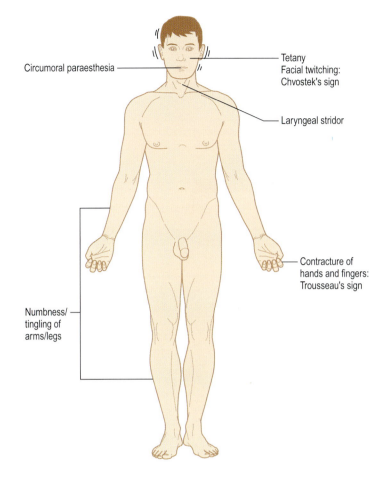

Fig. 6.26 Hypoparathyroidism.

Labels on figure: Circumoral paraesthesia; Tetany Facial twitching: Chvostek's sign; Laryngeal stridor; Contracture of hands and fingers: Trousseau's sign; Numbness/tingling of arms/legs

HYPOPARATHYROIDISM

General aspects

The most frequent cause of hypoparathyroidism is thyroidectomy, but it is relatively transient and typically resolves when the remaining parathyroid tissue undergoes compensatory hyperplasia. Rare cases of idiopathic hypoparathyroidism are congenital.

Clinical features

Low plasma calcium leads to muscle irritability and tetany, with facial twitching (Chvostek's sign; contracture of the facial muscles upon tapping over the facial nerve); carpopedal spasms (Trousseau's sign; contracture of the hand and fingers (*main d'accoucheur* – obstetrician's hand) on occluding the arm with a cuff); numbness and tingling of arms and legs; and even laryngeal stridor (Box 6.9 and Fig. 6.26).

Rare cases of idiopathic hypoparathyroidism may be associated with CATCH 22 (Ch. 37), or other endocrine defects – especially hypoadrenocorticism – associated with multiple autoantibodies (see Table 6.22) and cataracts, calcification of the basal ganglia, defects of the teeth and, sometimes, chronic mucocutaneous candidosis.

Pseudohypoparathyroidism is characterized by normal or raised PTH secretion but unresponsive tissue receptors, and has clinical features similar to idiopathic hypoparathyroidism, but there is short stature and small fingers and toes, with a liability to develop cataracts, and no dental defects. Similar appearance in patients with normal biochemistry is termed pseudo-pseudohypoparathyroidism.

General management

Diagnosis is from low plasma calcium; phosphate is often raised (see Table 6.21). Replacement therapy includes vitamin D and calcium supplements.

Dental aspects

There may be facial paraesthesia and facial twitching caused by tetany (Chvostek's sign). Idiopathic (congenital) hypoparathyroidism may feature enamel hypoplasia, shortened roots with osteodentine formation, delayed eruption and sometimes chronic mucocutaneous candidosis (see Box 6.9).

LA is satisfactory. CS can be given, preferably after replacement therapy. Dental management may be complicated by tetany, seizures, psychiatric problems or learning disability, hypoadrenocorticism, diabetes mellitus or other endocrinopathies or arrhythmias.

HYPERPARATHYROIDISM

General aspects

Primary hyperparathyroidism is usually caused by a parathyroid adenoma and is seen in postmenopausal women. Rare causes include carcinoma of the parathyroids.

Secondary hyperparathyroidism is a response to low plasma calcium caused by chronic renal failure or prolonged dialysis, or by severe malabsorption, and is rising in frequency.

Tertiary hyperparathyroidism follows prolonged secondary hyperparathyroidism, which has become autonomous.

Clinical features

The main features (Box 6.10) include hypercalcaemia and renal disease (most patients have renal calcifications), skeletal disease (bone pain, pathological fractures, giant cell tumours, bone rarefaction), peptic ulceration, pancreatitis, hypertension and arrhythmias (Fig. 6.27). Therefore, the expression 'stones, bones and abdominal groans' sometimes applies.

Hyperparathyroidism may occasionally be familial and associated with tumours of other endocrine glands (MEA I, II and III).

Box 6.10 *Hyperparathyroidism: clinical features*

- Bone resorption
- Nephrocalcinosis
- Peptic ulcer: pain
- Polyuria
- Psychiatric disorders
- Renal stones

Table 6.22 *Multiple endocrine adenoma (MEA) syndromes*

	MEA type I	MEA type II (IIa)	MEA type III (IIb)
	Werner syndrome	Sipple syndrome	Schmidt syndrome
Genetics	*Menin* gene	*Ret* gene	*Ret* gene
Adrenals	Adenoma	Phaeochro-mocytoma in 33%	Phaeochro-mocytoma in 70%
Pancreas	Nesidioblastoma, Zollinger–Ellison syndrome, insulinoma	–	–
Parathyroid	Hyperplasia	Hyperplasia	Hyperplasia
Pituitary	Adenoma (usually prolactinoma)	–	–
Thyroid	±	Medullary cell carcinoma in 75–100%[a] (calcitonin-secreting)	Medullary cell carcinoma in up to 80–100% (calcitonin-secreting)
Others	Carcinoid, lipomas, gastrinoma	Dermal neuroma	Oral mucosal neuromas, Marfanoid skeletal anomalies, visual disturbances

[a]Causes raised serum calcitonin levels and low serum calcium levels.

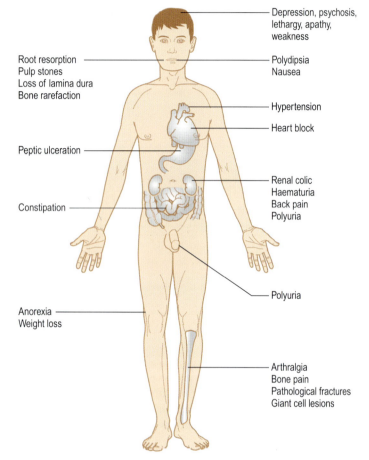

Depression, psychosis, lethargy, apathy, weakness

Root resorption
Pulp stones
Loss of lamina dura
Bone rarefaction

Polydipsia
Nausea

Hypertension

Heart block

Peptic ulceration

Renal colic
Haematuria
Back pain
Polyuria

Constipation

Polyuria

Anorexia
Weight loss

Arthralgia
Bone pain
Pathological fractures
Giant cell lesions

Fig. 6.27 Hyperparathyroidism ('stones, bones and abdominal groans').

General management

The diagnosis in primary hyperparathyroidism is confirmed by raised PTH levels, raised serum calcium, low or normal phosphate level, and normal or raised alkaline phosphatase. *Primary hyperparathyroidism* is treated by parathyroidectomy, but medical treatment such as active vitamin D hormone (1,25-dihydroxycholecalciferol; 1,25-DHCC) is useful in those with severe bone disease. *Secondary hyperparathyroidism* often responds to 1,25-DHCC but not to dietary vitamin D (cholecalciferol). Parathyroidectomy may be needed. *Tertiary hyperparathyroidism* requires parathyroidectomy.

Calcimimetics, drugs which bind to the calcium-sensing receptors of the parathyroid glands and lower the sensitivity for receptor activation by extracellular calcium, diminish PTH release, and may become useful for the treatment of primary and secondary hyperparathyroidism.

Dental aspects

Dental changes in hyperparathyroidism include loss of the lamina dura and generalized bone rarefaction, but giant cell lesions are late

and uncommon. Giant cell lesions of hyperparathyroidism (brown tumours) are rare but histologically indistinguishable from central giant cell granulomas of the jaws. If, therefore, a giant cell lesion is found, particularly in a middle-aged patient or in a patient with renal failure, parathyroid function should be investigated.

LA is the main means of pain control, especially if hypertension and arrhythmias are present. CS is preferably carried out with nitrous oxide and oxygen. GA may be challenging because of cardiovascular complications and sensitivity to muscle relaxants. Dental treatment in hyperparathyroidism may be complicated by renal disease, peptic ulceration, bone fragility or pluriglandular disease.

MULTIPLE ENDOCRINE ADENOMA SYNDROMES

Multiple endocrine adenoma (MEA) syndromes, also known as the multiple endocrine neoplasia (MEN) syndromes, are rare autosomal dominant diseases affecting several endocrine glands, often with *hyperfunction* (Table 6.22); they are distinct from polyglandular autoimmune syndromes (see below). All MEA syndromes feature parathyroid hyperplasia and hypercalcaemia. Type III is most relevant to dentistry. In the latter, numerous small plexiform neuromas form in the oral mucosa, lips, eyelids and skin. The patient may also have a Marfanoid habitus and diarrhoea.

POLYGLANDULAR AUTOIMMUNE SYNDROMES

Polyglandular autoimmune syndromes feature multiple endocrine *deficiencies*, due to autoantibodies to the glands, most commonly Addison disease and hypoparathyroidism.

As shown in Table 6.23, chronic mucocutaneous candidosis is a very frequent feature in type 1. Its onset is frequently in infancy and it can precede any glandular deficiencies by 10 or more years. Occasionally this sequence is reversed but, in either case, treatment of the glandular deficiency has no effect on the candidosis and vice versa.

Treatment of the hormone deficiencies is as described earlier.

Table 6.23 *Polyglandular autoimmune disease, type I and type II*

	Type I	Type II
Female:male ratio	1.5:1	1.8:1
Human leukocyte antigen (HLA) associations	Not constant	B8 (A1)
Addison disease	100%	100%
Hypoparathyroidism	76%	–
Chronic mucocutaneous candidosis	73%	–
Alopecia	32%	0.5%
Malabsorption syndromes	22%	–
Gonadal failure	17%	3.6%
Pernicious anaemia	13%	0.5%
Chronic active hepatitis	13%	–
Autoimmune thyroiditis	11%	69%
Type 1 diabetes	4%	52%

HORMONE PRODUCTION BY TUMOURS

Tumours, especially bronchogenic carcinoma, can occasionally produce polypeptide hormones or other biologically active substances ectopically (Appendix 6.1: see also ch. 22).

GONADS

See Chapter 30.

KEY WEBSITES

(Accessed 27 May 2013)
British Medical Journal <http://www.bmj.com/specialties/diabetes>
Centers for Disease Control and Prevention. <http://www.cdc.gov/diabetes/>
National Institute of Diabetes and Digestive and Kidney Diseases, National Institutes of Health. <http://diabetes.niddk.nih.gov/>
National Institutes of Health. <http://health.nih.gov/topic/Diabetes>

USEFUL WEBSITES

(Accessed 27 May 2013)
Diabetes UK. <http://www.diabetes.org.uk/>
DIABETESNET.COM. <http://www.diabetesnet.com/about-diabetes/insulin>
endocrineweb. <http://www.endocrineweb.com/>
Glycosmedia. <http://www.glycosmedia.com/>
MedlinePlus. <http://www.nlm.nih.gov/medlineplus/ency/article/001214.htm>

FURTHER READING

Alexander, R.E., Throndson, R.R., 2000. A review of perioperative corticosteroid use in dentoalveolar surgery. Oral Surg. Oral Med. Oral Pathol. Oral Radiol. Endod. 90, 406.

Auluck, A., 2007. Diabetes mellitus: an emerging risk factor for oral cancer? J. Can. Dent. Assoc. 73, 501.
Barnett, A., 2007. Exenatide. Expert Opin. Pharmacother. 8, 2593.
Blase, E., et al. 2005. Pharmacokinetics of an oral drug (acetaminophen) administered at various times in relation to subcutaneous injection of exenatide (exendin-4) in healthy subjects. J. Clin. Pharmacol. 45, 570.
Combettes, M., Kargar, C., 2007. Newly approved and promising antidiabetic agents. Therapie 62, 293.
Consensus Statement on the Worldwide Standardization of the Hemoglobin A1C Measurement: The American Diabetes Association, 2007. European association for the study of diabetes, international federation of clinical chemistry and laboratory medicine, and the international diabetes federation. Diabetes. Care 30, 2399.
Fiske, J., 2004. Diabetes mellitus and oral care. Dent. Update 31, 190.
Gibson, N., Ferguson, J.W., 2004. Steroid cover for dental patients on long-term steroid medication: proposed clinical guidelines based upon a critical review of the literature. Br. Dent. J. 197, 681.
Greenwood, M., Meechan, J.G., 2003. General medicine and surgery for dental practitioners. Part 6: The endocrine system. Br. Dent. J. 195, 129.
Keene, J.R., et al. 2002. Treatment of patients who have type 1 diabetes mellitus: physiological misconceptions and infusion pump therapy. J. Am. Dent. Assoc. 133, 1088.
Khalaf, M.W., et al. 2013. Risk of adrenal crisis in dental patients: results of a systematic search of the literature. J. Am. Dent. Assoc. 144 (2), 152. PubMed PMID: 23372131.
Lorenzo-Calabria, J., et al. 2003. Management of patients with adrenocortical insufficiency in the dental clinic. Med. Oral 8, 207.
Manfredi, M., et al. 2004. Update on diabetes mellitus and related oral diseases. Oral Dis. 10, 187.
McKenna, S.J., 2006. Dental management of patients with diabetes. Dent. Clin. North. Am. 50, 591.
Mealey, B.L., Ocampo, G.L., 2000. Diabetes mellitus and periodontal disease. Periodontology 2007 (44), 127.
Mealey, B.L., Rose, L.F., 2008. Diabetes mellitus and inflammatory periodontal diseases. Curr. Opin. Endocrinol. Diabetes. Obes. 15, 135.
Nicholson, G., et al. 1998. Peri-operative steroid supplementation. Anaesthesia 53, 1091.
Perry, R.J., et al. 2003. Steroid cover in dentistry: recommendations following a review of current policy in UK dental teaching hospitals. Dent. Update 30, 45.
Pinto, A., Glick, M., 2002. Management of patients with thyroid disease: oral health considerations. J. Am. Dent. Assoc. 133, 849.
Scully, C., Chaudhry, S., 2007. Aspects of human disease 10. diabetes. Dent. Update 34, 189.
Scully, C., 2009. Aspects of human disease 33, pregnancy. Dent. Update 36, 253.
Scully, C., 2009. Aspects of human disease 35, hyperthyroidism. Dent. Update 36, 381.
Scully, C., et al. 2007. Special care in dentistry: handbook of oral healthcare. Elsevier, Edinburgh.
Seymour, R.A., 2003. Dentistry and the medically compromised patient. Surgeon 1, 207–214.
Skamagas, M., Breen, T.L., LeRoith, D., 2008. Update on diabetes mellitus: prevention, treatment, and association with oral diseases. Oral Dis. 14, 105–114.
Soon, D., Kothare, P.A., Linnebjerg, H., 2006. Effect of exenatide on the pharmacokinetics and pharmacodynamics of warfarin in healthy Asian men. J. Clin. Pharmacol. 46, 1179–1187.
Vairaktaris, E., Spyridonidou, S., Goutzanis, L., et al. 2007. Diabetes and oral oncogenesis. Anticancer. Res. 27, 4185–4193.
Vernillo, A.T., 2001. Diabetes mellitus: relevance to dental treatment. Oral Surg. Oral Med. Oral Pathol. Oral Radiol. Endod. 91, 263–270.

APPENDIX 6.1 ENDOCRINE AND METABOLIC EFFECTS OF SOME CANCERS

Substance released	Tumours most commonly responsible[a]	Disease resulting	Features
Adrenocorticotropic hormone (ACTH)	Bronchial, carcinoid, pancreatic, parotid, phaeochromocytoma	Cushing syndrome	See text
Antidiuretic hormone (ADH)	Bronchial, Hodgkin disease, pancreatic	Syndrome of inappropriate ADH secretion (SIADH)	See text
Catecholamines	Adrenal medulla	Phaeochromocytoma	Facial flushing
Erythropoietin	Adrenal, breast, bronchial, fibroids, hepatoma, phaeochromocytoma	Polycythaemia	See Ch. 12
Gastrin	Pancreatic	Zollinger–Ellison syndrome	Diarrhoea, multiple small intestinal ulcers
Human chorionic gonadotropin (HCG)	Breast, hepatoblastoma, pancreatic	Precocious puberty	–
Oestrogens	Adrenal, lung, testicular	Gynaecomastia	Gynaecomastia
Parathyroid hormone (PTH) and prostaglandins	Renal, almost any squamous cell carcinoma	Hypercalcaemia	Polyuria, polydipsia, psychosis, constipation, abdominal pain
Serotonin (5-hydroxytryptamine) and other vasoactive substances	Bronchial, ileocaecal	Carcinoid syndrome	Symptoms mainly if there are hepatic metastases, facial flushing, bronchospasm, diarrhoea. Right-sided valvular heart lesions (especially pulmonary stenosis)
Testosterone	Adrenal, ovarian	–	Hirsutism
Thyroid-stimulating hormone (TSH)	Trophoblastic	Hyperthyroidism	See text
Transforming growth factor (TGF)	Abdominal, breast	Acanthosis nigricans	See text

[a]Carcinomas unless otherwise stated.

THE OESOPHAGUS

The oesophagus has the single important function of carrying food, liquids and saliva from the mouth to the stomach, achieved by an automatic process of coordinated contractions of its muscular lining (peristalsis), termed deglutition (swallowing). Deglutition involves a complex and coordinated process initiated by sensory impulses from stimulation of receptors on the fauces, tonsils, soft palate, base of the tongue and posterior pharyngeal wall to the brainstem primarily through cranial nerves VII, IX and X. Cricopharyngeal sphincter opening is reflexive and starts when the bolus reaches the posterior pharyngeal wall before reaching this sphincter. The efferent (motor) function of swallowing is mediated by cranial nerves IX, X and XII. Swallowing has three phases; the first is voluntary, the others are involuntary:

- *Phase one* is collection and swallowing of the masticated food bolus.
- *Phase two* is passage of food through the pharynx into the oesophagus.
- *Phase three* is the passage of food down into the stomach.

Swallowing and respiration are inextricably linked. Neurological damage, such as from a stroke, can lead to disturbed swallowing (dysphagia) and the risk of aspiration into the lungs.

The oesophagus is generally examined by endoscopy. The current 'gold standard' examination of swallowing is videofluoroscopy but this is time-consuming and carries a small radiation risk.

REFLUX OESOPHAGITIS (GASTRO-OESOPHAGEAL REFLUX DISEASE)

General aspects

Gastro-oesophageal reflux disease (GORD) is the term used to describe a backflow of acid from the stomach into the oesophagus. One of the most common kinds of dyspepsia, GORD is predisposed to by gastrointestinal disorders (e.g. high acidity of gastric contents; impaired gastro-oesophageal motility) or extragastrointestinal conditions (obesity, stooping, large meals, smoking, alcohol). Although it was at one time considered to be a result of hiatus hernia (diaphragmatic hernia), the relationship between the symptoms and appearances on barium swallow is inconsistent. Hiatal hernias are found in about 25% of all people over age 50 – particularly in women and those who are overweight. They form at the opening (hiatus) in the diaphragm where the oesophagus joins the stomach. The muscle tissue around the hiatus weakens, allowing the upper stomach to herniate through the diaphragm into the chest cavity. Most hernias cause no symptoms but larger ones may allow food and acid to regurgitate into the oesophagus, which can cause chest pain ('heartburn').

Clinical features

The usual symptom is an uncomfortable burning sensation behind the sternum, most commonly felt after a meal ('heartburn'). Acid taste is common. Rare complications may include stricture and iron-deficiency anaemia.

General management

Diagnosis can be confirmed by oesophageal pH monitoring. Conditions to differentiate include candidal oesophagitis, or chemical burns from acids or alkalis, non-steroidal anti-inflammatory drugs (NSAIDs), potassium chloride or tetracyclines. Symptoms can often be effectively relieved by losing weight, raising the head of the bed by at least 10 cm at night and taking frequent small meals with antacids. Proton-pump inhibitors such as omeprazole or lansoprazole are effective but H2-blockers (cimetidine, ranitidine) are often used.

Dental aspects

Gastric contents can have a pH as low as 1 and regurgitation, if chronic, can thus cause dental erosion, typically of the palatal aspects of the upper anterior teeth and premolars; this may be worse if there is impaired salivation. Some patients are convinced that other oral symptoms or diseases are caused by 'acid' but, apart from the few genuine cases with persistent regurgitation of gastric contents, this is no more than a folk myth, probably fostered by advertisements for antacids. Other causes of erosion include anorexia nervosa, bulimia (Ch. 27) and alcoholism (Ch. 34).

POST-CRICOID WEB

The association of post-cricoid dysphagia, upper oesophageal webs and iron-deficiency anaemia is known as the Paterson–Brown-Kelly syndrome in the UK and the Plummer–Vinson syndrome (PVS) in the USA. The term sideropenic dysphagia has also been used, since the syndrome can feature iron deficiency (sideropenia) but no anaemia. Postulated aetiopathogenic mechanisms include iron and nutritional deficiencies, genetic predisposition and autoimmune factors. The improvement in dysphagia after iron therapy provides evidence for an association between iron deficiency and post-cricoid dysphagia. Moreover, the decline in Paterson–Brown-Kelly syndrome seems to parallel an improvement in nutritional status, including iron supplementation. However, population-based studies have shown no relationship between post-cricoid dysphagia and anaemia or sideropenia.

If a web is suspected, endoscopy should be carried out carefully under direct vision through the upper oesophageal sphincter. The web typically appears as a thin mucosal membrane covered by normal squamous epithelium. Although reports are inconsistent, patients with Paterson–Brown-Kelly syndrome seem to be at greater risk for hypopharyngeal, oesophageal and oral cancers. Patients with

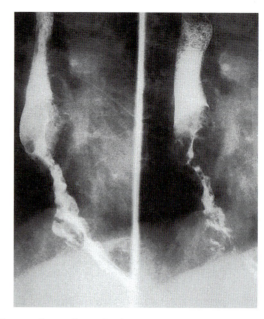

Fig. 7.1 Barium swallow radiography showing oesophageal carcinoma.

Paterson–Brown-Kelly syndrome usually respond well to iron therapy, diet modification and, if necessary, oesophageal dilatation.

CANCER OF THE OESOPHAGUS

General aspects

Oesophageal cancer is usually squamous cell carcinoma in the upper and middle part of the oesophagus, or adenocarcinoma in the lower third. It is more frequent in older people and in men. Risk factors are shown in Box 7.1.

Clinical features

Early oesophageal cancer usually causes few or no symptoms but later features may include dysphagia, weight loss, pain (in the throat or back, behind the sternum or between the shoulder blades), hoarseness, chronic cough, vomiting or haemoptysis (coughing up blood).

Metastases are typically in the lymph nodes, liver, lungs, brain and bones.

General management

Diagnosis is confirmed by chest radiography, barium swallow (Fig. 7.1), oesophagoscopy (endoscopy), computed tomography (CT), magnetic resonance imaging (MRI) and biopsy. Bone scan and bronchoscopy may be needed.

Surgery is the most common treatment (oesophagectomy). Laser therapy or photodynamic therapy is sometimes used. A stent may be used for palliation; alternatively, a plastic tube or part of the intestine is used to reconnect with the stomach. Radiation therapy may be used alone or with chemotherapy as primary treatment or to shrink the tumour before surgery.

Dental aspects

Patients who have had oesophageal cancer have a greater chance of developing a second cancer in the head and neck area. Paterson–Brown-Kelly syndrome may be associated with a high risk of oral cancer. Rare patients have tylosis and oral leukoplakia.

THE STOMACH AND INTESTINES

Common features of gastrointestinal disorders include nausea and vomiting, diarrhoea and constipation, though none of these is specific and all have a wide range of causes (Ch. 4).

THE STOMACH

Gastric products include hydrochloric acid (secreted by parietal cells), pepsin (secreted by chief or peptic cells) and intrinsic factor (secreted by parietal cells). Gastric mucus contains several glycoproteins, which, with bicarbonate, are produced by surface cells and protect the mucosa against erosion.

Hydrochloric acid secretion is stimulated by: hypoglycaemia and mediators including acetylcholine (muscarinic-type receptor); gastrin (from G cells) and synthetic analogues of gastrin (pentagastrin); and histamine (from histaminocytes). Hydrochloric acid secretion is inhibited from higher centres and by low gastric pH and hormones – cholecystokinin, gastric inhibitory peptide (GIP) and secretin (Table 7.1).

Gastric acid secretion in response to various stimuli can be assessed by passing a nasogastric tube and measuring the volume, pH and acid concentration of the aspirate. The response to a meal is regulated by complex hormonal and neural (vagal) mechanisms (see Table 7.1).

Peptic ulcer

General aspects

An ulcer is a break in the continuity of an epithelial surface. Peptic ulcer disease (PUD) develops in or close to acid-secreting areas in the stomach (gastric ulcer) or proximal duodenum (duodenal ulcer). It affects up to 15% of the population, mostly men over the age of 45 years.

Helicobacter pylori, a spiral bacterium that lives in the stomach and duodenum, is the most common contributory cause to peptic ulcers. In the developed world, some 20–50% of normal adults are infected, but the figure is much higher in poor socioeconomic circumstances. Few carriers have disease, but *H. pylori* can cause increased gastric acid secretion, loss of the mucous protective layer, increased secretion of pepsinogen and increased gastrin release. *H. pylori* survives in the mucous lining, and resists gastric acid via the enzyme urease, which converts urea (abundant in the stomach from saliva and gastric juices) into bicarbonate and ammonia – both strong bases. This reaction of urea hydrolysis is important for the diagnosis of *H. pylori* by the 'breath test'. *H. pylori* has another defence, in that the immune response cannot reach it, and the polymorphs may release their destructive superoxide radicals on to the stomach-lining cells, causing

Table 7.1 *Gastrointestinal hormones*

Part of gastrointestinal tract	Source	Hormones	Stimulus	Effects
Stomach	G cells	Gastrin	Gastric distension, amino acids	Secretion of gastric acid, pepsin, intrinsic factor
Small intestine	Duodenum and jejunum	Cholecystokinin (pancreozymin)	Fats, amino acids, peptides	Pancreatic secretion, gallbladder contraction, delay in gastric emptying
	Duodenum and jejunum	Gastric inhibitory peptide (GIP)	Glucose, fats, amino acids	Inhibition of gastric acid secretion, release of insulin, reduction of gut motility
	Duodenum and jejunum	Motilin	Acid	Increase in gut motility
	Duodenum and jejunum	Secretin	Acid	Pancreatic bicarbonate secretion, delay in gastric emptying
	Jejunum	Vasoactive intestinal peptide (VIP)	Neural stimulation	Inhibition of gastric acid and pepsin secretion, stimulation of pancreatic and intestinal secretion
Pancreas	D cells	Somatostatin	Neural stimulation	Inhibition of gastric and pancreatic secretion
	Pancreatic polypeptide cells	Pancreatic polypeptide	Proteins	Inhibition of biliary and pancreatic secretion

gastritis and perhaps eventually a peptic ulcer. *H. pylori* is found in the mouth, especially the gingival sulcus, and believed to be transmitted orofaecally. It is possible that *H. pylori* could be transmitted from the stomach to the mouth through gastro-oesophageal reflux and then be transmitted through oral contact.

PUD is also associated with raised gastrin levels, as in Zollinger–Ellison syndrome (a gastrin-producing tumour; high serum calcium provokes gastrin release) and chronic renal failure (poor gastrin metabolism). Other factors that predispose to peptic ulceration include NSAIDs, corticosteroids, smoking, alcohol, diet and stress. There are genetic influences: first-degree relatives have a threefold risk and there is an association with blood group O.

Clinical features

The main feature of PUD is epigastric pain, often relieved by antacids. Many of those affected have no symptoms and the first sign may be one of the complications – haemorrhage, perforation or pyloric obstruction (stenosis) with vomiting.

General management

Patients less than 45 years old who present with typical ulcer symptoms should be screened for *H. pylori*. Four tests are used to detect the bacterium:

- Blood test for antibodies to *H. pylori* – shows past or present infection
- Urea breath test – shows *H. pylori* infection
- Stool antigen test – tests for the presence of *H. pylori* antigens in faeces (stool)
- Stomach biopsy.

Studies of gastric acid or serum gastrin levels may be helpful and, if gastric outlet obstruction is suspected, a barium meal may be diagnostically useful (Fig. 7.2). Management of PUD involves conservative measures: dietary modification (frequent small meals with no fried foods); smoking cessation; alcohol moderation; and treatment of any *H. pylori*. Individuals who are *H. pylori*-positive should be given 'triple therapy', usually for 7 days, to eradicate infection. This normally is effective in over 90% with little risk of relapse and consists of a proton-pump inhibitor (esomeprazole, lansoprazole, omeprazole, pantoprazole or rabeprazole) and antibiotics (amoxicillin, clarithromycin and metronidazole). An additional reason to treat *H. pylori* infection is that it may lead to gastric cancer or mucosa-associated lymphoid tissue (MALT) lymphomas.

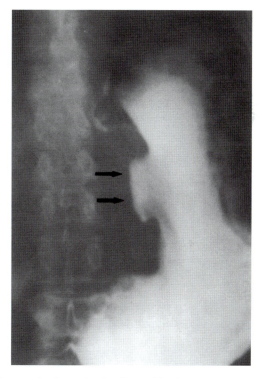

Fig. 7.2 Barium meal radiography showing gastric ulcer.

PUD that is *H. pylori*-negative is usually associated with NSAID use. Drugs that block histamine (H2) receptors, such as cimetidine and ranitidine, are therefore used to reduce gastric acid secretion. Prostaglandin analogues such as misoprostol promote healing in PUD and are indicated in patients from whom NSAIDs cannot be withdrawn. Surgery is usually reserved for those with complications; gastric ulcers may be managed by antrectomy with gastroduodenal anastomosis or partial gastrectomy, while duodenal ulcers are managed with vagotomy and pyloroplasty (rarely).

Dental aspects

Gastric acid regurgitation can cause severe dental erosion (perimylolysis), typically of the palatal aspects of the upper anterior teeth and premolars. *H. pylori* may be transmitted in saliva but dental healthcare professionals do not appear to be at particular risk from infection. There are conflicting findings as to whether dental plaque or dentures

- Achlorhydria
- Atrophic gastritis
- Blood group A
- Diet (smoked foods, salted fish and meat, and pickled vegetables; nitrates and nitrites are substances commonly found in cured meats)
- Genetic influences (carcinoma is common in Japanese and where there is a positive history in first-degree relatives). The E-cadherin/*CDH1* gene is responsible. Hereditary non-polyposis colorectal cancer (HNPCC; Lynch syndrome) and familial adenomatous polyposis (FAP) are genetic disorders with a greatly increased risk of colorectal cancer and a slightly increased risk of stomach cancer. People with mutations of the inherited breast cancer genes *BRCA1* and *BRCA2* may also have a higher rate of stomach cancer
- *Helicobacter pylori*
- Male gender
- Ménétrier disease (hypertrophic gastropathy)
- Obesity
- Occupations – workers in coal, metal and rubber industries
- Older age
- Pernicious anaemia
- Previous stomach surgery
- Tobacco

are an important reservoir for *H. pylori* and significant in transmission of the organism. There may be an association with halitosis.

Gastric surgery may result in attacks of hypoglycaemia. After resection, deficiencies of vitamin B_{12}, folate or iron may cause ulcers, sore tongue or angular stomatitis. Drugs such as aspirin and other NSAIDs and corticosteroids that cause gastric irritation, or promote bleeding, and should not be given to patients with peptic ulcers.

Labial vascular anomalies may be associated with PUD.

Oral adverse effects from medications may include:

- dry mouth from proton-pump inhibitors, pirenzepine and sucralfate
- erythema multiforme from ranitidine
- loss of taste or erythema multiforme from omeprazole.

Antacids impede absorption of ciprofloxacin, erythromycin, metronidazole and tetracyclines. Cimetidine and omeprazole may delay clearance of lidocaine and benzodiazepines but the effect is rarely clinically significant.

Cancer of the stomach

General aspects

Stomach cancer, usually adenocarcinoma, is common. Men are affected nearly twice as often as women. The aetiology of gastric cancer is unclear (Box 7.2).

Clinical features

Early symptoms of gastric cancer may closely mimic those of peptic ulcer – indigestion or vague upper abdominal pain. Later, there may be anorexia, loss of weight, nausea, vomiting, haematemesis or melaena (black and tarry stools with blood). Anaemia may develop. The tumour spreads locally later and leads to pain, and may obstruct the intestine to cause vomiting, or the bile duct to cause jaundice. Metastases are mainly to liver, peritoneum (causing ascites), lungs, bones or brain.

General management

The lesion may show on barium imaging and the diagnosis is usually confirmed by gastroscopy and biopsy, but is often delayed by the lack of early symptoms.

Most patients are treated by surgery but frequently this is only palliative. The prognosis is poor, with about a 7% 5-year survival rate (Ch. 22).

Dental aspects

Anaemia or obstructive jaundice may complicate dental treatment. Oral effects of anaemia (glossitis, ulcers, angular stomatitis) can be an initial sign. It is important to remember that iron deficiency usually results from chronic haemorrhage, in a male often from the gastro-intestinal tract, and then sometimes due to an ulcer or neoplasm in the stomach or large bowel.

Orofacial metastases from gastric carcinoma are rare, usually in the body of the mandible, and may cause swelling, pain, paraesthesia, loosening of teeth or sockets that fail to heal; they may be found as ragged radiolucent areas, sometimes with tooth root resorption. Occasionally, metastases may be first detected in a lower cervical (supraclavicular, or Virchow) lymph node, usually on the left side (Troisier sign).

THE SMALL INTESTINE

The small intestine is the main site of food digestion, which depends on intestinal and pancreatic enzymes acting on food previously exposed to salivary amylase, gastric acid and pepsin. This is where food absorption chiefly occurs.

Iron and folate are absorbed in the duodenum, most other substances in the jejunum. Bile salts facilitate the absorption of fats and the fat-soluble vitamins (A, D, E and K). Gastric intrinsic factor from the stomach parietal cells is needed for vitamin B_{12} absorption, which occurs in the terminal ileum.

Small intestine disease causes malabsorption, with diarrhoea or steatorrhoea (fatty stools), sometimes abdominal discomfort, and deficiency states leading to lassitude, weakness, loss of weight or failure to thrive, and anaemia.

Diseases of the small intestine of most significance include coeliac disease and Crohn disease. Other causes of problems include surgery, infestations and drugs. For example, olmesartan can cause a sprue-like disease (diarrhoea, weight loss and villous atrophy, which resolves after discontinuation of the drug).

Coeliac disease

Coeliac disease (CD; gluten-sensitive enteropathy; coeliac sprue, non-tropical sprue) is the most common genetic disease in Europe, where up to 1 in 250 people have it. It is rare in Africans, Chinese or Japanese. CD is strongly associated with genes on chromosome 6, on a genetic background of HLA-DQw2 or DRw3, and may have a familial tendency.

CD is a hypersensitivity or toxic reaction of the small intestine mucosa to the gliadin component of gluten (prolamine), a group of proteins found in all forms of wheat (including durum, semolina, spelt, kamut, einkorn and faro), related grains (rye, barley, triticale) and possibly oats. Ingestion of gluten causes destruction of jejunal villi (villous atrophy) and inflammation, leading to malabsorption. Coeliac disease may be associated with autoimmune disorders (Box 7.3). Other food sensitivities or lactose intolerance may also be associated.

Clinical features

CD is one of the great mimics in medicine. It may present at any age and many affected individuals are asymptomatic, but CD can result

- Dermatitis herpetiformis
- Diabetes mellitus type 1
- Immunoglobulin A (IgA) deficiency
- IgA nephropathy
- Primary biliary cirrhosis
- Systemic lupus erythematosus
- Thyroid disease

Table 7.2 *Serum antibodies, and antigens, in coeliac disease*

	Antigens	Antibodies
Endomysium	Connective tissue stroma covering muscle fibres	Immunoglobulin (Ig) A class antibodies present in those with severe mucosal damage
Gliadin (gliaden)	Prolamins (glycoproteins) in wheat and several other cereals in the grass genus *Triticum*	ELISA test for gliadin antibodies is a reliable screening tool. IgG antibody detection is more sensitive but less specific than IgA antibodies. Antigliadin antibodies lose specificity with age
Reticulin	Fibres composed of type III collagen	IgA class reticulin antibodies found in 60% of patients. IgG class reticulin antibodies occasionally also found in bullous dermatoses and in some normal subjects
Transglutaminase	Tissue transglutaminase – the protein cross-linking enzyme – is the endomysial antigen	IgA anti-tissue transglutaminase is 85% sensitive and 97% specific – and the diagnostic gold standard

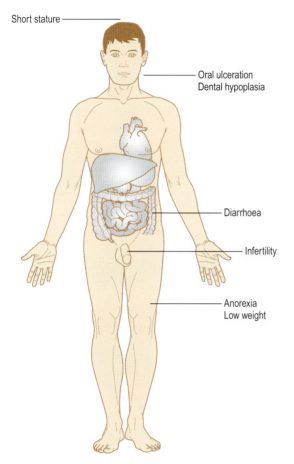

Short stature

Oral ulceration
Dental hypoplasia

Diarrhoea

Infertility

Anorexia
Low weight

Fig. 7.3 Coeliac disease.

in malabsorption (leading to growth retardation, vitamin and mineral deficiencies, which may in turn lead to anaemia, osteomalacia, bleeding tendencies and neurological disorders), abdominal pain, steatorrhoea and behavioural changes (Fig. 7.3). Intestinal lymphomas arise in about 6% of individuals.

General management

It is important to diagnose CD and to institute a gluten-free diet as early as possible, even in those with minimal symptoms, in order to prevent long-term complications (especially intestinal lymphoma). Investigations needed to establish the diagnosis include full blood count (anaemia is present in 50%); haematinics (ferritin, vitamin B_{12} and folate levels may be low secondary to malabsorption); stool examination (24-hour weight of stool – abnormal if greater than 300 g – and the presence of excess fat – more than 6% of the fat consumed). Tolerance or measure-of-digestion/absorption investigations include lactose tolerance and D-xylose tests. Serum antibody screening is indicated (Table 7.2). Endoscopic biopsy of jejunal mucosa shows

villous atrophy if positive, and is repeated after a gluten-free diet has been maintained for 3 months. In children the same procedure is used, except that an additional biopsy is carried out after a test challenge of gluten, as it is essential to establish the diagnosis with certainty from the outset, in order to encourage normal growth and to eliminate such conditions as post-infectious gastroenteritis, which can cause a histologically similar lesion. Similar jejunal changes are also seen in dermatitis herpetiformis.

Treatment of CD includes rectifying nutritional deficiencies, and adhering to a gluten-free diet for life. Instead of wheat flour, potato, rice, soy or bean flour and gluten-free bread, pasta and other products are used. Patients require continued supervision, as it is often difficult to comply with such a diet, especially if eating away from home.

Dental aspects

Short stature, associated with diarrhoea and enamel defects, is particularly suggestive of early-onset CD. Anaemia may predispose to oral lesions, notably glossitis, burning mouth, angular stomatitis and ulcers. CD may be found in up to 5% of patients with aphthous-like ulcers and should be suspected if there are any other symptoms suggesting small intestine disease.

Some untreated patients may have a bleeding tendency. Anaemia may complicate general anaesthesia (GA).

Inflammatory bowel disease

Inflammatory bowel disease (IBD) is a collective term for diseases that cause inflammation in the intestines and encompasses the spectrum of disease seen in Crohn disease and ulcerative colitis (UC; Table 7.3). The differential diagnosis includes infectious colitis, microscopic colitis, segmental colitis associated with diverticula, ischaemic colitis, and even cancers. These diseases are seen mainly in northern Europe and USA and in Caucasians.

Genetic factors appear to influence disease susceptibility and patterns but environmental, dietary, and infective factors may be at play. In Crohn disease, all layers of the intestine may be involved and there can be normal healthy bowel between patches of diseased bowel. The

Table 7.3 *Crohn disease and ulcerative colitis compared*

	Crohn disease	Ulcerative colitis
Main site affected	Ileum	Colorectum
Other sites affected	Any part of the gastrointestinal tract, including the mouth	Terminal ileum
Pathology	Transmural granulomatous inflammation	Superficial inflammation
Abdominal pain	Prominent	Less prominent
Bloody diarrhoea	Less common	Prominent
Fistulae and abscesses	Possible	Rare
Colonic carcinoma risk	Increased	High
Iron deficiency	Common	Common
Folate deficiency	Common	Common
Other deficiencies	Vitamin B_{12} deficiency	Rare

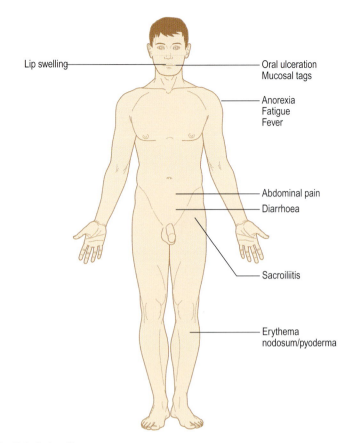

Fig. 7.4 Crohn disease.

aetiology is unknown but available evidence suggests that a deregulated immune response towards commensal bacterial flora is responsible for intestinal inflammation in genetically predisposed individuals. Antigens from commensal microorganisms appear to trigger and maintain inflammation in a number of ways, with effector T cells (Th1, Th2, Th17) predominating and releasing interferon-gamma and interleukin-12 (IL-12); other cytokines, such as tumour necrosis factor alpha (TNFα), IL-1 and IL-6, are produced in response, by macrophages. IL-23 promotes expansion and maintenance of Th17 cells, which secrete the proinflammatory cytokine IL-17. IL-23 also acts on cells of the innate immune system that can contribute to inflammatory cytokine production and tissue inflammation. Natural killer (NK) cells also contribute directly and via IL-13. Chemoattractants, such as IL-8, macrophage inhibitory protein 1 (MIP1) and RANTES (regulated on activation normal T cells as secreted), recruit immunocytes to the area. Interactions between the nervous and immune systems may also play a role: activation of the enteric nervous system may reduce intestinal epithelial permeability, via several mediators including substance P, histamine, neurokinin, serotonin, vanilloids, S-nitrosoglutathione and vasoactive intestinal peptide (VIP).

Emerging biological therapies are thus aimed at cytokines (e.g. adalimumab, certolizumab, infliximab), T-cell activation receptors (abatacept, visilizumab) or adhesion molecules (alicaforsen, MLN-02, natalizumab).

Crohn disease (regional enteritis or ileitis)

General aspects

Crohn disease appears to be a heterogeneous group of chronic inflammatory disorders seen mainly in Caucasians. About 20% of people with Crohn disease have a blood relative with some form of IBD, most often a brother or sister and sometimes a parent or child.

Microscopically, there is submucosal chronic inflammation with many mononuclear, IL-1–producing cells and non-caseating granulomas in the submucosa and lymph nodes. The inflammatory response is probably mediated by factors such as TNFα. Susceptibility appears to be related in 15% to the *CARD15* gene with a locus on chromosome 16, and it has been hypothesized that Crohn disease involves augmentation of the Th1 response in inflammation. The microorganisms involved are unknown but many have been implicated. *Mycobacterium avium* subspecies *paratuberculosis* has been incriminated, but is probably one of a variety of microorganisms simply taking advantage of the damaged mucosa and inability to clear bacteria from the intestinal walls. Other workers have suggested that a lack of *Faecalibacterium*

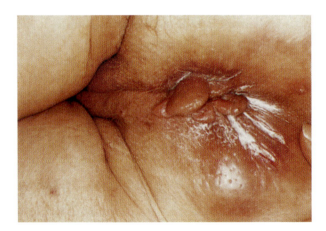

Fig. 7.5 Perianal tags in Crohn disease.

prausnitzii might be responsible. Diet, oral contraceptives, NSAIDs, isotretinoin and smoking have also been incriminated.

Clinical features

Crohn disease can affect any part of the gastrointestinal tract from mouth to anus (top to tail) but affects especially the ileocaecal region, typically with ulceration, fissuring and fibrosis of the wall. The manifestations depend on its severity and the site affected. Small-intestinal Crohn disease may cause abdominal pain that often mimics appendicitis, with malabsorption or abnormal bowel habits (Fig. 7.4). Features include persistent diarrhoea (loose, watery or frequent bowel movements), cramping abdominal pain, fever and, at times, rectal bleeding. Sometimes deep ulcers turn into tracts – fistulae with tags (Fig. 7.5). Patients may also malabsorb and develop a shortage of proteins, calories or vitamins. Loss of appetite and weight loss may also occur.

Fatigue is another common complaint. The most common complication of Crohn disease is intestinal blockage due to swelling and scar tissue, presenting with cramping pain, vomiting and bloating. Patients have an increased risk of colon cancer, and Crohn disease can also affect the joints, eyes, skin, liver and mouth.

General management

The major differential diagnoses include ulcerative colitis, tuberculosis, ischaemic colitis, infections, infestations such as giardiasis, and lymphoma. There are no specific diagnostic tests for Crohn disease. Investigations may include: faecal calprotectin – now used as a diagnostic marker indicator for IBD (replacing isotope leukocyte intestinal scans); blood count (anaemia is common); serum potassium, zinc and albumin (usually depressed); erythrocyte sedimentation rate (ESR), C-reactive protein (CRP) and seromucoid (often raised); small bowel MRI; plain-film and contrast radiography (barium enemas of large and small bowel, or barium meal and follow-through); ultrasound and CT; and endoscopy (sigmoidoscopy, colonoscopy) with mucosal biopsy (often shows typical granulomas).

A high-fibre diet is indicated and anaemia needs treatment. Treatment of Crohn disease includes:

- aminosalicylates (5-ASA) or newer 5-aminosalicylates (mesalazine or olsalazine)
- antibiotics (metronidazole, ampicillin, ciprofloxacin, others)
- immune modifiers (local [prednisolone/prednisone, budesonide] or systemic corticosteroids, azathioprine, 6-mercaptopurine [6-MP] or methotrexate; everolimus in unresponsive patients; biological therapy [monoclonal antibodies directed against TNFα – adalimumab, certolizumab pegol or infliximab]); thiopurines (such as 6-MP and azathioprine) unfortunately can increase a patient's risk of non-Hodgkin lymphoma
- surgery when medications can no longer control the symptoms – two-thirds to three-quarters of patients will require surgery at some point during their lives.

Dental aspects

Dental management may be complicated by any of the problems associated with malabsorption or by corticosteroid or other immunosuppressive treatment. NSAIDs should be avoided. Antibiotics that could aggravate diarrhoea should not be used; these include amoxicillin–clavulanic acid (co-amoxiclav) erythromycin and clindamycin.

Oral lesions may be caused by Crohn disease itself or by associated nutritional defects, and may include ulcers, facial or labial swelling (Fig. 7.6), mucosal tags or 'cobblestone' proliferation of the mucosa, and angular stomatitis. Patients with atypical ulcers, especially when they are large, linear and ragged, or those with recurrent facial swellings, should have biopsy of the mucosa. Melkersson–Rosenthal syndrome (facial swelling, facial palsy and fissured tongue), cheilitis granulomatosa and orofacial granulomatosis may also be incomplete manifestations of Crohn disease, and some of these patients may have asymptomatic intestinal disease or develop intestinal disease later.

A high prevalence of caries and periodontitis in Crohn disease has also been reported.

Orofacial granulomatosis

Orofacial granulomatosis (OFG) is the term given to granulomatous lesions similar to those of Crohn disease and found on oral biopsy but without detectable systemic Crohn disease, though this may be detected later. Th1 immunocytes produce IL-12 and RANTES/MIP1α, and the granulomas. HLA typing may show HLA-A2 or HLA-A11.

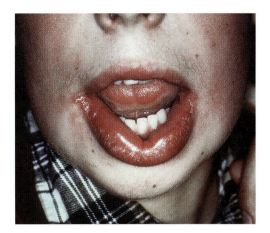

Fig. 7.6 Facial and labial swelling in Crohn disease.

Table 7.4 *Factors that have been implicated in orofacial granulomatosis*

Foods/additives	Chemicals/metals	Microorganisms
Benzoic acid	Cobalt	*Borrelia burgdorferi*
Butylated hydroxyanisole	Colophony	*Mycobacterium paratuberculosis*
	Eugenol	
Carbone piperitone	Formaldehyde	*Saccharomyces cerevisiae*
Carvone	Isoeugenol	Spirochaetes
Chocolate	Nickel	
Cinnamaldehyde or cinnamyl alcohol	Oak moss absolute	
	Sodium metabisulfite	
Cocoa		
Dairy products		
Eggs		
Monosodium glutamate or glutamic acid		
Peanuts		
Piperitone		
Sorbic acid		
Sun yellow		
Tartrazine		
Wheat		

OFG may sometimes result from reactions to some foods or medicaments, such as cinnamaldehyde and benzoates; up to 40% of patients may be positive to patch tests and half of these may respond to exclusion of dietary antigens (Table 7.4).

Oral lesions of OFG include ulcers, facial or labial swelling, mucosal tags or 'cobblestone' proliferation of the mucosa. Gut Crohn disease and reactions to foods should be excluded by gastrointestinal investigations, and allergy tests are often indicated. If systemic Crohn disease can be excluded, patients still need to be kept under observation for its possible development later.

Exclusion of offending substances can be difficult but may help facial swelling resolve. Clofazimine, dapsone, thalidomide, anti-TNF biological therapies or intralesional injection of corticosteroids may also be needed.

Short bowel syndrome

Short bowel syndrome, in which the small intestine is short, may be congenital or caused by surgery. Numerous metabolic defects, particularly vitamin and mineral deficiencies leading to osteomalacia and fractures, may result. Patients on home parenteral nutrition due to short bowel syndrome seem to have a high risk of developing systemic osteoporosis, including the jaws, but do not have a higher risk for deterioration of the dental or periodontal state.

THE LARGE INTESTINE

The large intestine has two main functions: recovery of water and electrolytes (sodium and chloride), and the formation, storage and expulsion of faeces (stools). The large intestine lies between the terminal ileum and anus, and consists of the caecum – a blind-ended pouch that carries a worm-like extension (the appendix) in humans; the colon, which forms most of the length of the large intestine and comprises ascending, transverse and descending segments; and the rectum – the short, terminal segment continuous with the anal canal.

Appendicitis

General aspects

Appendicitis is inflammation of the appendix, the cause of which is usually unknown; it may follow a viral infection or obstruction. Appendicitis is most common in people aged 10–30.

Clinical features

Not all appendicitis causes symptoms but features may include pain in the right abdomen, nausea, vomiting, constipation, diarrhoea, abdominal swelling, anorexia and low fever that begins later. The pain usually begins near the umbilicus and moves down and into the right iliac fossa. The pain becomes worse when moving, taking deep breaths, coughing, sneezing and being touched (McBurney point).

General management

Diagnosis is based upon symptoms, examination, blood tests, such as a leukocyte count to check for infection, and urine tests to rule out a urinary tract infection. If untreated, an inflamed appendix can burst, causing peritonitis and even death, and is thus considered an emergency.

If a diagnosis of appendicitis is definite, surgery (appendicectomy) is indicated, sometimes via laparoscopic surgery. If the diagnosis of appendicitis is not certain, the patient may be watched and sometimes treated with antibiotics.

Irritable bowel syndrome

Irritable bowel syndrome (IBS; spastic colon; mucous colitis) may affect up to 30% of the population and is the most common cause of referrals to gastroenterologists. IBS causes recurrent abdominal pain together with increased tone and activity of the colon, abnormal bowel habits and other symptoms. It may occur at any age and has a slight female predominance.

The cause of IBS is unclear but it may begin after an infection or stressful life event; there is often a positive family history, anxious personality type and history of migraine or psychogenic symptoms (Ch. 10). The protozoan *Dientamoeba fragilis* has been implicated by some researchers. Cytokines (IL-1, IL-6 and TNF) and serotonin have also been cited as causes.

Clinical features

IBS leads to crampy abdominal pain, flatulence, bloating and changes in bowel habit – constipation or diarrhoea, often with urgency (tenesmus). Additional gynaecological and urinary symptoms may be reported. Episodes may be precipitated by stressful life events or foods such as chocolate, caffeine, milk products or large amounts of alcohol.

Examination may reveal some abdominal distension and tenderness. However, guarding or rebound tenderness of the abdomen, along with blood or mucus per rectum, suggests other organic disease.

General management

IBS is a diagnosis of exclusion. Investigations are tailored to rule out coeliac disease, IBD or colonic cancer (full blood count and haematinics; inflammatory markers (ESR); contrast radiography; endoscopy and mucosal biopsy).

Stress reduction and a high-fibre diet may control symptoms. Antispasmodics (mebeverine, loperamide or an antimuscarinic such as dicycloverine, or peppermint oil) may help. Probiotics may have a role. Cognitive behavioural therapy or antidepressants may be of benefit for patients with IBS who are clinically depressed. For severe cases that fail to respond to the above measures, it is important to reconsider the diagnosis and re-evaluate the patient's history and presentation; coeliac disease or IBD can easily be missed.

Dental aspects

Local anaesthesia (LA) is satisfactory for pain control. Conscious sedation (CS) may be needed because of these patients' anxious personalities. Orofacial manifestations may include psychogenic oral symptoms such as pain dysfunction syndrome, sore tongue or atypical facial pain.

Loperamide or dicycloverine may cause dry mouth.

Diverticular disease

General aspects

Diverticular disease includes both diverticulosis (small colonic pouches – diverticula – that bulge out through weak spots of the large intestine wall) and diverticulitis (inflammation of these diverticula). Diverticular disease is most common in developed or industrialized countries, where it affects over 50% of those over 60 years. It may result from a low-fibre diet.

Clinical features

Left-sided diverticular disease (involving the sigmoid colon) is most common in the West, while right-sided diverticular disease is more prevalent in Africa and Asia. It may be asymptomatic but is often accompanied by dyspepsia, abdominal pain, constipation and flatulence. Complications include pericolic abscess, perforation and peritonitis, or fistula.

General management

Conditions to be excluded include IBD, IBS, cancer, and urological and gynaecological disorders. Management includes a high-fibre diet and reassurance. Antibiotics and surgery may be needed.

Dental aspects

There are no specific management problems in dentistry, although codeine should be avoided as it worsens constipation.

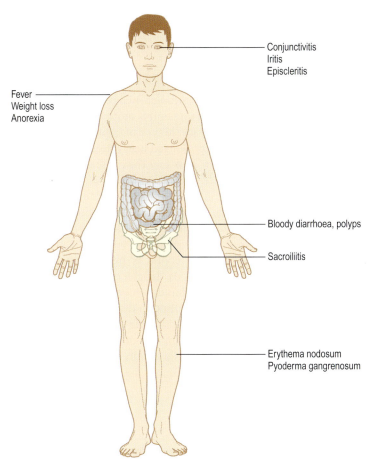

Conjunctivitis
Iritis
Episcleritis

Fever
Weight loss
Anorexia

Bloody diarrhoea, polyps

Sacroiliitis

Erythema nodosum
Pyoderma gangrenosum

Fig. 7.7 Ulcerative colitis.

and pyoderma gangrenosum), liver disease (especially primary sclerosing cholangitis), gallstones and renal calculi. Overproduction of platelets and some clotting factors may lead to thromboembolism.

General management

There are no specific diagnostic tests. Investigations include full blood count and haematinics; inflammatory markers (ESR); contrast radiography (barium studies); endoscopy and mucosal biopsy.

A high-fibre diet is indicated and any anaemia needs treatment. Medical therapy includes conservative measures (nutritional support) and drug therapy (Box 7.4). Vedolizumab is a humanized monoclonal antibody to alpha4 beta7 integrin that appears beneficial.

The surgical options in UC depend on the extent of disease but generally consist of colectomy (excision of diseased bowel with either re-anastomosis or ileostomy construction) if symptoms are severe, the response to medical treatment is poor, complications such as pyoderma gangrenosum or haemorrhage develop, or there is a risk of malignant change. Unlike in Crohn disease, surgery can be curative.

Dental aspects

Drugs that should be avoided include NSAIDs and antibiotics including amoxicillin–clavulanic acid (co-amoxiclav), erythromycin and clindamycin, which could aggravate diarrhoea.

LA is satisfactory and there are no objections to CS if needed. Management complications may include anaemia and those associated with corticosteroid therapy.

Oral manifestations in UC are rare but include pyostomatitis gangrenosum (chronic ulceration), pyostomatitis vegetans (multiple intraepithelial microabscesses), discrete haemorrhagic ulcers or lesions related to anaemia. Since uveitis, skin lesions and mouth ulcers can be found in UC, it is important to differentiate it from Behçet disease (Ch. 11).

Ulcerative colitis

General aspects

Ulcerative colitis (UC) is an IBD affecting part or the whole of the large intestine – most frequently the lower colon and rectum. It causes inflammation and ulcers in the superficial layers of the mucosa, followed by formation of pseudopolyps, which may be pre-malignant. It most often affects people between the ages of 15 and 40 years.

The aetiology is unknown but autoimmunity, diet, sulphate-reducing bacteria, drugs such as isotretinoin and a genetic basis have been suggested. A role for the *RUNX3* gene on chromosome 1 has been suggested but chromosomes 6, 16, 12, 14, 5, 19 and 3 have also been implicated. Psychosomatic symptoms are often associated.

Clinical features

Typical features are pain and diarrhoea with stools containing intermixed mucus, blood and pus, sometimes with systemic toxicity (fever, anorexia, weight loss, anaemia and raised ESR and CRP; Fig. 7.7). Disease with less than six bloody stools daily but no systemic toxicity is termed 'mild'; if there is toxicity, disease is termed 'moderate'; and the term 'severe ulcerative colitis' is applied when there are more than six bloody stools daily plus toxicity. Disease extension through the muscular layers may result in life-threatening toxic megacolon (the colon dilates and can perforate). The most serious complication is carcinoma of the colon, which is up to 30 times more frequent than in the general population and most likely to develop in patients with early-onset colitis or with disease persisting for more than 10 years.

Non-gastrointestinal features include arthralgia, conjunctivitis, uveitis, iritis, finger-clubbing, sacroiliitis, skin disease (erythema nodosum

Familial polyposis coli

Familial polyposis coli (FPC) is an autosomal dominant disease in which multiple adenomatous polyps affect the rectum and colon; carcinomatous change usually supervenes. FPC is a feature of Gardner syndrome, along with multiple exostoses and osteomas of the jaws. These bone lesions also appear to be more common in patients with non-familial colorectal cancer than in the general population. Colectomy is indicated.

Carcinoma of the colon

General aspects

Carcinoma of the colon (colorectal cancer) is common. The peak incidence is in the sixth or seventh decade and the tumour usually forms in the

- Cholecystectomy
- Diet low in fibre, fruit and vegetables, and high in red meat and fat
- Heredity; familial polyposis coli
- Inflammatory bowel disease
- Tobacco

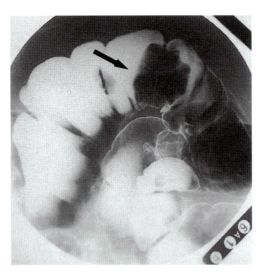

Fig. 7.8 Barium enema radiography showing colorectal carcinoma.

rectum or pelvic (sigmoid) colon. A series of gene alterations can lead to adenomas and eventually, in some patients, to carcinoma. Risk factors are shown in Box 7.5. Long-term aspirin use lowers the risk of colonic cancer.

Clinical features

Carcinoma of the colon may cause abdominal pain, change in bowel habit, melaena, weight loss or complications such as anaemia, intestinal obstruction or perforation.

General management

Abdominal examination may reveal a mass. Sigmoidoscopy and sometimes faecal occult blood testing (stool guaiac), MRI, ultrasound, barium enema (Fig. 7.8) and colonoscopy may be required. Methylated septin 9 (SEPT9), a plasma test to screen for colorectal cancer, has a sensitivity and specificity similar to those of stool guaiac or faecal immune tests (immunochemical faecal occult blood test).

Surgical resection is the usual treatment. Spread is frequently to the liver. The 5-year survival rate is overall about 30% (Ch. 22). Radiotherapy may be useful for dealing with pain from recurrences. Chemotherapy may be used in advanced cancer: capecitabine, irinotecan, oxaliplatin, raltitrexed and possibly cetuximab. Serial monitoring for serum carcino-embryonic antigen or serum or faecal M2-pyruvate kinase (M2-PK) antigen may help detect recurrences (Ch. 22). Metastatic carcinoma may be treated with bevacizumab, cetuximab or antiangiogenesis agents, such as aflibercept, in combination with chemotherapy.

Dental aspects

LA is satisfactory and acceptable. CS can be given if needed. GA must be given by a specialist, particularly if complications have developed.

Anaemia resulting from chronic intestinal haemorrhage can complicate dental management or cause oral signs or symptoms.

Mandibular osteomas may be markers of an enhanced risk of colorectal cancer.

Antibiotic-associated (pseudomembranous) colitis

Most of the orally administered antimicrobials can cause diarrhoea, but clinically significant colitis is rare and is more likely to affect older or debilitated patients. The most severe type of colitis is staphylococcal enterocolitis, usually caused by prolonged heavy doses of tetracyclines, particularly after bowel surgery; now that the cause is recognized, this type of colitis has become rare. Pseudomembranous colitis is caused more frequently by lincomycin and clindamycin than by other antibiotics, as a result of proliferation of toxigenic strains of clostridia, particularly *Clostridium difficile*, which are resistant to low concentrations of these antibiotics.

Clinically, antibiotic-associated colitis is characterized by painful diarrhoea and passage of mucus. In elderly debilitated patients especially, there is passage of blood and pseudomembranous material (necrotic mucosa), occasionally resulting in death. The diagnosis cannot be made from the presence of *C. difficile* in the stool, as 1–9% of hospital patients carry the bacterium, but only from sigmoidoscopy and biopsy. Pseudomembranous colitis usually responds to metronidazole or oral vancomycin, plus cessation of the causal antibiotic.

ANAL DISEASES

Because of the widespread habit of anal intercourse, the anus can show the signs of many sexually shared infections. It is also a particularly important portal of entry for human immunodeficiency virus (HIV) infection because of the delicate lining of the anal canal. Carcinoma of the anus is rare, but more common in patients with HIV/acquired immunodeficiency syndrome (AIDS) and often associated with human papillomavirus infection.

Haemorrhoids

General aspects

Haemorrhoids is a term that refers to a condition in which the veins around the anus or lower rectum are swollen and inflamed. Haemorrhoids may result from straining to pass stool; contributory factors include pregnancy, ageing, chronic constipation or diarrhoea, and anal intercourse.

Clinical features

The most common symptom of internal haemorrhoids is bright red blood covering the stool, on toilet paper, or in the WC pan. Symptoms of external haemorrhoids may include irritation around the anus. Bleeding and/or itching, a painful swelling or hard lumps from thrombosed external haemorrhoids are other effects.

General management

Sigmoidoscopy or colonoscopy may be needed to rule out other causes of gastrointestinal bleeding such as colorectal cancer. A softer stool makes emptying the bowels easier and lessens the pressure on haemorrhoids, as does diltiazem to relieve tension; application of a haemorrhoidal cream or suppository to the affected area relieves symptoms. Surgery may be needed, such as sclerotherapy, rubber band ligation, infrared coagulation or haemorrhoidectomy. Dental care should be deferred until the patient can sit normally.

PERITONITIS

The peritoneal cavity normally holds only 50 mL of fluid, which contains complement factors but few leukocytes, circulates in the peritoneal space and drains via the lymphatics. Acute peritonitis is fairly uncommon but is usually a serious infection with inflammation of the peritoneum that follows rupture of a viscus (e.g. appendix) or trauma. Chronic peritonitis develops in patients on continuous ambulatory peritoneal dialysis and in some intensive care patients.

Spontaneous bacterial peritonitis is an infection of ascites fluid in patients with cirrhosis, in which the source of the infection is not known. Although *Streptococcus pneumoniae* is the most common pathogen, there is rarely any obvious source.

Clinical features

Severe and generalized abdominal pain, vomiting, pyrexia, a rigid/board-like and tender abdomen and no bowel sounds are the main features. Peritonitis can lead rapidly to hypovolaemic shock and death.

General management

Diagnosis is clinical, supported by imaging and culture. Treatment includes urgent fluid administration, antibiotics and laparotomy/surgical debridement/drainage as required.

THE PANCREAS

The pancreas is intimately associated with the common bile duct and performs exocrine and endocrine functions (Fig. 7.9). The exocrine pancreas produces digestive juices and the enzymes trypsinogen, chymotrypsinogen, amylase and lipase, which enter the common bile duct via the pancreatic duct, and then pass from the common bile duct to the small intestine. The endocrine function is performed by the pancreatic islets of Langerhans, which secrete insulin and glucagon–regulating glucose metabolism – along with pancreatic polypeptide and somatostatin, which help control the function of other endocrine hormones (Ch. 6).

ACUTE PANCREATITIS

General aspects

Acute pancreatitis is mainly caused by gallstone disease but may be precipitated by alcoholism, trauma, hypercalcaemia, hyperlipidaemia, viral infections such as mumps, endoscopic retrograde cholangiopancreatography (ERCP) or various drugs such as azathioprine, contraceptive pills, corticosteroids, furosemide or phenothiazines.

Clinical features

Acute pancreatitis causes acinar damage and activation of enzymes, leading to local fat necrosis. Mild pancreatitis usually resolves in a few days but in fulminating pancreatitis the patient is severely ill with retroperitoneal haemorrhage, pleural effusion and paralytic ileus. Systemic effects include severe abdominal pain, nausea, vomiting, hypotension and shock. Possible complications are wide-ranging (Box 7.6). The mortality rate is 15–25%.

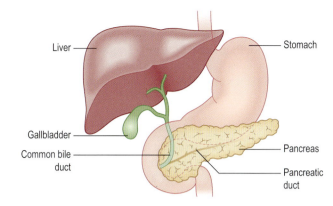

Fig. 7.9 Pancreatic anatomy.

Box 7.6 *Complications of acute pancreatitis*

- Abscess
- Acute renal failure
- Disseminated intravascular coagulopathy
- Metabolic (hypocalcaemia, hyperbilirubinaemia and hyperglycaemia)
- Respiratory distress
- Splenic vein thrombosis

General management

Raised serum levels of alkaline phosphatase, the transaminases, amylase and lipase, and radiology, MRI and ultrasonography aid the diagnosis. Shock, metabolic complications and pain must be urgently treated.

Dental aspects

LA is suitable if emergency treatment is required. CS and GA are not feasible until after resolution.

CHRONIC PANCREATITIS

General aspects

Causes include gallstone disease and alcoholism particularly. Malnutrition, hyperparathyroidism, haemochromatosis, hyperlipidaemia, carcinoma, cystic fibrosis and other factors may sometimes be implicated.

Clinical features

Chronic pancreatitis results in acinar atrophy and deterioration in both exocrine and endocrine function. Exocrine dysfunction causes a decline in the volume, bicarbonate content and enzyme content of pancreatic secretions. Endocrine dysfunction often includes abnormal glucose tolerance or frank diabetes. Chronic dull abdominal pain is punctuated by episodes of acute pancreatitis. Weight loss is common, as are nausea, vomiting and pruritus (from bile salt accumulation).

General management

Diagnosis is assisted by finding raised serum levels of amylase and lipase. Pancreolauryl and para-aminobenzoic acid testing are used to assess exocrine function. Pancreatic steatorrhoea is suggested by high faecal fat and undigested meat fibres. Faecal levels of chymotrypsin are depressed. CT demonstrates pancreatic calcification, especially in alcoholic pancreatitis. Barium meal, duodenography, cholangiography and endoscopy (ERCP) are diagnostically helpful.

Management includes analgesics, treatment of diabetes and the oral administration of pancreatic enzymes to aid digestion.

Dental aspects

Factors predisposing to or resulting from pancreatitis that might influence dental management include bleeding due to vitamin K malabsorption (Ch. 8), alcoholism (Ch. 34), diabetes mellitus (Ch. 6), hyperparathyroidism (Ch. 6), cystic fibrosis (Ch. 15) or narcotic abuse because of severe pain.

LA is satisfactory for pain relief. CS may be given for control of anxiety. Oral ulceration can result from holding pancreatic enzyme in the mouth.

Pancreatitis has *rarely* arisen from an oral source of infection.

PANCREATIC TUMOURS

General aspects

Most pancreatic tumours originate in the exocrine duct (acinar cells); nearly 95% are adenocarcinomas, usually involving the head of the pancreas. They appear to be rising in incidence and are now one-tenth as common as bronchogenic carcinoma. A minority (less than 10%) of pancreatic cancers result from an inherited tendency; there is a higher incidence of the familial tendencies in people with familial adenomatous polyposis, non-polyposis colonic cancer and familial breast cancer associated with the *BRCA2* gene. Known risk factors are shown in Box 7.7; periodontal inflammatory disease has also been implicated.

Tumours that begin in the islet cells (endocrine tumours) are rare but these and others may release hormones (Table 7.5).

Clinical features

Pancreatic carcinoma frequently invades to cause biliary obstruction (jaundice), pancreatitis and diabetes mellitus. Extrapancreatic complications, such as peripheral vein thrombosis (thrombophlebitis migrans), pruritus, nausea and vomiting, are common.

General management

Plain radiography, CT, MRI, ultrasound, endoscopy (ERCP) or percutaneous transhepatic cholangiography may be diagnostically helpful.

Pancreatic carcinoma is usually treated surgically, often with a bypass to relieve obstructive jaundice. Stenting may be used to relieve jaundice for as long as possible. Gemcitabine may help delay progress of advanced carcinoma. Pancreatic carcinoma has the worst prognosis of any cancer, with a 1-year survival of 10% and a 5-year survival of 3% (see Ch. 22).

Dental aspects

In many cases the poor prognosis of pancreatic cancer may significantly influence the dental treatment plan. Biliary obstruction may lead to bleeding tendencies, especially if there are hepatic metastases. Diabetes mellitus may be an added complication. Local anaesthesia is satisfactory. Conscious sedation may be given to relieve excessive anxiety. GA should not usually be considered because of the poor overall prognosis.

Box 7.7 *Risk factors for pancreatic cancer*

- Alcohol abuse
- Betel chewing
- Chronic exposure to petroleum compounds
- Chronic pancreatitis (often alcohol-induced)
- Diets high in animal fat and low in fruits and vegetables
- Heredity
- Obesity and physical inactivity
- Tobacco (responsible for at least 30%)

Table 7.5 *Hormone-secreting pancreatic tumours*

Tumour	Hormone released	Comments
Glucagonomas	Glucagon	Hyperglycaemia and abnormal glucose tolerance. Tumours are frequently malignant. Estimation of plasma glucagon levels differentiates glucagonomas from diabetes mellitus. Glucagon levels may also be raised in patients taking danazol. A major clinical feature is distinctive bullous or pustular skin and mouth lesions. There is often weight loss, anaemia and hypercholesterolaemia too
Insulinomas	Insulin	Hypoglycaemia – the most common cause in those not taking insulin
Watery diarrhoea, hypokalaemia and achlorhydria (WDHA) syndrome	Vasoactive peptides	Hyperglycaemia accompanies the watery diarrhoea, hypokalaemia and achlorhydria
Zollinger–Ellison syndrome	Gastrin	Diarrhoea and duodenal ulceration. May be part of the multiple endocrine adenoma syndrome (MEA I; Ch. 6).

PANCREATIC TRANSPLANTATION AND SIMULTANEOUS PANCREAS–KIDNEY TRANSPLANTATION

General aspects

Pancreas transplantation is used to ameliorate type 1 diabetes and provide complete insulin independence. The pancreas usually comes from a cadaveric organ donor but living donor pancreas transplants have been carried out. About 85% of pancreatic transplants are performed along with a kidney transplant (both organs from the same donor) in diabetic patients with renal failure; this is called a simultaneous pancreas–kidney transplant. About 10% of cases are performed after a previously successful kidney transplant (called a pancreas-after-kidney transplant); 5% are performed as pancreas transplant alone in non-uraemic patients with very labile and problematic diabetes.

General management

All transplant recipients require lifelong immunosuppression to prevent a T-cell alloimmune rejection response.

Dental aspects

A meticulous oral assessment is required before surgery, and dental treatment should be undertaken with particular attention to establishing optimal oral hygiene and eradicating sources of potential infection.

Dental treatment should be completed before surgery. For 6 months after surgery, elective dental care is best deferred. If surgical treatment is needed during that period, antibiotic prophylaxis is probably warranted. See also Chapter 35.

KEY WEBSITES

(Accessed 27 May 2013)
British Medical Journal. <http://www.bmj.com/specialties/gastroenterology>
Centers for Disease Control and Prevention. <http://www.cdc.gov/ibd/>
MedlinePlus. <http://www.nlm.nih.gov/medlineplus/digestivediseases.html>
NHS Choices. <http://www.nhs.uk/conditions/Inflammatory-bowel-disease/Pages/Introduction.aspx>

USEFUL WEBSITES

(Accessed 27 May 2013)
Mayo Clinic. <http://www.mayoclinic.com>
Medscape Reference. Cheilitis granulomatosa. <http://emedicine.medscape.com/article/1075333-overview>
National Institutes of Health: National Digestive Diseases Information Clearinghouse (NDDIC). <http://digestive.niddk.nih.gov/>
Celiac disease. <http://digestive.niddk.nih.gov/ddiseases/pubs/celiac/index.aspx>
Crohn's disease. <http://digestive.niddk.nih.gov/ddiseases/pubs/crohns/index.htm>
Ulcerative colitis. <http://digestive.niddk.nih.gov/ddiseases/pubs/colitis/index.htm>

FURTHER READING

Baumgart, D.C., Sandborn, W.J., 2007. Inflammatory bowel diseases: cause and immunobiology. Lancet 369, 1627.
Baumgart, D.C., Sandborn, W.J., 2007. Inflammatory bowel diseases: clinical aspects and established and evolving therapies. Lancet 369, 1641.
Cornish, J.A., et al. 2008. The risk of oral contraceptives in the etiology of inflammatory bowel disease: a meta-analysis. Am. J. Gastroenterol. 103, 2394.
Geremia, A., Jewell, D.P., 2012. The IL-23/IL-17 pathway in inflammatory bowel disease. Expert. Rev. Gastroenterol. Hepatol. 6 (2), 223.
Hegarty, A., et al. 2003. Thalidomide for the treatment of recalcitrant oral Crohn's disease and orofacial granulomatosis. Oral Surg. Oral Med. Oral Pathol. Oral Radiol. Endod. 95, 576.
Kang, X., et al. 2008. Prohibitin: a potential biomarker for tissue-based detection of gastric cancer. J. Gastroenterol. 43, 618.
Katz, J., et al. 2003. Oral signs and symptoms in relation to disease activity and site of involvement in patients with inflammatory bowel disease. Oral Dis. 9, 34.
MacDonald, J.K., McDonald, J.W.D, 2006. Natalizumab for induction of remission in Crohn's disease. Cochrane. Database Syst. Rev. 3, 1465.
Miyagaki, H., et al. 2008. The significance of gastrectomy in advanced gastric cancer patients with non-curative factors. Anticancer Res. 28 (4C), 2379.
Moshkowitz, M., et al. 2007. Halitosis and gastroesophageal reflux disease: a possible association. Oral Dis. 13, 581.
Rigoli, L., et al. 2008. Clinical significance of NOD2/CARD15 and Toll-like receptor 4 gene single nucleotide polymorphisms in inflammatory bowel disease. World J. Gastroenterol. 14, 4454.
Scheper, H.J., Brand, H.S., 2002. Oral aspects of Crohn's disease. Int. Dent. J. 52, 163.
Schønnemann, K.R., et al. 2008. Phase II study of short-time oxaliplatin, capecitabine and epirubicin (EXE) as first-line therapy in patients with non-resectable gastric cancer. Br. J. Cancer. (Epub ahead of print)
Scully, C., 2001. Gastroenterological diseases and the mouth. Practitioner 245, 215.
Scully, C., Chaudhry, S., 2007. Aspects of human disease 11. Peptic ulcer disease (PUD). Dent. Update 34, 253.
Scully, C., Chaudhry, S., 2007. Aspects of human disease 12. Inflammatory bowel disease (IBD). Dent. Update 43, 317.
Scully, C., Chaudhry, S., 2007. Aspects of human disease 13. Coeliac disease (gluten-sensitive enteropathy). Dent. Update 43, 381.
Scully, C., Chaudhry, S., 2007. Aspects of human disease 14. Irritable bowel syndrome (IBS). Dent. Update 43, 453.
Silva, M.A.G.S., et al. 2001. Gastroesophageal reflux disease: new oral findings. Oral Surg. 91, 301.
Tilakaratne, W.M., et al. 2008. Orofacial granulomatosis: review on aetiology and pathogenesis. J. Oral. Pathol. Med. 37, 191.

8 Haematology

HAEMOSTASIS

Normal haemostasis (bleeding cessation) depends on the interaction of blood vessels, platelets, fibrin coagulation and deposition, and fibrinolytic proteins (Fig. 8.1). Three reactions – primary, secondary and tertiary haemostasis – act simultaneously. Excessive blood clotting is prevented by the endothelium, which provides a physical barrier and secretes products that inhibit platelets (e.g. nitric oxide and prostaglandin I_2 [prostacyclin]). Inhibitors limit haemostasis to the site of injury and prevent overproduction of the clot – which could lead to pathological thrombosis.

PRIMARY HAEMOSTASIS (VASCULAR AND PLATELET ACTIVITY)

Primary haemostasis is by vasoconstriction after injury, which retards blood loss, slows local blood flow, enhances platelet adherence to subendothelial surfaces and activates coagulation.

The endothelial lining of the vessel wall is a barrier between the circulating platelets and the prothrombotic subendothelial matrix. Upon vessel injury, the endothelial layer is disrupted and the circulating platelets interact with the subendothelium through adhesive receptors, such as glycoprotein (GP) Ib-IX-V receptors, that mediate rolling and tethering of the platelets to von Willebrand factor (vWF) at the site. Platelet collagen receptors $\alpha_2\beta_1$ and GP VI then mediate more firm adhesion and further platelet activation, causing release of platelet dense granules contents; these contain agonists such as adenosine diphosphate (ADP), and α-granules, which contain fibrinogen, factor V and P-selectin. The platelet generates lipid mediators such as thromboxane A_2. ADP elicits its effects on the platelet through the $P2Y_1$ and $P2Y_{12}$ receptors, whereas thromboxane A_2 activates the thromboxane-prostanoid (TP) receptor on the platelet surface. The release of the granule contents also triggers the blood coagulation response as a result of the release of clotting factor V, and the inflammatory response through the exposure of P-selectin on the platelet surface. Also, tissue factor is exposed, which initiates the coagulation response that results in formation of thrombin. Thrombin activates platelets via interactions with the proteinase-activated receptor-1 (PAR1) and PAR4 receptors and also cleaves fibrinogen to form fibrin. Fibrin further stabilizes the accumulating platelet plug at the site of injury, resulting in a stable haemostatic plug.

Platelet activation in response to vessel injury is thus important for the arrest of bleeding (Fig. 8.2), but activation during disease states leads to vascular occlusion and ischaemic damage. The $P2Y_{12}$ receptor,

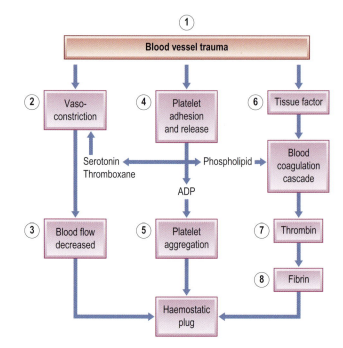

Fig. 8.1 Haemostasis. ADP = Adenosine diphosphate.

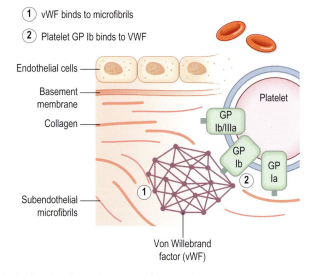

Fig. 8.2 Platelet plug formation. GP = glycoprotein.

activated by ADP, plays a central role in platelet activation and is the target of $P2Y_{12}$ receptor therapeutic antagonists such as clopidogrel (antiplatelets).

Abnormalities in primary haemostasis

Abnormalities in primary haemostasis (abnormal platelet number or function, abnormal vWF or defects in the blood vessel wall) lead to haemorrhage from mucosal surfaces (epistaxis, gingival bleeding, melaena, haematuria), and into skin and mucosae (petechial or ecchymotic haemorrhages). Prolonged bleeding from wounds is usually

Table 8.1 *Blood coagulation factors*

Factor	Name
I	Fibrinogen
II	Prothrombin
III	Thromboplastin
IV	Calcium
V	Proaccelerin
VI	–
VII	Proconvertin
VIII	Antihaemophilic factor
IX	Christmas factor (plasma thromboplastin component)
X	Stuart–Prower factor
XI	Plasma thromboplastin antecedent
XII	Hageman factor
XIII	Fibrin-stabilizing factor
Fitzgerald factor	High-molecular-weight kininogen
Fletcher factor	Prekallikrein

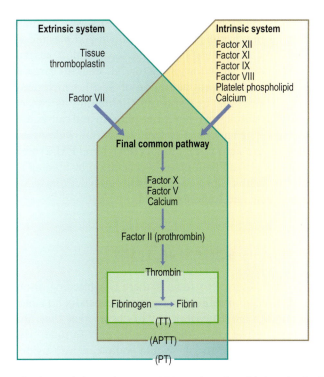

Fig. 8.3 Blood coagulation and assays. APTT = activated partial thromboplastin time; PT = prothrombin time; TT = thrombin time.

restricted by blood coagulation. However, if the defect is severe, more pronounced bleeding can result (e.g. intracavity haemorrhage).

Primary haemostasis inhibitors are the natural inhibitors of platelet function, such as bradykinin, prostacyclin and nitric oxide, released by endothelial cells. Acquired inhibitors of platelet function are rare, whereas acquired inhibitors of vWF (platelet GP Ib) form in a variety of diseases and result in acquired von Willebrand disease (avWD).

More commonly, platelet function is inhibited intentionally by the administration of agents such as aspirin or clopidogrel for the prevention of thrombosis.

SECONDARY HAEMOSTASIS (BLOOD COAGULATION OR CLOTTING)

Secondary haemostasis is the formation of fibrin through the coagulation cascade (Table 8.1, Fig. 8.3), which is traditionally separated into three pathways (extrinsic, intrinsic and common) involving blood coagulation factors acting as enzymes, which require activation and cofactors.

The *extrinsic* pathway is the main pathway. It is initiated by the generation/exposure of tissue factor (factor III), with expression being upregulated by cytokines (tumour necrosis factor alpha [TNFα], interleukin [IL]-6), and the tissue factor–factor VII complex, the latter activating factor X.

The *intrinsic* pathway amplifies coagulation, is stimulated by thrombin, through activation of factor XI, and involves high-molecular-weight kininogen, prekallikrein, factors XII, XI and IX, and factor VIII, which acts as a cofactor (with calcium and platelet phospholipid) for the factor IX-mediated activation of factor X. A minor route of stimulation of the intrinsic pathway (the alternative pathway) is the direct activation of factor IX by the tissue factor–factor VII complex.

The *common* pathway involves the factor X-mediated generation of thrombin from prothrombin (facilitated by factor V, calcium and platelet phospholipid ['prothrombinase complex']). Thrombin then activates factors XI and VIII, amplifying the coagulation cascade. Activated factor IX, together with activated factor VIII, calcium and phospholipid ('tenase complex'), amplify the activation of factor X, generating large amounts of thrombin.

Thrombin cleaves fibrinogen to form soluble fibrin monomers, which spontaneously polymerize to soluble fibrin polymer; thrombin also activates factor XIII, which, together with calcium, cross-links

and stabilizes the soluble fibrin polymer, resulting in cross-linked (insoluble) fibrin. Thrombin also promotes coagulation by promoting platelet aggregation, and activating factors V and VIII – necessary cofactors for the 'prothrombinase' and 'tenase' complexes, respectively. Thrombin also activates factor XIII, essential for the cross-linking of the fibrin polymer, and inhibits fibrinolysis by generation of a thrombin-activatable fibrinolytic inhibitor (TAFI).

Drugs that act as anticoagulants include warfarin, new oral anticoagulants (NOACs), heparin and hirudin.

Abnormalities in the coagulation cascade

These cause more serious bleeding than do defects of primary haemostasis, resulting in bleeding into cavities (chest, joints and cranium) and subcutaneously (haematomas). Petechial haemorrhages are rare. The main *coagulation inhibitor* is antithrombin (AT; also called antithrombin III, or ATIII), a liver alpha$_2$-globulin that inhibits thrombin (factor IIa) and many activated coagulation proteins (including factors II, IX, X, XI and XII). Heparin, produced *in vivo* by degranulated mast cells or basophils, enhances antithrombin binding to thrombin, and this is the basis for its use as an anticoagulant.

Protein C, a vitamin K-dependent protein produced in the liver, inactivates factors V and VIII. Protein S (named after Seattle), another vitamin K-dependent protein synthesized in endothelial cells, megakaryocytes and hepatocytes, facilitates the action of protein C.

TERTIARY HAEMOSTASIS (FIBRINOLYSIS)

Tertiary haemostasis is the formation of plasmin from plasminogen via tissue-type plasminogen activators (t-PAs); other plasminogen activators include urokinase, factor XII and kallikrein. Plasmin lyses both fibrinogen and fibrin, releasing fibrin(ogen) degradation products (FDPs). Activation of fibrinolysis is triggered by fibrin and t-PA, a process regulated by haemostasis inhibitors.

Haemostasis inhibitors (inhibitors of fibrinolysis) include TAFI, alpha$_2$-antiplasmin, histidine-rich glycoprotein and plasminogen activator inhibitors. Amplification of the coagulation cascade from thrombin-mediated activation of factor XI leads to large amounts of thrombin and subsequent activation of TAFI, which prevents the binding of plasminogen to fibrin, thus inhibiting its conversion to plasmin. Alpha$_2$-antiplasmin binds free plasmin and causes its removal by the monocyte–macrophage system, preventing widespread fibrinolysis. Plasminogen activator inhibitors (PAI-1 and PAI-2) are released by endothelial cells and limit plasmin generation by binding to t-PA.

Drugs that inhibit fibrinolysis (antifibrinolytics) include epsilon aminocaproic acid and tranexamic acid.

HAEMOSTASIS SCREENING TESTS

Screening tests are done to show if there is a bleeding disorder, but further tests needed to define the disorder (Appendix 8.1) must follow consultation with the haematologist to ensure that they are appropriate. All that is needed on the request form is to state: 'History of prolonged bleeding' and to ask 'Would you please investigate haemostatic function?', giving as much clinical detail as possible. The blood sample should be adequately labelled and sent immediately for testing, together with relevant clinical information. Tests may need to be repeated before an accurate diagnosis can be made because levels of factors vary over time as a result of stress, pregnancy and infections.

Essential tests usually include:

- *full blood count, film.* A routine 'blood count' [full blood picture] cannot identify a clotting defect but might show platelet deficiency
- *activated partial thromboplastin time (APTT).* The APTT measures the intrinsic pathway and factors V, VIII, IX, X and XI (Table 8.2). Normal APTT values range between 25 ± 10 seconds. The APTT was sometimes known as PTT or kaolin cephalin PTT. It is prolonged in heparin treatment, liver disease, haemophilias, disseminated intravascular coagulation (DIC), massive transfusion and some autoimmune disorders
- *prothrombin time (PT) and international normalized ratio (INR).* The activity of the extrinsic coagulation pathway (factors II, V, VII and X) is measured by the PT, normal values ranging between 12 and 15 seconds. The PT will vary with the type of thromboplastin (e.g. rabbit, human, bovine, etc.) used in the assay, so therefore the INR is used. The INR is the PT ratio of a test sample compared to a normal PT corrected for the sensitivity of the thromboplastin used. Normal INR values are about 1.0. An INR above 1 indicates that clotting will take longer than normal. An INR of 2–3 is the usual therapeutic range for patients on anticoagulants used to treat deep vein thrombosis, and an INR of up to 3.5 is required for patients with prosthetic heart valves. The INR (and PT) is prolonged in warfarin treatment, liver disease, vitamin K deficiency, and DIC (Table 8.3). The INR may be quite stable or erratic in an individual but, in any event, is best assayed less than 24 hours preoperatively, though less than 72 hours may suffice. A normal PT does not necessarily exclude a significant underlying coagulopathy; for example, the PT is normal in severe haemophilias A and B and in factor XI deficiency
- *thrombin time* (TT) (citrated sample)
- *platelet count.* In the tourniquet test (Hess test), the appearance of more than a few petechiae on the forearm when a

Table 8.2 *Interpretation of activated partial thromboplastin time (APTT) results*

APTT	Interpretation
Isolated prolonged	Acquired clotting factor inhibitors – usually directed against factor VIII (e.g. acquired haemophilia A)
	Congenital deficiencies of factor XII, XI, IX or VIII (in general, the factor has to be lower than 20–40% of normal before APTT is prolonged)
	Lupus anticoagulant (LA) – targets phospholipid
Prolonged + prolonged PT	Combined clotting factors deficiency
	Disseminated intravascular coagulation (DIC)
	Liver disease
	Massive blood transfusion – dilutional coagulopathy
	Thrombin inhibitors (hirudin, argatroban and dabigatran)
	Thrombolytic therapy
	Vitamin K deficiency
Increased ± prolonged PT	Unfractionated heparin [UFH] significantly prolongs APTT but PT usually shows little prolongation Antiphospholipid antibodies
	Acquired clotting factor inhibitors, e.g. factors V, X
Prolonged ± prolonged PT	Warfarin overdose
Short	An acute phase response with high factor VIII

Table 8.3 *Interpretation of international normalized ratio (INR) and prothrombin time (PT) results*

PT or INR	Interpretation
Prolonged alone	Factor VII deficiency
Prolonged, along with other coagulation abnormalities	Afibrinogenaemia and dysfibrinogenaemia
	Dilutional coagulopathy, e.g. massive blood transfusion
	Direct thrombin inhibitors, e.g. lepirudin
	Liver disease
	Malabsorption (leads to vitamin K deficiency)
	Multiple clotting factor deficiencies
	Unfractionated heparin
	Vitamin K deficiency
	Vitamin K antagonists (e.g. warfarin, phenindione)
Shortened	Treatment with recombinant factor VIIa

sphygmomanometer cuff is inflated suggests a platelet or vascular defect, but the clinical test is neither sensitive nor specific. The 'bleeding time' is also rarely used, as it is not completely reliable. Thus to exclude platelet defects, a platelet count is essential and platelet function assays may be indicated. A normal platelet count should be 100 000–400 000 cells/mm^3 (Fig. 8.4); a count of less than 100 000 cells/mm^3 (thrombocytopenia) can be associated with major postoperative bleeding

- *serum for blood grouping and cross-matching.* This should be done if an operation is planned.

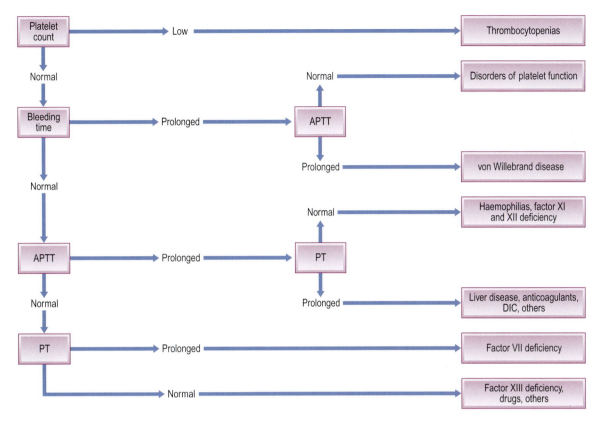

Fig. 8.4 Protocol for investigation of a bleeding disorder. DIC = disseminated intravascular coagulation.

Once the haemostasis screening tests have indicated that there is a bleeding disorder, other, more specific tests are required, such as:

- *factor VIII clotting activity* – to measure factor VIII amount
- *vWF antigen* – to measure vWF amount
- *ristocetin cofactor activity* – to measure vWF function
- *vWF multimers* – to measure vWF structure
- *platelet aggregation tests* – before assessing platelet function using *in vitro* tests of platelet adhesion and aggregation, aspirin, non-steroidal inflammatory drugs (NSAIDs) and antiplatelet drugs should be avoided for at least 7 days. The average lifespan of a platelet ranges from 7 to 12 days. Platelet aggregation can be measured using aggregating agents such as ristocetin but, unfortunately, such tests are difficult to standardize and do not identify all platelet disorders; the clinical features are often more important.

A practical guide to laboratory haemostasis is provided at: http://www.practical-haemostasis.com/Screening%20Tests/tt.html (accessed 30 September 2013).

BLEEDING (HAEMOSTATIC) DISORDERS

General aspects

Bleeding disorders manifest with common bleeding features, including epistaxis and gingival bleeding, and may occur after wounds and surgery; these are often the first indications of a haemostatic defect. Defects in haemostasis can comprise abnormalities in platelet activation and function, contact activation or with clotting proteins, or may signal excess antithrombin function. The more common causes of a bleeding tendency include:

- aspirin (one tablet impairs platelet function for almost 1 week but this rarely causes significant postoperative haemorrhage), NSAIDs and other antiplatelet drugs

- warfarin (the most common anticoagulant, which interferes with clotting factor production via vitamin K blockage)
- von Willebrand disease (the most common inherited bleeding disorder).
- acquired bleeding tendencies, such as:
  - bone marrow disease
  - immune disorders
  - liver disease
  - renal disease.

Clinical features

Examination may reveal signs of purpura in the skin or mucosae (Fig. 8.5). Signs of underlying disease – such as anaemia and lymphadenopathy in leukaemia, for example – must also be sought. Joint deformities from haemarthroses, characteristic of haemophilia, should also be looked for but are infrequently seen now (Fig. 8.6).

Alternatively, purpura may be localized to the mouth (sometimes grandiloquently termed 'angina bullosa haemorrhagica') and not associated with any abnormal bleeding tendencies. People with *senile purpura* (an age-related condition) bruise easily with minimal trauma, often without any other apparent underlying cause, and generally on the forearms and tops of the hands. The resulting dark purplish-red splotches fade gradually, often leaving a yellow/brown stain, which may disappear completely or remain. Such purpura can be caused by excessive sun exposure; drugs, such as aspirin and steroids (*steroid purpura*); diabetes; vascular diseases; thrombocytopenia; scurvy; and connective tissue diseases. There is no treatment available.

General management

Patients may already be aware of having a bleeding disorder and may carry an appropriate warning card, bracelet or wristband. Otherwise,

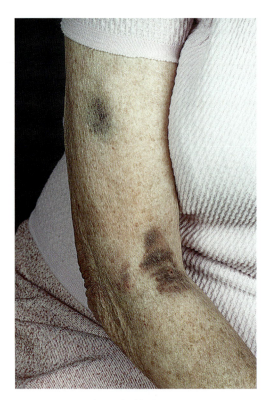

Fig. 8.5 Purpura in a patient with myeloid leukaemia.

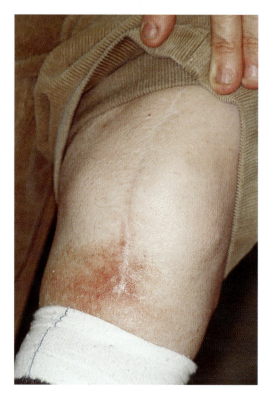

Fig. 8.6 Haemarthrosis in an older haemophiliac has caused crippling arthritis. His five brothers all succumbed to haemophilia at a time when factor VIII was unknown.

Table 8.4 *Comparative features of bleeding disorders*

	Platelet defects[a]	Coagulation defects
Gender affected	Females mainly	Males
Family history	Rarely	Usually positive
Nature of bleeding after trauma	Immediate	Delayed
Effect when locally applied pressure removed	May stop bleeding	Bleeding recurs
Spontaneous bleeding into skin or mucosa, or from mucosa or gingivae	Common	Uncommon
Bleeding from minor superficial injuries (e.g. needle prick)	Common	Uncommon
Deep haemorrhages or haemarthroses	Rare	Common
Bleeding time	Prolonged	Normal
Tourniquet (Hess) test	Positive	Negative
Platelet count	Often low	Normal
Clotting function	Normal	Abnormal

[a]Purpura is rarely vascular.

Table 8.5 *Typical laboratory findings in platelet disorders*

Disorder	Bleeding time	Platelet count	Clot retraction	Platelet aggregation	Platelet factor III activity
Thrombocytopenia	↑	↓	↓	–	–
Thrombasthenia	↑	N	↓	↓	↓
Storage pool deficiency	↑	N	N	N or ↓	↓
Aspirin/von Willebrand disease	↑	N	N	↓ (only with ristocetin)	N
Thrombocythaemia	↑	↑	N or ↓	N or ↓	N or ↓

N = normal.

an adequate history is the single most important part of evaluation; physical examination is necessary and laboratory tests are needed to confirm the diagnosis. Table 8.4 shows comparative features of coagulation defects and platelet defects, and Table 8.5 lists typical laboratory findings in platelet disorders.

A history with any suggestion of a haemorrhagic tendency must be taken seriously. Nevertheless, patients can be remarkably capricious as to the information they provide and, in any case, cannot always be expected to know when bleeding can legitimately be regarded as 'abnormal'. Previous dental extractions provide a useful guide, but

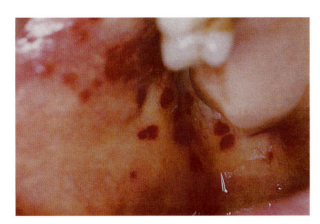

Fig. 8.7 Oral purpura.

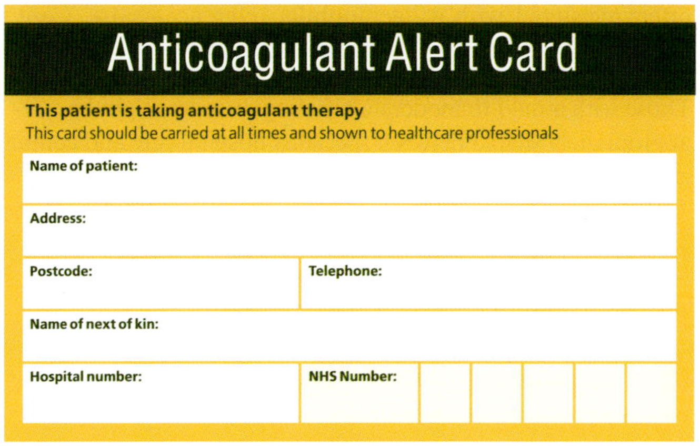

Anticoagulant Alert Card

This patient is taking anticoagulant therapy
This card should be carried at all times and shown to healthcare professionals

Name of patient:	
Address:	
Postcode:	Telephone:
Name of next of kin:	
Hospital number:	NHS Number:

Fig. 8.8 Oral anticoagulant therapy warning card.

prolonged bleeding (up to 24–48 hours) as an isolated episode is usually the result of local factors, especially excessive trauma. It should be stressed again that a history of previous haemorrhagic episodes is the most important feature since screening tests of haemostasis do not always detect mild defects.

Special emphasis must be placed on the following, which are suggestive of a bleeding disorder:

- Deep haemorrhage into muscles, joints or skin – suggests a clotting defect
- Bleeding from and into mucosae – suggests purpura (Fig. 8.7).

Females often 'bruise easily' but any such bruises are usually insignificant and small. Excessive menstrual bleeding is also rarely due to a bleeding disorder.

Most significant congenital bleeding disorders become apparent in childhood and patients may carry a warning card. However, people with mild bleeding tendencies can escape recognition until adult life if they manage to avoid injury or surgery, but can then present with oozing from an extraction socket for 2–3 weeks despite local haemostatic measures such as suturing. Patients who have had tonsillectomy or dental extractions without trouble, or previous dental bleeding that was controlled by local measures, are unlikely to have a serious congenital haemorrhagic disease. On the other hand, admission to hospital and blood transfusion or comparable measures have obvious implications. Haemorrhagic disease in a blood relative is also strongly suggestive of a clotting defect. Many drugs, such as anticoagulants (Fig. 8.8), NSAIDs and antiplatelet drugs, may cause bleeding tendencies, as may hepatic, renal, human immunodeficiency (HIV) and other disease. Some herbal products may also impair platelet aggregation and prolong bleeding (Ch. 26).

Precise characterization of a congenital clotting defect depends on assay of the individual factors, and a wide range of other investigations may be indicated according to the type of case. For example, the assays usually used in the diagnosis of haemophilia A are the APTT and the factor VIII coagulant (FVIIIC) activity. The bleeding time and whole-blood clotting time are uninformative and obsolete.

It is important also to investigate patients with a suspected bleeding tendency for anaemia. This is because:

- anaemia is an expected consequence of repeated haemorrhages
- any further bleeding as a result of surgery will worsen the anaemia, or the anaemia may need to be treated before surgery can be carried out
- anaemia may be an essential concomitant of the haemorrhagic tendency – as in leukaemia.

Patients may also need to be screened for liver disease and for blood-borne infections, particularly HIV and hepatitis viruses.

Individuals with bleeding disorders may need to be treated with replacement of the missing factor. Earlier, use of blood or blood fractions sometimes resulted in the transmission of blood-borne viruses and other infections. In many countries, blood is now collected from donors under careful precautions, and screened to exclude antibodies to infections such as HIV, hepatitis B, hepatitis C, syphilis or cytomegalovirus. In developed countries, all cellular blood products are leukodepleted to limit the risk of transmission of prions and some other infections. Leukocytes in erythrocyte and platelet concentrates are now considered as a contaminant since they can cause many other adverse effects, such as the transmission of other cell-associated infectious agents (e.g. herpesviruses and *Toxoplasma*), febrile non-haemolytic reactions, graft-versus-host disease and immunosuppression. Recombinant factors are thus preferred for factor replacement.

Dental aspects

Prolonged post-operative bleeding is defined if any of the following appertains:

- Bleeding continues for 12 hours.
- Bleeding causes the patient to return for attention.
- Bleeding causes a large haematoma/ecchymosis.
- The patient needs a transfusion.

All dental professionals encounter patients who experience prolonged bleeding following operative procedures, often a dental extraction. Saliva contains fibrinolytic agents that may aggravate the situation. In most cases, the cause is local, and bleeding can be managed using simple local haemostatic measures such as applying pressure to the wound with sterile pads (moistened with water, normal saline or 5% tranexamic acid solution), using absorbable oxidized cellulose sponges, and suturing, as well as giving postoperative instructions verbally and in writing.

A bleeding tendency can be encountered in patients with congenital haemostatic defects such as haemophilias or some rare platelet defects; or acquired disorders such as may arise in liver disease, renal disease, bone marrow disease, immune disorders or with some drugs. In vascular or platelet disorders, postoperative problems following an extraction usually present as prolonged bleeding *immediately* after the event; in coagulation defects, the bleeding typically begins *after some delay*. Patients with a bleeding tendency may require prophylactic measures preoperatively, special precautions perioperatively and careful management postoperatively. Patients with hereditary bleeding disorders are often registered with a haemophilia reference centre. Care is as follows:

- Those with a mild to moderate bleeding disorder might be appropriately shared between specialist hospital care and community and/or primary care dental services for different procedures.
- Those with a severe bleeding disorder managed from home with appropriate medication may possibly be treated in primary care under the direction of the haemophilia reference centre.
- Those with a severe bleeding condition with associated complications such as HIV, hepatitis C or inhibitors, or those requiring surgery, are often more appropriately cared for in a hospital care setting.

Some known haemophiliacs have neglected oral health because of barriers to accessing care, including travel to specialist centres, waiting times, increased treatment needs and cost, or fear of bleeding from dental procedures. They may require more complex treatment and management by the time that they present.

Surgery should ideally be planned and done where appropriate after suitable measures to correct the bleeding tendency, such as blood clotting factor or platelet replacement or, where drugs are responsible, by modifying drug doses provided that the risk of subsequent thromboembolism is not a contra-indication:

- at the beginning of the day – this allows more time to deal with immediate rebleeding problems
- early in the week – this allows for delayed rebleeding episodes occurring after 24–48 hours to be dealt with during the working week.

VASCULAR DISORDERS

Vascular purpura rarely causes serious bleeding; any bleeding into mucous membranes or skin starts immediately after trauma but stops within 24–48 hours. Vascular disorders are a rare cause of bleeding problems; they include Marfan, Ehlers–Danlos (Ch. 16) and Osler–Rendu–Weber syndromes.

OSLER–WEBER–RENDU SYNDROME (HEREDITARY HAEMORRHAGIC TELANGIECTASIA [HHT/HHT1])

General aspects

Hereditary haemorrhagic telangiectasia (HHT) is an autosomal dominant condition with a high penetrance, as 97% of people affected exhibit symptoms. There is vascular dysplasia leading to telangiectasia and arteriovenous malformations in the skin, mucosa and viscera. There may be associated immunoglobulin A (IgA) deficiency or, rarely, vWD (see below).

Clinical features

Interestingly, HHT usually presents in adolescence. Telangiectasia on the skin or any part of the oral, nasal, conjunctival, respiratory, gastrointestinal or urogenital mucosa, or brain and liver (Fig. 8.9), leads to bleeding. Most people (62%) are diagnosed by the age of 16, with over 90% of cases presenting with recurrent epistaxis, not present until adult life. Other associated features include:

- haemorrhage of the gastrointestinal tract, which can result in iron deficiency anaemia

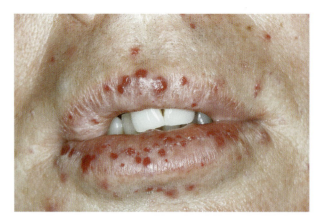

Fig. 8.9 Hereditary haemorrhagic telangiectasia.

- respiratory arteriovenous malformations, which can present as dyspnoea, cyanosis or finger-clubbing. Paradoxical cerebral emboli can cause stroke or cerebral abscess. Care must be taken when prescribing midazolam sedation or general anaesthesia for these patients
- liver arteriovenous malformations that can cause cirrhosis, which can further exacerbate the bleeding tendency, and high-output cardiac failure.

General management

Investigations include capillary microscopy, computed tomography (CT), magnetic resonance imaging (MRI) and angiography. Treatment is by cryosurgery or argon laser treatment, if the telangiectases have bled significantly or are cosmetically unacceptable.

Dental aspects

Telangiectases may be seen in any part of the mouth and may be conspicuous on the lips and tongue. Bleeding from oral surgery is unlikely to be troublesome. Rarely, brain abscesses or other infections have followed oral procedures that cause bacteraemias but there is no consensus as to the need for antibacterial prophylaxis.

Regional local anaesthesia (LA) should be avoided because of the risk of deep bleeding. Conscious sedation (CS) can be given if required. In general anaesthesia (GA), nasal intubation is best avoided and close postoperative observation is advisable.

LOCALIZED ORAL PURPURA ('ANGINA BULLOSA HAEMORRHAGICA')

Blood blisters are occasionally seen, typically in older persons, in the absence of obvious trauma, generalized purpura, any other bleeding tendency or evidence of any systemic disease. These blood blisters are often in the palate and may sometimes be a centimetre or more in diameter; after rupture, they may leave a sore area for a few days. When a large blood blister of this type is in the pharynx, it can cause an alarming choking sensation and was therefore originally termed 'angina bullosa haemorrhagica'. However, almost any site in the mouth can be affected.

Before the diagnosis of localized oral purpura can be made confidently and the patient reassured, other causes of blood blisters in the mouth must be excluded. These include: platelet disorders, amyloidosis (causing factor X deficiency), leukaemia, infectious mononucleosis, HIV or rubella; trauma; corticosteroid inhalers; or bleeding into subepithelial blisters, such as in mucous membrane pemphigoid (Ch. 11).

Table 8.6 *Platelet defects*

	Defect	Manifestations	Management
Thrombasthenia (Glanzmann syndrome)	Defective platelet aggregation due to defective membrane protein	Severe bleeding tendency	Platelet infusions needed preoperatively
Bernard–Soulier syndrome	Giant platelets with defect in platelet glycoprotein which acts as receptor for von Willebrand factor	Heritable disorder resembling von Willebrand disease but considerably more rare	Platelet infusions needed preoperatively
Storage pool deficiency	Platelets lack capacity to store serotonin and adenine nucleotides, and consequently fail to aggregate	Usually congenital with autosomal inheritance. If associated with albinism, is termed Hermansky–Pudlak syndrome	Platelet infusion or cryoprecipitate corrects the bleeding tendency
HIV infection	Purpura is a relatively common feature of HIV infection. May be autoimmune but there appears also to be a platelet defect resulting from the infection; drugs such as zidovudine or some protease inhibitors and bone marrow disease may also contribute	Oral purpura in HIV infection may closely mimic oral lesions of Kaposi sarcoma (Ch. 20)	See Ch. 20
Chronic renal failure	Ch. 12		
Drugs: heparin, dextrans	See later in this chapter		
Dysproteinaemias	See later in this chapter		
Myelodysplastic syndrome	See later in this chapter		

PLATELET DISORDERS

Platelets originate from bone marrow megakaryocytes and have a life span of about 1 week, before they are destroyed in the spleen. Thrombopoietin, the megakaryocyte-stimulating hormone is produced in the liver and kidneys, so liver, kidney or bone marrow disease can each cause thrombocytopenia. Platelet numbers or function, if impaired, can cause a bleeding tendency, purpura and abnormal laboratory investigation results (Tables 8.5 and 8.6). Drugs, bone marrow invasion, autoimmune diseases and other disorders can reduce platelet numbers (if the platelet count falls below 100×10^9/L, a patient has thrombocytopenia). Thrombocytopenia may arise from (Fig. 8.10):

- *decreased megakaryocyte production/maturation.* Most thrombocytopenia is idiopathic (autoimmune thrombocytopenia), but can be caused by viruses such as human parvovirus B19, rubella, Epstein–Barr, cytomegalovirus and HIV, as well as drugs such as cytotoxics. Infiltration of the bone marrow by leukaemia, myeloma or carcinoma leads to bone marrow suppression and thrombocytopenia plus anaemia. Vitamin B_{12} and folate deficiency leads to inadequate megakaryocyte maturation
- *increased platelet destruction.* This is seen in *idiopathic thrombocytopenic purpura* (ITP), *haemolytic uraemic syndrome* (HUS) and *thrombotic thrombocytopenic purpura* (TTP) – see below. *DIC* (see later) leads to consumption of platelets and to thrombocytopenia
- *sequestration of platelets.* An enlarged spleen (splenomegaly) is usually responsible for platelet sequestration which may be, therefore, caused by:
    portal hypertension, e.g. cirrhosis
    haematological disorders, e.g. myeloproliferative disorders
    infections, e.g. malaria, leishmaniasis, Epstein–Barr virus
    storage disorders, e.g. Gaucher disease, Niemann–Pick disease
    inflammatory disorders, e.g. systemic lupus erythematosus (SLE), Felty syndrome.

Inherited platelet abnormalities tend to affect platelet function rather than number. *Abnormal platelet function* is seen in Glanzmann disease and dysproteinaemias. Platelet function can also be impaired

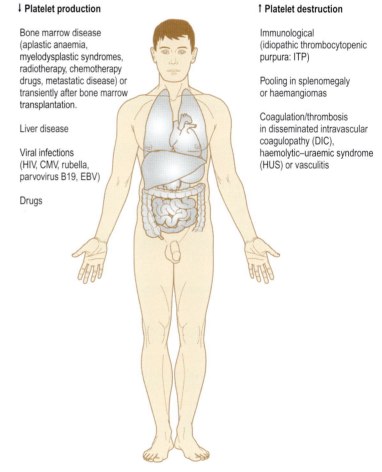

↓ Platelet production

Bone marrow disease (aplastic anaemia, myelodysplastic syndromes, radiotherapy, chemotherapy drugs, metastatic disease) or transiently after bone marrow transplantation.

Liver disease

Viral infections (HIV, CMV, rubella, parvovirus B19, EBV)

Drugs

↑ Platelet destruction

Immunological (idiopathic thrombocytopenic purpura: ITP)

Pooling in splenomegaly or haemangiomas

Coagulation/thrombosis in disseminated intravascular coagulopathy (DIC), haemolytic–uraemic syndrome (HUS) or vasculitis

Fig. 8.10 Thrombocytopenia. CMV = cytomegalovirus; EBV = Epstein–Barr virus.

due to an increase in numbers (thrombocytosis). *Abnormal platelet distribution* is seen in splenomegaly or transfusion of stored blood.

IDIOPATHIC THROMBOCYTOPENIC PURPURA (ITP)

This involves autoantibody-mediated platelet destruction, the most common antibody being directed against the platelet GPIIb–IIIa receptor. Features include petechiae, ecchymoses and postoperative haemorrhage. Full blood picture and platelet counts are indicated. Corticosteroids or other immunosuppressives are the main treatments. Splenectomy or splenic irradiation, followed by thrombopoietin therapy is sometimes needed. Eltrombopag and romiplostin are thrombopoietin receptor agonists which stimulate platelet production and used to treat ITP. Dental extractions can be covered by these agents.

HAEMOLYTIC URAEMIC SYNDROME (HUS) AND THROMBOTIC THROMBOCYTOPENIC PURPURA (TTP)

These conditions are caused by small-vessel wall damage, leading to fibrin and platelet deposition and haemolysis. HUS predominantly affects the kidneys and TTP the brain. *Escherichia coli* O157 gastroenteritis may cause HUS in children, but in adults more commonly causes TTP.

GLANZMANN DISEASE (GLANZMANN THROMBASTHENIA)

Glanzmann disease is a rare autosomal recessive disorder caused by either deficient or abnormal glycoprotein platelet receptors. Defects in the GP IIb/IIIa complex lead to defective platelet aggregation and subsequent bleeding, usually presenting in infancy or early childhood, with bruising or petechiae following minimal or unrecognized trauma, or epistaxis. The platelet count is normal but platelet aggregation defective.

Management includes avoiding trauma and avoiding analgesics such as aspirin. Minor bleeding intraorally can be managed with tranexamic acid. Major bleeding may require platelet transfusion. Recombinant human-activated factor VII (rFVII) has been used in patients with antibodies to GP IIb/IIIa and/or human leukocyte antigen (HLA) that render transfusions ineffective.

BERNARD–SOULIER SYNDROME

Bernard–Soulier syndrome is a rare congenital disorder with large platelets that lack platelet membrane glycoproteins – resulting in defective platelet adhesion. Clinical features resemble those of Glanzmann disease. A full blood count reveals giant platelets. Platelets fail to aggregate in response to vWF.

Management is as for Glanzmann disease.

RENAL FAILURE

High serum urea levels directly inhibit platelet function and there may also be thrombocytopenia. Desmopressin (deamino-8-D-arginine vasopressin; DDAVP) may be used to boost vWF levels in order to treat mild bleeding episodes. In severe bleeding, cryoprecipitate or platelet transfusion may be required.

ANTIPLATELET DRUGS

Platelets may pathologically aggregate intravascularly as arterial thrombi in response to haemorrhage into atherosclerotic plaques, and this is potentially lethal. Antiplatelet drugs prevent and/or reverse platelet aggregation in arterial thromboses, and help prevent clotting in patients who have had a myocardial infarct, unstable angina, ischaemic strokes, transient ischaemic attacks (TIAs or 'little strokes') and other forms of cardiovascular disease. In practice, a favourable balance between the beneficial and harmful effects of antiplatelet therapy is achieved by treating patients whose thrombotic risk outweighs their risk of bleeding complications.

Commonly used antiplatelet agents include:

- aspirin
- GP IIb/IIIa inhibitors (abciximab, eptifibatide and tirofiban)
- phosphodiesterase inhibitors (e.g. dipyridamole)
- thienopyridines (e.g. clopidogrel, prasugrel and ticlopidine).

Aspirin

Aspirin is an irreversible inhibitor of platelet cyclo-oxygenase (COX) enzymes, which catalyse the production of thromboxane A_2 (an important platelet aggregator) from arachidonic acid. Low-dose aspirin is the usual first-line treatment for thrombosis and myocardial infarction. The most common adverse effect of aspirin is gastrointestinal bleeding, which can be minimized by using the lowest effective dose (often 75 mg daily), advising patients to take aspirin with food, and, where indicated, co-prescribing a proton pump inhibitor (PPI).

GP IIb/IIIa inhibitors

These drugs prevent cross-linking of platelets. *Abciximab* is a chimeric human–murine GP IIb/IIIa antibody; the peptide derivatives, *eptifibatide* and *tirofiban*, are more selective towards the GP IIb/IIIa receptor and have a shorter effect than abciximab. These agents are used parenterally in acute coronary syndromes, but only by specialists. Serious adverse effects of GP IIb/IIIa antagonists include major bleeding, intracerebral haemorrhage and thrombocytopenia.

Phosphodiesterase inhibitors

Phosphodiesterase inhibitors include *dipyridamole* – a vasodilator and antiplatelet agent that inhibits adenosine uptake and cyclic guanosine monophosphate (cGMP) phosphodiesterase activity, thus decreasing platelet aggregability. Dipyridamole is used with aspirin or warfarin in the prophylaxis of thromboembolic disorders.

Thienopyridines

Thienopyridines act via inhibition of platelet activation by the ADP-dependent pathway without a direct effect on prostaglandin metabolism. *Ticlopidine* is the oldest thienopyridine available and is approved for secondary prevention of thrombotic strokes in aspirin-intolerant patients, and in combination with aspirin for prevention of coronary stent thrombosis. Serious adverse effects are mainly haematological (neutropenia, thrombocytopenia and TTP). *Clopidogrel* has a better safety profile than ticlopidine and is often reserved for those with true aspirin hypersensitivity or intolerance, and for prevention of atherosclerotic events following recent myocardial infarction, stroke or established peripheral arterial disease. It is also approved for use in acute coronary syndromes that are treated with either percutaneous coronary intervention (PCI) or coronary artery bypass grafting (CABG). Dual therapy with aspirin and clopidogrel increases the risk of gastrointestinal bleeding and is thus usually restricted to patients following PCI or acute coronary syndromes. *Prasugrel* is a more rapid-acting and potent platelet aggregation inhibitor and may be used together with aspirin in the setting of high-risk or urgent PCI.

Dental aspects of platelet disorders

The main danger of platelet disorders is haemorrhage but this is rarely as severe as in clotting disorders. Regional LA block injections can

Table 8.7 *Thrombocytopenia: manifestations and management of oral surgery*

Platelet count (× 10⁹/L)	Severity of thrombocytopenia	Manifestations	Management in relation to type of surgery	
			Dentoalveolar	Maxillofacial
100–150	Mild	Mild purpura sometimes. Slightly prolonged postoperative bleeding	No platelet transfusion. Local haemostatic measures.ᵃ Observe	Consider platelet transfusion. Local haemostatic measures.ᵃ Observe
50–100	Moderate	Purpura, postoperative bleeding	Platelets may be needed. Local haemostatic measures.ᵃ Consider postoperative tranexamic acid mouthwash for 3 days	Platelets needed. Local haemostatic measures.ᵃ Postoperative tranexamic acid mouthwash for 3 days
30–50	Severe	Purpura, postoperative bleeding, even from venepuncture	Platelets needed. Local haemostatic measures.ᵃ Postoperative tranexamic acid mouthwash for 3 days	Platelets needed. Local haemostatic measures.ᵃ Avoid surgery where possible. Postoperative tranexamic acid mouthwash for 3 days
<30	Life-threatening	Purpura, spontaneous bleeding	Platelets needed. Local haemostatic measures.ᵃ Avoid surgery where possible. Postoperative tranexamic acid mouthwash for 3 days	Platelets needed. Local haemostatic measures.ᵃ Avoid surgery where possible. Postoperative tranexamic acid mouthwash for 3 days

ᵃLocal haemostatic measures comprise compressive packing, sutures, and microfibrillar collagen or oxidized cellulose.

be given if the platelet levels are above 30×10^9/L. Haemostasis after dentoalveolar surgery is usually adequate if platelet levels are above 50×10^9/L. Major surgery requires platelet levels above 75×10^9/L. CS can be given but if it is delivered by the intravenous route, care must be taken not to damage the vein. GA can be given in hospital but expert intubation is needed to avoid the risk of submucous bleeding into the airway.

Platelets can be replaced or supplemented by platelet transfusions (1 unit of platelets should raise the count by around 10×10^9 platelets/L), but sequestration of platelets is very rapid. Platelet transfusions are therefore best used for controlling already established thrombocytopenic bleeding. When given prophylactically, platelets should be given in the following way: half just before surgery to control capillary bleeding, and half at the end of the operation to facilitate placement of adequate sutures. Platelets should be used within 6–24 hours of collection. Suitable preparations include platelet-rich plasma (PRP), which contains about 90% of the platelets from a unit of fresh blood in about half this volume, and platelet-rich concentrate (PRC), which contains about 50% of the platelets from a unit of fresh whole blood in a volume of only 25 mL. PRC is thus the best source of platelets. Platelet infusions carry the risk of isoimmunization, infection with blood-borne agents and, rarely, graft-versus-host disease. Where there is immune destruction of platelets (e.g. in ITP), platelet infusions are less effective. The need for platelet transfusions can be reduced by local haemostatic measures and use of desmopressin (DDAVP) or tranexamic acid or topical administration of platelet concentrates. Absorbable haemostatic agents, such as oxidized regenerated cellulose (Surgicel), synthetic collagen (Instat) or microcrystalline collagen (Avitene), may be put in the socket to assist clotting.

Splenectomy predisposes to infections, typically with pneumococci, and especially within the first 2 years. Systemic infection post-splenectomy, involving oral streptococci, is rare and antimicrobial prophylaxis is not therefore generally recommended before invasive dental procedures.

Long-term corticosteroids can cause well-recognized problems (Ch. 6). Perioperative management is summarized in Tables 8.6 and 8.7 and Figure 8.11. Drugs such as aspirin and other NSAIDs that damage platelets should be avoided (Table 8.8). The effects of aspirin are *not* dose-dependent; even a single tablet can affect platelet COX

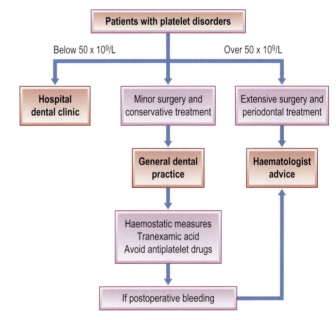

Fig. 8.11 Dental management in platelet disorders.

irreversibly for about a week. Other NSAIDs may have a reversible effect and act for up to 48 hours only. COX-2 inhibitors have no such effect on platelets.

When prescribed as primary prevention, *antiplatelet agents* may be safely withdrawn 7 days before surgery, but any decision to stop antiplatelet therapy used for secondary prevention must balance the risk of thrombosis and ischaemia against bleeding. There is no evidence that continuing antiplatelet monotherapy causes major bleeding problems during or after minor surgery such as dental extractions. The risk of bleeding is greater with aspirin–clopidogrel or prasugrel–aspirin combinations, but patients taking these drugs are generally already at a higher risk of thromboembolic events; therefore, advice from a specialist should be sought before withholding treatment, or the patient may need to be referred to a hospital setting for the procedure. There is no suitable test available to assess the increased risk of bleeding in patients taking antiplatelet medications.

Table 8.8 *Some drugs that may impair platelets or their function*

Class	Examples
Alcohol	
Analgesics and other platelet inhibitors	Aspirin and other NSAIDs
	Clopidogrel
Antibiotics	Amoxicillin
	Ampicillin and derivatives
	Azithromycin
	Benzylpenicillin (penicillin G)
	Carbenicillin
	Cephalosporins
	Gentamicin
	Meticillin
	Rifampicin
	Sulphonamides
	Trimethoprim
Antidiabetics	Tolbutamide
Cardiovascular drugs	Digitoxin
	Heparin
	Methyldopa
	Oxprenolol
	Quinine
Cytotoxic drugs	Many
Diuretics	Acetazolamide
	Chlorothiazide
	Furosemide
General anaesthetic agents	Halothane
Psychoactive drugs	Antihistamines (some)
	Chlorpromazine
	Diazepam
	Haloperidol
	Tricyclic antidepressants
	Valproate

Table 8.9 *Drug effects on bleeding tendency*

Drug	Effect on bleeding
Alcohol	Warfarin enhanced by large amounts of alcohol
Analgesics	Bleeding enhanced by aspirin effect on platelets
Antibacterials	Warfarin enhanced by cephalosporins, erythromycin and metronidazole. Ampicillin and amoxicillin may increase bleeding
Antifungals	Warfarin enhanced by azoles, including miconazole topically
Anti-inflammatories	Bleeding enhanced by antiplatelet activity of NSAIDs; warfarin may also be enhanced. Corticosteroids may alter warfarin activity

Box 8.1 *Main coagulation defects*

- Anticoagulants and thrombolytic agents
- Chronic renal failure
- Deficiencies of factors XII and XIII and others
- Disseminated intravascular coagulation
- Dysproteinaemias, especially multiple myeloma
- Haemophilia
- Liver disease, including obstructive jaundice
- Lupus erythematosus
- Von Willebrand disease

Patients who should *not* have their medications stopped or altered prior to dental surgical procedures in primary care include those taking:

- low-dose aspirin
- clopidogrel
- dipyridamole.

Patients are more at risk of permanent disability or death from thromboembolic episodes if they stop antiplatelet medications prior to a surgical procedure than if they continue them. Although the risk is low, the outcome is serious, so antiplatelet medications should only be discontinued in the perioperative period when the haemorrhagic risk of continuing them is definitely greater than the cardiovascular risk associated with their discontinuation. Bleeding complications, while inconvenient, do not carry the same risks as thromboembolic complications. Patients taking antiplatelet medications will have a prolonged bleeding time but this may not be clinically relevant and postoperative bleeding after dental procedures can usually be controlled using local haemostatic measures.

Consensus, then, is that for dentoalveolar surgical procedures, antiplatelet medications should not be stopped nor doses altered, but that local haemostatic measures should be used to control bleeding. The following patients taking antiplatelet medication, however, should

not be treated in primary care without medical advice – or should be referred to a dental hospital or hospital-based dental clinic:

- Those with liver impairment and/or alcoholism
- Those with renal failure
- Those with thrombocytopenia, haemophilia or other disorder of haemostasis
- Those currently receiving a course of cytotoxic medication.

Dentoalveolar surgical procedures likely to be carried out in primary care will be classified as minor, e.g. simple extraction of up to three teeth, gingival surgery, crown and bridge procedures, dental scaling and the surgical removal of teeth. When more than three teeth need to be extracted, multiple visits will be required. Extractions may be planned to remove two or three teeth at a time, by quadrants, or singly at separate visits. Scaling and gingival surgery should initially be restricted to a limited area to assess whether bleeding is problematic. Patients requiring major surgery should usually be treated in a secondary care setting.

BLOOD COAGULATION DISORDERS

Blood coagulates via a number of liver-synthesized serum proteins (coagulation factors), activated by a cascade of enzymatic reactions. Two pathways of coagulation – the intrinsic and extrinsic – have a common end-point at the formation of thrombin, which then catalyses the formation of fibrin from fibrinogen. Coagulation disorders – typically from drugs (e.g. warfarin), liver failure and renal failure – are the main causes of such a bleeding tendency.

Coagulation disorders are due mainly to genetic defects of clotting factors (vWD but also other haemophilias), to anticoagulant or other drug therapy (Table 8.9), or to a range of diseases, especially those affecting the liver or kidney (Box 8.1). These cause a range of changes in the results of laboratory investigations (Table 8.10).

Table 8.10 *Laboratory findings in clotting disorders*

Disorder	Prothrombin time (PT)	Activated partial thromboplastin time (APTT)	Thrombin time (TT)	Fibrinogen level	Fibrin(ogen) degradation products (FDP)
Haemophilia A; haemophilia B; von Willebrand disease; deficiency of factors XI and XII	N	↑	N	N	N
Warfarin or other coumarin therapy; obstructive jaundice or other causes of vitamin K deficiency; deficiency of factor V or X	↑	↑	N	N	N
Heparin therapy; disseminated intravascular coagulation	↑	↑	N	N	N
Parenchymal liver disease	↑	↑	↑	↓	↑
Deficiency of factor VII	↑	N	N	N	N

N = normal.

Table 8.11 *Blood coagulation factor defects in descending order of frequency*

Factor deficient	Inheritance	Incidence (1 in)
VIII	X-linked	10 000
IX	X-linked	60 000
VII	Autosomal recessive	500 000
V	Autosomal recessive	1 million
X	Autosomal recessive	1 million
XI	Autosomal recessive	1 million
XIII	Autosomal recessive	1 million
Fibrinogen	Autosomal recessive	1 million
Prothrombin	Autosomal recessive	2 million

CONGENITAL COAGULATION (CLOTTING) DISORDERS (COAGULOPATHIES)

These are usually due to a deficiency or lack of a specific blood-clotting factor. The vascular and platelet haemostatic responses usually mask any problem initially, and patients usually complain of a delayed blood oozing from the area, such as a tooth extraction socket.

The most important hereditary bleeding disorder in terms of prevalence and severity is von Willebrand disease, but haemophilia A and B (Christmas disease) are the other most common coagulopathies. Haemophilia A and B are hereditary X-linked recessive disorders characterized by deficiencies in blood clotting factors VIII and IX, respectively. Factor XI deficiency is also important. Less common disorders are summarized in Table 8.11 and Appendix 8.2.

HAEMOPHILIA A

Haemophilia A affects approximately 1 in 5000 males.

General aspects

Haemophilia A is an X-linked disorder resulting from a deficiency in blood clotting factor VIII, a key component of the coagulation cascade. Haemophilia A thus affects males. Sons of carriers have a 50:50 chance of developing haemophilia, while daughters of carriers have a 50:50 chance of being carriers. All daughters of an affected male are carriers but sons are normal. Carriers rarely have a clinically manifest bleeding tendency. The female carrier will transmit the disorder to half of her sons and the carrier state to half of her daughters. The affected males will not transmit the disorder to their sons because their Y chromosome cannot carry the haemophilic gene.

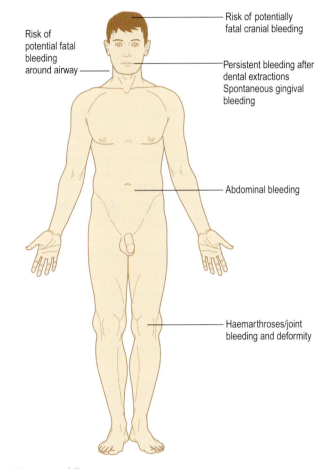

Fig. 8.12 Haemophilia.

Haemophilia A is about ten times as common as haemophilia B, except in some Asians, in whom frequencies are almost equal. Haemophilia A arises from a variety of mutations; some 150 different point mutations have been characterized but a family history can be obtained in only about 65% of cases.

Clinical features

Haemophilia is characterized by excessive bleeding, particularly after trauma and sometimes spontaneously. Haemorrhage appears to stop immediately after the injury (due to normal vascular and platelet haemostatic responses) but intractable oozing with rapid blood loss soon follows. Haemorrhage is dangerous either because of acute blood loss or due to bleeding into tissues, particularly the brain, larynx, pharynx, joints and muscles (Fig. 8.12). Abdominal haemorrhage may simulate

Table 8.12 *Severity of haemophilia*

	% factor VIII	Clinical features
Severe	<1	Spontaneous bleeding, typically from childhood, with bleeding into muscles or joints (haemarthroses), easy bruising and prolonged bleeding from minor injuries
Moderate	1–5	Comparatively minor trauma may still lead to significant blood loss
Mild	>5–25	Comparatively minor trauma may still lead to significant blood loss. Bleeding after dental extractions is sometimes the first or only sign of mild disease
Very mild	>25	Patient can generally lead a normal life and may remain undiagnosed but there can be prolonged bleeding after trauma or surgery. Some may not bleed excessively even after a simple dental extraction, so that the absence of post-extraction haemorrhage cannot reliably be used to exclude haemophilia. Most will, however, bleed excessively after more traumatic surgery, such as tonsillectomy

Box 8.2 *Laboratory findings in haemophilias*

- Normal prothrombin time (PT and INR)
- Prolonged activated partial thromboplastin time (APTT)
- Reduced factor VIII:C level (haemophilia A)
- Reduced factor IX level (haemophilia B)
- Normal levels of von Willebrand factor (vWF)

an 'acute abdomen'. Haemarthroses can cause joint damage and cripple the patient.

Dental extractions lead to prolonged bleeding and, in the past, have been fatal. Abnormal bleeding after extractions has sometimes led to recognition of haemophilia. The severity of bleeding in haemophilia A correlates with the level of factor VIII:coagulant (VIII:C) activity and degree of trauma (Table 8.12). Normal plasma contains 1 unit of factor VIII per millilitre, a level defined as 100%.

Haemophilia should be suspected in males presenting with a history of:

- easy bruising in early childhood
- 'spontaneous' bleeding (bleeding for no apparent/known reason), particularly into the joints, muscles and soft tissues
- excessive bleeding following trauma or surgery.

Unlike platelet disorders, which present as bleeding into and from mucous membranes, haemophilia presents mainly as bleeding into muscle or joints (haemarthrosis). More seriously, a cerebral bleed can be a fatal complication. Bleeding around the larynx or pharynx after inferior alveolar nerve block administration or floor-of-mouth infiltration can obstruct the airway. While the history of bleeding is usually life-long, some children with severe haemophilia may not have bleeding symptoms until later, when they begin walking or running. Patients with mild haemophilia may not bleed excessively until they experience trauma or surgery. The severity of bleeding in haemophilia is generally correlated with the clotting factor level:

- Severe – spontaneous bleeding into joints or muscles, predominantly in the absence of identifiable haemostatic challenge
- Moderate – occasional spontaneous bleeding; prolonged bleeding with minor trauma or surgery
- Mild – severe bleeding with major trauma or surgery; spontaneous bleeding is rare.

General management

Diagnosis

The diagnosis of haemophilias is based upon the clinical presentation, a positive family history, coagulation studies and clotting factor assays. Typical findings are shown in Box 8.2. In haemophilia, the various factors are:

- factor VIIIc – which participates in the clotting pathway

- factor VIIIR:Ag – von Willebrand factor – which binds to platelets and is the carrier for factor VIIIc
- factor VIIIR:Co – a cofactor which aids platelet aggregation.

Diagnostic laboratory findings can be summarized as:

- a prolonged APTT
- a normal PT
- low factor VIIIc.

Factor VIII assay is generally required, as even the APTT may be normal or mild in some cases. A definitive diagnosis depends on factor assay to demonstrate a deficiency of factor VIII. The severity of haemophilia A is associated with factor VIIIc activity, measured by the factor VIII plasma level. People with factor VIII levels below 25% lead relatively normal lives.

Management

Haemophiliacs should be under the care of recognized haemophilia reference centres, where the primary aim is to prevent and treat bleeding with the missing clotting factor, using a specific factor concentrate. Factor VIII must be replaced to adequate levels during episodes of bleeding and this must be ascertained preoperatively.

To facilitate appropriate management in emergency situations, all patients should carry easily accessible identification, indicating the diagnosis, severity of the bleeding disorder, inhibitor status, type of treatment product used, initial dosage for treatment of severe, moderate and mild bleeding, and contact information for the treating physician/clinic.

Patients usually recognize early symptoms of bleeding, even before the manifestation of physical signs. This is often described as a tingling sensation or 'aura'. During an episode of acute bleeding, an assessment should be performed to identify the bleeding site (if not clinically obvious) and appropriate clotting factor should be administered. Acute bleeds should be treated as quickly as possible, preferably within 2 hours. In severe bleeding episodes that are potentially life-threatening, especially those in the head, neck, chest and gastrointestinal tract, factor treatment should be initiated immediately, even before diagnostic assessment is complete.

Desmopressin (DDAVP) can raise factor VIII level adequately (3–6 times baseline levels) to control bleeding in patients with mild, and possibly moderate, haemophilia A.

Veins must be treated with care. They are lifelines for a person with haemophilia:

- Use of 23- or 25-gauge butterfly needles is recommended.
- It is advisable never to cut down into a vein, except in an emergency.
- Pressure should be applied for 3–5 minutes after venepuncture.
- Venous access devices should be avoided whenever possible, but may be required in some children.

Adjunctive therapies can be used to control bleeding, particularly in the absence of clotting factor concentrates, and may decrease the need for factor. If bleeding does not resolve despite adequate treatment, clotting factor levels should be measured. Inhibitor testing should be performed if the level is unexpectedly low. Prevention of bleeding can be achieved by prophylactic factor replacement. Factor levels should be raised to appropriate levels prior to any invasive procedure.

Patients should avoid:

- activities likely to cause trauma
- drugs that affect platelet function, particularly aspirin and NSAIDs, except certain COX-2 inhibitors; paracetamol (acetaminophen) is a safe alternative for analgesia.

For persons with haemophilia, good oral hygiene is essential to prevent periodontal disease and dental caries. Dental examinations should be regular, starting as the primary teeth start to erupt. Teeth should be brushed twice a day with a medium-texture brush. In view of the liability to gingival haemorrhage, careful cleaning with a powered brush that can be positioned to avoid gingival trauma can be helpful. Dental floss or interdental brushes should be used wherever possible. Airfloss or ultrasonic brushes may help. Toothpaste containing fluoride should be used in areas where natural fluoride is not present in the water supply. Fluoride supplements may also be prescribed if appropriate. An orthodontic assessment should be considered for all patients between the ages of 10 and 14. Close liaison between the dental surgeon and the haemophilia team is essential to provide good comprehensive dental care.

Infiltration and intrapapillary and intraligamentary injections are often done under factor cover (20–40%), although it may be possible for those with adequate experience to administer these injections without it. Treatment from the haemophilia unit may be required before an inferior alveolar nerve block or lingual infiltration.

Dental extraction or surgical procedures carried out within the oral cavity should be performed with a plan in place for haemostasis management, in consultation with the haematologist.

Tranexamic acid or epsilon aminocaproic acid (EACA) is often used after dental procedures to reduce the need for replacement therapy.

Oral antibiotics should only be prescribed if clinically necessary.

Local haemostatic measures may also be used whenever possible following a dental extraction. Typical products include oxidized cellulose and fibrin glue.

Following a tooth extraction, the patient should be advised to avoid hot food and drinks until normal feeling has returned. Smoking should be avoided, as this can cause problems with healing. Regular warm saltwater mouthwashes (1 teaspoon of salt in a glass of warm water [50°C]) should begin the day after treatment and continue for 5–7 days or until the mouth has healed.

Prolonged bleeding and/or difficulty in speaking, swallowing or breathing following dental manipulation should be reported to the haematologist/dental surgeon immediately.

The presence of blood-borne infections should not affect the availability of dental treatment.

Prevention of bleeding at the time of dental procedures in patients with inhibitors to factor VIII requires careful planning.

Synthetic vasopressin (desmopressin, DDAVP) acts to increase factor VIII levels and may be used in very mild haemophilia. 'Gene therapy' and 'gene-delivery systems' raise the possibility of a potential cure for haemophilia in the future.

Rarely, vWD may mimic haemophilia and, though the history may help to distinguish the two conditions, laboratory testing is essential (see later).

Factor VIII must be replaced to a level adequate to ensure haemostasis if bleeding starts or is expected. The following tests are typically required:

- Full blood count, APTT, PT, factor VIII assay
- Specific factor VIII antibody test
- Hepatitis B, hepatitis C, HIV tests
- Liver function tests
- Blood grouping and cross-matching in case of emergency, when surgery is contemplated.

The main aim of providing coagulant cover is to raise the existing factor VIII levels to normal to achieve adequate haemostasis (Table 8.13). Normal factor VIII levels can be achieved by the following measures:

- Desmopressin (DDAVP) may produce a two- to threefold rise in factor VIII activity after 90 minutes, and has a mean half-life of 9.4 hours. DDAVP can be taken as a nasal spray by some patients; in this case, the intranasal spray is delivered as 1.5mg desmopressin (DDAVP) per mL. Each 0.1mL pump spray delivers 100–150mcg dosage. It can also be given subcutaneously. DDAVP is more appropriate for mild cases and can only be

Table 8.13 *Dental care in haemophilias*

Severity	Factor VIII levels	Symptoms	Dental treatment	Treatment options
Severe	>1% (1IU/dL)	Spontaneous bleeding usually in childhood	Scale and polish	DDAVP (desmopressin; subject to response test)
		Bleeding into muscles/joints (haemarthrosis)	Conservation	Factor VIII
		Easy bruising	Inferior dental nerve block injection	Factor VIII and tranexamic acid
		Prolonged bleeding following minor injuries/trauma	Extractions	
Moderate	1–5% (FVIIIC >5IU/dL)	Prolonged bleeding following mild to moderate trauma/surgery/extractions	Scale and polish	DDAVP (subject to response test)
			Conservation	DDAVP and tranexamic acid
			Inferior dental nerve block injection	
			Extractions	
Mild	>5% (FVIIIC >5IU/dL)	Prolonged bleeding following mild trauma	Scale and polish	Nil
			Conservation	Nil for buccal infiltrations
			Inferior dental nerve block injections	DDAVP (subject to a response test)
			Extractions	DDAVP and postoperative tranexamic acid

repeated after 48 hours; therefore, factor VIII might be more suitable for the management of postoperative surgical cases. Multiple DDAVP infusions have been associated with a reduced response.

- Antifibrinolytic agents include tranexamic acid (Cyklokapron), a synthetic derivative of the amino acid lysine, which acts by reversibly blocking lysine-binding sites on plasminogen. This can be used systemically in a dose of 1 g (30 mg/kg) orally 4 times daily, starting 1 hour before the procedure, or as an infusion in a dose of 10 mg/kg in 20 mL normal saline over 20 minutes (child's dose is 20 mg/kg). However, nausea is a common adverse effect and antifibrinolytics must not be used systemically where residual clots are present (e.g. in the urinary tract or intracranially). Tranexamic acid significantly reduces blood loss after surgery in patients with haemophilia and can be used topically or systemically. Topical tranexamic acid as a 5% solution is used as a mouthwash in a dose of 10 mL 4 times daily for 1–2 weeks after scaling or dental extractions; it may also be applied on gauze swabs placed over the extraction sockets. Tranexamic acid is not approved for use in the USA by the Food and Drug Administration (FDA), where EACA is an alternative.
- Recombinant factor VIII. Factor VIII levels of 50–75% are required for minor surgery such as dental extractions. Patients can be helped postoperatively with tranexamic acid and local measures. For any persistent bleeding, factor VIII must be administered to manage the problem. For patients having a general anaesthetic, replacement factor VIII must be given to prepare for endotracheal intubation, which is likely to cause bleeding due to nasal trauma. Any major maxillofacial surgery must be carried out in a hospital setting; a bed should be arranged where appropriate in close consultation with the haemophilia reference centre.
- Many haemophiliacs with mild to moderate levels of factor VIII can manage their coagulant cover prior to dental treatment through their haemophilia reference centre. In mild to moderate haemophiliacs, non-surgical dental treatment can usually be carried out by using tranexamic acid and regional LA. Any surgical procedures in patients with mild to moderate haemophilia usually require at least DDAVP and tranexamic acid. Any major procedures must be carried out in a hospital setting in close consultation with the haemophilia reference centre.
- Haemophiliacs who manage their own factor VIII cover may well be able do so for their dental treatment in a primary care setting. Any dental treatment should still be as atraumatic as possible. Any major procedures must be carried out in a hospital setting in close consultation with the haemophilia reference centre.
- Severe haemophiliacs often self-administer factor VIII prophylactically to prevent joint damage, this needing injections three times weekly. The factor VIII half-life is around 12 hours. This has huge cost implications, as well as presenting the problem of antibody (inhibitor) formation.

In mild haemophilia, desmopressin (DDAVP) and antifibrinolytics such as tranexamic acid may be adequate (see later).

Recombinant factor VIII is used to treat patients acutely for bleeding episodes. (Pooled factor VIII from donor serum, fresh-frozen plasma, cryoprecipitate, or fractionated human factor concentrates from pooled blood sources were used for many years but allowed transmission of blood-borne viral infections, such as hepatitis B virus (HBV), hepatitis C virus (HCV) and HIV.) Many older adult haemophiliacs are HCV-positive; many have been exposed to HBV (a proportion of whom are carriers); and some are HIV-infected. Replacement of the missing clotting factor is therefore achieved with porcine factor VIII or recombinant factor VIII. Regular prophylactic replacement of factor VIII is used when possible but necessitates daily injections as the half-life is around 12 hours, and its use may be complicated by antibody formation.

Desmopressin (DDAVP) is a synthetic analogue of vasopressin that induces the release of factor VIIIC, vWF and tissue plasminogen activator from storage sites in endothelium. Desmopressin cover just before surgery, repeated 12-hourly if necessary for up to 4 days, is useful to cover minor operations in some very mild haemophiliacs, but factor VIII cover may be needed if there is any doubt about haemostasis. Desmopressin can be given as an intranasal spray of 1.5 mg desmopressin per mL with each 0.1 mL pump spray, or as a slow intravenous infusion over 20 minutes of 0.3–0.5 mcg/kg.

Although females may be carriers of haemophilia only, they may still exhibit symptoms of haemophilia. Depending on their factor VIII levels, they may need haematological management through a haemophilia reference centre prior to any invasive dental procedures requiring surgery or extractions.

Management challenges

- *Impaired mobility and access.* Joint problems are common in severe haemophiliacs.
- *Infections.* The stigma associated with infection by blood-borne viruses may constitute a barrier to care because of infection, increased bleeding due to liver damage or thrombocytopenia, delayed healing, impaired drug metabolism associated with hepatitis or adverse effects of medications. People who received British blood products between 1980 and 2001 may be at risk of variant Creutzfeld–Jakob disease (vCJD) transmitted in factor VIII concentrates.
- *Inhibitors.* Factor VIII antibodies/inhibitors are autoantibodies to factor VIII that may arise in people with severe haemophilia, and can constitute a major complication. Traumatic procedures must be avoided unless absolutely they are necessary. The haematologist must always be consulted and patients with inhibitors treated with caution when inferior dental nerve block injections are administered or surgery is carried out. In individuals requiring invasive treatment, human factor VIII inhibitor bypassing fractions (FEIBA) can be administered intravenously beforehand; FEIBA are usually either non-activated prothrombin complex concentrates (PCC) or activated prothrombin complex concentrates (APCC) that exert their effect by activating factor X, thus altogether bypassing the intrinsic clotting pathway. PCC contains factors II, IX, VII and X. Unfortunately, these products can cause uncontrolled coagulation and thromboses. An alternative is to administer 1 000 000 units of activated factor VIIa, which directly acts on the surface of platelets. Adjuncts such as Tisseel, a highly concentrated combination of fibrinogen, thrombin and factor XIII, aid cross-linking of the clot and, together with topical tranexamic acid, help to stabilize the clot postoperatively. Platelets may also be given.
- Some people who received British blood products between 1980 and 2001 may be at risk of variant CJD.

Dental aspects of haemophilia A

Many of the coagulation defects present a hazard to surgery and to LA injections, but in general the teeth erupt and exfoliate without problems, and non-invasive dental care is safe. Close cooperation is needed between the physician and dentist to plan safe, comprehensive dental care.

Prevention of dental disease

Haemophiliacs form a priority group in whom the need for dental operative intervention should be minimized, as it can cause severe, or occasionally fatal, complications. Early prevention will reduce the need for future dental treatment and for repeated cover, which is not only uncomfortable but also costly, and can lead to the formation of inhibitors. Education of patients or parents and preventive dentistry should be started as early as possible in the young child, when the teeth begin to erupt. Caries must be minimized or avoided. Prevention of periodontal disease is also imperative. It is important to institute the use of fluorides from childhood, to use fissure sealants/preventive resin restorations, and to emphasize the importance of dietary sugar restriction, good oral hygiene and regular dental check-ups. An orthodontic assessment should also be carried out at an early stage to predict any future problems such as overcrowding, which might be avoided. In adults, long term-prevention and routine care are also essential.

Pain and anxiety control

Anxiety and drug dependence can be barriers to managing patients.

- *LA.* There is an 80% chance of haematomas developing in haemophiliacs not treated with cover prior to mandibular block injection; infiltrations and intraligamentary, intraosseous and pulpal injections are safer. LA as an inferior dental nerve block, posterior superior alveolar nerve block, lingual infiltration or injections in the floor of the mouth must always be appropriately covered prior to dental treatment. Failure to achieve this can result in the life-threatening complication of haemorrhage, which can compromise the airway. Infiltration anaesthesia is safe without factor replacement, except for lingual infiltration where blood can track down into lingual spaces. Alternative methods of achieving LA must be tried, such as intraligamentary anaesthesia, or infiltrations using articaine where appropriate. Buccal infiltration of the mandibular first molar with 4% 1:100000 adrenaline (epinephrine) has resulted in a higher success rate than 2% lidocaine with 100000 epinephrine in non-haemophiliac patients. It is also more comfortable compared with inferior dental nerve block injection. However, it is less successful with mandibular second and third molar teeth because of the presence of denser cortical bone. Depending on their inhibitor titre, patients who have inhibitors must always be monitored postoperatively despite having cover.
- *CS.* Conscious sedation using inhalation sedation or midazolam is usually safe in selected cases, depending on the American Society of Anesthesiology (ASA) classification, and providing that appropriate cover is given by the haematologist. There should be no problems with haematoma formation at the cannulation site if there is a mild to moderate haemophilia or if the patient has received factor VIII cover.
- *GA.* A thorough preoperative assessment, with the anaesthetist, haematologist and dentist in close consultation, is essential. Nasal intubation should be avoided if possible. Overnight stay and postoperative follow-up should be considered, especially for those patients with added complications who have hepatitis, HIV or inhibitors. Individuals with severe haemophilia may also benefit from an overnight stay, depending on the treatment being carried out and the haematologist's advice.

Conservation and fixed prosthodontics

Careful placement of rubber dams and matrix bands can minimize bleeding. Trauma from high-speed suction or a saliva ejector can be avoided by placing gauze beneath it. Fissure sealants should be considered at an early stage as part of the prevention regime. Use of

atraumatic restorative technique (ART) or air abrasion/Carisolv gel may be appropriate. Any sharp-edged restorations or dentures must be smoothed. Conservative extension of gingival margins and supragingival crown preparations should be considered. Tranexamic acid can be used topically to control any local bleeding. Non-metal impression trays can minimize soft-tissue trauma. Endodontic treatment should be appropriately covered, the main concern being to avoid instrumentation through the apex (use an apex locator). Intrapulpal anaesthesia may also reduce the bleeding risk.

Periodontology

In mild haemophiliacs, scaling can usually be carried out using tranexamic acid cover; if in doubt, seek advice from the haematologist. In moderate haemophiliacs, DDAVP as well as tranexamic acid might be required. Severe haemophiliacs may require factor VIII and tranexamic acid cover. Any additional treatment, such as conservation, should also be carried out at the same visit to avoid the need for repeated cover. Periodontal surgery, as any surgery, requires appropriate cover, depending on the severity of the condition – at least to a level of factor VIII at 50–75%.

Orthodontic treatment

There is no contraindication to orthodontic treatment. Care must be taken with any sharp edges to orthodontic appliances or wires.

Exodontia/dentoalveolar surgery/maxillofacial surgery

Tooth extractions must be carefully planned in close communication with the haematologist, weighing up the risk of repeated factor VIII cover and managing bleeding. Factor VIII levels should be between 50 and 75%. When maxillofacial surgery is scheduled, factor VIII replacement is necessary for *all* haemophiliacs at a level of 75–100% and is required 1 hour postoperatively.

Lingual tissues should be left undisturbed when raising mucoperiosteal flaps to prevent blood from tracking down the mediastinum. Local measures must be implemented such as: minimal trauma to both soft tissues and bone, good wound cleaning, and placement of resorbable sutures to reduce the risk of further bleeding on removal. Polyglactin (Vicryl) sutures are preferable to stabilize the gum flap, as they remain in situ for about 4 days. In addition to the application of continuous pressure (i.e. gentle hand pressure, additional stitches), cooling of the site (i.e. with an ice pack) and use of vasoconstrictors, there are usually other materials that could be applied to the site in order to reduce or even stop the bleeding. These include: oxidized cellulose, absorbent gelatin sponge, collagen sponge, resorbable gelatin sponge, topical thrombin, EACA, tranexamic acid, fibrin sealant and many others (Table 8.14). Due to a concern regarding vCJD, recombinant fibrin glues are becoming more easily available.

Table 8.14 *Topical haemostatic agents*

Agent	Main constituent	Source
Avitene	Collagen	Bovine
Beriplast	Fibrin	Various
CollaCote	Collagen	Bovine
Cyklokapron	Tranexamic acid	Synthetic
Gelfoam	Gelatin	Bovine
Helistat	Collagen	Bovine
Instat	Collagen	Bovine
Surgicel	Cellulose	Synthetic
Thrombinar	Thrombin	Bovine
Thrombogen	Thrombin	Bovine
Thrombostat	Thrombin	Bovine

Patients should be instructed to take a soft diet for a week after surgery. Antimicrobials might be indicated. The patient should be warned to report any swelling, dysphagia or hoarseness, as this may indicate haematoma formation and risk to the airway. For postoperative pain management, paracetamol (acetaminophen) or a combination of codeine/paracetamol may be suitable; NSAIDs and aspirin should be avoided, and care should be taken when prescribing opioids, due to the enhanced sedative effects following sedation or GA on the same day.

LA injections or surgery can be followed by persistent bleeding for days or weeks; the haemorrhage cannot be controlled by pressure alone and the problem may be life-threatening. Management of haemophiliacs should take consideration of the factors listed in Box 8.3.

The bleeding tendency can be aggravated by NSAIDs. It may also be worsened by other factors, such as liver damage after hepatitis, HIV disease, thrombocytopenia and the effects of drugs such as protease inhibitors. Paracetamol (acetaminophen), codeine and COX-2 inhibitors are safer.

An outline of management of haemophiliacs needing surgery is given in Table 8.15.

Local use of fibrin glue and swish-and-swallow rinses of tranexamic acid before and after severe anaemia, neutropenia and thrombocytopenia, which predispose to oral manifestations.

Haemophiliacs with inhibitors

The haematologist must always be consulted. Factor VIII inhibitor levels should be checked preoperatively and, in general, patients with

low-titre inhibitors can have dental treatment in the same way as those who have no antibodies.

Those with high-titre inhibitors need special care. In this group, traumatic procedures must be avoided, unless absolutely essential. Human FEIBA can often be effective; these are usually either non-activated PCC or APCCs, which act by activating factor X, directly bypassing the intrinsic pathway of blood clotting. The danger with these products is that of uncontrolled coagulation with thromboses. The real choice lies between either prothrombin-complex concentrates (e.g. FEIBA) or recombinant factor VIIa. In some cases, desmopressin (DDAVP) is an effective alternative, and antifibrinolytics may help.

CS can be given but, if intravenous, great care must be taken to avoid damaging the vein. If GA is needed, nasal intubation should be avoided.

HAEMOPHILIA B (CHRISTMAS DISEASE)

General and clinical aspects

Haemophilia B (Christmas disease; factor IX deficiency) is clinically identical to haemophilia A and inherited in the same way; it also affects males only but is about one-tenth as common as haemophilia A, except in some Asians, in whom frequencies are almost equal. Female carriers of haemophilia B (unlike haemophilia A) often have a mild bleeding tendency.

General management

The APTT is prolonged with a normal PT, and factor IX levels are low. Treatment is with synthetic factor IX concentrate, which is more stable than factor VIII with a half-life that is usually 18 hours but often up to 2 days, so that replacement therapy can sometimes be given at longer intervals than in haemophilia A. A dose of 20 units of factor IX per kilogram body weight is given intravenously 1 hour preoperatively.

Dental aspects

Comments on dental management in haemophilia A apply to patients with haemophilia B, apart from using factor IX and not using desmopressin (DDAVP).

Box 8.3 *Factors to consider in haemophilia management*

- Aggravation of bleeding by drugs
- Anxiety
- Dental neglect necessitating frequent dental extractions
- Drug dependence as a result of chronic pain
- Factor VIII inhibitors
- Hazards of anaesthesia, nasal intubation and intramuscular injections
- Hepatitis and liver disease
- HIV infection
- Trauma, surgery and subsequent haemorrhage

Table 8.15 *Outline of management of haemophiliacs requiring surgery*

Operation	Factor VIII level required	Preoperative regimen	Postoperative schedule
Dental extraction, dentoalveolar or periodontal surgery	Minimum of 50% at operation	Factor VIII i.v.[a] Tranexamic acid 1 g i.v. (or by mouth starting 24 h preoperatively)	Local haemostatic measures[b]
Maxillofacial surgery	75–100% at operation; at least 50% for 7 days postoperatively	Factor VIII i.v.[c]	Local haemostatic measures[b]
			Rest as inpatient for 7 days unless resident close to centre (then 3 days)
			Soft diet
			For 10 days give tranexamic acid 1 g 4 times daily and penicillin V 250 mg 4 times daily
			If there is bleeding during this period:
			Give repeat dose of factor VIII[a]
			Rest inpatient for 10 days
			Soft diet
			Twice-daily i.v. factor VIII[a] for 7–10 days

[a]Factor VIII dose in units = weight in kilograms × 25 given 1 h preoperatively.
[b]See Table 8.14.
[c]Factor VIII dose in units = weight in kilograms × 50 given 1 h preoperatively.

Table 8.16 *Types of von Willebrand disease (vWD)*

Type	Type of vWD defect	Percentage of cases	Comments	Factor VIIIc levels	Benefit from factor VIII replacement	Desmopressin (DDAVP)
1	Partial quantitative	80	Autosomal dominant inheritance. Disease is mild and characterized by bleeding from mucous membranes – nosebleeds, gingival haemorrhage and gastrointestinal blood loss	May be normal	–	Used as nasal spray
2A	Qualitative	15		Reduced	+	Used as nasal spray
2B	Qualitative	Rare		Reduced	+	Contraindicated
2C	Qualitative	Rare		Reduced	+	Used as nasal spray
2M	Qualitative	Rare		Reduced	+	Contraindicated
2N	Qualitative	Rare		Reduced	+	Used as nasal spray
3	Complete lack of vWF	5	Bleeding is more severe than in types 1 and 2 but joint and muscle bleeds characteristic of haemophilia are rare	Reduced	+	Contraindicated

VON WILLEBRAND DISEASE (VWD)

General aspects

vWD is the most common inherited bleeding disorder and is caused by von Willebrand factor (vWF) deficiency. Inheritance is usually autosomal dominant and disease affects males or females. vWF is a protein expressed in both platelets and blood vessel endothelial cells; it is synthesized in the endothelium and megakaryocytes, and has binding sites for collagen and for platelet glycoprotein (GP) receptors. vWF normally acts in two ways:

- It normally binds to GP Ib and acts as a carrier for factor VIII, increasing factor VIII half-life by protecting it from proteolytic degradation; thus a deficiency of vWF also leads to a low factor VIII concentration in the blood.
- vWF also mediates platelet adhesion to damaged vascular endothelium, enhancing platelet aggregation. Thus a deficiency of vWF leads to defective platelet adhesion, which in turn causes a secondary deficiency in factor VIII.

Clinically significant vWD affects approximately 1% of the population and 6% of women with menorrhagia – a frequency at least twice that of haemophilia A. vWD may occasionally be inherited as a sex-linked recessive trait like true haemophilia. Rarely, vWD may be acquired, particularly in patients with autoimmune or lymphoproliferative diseases.

Clinical features

The types of vWD are shown in Table 8.16.

vWD causes bleeding that has features similar to those caused by platelet dysfunction; if severe, however, it can resemble haemophilia (Table 8.17). The common pattern is bleeding from, and purpura of, mucous membranes and the skin. Gingival haemorrhage is more common than in haemophilia. Postoperative haemorrhage can be troublesome; excessive haemorrhage may occur after dental treatment and surgery. Excessive menstrual bleeding is common in females. Haemarthroses are possible but rare.

The severity also varies from patient to patient and from time to time. Some patients have a clinically insignificant disorder, while others have factor VIII levels low enough to cause severe clotting defects as well as a prolonged bleeding time. However, severity does not correlate well with factor VIII level. Pregnancy and the contraceptive pill may cause transient amelioration.

The pattern of clinical features in vWD is distinct from that of haemophilia. Bruising, epistaxis and prolonged bleeding during surgical or dental procedures are the most common features but menorrhagia or gastrointestinal haemorrhage also occur frequently. The amount of bleeding depends on the type and severity of vWD but manifests with:

- frequent or hard-to-stop nosebleeds:
  - start without injury (spontaneous)
  - occur often, usually five times or more in a year
  - last more than 10 minutes
  - need packing or cautery to stop the bleeding
- easy bruising:
  - occurs with very little or no trauma or injury
  - occurs often (1–4 times per month)
  - is larger than the size of a 10 pence coin (or a US quarter)
  - is not flat and has a raised lump
- heavy menstrual bleeding:
  - involves the passing of clots larger than the size of a penny
  - soaks more than one pad through every 2 hours
  - is diagnosed as anaemia as a result of bleeding from heavy periods
- longer-than-normal bleeding after injury, surgery, childbirth or dental care:
  - lasts more than 5 minutes after a cut to the skin

Table 8.17 *Differentiation of haemophilia A and von Willebrand disease[a]*

	Haemophilia A	Von Willebrand disease
Dominant inheritance	Sex-linked recessive	Autosomal
Haemarthroses/deep haematomas	Common	Rare
Epistaxes	Uncommon	Common
Gastrointestinal bleeding	Uncommon	Common
Haematuria	Common	Uncommon
Menorrhagia	None (males)	Common
Post-extraction bleeding	Starts 1–24h after trauma, lasts 3–40 days and is not controlled by pressure	Starts immediately, lasts 24–48h and is often controlled by pressure
Bleeding time	Normal	Prolonged
Factor VIII coagulant activity	Low	Low
Factor VIIIR:RCo (plasma factor VIII complex; ristocetin cofactor)	Normal	Low

[a]Severe von Willebrand disease is occasionally identical to haemophilia.

- ◆ involves heavy or longer bleeding after surgery; bleeding sometimes stops but starts up again hours or days later
- ◆ involves heavy bleeding during or after childbirth
- ◆ involves heavy bleeding during or after dental surgery
- ◆ leads to oozing of blood from the surgery site longer than 3 hours after the dental surgery
- ◆ means that the dental surgery site needs packing or cautery to stop the bleeding
- ■ other common bleeding events, including:
  - ◆ blood in the stool (faeces) from bleeding into the stomach or intestines
  - ◆ blood in the urine from bleeding into the kidneys or bladder
  - ◆ bleeding into joints or internal organs in severe cases (type 3).

Expression is variable, with some patients experiencing bleeding only after surgery or major trauma and others suffering from frequent spontaneous bleeding of the mucosal surfaces. Patients also present with deep-seated haemorrhages caused by factor VIII deficiency.

Type 1

This is the most common form of VWD and the mildest. Inherited in autosomal dominant fashion, it is usually confirmed by a combination of:

- ■ abnormal platelet function
- ■ decreased vWF antigen
- ■ proportional decrease in factor VIII.

Type 2

There are normal amounts of vWF but it is dysfunctional. Type 2 contains subtypes 2A, 2B, 2C, 2M and 2N, and treatment is different for each type. Platelet-type vWD, also known as pseudo-vWD, is an autosomal dominant condition inherited by gain-of-function mutations of the vWF receptor on platelets. It is similar to type 2B vWD.

Type 3

This is the most severe form of vWD, in which a person has no vWF and also low levels of factor VIII. The presentation usually resembles haemophilia.

Rarely, aortic stenosis (Heyde syndrome), hereditary haemorrhagic telangiectasia, IgA deficiency, mitral valve prolapse or factor XII deficiency may be associated with vWD.

General management

vWD is characterized by the laboratory findings shown in Box 8.4. The PT is normal and the APTT often normal (factor VIII levels are often adequate for a normal APTT). vWF levels are, however, reduced. Platelet count is usually normal. Factor VIII assay is usually reduced while the tourniquet test may be positive in most cases.

Before surgery, patients with vWD need treatment to reduce the risk of haemorrhage (Table 8.18). Essentially, management is the same as for haemophilia A. The following should be discussed with the haematologist:

- ■ The severity of the disease
- ■ The procedures planned and the nature of the bleeding risk
- ■ The patient's response to previous treatment, surgery and trauma
- ■ The patient's response to various types of systemic therapy.

Dental aspects

The treatment prescribed for vWD depends on the type and severity of the disease. For minor bleeds, treatment might not be needed. The most commonly used types of treatment are:

Box 8.4 *Laboratory findings in von Willebrand disease*

- • Prolonged activated partial thromboplastin time
- • Low levels of von Willebrand factor (factor VIIIR:Ag)
- • Low factor VIIIC levels
- • Reduced platelet aggregation in the presence of ristocetin

---

Table 8.18 *von Willebrand disease: haemostatic prophylaxis for surgery*[a]

von Willebrand disease type	Desmopressin	Factor VIII replacement
1	Nasal spray typically effective	–
2A	Nasal spray may be effective: check response with trial dose	±
2B	Contraindicated	+
2C	Nasal spray useful	±
2M	Contraindicated	+
2N	Unlikely to be of value	±
3	Contraindicated	+

[a]Plus local haemostatic measures (see Table 8.14).

- ■ desmopressin acetate (DDAVP) nasal spray – this acts by boosting levels of vWF and factor VIII and is used to treat people with some milder forms of vWD. DDAVP acts by boosting levels of vWF and factor VIII, and is sometimes injected intravenously to treat some forms of vWD (mainly type 1)
- ■ vWF factor replacement – human plasma rich in vWF and factor VIII is used to treat more severe forms of vWD, or people with milder forms of vWD who do not respond well to nasal DDAVP. Recombinant vWF is unavailable, and recombinant factor VIII has no beneficial effect.
- ■ antifibrinolytic drugs – these are either injected or taken orally to help slow or prevent blood clot breakdown.

In type 1 vWD, desmopressin (DDAVP) may be used to increase vWF levels acutely.

DDAVP may be effective in type 2A and it is often helpful to give patients a trial dose to ascertain the response.

In some type 2B vWD, DDAVP is contraindicated, as it can stimulate release of dysfunctional vWF, which leads in turn to platelet aggregation and severe, though transient, thrombocytopenia.

DDAVP is contraindicated in type 3 vWD, as there is an almost complete lack of vWF; patients are managed as for severe haemophilia A.

Clotting factor replacement is needed. Intermediate-purity factor VIII, cryoprecipitate and fresh-frozen plasma are effective. Human plasma does contain vWF and is usually effective in treating severe vWD. In more severe cases, vWF concentrate may be needed. However, recombinant factor VIII lacks vWF and is thus a non-viable treatment for vWD.

In all types, aspirin and NSAIDs should be avoided. Infiltration or intraligamentary LA should generally be used. CS can be given, but care must be taken not to damage the vein. GA must be given in hospital, where expert attention is available. Intubation is a possible hazard because of the risk of submucosal bleeding in the airway.

All invasive procedures, such as extractions, minor oral/periodontal surgery, implants and deep scaling, require haematological cover, depending on the severity of disease.

Following dental treatment, antiplatelet medications for analgesia, such as aspirin or ibuprofen, are contraindicated. Paracetamol

Table 8.19 *Inherited disorders in fibrinogen*

Condition	Definition	Inheritance	Features
Afibrinogenaemia	Complete lack of fibrinogen	Autosomal recessive	Neonatal umbilical cord haemorrhage, ecchymoses, mucosal haemorrhage, internal haemorrhage and recurrent abortion
Hypofibrinogenaemia	Low levels of fibrinogen below 100 mg/dL (normal is 250–350 mg/dL)	Acquired or inherited	Symptoms similar to but less severe than afibrinogenaemia
Dysfibrinogenaemia	Dysfunctional fibrinogen	Inherited	Haemorrhage, spontaneous abortion and thromboembolism
Hypoplasminogenaemia	Plasminogen deficient or defective	Inherited	Fibrin deposits with gingival swelling and sometimes ligneous conjunctivitis

(acetaminophen) is the usual drug of choice, or combination analgesia, such as co-codamol, may be given for further pain relief.

FACTOR XI DEFICIENCY ('HAEMOPHILIA C')

Common in Ashkenazi Jews, factor XI deficiency is inherited as an autosomal disorder with either homozygosity or compound heterozygosity.

Patients with factor XI deficiency cannot activate thrombin-activatable fibrinolytic inhibitor (TAFI); this results in rapid fibrinolysis, which is responsible for the bleeding tendency seen in this disorder. Fresh-frozen plasma or factor XI is required.

FACTOR XII DEFICIENCY

Factor XII (the first component of the intrinsic pathway) is more important for the generation of bradykinin and stimulation of fibrinolysis than for initiation of coagulation. Patients with factor XII deficiency rarely show signs of haemorrhage.

FACTOR XIII DEFICIENCY

Factor XIII, the pro-enzyme of plasma transglutaminase, is normally activated by thrombin in the presence of calcium to catalyse the cross-linking of fibrin monomers.

Factor XIII deficiency leads to neonatal umbilical cord bleeding, intracranial haemorrhage and soft-tissue haematomas. Primary haemostasis is normal but delayed bleeding is seen.

FIBRINOGEN DISORDERS

Inherited disorders in fibrinogen are rare (Table 8.19). In contrast, raised plasma fibrinogen levels are found in coronary artery disease, diabetes, hypertension, peripheral artery disease, hyperlipoproteinaemia, hypertriglyceridaemia, pregnancy, menopause, hypercholesterolaemia, use of oral contraceptives and smoking.

ACQUIRED COAGULATION DEFECTS

Acquired haemorrhagic disorders are far more prevalent than congenital diseases but, except in anticoagulant therapy or liver disease, are usually less severe. Important causes include anticoagulant therapy and liver disease, vitamin K deficiency or malabsorption, disseminated intravascular coagulation, fibrinolytic states, amyloidosis (deficiency of factor X) and autoimmune disorders (e.g. acquired haemophilia). Some patients also have clinical bleeding tendencies but no defect detectable by current laboratory methods.

LIVER FAILURE

Liver failure leads to impaired synthesis of vitamin K-dependent clotting factors, such as factors II, VII, IX, X and fibrinogen – leading to prolonged PT and INR. Patients with liver failure may also have oesophageal varices associated with portal hypertension, and serious bleeding from these is possible. During bleeding, fresh-frozen plasma (contains all clotting factors) may be needed. Treatment with regular high-dose vitamin K increases levels of these clotting factors.

DRUGS

Anticoagulants are given to prevent and treat thromboembolic disease but have many uses. They are used to treat atrial fibrillation, cardiac valvular disease, ischaemic heart disease and post-myocardial infarction (sometimes), deep venous thrombosis (DVT), pulmonary embolism, cerebrovascular accident and many other conditions, and are used when there are heart valve replacements or renal dialysis.

Commonly used anticoagulants are the coumarin warfarin for long-term treatment and heparin for short-term treatment. Because it takes several days for the maximum effect of warfarin to be realized, heparin is normally given first.

Warfarin, a 4-hydroxycoumarin derivative, is the most commonly used oral anticoagulant. It is a vitamin K antagonist, which acts by inhibiting the post-translational glutamate carboxylation of blood coagulation factors II, VII, IX and X. Warfarin also inhibits glutamate carboxylation of the proteins C and S. The anticoagulant effect of warfarin results predominantly from reduction in factor II.

Warfarin is most frequently prescribed to control and prevent thromboembolic disorders in atrial fibrillation, after cardiac surgery or organ transplants, after cerebrovascular accident, or in DVT or pulmonary embolism.

Warfarin effects begin after 8–12 hours, are maximal at 36 hours, and persist for 72 hours, prolonging the INR – the ratio of the patient's prothrombin time to a standardized control. An INR above 1 indicates that clotting will take longer than normal. The management of patients on warfarin should take into consideration the type of dental procedure, the INR value, the underlying condition for which anticoagulation is used and other risk factors (e.g. hepatic disorders or local inflammation). Surgery is the main oral health-care hazard to the patient on warfarin (see below).

The plasminogen activators, such as t-PA (alteplase) or streptokinase, also are useful for controlling coagulation, in particular during the short period after myocardial infarction (Ch. 5). Because t-PA is highly selective for the degradation of fibrin in clots, it is extremely helpful in restoring the patency of the coronary arteries after thrombosis. Streptokinase (an enzyme from streptococci) is another plasminogen activator that is useful from a therapeutic standpoint but it is less selective than t-PA, being able to activate circulating plasminogen as well as that bound to a fibrin clot.

Aspirin, by virtue of inhibiting the activity of the COX enzyme, depresses the production of thromboxane (TXA_2) and prostacyclin (PGI_2), and inhibits platelet aggregation.

Commonly prescribed anticoagulants include:

- dalteparin (Fragmin)
- danaparoid (Orgaran)
- enoxaparin (Lovenox)
- heparin (various)
- tinzaparin (Innohep)
- warfarin (Coumadin).

Warfarin

Surgery is the main oral health-care hazard to the patient on warfarin and thus the possibility of alternatives, e.g. endodontics, should always be considered. The INR is used as a guideline to care and should be checked on the day of operation or, if that is not possible, within the 24 hours prior to surgery.

Anticoagulant treatment should not be altered without the agreement of the clinician in charge, and stopping it preoperatively is rarely the best policy, since it does not necessarily reduce bleeding significantly; in contrast, it may cause hypercoagulability and rebound thrombosis – which has damaged prosthetic cardiac valves and even caused thrombotic deaths in dental patients. Hospital or specialist referral is indicated in the presence of:

- an INR of more than 4.0
- the need for more than a simple surgical procedure
- the presence of additional bleeding risk factors or logistical difficulties
- drug interactions with warfarin.

LA regional block injections, or those in the floor of the mouth, may be a hazard, since bleeding into the fascial spaces of the neck can threaten airway patency.

If surgery is to be limited, such as the uncomplicated forceps extraction of 1–3 teeth, and the INR is below 4.0, with no other risk factors (additional bleeding risk factors or logistical difficulties; drug interactions with warfarin) present, local haemostatic measures alone should suffice. Postoperative bleeding may be minimized by the use of oxidized cellulose, collagen sponges and sutures. If surgery is not to be simple or minor, the INR is over 4.0 or other risk factors are present, the patient should be treated in a hospital or other specialist centre. Topical antifibrinolytic agents, such as tranexamic acid (10 mL of a 5% w/v solution used as a mouthwash for 2 minutes, four times daily for 7 days), may help. Postoperatively, airway patency must always be ensured.

Warfarin may be enhanced by drugs such as NSAIDs, some antibiotics and azole antifungal agents (Table 8.20). Paracetamol (acetaminophen) is the analgesic of choice since it does not affect platelets. Codeine is a suitable alternative in adults. Penicillin V and clindamycin are the antibiotics of choice.

As we have seen, warfarin is orally administered and acts by inhibiting the vitamin K activation of clotting factors II, VII, IX and X. It prolongs the INR and PT, but it takes 2–3 days for warfarin's full anticoagulant effects to manifest and several days for its effects to abate. INR monitoring must be performed regularly for all patients so that the dose of warfarin may be adjusted appropriately. If more rapid reversal of anticoagulation is needed, protamine or APCC can be used.

Table 8.20 *Drug use in patients on warfarin*[a]

Drug group	Avoid: warfarin effect is enhanced	Alternatives that can probably be used safely[b]
Analgesics	Aspirin and other NSAIDs	Paracetamol (acetaminophen)
	Tramadol	Celecoxib
		Codeine
Antibacterials	Amoxicillin	Azithromycin
	Amoxicillin plus clavulanic acid	Cephalosporins (others)
	Ampicillin	Clindamycin
	Benzylpenicillin	Erythromycin
	Cephalosporins (2nd, 3rd generation)	Penicillins (others)
	Ciprofloxacin	
	Clarithromycin	
	Co-trimoxazole (and other sulphonamides)	
	Doxycycline	
	Isoniazid	
	Metronidazole	
	Neomycin	
	Quinolones	
	Tetracyclines	
Antidepressants	Selective serotonin reuptake inhibitors (Ch. 10)	Tricyclic antidepressants (Ch. 10)
Antifungals	Azoles (fluconazole, itraconazole, ketoconazole, miconazole)	Amphotericin
	Griseofulvin	Nystatin
Antivirals	Ritonavir	
	Saquinavir	

[a]Warfarin effect may be enhanced by several drugs but where a single dose of amoxicillin is required there should be no problem. If infection is present, no elective surgery should be done until the patient has been treated with antibiotics and is free from acute infection. In case of emergency, careful haemostatic control should suffice.
[b]Patients should still be advised to be vigilant for excessive bleeding.

Medication and dietary interactions with warfarin

Warfarin's effect may be changed by several drugs (see Table 8.20). Even *topical* miconazole gel has led to bleeding. Aspirin and other NSAIDs can also interfere with platelet function and cause gastric bleeding.

Of greater significance is the increased risk of intracranial haemorrhage from the concurrent administration of warfarin and aspirin.

For postoperative pain management, paracetamol (acetaminophen; an intake of four 500-mg tablets per day for up to 5 days) is recommended as the general analgesic and antipyretic of choice for short-term use in patients on oral anticoagulant therapy. Paracetamol is preferred over NSAIDs because it does not affect platelets, but excessive and prolonged administration can enhance warfarin activity. An intake of fewer than six tablets of 325 mg of paracetamol per week has little effect on INR; however, four tablets a day for a week significantly affects the INR. The concurrent administration of warfarin and paracetamol at a dose of four 325-mg tablets a day for 7 days will raise the INR and risk of haemorrhage because one of the metabolites inhibits a key enzyme in the vitamin K cycle that is required for the liver to produce coagulation factors. Paracetamol will affect the INR within 18–48 hours of administration.

Codeine may be prescribed with the paracetamol to enhance the analgesic effect. COX-2–selective NSAIDs (celecoxib and rofecoxib),

Table 8.21 *Novel oral anticoagulants compared with warfarin*

	Warfarin	Dabigatran	Rivaroxaban
Targets	Factors II, VII, IX and X Proteins C and S	Thrombin (inhibits)	Factor Xa (inhibits)
Effective half-life	20–60 h (mean ~40 h)	Adult 12–17 h; older people 14–17 h (assuming no renal impairment)	Young people 5–9 h; older people 11–13 h
Food and other effects on absorption	Food may delay rate	Acidic environment needed. Absorption may be reduced by drugs such as proton pump inhibitors and antacids	Food increases rate and extent of absorption by 25–35%
Need for routine monitoring of coagulation	Yes (PT/INR)	No	No
Antidote/reversal agent available	Yes (vitamin K)	No	No
Drug and food interactions: increased anticoagulation			
Antifungals	Miconazole, ketoconazole, fluconazole (itraconazole to a lesser degree)	Ketoconazole, itraconazole	Ketoconazole, itraconazole (miconazole if renal function impaired)
Antibiotics	Erythromycin, clarithromycin, (metronidazole possibly), azithromycin, tetracycline, doxycycline, cephalosporins, levofloxacin	Erythromycin, clarithromycin	–
Analgesics	NSAIDs, (antiplatelet agents: aspirin, clopidogrel), ibuprofen, diclofenac, paracetamol (acetaminophen; prolonged regular use)	NSAIDs (antiplatelet agents: aspirin, clopidogrel), ketorolac (diclofenac appears not to interact)	NSAIDs (antiplatelet agents: aspirin, clopidogrel)
Food/herbs:	Cranberry juice, St John's wort, alcohol, many dietary supplements	Alfalfa, anise, bilberry	Grapefruit juice, alfalfa, anise, bilberry
Drug and food interactions: decreased anticoagulation	Green leafy vegetables (Vitamin K), vitamin E	Dexamethasone Carbamazepine Rifampicin St John's wort	Phenytoin Rifampicin St John's wort

which were potential alternatives, are contraindicated because of cardiotoxicity. Tramadol occasionally interferes with warfarin and raises the INR.

When taken over a number of days concurrently with warfarin, certain other medications may increase the patient's INR value and risk of haemorrhage unless the warfarin dosage is adjusted. Warfarin's anticoagulation effect is derived as discussed, from its ability to prevent the metabolism of vitamin K to its active form, which is needed for the liver to synthesize clotting factors II, VII, IX and X. Some antimicrobials (tetracylines, broad-spectrum penicillins – amoxicillin, ampicillin) further decrease available vitamin K because they destroy some of the normal intestinal bacteria that produce it. The INR and risk of haemorrhage may also be increased by antimicrobials such as metronidazole and the macrolides (erythromycin, azithromycin, clarithromycin) because they inhibit the normal metabolism of warfarin. If a full antimicrobial course is indicated, the narrow-spectrum penicillin V (or clindamycin for those allergic to penicillin) is the preferred medication. Azole antifungals, such as ketoconazole, fluconazole, clotrimazole, itraconazole and miconazole, may also increase the INR by inhibiting the hepatic metabolism of warfarin.

Other medications that may adversely interact include dicloxacillin, nafcillin, phenobarbital and chloral hydrate, which can induce enzyme systems to metabolize warfarin rapidly.

Warfarin's effect can also be influenced by irregular tablet-taking. Diets high in vitamin K (avocado, sugar beet/beetroot, broccoli, Brussels sprouts, cabbage, chick peas, green peas, green tea, kale, lettuce, liver, spinach and turnips) can lower the INR. Alcohol can inhibit warfarin but may have the converse effect if there is liver disease. Disorders such as diarrhoea, liver disease and malignant disease can

raise the INR. Cranberry juice (*Vaccinium macrocarpon*), popularly used to prevent cystitis, may enhance warfarin activity.

Novel oral anticoagulants (NAOCs)

Novel oral anticoagulants (NOACs), such as direct thrombin inhibitors (DTIs; gatrans) and anti-factor Xa (xabans), target the single coagulation enzymes thrombin (dabigatran) or factor Xa (apixaban, rivaroxaban and edoxaban) (Table 8.21). In contrast to warfarin, NOACs have minimal food and drug interactions. Moreover, NOACs do not require monitoring and, compared with warfarin, have fewer thrombotic events and lower rates of major bleeding events. NOACs are thus poised to replace vitamin K antagonists for many patients with atrial fibrillation and may have a role after acute coronary syndromes. It is possible that two anticoagulants will eventually replace warfarin. The National Institute for Health and Care Excellence (NICE) has recommended dabigatran etexilate as a possible treatment to prevent stroke and systemic embolism in people with atrial fibrillation. The FDA has also approved rivaroxaban.

Dabigatran and rivaroxaban are both quickly absorbed (dabigatran action starts within 30 minutes to 2 hours of oral administration) and have short half-lives compared to warfarin, and so, in the event of excessive anticoagulant activity, discontinuing the drug is usually sufficient. They have no antidotes. There is no need for routine coagulation monitoring using the prothrombin time or INR.

Concomitant administration of potent permeability glycoprotein (P-gp) enzyme inducers (such as rifampicin, St John's wort, carbamazepine and phenytoin) can decrease dabigatran plasma concentrations and should be avoided. Co-administration of potent P-gp inhibitors, such as quinidine, ketoconazole, amiodarone and verapamil, can increase plasma concentrations of dabigatran by enhancing its reabsorption via P-gp into the gastrointestinal tract. The anti-arrhythmic dronedarone should not be co-administered with dabigatran. As rivaroxaban is metabolized via CYP3A4 and CYP2J2, and is a substrate of P-gp, it is not recommended in patients receiving strong inhibitors of both CYP3A4 and P-gp, such as azole antimycotics and HIV protease inhibitors.

The known drug interaction profiles of both dabigatran and rivaroxaban, as regards antimicrobials and analgesics, are less restrictive than those of warfarin. It may be better to confine analgesic use to paracetamol (acetaminophen) since NSAIDs have antiplatelet effects. Table 8.21 shows data relevant to dental health care. Most dental situations, such as removal of a small number of teeth, would be comparable to treating a patient with an INR of 4 or below, relying on local haemostatic measures.

Surgery and oral anticoagulants

Vitamin K antagonists (VKAs), such as warfarin, should be continued in patients undergoing selected minor procedures. In major procedures that necessitate warfarin interruption, however, heparin bridging therapy, either with unfractionated heparin (UFH) or low-molecular-weight heparin (LMWH), should be considered in patients at high thromboembolic risk and in a minority of those at moderate risk of thromboembolism. The emergence and anticipated routine clinical use of NOACs, such as the direct factor IIa (thrombin) inhibitor dabigatran and the direct factor Xa inhibitors rivaroxaban and apixaban, have the potential to simplify periprocedural anticoagulant management greatly. Minor dental procedures include tooth extractions, endodontic (root canal) and minor reconstructive procedures.

Clinical data support two approaches:

■ Continuation of VKA and the use of a prohaemostatic agent (e.g. oral tranexamic acid mouthwash with local application and expectoration)
■ Partial interruption of VKA therapy 2–5 days before the procedure.

Both approaches are associated with a low risk of clinically relevant bleeding (<5%) and rare thromboembolic outcomes (<0.1%), although minor bleeding (such as oozing from gingiva) may be common.

In patients on dabigatran who are undergoing relatively minor procedures (dental, skin, cataract; Box 8.5) or coronary angiography, it may be reasonable to continue dabigatran in the same circumstances in which warfarin can be safely continued. However, clinical data to support this approach are lacking, to date.

For major procedures or those involving a high bleed risk that necessitate the interruption of oral anticoagulant therapy, heparin bridging therapy using a standardized protocol should be reserved for patients at high thromboembolic risk and for a minority of patients at intermediate thromboembolic risk. Depending on procedural bleed risk and haemostasis, postprocedure initiation of bridging therapy for most major surgeries should delay resumption of treatment-dose therapy for a full 48–72 hours, using a stepwise approach moving from prophylactic to treatment doses; alternatively, bridging therapy should be avoided altogether during reinitiation of warfarin. For the NOACs, the timing of postprocedural reinitiation should also depend on procedural bleed risk, haemostasis and renal function (especially in the case of dabigatran), with either delayed resumption of full-dose therapy or stepwise resumption moving from prophylactic to full dose in the case of high-bleed-risk procedures. Given the pharmacokinetic profiles of the NOACs, heparin bridging therapy is unlikely to be useful, except in cases where patients cannot tolerate oral medications postoperatively.

Box 8.5 *Procedural bleeding risks[a]*

High (2-day risk of major bleed 2–4%)

- Heart valve replacement
- Coronary artery bypass
- Abdominal aortic aneurysm repair
- Neurosurgical/urological/*head and neck*/abdominal/breast cancer surgery
- Bilateral knee replacement
- Laminectomy
- Transurethral prostate resection
- Kidney biopsy
- Polypectomy, variceal treatment, biliary sphincterectomy, pneumatic dilatation
- *Percutaneous endoscopic gastrostomy (PEG) placement*
- Endoscopically guided fine-needle aspiration
- *Multiple tooth extractions*
- Vascular and general surgery
- Any major operation (procedure duration < 45 min)

Low (2-day risk of major bleed 0–2%)

- Cholecystectomy
- Abdominal hysterectomy
- Gastrointestinal endoscopy, biopsy, enteroscopy, biliary/pancreatic stent without sphincterotomy, endosonography without fine-needle aspiration
- Pacemaker and cardiac defibrillator insertion and electrophysiological testing
- *Simple dental extractions*
- Carpal tunnel repair
- Knee/hip replacement and shoulder/foot/hand surgery and arthroscopy
- Dilatation and curettage
- *Skin cancer excision*
- Abdominal hernia repair
- Haemorrhoidal surgery
- Axillary node dissection
- Hydrocoele repair
- Cataract and non-cataract eye surgery
- Non-coronary angiography
- Bronchoscopy/biopsy
- Central venous catheter removal
- Cutaneous and bladder/prostate/thyroid/breast/*lymph node biopsies*

Adapted from Spyropoulos AC, Douketis JD. How I treat anticoagulated patients undergoing an elective procedure or surgery. *Blood* 2012 11 Oct; 120(15):2954.

[a]Italics show the most relevant risks.

Several oral direct thrombin inhibitors (DTIs) and factor Xa (FXa) inhibitors have received recent FDA approval or are under investigation in late-stage clinical trials for the prevention and treatment of thromboembolic events. Rapid reversal of anticoagulation is typically recommended in patients with severe or life-threatening bleeding and in those requiring surgery or invasive procedures. However, no antidote exists for DTIs or FXa inhibitors, though replacement of coagulation factors using clotting factor concentrates is routinely considered in some clinical scenarios. Clotting factor concentrates available in the United States include prothrombin complex concentrate, activated prothrombin complex concentrate, and recombinant factor VII, activated. Coagulation tests to confirm adequate reversal of anticoagulation should be considered and commonly include APTT and TT for DTIs, and chromogenic FXa assay and TT for FXa inhibitors.

Monitoring of coagulation tests should continue for 1–2 days after achievement of haemostasis, since the duration of the clotting factor

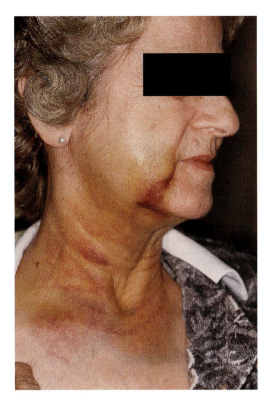

Fig. 8.13 Ecchymosis tracking to mediastinum after oral surgery.

concentrate may be shorter than that of the oral anticoagulant, especially in patients with organ dysfunction.

Dental aspects of oral anticoagulants

Some patients on anticoagulant drugs have a tendency to bleed excessively after trauma or surgery. Dental preventive care is especially important in order to minimize the need for surgical intervention. Alternatives, such as endodontics, should always be considered. Patients must be warned of the risk of intra- and postoperative bleeding and intra-/extraoral bruising (Fig. 8.13). Systemic conditions that may aggravate the bleeding tendency include coagulopathies, thrombocytopenias, vascular disorders such as Ehlers–Danlos syndrome, liver disease, renal disease, malignancy and HIV infection. Drugs that might worsen the bleeding tendency (aspirin and other NSAIDs) should be avoided (see later), as should intramuscular injections. Regional block LA injections may also be a hazard. Bleeding into the fascial spaces of the neck can threaten airway patency. Intraligamentary or intrapapillary injections are safer. CS can be given but, if intravenous, care must be taken not to damage the vein. GA requires expert attention in hospital.

In general, anticoagulation should not be stopped, except for very good reasons, because it does not necessarily reduce bleeding significantly; in contrast, stopping anticoagulation may cause hypercoagulability and rebound thrombosis, which has damaged prosthetic cardiac valves and even caused thrombotic deaths in dental patients. Certainly, anticoagulant treatment should not be altered without the agreement of the clinician in charge.

Warfarin does not usually need to be stopped before primary-care dental surgical procedures. *Minor dental procedures*, such as the administration of infiltration LA, restoration placement, fabrication of fixed and removable prosthetic appliances, and supragingival scaling and polishing, do not usually require consideration of the INR, but the prudent dentist will consult with the physician responsible for the patient's warfarin therapy before performing *more invasive procedures*.

Such potentially invasive procedures as the administration of LA via an inferior alveolar nerve block, dentoalveolar surgery (tooth extractions, periodontal surgery, implant placement, biopsies) and subgingival scaling, as well as the prescribing of certain medications, may need modification. The discussion should include the patient's recent INR values, access to the patient's INR value on the day of surgery, consideration of optimizing blood pressure control to minimize intraoperative bleeding, and an assurance that the patient is not also receiving antiplatelet agents (such as aspirin and/or clopidogrel). Although it is not uncommon for the physician to concur with or support the guidelines that permit interruption of anticoagulation for a period of up to 1 week for surgical procedures that carry a risk of bleeding (e.g. those of the American Heart Association [AHA]), the dentist should alert the physician to more recent guidelines (such as those of the American Dental Association Council on Scientific Affairs [ADA/SCA]), as these recognize that, while the older guidelines may be relevant for patients undergoing major surgery, they are not applicable for patients having dentoalveolar surgery. The dentist can emphasize that the ADA/SCA, the British Dental Association, the National Patient Safety Agency and the Haemostasis and Thrombosis Task Force of the British Committee for Standards in Haematology, having reviewed the scientific literature, have concluded that warfarin therapy should *not* be discontinued for patients having routine dentoalveolar surgery if the INR is below 4. This is due to the difficulty in predicting the drop in the INR value in any given patient and because the risk of experiencing a thromboembolism (which may be fatal) outweighs the risk of excessive postoperative oral bleeding. These conclusions should be reassuring to the physician because this level of anticoagulation is far in excess of the 2.0–3.0 range (2.5 target) typically prescribed for patients with atrial fibrillation and thus provides an even greater margin of safety. The guidelines from the National Patient Safety Agency are available at http://www.nrls.npsa.nhs.uk/resources/?entryid45=59814 (accessed 30 September 2013). Note, however, that there are no studies to date involving significant numbers of patients having more extensive surgeries, such as more than six extractions, removal of impacted teeth, alveolectomies and tori removal.

Previously published studies have identified certain procedures or precautions that may limit intraoperative and postoperative haemorrhage when performing oral surgery for these patients. The administration of LA agents containing vasoconstrictors assists in maintaining a dry surgical field, and intraligamentary and intrapapillary injections are preferred over regional blocks if the INR is above 4.0 because of an anecdotal risk of bleeding into the floor of mouth and fascial planes of the neck with consequent obstruction of the airway.

To minimize the risk and extent of postoperative bleeding, the number of teeth to be extracted at any one sitting should be limited and, when required, teeth should be sectioned so as to limit the need for bone removal. When needed, subperiosteal tension-free flaps should be raised and minimal bone removed so as to enhance clot stabilization. Resorbable gelatin or oxidized cellulose materials should be placed in the socket; the bony wound should be compressed; soft tissues should be closely apposed; and tight multiple interrupted sutures should be placed. The patient should be requested to bite on saline-soaked gauze compresses for 30 minutes and advised not to exercise or to rinse their mouth for 24 hours or to take anything other than a cold liquid diet for 48 hours. Some clinicians augment the above by also asking the patient to rinse their mouth with an antifibrinolytic, such as EACA (or tranexamic acid), four times per day for 2 minutes.

When more complex and invasive maxillofacial surgical procedures are planned, such as an extraoral open reduction of facial fractures, which is associated with extensive bleeding, for patients without a history of prior stroke, transient ischaemic attack, systemic embolisms or

Table 8.22 *Warfarin therapy and surgery*

	Prothrombin time(s)	Thrombotest	INR
Normal level	<1.3	>70%	1
Therapeutic range	2–4.5	5–20%	2–5
Levels at which dentoalveolar surgery can be carried out[a]	<2.5	>15%	<4

[a]Uncomplicated forceps extraction of 1–3 teeth.

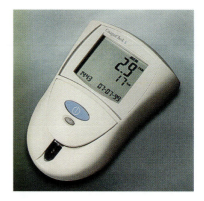

Fig. 8.14 CoaguChek for measuring INR.

mechanical heart valve, the AHA's guidelines may be applicable. The warfarin therapy should be managed with the patient's physician and the INR must be evaluated on the day of surgery. Older individuals are slower to normalize an elevated INR and may experience warfarin-related bleeding events at lower INRs than do younger individuals. In some instances, the physician may prescribe 'bridging anticoagulation' of subcutaneous LMWH in order to shorten the time that the patient is unprotected from thromboembolism. Typically, the last preoperative dose of LMWII is administered 24 hours before surgery. The first postoperative dose is given no earlier than 24 hours after surgery, and commonly on the second postoperative day when haemostasis has been secured. Warfarin therapy may be reinstituted on the evening of surgery if haemostasis has been assured; if not, then it is started 24 hours postoperatively.

Most cases of postoperative bleeding are easily treated with local measures, such as packing with a haemostatic dressing, suturing and pressure.

For patients awaiting elective dental procedures who are taking warfarin for a limited period (e.g. 6 months for a DVT), the procedure should be postponed until the warfarin has been stopped.

UK Medicines Information (UKMI) summarizes these guidelines as follows:

- An INR should be measured within 24–72 hours of undertaking the procedure.
- The UKMI recommends that no individuals should have a dental procedure in primary care if they have an INR of more than 4.0; however, the British Committee for Standards in Haematology guidelines recommend that the INR should be no greater than 2 at the time of the procedure.
- The UKMI also recommends that warfarin patients with renal or hepatic disease or those on chemotherapy or cytotoxics should have dental procedures in hospital.

The management of patients on anticoagulants (Table 8.22) should consider: the type of procedure; the INR value, which can be tested approximately if necessary with a bedside machine (Fig. 8.14); the underlying condition for which anticoagulation is used; and other risk factors.

The INR should be checked on the day of operation or, if that is not possible, the day before. For patients with a constant INR level of up to 2.5 who need emergency surgery, an INR level determined within the week before surgery can be used. A bedside device, such as the CoaguChek (Roche Diagnostics), may be used. It appears that there may be statistically significant INR differences between CoaguChek and the international reference preparations, but these test strips achieve a clinically acceptable level of accuracy.

Medico-legal and other considerations suggest that one should err on the side of caution and fully inform and discuss treatment with the patient, take medical advice in any case of doubt, and arrange adjustment of warfarin for patients with INR greater than 4.0, or greater than 3.0 if the procedure is not minor.

Table 8.23 *Protocol for warfarinized patients having oral surgery*

Preoperatively	Perioperatively	Postoperatively for 24 h
Check INR within 24 h of operation	Minimize trauma	Rest
If INR <3.5 (some suggest <3), and no liver disease, do not change warfarin	Use regional block LA only if essential	No mouth-rinsing
If INR <3.5, and liver disease, or if INR >4, consult physician about reducing warfarin	Local haemostatic measures[a]	No hot food or drink
No NSAIDs	No NSAIDs	No chewing

[a]Local haemostatic measures (see Table 8.14).

Always refer patients to hospital for care in the presence of any of the following conditions: INR of more than 4; the need for more than simple surgical procedures; the presence of additional bleeding risk factors or logistical difficulties; and drug interactions with warfarin.

If surgery is to be more than simple or minor, or the INR is over 4.0, or other risk factors are present, the patient should be treated in hospital and consideration given to whether the anticoagulation will need to be modified, possibly changing to heparin during the preoperative period (Table 8.23). If anticoagulants are to be continued after the operation, vitamin K should be avoided, as it makes subsequent anticoagulation difficult. Usually, it is simply best to discontinue the warfarin for 2 or 3 days preoperatively. A 2-day suspension appears to be a simple and safe policy for patients with prosthetic heart valves who are anticoagulated. If necessary, LMWHs can be used. To prevent postoperative bleeding, an antifibrinolytic agent (tranexamic acid; see later) can be used topically to control haemorrhage. Warfarin therapy should be restarted simultaneously with heparin unless a contraindication exists or the patient is suspected of having a hypercoagulable state. Heparin should be stopped once the INR reaches the required therapeutic level. Generally, heparin and warfarin overlap for approximately 4 days. Follow-up INR with the patient's physician should be arranged for 3 days after discharge.

Whenever possible, potentially problematic surgical procedures are best carried out in the morning, allowing more time for haemostasis before nightfall, and early in the week, to avoid problems at the weekend when staffing may be less intense. Unless the patient is also an active cocaine abuser, 2% lidocaine with 1:80000 or 1:100000 adrenaline (epinephrine) should be used. Adrenaline should then be avoided.

Bleeding should be assessed intraoperatively and, if there is concern, an absorbable haemostatic agent such as oxidized regenerated cellulose, resorbable gelatin sponge or collagen (synthetic or micro-crystalline or porcine) can be placed in the socket. Cyanoacrylate or fibrin glues provide rapid haemostasis, as well as tissue sealing and adhesion. Recombinant fibrin products are preferred.

Suturing is desirable to stabilize flaps and to prevent postoperative disturbance of wounds by eating. Resorbable sutures are preferred since they retain less plaque. Gauze pressure (a gauze soaked with tranexamic acid helps; see later), asking the patient to bite on the gauze for 10 minutes, helps haemostasis. If bleeding is controlled, the patient should be dismissed and given a 7-day follow-up appointment and the phone number of the surgery, with instructions to call if bleeding starts. Additional risk factors for bleeding should prompt the treating clinician to be more cautious (i.e. to place more sutures and to prescribe in advance an antifibrinolytic drug such as topical 4.8% tranexamic acid, for up to 7 days).

Postoperatively, the patency of the airway must be ensured. Care should be taken to watch for haematoma formation, often signified by swelling, dysphagia or hoarseness.

Many patients can be managed postoperatively with antifibrinolytic agents given topically as mouthwashes during the first 7–10 days. Systemic tranexamic acid does not result in therapeutic concentrations in saliva. Topical tranexamic acid is effective, even when anticoagulant therapy remains unchanged. Controlled studies have shown the efficacy and safety of tranexamic acid mouthwashes, and their lack of unwanted systemic effects. Overall, tranexamic acid reduces bleeding complications to 0–7% from 13–40% in controls. It is given topically as 10 mL of a 4.8–5% w/v solution, used as a mouthwash for 2 minutes, four times daily for 7 days.

Infection also appears to induce fibrinolysis and therefore antimicrobials, such as oral penicillin V 250–500 mg four times daily, or clindamycin, should be given postoperatively for a full course of 7 days if there is risk of secondary haemorrhage. Metronidazole is contraindicated, and amoxicillin and erythromycin are less appropriate because of possible drug interactions with warfarin, which may enhance bleeding.

For postoperative pain management, paracetamol is the analgesic and antipyretic of choice for *short-term use* in patients on oral anticoagulant therapy. It is preferred over NSAIDs since it does not affect platelets. Codeine is a suitable alternative analgesic. A diet of cool liquid and minced solids should be taken for several days.

Postoperative prolonged bleeding should be controlled by biting on a moist gauze, a gauze pad soaked in tranexamic acid, or a moist tea bag with firm pressure for 30 minutes. Faced with persistent bleeding, the dentist must establish whether the situation is urgent, when the patient will require admission for intravenous fluids or reversal of anticoagulation. This may be needed if the patient is losing large quantities of blood or is hypotensive (hypovolaemic).

To stop oral bleeding, an LA injection containing adrenaline (epinephrine) should be given and a sterile gauze pad soaked with tranexamic acid should be pressed over the extraction socket for 10–15 minutes. The socket edges should be approximated by squeezing with the fingers. The socket should then be sutured using black silk sutures to ensure tight closure. A resorbable haemostatic preparation may be placed in the socket before suturing. If the patient continues to bleed, consult the physician about possible use of vitamin K.

In people at high risk of bleeding or undergoing major surgery in which normal haemostasis is required, NOACs such as dabigatran etexilate should be stopped 2–5 days before surgery. If surgery is elective and the patient has normal renal function, two doses of the drug can be missed; if renal function is abnormal, the patient should miss three or four doses of dabigatran. Warfarin remains the treatment of choice for patients with a low creatinine clearance below 15 mL/min.

Heparins

Heparin acts by potentiating antithrombin III, which inhibits the activation of clotting factors II, IX, X and XI and prolongs the APTT. Use for more than 5 days can induce thrombocytopenia.

Unfractionated heparin (UFH) is given via intravenous infusion, with the dose titrated according to the APTT. The half-life of UFH is 1 hour, making it useful where rapid normalization of anticoagulation is required: for example, before surgery. If more rapid reversal of anticoagulation is needed, protamine can be used.

Low molecular weight heparins (LMWHs; ardeparin, dalteparin, danaparoid, enoxaparin, nadroparin, reviparin, tinzaparin) act more specifically on inhibition of factor X activation and the APTT is therefore normal. A factor Xa assay can be used to monitor the anticoagulant effect of LMWH but this is not routinely required. LMWH is at least as safe and effective as UFH in the treatment of uncomplicated DVT. Overlapping the initiation of warfarin permits long-term anticoagulation. Advantages include a decreased incidence of heparin-induced thrombocytopenia and fewer bleeding episodes.

General aspects

Heparin is a natural product, abundant in granules of the mast cells that line the vasculature, and is released in response to injury. It is also used as a parenteral anticoagulant given subcutaneously or intravenously, for acute thromboembolic episodes or for hospitalization protocols that include significant surgical procedures, to prevent DVT and pulmonary emboli. Heparin is a sulphated glycosaminoglycan and was originally obtained from liver (hence *heparin*). It acts immediately on blood coagulation to block the conversion of fibrinogen to fibrin, mainly by inhibiting the thrombin–fibrinogen reaction via its binding to and catalysing of antithrombin III, which then inhibits the serine proteases of the coagulation cascade to inactivate thrombin. Heparin also acts on activated factors IX–XII and increases platelet aggregation but inhibits thrombin-induced activation. The anticoagulant effect of standard or unfractionated heparin has an immediate action on blood clotting, which is usually lost within 6 hours of stopping it.

The PT, APTT and TT are prolonged. Most patients are monitored with the APTT and are maintained at 1.5–2.5 times the control value (the therapeutic range). Large doses of heparin can also prolong the INR. Platelet counts should also be monitored if heparin is used for more than 5 days, since it can cause thrombocytopenia. Autoimmune thrombocytopenia is possible within 3–15 days, or sooner if there has been previous heparin exposure.

Heparin is available as standard or unfractionated heparin or LMWHs. The latter, such as certoparin, interact with factor Xa but do not affect standard blood test results. Low-dose heparin therapy, such as Minihep, is used to reduce the risk of DVT. Some heparins are also being used for other effects, such as immunosuppression.

LMWHs have more predictable pharmacokinetic and pharmacodynamic properties than the largely replaced UFH. Antifactor Xa monitoring is superior to measurement of APPT, and is prudent in patients with severe obesity or renal insufficiency, and UFH infusion is preferable to LMWH injection in patients with renal failure. Protamine may help reverse bleeding related to LWMH. The synthetic pentasaccharide fondaparinux is a promising new antithrombotic agent. Exclusion criteria for outpatient therapy with LMWH are shown in Box 8.6.

Dental aspects of heparin anticoagulation

For uncomplicated forceps extraction of 1–3 teeth, there is usually no need to interfere with heparin or LMWH anticoagulation.

- Clinical evidence of pulmonary embolism or suspected embolism
- Conditions that increase the risk of bleeding:
  - Recent surgery
  - Peptic ulcer disease
  - Malignant hypertension
  - Increased risk of falling
- High risk of recurrent thrombosis:
  - Extensive proximal deep venous thrombosis
  - Recurrent deep venous thrombosis
- Pregnancy
- Protein C or S deficiency
- Likelihood of non-compliance
- Unavailability for follow-up
- Inadequate home support system

Table 8.24 *Other parenteral anticoagulant agents*

Antiplatelets	Heparinoids	Hirudins	Low-molecular-weight heparins	Prostacyclin
Abciximab	Danaparoid	Desirudin	Certoparin	Epoprostenol
Aspirin		Lepirudin	Dalteparin	
Clopidogrel			Enoxaparin	
Dipyridamole			Reviparin	
Eptifibatide			Tinzaparin	
Ticlopidine				
Tirofiban				

Other drugs affecting haemostasis

Other parenteral agents influencing haemostasis include *heparinoids*, such as danaparoid; and *hirudins*, such as lepirudin and desirudin (see Table 8.24). The physician should be consulted before any major surgical procedure but dentoalveolar surgery is usually uncomplicated.

VITAMIN K DEFICIENCY AND MALABSORPTION

General aspects

Vitamin K is a fat-soluble vitamin present in the diet and also synthesized by the gut flora. It is absorbed in the small gut, in the presence of bile salts. After transport to the liver, vitamin K is used for the synthesis of factors II (prothrombin), VII, IX and X. Haemorrhagic disease may, therefore, result from interference with vitamin K use by:

- anticoagulants
- malabsorption
- obstructive jaundice
- severe liver disease.

General management

In liver disease, many haemostatic functions are severely impaired and vitamin K is of little or no value (Box 8.7).

Dental aspects

Dental management in vitamin K deficiency may be complicated by the clotting defect and the underlying disorder, particularly obstructive jaundice (Ch. 9). The latter may be caused by gallstones, viral hepatitis or carcinoma of the head of the pancreas.

The underlying disorder should preferably be corrected but vitamin K can be given if surgery is urgent. Phytomenadione (5–25 mg) is the most potent and rapidly acting form and should preferably be given intravenously. The PT should be monitored after 48 hours; if the defect has not been corrected by then, this suggests parenchymal liver disease.

Liver disease is an important cause of bleeding disorders related to: impaired vitamin K metabolism; excessive fibrinolysis; failure of synthesis or overconsumption of normal clotting factors; synthesis of abnormal clotting factors; and thrombocytopenia.

Haemorrhage can be severe and difficult to manage because of the complexity of these defects.

Antifibrinolytic treatment and fresh-frozen plasma may sometimes be effective. If there is an obstructive element to the disease, vitamin K may be effective, but only if parenchymal disease is mild (Ch. 9).

Before more advanced surgery in a heparin-treated patient, medical advice should be sought. Heparin has an immediate effect on blood clotting but acts for only 4–6 hours and no specific treatment is therefore needed to reverse its effect. The effect of heparin is best assessed by the APTT. Withdrawal of heparin is adequate to reverse anticoagulation where this is necessary. In an emergency, anticoagulation can be reversed by intravenous protamine sulfate given in a dose of 1 mg per 100 IU heparin, but a medical opinion should be sought first. Where heparin has been stopped, any surgery can safely be carried out after 6–8 hours. In renal dialysis patients, or those having cardiopulmonary bypass or other extracorporeal circulation with heparinization, surgery is best carried out on the day after dialysis. The effects of heparinization have then ceased and there is maximum benefit from dialysis.

LMWHs may have little effect on postoperative bleeding, despite their longer activity (up to 24 hours). However, the advice of the haematologist should be sought before surgery.

Aspirin and antiplatelet drugs

These include clopidogrel and glycoprotein IIb/IIIa inhibitors (abciximab, eptifibatide and tirofiban; Table 8.24). They can affect the APTT and postoperative bleeding.

Aspirin irreversibly impairs platelet aggregation and is used long-term in the prevention of cardiovascular events and stroke in patients at risk. In large doses, aspirin may also cause hypoprothrombinaemia. Even small doses prolong the bleeding time and impair platelet adhesiveness. Aspirin may worsen bleeding tendencies if there are other anticoagulation medications or other bleeding disorders, such as uraemia.

In patients with no other cause for a bleeding tendency who are receiving up to 100 mg aspirin daily, in general, for uncomplicated forceps extraction of 1–3 teeth, there is no need to interfere with aspirin treatment. Suturing and packing the socket with resorbable gelatin sponge, oxidized cellulose or microfibrillar collagen can be carried out if necessary.

In patients with no other cause for a bleeding tendency who are receiving doses of aspirin higher than 100 mg daily, if there is concern, the current value of the bleeding time should be established. If it is over 20 minutes, surgery should be postponed.

In practice, aspirin rarely interferes significantly with dental surgical procedures.

- Lack of vitamin K synthesis in the gut
- Broad-spectrum antibiotics used for prolonged periods
- Parenteral feeding in inpatients
- Poor absorption
- Malabsorption syndromes
- Blind loop syndrome
- Obstructive jaundice
- Failure of utilization
- Oral anticoagulant treatment
- Liver failure
- Viral hepatitis (has an obstructive component)

[a]Deficiency responds to parenteral vitamin K.

FIBRINOLYTIC DRUGS

Fibrinolytic drugs, such as streptokinase, may cause abnormal bleeding and dental surgery should be deferred where possible.

ACQUIRED HAEMOPHILIA

Acquired haemophilia is a rare disorder caused by circulating antibodies to factor VIII; these typically are of unknown origin but may rarely form in autoimmune disorders such as rheumatoid arthritis, drug therapy (especially with penicillin), and pregnancy or the puerperium. In contrast to congenital haemophilia, females are affected just as frequently as males.

Specialist haematological attention is required before any operative treatment is considered.

OTHER DISORDERS ASSOCIATED WITH BLEEDING TENDENCIES

These may include:

- the period after massive transfusions
- antibodies to clotting factors
- chronic renal failure (Ch. 12)
- cyanotic congenital heart disease (Ch. 5)
- disseminated intravascular coagulopathy
- Gram-negative shock
- head injuries (Ch. 24)
- hypertension
- myelofibrosis, leukaemia or lymphoma (see later)
- polycythaemia vera (see later).

POSTOPERATIVE BLEEDING

Plasminogen and plasminogen activator are present in the oral environment, since plasminogen is secreted into the saliva and t-PA arises from oral epithelial cells and gingival crevicular fluid. Oral surgery induces changes of fibrinolysis; initially, the fibrinolytic activity of saliva is weakened, due to inhibitors of fibrinolysis originating from the blood and the wound exudates, but when the bleeding and exudation abate, the fibrinolytic activity of saliva increases. This may contribute to bleeding.

Prolonged bleeding after dental extraction is, however, one of the most common signs of haemorrhagic disease and may amount to a haemorrhagic emergency. It is sometimes how the bleeding tendency is first recognized.

Faced with a bleeding patient, the dentist must establish whether the situation is urgent; whether there could be a bleeding tendency; or if the patient is losing large quantities of blood, whether the patient is hypotensive (hypovolaemic) or bleeding internally.

MANAGEMENT OF POSTOPERATIVE BLEEDING

The precise site or origin of the bleeding must be discovered by cleaning out the mouth with swabs. Pressing firmly with a gauze pad over the socket for 10–15 minutes will usually stop the bleeding, even in some bleeding tendencies, but this is often only temporary. A quicker and more effective means is to suture the socket under LA. If the bleeding persists, consider a systemic cause such as ascertaining whether there are:

- acquired deficiencies of haemostasis, such as those caused by anticoagulants or thrombocytopenia
- hereditary deficiencies of clotting factors (e.g. vWD and haemophilia).

There could be a bleeding tendency if the bleeding is unexplained by the degree of trauma or there is a previous or family history of excessive bleeding, such as:

- a previous diagnosis of a bleeding tendency
- bleeding for more than 36 hours or restarting more than 36 hours after operation (however, this could indicate an infection)
- admission to hospital to arrest bleeding
- blood transfusion for bleeding
- spontaneous bleeding (e.g. haemarthrosis, deep bruising or menorrhagia from little obvious cause)
- a convincing family history of one of the above, combined with a degree of personal history
- treatment with significant drugs such as anticoagulants.

In emergencies, an intravenous line must be established and plasma expanders or blood given. Blood transfusions used to be refused by Jehovah's Witnesses, but their principles are being reconsidered and alternatives to allogeneic blood are becoming available. In this group, blood loss may be minimized by using aprotinin and tranexamic acid. Recombinant blood coagulation factors are acceptable to Jehovah's Witnesses (Ch. 30). Erythropoietin is acceptable, as often is intraoperative salvage of blood or acute normovolaemic haemodilution (ANH; the preoperative removal of blood and its replacement by crystalloid or colloid, followed by reuse of the patient's blood at operation). Some will accept the use of Hemopure, a polymerized bovine haemoglobin.

Transfusions carry the risk of blood-borne viral infections (Chs 9 and 21) and circulatory overload.

BLOOD TRANSFUSION

Blood can supply a range of products useful in a variety of situations (Fig. 8.15). Perioperative blood loss and anaemia is best dealt with by reducing the amount of blood lost at surgery through minimizing trauma, improving mechanical haemostasis, limiting phlebotomy to essential diagnostic tests, using microsample laboratory techniques; and giving antifibrinolytics, such as EACA or tranexamic acid (or, for high-risk procedures, aprotinin). Erythropoietin can also help where blood has been lost but the replacement of blood by transfusion can be essential after severe haemorrhage and in some other circumstances. Allogeneic blood transfusion (from a genetically similar but not identical donor) may carry hazards of:

- incompatibility
- fluid overload

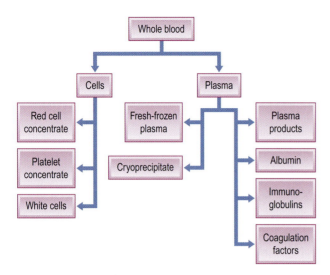

Fig. 8.15 Blood products.

Box 8.8 *Diseases known to be transmitted via allogeneic blood transfusion*

- Bacterial infections (various)
- Chagas disease
- Cytomegalovirus infection
- Hepatitis A virus infections
- Hepatitis B virus infections
- Hepatitis C virus infections
- Human immunodeficiency virus (HIV-1 and HIV-2) infection
- Human T-lymphotropic viruses (HTLV-1 and HTLV-2) infection
- Malaria
- *Treponema pallidum* infection
- West Nile virus infection
- Variant Creutzfeldt–Jakob disease (prions)

- transmission of infections (Box 8.8)
- post-transfusion purpura
- transfusion-associated graft-versus-host disease
- transfusion-associated acute lung injury (TRALI).

In the UK, therefore, blood is now screened and leukodepletion also used, as this reduces the risk of infection and also of acute non-haemolytic transfusion reactions and transfusion-associated graft-versus-host disease.

Some medications may be transmitted, and this is especially a concern with pregnant women and prostatic medications such as dutasteride and finasteride (Ch. 25). Allogeneic transfusion may lead to an increased risk of postoperative bacterial infections and multiorgan failure.

Autologous transfusion (obtained from the same individual) reduces the need for allogeneic transfusion and is most widely used in elective surgery. The three main techniques are pre-deposit transfusion, intraoperative haemodilution, and intraoperative and postoperative salvage. Autologous transfusion is more cost-effective than allogeneic transfusion and clinical outcomes are improved.

If blood transfusion is needed:

- establish an intravenous line
- take blood for grouping and cross-matching
- seek a surgical opinion and begin a thorough secondary survey
- organize quarter- or half-hourly observations of pulse rate, blood pressure, respiratory rate, daily urine output and fluid balance (usually daily).

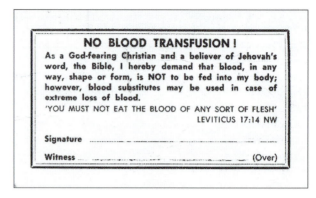

Fig. 8.16 Jehovah's Witness declaration.

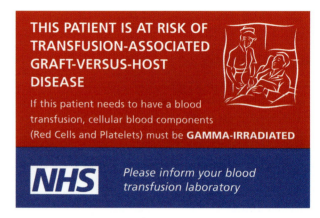

Fig. 8.17 Transfusion-associated graft-versus-host disease warning card.

Blood transfusion is not needed to replace losses of less than 500 mL in an adult, unless there was pre-existing anaemia or deterioration of the general condition warrants transfusion. Blood should therefore never be given unless warranted. In people belonging to some faiths, such as Jehovah's Witnesses, transfusion is not permissible (Fig. 8.16 and Ch. 30), as discussed above.

Transfusion-associated graft-versus-host disease

Transfusion-associated graft-versus-host disease is a rare but serious complication of blood transfusion. People at risk include those who have:

- received blood transfusions from HLA-matched donors, including family members
- had a stem-cell transplant
- inherited immune defects
- acquired immune defects, such as Hodgkin disease
- been treated with purine analogues, such as fludarabine, cladribine or deoxycoformycin.

Transfusion-associated graft-versus-host disease results from transfused leukocytes; gamma irradiation of the transfused blood will obviate the reaction.

Patients should be pre-warned and should carry a warning card themselves (Fig. 8.17).

THROMBOTIC DISORDERS

Superficial vein thrombosis may complicate intravenous injections, particularly of diazepam, but does not lead to pulmonary embolism. Treatment

Table 8.25 *Disorders predisposing to thromboses*

Factor involved	Genetic forms	Acquired forms	Management
Antithrombin deficiency	Autosomal dominant Affects ~1 per 2000 of population	Eclampsia, disseminated intravascular coagulation (DIC), nephrotic syndrome	Resistant to heparin anticoagulation – use oral anticoagulants or fresh-frozen plasma
Factor V Leiden	Autosomal dominant Affects ~5% of population	Liver transplantation	Warfarin
Platelets (thrombocytosis and thrombocythaemia)	–	Exercise, pregnancy, trauma, post-splenectomy, chronic inflammatory disease, malignancy	Treat underlying cause. Preoperative aspirin, dipyridamole or heparin
Protein C deficiency	Autosomal dominant	Warfarin, liver disease, vitamin K deficiency, sepsis, DIC, thrombosis, asparaginase (crisantaspase)	Protein C concentrate or anticoagulation
Protein S deficiency	Genetic	Liver disease, DIC	Management takes place in the event of acute venous thromboembolism or in patients with asymptomatic carrier states without a thrombotic event. Heparin therapy and then warfarin

of acute episodes of thrombosis is by subcutaneous injection or infusion of heparin (for 5–7 days), followed by oral anticoagulant therapy.

DEEP VEIN THROMBOSIS AND THROMBOEMBOLIC DISEASE

General aspects

Blood contains natural anticoagulants, mainly antithrombin, which inhibits several activated coagulation factors, including thrombin, factor IXa and factor Xa, by forming a stable complex with the various factors. Heparin and heparan sulphates increase the activity of antithrombin at least 1000 fold. Other natural anticoagulants include protein S and protein C, which inhibit activated factor V (Table 8.25).

Deep vein thrombosis (DVT) and subsequent pulmonary embolism (PE) are important sequelae and causes of death or significant morbidity, especially in older, bedridden and postoperative patients as a consequence of immobility and pressure on the calf from prolonged bed rest; there is also increased blood coagulability in pregnancy. They may also follow GA and surgery. Several other factors may contribute, including, sometimes, dehydration or oral contraceptives (Fig. 8.18).

About 30% of people who have had a DVT or PE are at risk for another episode. Factors that increase the risk of thrombosis include:

- injury to a vein:
  - fractures
  - muscle injury
  - major surgery (particularly involving the abdomen, pelvis, hip or legs)
- slowed blood flow:
  - confinement to bed or a chair
  - limited movement (e.g. after surgery or a plaster cast on a leg)
  - paralysis
- increased oestrogen:
  - hormonal contraceptives
  - hormone replacement therapy
  - pregnancy
- coagulation disorders:
  - factor V Leiden
  - prothrombin
  - antithrombin III deficiency
  - protein C deficiency
  - protein S deficiency
  - antiphospholipid syndrome
  - hyperhomocysteinaemia

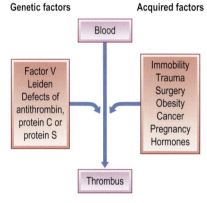

Fig. 8.18 Deep vein thrombosis causes.

- chronic medical disorders:
  - heart disease
  - lung disease
  - cancer
  - inflammatory bowel disease (Crohn disease or ulcerative colitis)
- other factors:
  - advancing age
  - central vein catheter
  - DVT or PE previously or positive family history
  - hypertension
  - obesity
  - smoking.

Hypercoagulability (thrombophilia) is when there is a risk of thrombosis under circumstances that would not cause thrombosis in a normal person and is common postoperatively, during long-haul air flights ('economy class syndrome') and in obesity. Oestrogen use, malignant and myeloproliferative disease, congestive cardiac failure, homocystinuria and systemic lupus erythematosus (anticardiolipin antibodies) also lead to a hypercoagulable state.

Activated protein C (APC) normally inactivates coagulation factor V, slowing down the clotting process and prevents clots from growing. Defects of protein C or other natural anticoagulants (antithrombin or protein S), as well as impaired fibrinolysis or Leiden factor (Table 8.26), can cause thrombosis.

Factor V Leiden thrombophilia is an inherited increased clotting tendency seen in about 5% of Europeans, who have an abnormal blood clotting factor V (termed factor V Leiden) that cannot be inhibited by protein C. These individuals are predisposed to blood clotting, with a

Table 8.26 *Medications used as prophylaxis for thromboses*

Antiplatelet agents	Heparins	Hirudins	Oral anticoagulants
Aspirin	Dalteparin	Lepirudin	Apixaban
Clopidogrel	Danaparoid		Dabigatran
Dipyridamole	Enoxaparin		Warfarin
Ticagrelor	Heparin sodium		
	Tinzaparin		

higher than average risk of DVT (most often in the legs but also the brain, eyes, liver and kidneys), pulmonary emboli and increased risk of pregnancy loss (miscarriage).

Clinical features of DVT

About half of people with DVT have no symptoms. Venous thrombosis usually affects the deep calf veins and there the most common symptoms include:

- pain, especially on flexing the ankle (Homan sign) – characteristic but its absence should certainly not be relied upon to exclude the diagnosis
- swelling
- tenderness
- redness.

About 30% of people who have a DVT develop complications (post-thrombotic syndrome [PTS]), caused by damage to the vein valves. PTS manifests with swelling, pain, discolouration, scaling or ulcers in the affected part. In some cases, PE may ensue and can be lethal.

General management of DVT

Prophylaxis against venous thromboembolism is important but not reliably effective. Consideration should be given to stopping the contraceptive pill preoperatively.

The calves must not rest on hard objects during surgery and stasis may be eliminated by calf contractions stimulated electrically, by use of compression hosiery or by pneumatic compression. Early mobilization and leg movements postoperatively must be encouraged. Heparin anticoagulation is the most effective method of preventing thromboembolism but must be balanced against the risks of haemorrhage. However, low-dose heparin, sufficient to provide an INR between 1.5 and 2, protects against DVT without inducing a significant risk of bleeding. Fondaparinux sodium (which blocks factor X) is an alternative.

DVT is often diagnosed clinically but confirmed using:

- duplex ultrasound to evaluate the vein blood flow
- venography
- blood D-dimer test – indicates abnormally high levels of fibrin degradation products, suggesting thrombosis. A negative d-dimer test virtually rules out DVT. D-dimers are breakdown products of a fibrin mesh stabilised by factor XIII.

Less frequently used tests include:

- MRI
- CT.

While DVT and PE are common clinically, they are rare in the absence of elevated blood D-dimer levels and certain specific risk factors. Imaging, particularly CT pulmonary angiography, is a rapid, accurate and widely available test but has limited value in patients who are very unlikely, based on serum and clinical criteria, to have significant risk.

Treatment of DVT is by heparin, starting with at least 5000 units intravenously, then continuous infusion at 1000 units per hour or 15000 units subcutaneously every 24 hours, with APTT monitoring. Patients with acute DVT have traditionally been treated with UFH followed by oral anticoagulation. In severe cases, the clot might need surgical removal.

Compression stockings may help relieve pain and swelling. These might need to be worn for 2 years or more after having DVT.

Clinical features of PE

PE can occur without any symptoms of a DVT but features can include:

- dyspnoea
- arrhythmias
- chest pain, which worsens with a deep breath or coughing
- anxiety
- haemoptysis or pleurisy
- low blood pressure, light-headedness or fainting.

PE may gradually cause pulmonary hypertension and right-sided heart failure, or may be fatal as a result of sudden circulatory collapse.

General management of PE

Massive PE with collapse and cardiac arrest requires emergency care and early treatment with thrombolytics and anticoagulants:

- external cardiac massage, which may break up the embolus
- oxygen
- intravenous heparin
- a thrombolytic agent, such as streptokinase.

Minor PE usually resolves spontaneously but anticoagulants should be given. Tests to find the location of the embolus and the damage it has caused to the lungs include imaging with MRI or CT, angiography, or lung ventilation/perfusion scan ({Vdot}/{Qdot} scan).

Dental aspects of thromboses

Venous thrombosis may affect the deep calf veins as a consequence of immobility, pressure on the calf and increased blood coagulability, which follows GA and surgery (see earlier).

Thrombophilia and hypofibrinolysis may possibly underlie so-called neuralgia-inducing cavitational osteonecrosis (NICO) or Ratner bone cavities, which may cause severe pain. NICO appears to be due to resistance to activated protein C or to low protein C levels, or low levels of stimulated t-PA. Bone sites most frequently involved, in decreasing order of prevalence, are mandibular molars, maxillary molars and maxillary canines/lateral incisors. Third molar sites account for 45% of all jawbone involvement. Unlike abscesses, cysts or periapical lesions, the cavities in NICO are often not apparent on radiographs, though thin-slice CT scanning may show the areas. They may be detectable by technetium-99 methylene diphosphonate radioisotope scanning or ultrasonography.

DISSEMINATED INTRAVASCULAR COAGULATION

Disseminated intravascular coagulation (DIC; consumption coagulopathy or defibrination syndrome) is an uncommon, complex process with potentially fatal activation of the haemostasis-related

Causes

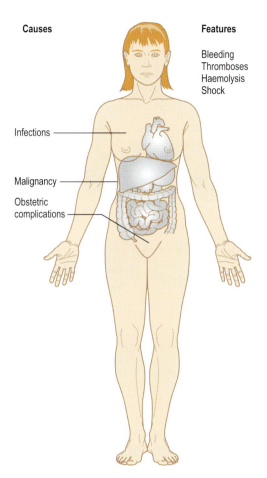

Features

Bleeding
Thromboses
Haemolysis
Shock

Infections

Malignancy

Obstetric
complications

Fig. 8.19 Disseminated intravascular coagulopathy.

mechanisms within the circulation. Uncontrolled consumption of clotting factors and intravascular deposition of platelets may result in serious coagulopathy and thrombocytopenia.

DIC may be caused by many conditions, including sepsis, adenocarcinoma, acute myeloid leukaemia (M3 variant), obstetric complications such as amniotic fluid embolus, incompatible blood transfusions, burns, cancers or severe trauma. In one series of head injuries, a minor degree of DIC was found in 57%. Brain ischaemia by vascular occlusion may therefore complicate head injury, as a result of DIC.

DIC can lead to bleeding, thrombosis, haemolysis and shock (Fig. 8.19). Haemorrhagic tendencies result from the consumption of platelets and clotting factors internally and from activation of the fibrinolytic system. Purpura and bleeding from sites such as the gastrointestinal tract and gingivae can result. In the case of head injuries, DIC may lead to intracranial haemorrhage. Thrombotic phenomena include clotting in capillaries, which can damage any organ, but the kidneys, liver, adrenals and brain are particularly vulnerable. Red cells also become damaged as a result of the changes in the capillaries (microangiopathic haemolysis). Shock may be caused by adrenal damage or obstruction of the pulmonary circulation by fibrin deposition and other factors.

Symptoms suggestive of DIC include bleeding from the gingiva, nausea, vomiting, muscle and abdominal pain, seizures and oliguria. PT, APTT and FDPs and the D-dimer test are increased but, due to fibrin consumption, there are low levels of fibrinogen.

DIC is an acute emergency; the underlying cause and any hypoxia or acidosis should be corrected, and heparinization, replacement of clotting factors and platelets, or antifibrinolytic therapy given as appropriate. The management of DIC is controversial and must, in any case, depend on the cause and the pathological changes taking place. No single programme of treatment is effective for all cases.

Dental aspects

The main importance of DIC is in relation to head injuries, as discussed earlier. Gingival bleeding may be seen.

PLASMINOGEN DEFICIENCY (HYPOPLASMINOGENAEMIA)

In health, body fluid fibrinolytic activity clears fibrin deposits but does not cause systemic fibrinolysis.

Plasminogen can be activated by tissue plasminogen activator, kallikrein or drugs such as streptokinase. Tissue plasminogen activator is produced by damaged endothelial cells and activates plasminogen to plasmin when it is bound to fibrin. If plasminogen is deficient, this mechanism fails, leading to fibrin deposition.

Some patients develop gingival swelling, corneal involvement and blindness; others may also develop congenital occlusive hydrocephalus. Whether therapy with topical heparin or intravenous purified plasminogen concentrate will effectively control the lesions remains to be established.

Dental aspects

Plasminogen deficiency may rarely underlie ligneous conjunctivitis, an idiopathic form of chronic membranous conjunctivitis associated with fibrin deposits and often with lesions in the larynx, nose, cervix and gingivae.

ERYTHROCYTES (RED BLOOD CELLS)

Erythrocytes are responsible for oxygen (O_2) carriage from the lungs to the tissues. They are produced (*erythropoiesis*) in the bone marrow from nucleated stem cells (undifferentiated *pluripotent* stem cells), via immature intermediate cells (*reticulocytes*), which retain their organelles, have nuclear remnants and can still divide. Reticulocytes are prematurely released into the blood (reticulocytosis) when demand is high. Erythropoiesis is triggered by *erythropoietin* released from the kidney when low O_2 levels are detected, and this stimulates the pluripotent stem cells. Erythrocytes, when mature, contain only haemoglobin (Hb) – the molecule responsible for the transport of O_2 and carbon dioxide (CO_2). Hb production requires iron, protoporphyrin and globin chains. Hb is a heterogeneous group of proteins consisting of four globin chains and four haem groups. In adults, the normal haemoglobins are HbA, HbA_2 and HbF. Effete erythrocytes are broken down largely in the spleen, and Hb is degraded to haem and then bilirubin in the liver (Fig. 8.20).

ANAEMIA

General aspects

Anaemia is defined as an Hb level below the norm for the age, gender and ethnic background of the individual and may be due to insufficient red blood cell (RBC) numbers or Hb content. Up to puberty, an Hb level below 11.0 g/dL is the hallmark of anaemia; the corresponding figure in adult females is below 11.5 g/dL, and in adult males below 13.5 g/dL. The effect of anaemia is to lower the oxygen-carrying capacity of the blood. Its causes are outlined in Tables 8.27 and 8.28, and in Figure 8.21. Although common, anaemia is not a disease in itself but it may be a feature of many diseases (Fig. 8.22).

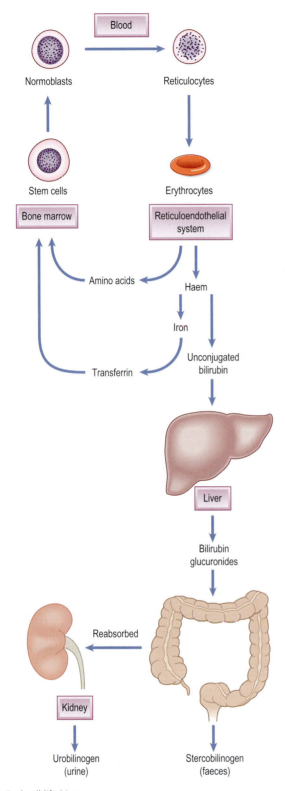

Fig. 8.20 Red-cell life history.

Table 8.27 *Causes of anaemia*

Nature of anaemia	Cause
Increased red blood cell (RBC) loss	Menstrual blood loss
	Gastrointestinal blood loss
	Haemolysis
Reduced RBC production	Haematinic deficiency
	Bone marrow infiltration
Increased tissue requirements	Puberty
	Pregnancy
Decreased tissue requirements	Hypothyroidism

Table 8.28 *Types of anaemia*

Cause	Examples
Poor intake of haematinics (uncommon)	Socioeconomic factors
	Dietary fads
	Dysphagia
Impaired absorption of haematinics	Diseases of small intestine in particular (e.g. coeliac disease)
Increased demands for haematinics	Pregnancy and haemolysis especially
Impaired erythropoiesis	Aplastic anaemia and leukaemia
	Drugs
	Chronic disease (e.g. rheumatoid arthritis)
	Viral infections
Haemolytic anaemias	Sickle cell and thalassaemia mainly
Blood loss (most common cause)	Menorrhagia
	Any gastrointestinal lesion (ulcers or carcinoma)
	Lesions of the urinary tract
	Trauma

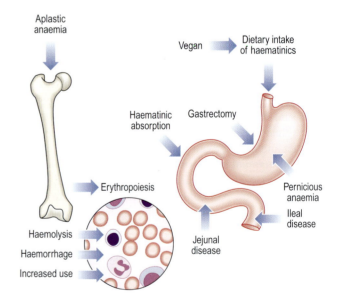

Fig. 8.21 Main causes of anaemia.

The most common cause of anaemia in developed countries is chronic blood loss and consequent iron deficiency, usually from heavy menstruation in women. Folate and vitamin B_{12} (cobalamin) deficiencies are the next most common causes.

Anaemia is classified on the basis of red-cell size as microcytic (small), macrocytic (large) or normocytic (normal-size erythrocytes; Table 8.29).

Microcytic anaemia is the most common and is usually due to iron deficiency, or occasionally to thalassaemia or chronic diseases. The mean corpuscular (cell) volume (MCV) falls below 78 fl.

Macrocytic anaemia (MCV more than 99 fl) is caused usually by vitamin B_{12} or folate deficiency (not infrequently in alcoholics); sometimes by the consumption of folate and vitamin B_{12} in chronic haemolysis, pregnancy or malignancy; and sometimes by drugs (methotrexate,

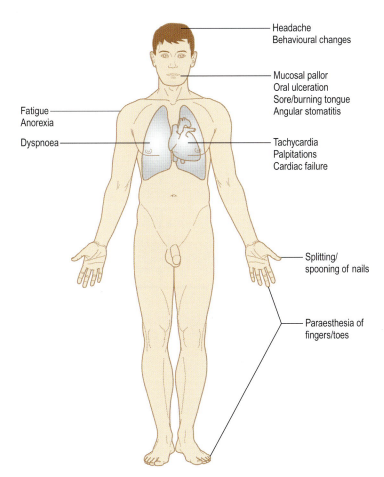

Headache
Behavioural changes

Mucosal pallor
Oral ulceration
Sore/burning tongue
Angular stomatitis

Fatigue
Anorexia

Dyspnoea

Tachycardia
Palpitations
Cardiac failure

Splitting/
spooning of nails

Paraesthesia of
fingers/toes

Fig. 8.22 Anaemia – features.

Clinical features

Patients with anaemia are commonly symptomless in the early stages or if the onset is slow. However, as the anaemia worsens and the oxygen-carrying capacity of the blood falls, cardiac symptoms and signs develop (tiredness, dyspnoea, palpitations, tachycardia, flow murmurs and eventual cardiac failure). Pallor of the oral mucosa, conjunctiva or palmar creases suggests severe anaemia but skin colour can be misleading. Anaemia may worsen the symptoms of pre-existing coronary, peripheral and cerebrovascular disease. The different types of anaemia have many clinical features in common (Box 8.9).

General management

Anaemia is diagnosed from the Hb level but the precise nature and underlying cause must be established. The key to management of anaemia is the establishment and treatment of the underlying cause. Depending on the clinical presentation, the following investigations may be indicated:

- Full blood count – to ascertain the Hb level and RBC indices; it is important to include a reticulocyte count
- Blood film – to demonstrate abnormal RBC forms (sickle cells in sickle cell disease and pencil cells in iron-deficiency anaemia; Figs 8.23 and 8.24)
- Erythrocyte sedimentation rate (ESR) or plasma viscosity (PV) – the latter is better, since it changes earlier in disease and is unaffected by drugs
- Hb electrophoresis – for haemoglobinopathy screening
- Haematinics – serum vitamin B_{12}, folate and ferritin levels; the ferritin is also an acute-phase reactant and can rise in inflammatory states
- Endoscopy – to identify sources of gastrointestinal blood loss
- Bone marrow biopsy – to exclude bone marrow infiltration and disease

Table 8.29 *Main types of anaemia*

Type of anaemia	Examples	Comments
Microcytic hypochromic	Iron deficiency	Blood loss (e.g. from menstruation or occult – gastrointestinal or genitourinary – sources)
	Thalassaemia	Malabsorption (post-gastrectomy)
Macrocytic	Vitamin B_{12} deficiency	Malabsorption (post-gastrectomy)
	Folate deficiency	
	Haemolysis	
	Hypothyroidism	
	Liver disease	
	Aplastic anaemia	
Normocytic anaemia	Chronic diseases	
	Renal failure	
	Haemolysis	
	Hypothyroidism	

azathioprine, cytosine or hydroxycarbamide). Macrocytic anaemia may also be caused by liver disease, myxoedema or, sometimes, aplastic anaemia.

Normocytic anaemia (MCV between 79 and 98 fl) may result from chronic diseases such as leukaemia, chronic inflammatory disease, liver disorders, renal failure, infection, malignancy and sickle cell disease.

Haematinic deficiency states must be corrected with iron, folic acid and/or vitamin B_{12} supplements. If the onset of anaemia has been rapid, blood transfusion may be indicated so as to prevent worsening of

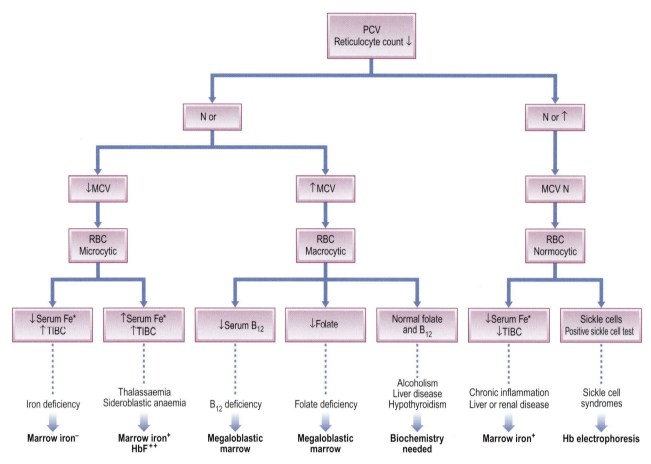

Fig. 8.23 Laboratory investigations for the cause of anaemia. HbF = fetal haemoglobin; MCV = mean cell volume; N = normal; PCV = packed cell volume; RBC = red blood cell; TIBC = total iron-binding capacity; *Fe = ferritin.

ischaemic symptoms. In end-stage renal failure, the hormone erythropoietin may be administered regularly to encourage haemopoiesis.

Automated examination of blood provides a quick and reliable Hb estimation and count of all the blood cells. It also shows important cytological features of red cells, such as red cell distribution width (RDW), MCV and Hb content. The laboratory investigation of the common anaemias is summarized in Figure 8.23. A blood film may also be required, especially as a mixed macro- and microcytic picture may sometimes not be revealed by an automated counter (a mix of large and small cells may produce an average within the normal range) and other abnormalities may be seen. For this purpose, a sample of EDTA-anticoagulated blood should be sent, with as much clinical information as possible, to the haematologist. The terminology used to describe examination of a stained blood film is shown in Figure 8.24.

Special investigations are discussed under the specific diseases.

Hb can be replaced by blood transfusions, haematinics or occasionally the hormone erythropoietin to encourage natural haemopoiesis. It is better to treat with haematinics such as iron or folic acid. Blood transfusions should be used only when absolutely necessary, if the Hb concentration has fallen below 7 g/dL, since they may carry the risk of infection, circulatory overload and allergic reactions. Erythropoietin is mainly used in the treatment of anaemia of chronic renal failure or cytotoxic therapy.

Dental aspects

LA is usually satisfactory for pain control. CS may be given only if there is supplemental oxygen. Deeper levels of sedation are more likely to lead to hypoxia. Nitrous oxide is theoretically contraindicated

in vitamin B$_{12}$ deficiency (see later). When GA is given, it is vital to ensure full oxygenation. Nevertheless, the myocardium may be unable to respond to the demands of anaesthesia. Whenever possible, therefore, the anaemia should be corrected preoperatively and the Hb level must be raised, if necessary by transfusion. Anaemia of sickle cell disease can make GA especially hazardous (see later). Elective operations under GA should not usually be carried out when the Hb is less than 10 g/dL (male). In an emergency, anaemia can be corrected by whole blood transfusion, but this should only be given to a young and otherwise fit patient. Packed red cells avoid the risk of fluid overload and can be given in an emergency to older patients or those with incipient congestive cardiac failure. A diuretic given at the same time further reduces the risk of congestive cardiac failure. The patient should be stabilized at least 24 hours preoperatively and it should be noted that Hb estimations are unreliable for 12 hours post-transfusion or after acute blood loss.

Some anaemias can also cause oral lesions, such as ulcers, glossitis or angular stomatitis (Fig. 8.25).

DEFICIENCY ANAEMIAS

Iron-deficiency anaemia

General aspects

Dietary iron is found mainly as iron salts, partly as haem from the myoglobin and Hb in meat. Dietary iron exists as haem iron only in animal tissues; in plant foods it is present as non-haem iron, which is less easily absorbed. In a mixed omnivorous diet, around 25% of dietary iron is non-haem iron. The amount of iron absorbed from

Red cell abnormalities		Causes	Red cell abnormalities		Causes
⊙	Microcyte	Iron deficiency, haemoglobinopathy	◯	Spherocyte	Hereditary spherocytosis, autoimmune haemolytic anaemia, septicaemia
◯	Macrocyte	Liver disease, alcoholism, megaloblastic anaemia	◳	Fragments	DIC, microangiopathy, HUS, TTP, burns, prosthetic valves
◎	Target cell	Iron deficiency, liver disease, haemoglobinopathies, post-splenectomy	◺	Elliptocyte	Hereditary elliptocytosis
◗	Stomatocyte	Liver disease, alcoholism	◌	Tear drop poikilocyte	Myelofibrosis, extramedullary haemopoiesis
╲	Pencil cell	Iron deficiency	◔	Basket cell	Oxidant damage, e.g. G6PD deficiency, unstable haemoglobin
✶	Ecchinocyte	Liver disease, post-splenectomy	◉	Howell-Jolly body	Hyposplenism, post-splenectomy
✺	Acanthocyte	Liver disease, abetalipoproteinaemia, renal failure	⁙	Basophilic stippling	Haemoglobinopathy, lead poisoning, myelodysplasia, haemolytic anaemia
☾	Sickle cell	Sickle cell anaemia	⁖	Siderotic granules (Pappenheimer bodies)	Disordered iron metabolism, e.g. sideroblastic anaemia, post-splenectomy

Fig. 8.24 Red cell morphological changes. DIC = disseminated intravascular coagulation; G6PD = glucose-6-phosphate dehydrogenase; HUS = haemolytic–uraemic syndrome; TTP = thrombotic thrombocytopenic purpura.

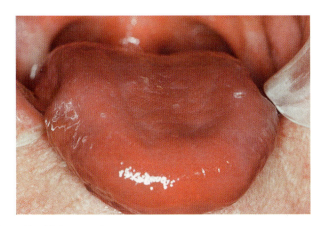

Fig. 8.25 Glossitis in anaemia.

various foods ranges from around 1–10% from plant foods to 10–20% from animal foods. Fibre, phytates, oxalates and phosphates present in plant foods, and tannin in tea, can inhibit iron absorption. Foods rich in vitamin C, including citrus fruits, green peppers and fresh leafy green vegetables, promote absorption of non-haem iron. Citric acid, sugars, amino acids and alcohol, as well as meat, poultry, fish and orange juice, also promote intestinal absorption of iron. Good sources of iron for vegetarians include wholegrain cereals and flours, leafy green vegetables, pulses such as lentils and kidney beans, and some dried fruits. Gastric acid is needed for the adequate conversion of iron salts from ferric to ferrous forms for their absorption from the proximal small intestine. Iron is stored in the bone marrow as haemosiderin.

The remainder is stored in the liver and spleen, and a small amount is present as myoglobin, which acts as an oxygen store in muscle tissue. Iron is required for synthesis of haem, respiratory cytochromes and myeloperoxidase. It also plays a vital role in many metabolic reactions (Fig. 8.26).

The most common causes of anaemia in developed countries are iron deficiency as a result of nutritional deficiencies or chronic blood loss, while in developing countries, malaria and chronic blood loss (Fig. 8.27) are the most frequent.

Excessive chronic menstrual or gastrointestinal blood loss is the main cause – women of childbearing age and older are mainly affected. About 5% of American women may have mild iron-deficiency anaemia and up to 25% may have low iron levels without anaemia. Neonates maintained on a milk diet may become iron-deficient. Very many older children are mildly iron-deficient because of the high demands for growth, especially during adolescence. By contrast, iron deficiency in an adult male almost invariably indicates blood loss, usually from the gastrointestinal or genitourinary tract. The same holds true for postmenopausal women.

Clinical features

The important features of iron-deficiency anaemia are summarized in Box 8.10. Impaired exercise capacity, koilonychia (Fig. 8.28) and beeturia (urine appearing red after eating beetroot) may be seen. In childhood, iron deficiency may also predispose to developmental or behavioural disorders. However, symptoms ascribed to iron deficiency do not always respond to iron replacement.

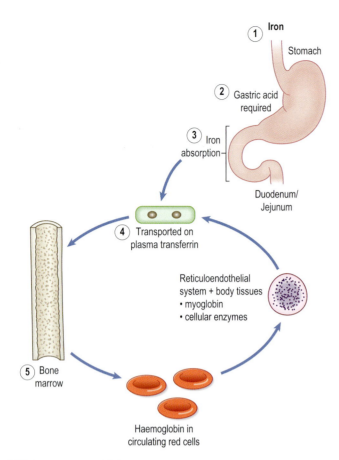

Fig. 8.26 Iron sources and fate.

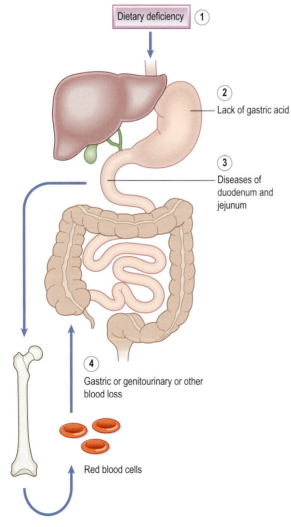

Fig. 8.27 Iron-deficiency anaemia.

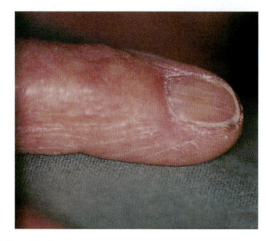

Fig. 8.28 Koilonychia.

Table 8.30 *Differential diagnosis of microcytosis*

Index	Iron deficiency	Heterozygous α- or β-thalassaemia trait	Lead poisoning
Haemoglobin	Low	Low	Normal[a]
Mean corpuscular (cell) volume (MCV)	Low	Low	Normal[a]
Red cell distribution width (RDW)	Raised	Normal	Normal
Free erythrocyte porphyrins (FEP)	Raised	Normal	Raised
Serum iron	Low	Normal	Normal
Total iron-binding capacity (TIBC)	Raised	Normal	Normal
Ferritin	Low	Normal	Normal

[a]May be low if the blood lead concentration is in excess of 100 mg/dL.

General management

Iron deficiency is the main cause of a microcytic anaemia (see Table 8.29). In the early stages, stainable iron is lost from the bone marrow (Table 8.30); deficiency only appears after stores are depleted. Erythrocyte size changes show as an abnormal RDW on automated red cell sizing, before the transport iron, serum iron and ferritin levels fall.

Falling serum ferritin levels are one of the most sensitive indices of iron deficiency, but this test is not universally available and the level rises in inflammation, as ferritin is an acute-phase protein. The serum iron-binding capacity rises and transferrin saturation (total iron-binding capacity/serum iron) falls; a value of less than 16% indicates iron deficiency. Declining erythrocyte size (microcytosis and a low MCV) follows, with rising red cell protoporphyrin concentrations. Later there is a fall in Hb and a hypochromic microcytic anaemia. Hypochromic microcytic anaemia with normal marrow iron stores is

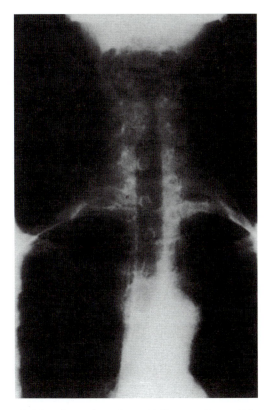

Fig. 8.29 Postcricoid carcinoma in patient with Paterson–Brown-Kelly. (Plummer–Vinson) syndrome.

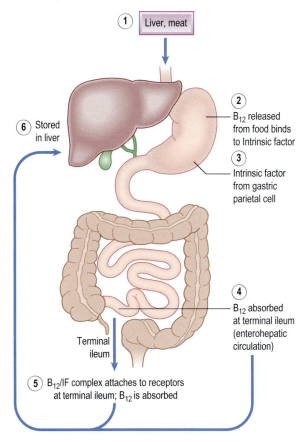

Fig. 8.30 Vitamin B_{12} sources and absorption.

not caused directly by iron deficiency but is a feature of thalassaemia and sideroblastic anaemia, as discussed later.

The cause of the iron deficiency must be sought and treated. The best treatment for iron deficiency is an iron salt such as ferrous sulfate 200 mg three times daily orally, which is better absorbed than ferric salts. Ferrous gluconate 250 mg/day can be given if ferrous sulfate is not tolerated. Nausea or constipation is fairly common. The stools are black whilst on oral iron therapy and this should not be mistaken for melaena. Oral iron may need to be given for 3 months or more after the Hb has reached normal levels, to replenish marrow iron stores. Parenteral iron does not raise the Hb level more rapidly than oral iron; it must be given intramuscularly and may cause reactions, including arrhythmias. Parenteral iron only has advantages when, for example, the patient cannot take iron by mouth or when inflammatory bowel disease is aggravated by oral iron.

Dental aspects

LA is satisfactory for pain control. CS can be given if full oxygenation is possible. For GA, see earlier.

A sore, physically normal tongue can develop before the Hb falls below the lower limit of normal. Atrophic glossitis – soreness of the tongue with depapillation or colour change – is the best-known effect of severe anaemia. It is seen much less frequently than in the past. The Paterson–Brown-Kelly (Plummer–Vinson) syndrome of glossitis and dysphagia with hypochromic (iron-deficiency) anaemia is uncommon. Women are mainly affected and the prevalence appears to be highest in northern Europe. There is a substantial risk of carcinoma in the postcricoid region or in the mouth (Fig. 8.29). Candidosis can be aggravated or precipitated by anaemia and may be the presenting feature. Angular stomatitis is a well-known sign of iron-deficiency anaemia but affects only a minority. Nowadays, it is more frequently caused by infection, mainly by *Candida albicans*, which may be promoted by the

anaemia itself. Occasionally, adequate treatment of anaemia alone, without antifungal treatment, relieves the infection. The majority of patients with chronic mucocutaneous candidosis, particularly the familial and diffuse types, are also iron-deficient and treatment with iron appears to improve the response to antifungal treatment.

Aphthous-like ulceration is sometimes associated with iron deficiency, which, if remedied, can sometimes bring about a cure. Deficiencies should be suspected, especially in patients of middle age or over who develop ulcers.

Staining of the teeth by iron can be prevented in children by using sodium iron edetate as the iron source, as it is also sugar-free and more palatable than ferrous sulfate. Some iron preparations can cause tooth erosion, as can chewable vitamin C.

Vitamin B_{12} (cobalamin) deficiency

General aspects

Vitamin B_{12} is needed by the body to synthesize and break down amino acids, and to synthesize deoxyribonucleic acid/ribonucleic acid (DNA/RNA). This is needed to build new cells, especially blood, skin and mucosal cells. Vitamin B_{12} is found in the diet in meat, especially liver.

Vitamin B_{12} is bound to gastric intrinsic factor secreted by parietal cells, and absorbed via the 'cubam receptor' in the terminal ileum. It is stored in the liver (Fig. 8.30). Vitamin B_{12} is a cofactor for only two enzymes – methionine synthase and l-methylmalonyl–coenzyme A mutase – and is necessary for development and myelination of the central nervous system (CNS), as well as for the maintenance of its normal function.

Deficiency of vitamin B_{12} is usually due to a defect in intrinsic factor (as a result of pernicious anaemia or gastrectomy), occasionally ileal disease or resection, or rarely a congenital ileal absorption defect, a

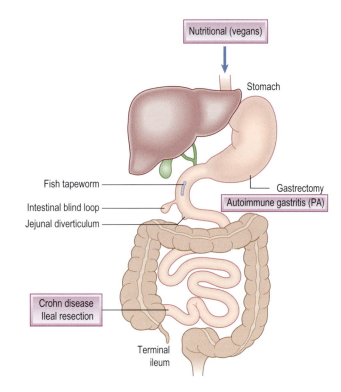

Fig. 8.31 Vitamin B$_{12}$ deficiency. PA = pernicious anaemia.

vegan diet or drugs (Box 8.11 and Fig. 8.31). Nitrous oxide can also interfere with vitamin B$_{12}$ metabolism and with neurological function if administration continues for 12 hours or more, or if it is used as a drug of abuse.

Lack of vitamin B$_{12}$ leads to accumulation of homocysteine (with a possible risk of cardiovascular disease) and methylmalonic acid. Pernicious (Addisonian) anaemia, the most common type of macrocytic anaemia, is caused by a specific defect of absorption of vitamin B$_{12}$, and is due to autoantibodies against gastric parietal cells and/or the intrinsic factor directed against the gastric hydrogen/potassium–adenosine triphosphatase (H/K–ATPase), which accounts for an associated achlorhydria. The underlying lesion is an atrophic gastritis causing failure of production of intrinsic factor by parietal cells and of gastric acid. There may be gastrointestinal symptoms and also a greater risk of stomach cancer. Ultimately, there is macrocytic (megaloblastic) anaemia with depressed production of all blood cells. Pernicious anaemia typically affects women in middle age or over, particularly those of northern European or African descent. It is sometimes seen with other autoimmune diseases, especially hypothyroidism, or less often as a feature of the autoimmune polyendocrinopathy syndrome (Ch. 6). Pernicious anaemia affects around 1 in 1000 of the northern European population and about 1% of females over age 70.

Clinical features

Deficiency of vitamin B$_{12}$ develops slowly since liver stores last up to 3 years. In addition to the usual signs and symptoms of anaemia, neurological symptoms – particularly paraesthesiae of the extremities – develop in about 10%. Early signs include loss of toe positional sense and diminished perception of the vibration of a tuning fork. These early neurological changes are reversible with treatment.

In the USA, 5% of persons over 50 appear to have low serum vitamin B$_{12}$ levels. Neurological damage can precede anaemia or even macrocytosis, and lead to subacute combined degeneration of the spinal cord and, ultimately, paraplegia. Absence of macrocytosis is occasionally due to concomitant iron deficiency, but in another study on 70 patients with very low (less than 100 ng/L) serum vitamin B$_{12}$ levels, anaemia was absent in 19% and macrocytosis was absent in 33%. In some of these cases, vitamin B$_{12}$ deficiency was manifested first as cerebral abnormalities and what has been termed 'megaloblastic madness'.

Premature greying of the hair is another well-recognized feature. Less common conditions associated with vitamin B$_{12}$ deficiency include malabsorption, infertility and thromboses (attributed to the marked hyperhomocysteinemia seen in severe vitamin B$_{12}$ deficiency).

General management

The diagnosis of B$_{12}$ deficiency depends on the clinical findings and low serum B$_{12}$ levels, together with autoantibodies against gastric parietal cells and/or intrinsic factor. If the patient consumes adequate vitamin B$_{12}$ but has clinically confirmed B$_{12}$ deficiency, malabsorption must be present. The Schilling test for impaired vitamin B$_{12}$ absorption is obsolete. Measurement of the raised serum levels of methylmalonic acid and homocysteine seen in B$_{12}$ deficiency appears to be more sensitive and specific for deficiency than assay of serum vitamin B$_{12}$ itself, though renal and other disorders may confuse the interpretation.

Most patients with vitamin B$_{12}$ deficiency have malabsorption and will require parenteral or high-dose oral replacement. Pernicious anaemia is treated for life with intramuscular hydroxycobalamin 1 mg five times at 3-day intervals to replete liver stores, and then at about 3-monthly intervals.

Dental aspects

LA is satisfactory. CS can be given if the Hb level is only moderately depressed and supplemental oxygen can be given. Nitrous oxide is (theoretically) contraindicated. GA should be postponed until low Hb has been remedied.

A physically normal but sore or burning tongue can be caused by early vitamin B$_{12}$ deficiency, often with normal Hb levels. It is important for these patients to undergo haematological examination. As

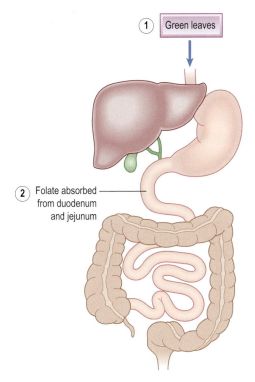

Fig. 8.32 Folate source and absorption.

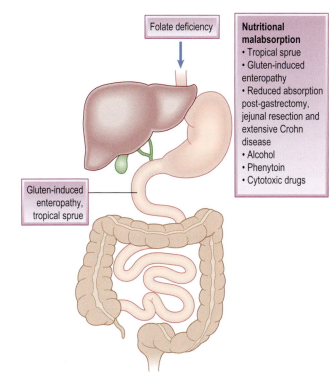

Fig. 8.33 Folate deficiency.

discussed earlier, anaemia or macrocytosis may be absent at this point. It can also, at this early stage, occasionally be associated with neurological disorders. In early B$_{12}$ deficiency, the tongue, rather than being sore, may show a pattern of red lines without depapillation; alternatively, red sore patches may form. These may come and go, and range from pinhead red spots to circular areas up to a centimetre across, which may resemble erythroplasia clinically; though they resolve with treatment of the anaemia, they may show dysplasia histologically.

Paterson–Brown-Kelly syndrome is rarely associated with a macrocytic anaemia.

Candidosis can be aggravated or precipitated by anaemia and may be the presenting feature. Angular stomatitis is uncommon. Aphthous stomatitis is occasionally the presenting feature and pernicious anaemia should be considered when ulceration starts in middle age or later.

Folate (folic acid) deficiency

General aspects

Folic acid is needed by the body to synthesize and break down amino acids, and to synthesize DNA/RNA, needed to build new cells, especially blood, skin and mucosal cells. Folic acid is found in fresh leafy and other vegetables, especially spinach, kale, Brussels sprouts and asparagus. Folic acid is absorbed from the proximal small intestine (Fig. 8.32). There are virtually no body stores of folic acid. Most folic acid deficiency is caused by dietary deficiency (Fig. 8.33). Some is caused by disease of the small intestine, such as coeliac disease, or drugs (Box 8.12), but occasionally no cause can be discovered.

Clinical features

The effects of folate deficiency are very similar to B$_{12}$ deficiency. Both cause megaloblastic changes in the marrow and macrocytic anaemia, defective DNA synthesis and impaired production of blood cells and, ultimately, of many other cells.

Box 8.12 *Causes of folate deficiency*

Poor intake

- Poverty
- Dietary ignorance
- Old age
- Alcoholism

Malabsorption

- Coeliac disease
- Crohn disease
- Other malabsorption states

Increased demands

- Infancy
- Pregnancy
- Chronic haemolysis (haemolytic anaemia)
- Malignant disease
- Exfoliative skin lesions
- Chronic dialysis

Drugs

- Alcohol
- Azathioprine
- Barbiturates
- Co-trimoxazole
- Methotrexate
- Oral contraceptives
- Pentamidine
- Phenytoin
- Primidone
- Pyrimethamine
- Sulfasalazine
- Triamterene
- Zidovudine

Folate deficiency in adults leads to anaemia. Folic acid deficiency in pregnancy appears to predispose to neural tube defects or cleft lip–palate in the fetus. Folic acid prophylaxis is thus recommended. Folate deficiency in adults does not lead to subacute combined degeneration of the cord, but does predispose to raised homocysteine levels and possibly ischaemic heart disease.

General management

The red-cell folate levels are low and serum B_{12} normal. Red-cell folate levels, when low, are unequivocal evidence of folate deficiency but may remain normal for a time in a few folate-deficient patients until older erythrocytes are replaced. Serum folate assays are considerably less reliable.

Once the cause has been found and rectified, treatment with folic acid (5 mg daily by mouth) rapidly restores the normal blood picture. Treatment is usually given for at least 4 months.

Dental aspects

LA, CS and GA considerations apply as for pernicious anaemia, but there is no contraindication to nitrous oxide.

Soreness of the tongue without depapillation or colour change can be caused by early deficiencies, often with normal Hb levels.

Atrophic glossitis is the best-known effect of severe anaemia but is much less frequently seen than in the past. Angular stomatitis is also a well-known sign but affects only a minority. Aphthous stomatitis is sometimes associated and, if remedied, can sometimes bring about a cure.

HAEMOLYTIC ANAEMIAS

General aspects

Haemolytic anaemia may result from: inherited abnormalities of Hb formation (the haemoglobinopathies); inherited abnormalities of erythrocyte structure or function (spherocytosis; glucose-6-phosphate dehydrogenase [G6PD] deficiency); or from damage to erythrocytes (autoimmune, drug-induced or infective). Worldwide, malaria is the most common cause.

Clinical features

Accelerated erythrocyte destruction leads to bilirubin overproduction and sometimes jaundice. The spleen may enlarge and increased red cell turnover raises the reticulocyte count and plasma lactate dehydrogenase (LDH), bilirubin and uric acid levels. This raises the demand for folic acid and may in turn cause macrocytic changes.

General management

The cause should be treated if possible. Folic acid may be required and, in some instances, blood transfusion, but this carries the possibility of iron overload.

Dental aspects

LA is the safest method of pain control. CS may be given, with supplemental oxygen if necessary. Any of the haemolytic anaemias may be a contraindication to GA but, in practical terms, sickle cell disease is by far the most important cause of difficulties in dental management.

Haemoglobinopathies

The fetus is normally born with fetal haemoglobin (HbF) as the main haemoglobin and, in infancy, this is replaced with adult haemoglobin (HbA) and a small amount of HbA_2. These haemoglobins differ in their peptide chain composition (Table 8.31).

Haemoglobinopathies are genetically determined disorders of Hb production. Each of the Hb peptide (globin) chains has a unique amino acid sequence, which can be altered as a result of DNA mutations. Qualitative defects in the production of Hb then lead to 'variant haemoglobins'. Quantitative defects in the production of globins lead to the thalassaemias.

Haemoglobinopathies are seen mostly in non-Caucasians. Sickling disorders are common in Afro-Caribbean, Mediterranean, Middle Eastern, Indian, Bangladeshi and Pakistani patients (Fig. 8.34). In the UK, about 1 in 10 Afro-Caribbeans and 1 in 100 Cypriots and Asians carry the sickle cell trait. Thalassaemias and G6PD deficiency are seen mainly in Mediterranean, Vietnamese, Cambodian, Laotian

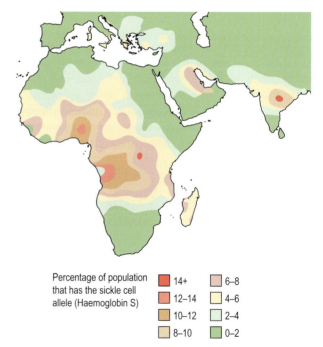

Percentage of population that has the sickle cell allele (Haemoglobin S)

- 14+
- 12–14
- 10–12
- 8–10
- 6–8
- 4–6
- 2–4
- 0–2

Fig. 8.34 Distribution of sickling.

Table 8.31 *Laboratory findings during development of iron-deficiency anaemia*

	Mean corpuscular (cell) volume (MCV)	Haemoglobin (Hb)	Mean corpuscular (cell) Hb concentration (MCHC)	Serum ferritin	Transferrin saturation[a]	Marrow iron stores
Normal	N	N	N	N	33%	N
Mild anaemia	↓	N or ↓	N	↓	<16%, <33%	↓
Moderate anaemia	↓	↓	↓	↓	<16%	↓
Severe anaemia	↓↓	↓↓	↓↓	↓↓	<16%	↓↓

N= normal.
[a]It is better to measure ferritin.

and Chinese peoples. In the UK, about 1 in 10 from the Indian subcontinent, about 1 in 30 Chinese and 1 in 50 Afro-Caribbeans have thalassaemia.

Haemoglobinopathies result in consequences ranging from significant morbidity and mortality in sickle cell disease, to no significant clinical effect as in haemoglobin E disease. Patients may have combinations of more than one haemoglobinopathy. Short stature, abnormal skeletal development and jaundice are often found, in addition to signs and symptoms of anaemia.

The diagnosis of haemoglobinopathy rests on the history, examination and laboratory investigations. A family history is especially important. A full blood picture and red cell indices should be obtained and blood should also be sent for electrophoresis (4 mL of EDTA-anticoagulated blood) and for assay of variant haemoglobins. Special tests, such as the Sickledex, may also be useful (see later).

The sickling disorders

General aspects

Amino acid substitution in the Hb globin chain results in changes in haemoglobin (HbS), which assumes a propensity to polymerize or precipitate, causing gross distortions in the shape of erythrocytes, with impaired deformability and membrane damage. The erythrocytes cause vascular occlusions in the microcirculation. Integrins on the erythrocyte surface bind to vascular endothelial adhesion molecules, which are upregulated by tumour necrosis factor (TNF) and other pro-inflammatory cytokines; thus obstruction is more common during infections.

The sickling disorders include the sickle cell anaemia or disease, and sickle cell trait (Table 8.32 and 8.33). Inheritance in the sickling disorders is autosomal. Sickling disorders mainly affect people of African heritage. In West Africa about 2% of the population have sickle cell disease and up to 30% have the trait. Sickle cell trait is many times more common than sickle cell anaemia in Britain and affects some 10% of people of Afro-Caribbean descent, and 20% of African descent.

Sickle cell *anaemia or disease* (HbSS is present in erythrocytes) is homozygous and is usually a serious disease with widespread complications (Box 8.13; Fig. 8.35). It frequently becomes apparent in about the third month of life.

Sickle cell *trait* (HbSA is present) is heterozygous and at least ten times as common. Sickle cell trait is frequently asymptomatic, but

sickle cell crises can be caused by low O_2 tension (see later; GA, high altitudes or unpressurized aircraft). At times, such patients may have renal complications causing haematuria or splenic infarcts. Sickle cell trait may be associated with another haemoglobinopathy.

Clinical features

Sickle cell disease presents six main clinical problems, as listed below.

Painful crises, which are usually due to infarction as a result of sickling, are brought on by infection, dehydration, hypoxia, acidosis or cold, and cause severe pain and pyrexia. Infarcts form mainly in the spleen (with eventual autosplenectomy), bones and joints, brain, kidneys, lungs, retinae and skin. Bone infarcts can cause inflammation and pain, especially in the hands and feet. Pulmonary infarcts cause chest pain and eventually lead to pulmonary hypertension and right-sided cardiac failure. The kidneys may also be affected, causing haematuria and a nephrotic syndrome. Ocular defects or cerebrovascular

---

Box 8.13 *Features of sickle cell anaemia*

- Anaemia
- Crises
  - Painful crises
  - Aplastic crises
  - Dactylitis – painful osteitis in the hands (Fig. 8.35)
  - Infarcts of central nervous system, lungs, kidney, spleen, bone
  - Skin ulcers
- Haemolysis
  - Jaundice
  - Gallstones
  - Reticulocytosis
- Impaired growth
- Skeletal deformities
- Susceptibility to infections

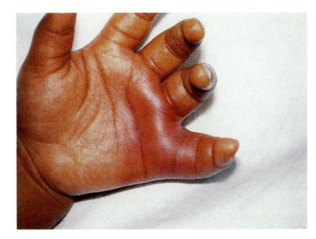

Fig. 8.35 Dactylitis showing painful red swellings.

Table 8.32 *Normal haemoglobins*

Haemoglobin	Alpha chain	Beta chain	Gamma chain	Delta chain
Fetal HbF	2		2	
Adult HbA	2	2		
HbA$_2$	2			2

Table 8.33 *The sickling disorders*

Disorder	Hb type	Origins of predominant ethnic groups affected	Clinical features
Sickle cell anaemia	SS	Africa, West Indies, Mediterranean, India	Severe anaemia
Sickle cell trait	SA	Africa, West Indies, Mediterranean, India	Usually asymptomatic
Sickle cell – HbC disease	SC	West Africa, South-East Asia	Variable anaemia
Sickle cell – HbD disease	SD	Africa, India, Pakistan	Moderately severe anaemia
Sickle cell – HbE disease	SE	South-East Asia	Moderately severe anaemia
Sickle cell – thalassaemia	SAF	Mediterranean, Africa, West Indies	Moderately severe anaemia

accidents – often with hemiplegia – are possible. Priapism is a sustained painful erection due to infarction in the corpora cavernosa. Abdominal crises may mimic a surgical emergency.

Haematological crises are caused by parvovirus infection and can be haemolytic, aplastic or related to sequestration.

Chronic anaemia may feature an Hb level that is often as low as 5–9 g/dL.

Chronic hyperbilirubinaemia predisposes to bile pigment gallstones.

Infections, particularly by pneumococci, meningococci, *Haemophilus* and salmonellae, represent the main cause of death in sickle cell disease. An immune defect results from splenic infarction and dysfunction. Most patients are kept on prophylactic phenoxymethyl penicillin.

Sequestration syndromes include sequestration of sickle cells in:

- the lungs, impeding gas exchange (chest syndrome)
- the spleen (septicaemia may result)
- the liver ('girdle syndrome'; may be associated with bowel dilatation).

Morbidity and early mortality rates are high in sickle cell disease. Most patients eventually succumb to cardiac failure, renal failure, overwhelming infection or stroke.

General management

Sickling disorders should be suspected in those with a positive family history and in any patient of African, West Indian or (less frequently) Asian or Mediterranean descent. Many already carry warning cards (Fig. 8.36).

In sickle cell *disease*, the Hb level is typically below 9 g/dL. Target cells, reticulocytosis of 5–25%, and sometimes sickled erythrocytes may be seen in a stained blood film. Hb electrophoresis shows mainly HbS and up to 15% HbF, but no HbA.

In sickle cell *trait*, haematological findings are often normal. Electrophoresis shows 40% HbS and up to 60% HbA.

Sickling may be demonstrated both in sickle cell *disease* and in *trait*, by tests relying on the low solubility of HbS (Sickledex; Fig. 8.37) or by the addition of a reducing agent (such as 10% sodium metabisulfite or dithionite) to a blood sample.

Patients with sickle cell *disease* need regular blood pictures, a comprehensive care programme, regular folic acid, and sometimes blood transfusions for cerebrovascular symptoms in early childhood or recurrent pulmonary thromboses. However, many patients retain moderate degrees of anaemia for most of their lives. Transfusions can and should usually be minimized, especially because of the risk of hepatitis virus and HIV infection. A growing number of patients with sickle cell disease survive into late middle age. Infections and thromboses are the main causes of death.

The main principles in patients with sickle cell *disease* are to prevent trauma, infection, hypoxia, acidosis or dehydration, all of which can precipitate a crisis. Infections must be treated early. Painful crises should be treated promptly with analgesics, such as diamorphine or pethidine, and hydration. Patients with sickle cell anaemia are treated with hydroxycarbamide (hydroxyurea), which raises the levels of HbF and iron-chelating agents (desferrioxamine, deferasirox or deferiprone).

Patients with sickle cell *trait* are less liable to complications from trauma, infection, hypoxia, acidosis or dehydration, but if severe, these can precipitate a crisis.

Dental aspects

All those at risk from sickling disorders should be investigated if GA is to be given. Sickle cell anaemia is probable if the Hb is less than 11 g/dL, and presents a hazard for GA. If the sickle cell test is positive, Hb electrophoresis is required to confirm the diagnosis.

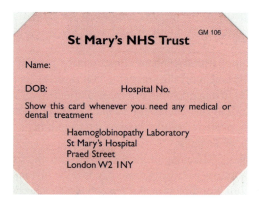

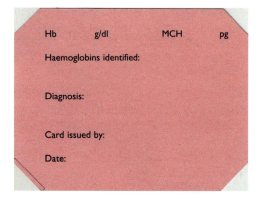

Fig. 8.36 Haemoglobinopathy card.

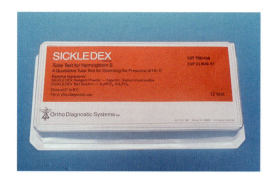

Fig. 8.37 Sickledex test.

Patients with sickle cell *trait* (HbSA) present few problems in management but, if GA is necessary, full oxygenation must be maintained.

For patients with sickle cell *disease* (HbSS), LA is the preferred mode of pain control. It may be preferable to avoid prilocaine, which may, in overdose, cause methaemoglobinaemia. Aspirin is best avoided as, in large doses, it may cause acidosis and precipitate a crisis; paracetamol (acetaminophen) and codeine are effective alternatives. CS with relative analgesia can be used safely. At least 30% O_2 is needed and, provided that there is no respiratory depression or obstruction, normal procedures can be used. Benzodiazepines are best avoided.

Elective surgery should be carried out in hospital and during a phase when haemolysis is minimal. Anaemia should be corrected before GA, and the Hb brought up to at least 10 g/dL. Exchange transfusion is occasionally required for major surgery but only in selected patients. It carries the risk of red cell alloimmunization in up to 20%. Blood should be available for transfusion. If a crisis develops, O2 is given and bicarbonate infused. A packed red cell transfusion may be required if the Hb falls below 50%.

Prophylactic antimicrobials (penicillin V or clindamycin) should be given for surgical procedures and infections must be treated vigorously, since the patient may be immunocompromised if the spleen is non-functional. As a consequence of multiple transfusions, some patients have become infected with blood-borne viruses. Drugs that can cause respiratory depression, including sedative agents, should not be given. Acidosis and hypotension must also be avoided.

Orofacial manifestations of sickle cell disease include painful infarcts in the jaws (which may be mistaken for toothache) or osteomyelitis. Pulpal symptoms are common in the absence of any obvious dental disease and pulpal necrosis has sometimes resulted. Lesions suggestive of bone infarction (dense radio-opacities) may be seen in the jaws and/or skull. Bone scans using technetium diphosphonate show stronger uptake in these areas. Radiographic findings include a 'stepladder' trabeculae pattern. Some patients have such severe pain during crises that they abuse analgesics and become addicts (Ch. 34). Hypercementosis may be seen. Bone marrow hyperplasia leads to an enlarged haemopoietic maxilla with excessive overjet, and overbite. Skeletal but not dental maturation is delayed. The skull is thickened but osteoporotic with a hair-on-end pattern to the trabeculae. The diploë are thickened, especially in the parietal regions, giving a tower skull appearance. Enamel hypomineralization and calcified pulp canals may be seen. The lamina dura is distinct and dense, and the permanent teeth may be hypomineralized, though neither caries nor periodontal disease is more severe.

The thalassaemias

Thalassaemias are autosomally dominant inherited disorders in which either alpha- or beta-globin chains are synthesized at a low rate, thereby lessening the production of HbA. The unaffected chains are produced in excess and precipitate within the erythrocytes to cause excessive erythrocyte fragility and haemolysis. Thalassaemias are characterized by a hypochromic microcytic anaemia, and are predominantly found in persons of Mediterranean, Middle Eastern or Asian descent. They may be severe (major; homozygous) or mild (minor; heterozygous), and may affect alpha-chain (alpha-thalassaemias) or beta-chain (beta-thalassaemias) production.

Alpha-thalassaemias

Alpha-thalassaemias result from deficient synthesis of alpha chains and are mainly found in Asians. There are four main subtypes, of varying degrees of severity. In alpha-thalassaemia major, there is no compensatory mechanism for the loss in alpha-chain production, so tetramers of the beta and gamma chains combine to form, respectively, HbH and Barts, both of which are ineffective O_2 carriers. Thus the condition is lethal *in utero* or infancy.

Beta-thalassaemias

General aspects Beta-thalassaemias (Mediterranean anaemia) result from the depressed production of beta chains. They mainly affect peoples from the Mediterranean littoral, Afro-Caribbeans, South-East Asians and Africans. In the homozygous form, they can be life-threatening. A relative increase in delta and gamma chains is associated with raised levels of HbA_2 and HbF. Homozygous beta-thalassaemia (Cooley anaemia; thalassaemia major) is characterized by failure to thrive, increasingly severe anaemia, hepatosplenomegaly and skeletal abnormalities. Heterozygotes for beta-thalassaemia may be asymptomatic.

Clinical features Homozygotes for thalassaemia suffer from chronic anaemia, marrow hyperplasia, skeletal deformities, splenomegaly, cirrhosis, gallstones and iron overload. There is no pubertal growth spurt. Affected children are susceptible to folate deficiency (as in other chronic haemolytic states) and also to infection.

Patients with homozygous beta-thalassaemia become overloaded with iron (haemosiderosis) from high gut absorption and from repeated transfusions. The iron damages the heart (cardiac haemosiderosis), causing cardiomyopathy and arrhythmias, which often result in death in early adult life. Iron deposits lead to liver and pancreas dysfunction, and deposits in salivary glands can cause a sicca syndrome. Some patients survive, probably because they have a milder variant, such as beta-thalassaemia with high levels of HbF.

Heterozygous beta-thalassaemia (thalassaemia minor or thalassaemia trait) is common and usually asymptomatic, except for mild hypochromic anaemia. Anaemia may be aggravated by pregnancy or intercurrent illness.

General management Diagnosis of beta-thalassaemia is confirmed by finding severe microcytic hypochromic anaemia with gross aniso- and poikilocytosis, target cells and basophilic stippling of erythrocytes, normal or raised serum iron and ferritin, and normal TIBC. There is a great increase in HbF and some increase in HbA_2.

The main treatment measures in beta-thalassaemia are blood transfusions, folic acid supplements and iron-chelating agents (desferrioxamine, deferasirox or deferiprone) and ascorbic acid. Hydroxycarbamide is now used but the side-effects can be a significant disadvantage. Splenectomy may be required if there is hypersplenism causing greater blood destruction, which leads to accumulation of iron elsewhere and other complications.

Dental aspects of thalassaemia

Hepatitis B or C, or HIV carriage, may be a complication in repeatedly transfused patients. Since splenectomy results in an immune defect, it may be prudent to cover surgical procedures with prophylactic antimicrobials.

LA is safe. CS may be given with oxygen levels not less than 30%. GA induction may be complicated by enlargement of the maxilla, which may cause difficulties in intubation, but in any event, the chronic severe anaemia and often cardiomyopathy are contraindications.

Orofacial manifestations include expansion of the diploë of the skull, causing a hair-on-end appearance that is frequently conspicuous on lateral skull radiographs. Enlargement of the maxilla is caused by bone marrow expansion (chipmunk facies); there is often spacing of the teeth and forward drift of the maxillary incisors, so that orthodontic treatment may be indicated. Alveolar bone rarefaction produces a chicken-wire appearance on radiography. Pneumatization of the sinuses may be delayed. Less common oral complications include painful swelling of the parotids and hyposalivation caused by iron deposition, and a sore or burning tongue related to the folate deficiency.

Sickle cell trait with another haemoglobinopathy

Persons who have sickle cell trait with another haemoglobinopathy, such as thalassaemia, or both sickle cell haemoglobin S and C (SC disease) are usually not as ill as those with isolated sickle cell disease. However, they are at about the same level of risk from GA as are those with sickle cell disease. Patients with other combined defects should be managed in the same way as those with sickle trait alone.

Other haemoglobin variants

Other Hb variants that can lead to haemolytic anaemia, particularly when certain drugs are given, include Hb Zurich (which causes acute haemolytic reactions when sulphonamides are given) and HbH (a relatively common variant in the Far East, in which oxidants cause acute haemolysis in homozygotes, similar to that in G6PD deficiency). Various drugs may worsen haemolysis and the physician must be consulted.

Erythrocyte membrane defects

General and clinical aspects

Hereditary spherocytosis (acholuric jaundice) is the main form of congenital haemolytic anaemia in Caucasians. It is an autosomal dominant trait characterized by haemolytic anaemia, jaundice, spleno-megaly, gallstones, haemochromatosis and skin ulcers. Episodes of haemolysis may be precipitated by infections.

Hereditary elliptocytosis (*ovalocytosis*) and *hereditary stomatocytosis* are similar autosomal dominant disorders characterized by chronic haemolytic anaemia.

General management

Splenectomy and folic acid treatment are almost invariably required.

Dental aspects

LA is safe. CS or GA may be given if there is optimal oxygenation.

Erythrocyte metabolic defects

The most common disorder of this type is glucose-6-phosphate dehy-drogenase deficiency; various drugs are contraindicated (Table 8.34).

Acquired haemolytic anaemias

Haemolysis can be caused by gross trauma, complement-mediated lysis, drugs, toxins, malaria and other factors. These may occasionally have dental relevance because of anaemia, corticosteroid treatment or haemorrhagic tendencies.

Microangiopathic haemolytic anaemia (MAHA) is caused by fibrin strands depositing in small vessels and damaging erythrocytes in: pre-eclampsia; DIC; malignant hypertension; TTP – usually caused by a defect in breakdown of vWF; and HUS, which is usually caused by *E. coli* O157 verotoxin (Ch. 21) or a defect in factor H – the complement regulatory protein.

OTHER ANAEMIAS

Aplastic anaemia

General aspects

Aplastic anaemia is pancytopenia with a non-functioning bone mar-row. It is a rare disease causing leukopenia, thrombocytopenia and refractory anaemia.

Chemicals such as benzene, drugs, hepatitis viruses, irradiation and graft-versus-host disease (GVHD) are important causes (Box 8.14) but many cases are idiopathic, though probably immunologically mediated.

Clinical features

The clinical manifestations are those of anaemia (normochromic, normocytic or macrocytic), together with abnormal susceptibility to infection and bleeding. Purpura is often the first manifestation.

Table 8.34 *Drugs in glucose-6-phosphate dehydrogenase (G6PD) deficiency*

Contraindicated	Possible risk
Dapsone	Aspirin – although up to 1 g daily is usually harmless
Methylthioninium chloride (methylene blue)	Chloroquine, quinidine and quinine
Nitrofurantoin and quinolones, including ciprofloxacin, moxifloxacin, nalidixic acid, norfloxacin and ofloxacin	Vitamin K analogues (e.g. menadione and water-soluble derivatives like menadiol sodium phosphate)
Prilocaine	
Primaquine – although 30 mg weekly for 8 weeks has been found not to have harmful effects in African and Asian people	
Sulphonamides, including co-trimoxazole – although some sulphonamides like sulfadiazine are not haemolytic in many with G6PD deficiency	
Sulphonylureas	

Box 8.14 *Causes of aplastic anaemia*

- Genetic
  - Fanconi anaemia
  - Dyskeratosis congenita
- Immunological
  - Autoimmune
  - Graft-versus-host disease
- Drugs
  - Allopurinol
  - Anticonvulsants
  - Antithyroids
  - Chloramphenicol
  - Cytotoxic agents
  - Gold
  - Non-steroidal anti-inflammatory drugs (NSAIDs)
  - Penicillamine
  - Phenylbutazone
  - Sulphonamides
- Chemicals
  - Benzene
  - Glue-sniffing
  - Heavy metals
  - Toluene
- Viruses
  - Hepatitis
- Irradiation

General management

The principles of management include removal of the cause (even when this is discoverable, as in the case of drugs such as chloram-phenicol, marrow damage may still be irreversible); isolation and antibiotics to control infection; bone marrow transplantation (BMT; haemopoietic stem cell transplantation, HSCT [Ch. 35]) after intense immunosuppression (this in turn may cause GVHD, which is often fatal [Ch. 35]); androgenic (anabolic) steroids, which may be of some value (corticosteroids are of questionable benefit); and blood transfu-sion – but this carries risks from iron overload or infection.

The prognosis is poor and 50% of patients die within 6 months, usually from haemorrhage or infection. Iron overload may result from repeated blood transfusions.

Dental aspects

Treatment modification needs to take into consideration:

- anaemia
- haemorrhagic tendencies
- susceptibility to infections
- effects of corticosteroid therapy (Ch. 6)
- hepatitis B and other viral infections (Ch. 9).

LA is satisfactory. CS and GA should be avoided because of the anaemia.

Oral manifestations of aplastic anaemia, and management, are somewhat similar to those of leukaemia, i.e. ulceration, haemorrhagic tendencies and susceptibility to infections. Oral lichenoid lesions, or a Sjögren-like syndrome, may develop if there is GVHD following marrow transplantation to relieve the anaemia (see later and Ch. 35). Gingival swelling may develop if ciclosporin is used.

Fanconi anaemia

Fanconi anaemia is a rare autosomal dominant disorder with bone marrow failure, absent radii and predisposition to malignant disease, including oral cancer. Birth defects occur in up to 75% of Fanconi anaemia patients, and complications include haemorrhages, infections, leukaemia, myelodysplastic syndrome, liver tumours and other cancers.

Pure red-cell aplasia

Pure red-cell aplasia is a rare disease that may be congenital or acquired. The latter is often associated with a thymoma and sometimes with chronic mucocutaneous candidosis. These patients need regular blood transfusions and are therefore at risk from hepatitis viruses and HIV infection.

Anaemia caused by bone marrow infiltration

Bone marrow infiltration by abnormal cells (metastases, leukaemias, myeloma or myelofibrosis) causes normocytic anaemia and often leukopenia or thrombocytopenia with a leukoerythroblastic peripheral blood picture. There may be extramedullary haemopoiesis in other organs. Dental care may be complicated by susceptibility to infections, haemorrhage (as in aplastic anaemia) or the underlying disease.

Anaemias associated with chronic systemic diseases

Anaemia of various types may be associated with chronic systemic disorders, which include chronic inflammation (infections, or connective tissue disease such as rheumatoid arthritis); neoplasms, particularly leukaemia; liver disease (Ch. 9); uraemia (Ch. 12); HIV infection (Ch. 20); or, rarely, endocrinopathies (hypothyroidism, hypopituitarism or hypoadrenocorticism (Ch. 6).

LEUKOCYTES (WHITE BLOOD CELLS)

Several types of leukocytes (white blood cells) exist, all derived from a multipotent bone marrow stem cell. Leukocytes are important defence cells found throughout the body and discussed in Chapter 20.

LEUKOPENIA

See Chapter 20.

MALIGNANT DISEASE OF LEUKOCYTES

Malignant diseases involving lymphoid cells (lymphoreticular malignancies – leukaemias and lymphomas) are potentially fatal. Lymphoid tissue is widely spread throughout the body, and thus lymphoreticular malignances have wide effects.

In most forms of malignant disease, some form of staging is used to assist treatment planning and in making a possible prognosis. Staging aims to determine the spread of the malignant neoplasm from its original site. It is based on history, physical examination and investigations, such as blood tests, biopsies (e.g. of lesions, lymph nodes, bone marrow) and imaging – radiography, CT and MRI scans, or ultrasound.

Treatment of malignant disease can be with surgery, radiotherapy, cytotoxic drugs singly or in combination, stem cell transplantation, immunotherapy (monoclonal antibodies and, on the horizon, vaccines) and gene therapy.

Quality of life is as important as, or more important than, simply extension of survival.

LEUKAEMIAS

General aspects

Leukaemias are potentially fatal diseases in which there is neoplastic proliferation of bone marrow white blood stem cells associated with specific gene mutations, deletions or translocations. The aetiology is unknown in most cases but may include:

- a genetic predisposition (e.g. in Down syndrome)
- ionizing radiation
- chemicals (e.g. benzene or formaldehyde)
- chemotherapy (e.g. certain of the alkylating agents and topoisomerase inhibitors, used to treat cancers)
- viruses (e.g. human T-cell leukaemia virus 1 [HTLV-1] infection – linked to T-cell leukaemia)
- myelodysplastic syndromes (formerly called 'pre-leukaemia').

Leukaemias are classified by:

- cell of origin – lymphoblast or non-lymphoblast
- cell maturity – immature (acute) or mature (chronic).

This classification allows a patient's prognosis to be assessed and has implications for treatment.

Acute leukaemias are characterized by primitive blast cells in the blood and bone marrow, account for nearly 50% of all malignant disease in children and are the most common cause of non-accidental death. A total of 85% of leukaemia in children is acute lymphoblastic leukaemia.

Chronic leukaemias are characterized by an excess of mature leukocytes in blood and bone marrow, are mainly diseases of adult life, and are chronic disorders but may progress to acute leukaemia.

Clinical features

Many of the manifestations of leukaemias arise from the crowding-out of normal blood cells from the marrow by the leukaemic cells, leading to:

- anaemia (fatigue, pallor, etc.)
- thrombocytopenia (purpura and a bleeding tendency)

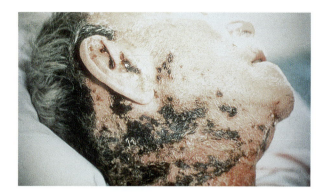

Fig. 8.38 Herpes zoster (shingles) of the upper cervical nerves in a patient dying from leukaemia.

Table 8.35 *Clinical features of leukaemia*

Site of disease	Clinical manifestation
Bone marrow failure	
Anaemia	Pallor, lethargy, dyspnoea
Neutropenia	Recurrent infection
Thrombocytopenia	Mucosal bleeding and bruising
Tissue infiltration	
Lymphatics	Lymphadenopathy
Liver and spleen	Hepatosplenomegaly
Mediastinum	Hilar lymphadenopathy
Gingiva and skin	Gingival and skin deposits
Meninges and brain	Meningitis-like syndrome
Bone	Bone pain and pathological fractures

- liability to infections (Fig. 8.38)
- lymphadenopathy, especially in lymphatic leukaemias.

The clinical features of leukaemia are variable but broadly reflect the degree of tissue infiltration by the leukaemic cells and the extent of bone marrow failure (Table 8.35).

Symptoms usually develop fairly quickly in acute leukaemias but gradually in chronic leukaemias (about 20% of people with chronic leukaemia do not have symptoms at the time of diagnosis). However, as leukaemic cells grow and eventually outnumber normal cells, the following events may occur:

- Leukocytes falter in combating infections. The leukaemic cells may also collect in certain parts of the body, such as the testicles, brain, lymph nodes, liver, spleen, digestive tract, kidneys, lungs, eyes and skin – in effect, virtually every tissue site – causing pain, swelling and other problems
- Erythrocytes are crowded out, producing anaemia
- Platelets are crowded out, producing a bleeding tendency.

The following symptoms may arise, many of which are non-specific and common to all leukaemias:

- Unexplained fevers
- Frequent infections
- Night sweats
- Fatigue and malaise
- Weight loss
- Easy bleeding and/or bruising
- Headaches
- Confusion
- Balance problems
- Blurred vision
- Painful lymph node swellings in the neck, axillae or groin
- Shortness of breath
- Nausea or vomiting
- Abdominal discomfort and/or swelling
- Testicular discomfort and/or swelling
- Pain in the bones or joints
- Weakness or loss of muscle control
- Seizures.

General management

The following investigations should be carried out:

- Blood tests: the leukocyte count is very high (although it is not uncommon for this to be normal in childhood acute lymphocytic leukaemia), whereas the platelet and erythrocyte counts are low

- Liver and kidney function tests
- Bone marrow biopsy: via an aspirate
- Lymph node excision
- Chest X-ray
- Genetic studies: help in classifying the various leukaemia types
- Lumbar puncture or spinal tap for the possible presence of leukaemic cells.

Staging

In general, in order to determine the most appropriate therapy, leukaemias are classified according to their genotypes rather than staged. Chronic myelocytic leukaemia is also classified by phase – chronic, accelerated and blast (or 'blast crisis') phases defined by the number of blasts (immature leukaemia cells) in the blood and bone marrow.

Treatment

Leukaemia treatment depends almost exclusively on the type. Modifying factors may be age, overall health, and prior therapy. General factors affecting outcomes include:

- age
- percentages of leukaemia cells in blood and bone marrow
- degree to which specific systems of the body are affected by leukaemia
- chromosome abnormalities in leukaemia cells.

Specific factors are associated with outcomes in each leukaemia type, and outlook is measured in terms of survival rates. The number of people who are still alive 5 years after treatment varies by type of leukaemia. After 5 years, more than 80% of patients without detectable disease are likely to maintain a lifelong remission. Patients in remission for longer than 15 years are considered unequivocal cures.

Leukaemia therapy includes measures to fight the cancer and treatments to relieve both the symptoms and the adverse effects of the treatment (supportive care).

Leukaemias vary in their response to treatment. In general:

- acute leukaemias respond well to treatment and can be cured. Others do not have such a positive outlook
- chronic leukaemias usually cannot be cured, but they can be controlled for long periods.

Chemotherapy

The most widely used antileukaemic treatment is chemotherapy; the goal is to cure the patient, meaning that blood tests and bone marrow biopsy show no evidence of leukaemia (i.e. a remission – no evidence of disease) and the leukaemia does not come back (relapse) over time. Only time can determine whether there will be disease-free survival (cure). Remission may be short-lived, thereby requiring administration of new, previously unseen therapy (second-line therapy).

Haematologists and oncologists often refer to phases of chemotherapy as:

- *induction*. The purpose of this first phase is to kill as many leukaemia cells as possible and bring about a remission
- *consolidation*. In this phase, the goal is to seek out and kill the residual leukaemia cells not destroyed by induction. Often, these cells are not detectable but they are assumed still to be present
- *maintenance*. The third phase is used to keep numbers of leukaemia cells low, i.e. to keep the disease in remission. The doses of chemotherapy are not as high as in the first two phases. This phase can last as long as 2 years.

However, only in certain leukaemia types are all three phases used.

Chemotherapy usually involves different combinations of drugs, and may be administered via a vein or by mouth. Many patients have a semi-permanent intravenous central line inserted. People who have leukaemia in their cerebrospinal fluid receive chemotherapy directly into the cerebrospinal canal (intrathecal chemotherapy); sometimes the therapy is inserted into a sac (Ommaya reservoir) placed in one of the brain ventricles.

Chemotherapy kills malignant cells or stops them from reproducing. Unfortunately, it also destroys rapidly growing healthy cells – leading to many of the adverse effects of treatment. These may include:

- common side-effects, such as nausea and vomiting, diarrhoea, hair loss and oesophagitis
- some effects similar to those of leukaemia itself: infections, anaemia and bleeding problems
- severe effects on the bone marrow, hair follicles and digestive system (from mouth to anus); occasionally, the nails may splinter, crack, develop ridges or cease growing
- effects on fertility
- an increase in the risk of developing cancer.

Chemotherapy is usually given in cycles, each cycle consisting of intensive treatment over several days, followed by a few weeks without treatment for rest and recovery from adverse effects caused by the therapy. The sequence is then repeated. Regimens may be administered for 2–6 cycles, depending on the leukaemia type. Blood and bone marrow examinations may be carried out prior to each cycle of chemotherapy and after completion of treatment.

Biological drug therapy

Biological drugs act in a similar way to the body's natural immune system; they include monoclonal antibodies, interferon or interleukins (see below).

Radiation therapy

Radiation is another treatment occasionally used in some types of leukaemia:

- A high-energy radiation beam is targeted at an organ, such as the brain, bones or spleen, where large numbers of leukaemia cells have collected.
- Radiation to the brain can have negative cerebral long-term effects, especially in children.

Table 8.36 *Examples of chemotherapy regimes for lymphoproliferative disorders*

Disease	Specific type	Agents
Acute leukaemias	Acute lymphoblastic leukaemia	Vincristine, prednisolone (prednisone), asparaginase (crisantaspase), daunorubicin
	Acute myeloblastic leukaemia	Daunorubicin and cytosine arabinoside
Chronic leukaemias	Chronic lymphoblastic leukaemia	Sometimes chlorambucil
	Chronic myeloblastic leukaemia	Hydroxycarbamide
Lymphomas	Hodgkin disease	ABVD or MOPP (see Table 8.45)
	Non-Hodgkin lymphomas	CHOP (see Table 8.45)

Stem cell transplantation

Haemopoietic stem cell transplantation (HSCT) uses high doses of chemotherapy along with total body irradiation in order to kill the leukaemic cells. After this, the immune system is essentially depleted, patients becoming at high risk of developing serious life-threatening infections; they are thus treated in specially designed, sterile, air-filtered marrow transplant rooms. Stem cells from a healthy, complete blood cell-matched donor (usually a sibling or, less commonly, a parent) are then transplanted allogeneically into a vein, whereupon they migrate to the marrow and grow and multiply before entering the circulation. This whole process may take 2–3 weeks to be completed. Marrow or stem cells from an identical twin are referred to as syngeneic. If an allogeneic donor is not available, the patient's own marrow cells, usually pretreated in order to remove residual, but otherwise unseen, leukaemic cells, are infused. This autologous approach is far less successful than the use of matched donor cells.

Prognosis and adverse effects of treatment

Diagnosis and prognosis of leukaemias are established by haematological examination (especially white cell count and blood film examination). This is supplemented by bone marrow biopsy, chest radiography, CT and MRI scans, and lumbar puncture. There is an excess of circulating white blood cells but there may be phases when few are released from the bone marrow (aleukaemic leukaemia). Cytochemistry, analysis of membrane markers and immunophenotyping are required for categorization of the cell type. Detection of chromosomal abnormalities may guide treatment and prognosis.

The treatment of leukaemia is dependent upon accurate diagnosis and generally involves combination chemotherapy with a variety of cytotoxic agents (Table 8.36). Induction of remission with cytotoxic drugs, singly or in combination, is increasingly followed by bone marrow transplantation (haemopoietic stem cell transplantation; Ch. 35). Post-remission treatment (consolidation) and, in some instances, maintenance therapy are indicated.

Newer treatments include retinoids, monoclonal antibodies, T-cell infusions, peptide vaccines and cytokines (such as granulocyte colony-stimulating factor [G-CSF]). Minimal residual disease (MRD) may remain and this guides further care. Prognosis of most leukaemias in the absence of treatment is very poor; few patients survive more than a year after diagnosis.

Cytotoxic chemotherapeutic drugs, given by intravenous, oral, intramuscular or intrathecal routes, damage all proliferating cells, including epithelium, bone marrow and reproductive tissues. Their toxic nature causes nausea and vomiting, impaired immunity, alopecia and mucositis. They are also teratogenic.

Table 8.37 *Synopsis of principles of oral health care in leukaemia*

Pre-chemotherapy	During induction chemotherapy	During remission	Long-term
Assessment	Continuation of preventive oral health care	Continuation of preventive oral health care	Continuation of preventive oral health care
Treatment planning			
Removal of unsaveable teeth	Antifungal prophylaxis (e.g. nystatin)		Monitoring of craniofacial and dental development
Treatment of caries	Antiviral prophylaxis (e.g. aciclovir)		
Dietary advice			
Initiation of fluoride prophylaxis			
Oral hygiene advice			
Initiation of chlorhexidine prophylaxis			

Patients are highly susceptible to infection during the induction of remission and may need to be isolated. Supportive care includes control of nausea, infections, haemorrhagic tendencies, anaemia, hyperuricaemia (gout) and renal malfunction. Nausea may be controllable with phenothiazines (prochlorperazine) or domperidone; if it is severe, 5-hydroxytryptamine (5HT) antagonists, such as granisetron, may be needed.

Dental aspects of leukaemias

Orofacial manifestations include mucositis, ulcers or gingival swelling and bleeding. Oral health care principles are summarized in Table 8.37.

Dental management can often be complicated by bleeding tendencies and susceptibility to infection. Septicaemias may spread from oral infections in these patients, as in other immunocompromised persons (Ch. 20).

Cytotoxic drugs are potentially hazardous to staff, who should only handle them wearing medical gloves and protective eyewear, should dispose of waste and sharps carefully, and should not handle them at all while pregnant.

The main types of leukaemia are:

- acute lymphocytic leukaemia (ALL) – accounts for 65% of childhood acute leukaemias but affects both children and adults
- chronic lymphocytic leukaemia (CLL) – almost twice as common as chronic myelocytic leukaemia and is essentially an adult disorder affecting older people
- acute myelocytic leukaemia (AML) – the most common acute leukaemia in adults
- chronic myelocytic leukaemia (CML) – most common in adults.

Less common types include hairy cell and human T-cell leukaemias.

Acute lymphocytic leukaemia (ALL)

General aspects

ALL is the most common childhood leukaemia; it has a peak incidence at 2–4 years but can affect any age group. Aetiological factors may include exposure to ionizing radiation or benzene. Electromagnetic radiation from power lines has little observable effect.

ALL presumably arises from malignant transformation of B- or T-cell progenitor cells and is characterized by the accumulation of malignant lymphoblasts, which proliferate and infiltrate the bone marrow (causing granulocytopenia, anaemia and thrombocytopenia), viscera, skin and nervous system. B- and T-cell lymphoblastic leukaemia cells express surface antigens that parallel their respective lineage developments. Precursor B-cell ALL cells typically express

Table 8.38 *Acute leukaemia: typical features*

General features	Features due to leukaemic infiltration of bone marrow	Features due to leukaemic infiltration of lymphoreticular system
Weight loss	Anaemia (pallor)	Lymphadenopathy
Weakness	Bone pain	Splenomegaly
Anorexia	Ineffective leukocytes (infections)	Thrombocytopenia (purpura and bleeding from mucous membranes)

B-cell surface markers CD10, CD19 and CD34, along with nuclear terminal deoxynucleotide transferase (TdT), while precursor T-cell ALL cells commonly express CD2, CD3, CD7, CD34 and TdT. ALL is associated with translocations that involve movement of the *c-myc* proto-oncogene to the immunoglobulin gene loci t(2;8), t(8;12) and t(8;22). Some patients with acute leukaemia may have a cytogenetic abnormality that is indistinguishable from the Philadelphia chromosome (Ph1). This occurs in 1–2% of patients with AML, but in about 20% of adults and a small percentage of children with ALL. In most children and more than one-half of adults with Ph1-positive ALL, the molecular abnormality is different from that in Ph1-positive CML. Ph1 is characterized by a *BCR-ABL* fusion gene.

Clinical features

Anaemia, lymphadenopathy, splenomegaly, infections, fever, bruising and bleeding tendencies are the main features. CNS involvement is not uncommon. ALL is clinically indistinguishable from non-lymphoblastic (myeloblastic) leukaemia (Table 8.38).

General management

Remission induction therapy over the first 3–4 weeks after diagnosis is designed to destroy most leukaemia cells, reduce symptoms and return blood counts to normal. During induction of remission, the child may need to be kept in isolation, such as in a laminar flow room, because of the high susceptibility to infection. Strict asepsis is indicated, live vaccines must not be given and infected persons should be kept away.

Specific treatments used may include:

- doxorubicin, cyclophosphamide or vincristine, by intravenous injection
- asparaginase (crisantaspase), given by injection
- dexamethasone or prednisolone (prednisone) orally
- methotrexate or cytarabine (Ara-C) by injection into the spinal fluid.

Chemotherapy for ALL in the *induction phase*, which normally lasts 3–8 weeks, may include:

- daunorubicin
- doxorubicin
- idarubicin
- mitoxantrone
- methotrexate
- asparaginase (crisantaspase)
- mercaptopurine
- cyclophosphamide
- vincristine.

Corticosteroids are often given as part of chemotherapy. Allopurinol or rasburicase helps to protect against uric acid-induced renal damage. Apart from the common chemotherapy adverse effects, some of the above drugs may affect heart muscle.

Intensification (*consolidation*) treatment usually lasts several months, involving the same drugs as used in induction, plus some of:

- cytarcytarabine (Ara-C)
- etoposide
- tioguanine.

Remission *maintenance* or continuation therapy is a less intensive chemotherapy course using mercaptopurine, methotrexate and vincristine. Steroids are usually continued in short courses. Some patients are given high-dose treatment with a stem cell transplant, with high doses of a chemotherapy drug such as etoposide or busulfan, and total body irradiation (TBI). Treatment is given both orally and intravenously over a 2–3-year period to keep the ALL from returning.

CNS prophylaxis, given directly into the spinal fluid by lumbar puncture and/or by vein, helps prevent the leukaemia spreading to the brain or spinal cord, and is often given in combination with radiation therapy to the head. Craniospinal irradiation is no longer routine in low-risk ALL patients but intrathecal methotrexate may be given.

Targeted therapy for ALL is recommended in addition to standard chemotherapy for patients with Philadelphia chromosome-positive ALL (Ph+ ALL). Such drugs include imatinib, dasatinib and nilotinib. Nelarabine targets T-cell ALL. Monoclonal antibodies such as rituximab target B-cell ALL.

The goal is a complete remission, which is achieved in about 95% of children and 75% of adults. The risk of relapse is greatest in the first 18 months and maintenance therapy is usually continued for 2–3 years. Relapse is higher in males, partly because of occult testicular or CNS disease. Bone marrow transplantation (haemopoietic stem cell transplantation; Ch. 35) may give better control if chemotherapy fails to prevent relapse.

Dental aspects

Dental treatment should only be carried out after consultation with the physician, as it may be affected by various aspects of management and the probable life expectancy.

Preventive oral health care is essential and, where indicated, conservative dental treatment may be possible. Surgery should be deferred (except for emergencies such as fractures, haemorrhage, potential airways obstruction or dangerous sepsis) until a remission phase.

The main dental management problems to consider in ALL are listed in Box 8.15.

Regional LA injections may be contraindicated if there is a severe haemorrhagic tendency. CS is usually possible. Anaemia may be a

---

Box 8.15 *Considerations in the care of acute lymphoblastic leukaemia*

- Abnormal susceptibility to infection – patient may be kept in isolation, such as in a laminar flow room, where strict asepsis is indicated. Antimicrobial cover is needed for surgery, particularly for those with indwelling atrial catheters
- Anaemia
- Bleeding tendencies
- Complications of bone marrow transplantation (haemopoietic stem cell transplantation; Ch. 35)
- Corticosteroid treatment (Ch. 6)
- Disseminated intravascular coagulopathy
- Hepatitis B or C (Ch. 9) and HIV infection (Chs 20 and 21; preoperative precautions include screening for hepatitis B and HIV in blood transfusions)
- Interaction between methotrexate and nitrous oxide (largely theoretical)

---

contra-indication to GA – intravenous sedation or relative analgesia may be used as alternatives. However, nitrous oxide, which interferes with vitamin B_{12} and hence folate metabolism, is possibly contraindicated if the patient is being treated with methotrexate. The toxic effects of the latter may be exacerbated.

Due to the dangers of haemorrhage and infections such as osteomyelitis or septicaemia, desmopressin (DDAVP) or platelet infusions or blood may be needed preoperatively, and antibiotics may be given until the wound has healed. Penicillin is the antibiotic of choice; intramuscular injections should be avoided because a haematoma may result. Sockets should not be packed, as this appears to predispose to infection. Operative procedures must be performed with strict asepsis and with the least trauma. Absorbable polyglycolic acid sutures are preferred.

Aspirin and other NSAIDs should not be given, since they can aggravate bleeding.

Oropharyngeal lesions can be the presenting complaint in over 10% of cases of acute leukaemia. Oral bleeding and petechiae are typical manifestations, together with mucosal pallor and sometimes gingival swelling (localized or generalized), mucosal or gingival ulceration, pericoronitis and cervical lymphadenopathy. Severe bleeding from the mouth, particularly from the gingival margins, may result from the thrombocytopenia. It needs treatment with desmopressin or even platelet transfusion. Gentle oral hygiene measures should control gingivitis, which otherwise aggravates the bleeding.

Herpetic oral and perioral infection is common and troublesome, as are varicella-zoster infections. They should be treated vigorously, usually with aciclovir. Varicella-zoster (VZV) and measles viruses can also cause encephalitis or pneumonia. Prophylactic aciclovir has greatly reduced the incidence, morbidity and mortality from VZV infections, including those secondary to bone marrow transplants.

Candidosis is particularly common in the oral cavity and the paranasal sinuses, and is usually caused by *Candida albicans*. Prophylactic antifungal therapy, such as nystatin mouthwashes or pastilles, or amphotericin lozenges, is therefore indicated. Fluconazole-resistant candidal species and a rising number of cases of infection with *Candida krusei* are seen.

Aspergillosis or mucormycosis can involve the maxillary antrum and be invasive.

Bacterial infections with Gram-negative species occasionally cause oral lesions, which can be a major source of septicaemia or metastatic infections in leukaemic patients. Lesions tend to become infected with bacteria such as *Pseudomonas* or *Escherichia*, or with *Candida* or *Aspergillus*. In severely immunosuppressed patients, over 50% of systemic infections result from oropharyngeal microorganisms. Microbiological investigations with care to obtain specimens for anaerobic culture are essential to enable appropriate antimicrobial therapy to be given. Meticulous oral hygiene should be carefully maintained, with regular frequent warm 0.2% aqueous chlorhexidine mouth rinses and the use of a soft nylon toothbrush.

Gram-negative bacteria can sometimes form a white adherent plaque on the tongue.

Other oral findings include tonsillar swelling, paraesthesiae (particularly of the lower lip), extrusion of teeth, and painful swellings over the mandible and of the parotid (Mikulicz syndrome).

Bone changes seen on radiography may include destruction of the crypts of developing teeth, thinning or disappearance of the lamina dura, especially in the premolar and molar regions, and loss of the alveolar crestal bone. Bone destruction near the apices of mandibular posterior teeth may also be seen. These bone changes may be reversible with chemotherapy.

Many of the cytotoxic drugs can precipitate mucositis with oral ulceration.

Adult acute lymphocytic leukaemia

Adult acute lymphoblastic leukaemia has a worse prognosis than childhood ALL but treatment schedules are similar.

Acute non-lymphocytic (myeloblastic) leukaemia (ANLL)

General aspects

ANLL is less common than ALL in children. Acute myeloblastic leukaemia (AML) is the most common of the seven subtypes described, and is the most common acute leukaemia of adults. The classification of AML has been revised by a group of pathologists and clinicians under the auspices of the World Health Organization (WHO). While elements of the French–American–British classification have been retained (i.e. morphology, immunophenotype, cytogenetics and clinical features), the WHO classification incorporates recent discoveries regarding genetics and clinical features of AML. Increased morbidity and mortality during induction appear to be directly related to age, CNS involvement, systemic infection, treatment-induced AML, and history of myelodysplastic syndromes or another antecedent haematological disorder. Patients with leukaemias that express the progenitor cell antigen CD34 and/or the P-glycoprotein (*MDR1* gene product) have a worse outcome. Deletions of the long arms or monosomies of chromosomes 5 or 7; translocations or inversions of chromosome 3, t(6; 9), t(9; 22); or abnormalities of chromosome 11q23 have particularly poor prognoses with chemotherapy. Cytogenetic abnormalities that indicate a good prognosis include t(8; 21), inv(16) or t(16;16), and t(15;17).

Although each criterion has prognostic and treatment implications, for practical purposes, current antileukaemic therapy is similar for all subtypes.

Clinical features

Anaemia, lymphadenopathy, splenomegaly, infections, fever, bruising and bleeding tendencies are the main features. CNS involvement is rare, though the disease occasionally causes cranial nerve palsies.

General management

AML (ANLL) treatment endeavours to achieve complete remission, since partial remission offers little survival benefit. Up to 70% of adults with AML can nowadays be expected to attain complete remission and about 45% of those can survive 3 or more years.

Chemotherapy drugs are usually given in combination. In some situations, high-dose chemotherapy plus stem cell or bone marrow transplant are used.

People who have acute promyelocytic leukaemia (APL) are treated with tretinoin (all trans-retinoic acid; ATRA) for up to 3 months alongside chemotherapy. ATRA has adverse effects, which can include:

- headaches
- nausea
- dry skin
- dry mouth
- dry eyes
- bone pain.

Induction chemotherapy is two cycles of one or more of:

- cytarabine (Ara-C)
- daunorubicin
- etoposide
- fludarabine
- idarubicin
- mitoxantrone.

Other agents used include clofarabine, everolimus, gemtuzumab, arsenic trioxide (for APL), midostaurin, lenalidomide, sorafenib, calicheamicin and tipifarnib. Consolidation chemotherapy usually involves cytarabine (Ara-C), etoposide, amsacrine and mitoxantrone.

Combination chemotherapy has greatly improved the prognosis in AML but is less successful than in childhood ALL. Remission can be obtained in up to 85% of patients but is rarely maintained. Whenever possible, bone marrow transplantation (haemopoietic stem cell transplantation; Ch. 35) is employed and 5-year survival rates of up to 60% are then reported.

Dental aspects of acute leukaemias

Treatment modifications are as provided earlier for ALL. Orofacial manifestations develop in 65–90% of cases (Box 8.16).

Box 8.16 *Oral and perioral manifestations of leukaemia*

- Lymph node enlargement
- Pallor
- Purpura, bleeding from gingivae
- Infections
  - Candidosis and other fungal infections
  - Herpesvirus infections
- Oral ulceration
  - Caused by herpesviruses, drugs and other factors
- Gingival swelling
  - Caused by leukaemic infiltrate
- Drug side-effects
  - Mucositis and ulceration (many of the cytotoxics)
  - Dry mouth (doxorubicin [Adriamycin])
  - Pigmentation (busulfan)
  - Candidosis (antimicrobials)

Oral bleeding and petechiae are typical manifestations, together with mucosal pallor and sometimes gingival swelling (localized or generalized), mucosal or gingival ulceration, pericoronitis and cervical lymphadenopathy. AML in particular may cause gingival swelling in 20–30% of patients. Gingival swelling results from an abnormal response to dental plaque, causing the tissues to be distended by dysfunctional white cells. Improvement in oral hygiene, aided by chlorhexidine, for example, can greatly ameliorate or abolish the swelling. ATRA, used in the treatment of APL, may also cause gingival swelling.

Chronic lymphocytic leukaemia (CLL)

General aspects

CLL is the most common type of leukaemia. In 10% there is a positive family history of the disease. Men are particularly affected but CLL is rare in Asians. CLL is almost invariably a B-cell neoplasm but there are several variants (Table 8.39).

Clinical features

Many patients with CLL are asymptomatic; some 60% of cases are detected coincidentally during a blood screen for an unrelated reason, and life expectancy may not be affected.

In others, CLL is insidiously progressive, with fatigue, fever, weight loss, anorexia, lymphadenopathy, haemorrhage and infections. Lymph nodes enlarge early, whereas the liver and spleen enlarge later. Other effects are anaemia and thrombocytopenia. Leukaemic infiltration of the skin is more common than in CML and may be a major manifestation. In some, autoimmune disorders – such as haemolytic anaemia or thrombocytopenia, or both (Evan syndrome) – may develop.

About 15% of patients with CLL undergo transformation to a more rapidly progressive form of leukaemia, or lymphoma (Richter syndrome).

General management

Asymptomatic patients may not need treatment. CLL patients may choose a watchful waiting approach but may need to start treatment, e.g. with biological drugs, when:

- the number of CLL cells spikes to much higher levels
- the number of non-cancerous cells drops precipitously
- lymph nodes become swollen
- the spleen becomes swollen.

Fludarabine is standard chemotherapy for CLL but pentostatin (2-deoxycoformycin) and cladribine are also used. Currently, the following combinations involve fludarabine often with:

- rituximab (FR)
- cyclophosphamide (FC)
- cyclophosphamide and rituximab (FCR).

Alternatives are rituximab with:

- pentostatin (2-deoxycoformycin) and cyclophosphamide (PCR)
- bendamustine (BR).

Chlorambucil and cyclophosphamide can be given orally, while cyclophosphamide can also be given intravenously, alone or with prednisolone (prednisone). Other monoclonal antibodies approved for CLL treatment include alemtuzumab and ofatumumab. Interferon, pentostatin (2-deoxycoformycin) and cladribine are used for hairy cell leukaemia.

Splenectomy may be needed. The 5-year survival of CLL is over 50%.

Chronic myeloid leukaemia (CML)

General aspects

CML is characterized by proliferation of myeloid cells in the bone marrow, peripheral blood and other tissues. A total of 90% of patients with CML have the Philadelphia chromosome and the *BCR-ABL* gene, which can aid diagnosis and treatment monitoring. Most patients with CML suffer from chronic granulocytic leukaemia (CGL) and are over 40 years of age, but there are several rare subgroups (Table 8.40).

Clinical features

Anaemia, weight loss, joint pains, splenomegaly and hepatomegaly are common but lymphadenopathy is rare.

After about a 4–5-year phase, CML transforms to an acute phase similar to AML (blast crisis). Fever, haemorrhage or bone pain is then common.

Table 8.39 Chronic lymphoid leukaemias[a]

Disorder	Particular features
Chronic lymphocytic leukaemia	Splenomegaly, skin lesions
	Prolonged survival possible
Sézary syndrome	Generalized lymph node enlargement; pruritus; exfoliating erythroderma, sometimes oral deposits
	Chemotherapy relatively ineffective
Hairy cell leukaemia	Splenomegaly; may be associated with HTLV-1 infection; predisposes to mycobacterial infection
	Relatively long survival
	Responds to interferon-alpha
Prolymphocytic leukaemia	Splenomegaly; resistant to chemotherapy and radiotherapy
Adult T-cell leukaemia–lymphoma	Resembles lymphocytic leukaemia
	Poor prognosis

HTLV = human T-cell lymphotropic virus.
[a]Most involve B cells, except for T-cell leukaemia and Sézary syndrome, which involve T cells.

Table 8.40 Chronic myeloid leukaemia

Disorder	Particular features
Chronic granulocytic leukaemia	Splenomegaly
	Positive for Philadelphia chromosome
	Fairly responsive to chemotherapy
Atypical chronic granulocytic leukaemia	Negative for Philadelphia chromosome
	Less responsive to chemotherapy
Juvenile leukaemia	Mainly young children
	Lymphadenopathy
	Poor response to chemotherapy
Chronic myelomonocytic leukaemia	Little response to chemotherapy
Chronic neutrophilic leukaemia	Difficult to differentiate from a benign leukocytosis
Eosinophilic leukaemia	Eventual cardiac damage

General management

Cytoreductive chemotherapy agents, such as busulfan and hydroxyurea, have been the mainstay, but the discovery of the Philadelphia chromosome and the identification of *BCR-ABL* have revolutionized treatment. Newer agents, such as imatinib mesylate, dasatinib, nilotinib and bosutinib, target leukaemia cells and inhibit the BCR-ABL enzyme, causing CML cells to die but only minimally affecting healthy cells. Radiotherapy may be useful later.

The prognosis of CML is variable, but sooner or later there is transformation to a blast crisis. In blast transformation, the same treatment is given as for AML, but the acute phase is usually refractory and the patient may die within a few months.

Dental aspects of chronic lymphocytic and myeloid leukaemia

The prognosis of chronic leukaemia is better than that for acute leukaemia and routine dental treatment is more likely to be required. Close cooperation with the haematologist is needed since there may be:

- bleeding tendencies
- liability to infection
- anaemia
- susceptibility to hepatitis B, C and HIV infection.

Side-effects of treatment include pulmonary fibrosis as a result of busulfan. In addition, ampicillin and amoxicillin may cause irritating rashes similar to those seen in infectious mononucleosis and unrelated to penicillin allergy. Gingival bleeding, oral petechiae or oral ulceration may also be features. Ulceration may be aggravated by cytotoxic therapy. Interferon-alpha can disturb taste and cause dry mouth. Herpes simplex or zoster, and candidosis, are common. Gingival swelling is less frequent than in the acute leukaemias. Palatal swelling (submucosal leukaemic nodules) may develop.

LA is satisfactory. CS can be given if required. GA must be carried out in hospital.

In CML, oral haemorrhage may result from platelet deficiency. Leukaemic infiltration can cause swelling of lacrimal and salivary glands (Mikulicz syndrome). Granulocytic sarcoma is a rare tumour-like proliferation of leukaemic cells, which can affect the jaws or soft tissues, and may rarely precede other manifestations or herald a blast crisis.

MYELODYSPLASTIC (PRE-LEUKAEMIC) SYNDROMES

General aspects

The myelodysplastic syndromes (MDSs; Box 8.17) are a group of diseases, found especially in the elderly, which originate in a bone marrow stem cell. Though the bone marrow is initially active, erythrodyspoiesis and dysplastic changes develop later.

There is a tendency to transform to AML. The poor quality of the blood cells means that a significant number of them are destroyed, leading to pancytopenia.

Clinical features

MDSs mainly affect males over the age of 60 who have neutropenia, macrocytic anaemia and/or thrombocytopenia.

The usual signs and symptoms are therefore excessive tiredness on exertion, breathlessness, bleeding, easy bruising, infection and enlargement of spleen or liver. Some patients succumb to marrow failure.

Box 8.17 *The myelodysplastic syndromes*

- Refractory anaemia alone (RA)
- Refractory anaemia with ring sideroblasts (RAS)
- Refractory anaemia with excess blasts (RAEB)
- Refractory anaemia with blasts in transformation (RABT)
- Chronic myelomonocytic leukaemia (CML)

General management

Diagnosis is from examination of blood and bone marrow. There is usually a monocytosis.

Treatment of MDSs is mainly supportive, since the majority of patients with these syndromes are too old to be eligible for a bone marrow transplant. This treatment includes erythrocyte and platelet transfusions, erythropoietin, G-CSF or granulocyte–macrophage colony-stimulating factor (GM-CSF), antibiotics, folic acid and vitamin B_6, and systemic corticosteroids.

Dental aspects

Dental management may be complicated by:

- bleeding tendencies due to thrombocytopenia
- anaemia
- neutropenia and a liability to infection, including hepatitis B and HIV (Ch. 20)
- corticosteroids (Ch. 6)
- gingival infiltration and oral ulceration; these may develop in CML but not in the other MDSs.

HYPEREOSINOPHILIC SYNDROME

Hypereosinophilic syndrome (HES) is an uncommon disorder in which there is hypereosinophilia in the absence of allergic disease. T-cell proliferation or parasitic infestation, together with disease of various organs, especially cardiomyopathy, and various rashes, are typical. Mucosal erosions and ulcers may be an early feature. HES is sometimes pre-lymphomatous.

Management is with systemic corticosteroids and usually hydroxycarbamide, or interferon.

MYELOPROLIFERATIVE DISORDERS

Myeloproliferative disorders, characterized by proliferation of bone marrow cells other than leukocyte stem cells, are regarded as separate entities from leukaemias but may progress to acute leukaemia. They have several common features and transition between them is common (Table 8.41). All are rare. Chronic granulocytic leukaemia is sometimes also included in this group.

Polycythaemia rubra vera

General aspects

Polycythaemia is an expansion mainly in the red cell population. It may be primary and idiopathic, and associated with normal erythropoietin levels. Polycythaemia rubra vera (PRV; Fig. 8.39) is mainly a disease of the elderly and of smokers; it has a slight male predominance and also causes proliferation of other blood cells.

Table 8.41 *Important laboratory findings in myeloproliferative diseases*

	Red blood cell count	White blood cell count	Platelet count	Alkaline phosphatase	Marrow fibrosis	Splenomegaly
Polycythaemia rubra vera	↑	↑	↑	↑	–	+
Agnogenic myeloid metaplasia	↓	↑	N or ↑	↑	+	++
Essential thrombocythaemia	N	N	↑↑↑	N	–	+

N = normal.

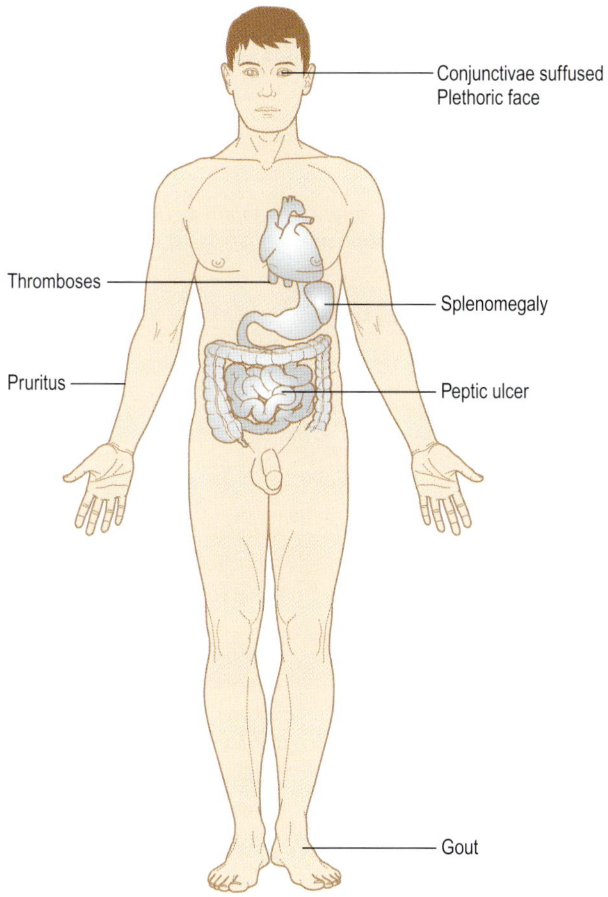

Conjunctivae suffused
Plethoric face

Thromboses

Splenomegaly

Pruritus

Peptic ulcer

Gout

Fig. 8.39 Polycythaemia.

Clinical features

Red cell overproduction leads to hyperviscosity syndrome (see later) and the risk of thromboses because of changes in platelets and clotting mechanisms. Stroke, myocardial infarction or less serious consequences can follow.

Granulocyte overproduction and excessive cell turnover may lead to hyperuricaemia, gout and renal damage. Platelet overproduction with platelet dysfunction leads to haemostatic defects, bruising or bleeding. Bone marrow replacement by erythropoietic tissue causes bone pain and there may eventually be myelofibrosis, and myeloid metaplasia in the liver and spleen.

General management

In the absence of treatment, few patients with PRV survive more than 2 years.

Repeated venesection shrinks the red cell mass and extends survival to more than 10 years. Phosphorus-32 is also a simple and effective method of depressing erythropoiesis but may increase the risk of

leukaemia. Cytotoxic agents (busulfan, chlorambucil or melphalan) may be given to suppress marrow activity, especially if there is thrombocytosis, but they also raise the risk of neoplasia. Cyproheptadine to control pruritus and allopurinol for gout may also be needed.

Dental aspects

The main dental management problems are susceptibility to thrombosis and haemorrhage. Venesection is especially important, if surgery is indicated, since postoperative morbidity and mortality are greatly increased by thrombotic complications.

LA regional blocks should be avoided. CS can be given. GA is a matter for expert attention in hospital.

There may be oral complications from cytotoxic chemotherapy.

Agnogenic myeloid metaplasia and myelofibrosis

General aspects

Myelofibrosis may be primary (agnogenic myeloid metaplasia) or it may be secondary to PRV, carcinomatosis or tuberculosis. Most patients are elderly.

Clinical features

Fibrosis of the bone marrow gradually depresses cell proliferation and extends throughout the reticuloendothelial system. There may be loss of weight, anaemia, thrombocytopenia purpura and bleeding tendencies, weakness, bone pain, splenomegaly, hepatomegaly and gout.

General management

Most patients require correction of anaemia and thrombocytopenia by transfusion. Bone pains and hyperuricaemia also need to be controlled. Corticosteroids are used occasionally. The median survival time is about 5 years, but less in myelofibrosis secondary to carcinomatosis or polycythaemia.

Dental aspects

Management problems may result from:

- anaemia
- haemorrhage
- possible hepatitis B and C or HIV carriage
- corticosteroid treatment.

Essential thrombocythaemia

General aspects

Thrombocythaemia (increased platelets) may be an isolated abnormality or associated with other myeloproliferative disorders.

Table 8.42 *Lymphomas*

	Hodgkin lymphoma	Non-Hodgkin lymphoma
Sites mainly affected	Lymphatic tissues	Lymphatic tissues
Clinical features	Swellings, fevers, chills, weight loss, night sweats, lack of energy, itching	Swellings, fevers, chills, weight loss, night sweats, lack of energy, itching
Prevalence	More common, especially in young adults 16–34 years of age and in older people ≥ 55 years	Less common; seen mainly in older people
Lymphocyte of origin	B	B or T
Subtypes	5 are microscopically distinct; typing is based on microscopic differences, as well as extent of disease	30 look similar but are functionally quite different and respond to different therapies
Main treatments	Early stage usually treated with chemotherapy before radiotherapy; chemotherapy is nearly always the main treatment when disease is more widespread	Chemotherapy
Staging	I–IV plus A or B	I–IV plus A or B
Survival	Greater	Lesser

Clinical features

The common effects are thromboses or haemorrhages. There is usually gross thrombocytosis with functionally defective, giant platelets.

General management

Radioactive phosphorus is the treatment of choice. If this fails, cytotoxic drugs are used. Aspirin and dipyridamole are useful for preventing thrombosis but heparin may be required.

Dental aspects

Surgery must be avoided until the disease is controlled, particularly because of the haemorrhagic tendencies.

LYMPHOMAS

General aspects

Lymphoma is a malignant transformation of either B or T lymphocytes or one of about 35 subtypes. The malignant lymphocytes multiply and may aggregate in, and enlarge, organs such as lymph nodes or other lymph tissues such as the spleen. Lymphomas fall into one of two major categories (Table 8.42):

- Hodgkin lymphoma (HL; previously termed Hodgkin disease)
- non-Hodgkin lymphomas (NHLs; all other lymphomas).

Most lymphomas (90%) are NHLs. About 10% of all lymphomas are Hodgkin disease, which can affect any age group but particularly males in their thirties. They are not reliably distinguishable clinically.

Lymphoma risk factors include:

- advancing age
- infections
  - HIV
  - HTLV-1
  - Epstein–Barr virus (EBV)
  - hepatitis B virus
  - hepatitis C virus
  - *Helicobacter pylori*
- immune disorders
  - autoimmune disease
  - immune suppressive therapy
  - immune defects such as HIV/AIDS
  - inherited immunodeficiency diseases (e.g. severe combined immunodeficiency, ataxia telangiectasia)

Table 8.43 *Revised European–American Lymphoma (REAL)/World Health Organization (WHO) classification of lymphomas*

Classical Hodgkin disease

Lymphocyte-rich

Nodular sclerosing

Mixed cellularity

Lymphocyte-depleted

Nodular lymphocyte predominant (some suggest this is NHL)

Non-Hodgkin lymphoma (NHL)

Nodular	Indolent course usually
Poorly differentiated lymphocytic	Most frequent; disseminated
Mixed cellular (lymphocytic and histiocytic)	Good response to chemotherapy
Histiocytic	Aggressive; behaves like diffuse
Diffuse	Aggressive course usually
Lymphocytic	Chronic if well differentiated
	Others disseminated
Mixed cellular	Disseminated
Histiocytic	Formerly called reticulum cell sarcoma
Lymphoblastic	50% develop acute lymphoblastic leukaemia
Burkitt lymphoma	Good response to chemotherapy

- chemicals
  - farm work or exposure to toxic chemicals such as pesticides, herbicides, or benzene and/or other solvents
  - hair dye
- genetics
  - family history of lymphoma.

Classification of lymphomas has been confusing; the European Organization for Research and Treatment of Cancer (EORTC) classification (1997) and the World Health Organization (WHO) classification of haematological malignancies (2000) – the Revised European–American Lymphoma (REAL) modification – are usually used (Table 8.43).

Clinical features

Lymphomas are mainly focused in lymphatic tissue but can spread to other tissues; lymphoma outside of lymphatic tissue is called extranodal disease.

Table 8.44 *Staging and treatment of lymphomas*

Stage[a]	Spread	Definition	Treatment
I	Early disease	Lymphoma located in a single lymph node region or in one area or organ outside the lymph node	Radiotherapy
II	Locally advanced disease	Lymphoma located in two or more lymph node regions, all located on the same side of the diaphragm, or in one lymph node region and a nearby tissue or organ	Radiotherapy
III	Advanced disease	Lymphoma affects two or more lymph node regions, or one lymph node region and one organ, on opposite sides of the diaphragm	Radiotherapy (IIIA) or quadruple therapy (IIIB)[b]
IV	Widespread or disseminated disease	Lymphoma is outside the lymph nodes and spleen, and has spread to another area or organ, such as the bone marrow, bone or CNS	Quadruple therapy[b]

[a]Both HL and NHL are further classified with the following letters:
- 'B' indicates that the person with lymphoma had symptoms such as fevers and/or weight loss at the time of diagnosis.
- 'A' indicates the absence of such symptoms.
- 'E' indicates that the tumour spread directly from a lymph node into an organ or that a single organ outside the lymphatic system is affected with no apparent lymphatic involvement.
- 'S' indicates that the spleen is involved.

[b]Quadruple therapy is combined chemotherapy, either MOPP or ABVD (see Table 8.45).

Often, the first sign of lymphoma is a painless lymph node enlargement – in the neck, under an arm or in the groin. Lymph nodes or lymphatic tissues elsewhere may also swell; the spleen, for example, often enlarges.

An enlarged lymph node sometimes causes pressure effects against a vein or lymphatic (swelling of an arm or leg), or a nerve (pain, numbness or tingling). Splenic enlargement may cause abdominal pain or discomfort. Many people have no other symptoms.

Non-specific symptoms of lymphoma may include:

- fevers
- chills
- weight loss
- night sweats
- lack of energy
- pruritus (most common in the lower extremity but can occur anywhere).

General management

Microscopic appearance, immunological characterization of the cell lineage and the clinical extent of the disease (staging) determine the treatment and prognosis (Tables 8.44–8.46): the higher the stage, the worse the prognosis.

Diagnosis depends on:

- blood tests
- liver and kidney function tests: high levels of LDH in NHL may indicate a more aggressive form of lymphoma
- biopsy
- imaging: a simple X-ray can sometimes detect lymphoma. CT may detect enlarged lymph nodes and other masses anywhere in the body. MRI gives three-dimensional images with excellent detail and provides better definition than CT in brain and spinal cord. The positron-emission tomographic (PET) scan is a newer alternative to the lymphangiogram and gallium scan
- bone marrow examination

Other tests include lumbar puncture and spinal tap.

Staging

Lymphoma staging is classification by size and spread; it is based on the results of imaging and related studies, and helps indicate appropriate treatment and prognosis.

Table 8.45 *Chemotherapeutic regimens*

Acronym	Regimen
ABVD	Doxorubicin (Adriamycin), bleomycin, vinblastine, dacarbazine
BEACOPP	Bleomycin, etoposide, doxorubicin (Adriamycin), plus COPP
ChlVPP	Chlorambucil, vinblastine, procarbazine and prednisolone (prednisone)
CHOP	Cyclophosphamide, doxorubicin (Adriamycin), vincristine (Oncovin), prednisolone (prednisone)
COPP	Cyclophosphamide, vincristine (Oncovin), procarbazine, prednisolone (prednisone),
CVP	Cyclophosphamide and vincristine (Oncovin) intravenously, and prednisolone (prednisone)
M-BACOD	Methotrexate, bleomycin, doxorubicin (Adriamycin), cyclophosphamide, vincristine (Oncovin), dexamethasone (Decadron)
MOPP	Mechlorethamine, vincristine (Oncovin), procarbazine, prednisolone (prednisone)
Pro-MACE-MOPP	Prednisolone (prednisone), methotrexate, doxorubicin (Adriamycin), cyclophosphamide, etoposide followed by MOPP
Pro-MACE-CytaBOM	Prednisolone (prednisone), methotrexate, doxorubicin (Adriamycin), cyclophosphamide, etoposide, cytarabine (Ara-C), bleomycin, vincristine (Oncovin), methotrexate
MACOP-B	Methotrexate, doxorubicin (Adriamycin), cyclophosphamide, vincristine (Oncovin), prednisolone (prednisone), bleomycin
PACEBOM	Prednisolone (prednisone), doxorubicin (Adriamycin), cyclophosphamide, etoposide, bleomycin, vincristine (Oncovin), methotrexate
Stanford V	Mustine, vinblastine, vincristine (Oncovin), bleomycin, doxorubicin (Adriamycin), etoposide and steroids

The newest classification system takes into account not only the microscopic appearance of the lymphoma but also its location in the body and genetic and molecular features. The staging, or evaluation of extent of disease, is similar for both HL and NHL (see Table 8.44). Grade is also an important component of the NHL classification:

- Low-grade lymphomas: often called 'indolent' because they grow slowly. They are often widespread when discovered but usually do not require immediate treatment unless organ function is compromised. They are rarely cured but can transform over time to a combination of indolent and aggressive types.

Table 8.46 *Factors predicting a poor outcome for lymphomas*

Hodgkin lymphoma	Non-Hodgkin lymphoma
Male sex	Age >60 years
Age ≥45 years	Stage III or IV disease
Stage IV disease	High lactate dehydrogenase
Albumin (blood test) <4.0 g/dL	More than one extranodal site
Hb <10.5 g/dL	Poor performance status (as a measure of general health)
Elevated white blood cell count (WBC) of 15 000/mL	
Low lymphocyte count <600/mL or less than 8% of total WBC	

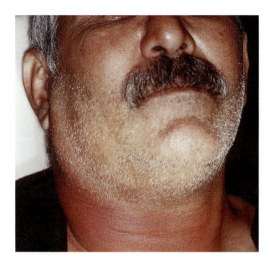

Fig. 8.40 Lymphoma.

- Intermediate-grade lymphomas: rapidly growing (aggressive) lymphomas that usually require immediate treatment but are often curable.
- High-grade lymphomas: rapidly growing aggressive lymphomas that require immediate, intensive treatment and are less often curable.

Several risk factors have been extensively evaluated and shown to play a role in treatment outcome (see Table 8.46). From these factors, the following risk groups have been identified:

- Low risk: one risk factor, 5-year lymphoma-free survival (LFS) of 70%
- Intermediate risk: 2–3 risk factors, 5-year LFS of 49–50%
- Poor risk: 4–5 risk factors, 5-year LFS of 26%.

Treatment

Treatment for lymphomas depends mainly on type and stage. Standard first-line therapy (primary therapy) for lymphoma includes radiation therapy for most early-stage lymphomas, or a combination of chemotherapy and radiation. For later-stage lymphomas, chemotherapy is primarily used, with radiation therapy added for control of bulky disease.

Dental aspects of lymphomas

Lymphomas often involve cervical lymph nodes and occasionally are seen in the mouth. Dental management may be complicated by corticosteroid or cytotoxic therapy, liability to infection, radiation or anaemia.

Hodgkin disease (lymphoma)

General aspects

Hodgkin lymphoma (HL) appears to originate in a cell of the monocyte–histiocyte series, and is defined by the presence of the Reed–Sternberg cell. It is usually classified using the REAL/WHO classification (see Table 8.43).

HL may be related to Epstein–Barr virus (EBV) infection, and the prevalence is greater in persons who are immunocompromised. Hodgkin disease pursues a more aggressive course in HIV/AIDS.

Clinical features

There is progressive involvement of lymphoid tissue, often beginning in the neck (Fig. 8.40). The lymph nodes become enlarged, discrete and rubbery, and can cause symptoms by pressure on other organs or ducts. Alcoholic drinks may cause pain in affected lymph nodes in nodular sclerosing Hodgkin disease.

Systemic symptoms, which indicate a poor prognosis, include pain, remittent fever, night sweats, weight loss, malaise, bone pain and pruritus. Anaemia is common late in the disease.

Cellular immunity is impaired so that fungal and viral infections are common and may disseminate.

General management

Treatment of HL includes chemotherapy and radiotherapy, depending on the staging. People with early-stage HL are usually given chemotherapy before radiotherapy (see Table 8.45), and when the disease is widespread, chemotherapy is nearly always the main treatment. If HL fails to respond well to standard chemotherapy, or recurs, high-dose chemotherapy with stem cell support may be used. The drug combinations most commonly used include:

- ABVD – doxorubicin (Adriamycin), bleomycin, vinblastine and dacarbazine (DTIC)
- ChlVPP – chlorambucil, vinblastine, procarbazine and prednisolone (prednisone)
- BEACOPP – bleomycin, etoposide, doxorubicin, cyclophosphamide, vincristine (Oncovin), procarbazine and prednisolone (prednisone)
- Stanford V – mustine, vinblastine, vincristine, bleomycin, doxorubicin, etoposide and steroids
- OEPA, COPP and COPDAC – the following drugs in varying combinations: vincristine, procarbazine, doxorubicin, etoposide, dacarbazine, cyclophosphamide and prednisolone (prednisone).

Radiotherapy, especially mantle radiotherapy, may be required but can lead to radiation damage to lungs (pneumonitis), heart (pericarditis) and thyroid (hypothyroidism), and predisposes to acute leukaemia.

The 5-year survival in HL in the earlier stages approaches 100%, and is over 60% even in more advanced Hodgkin disease. Those who relapse usually do so within the first 2 years.

Dental aspects

Hodgkin disease very rarely affects the mouth. When it does, it is not clinically distinguishable from NHL. Orofacial manifestations are as follows:

- Painless enlarged cervical lymph nodes – the initial complaint in 50%
- Oral infections – especially with viruses and fungi
- Mucositis and oral ulceration – caused by cytotoxic drugs

- Hyposalivation – from salivary gland irradiation damage
- Herpes zoster, herpetic stomatitis and oral candidosis – especially in those on cytotoxic or radiation therapy; zoster, secondary to immunodeficiency, may be the first sign of the disease.

Hodgkin disease of salivary glands is exceptionally rare and usually involves juxtaglandular lymphoid tissue.

The main problems from lymphomas that may influence oral health care are:

- anaemia
- corticosteroid therapy
- bleeding tendencies
- impaired respiratory function – pulmonary fibrosis due to irradiation
- mediastinal irradiation – may impair lung function or cause cardiac disease
- acute leukaemia – 7% of treated patients.

LA regional blocks should be avoided if there is any haemorrhagic tendency. CS may be given if required. GA is a matter for expert attention in hospital.

Non-Hodgkin lymphomas

General aspects

NHLs are more common than HL and have a variable but generally poor prognosis. European types of NHL (seen in Europe, the USA and Australia) are seen mainly in older persons, differ in age profile from NHL in other areas, and are growing in frequency.

Most NHLs are of B-cell origin. Most are Diffuse Large B Cell Lymphomas (DLBCL). They are found more commonly in association with immune defects such as HIV infection, in which NHL may be EBV-related and is second only to Kaposi sarcoma in frequency. Chronic immunosuppression or cytotoxic chemotherapy also predisposes to the condition. Post-transplantation lymphoproliferative disease is often NHL (Ch. 35).

NHLs are also more frequent in association with connective tissue diseases and may sometimes have a recognized microbial aetiology, such as EBV, hepatitis C virus, HTLV-1 or *Helicobacter pylori*.

A further strong risk factor is a family history of NHL, which entails a 3–4-fold greater risk to relatives. Weaker factors are occupational exposure, especially to pesticides and herbicides, and a slight, inconsistent association with hair dye use.

Clinical features

NHLs have a predilection for sites such as the gastrointestinal tract and CNS. They frequently involve the mesenteric lymph nodes and bone marrow, but often enlargement of cervical lymph nodes is the first sign. About one half NHL are extra-nodal and most of these affect the head and neck region.

General management

NHLs are broadly classified as either indolent (usually follicular types) or aggressive (usually diffuse). NHL is staged along the same lines as Hodgkin disease. In general, NHL is treated by multiple chemotherapy, since early dissemination is common. The most commonly used treatments include:

- CVP – cyclophosphamide and vincristine intravenously, and prednisolone (prednisone)

- CHOP– cyclophosphamide, doxorubicin (Adriamycin) and vincristine intravenously, and prednisolone (prednisone)
- chlorambucil – orally
- fludarabine – intravenously or as tablets, often given in combination with another chemotherapy drug
- bendamustine – intravenously.

In addition to chemotherapy, many indolent lymphomas are treated with the monoclonal rituximab; if chemotherapy and rituximab are given together, 'R' is added to the treatment name – for example, R-CVP or R-CHOP.

Dental aspects

The main problems from lymphomas that may influence oral health care are:

- oral infections, especially with viruses and fungi
- mucositis or oral ulceration caused by cytotoxic drugs
- anaemia
- corticosteroid therapy
- bleeding tendencies
- impaired respiratory function – pulmonary fibrosis due to irradiation
- acute leukaemia – 7% of treated patients
- painless enlarged cervical lymph nodes – the initial complaint in 50% of cases.

LA regional blocks should be avoided if there is any bleeding tendency. CS can be given if required. GA should be given in hospital.

Lymphomas rarely form in the oral cavity or oropharynx, but do so more frequently in HIV infection. Involvement of Waldeyer's ring is more common in NHL than in Hodgkin disease. Lesions appear as erythematous swellings, often with surface ulceration as a result of trauma. The jaws are rarely involved.

Herpes zoster, herpetic stomatitis and oral candidosis may be seen, especially in those receiving cytotoxic or radiation therapy.

NHL is one of the most common types of non-epithelial tumour of salivary glands in adults, but accounts for only about 5% of salivary gland tumours. Its diagnosis causes difficulties in this site because of possible confusion with benign lymphoepithelial lesion and Sjögren syndrome, and the fact that these may progress to lymphoma in about 20% of cases.

Other lymphomas

African Burkitt lymphoma is often EBV-related and is seen particularly in children, presenting mainly with jaw swellings but also frequently involving abdominal viscera (Fig. 8.41). It responds well to chemotherapy.

T-cell lymphomas are rare but are the cause of midline granuloma syndrome. The mouth may be involved by spread from the nasal cavity. Mycosis fungoides is the most common form of cutaneous T-cell lymphoma. Sézary's syndrome is a variant, in which the patient has more than 1000 per mm^3 atypical T lymphocytes in the blood – Sézary cells – CD4+ T lymphocytes with a convoluted and bizarre appearance. It is characterised by erythroderma, leukaemia, generalised lymphadenopathy and hepatosplenomegaly.

Nasopharyngeal (peripheral) T-cell lymphomas

Nasopharyngeal (peripheral) T-cell lymphomas can be clinically indistinguishable from Wegener granulomatosis in their early stages. If allowed to progress, they can cause mid-facial destruction; when

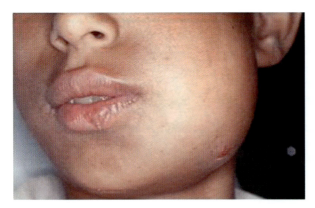

Fig. 8.41 Burkitt lymphoma.

this is neglected, it can be so severe as to open the cranial cavity to the exterior. In such cases, death from intercurrent infection was common.

Downward spread of the disease from the nasal cavity can lead to palatal necrosis and ulceration. In such cases, superimposed infection from the oral cavity can seriously confuse the microscopic picture and make diagnosis even more difficult. In uncomplicated cases, the microscopic picture is highly pleomorphic but typically characterized by angiocentric and angiodestructive changes, which mimic vasculitis.

T-cell lymphomas can have a highly variable course, sometimes with prolonged survival or even apparently spontaneous remissions. Wide dissemination follows sooner or later.

The optimal form of treatment is therefore uncertain, but radiotherapy and cytotoxic chemotherapy may be effective if the disease is not too far advanced.

Midline granuloma syndromes (fatal midline granuloma)

These 'idiopathic' diseases mainly affect adults between 40 and 50 years of age, males more than females, and are usually nasopharyngeal T-cell lymphomas (the so-called Stewart-type granuloma) or Wegener granulomatosis diseases, which are not reliably distinguishable clinically (Box 8.18). The diseases start in the nasal or paranasal tissues and can cause mid-facial destruction, sometimes of hideously disfiguring degree and often with a fatal systemic involvement (Table 8.47).

The most common upper respiratory tract symptoms are nasal stuffiness and crusting, and often discharge, which can be bloody.

PLASMA CELL DISEASES

Plasma cells derive from B lymphocytes. Plasma cell diseases are uncommon disorders, sometimes termed paraproteinaemias or monoclonal gammopathies, and are characterized by overproduction of a specific immunoglobulin detectable on electrophoresis, and often dominating other proteins (Box 8.19).

These homogeneous immunoglobulins (monoclonal immunoglobulins) are defective, leading to immunodeficiency); the rates of production of immunoglobulin light or heavy chains may be unbalanced, leading to overproduction of light chains appearing in the urine (Bence Jones protein) or heavy chains detectable in the serum and urine (Table 8.48).

Multiple myeloma (myelomatosis: Kahler disease)

General aspects

Multiple myeloma is a disseminated plasma cell neoplasm, predominantly causing bone lesions. The malignant plasma cells produce

Table 8.47 *Features of the main types of idiopathic midline granuloma syndrome*

	Wegener granulomatosis	Peripheral T-cell lymphomas
Destruction of facial skeleton and soft tissues	±	+++
Systemic involvement	Pulmonary cavitation Glomerulonephritis	Predominantly lymphatic spread. Liver, kidneys or other viscera may become involved
Biopsy findings	Necrotizing vasculitis, fibrinoid necrosis, multiple giant cells, ill-formed granulomas	Highly pleomorphic cellular picture, T cells recognizable by immunocytochemistry. Angiocentric and angiodestructive changes
Suggested treatment	Cyclophosphamide or azathioprine + prednisolone (prednisone)[a]	Radiotherapy + cytotoxic chemotherapy

[a]Or co-trimoxazole.

defective immunoglobulins and release osteoclast-activating factors, which cause bone resorption and pain.

Multiple myeloma is a disease mainly of the middle-aged and elderly. It has a slight predilection for males and is occasionally related to exposure to ionizing radiation or petroleum products.

Clinical features

Abnormal serum immunoglobulins form early and are occasionally detectable by chance during routine haematological examination, by a raised ESR, rouleaux formation or high plasma viscosity, or during serum protein investigations. Many years may elapse before symptoms appear.

Neoplastic proliferation of plasma cells in the bone marrow and their release of cytokines, such as IL-1, ultimately cause pain,

Table 8.48 *Paraproteins found in the serum and urine in plasma cell diseases*

	Serum	Bence Jones proteinuria
Heavy-chain disease	Alpha chain (or gamma or mu)	–
Idiopathic monoclonal gammopathy	IgG (or IgA or IgM)	–
Multiple myeloma	IgG (50%)	+
	IgA (25%)	
	IgD or IgE rarely	
Waldenström macroglobulinaemia	IgM	Rarely

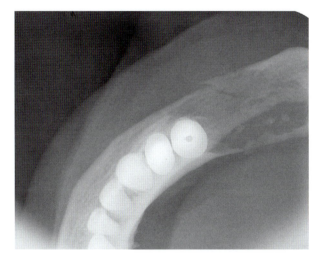

Fig. 8.42 Multiple myeloma in mandible, presenting with pathological jaw fracture.

osteolysis and bone destruction, hypercalcaemia, suppression of hae-mopoiesis, and other secondary effects. Circumscribed areas of bone destruction are seen (Fig. 8.42), typically in the vault of the skull. The defective immunoglobulins may lead to plasma hyperviscosity with a clotting or bleeding tendency, renal failure, liability to infections and neurological sequelae (Box 8.20).

General management

Diagnostic findings include those listed in Box 8.21.

Symptomatic patients, or those with progressive bone lesions or worsening paraproteinaemia, are treated by chemotherapy with melphalan, cyclophosphamide or chlorambucil plus corticosteroids. More complicated chemotherapeutic regimens have not been shown to be consistently superior, though relapses are probably best treated with vincristine, doxorubicin (Adriamycin) and dexamethasone (VAD). New treatments include interferon, thalidomide, lenalidomide (Revlimid), bortezomib, bone marrow transplantation (haemopoietic stem cell transplantation; Ch. 35) and haemopoietic growth factors. Bisphosphonates, such as pamidronate, help prevent pathological fractures.

The prognosis is variable but the survival of treated symptomatic patients averages 3 years. Anaemia, chronic renal failure, low serum albumin and high levels of serum beta$_2$-microglobulin in the absence of renal disease indicate a poor prognosis. A few patients treated with cytotoxic chemotherapy develop acute myelomonocytic leukaemia.

Box 8.20 *Multiple myeloma: clinical findings*

- Bone infiltration and destruction
- Bone pain (especially spinal)
- Pathological fractures
- Hyperviscosity syndrome
- Weakness
- Visual disturbances
- Bleeding tendencies
- Renal failure
- Anaemia
- Susceptibility to infections
- Neurological lesions
- Paraesthesiae
- Weakness

Box 8.21 *Multiple myeloma: investigational findings*

Biochemical

- Hypergammaglobulinaemia
- Bence Jones proteinuria
- Monoclonal immunoglobulin (Ig) G (less often IgA, rarely IgD or IgE) on electrophoresis of serum or urine (IgG in 55%, IgA in 25% and only light chains in 20%)
- Plasma cell proliferation on marrow biopsy
- Uraemia (in renal disease)
- Hypercalcaemia
- Hyperuricaemia (after treatment)

Haematological

- Normochromic anaemia
- Leukopenia
- Thrombocytopenia
- Erythrocyte sedimentation rate (ESR) very high

Skeletal radiographs or bone scanning

- Osteolytic lesions

A growing number of asymptomatic patients are found to have myelomatosis by electrophoretic evidence of hypergammaglobulin-aemia. Such patients must be followed and treatment started when appropriate.

Dental aspects

Dental treatment may be complicated by anaemia, infections, haemor-rhagic tendencies, renal failure or corticosteroid therapy.

The skull, especially the calvarium, is ultimately affected, with rounded, discrete (punched-out) osteolytic lesions in about 70%. Jaw lesions are seen less frequently but can be the first sign; small, punched-out, osteolytic lesions involving the posterior mandible are typical. Root resorption, loosening of teeth, mental anaesthesia and, rarely, pathological fractures are other possible effects. Rare complica-tions are gingival bleeding, oral petechiae, cranial nerve palsies and herpes simplex or zoster infections. Amyloid may be deposited in the oral soft tissues, causing local or more widespread swellings, such as macroglossia, the nature of which can be confirmed by biopsy.

Melphalan can cause severe mucositis. Bisphosphonates may cause osteonecrosis (Chapter 16).

Solitary plasmacytoma

Solitary plasmacytomas (localized myeloma) occasionally form in the jaws or soft tissues nearby, and are more likely than bone lesions to remain localized for a time. There is usually no abnormal immunoglobulin production but, even when present, levels are low.

Local radiotherapy may be useful, but cytotoxic chemotherapy is contraindicated. Patients should be kept under observation, as multiple myeloma develops in many, even after 20 years.

Waldenström macroglobulinaemia (primary macroglobulinaemia)

General aspects

Macroglobulinaemia is a rare disease in which B lymphocytes produce excessive amounts of monoclonal IgM.

Clinical features

The large monoclonal IgM molecules increase blood viscosity and cause hyperviscosity syndrome (see later).

There is usually also anaemia, recurrent infections, haemorrhagic tendencies and a wide variety of other possible manifestations, particularly lymphadenopathy and splenomegaly. In contrast to myeloma, foci of bone destruction and hypercalcaemia are not features, and renal involvement is uncommon.

The prognosis of macroglobulinaemia is slightly better than that of myeloma, but it may progress to lymphoma and a more rapid termination.

General management

The clinical course is very variable; nearly 25% of patients need no treatment for long periods and there is a median survival of over 3 years.

Dental aspects

The major problems of dental treatment are bleeding tendencies, corticosteroid therapy (Ch. 6) or anaemia. LA regional blocks should be avoided if there is a bleeding tendency. CS can be given if required. GA must be given in hospital.

Haemorrhagic tendencies may cause spontaneous gingival bleeding or post-extraction haemorrhage. Deep punched-out ulcers of the tongue, buccal mucosa or palate may form, but are rare.

Heavy-chain diseases

Heavy-chain diseases are rare disorders in which gamma, alpha or mu immunoglobulin heavy chains appear in serum and urine. Gamma-chain disease (Franklin disease) may cause palatal swelling due to lymphoid proliferation in Waldeyer's ring.

Benign monoclonal gammopathy

Benign monoclonal gammopathy or *m*onoclonal *g*ammopathy of *u*ndetermined *s*ignificance (MGUS) occurs when excessive amounts of monoclonal immunoglobulins are found in the serum of older patients, who appear otherwise healthy. MGUS occurs when particular plasma cells produce abnormally large amounts of a single type of antibody/immunoglobulin called a paraprotein (or M-protein). Clinical features may be absent (MGUS is usually found by chance), though occasionally people with MGUS have hypoaesthesia, paraesthesia or ataxia.

Table 8.49 *Differentiation of myeloma from monoclonal gammopathy*

	Myeloma	Benign monoclonal gammopathy
Plasma paraprotein level at presentation	High	Low
Plasma paraprotein levels observed over months and years	Rising	Stable
Other plasma immunoglobulin levels	Depressed	Normal
Imaging	Bone lesions	No evidence of lesions

'Benign' is only a relative term, since 20% ultimately develop myeloma and some others die from amyloid renal disease. Investigations such as urinalysis, serum protein electrophoresis, blood calcium, radiographs and marrow biopsy are needed to rule out myeloma (Table 8.49) but it is essential not to interpret monoclonal gammopathy as necessarily predicting myeloma. Amyloid deposition in the tongue may cause macroglossia. Further information on MGUS can be found at http://www.macmillan.org.uk/Canccrinformation/Causcsriskfactors/Precancerous/MGUS.aspx (accessed 30 September 2013).

Secondary macroglobulinaemia

Large amounts of serum IgM, which is often polyclonal and not a precursor to myeloma or macroglobulinaemia, can be an incidental finding on blood examination. It can be secondary to chronic disorders, such as connective tissue diseases, liver disease or lymphocytic leukaemia.

Hyperviscosity syndrome

General aspects

Hyperviscosity syndrome is caused by excessive amounts of high-molecular-weight plasma proteins, which adsorb to platelets and erythrocytes and cause excessive platelet adhesiveness and erythrocyte rouleaux formation.

Polycythaemia, Waldenström macroglobulinaemia and myeloma account for most cases.

Clinical features

Hyperviscosity syndrome is characterized by slowing of the peripheral circulation. The large protein molecules also activate clotting factors and complement, causing local thrombosis and inflammation.

General management

Venesection may be tried. Plasmapheresis reduces the viscosity but treatment should be aimed at the primary condition. Penicillamine is useful for a short period only, since the side-effects can be severe.

Dental aspects

Gingival or post-extraction haemorrhage, or taste loss and oral ulceration due to penicillamine, may be features.

CRYOGLOBULINAEMIA

Cryoglobulinaemia is a condition where cryoglobulins – immunoglobulins that precipitate when cooled below the normal body temperature – are formed.

Cryoglobulins are of three main types:

- Type I is monoclonal, and is a typical feature of lymphoproliferative and related diseases.

Table 8.50 *Langerhans cell histiocytoses*

	Age of onset	Bone lesions	Skin or mucosal lesions	Visceral lesions	Pituitary lesions	Treatment	Prognosis
Solitary eosinophilic granuloma	>10 y	+	+/−	−	−	Surgery Local radiotherapy	Good
Multifocal eosinophilic granuloma (Hand–Schuller–Christian disease)	<5 y	+	+	±	+	Chemotherapy	Variable
Letterer–Siwe disease	Infancy	+	+	+	+	Chemotherapy Steroids	Often fatal

■ Types II and III are typically associated with connective tissue diseases and infections, where the effects may result from immune complex formation.

Cryoglobulins can occasionally cause effects as a result of their physical properties, particularly Raynaud phenomenon. Occasionally, they cause peripheral thromboses and obstruction of small vessels. Purpura or bleeding tendencies may also result. Plasmapheresis may be beneficial.

LANGERHANS CELL HISTIOCYTOSIS (SOLITARY AND MULTIFOCAL EOSINOPHILIC GRANULOMA)

Langerhans cell histiocytosis is a group of tumours or tumour-like lesions of Langerhans cells, antigen-presenting counterparts of macrophages. This cell is recognizable on electron microscopy by the presence of rod-shaped Birbeck granules and by immunohistochemistry. The three main types of Langerhans cell histiocytosis are shown in Table 8.50.

Solitary eosinophilic granuloma

General aspects

Eosinophilic granuloma is an osteolytic lesion of bone with a predilection for the mandible.

Clinical features

Adults mainly are affected. Typical symptoms are pain, tenderness, swelling or bone destruction.

General management

Radiographs show a tumour-like area of rarefaction. A bone scan should be carried out to ensure that the disease is not multifocal. Diagnosis is confirmed by biopsy, which typically shows foamy histiocytes and eosinophils with an ill-defined, somewhat fibrillar background and areas of necrosis.

Eosinophilic granuloma is relatively benign and sometimes resolves spontaneously. Otherwise, it responds to curettage or, if recurrent, to modest doses of irradiation or to chemotherapy.

Dental aspects

Eosinophilic granuloma is an osteolytic lesion of bone with a predilection for the mandible. It can produce a characteristic form of periodontal destruction with gross gingival recession and alveolar bone loss, typically involving a small group of teeth and often exposing the roots of the teeth, with a 'teeth floating in air' appearance on radiography.

Eosinophilic granuloma can also affect the oral soft tissues, but less frequently than the mandible. However, a lesion that is histologically somewhat similar (eosinophilic granuloma or ulcer) can be traumatic in origin or reactionary without any history of trauma, and there is some doubt about the nature of eosinophilic granulomas of soft tissues reported in the past. 'Traumatic' eosinophilic granuloma eventually resolves spontaneously, though it may need to be excised for cosmetic reasons. Alternatively, the lesion may be excised because of its clinical resemblance to a tumour.

Multifocal eosinophilic granuloma and Hand–Schuller–Christian disease

General aspects

These lesions are the same histologically as the solitary eosinophilic granuloma and are sometimes referred to indifferently as Hand–Schuller–Christian disease.

Clinical features

Multifocal eosinophilic granuloma most frequently develops before the age of 5 years.

Hand–Schuller–Christian disease, strictly speaking, comprises osteolytic lesions of the skull, exophthalmos and diabetes insipidus; it is a variant of multifocal eosinophilic granuloma but develops in only 25%.

Flat bones, including the mandible, are the main sites. Soft tissues also become involved. Lymphadenopathy and hepatosplenomegaly may develop in up to 50%. Malaise, fever and infections of the ear, mastoid and respiratory tract are common.

General management

Diagnosis is by biopsy (which shows essentially the same features as solitary eosinophilic granuloma) and skeletal radiography or bone scans (show the disease extent).

In approximately 50%, the lesions gradually resolve spontaneously over the course of years but can leave residual disabilities as a result of limb lesions or diabetes insipidus. To reduce such complications, or in refractory cases, chemotherapy in relatively modest doses may be given as for solitary lesions. The mortality may be 25–30%; the younger the patient and the more widespread the disease, the worse the prognosis.

Dental aspects

Complications can arise from radiotherapy to the oral or para-oral regions, or chemotherapy with corticosteroids or cytotoxic agents.

Multifocal eosinophilic granuloma of childhood or Hand–Schuller–Christian disease rarely has initial manifestations in the jaws. However, it can produce a characteristic form of periodontal destruction like that seen in solitary eosinophilic granuloma.

Letterer–Siwe disease

General aspects

Letterer–Siwe disease typically affects children between the ages of 2 and 3 years.

Clinical features

The main features of Letterer–Siwe disease are lymphadenopathy, hepatosplenomegaly and bone and skin lesions. Fever, infections and bleeding tendencies are secondary to pancytopenia, which results from marrow displacement by the histiocyte-like cells.

It sometimes follows a rapidly fatal course. Rarely, death follows within a week of diagnosis.

General management

Diagnosis is by biopsy, showing infiltration of the tissues by proliferating histiocyte-like cells. Treatment is with radiotherapy, corticosteroids and cytotoxic drugs, and may be successful. Occasionally, the course of the disease is less acute and recoveries are possible.

Dental aspects

In view of the age group mainly affected and the rapidity of the course, patients are unlikely to be seen by dentists. In the few older patients with a more chronic form of the disease, the features relevant to dentistry are essentially those of severe types of multifocal eosinophilic granuloma. Corticosteroid or cytotoxic treatment may complicate dental management.

MASTOCYTOSIS

Proliferation of mast cells with release of their mediators may result in urticaria pigmentosa, pruritus, flushing, diarrhoea, bone pain and neuropsychiatric problems. The condition is treated with steroids and antihistamines. Trauma, stress, extremes of temperature and various drugs (NSAIDs, codeine, opiates, radiographic media and some GA agents) may precipitate exacerbations.

BONE MARROW TRANSPLANTATION (HAEMOPOIETIC STEM CELL TRANSPLANT

See Chapter 35.

GRAFT-VERSUS-HOST DISEASE

See Chapter 35.

KEY WEBSITES

(Accessed 27 May 2013)
British Committee for Standards in Haematology. Guidelines for the management of patients on oral anticoagulants requiring dental surgery. Search on 'oral anticoagulants' at: <http://www.bcshguidelines.com/4_HAEMATOLOGY_GUIDELINES.html>.
Centers for Disease Control and Prevention. <http://www.cdc.gov/ncbddd/blooddisorders/index.html>.
National Institutes of Health: National Heart, Lung, and Blood Institute. <http://www.nhlbi.nih.gov/health/public/blood/index.htm>.
NHS: National Patient Safety Agency. <http://www.nrls.npsa.nhs.uk/resources/?EntryId45=61777>.

USEFUL WEBSITES

(Accessed 27 May 2013)
Introduction to G6PD Deficiency. <http://www.g6pd.org>.
Leukemia & Lymphoma Society. <http://www.lls.org/>.
MedlinePlus. <http://www.nlm.nih.gov/medlineplus/healthtopics.html>.
Merck Manual for Health Care Professionals. <http://www.merckmanuals.com/professional/index.html>.
National Cancer Institute. <http://www.cancer.gov/cancertopics>.

FURTHER READING

Aframian, D.J., et al. 2007. Management of dental patients taking common hemostasis-altering medications. Oral Surg. Oral Pathol. Oral Radiol. Endod. 103 (Suppl.), S45.e1.

Al-Mubarak, S., et al. 2006. Thromboembolic risk and bleeding in patients maintaining or stopping oral anticoagulant therapy during dental extraction. J. Thromb. Haemost. 4, 689.

Al-Mubarak, S., et al. 2007. Evaluation of dental extractions, suturing and INR on postoperative bleeding of patients maintained on oral anticoagulant therapy. Br. Dent. J. 203, 1.

Baker, R.I., et al. 2004. Warfarin reversal: consensus guidelines, on behalf of the Australasian Society of Thrombosis and Haemostasis. Med. J. Aust. 181, 492.

Becker, W., 2007. Postoperative bleeding and oral anticoagulants. Br. Dent. J. 203, 410.

Beirne, O.R., 2005. Evidence to continue oral anticoagulant therapy for ambulatory oral surgery. J. Oral Maxillofac. Surg. 63 (4), 540.

Bolden, J.E., et al. 2006. Anticancer activities of histone deacetylase inhibitors. Nat. Rev. Drug Discov. 5, 769.

Brennan, M.T., et al. 2002. Relationship between bleeding time test and postextraction bleeding in a healthy control population. Oral Surg. Oral Med. Oral Pathol. Oral Radiol. Endod. 94, 439.

Brewer, A.K., 2009. Continuing warfarin therapy does not increase the risk of bleeding for patients undergoing minor dental procedures. Evid. Based Dent. 10, 52.

Chou, W.C., Dang, C.V., 2004. Acute promyelocytic leukaemia: recent advances in therapy and molecular basis of response to arsenic therapies. Curr. Opin. Hematol. 12, 1.

Chugani, V., 2004. Management of dental patients on warfarin therapy in a primary care setting. Dent. Update 31 (379), 384.

Daniel, N.G., et al. 2002. Antiplatelet drugs: is there a surgical risk? J. Can. Dent. Assoc. 68, 683.

De Araujo, M.R., et al. 2007. Fanconi's anaemia: clinical and radiographic oral manifestations. Oral Dis. 13, 291.

Delaney, J.A., et al. 2007. Drug interactions between antithrombotic medications and the risk of gastrointestinal bleeding. CMAJ 177, 347.

Downing, J.R., 2008. Targeted therapy in leukaemia. Mod. Pathol. 21, S2.

Estey, E., Dohner, H., 2006. Acute myeloid leukaemia. Lancet 368, 1894.

Evans, I.L., et al. 2002. Can warfarin be continued during dental extraction? Results of a randomized controlled trial. Br. J. Oral Maxillofac. Surg. 40, 248.

Fang, M.C., et al. 2007. Death and disability from warfarin-associated intracranial and extracranial hemorrhages. Am. J. Med. 120, 700.

Ferrieri, G.B., et al. 2007. Oral surgery in patients on anticoagulant treatment without therapy interruption. J. Oral Maxillofac. Surg. 65 (6), 1149.

Gómez-Moreno, G., et al. 2005. Hereditary blood coagulation disorders: management and dental treatment. J. Dent. Res. 84, 978.

Goodchild, J., Donaldson, M., 2009. An evidence-based dentistry challenge: treating patients on warfarin. Dent. Implantol. Update 20, 1.

Harris, M., 2004. Monoclonal antibodies as therapeutic agents for cancer. Lancet Oncol 5, 292.

Holbrook, A.M., et al. 2005. Systematic overview of warfarin and its drug and food interactions. Arch. Intern. Med. 165, 1095.

Jaffer, A.K., 2006. Anticoagulant management strategies for patients on warfarin who need surgery. Cleve. Clin. J. Med. 73 (Suppl. 1), S100.

Jafri, S.M., 2004. Periprocedural thromboprophylaxis in patients receiving chronic anticoagulation therapy. Am. Heart J. 147, 3.

Jeske, A.H., Suchko, G.D., 2003. Lack of scientific basis for routine discontinuation of oral anticoagulation therapy before dental treatment. J. Am. Dent. Assoc. 134, 1492.

Juurlink, D.N., 2007. Drug interactions with warfarin: what clinicians need to know. CMAJ 177, 369.

Levis, M., Small, D., 2005. FLT3 tyrosine kinase inhibitors. Int. J. Hematol. 82, 100.

Little, J.W., 2012. New oral anticoagulants: will they replace warfarin? Oral Surg. Oral Med. Oral Pathol. Oral Radiol. 113 (5), 575. Epub 2012.

Lockhart, P.B., et al. 2003. Dental management considerations for the patient with an acquired coagulopathy. Part 1: Coagulopathies from systemic disease. Br. Dent. J. 195, 439.

Mancl, E.E., et al. 2012. Contemporary anticoagulation reversal: focus on direct thrombin inhibitors and factor Xa inhibitors. J. Pharm. Pract. 16 November 10.1177/0897190012465989.

Merritt, J.C., Bhatt, D.L., 2002. The efficacy and safety of perioperative antiplatelet therapy. J. Thromb. Thrombolysis 13, 97.

Nash, M.J., Cohen, H., 2004. Management of Jehovah's Witness patients with haematological problems. Blood Rev. 18, 211.

Nebbioso, A., et al. 2005. Tumour-selective action of HDAC inhibitors involves TRAIL induction in acute myeloid leukaemia cells. Nat. Med. 11, 77.

Nematullah, A., et al. 2009. Dental surgery for patients on anticoagulant therapy with warfarin: a systematic review and meta-analysis. J. Can. Dent. Assoc. 75 (1), 41.

Perry, D.J., et al. 2007. Guidelines for the management of patients on oral anticoagulants requiring dental surgery. Br. Dent. J. 203, 389.

Randall, C., 2005. Surgical management of the primary care dental patient on warfarin. Dent. Update 32, 414.

Rice, P.J., et al. 2003. Antibacterial prescribing and warfarin: a review. Br. Dent. J. 194, 411.

Richards, D., 2008. Guidelines for the management of patients who are taking oral anticoagulants and who require dental surgery. Evid. Based Dent. 9, 5.

Sacco, R., et al. 2006. Oral surgery in patients on oral anticoagulant therapy: a randomized comparison of different INR targets. J. Thromb. Haemost. 4, 688.

Salam, S., et al. 2003. Bleeding after dental extractions in patients taking warfarin. Br. J. Oral Maxillofac. Surg. 45, 463.

Scully, C., Chaudhry, S., 2007a. Aspects of human disease 16. Chronic renal failure (CRF). Dent. Update 43, 597.

Scully, C., Chaudhry, S., 2007b. Aspects of human disease 17. Anaemia. Dent. Update 43, 661.

Scully, C., Chaudhry, S., 2008a. Aspects of human disease 18. Von Willebrand's disease (vWD). Dent. Update 35, 69.

Scully, C., Chaudhry, S., 2008b. Aspects of human disease 19. Haemophilia. Dent. Update 35, 69.

Scully, C., Chaudhry, S., 2008c. Aspects of human disease 20. Leukaemia. Dent. Update 35, 141.

Scully, C, Gokbuget, A., 2007. Hypoplasminogenaemia, gingival swelling and ulceration. Oral Dis. 13, 515.

Scully, C., Wolff, A., 2002. Oral surgery in patients on anticoagulant therapy. Oral Surg. Oral Med. Oral Pathol. Oral Radiol. Endod. 94, 57.

Scully, C., et al. 2002. Complications in HIV-infected and non-HIV-infected hemophiliacs and other patients after oral surgery. Int. J. Oral Maxillofac. Surg. 31, 634.

Scully C., et al. Oral health care in hemophilia and other bleeding tendencies. World Federation on Hemophilia Treatment of Hemophilia Monograph Series 2002; 27.

Scully, C., et al. 2004a. Oral health care in patients with the most important medically compromising conditions 1. Platelet disorders. CPD Dent. 5, 3.

Scully, C., et al. 2004b. Oral health care in patients with the most important medically compromising conditions 2. Congenital coagulation disorders. CPD Dent. 5, 8.

Scully, C., et al. 2004c. Oral health care in patients with the most important medically compromising conditions 3. Anticoagulated patients. CPD Dent. 5, 47.

Scully, C., et al. 2004d. Oral health care in patients with the most important medically compromising conditions 4. Patients with cardiovascular problems. CPD Dent. 5, 50.

Scully, C., et al. 2004e. Oral health care in patients with the most important medically compromising conditions 5. Patients at risk for endocarditis. CPD Dent. 5, 75.

Shalom, A., Wong, L., 2003. Outcome of aspirin use during excision of cutaneous lesions. Ann. Plast. Surg. 50, 296.

Spyropoulos, A.C., Douketis, J.D., 2012. How I treat anticoagulated patients undergoing an elective procedure or surgery. Blood 120 (15), 2954.

Srivastava, A., et al. 2013. Guidelines for the management of hemophilia. Haemophilia 19 (1), 1.10.1111/j.1365-2516.2012.02909.x Epub 2012 July 6.

Stabler, S.P., 2013. Vitamin B_{12} deficiency. N. Engl. J. Med. 368, 149.

Tallman, M.S., et al. 2005. Drug therapy for acute myeloid leukaemia. Blood 4, 1154.

Thijssen, H.H., et al. 2004. Paracetamol (acetaminophen) warfarin interaction: NAPQI, the toxic metabolite of paracetamol, is an inhibitor of enzymes in the vitamin K cycle. Thromb. Haemost. 92, 797.

Vanderlinde, E.S., et al. 2002. Autologous transfusion. BMJ 324, 772.

Ward, B.B., Smith, M.H., 2007. Dentoalveolar procedures for the anticoagulated patient: literature recommendations versus current practice. J. Oral Maxillofac. Surg. 65, 1454.

APPENDIX 8.1 EXAMPLES OF HAEMOSTASIS DEFECTS

Vascular phase of haemostasis		Platelet phase of haemostasis		Coagulation phase of haemostasis	
Congenital	Acquired	Congenital	Acquired	Congenital	Acquired
Hereditary haemorrhagic telangiectasia	Senile purpura	Bernard–Soulier syndrome	Bone marrow diseases	Haemophilias	Warfarin
	Steroid purpura		Chronic kidney disease	Von Willebrand disease	Heparins
Ehlers–Danlos syndrome			Aspirin		Liver disease
			Antiplatelet agents		

APPENDIX 8.2 RARE GENETIC COAGULATION-RELATED FACTOR DEFECTS

Coagulation factor defect	Bleeding tendency	APTT	PT	Basic defect
V	+	−	−	AR, streptomycin, liver disease, others
VII	+	−	−	AR, liver disease, anticoagulants, many others
X Stuart–Power factor	+ usually	−	−	AR, primary amyloid, others
XI Plasma thromboplastin antecedent	+	−	−	High frequency in Ashkenazi Jews
XII Hageman factor	−	−	−	AR, liver disease
XIII Fibrin-stabilizing factor	+	−[a]	−[a]	AR
α-Antiplasmin (Miyasato disease)	+	−	−	AR, many others
Fibrinogen	+	−	−	AR
Prekallikrein (Fletcher factor)	−	−		AR, nephritic syndrome, liver disease

AR = autosomal recessive.
[a] Assay by clot solubility.

9 Hepatology

KEY POINTS

- Alcoholic liver disease is increasing, as are deaths from liver disease
- Viral hepatitis is common, increasing and transmissible in health-care facilities
- Health-care professionals must be immunized against hepatitis B virus
- Liver disease can lead to bleeding and drug intolerance

Life is impossible without the liver. The liver (*hepar*) consists of hepatocytes, organized for optimal contact with sinusoids (blood vessels) and bile ducts. It makes and breaks down sugar, proteins and fats; stores nutrients; produces bile; and removes metabolic products and other toxins from the blood. Bile drains to the gallbladder and, via the bile duct, to the small intestine, at which point it is intimately associated with the head of the pancreas, swelling of which may cause biliary obstruction and jaundice (Fig. 9.1).

The liver, through the function of the Kupffer cells (mononuclear phagocytes) that line the sinusoids forms part of the lymphoreticular system (along with macrophages in the lymphoid tissue and spleen) and plays an important role by capturing and digesting bacteria, fungi, parasites, effete blood cells, and cellular debris. The liver turns glucose into glycogen (stored in the liver). This is converted back into glucose when required, maintaining stable blood glucose levels. Excess carbohydrates and protein are converted to fat. The liver also makes proteins – blood proteins (e.g. most blood-clotting factors using vitamin K metabolites), and albumin, hormones, transporter proteins and complement. The liver underlies normal haemostasis, since it produces blood clotting factors I, II, VII, IX, X and XI; bile salts which aid vitamin K absorption (needed for clotting factors); and the hormone thrombopoietin which stimulates the bone marrow megakaryocyte production of platelets. The liver also forms bile essential for fat digestion and absorption of fat-soluble vitamins (A, D, E and K), and produces or stores these vitamins and vitamin B$_{12}$; it also stores minerals (e.g. copper and iron). Bile (gall) is made up of water, cholesterol, phospholipids, bicarbonate, bile pigments and bile salts; it is a bitter yellow or green fluid secreted by hepatocytes, stored in the gallbladder between meals, and discharged into the duodenum upon eating, being required for fat and fat-soluble vitamin absorption. The bile salts sodium glycocholate and sodium taurocholate are produced by the liver from cholesterol; they help emulsify fats for their absorption and facilitate the activity of pancreatic lipase.

The breakdown of haemoglobin, cholesterol, proteins, sex steroids and many drugs occurs, at least partly, in the liver. The enzyme haem oxygenase acts on haem to form biliverdin, which in turn is converted into bilirubin. Biliverdin and bilirubin are termed bile pigments. Bilirubin is not water-soluble (unconjugated bilirubin) and needs a carrier (albumin) to be transported. In the liver, bilirubin is conjugated by combining with glucuronic acid and becomes water-soluble *conjugated* bilirubin. This then enters the bile, and flows into the bile duct and finally the intestine, where it can be excreted in, and colours, the stool after being changed into urobilinoids. Alternatively, the process of conjugation can be reversed by beta-glucuronidase, which converts the conjugated bilirubin back into unconjugated bilirubin. Unlike conjugated bilirubin, unconjugated bilirubin can be reabsorbed from the

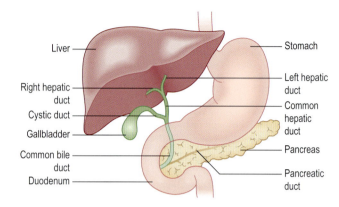

Fig. 9.1 Liver anatomy.

Table 9.1 *Some drugs metabolized by the liver*

Local anaesthetics	Bupivacaine, lidocaine, mepivacaine, prilocaine, articaine
Analgesics	Paracetamol (acetaminophen), aspirin, codeine, ibuprofen, meperidine
Antimicrobials	Ampicillin, azole antifungals, clindamycin, metronidazole, tetracyclines, vancomycin
Sedatives	Diazepam

intestine back into the blood (enterohepatic recirculation). Conjugated bilirubin can also be excreted in the urine, which it darkens. Increased levels of bilirubin in the blood can cause the body, especially the sclerae of the eyes, to appear yellow (jaundice).

Water-soluble toxins and waste products can be eliminated via the kidneys in the urine, but non–water-soluble toxins need to be chemically modified by the liver to allow this process to occur. Digested proteins in the form of amino acids are broken down further in the liver, a process known as deamination. Nitrogenous products such as ornithine and arginine are converted to urea, which is excreted into the urine by the kidneys. Sex steroids, such as the masculinizing hormone testosterone and the feminizing hormone oestrogen, are inactivated in the liver.

Most drugs, including alcohol, are metabolized/excreted via the liver (Table 9.1). In particular, oral drugs are absorbed by the gut and transported via the portal circulation to the liver. In the liver, these drugs may undergo first-pass metabolism, in which they are modified, activated or inactivated before they enter the systemic circulation.

The diagnosis of liver disease depends on the history, physical examination and evaluation of liver function tests (Table 9.2). Apart from bilirubin, liver enzyme levels may also be increased in the blood in various disorders. Aminotransferase levels are sensitive indicators of liver-cell injury (Table 9.3).

Alkaline phosphatase levels may be raised if there is biliary obstruction, but also vary with age. Rapidly growing adolescents can have serum alkaline phosphatase levels that are twice those of healthy adults as a result of the leakage of bone alkaline phosphatase into blood. Also, serum alkaline phosphatase levels normally increase gradually between the ages of 40 and 65 years, particularly in women.

Table 9.2 *Liver function tests*[a]

Serum test	Comments
Bilirubin	Positive in urine in most patients with jaundice, except unconjugated hyperbilirubinaemia. Bilirubin rises in serum because of overproduction or obstruction. In liver disease, the total serum bilirubin may rise (hyperbilirubinaemia). The total bilirubin includes that which has undergone conjugation (the direct or conjugated bilirubin) plus the portion of bilirubin that has not been metabolized (unconjugated bilirubin). When the direct bilirubin fraction is elevated, the cause is typically gallstones. If the direct bilirubin is low while the total bilirubin is high, this reflects liver cell damage or bile duct damage within the liver itself
Hyaluronic acid (HA)	Raised serum levels in liver fibrosis; marker of pre-cirrhosis
Alanine aminotransferase (ALT)	Leaks from damaged liver. Most sensitive marker of any form of hepatocyte damage. Also known as serum glutamic–pyruvic transaminase (SGPT)
Aspartate aminotransferase (AST)	Leaks from damaged liver, heart or muscle. Rises in liver, heart or muscle damage. Also known as serum glutamic–oxaloacetic transaminase (SGOT)
5′-Nucleotidase	Found in liver, thyroid and bone. Rises in biliary obstruction
Gamma-glutamyl transferase (GGT or GGTP)	Found in liver, kidneys, pancreas, prostate. Rises in obesity, alcoholism, most liver diseases, pancreatitis, diabetes, myocardial infarct and with some drugs. Medications commonly cause GGT to be elevated but alcohol is the main drug cause of an increase in the GGT
Alkaline phosphatase	Found in biliary canaliculi, osteoblasts, intestinal mucosa and placenta. Rises in pregnancy, liver disease, gallstones and bone disease
	Renal or intestinal damage can also cause the alkaline phosphatase to rise. One way to assess the aetiology of a raised level is to examine isoenzymes
Albumin	Low albumin (hypoalbuminaemia) may indicate that the synthetic function of the liver has been markedly diminished, such as in cirrhosis. Falls in malnutrition, nephrotic syndrome and gastrointestinal disease
Prothrombin time (and international normalized ratio [INR])	Prolonged in liver disease, malnutrition (decreased vitamin K ingestion)

[a]Statins and other drugs can disturb liver function tests.

Table 9.3 *Causes of raised aminotransferase levels*

Causes	Examples
Hepatic	Alcohol abuse
	Alpha-antitrypsin deficiency
	Autoimmune hepatitis
	Chronic hepatitis B
	Chronic hepatitis C
	Drugs
	Haemochromatosis
	Steatosis and non-alcoholic steatohepatitis
	Wilson disease
Non-hepatic	Acquired muscle diseases
	Coeliac sprue
	Inherited disorders of muscle metabolism
	Strenuous exercise
	Drugs
	Antibiotics
	Synthetic penicillins
	Ciprofloxacin
	Nitrofurantoin
	Ketoconazole and fluconazole
	Isoniazid
	Antiepileptic drugs
	Phenytoin
	Carbamazepine
	Inhibitors of hydroxymethylglutaryl–coenzyme A reductase
	Simvastatin
	Pravastatin
	Lovastatin
	Atorvastatin
	Non-steroidal anti-inflammatory drugs (NSAIDs)
	Sulphonylureas for hyperglycemia
	Glipizide
	Herbs and homeopathic treatments
	Alchemilla (lady's mantle)
	Chaparral
	Chinese herbs
	Ephedra (ma huang)
	Gentian
	Germander
	Jin bu huan
	Scutellaria (skullcap)
	Senna
	Shark cartilage
	Drugs and substances of abuse
	Anabolic steroids
	Chloroform
	Cocaine
	Ecstasy
	Phencyclidine
	Glues and solvents
	Glues containing toluene
	Trichloroethylene

Raised levels of gamma-glutamyl transferase (GGT) have been reported in a wide variety of clinical conditions, including pancreatic disease, myocardial infarction, renal failure, chronic obstructive pulmonary disease, diabetes and alcoholism. High serum GGT levels are also found in patients who are taking medications such as phenytoin and barbiturates.

CONGENITAL LIVER DISEASE

General and clinical aspects

Transient neonatal jaundice is common, usually due to the normal breakdown of haemoglobin around birth, and is of little consequence. Severe neonatal jaundice can be caused by prematurity, or haemolysis such as in rhesus incompatibility, biliary atresia or hepatic disease; it can lead to kernicterus (damage to the brain basal ganglia), which can be fatal, or cause epilepsy or choreoathetosis (with or without learning impairment) and deafness. Rare familial liver enzyme disorders that can cause jaundice are shown in Appendix 9.1.

Dental aspects

Disorders associated with an early rise in serum levels of conjugated bilirubin (mainly biliary atresia and haemolysis, such as in rhesus disease) can cause a greenish discolouration of the teeth and dental hypoplasia.

ACQUIRED LIVER DISEASE

Liver disease is increasing, due especially to alcohol use, obesity and infections; in the decade to 2009 in the UK, liver-associated deaths increased by one-fifth. A bleeding tendency, dangers from certain drugs, liability to infections and sometimes infectious hazards are factors to consider in the dental patient with liver disease.

HEPATITIS

The liver has some powers of regeneration but this capacity can be exceeded by repeated or extensive damage by infective agents, alcohol, drugs or poisons. The word 'hepatitis' means inflammation of the liver and also often refers to a group of viral infections that affect the liver, but hepatitis can also be caused by drugs or autoimmune disorders. The most common types of viral infection are hepatitis A, hepatitis B and hepatitis C. Alcohol abuse is the major drug causing acute hepatitis.

Chronic hepatitis is the term for hepatitis that persists longer than 6 months; it may follow acute hepatitis (or appear without warning) and may progress to cirrhosis. The most important causes of chronic hepatitis are hepatitis C virus, alcohol, drugs and autoimmune hepatitis (Table 9.4). Chronic liver disease includes chronic hepatitis, and cirrhosis.

Excessive alcohol intake, viral hepatitis and drugs also account for the majority of cases of cirrhosis (Box 9.1). Liver diseases can have many effects, according to the degree of liver damage – including jaundice, a bleeding tendency, and impaired drug and metabolite degradative and excretory activities (Table 9.5). Many patients with liver disease are asymptomatic and the problem frequently remains subclinical for years or decades. Malaise, anorexia and fatigue are common, sometimes with low-grade fever and upper abdominal discomfort.

Bilirubin ester is normally excreted in bile and is one of the factors that colour the faeces. If bilirubin is not conjugated (enzyme defect or parenchymal liver disease) or excreted (biliary obstruction), it accumulates in the body and colours the skin and mucous membranes (jaundice) and the whites of the eyes (icterus); it is detectable clinically at levels greater than 40 micromol/L, and the urine darkens.

Jaundice is often caused by liver disease but may also result from haemolysis, abuse of alcohol or other drugs, or infection (Table 9.6).

Pale, fatty faeces and malabsorption result from failure of bile salts to reach the intestine (obstructive diseases), causing malabsorption of fats, and of the fat-soluble vitamins (e.g. vitamin K) needed for clotting-factor synthesis. Bile salts accumulating in the blood may cause itching, nausea, anorexia and vomiting.

A bleeding tendency results from depressed synthesis of blood-clotting factors and excess fibrinolysins. Prothrombin time (PT), the international normalized ratio (INR) and activated partial

---

Table 9.4 *Causes of chronic hepatitis*

Hepatitis	Drugs	Autoimmune	Inflammatory bowel disease	Metabolic
Hepatitis B or C virus	Alcohol			Alpha$_1$-antitrypsin deficiency
	Aspirin			
	Cytotoxics			Wilson disease
	Halothane			
	Isoniazid			
	Methyldopa			
	Nitrofurantoin			
	Paracetamol (acetaminophen)			

Box 9.1 *Causes of chronic liver disease*

- Alcoholic and drug-induced liver disease
- Autoimmune hepatitis
- Gaucher disease
- Haemochromatosis
- Portal hypertension
- Primary biliary cirrhosis
- Primary sclerosing cholangitis
- Sarcoidosis
- Viral hepatitis
- Wilson disease
- Zellweger syndrome (cerebrohepatorenal syndrome; a rare congenital leukodystrophy)

Table 9.5 *Manifestations of liver diseases*

Impaired	Main causes	Consequences	Clinical features
Bilirubin metabolism	Congenital hyperbilirubinaemia	Hyperbilirubinaemia	Jaundice
Bilirubin excretion	Hepatocellular disease	Hyperbilirubinaemia	Jaundice
	Extrahepatic obstruction	Bilirubinuria	Dark urine
			Pale stools
Excretion of bile salts	Extrahepatic obstruction	Rise in serum alkaline phosphatase and 5′-nucleotidase	Pruritus
	Hepatocellular disease	Malabsorption of fats and fat-soluble vitamins (especially vitamin K), causing prolonged prothrombin time	Fatty stools Bleeding tendencies
Liver cell function	Hepatocellular disease	Impaired clotting factor synthesis and prolonged prothrombin time	Bleeding tendencies Oedema
		Impaired albumin synthesis	Coma or neurological disorders
		Impaired drug metabolism	Bleeding from oesophageal varices
		Rise in serum transaminases	
		Portal venous hypertension	
		Disorganized liver structure	
		Cirrhosis	

Table 9.6 *Causes of jaundice*

| Congenital | Acquired | | |
	Hepatocellular disease (parenchymal liver disease)	Extrahepatic biliary obstruction	Haemolysis
Haemolysis, such as in rhesus incompatibility	Viral hepatitis	Gallstones	Malaria
Prematurity	Drug-induced hepatitis	Carcinoma of pancreas	Yellow fever
Gilbert syndrome (Appendix 9.1)	Cirrhosis (often alcoholic)	Biliary atresia	Sickle cell diseases
Various rare syndromes (Appendix 9.1)	Primary biliary cirrhosis	Others	Incompatible transfusion
Others	Chronic hepatitis		
	Others		

thromboplastin time (APTT) are all increased. Chronic bleeding may cause anaemia.

Drugs (e.g. alcohol and barbiturates) that can induce the hepatic cytochrome P450 system can lead to diminished effects of other drugs, such as the contraceptive pill, phenytoin or warfarin. By contrast, some drugs (e.g. cimetidine, omeprazole, sulphonamides and valproate) impair P450 activity, causing enhanced activity of drugs such as carbamazepine, ciclosporin, phenytoin or warfarin (Table 9.7).

Cirrhosis chiefly affects the middle-aged or elderly, and is frequently asymptomatic in its earlier stages. Anorexia, malaise and weight loss are common, and effects can be widespread (Box 9.2; Fig. 9.2).

VIRAL HEPATITIS

Many viruses cause hepatitis (Table 9.8). The term 'viral hepatitis' used in health care usually refers to infection by hepatitis B, D or C viruses (HBV, HDV, HCV), which are transmitted parenterally (Table 9.9). Jaundice during childhood is often caused by hepatitis A virus (HAV) and typically is of little consequence; hepatitis B and C are the most relevant to health care, since the delivery of health care has the potential to transmit viral hepatitis to both health-care professionals (HCPs) and patients. Outbreaks have occurred in outpatient settings, haemodialysis units, long-term care facilities, and hospitals, primarily as a result of unsafe injection practices; reuse of needles, fingerstick devices and syringes; and other lapses in infection control.

Jaundice in the teenager or young adult may be due to viral hepatitis A, B, C, D or E. Several of these viruses, particularly HAV and hepatitis E virus (HEV), are transmitted faeco–orally. Some, especially HAV and HBV, and probably HCV, can be spread sexually. Hepatitis A and E are more of a problem in resource-poor areas and are transmitted faeco–orally; hepatitis E is more severe among pregnant women, especially in the third trimester.

Hepatitis B has long been of greatest importance but, in the absence of a vaccine, hepatitis C has become a more serious problem. Standard (universal) precautions against transmission of infection must always be employed, since these viruses, particularly HBV, HCV and HDV can be transmitted in blood and blood products and in other body fluids; they may be passed on by practices in which infection control is lacking, particularly in intravenous drug use where there is needle- or syringe-sharing. Any practice in which there is a skin breach, such as body-piercing or tattooing (Fig. 9.3), can also constitute a risk. Co-infection with other blood-borne agents, such as the human immunodeficiency virus (HIV), is common, particularly in intravenous drug users.

All hepatitis viruses can cause acute, or short-term, illness, and jaundice is common (Fig. 9.4). Some hepatitis viruses, particularly HCV and HBV, also have a small acute mortality. HBV, HCV and HDV can also cause chronic hepatitis, in which the infection is prolonged – sometimes lifelong – and may be associated with virus carriage, chronic liver disease and liver cancer (hepatoma; hepatocellular cancer); they can also be responsible for aplastic anaemia and other extrahepatic manifestations. The clinical and laboratory features of viral hepatitis are summarized in Table 9.10.

Hepatitis A ('infectious hepatitis')

General aspects

Hepatitis A is caused by HAV and is rarely serious. Hepatitis A is endemic throughout the world, seen particularly where socioeconomic and living conditions are poor and, in those areas, infection (and consequent immunity) is common in childhood (Fig. 9.5). In the developed world, many people reach adulthood without infection and have no immunity, and therefore are at risk from infection if they travel to endemic areas.

Spread of hepatitis A is largely faeco–oral, by consumption of contaminated water or food, particularly raw shellfish. For example, nearly 300 000 persons were infected in one outbreak in Shanghai, originating from contaminated clams. Hepatitis A can also be transmitted sexually and by close person-to-person contact, and in body fluids including saliva. Persons in the armed forces, food handlers, HCPs, sewage workers, travellers to areas of high endemicity, children and employees at day-care centres, promiscuous individuals who do not practise safe sex, and injecting drug users are at greatest risk.

Clinical features

The incubation period is 2–6 weeks. The disease is frequently subclinical or anicteric, but clinical features are similar to those of other forms of viral hepatitis (though muscle pains, rashes and arthralgia are rare); they include fatigue, nausea and vomiting, abdominal pain or discomfort, loss of appetite, low-grade fever, jaundice and itching. Recovery is usually uneventful. Blood and faeces become non-infective during or shortly after the acute illness. There is no evidence of either a carrier state or progression to chronic liver disease. About 15% have relapses over a 6–9-month period but the mortality is less than 0.1%. Hepatitis A can be lethal, however, if the patient is also infected with HBV/HCV. Hepatitis A gives long-lasting immunity.

General management

The diagnosis of hepatitis A can be confirmed if necessary by demonstrating serum antibodies to the virus (HAAb). No specific treatment

Table 9.7 *Drugs contraindicated and alternatives in liver disease*

Type of drug	Drugs contraindicated	Alternatives to use
Analgesics	Aspirin	Oxycodone
	Codeine	Paracetamol (acetaminophen)[a]
	Dextropropoxyphene	
	Indometacin	
	Mefenamic acid	
	Meperidine[a]	
	Non-steroidal anti-inflammatory drugs (NSAIDs)	
	Opioids	
	Pentazocine	
Antimicrobials	Aminoglycosides	Amoxicillin
	Azithromycin	Ampicillin, cephalosporins
	Azole antifungals (miconazole, ketoconazole, itraconazole)	Nystatin, fluconazole
	Clarithromycin[a]	Erythromycin stearate
	Clindamycin[a]	Imipenem
	Co-amoxiclav	Penicillin
	Co-trimoxazole	Nystatin
	Doxycycline	Penicillin
	Erythromycin estolate	Tetracycline
	Flucloxacillin	Penicillin
	Metronidazole[a]	
	Minocycline	
	Moxifloxacin	
	Roxithromycin	
	Talampicillin	
	Tetracyclines	
Corticosteroids	Prednisone	Prednisolone
Antidepressants	Monoamine oxidase inhibitors (MAOIs)	Selective serotonin reuptake inhibitors (SSRIs)
	Tricyclics[a]	
Muscle relaxants	Suxamethonium	Atracurium, cisatracurium, pancuronium, vecuronium
Local anaesthetics	Lidocaine[a]	Articaine, prilocaine
General anaesthetics	Halothane	Desflurane
	Methohexitone	Isoflurane
	Propofol[a]	Sevoflurane
	Thiopental	
Anxiolytics/ sedatives	Barbiturates	Lorazepam[a]
	Diazepam[a]	Oxazepam[a]
	Midazolam[a] (and flumazenil)	Pethidine[a]
	Phenothiazines	
	Promethazine	
Anticonvulsants	Carbamazepine	
	Lamotrigine	
	Phenytoin	
Others	Anticoagulants	
	Biguanides	
	Diuretics	
	Etretinate	
	Liquid paraffin	
	Co-phenotrope (Lomotil)	
	Methyldopa	
	Oral contraceptives	
	Pilocarpine	
	Sumatriptan	

[a]Or given in lower doses than normal. In a variety of liver diseases there is no evidence of increased risk of hepatotoxicity at currently recommended doses. Therefore, paracetamol/acetaminophen can be used safely in patients with liver disease and is a preferred analgesic/antipyretic because of the absence of the platelet impairment, gastrointestinal toxicity, and nephrotoxicity associated with nonsteroidal antiinflammatory drugs.

Box 9.2 *Cirrhosis: clinical features*

- Jaundice
- Oedema
- Ascites
- Swollen ankles
- Gastrointestinal haemorrhage
- Mental confusion
- Hepatomegaly
- Splenomegaly
- Finger-clubbing
- Skin manifestations
- Spider naevi
- Palmar erythema
- Opaque nails
- Sparse hair

Other occasional manifestations

- Parotid swelling (sialosis)
- Gynaecomastia
- Bleeding (liver failure)
- Portal hypertension and varices

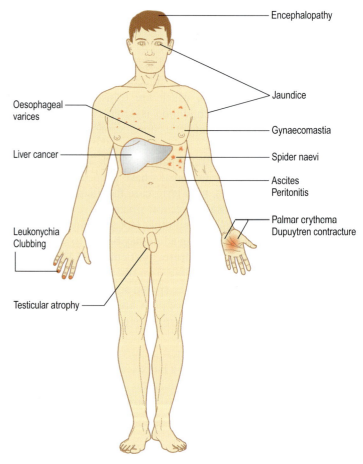

Fig 9.2 Cirrhosis.

is usually needed; normal human immunoglobulin may prevent or attenuate the clinical illness and is used mainly in sporadic outbreaks.

HAV vaccine is available, especially for prophylaxis in travellers to high-risk endemic areas such as Asia, South America and Africa. A combined vaccine against HAV and HBV may also be used.

Dental aspects

Patients are unlikely to seek dental treatment during the acute phase. There appears to be no risk of transmission of hepatitis A during dentistry that is conducted properly.

Table 9.8 *Viral causes of hepatitis*

Hepatitis viruses	Herpesviruses	Others
Hepatitis A virus	Cytomegalovirus	Coxsackie B virus
Hepatitis B virus	Epstein–Barr virus	Yellow fever
Hepatitis C virus	Herpes simplex virus	
Hepatitis D virus		
Hepatitis E virus		
Hepatitis G virus		
SEN viruses		
Transfusion-transmitted virus (torque teno virus; TTV)		

Hepatitis B

General aspects

Hepatitis B (serum hepatitis; homologous serum jaundice) is caused by HBV and is a serious disease. Genotype A is most common in the UK. HBV can cause lifelong infection, cirrhosis (scarring) or cancer of the liver, liver failure and occasionally fulminant hepatitis and death. Hepatitis B affects one-third of the world population, and one-quarter of those infected at birth die from liver disease.

Hepatitis B infection is endemic throughout the world, especially in institutions (such as those for custodial care), in cities and in poor socioeconomic conditions. It is especially common in the developing world; sub-Saharan Africa, the Pacific Basin, South-East Asia, Central Asia, parts of the Middle East, South America's Amazon Basin and some Eastern European countries are the areas of highest endemicity. Over 75% of some populations such as Australian aboriginals (hence the older term 'Australia antigen') are carriers. In parts of sub-Saharan Africa, Asia and the Pacific, nearly all children are infected. The prevalence is low (under 2%) in north-western Europe, North America and the Antipodes. Intermediate levels (2–8%) are found in Mediterranean countries, the Middle East, the Indian subcontinent and Japan.

Spread of HBV is mainly parenteral (via unscreened blood or blood products, particularly by intravenous drug abuse and by tattooing/body-piercing), sexual (especially among promiscuous individuals who do not practise safe sex) and perinatal. HBV is a robust virus, surviving for a week or more in dried blood on surfaces, and has been

Table 9.9 *Comparative features of more common forms of viral hepatitis*

	Hepatitis virus					
	A	B	C	D	E	G
Alternative terminology	Infectious	Serum	Non-A non-B	Delta agent	Non-A non-B[a]	Non-A non-B[a]
Prevalence in developed world	Common	Uncommon; about 5–10%	Uncommon; about 1–5%	In countries with low prevalence of chronic HBV infection, HDV prevalence is low among both HBV carriers (<10%) and patients with chronic hepatitis (<25%)	Rare except in endemic areas in Far East	Uncommon; about 1–2% of general population
						Associated with some cases of acute or chronic non-A, non-B, non-C, non-D, non-E hepatitis
Type of virus	Picornaviridae (RNA)	Hepadnaviridae (DNA)	Flaviviridae (RNA)	Circular RNA similar to plant viroid Delta virus	Similar to calcivirus (RNA)	Flaviviridae (RNA)
Incubation	2–6 weeks	2–6 months	2–22 weeks	3 weeks–2 months	2–9 weeks	?
Main route of transmission	Faecal–oral	Parenteral	Parenteral	Parenteral	Faecal–oral	Parenteral
Severity	Mild	May be severe	Moderate	Severe	May be severe	No consequences known
Carrier states	–	+	+	+	–	–
Complications	Rare Acute mortality 0.1%	Chronic liver disease in 10–20% Hepatoma Polyarteritis nodosa Chronic glomerulonephritis Acute mortality 1–2%	Many Chronic liver disease in >70% Hepatoma	Can cause fulminant hepatitis	Rare except in pregnancy	–
Vaccine available	+	+	–	–	–	–

[a]Several forms of enteric non-A non-B (NANB) exist (E, G).

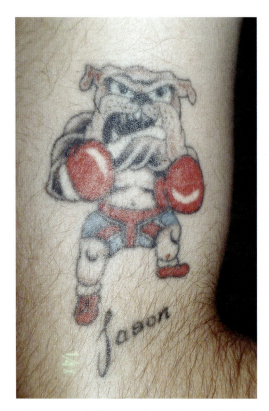

Fig. 9.3 Tattoo. Tattoos are safe if done under aseptic conditions, but can otherwise transmit blood-borne infections such as hepatitis viruses or human immunodeficiency virus.

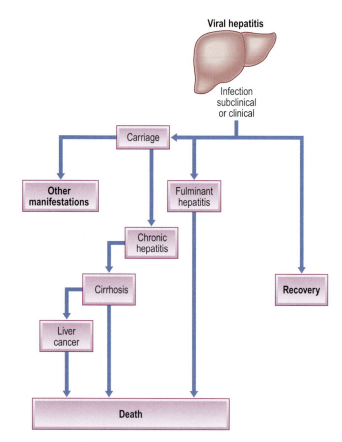

Fig. 9.4 Outcomes of infection with blood-borne viruses such as hepatitis B, C or D.

Table 9.10 *Acute viral hepatitis: clinical and biochemical features*

Stage	Clinical features	Serum bilirubin	AST	ALT	Alkaline phosphatase
Prodrome	Anorexia, lassitude, nausea, abdominal pain	N or ↑	↑	↑↑	N or ↑
Clinical hepatitis	As above plus jaundice, pale stools, dark urine, pruritus, fever, hepatomegaly	↑	↑	↑↑↑	N or ↑

N = normal.

transmitted to patients and staff in health-care facilities and between patients in a dental setting. HCPs in the past were not infrequently infected, but adherence to standard infection control procedures, and immunization, have resulted in a decline in infections. Nevertheless, in the USA, 91 HCPs were known to have transmitted HBV to patients in the health-care setting over the decade to 2006. Apart from HCPs, those in the armed forces, missionaries, aid workers, and persons travelling to the developing world are at risk (Box 9.3).

Clinical features

The incubation period for HBV is 2–6 months and the acute mortality rate is less than 2%. About 30% have no signs or symptoms, and most patients with clinical hepatitis recover completely with no untoward effect, apart perhaps from some persistent malaise. The effects of HBV infection, therefore, range from subclinical infections without jaundice (anicteric hepatitis) to fulminating hepatitis, acute hepatic failure and death.

The prodromal period of 1–2 weeks is characterized by anorexia, malaise and nausea. Hepatitis B viraemia usually precedes the clinical illness by weeks or months and lasts for some weeks before clearing completely.

As jaundice becomes clinically evident, the stools become pale and the urine dark due to bilirubinuria. The liver is enlarged and tender, and pruritus may be troublesome (see Table 9.10). Muscle pains, arthralgia and rashes are more common in hepatitis B than hepatitis A, and there is often fever.

Complications of hepatitis B include a carrier state, chronic infection, cirrhosis, liver cancer, polyarteritis nodosa or death. A carrier state, in which HBV persists within the body for more than 6 months, develops in 5–10% of people with chronic HBV infection and has the following phases:

- immune tolerance
- immune clearance
- low replication
- reactivation.

A carrier state is more frequent in anicteric infections or those contracted early in life. Although 5–10% of carriers lose the hepatitis antigen each year, carriage may persist for up to 20 years and may be asymptomatic. Some patients, especially those who have received blood products, those infected with HDV and those who have immune defects, are 'high-risk' and predisposed to the carrier state. Most carriers are healthy but others, especially those with persistently abnormal liver function tests, develop chronic liver disease (see later) and 15–25% of these patients die from it.

Infection with HBV confers immunity. Active immunity can therefore be acquired naturally. In the past, a high proportion of health-care staff working in developing countries or in institutions were not immunized and developed antibody to hepatitis B, despite a low incidence of overt hepatitis. However, rarely, where there has been co-infection with HDV, the death rate from HBV has been as high as 30%.

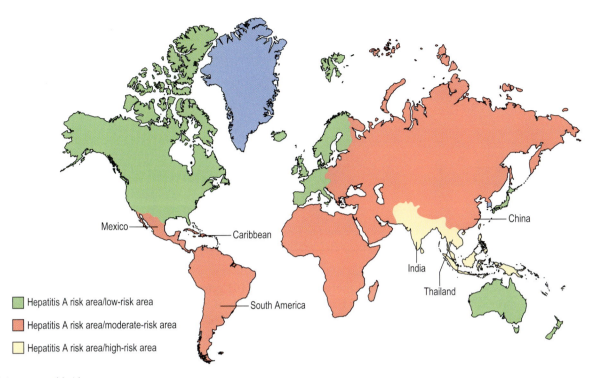

Fig. 9.5 Hepatitis A is seen worldwide.

- Hepatitis A risk area/low-risk area
- Hepatitis A risk area/moderate-risk area
- Hepatitis A risk area/high-risk area

Mexico
Caribbean
China
India
Thailand
South America

- Patients (e.g. haemophiliacs, thalassaemics) who have received unscreened blood products or multiple plasma or blood transfusions, especially in the Far East or Africa
- Patients receiving haemodialysis for end-stage renal disease
- Immunosuppressed or immunodeficient patients (e.g. those who are HIV-infected, have received a transplant or have malignant disease)
- Residents and staff of long-stay institutions, particularly prisons
- Persons in occupations that involve exposure to human blood – health-care and laboratory personnel (especially surgeons)
- Intravenous drug abusers
- Sexually active individuals, especially promiscuous individuals who do not practise safe sex
- Patients from the developing world, especially Africa and Asia
- Tattooing and acupuncture, especially in the Far East
- Individuals travelling to regions with high infection rates of hepatitis B virus (HBV), such as sub-Saharan Africa, South-East Asia, the Amazon Basin, the Pacific Islands and the Middle East
- People with certain other disorders (e.g. Down syndrome, polyarteritis nodosa)
- Partners of patients with hepatitis or any of the above groups
- Patients with some chronic liver diseases
- Household contacts of someone who has a chronic HBV infection
- Newborns whose mothers are infected with HBV – at high risk, as are infants and children whose parents were born in areas where HBV infection is widespread

General management

Electron microscopy of serum from HBV-infected patients shows three types of particle:

- The Dane particle, which probably represents intact HBV, and consists of an inner core containing DNA and core antigens (HBcAg), and an outer envelope of surface antigen (HBsAg)
- Smaller spherical forms and the tubular forms, which represent excess HBsAg.

Initial tests for HBV infection include serological tests for HBV surface antigen, surface antibody and core antibody. A positive test for surface antibody and core antibody indicates the presence of immunity to HBV. A positive test for surface antigen and core antibody indicates the presence of infection. Tests to determine whether there is viral replication, including serological tests for HBV e antigen, HBV e antibody and HBV DNA, should be undertaken. In patients with positive tests for HBV DNA and e antigen, liver biopsy and treatment should be considered. Serum enzyme estimations are useful; aspartate transaminase (AST) and alanine transaminase (ALT) are raised in proportion to the severity of acute hepatitis. Alkaline phosphatase, alpha-fetoprotein and serum bilirubin levels are also raised.

Diagnosis and prognosis depend, however, on serological markers. HBsAg (Australia antigen, hepatitis-associated antigen, hepatitis B antigen) is a non-infectious protein found transiently in those with acute hepatitis B, and persists in the serum in carriers and in some who are non-infectious. In a typical case, HBsAg develops 20–100 days after exposure, is detectable in the serum for 1–120 days and then disappears. The serum becomes negative for HBsAg about 6 weeks after the onset of clinical jaundice. Persistence of HBsAg beyond 13 weeks of the clinical illness often implies that a carrier state is developing. Hepatitis B surface *antibody* (anti-HBs) develops after infection or vaccination and, in the absence of HBsAg, implies immunity.

HBcAg is found in liver biopsies in acute hepatitis B. Hepatitis B core *antibody* is a sensitive marker of viral replication, indicating either current or recent infection. Anti-HBc associated with anti-HBs appears to indicate recovery and immunity to hepatitis. However, if anti-HBs is absent, anti-HBc suggests the carrier state or chronic hepatitis.

Hepatitis B e antigen (HBeAg) and its antibody, anti-HBe, are useful markers to determine the likelihood of spread of HBV (transmissibility) by persons affected with chronic hepatitis B viral infection; the presence of HBeAg means ongoing viral activity and the ability to infect others, whereas the presence of anti-HBe signifies a more inactive state of the virus and less risk of transmission. HBeAg indicates high infectivity and is found only in serum that is also HBsAg-positive, but in only about 25% of those who are HBsAg-positive. If HBeAg persists beyond

Table 9.11 *Hepatitis B serum markers in relation to disease progress*

Marker	HBsAg	Anti-HBs	Anti-HBc (total)	Anti-HBc IgM	HBeAg	Anti-HBe	HBV DNA
Acute infection – early phase	+	–	+	+	+	+	+
Acute infection – mid-phase	+	–	+	+	–	+	–
Acute infection – later phase	–	–	+	+	–	+	–
Recovery and immunity	–	+	+	–	–	–	–
Successful vaccination	–	+	–	–	–	–	–
Chronic infection with active reproduction	+	–	+	–	+ or –	–	+
Chronic infection in the inactive phase	+	–	+	–	–	+	–
Recovery, false positive or chronic infection	–	–	+	–	–	+ or –	–

Anti-HBc = hepatitis B core antibody; anti-HBs = hepatitis B surface antibody; anti-HBe = hepatitis B e antibody; HBeAg = hepatitis B e antigen; HBsAg = hepatitis B surface antigen; IgM = immunoglobulin M.

about 4 weeks after the onset of symptoms, the patient will probably remain infectious and develop chronic liver disease. Absence of HBeAg has usually indicated low infectivity. However, in some individuals infected with HBV, the genetic material for the virus has undergone a particular structural change, called a pre-core mutation, which results in an inability of the HBV to produce HBeAg, even though it is actively reproducing. This means that, even though no HBeAg is detected in the blood, HBV is still active in these persons and they can infect others.

Anti-HBe usually indicates complete recovery and loss of infectivity, provided HBeAg is lost. Asymptomatic HBsAg carriers often possess anti-HBe, and are usually at lower infective risk than those with HBeAg and DNA polymerase (supercarriers). The most specific marker of HBV reproduction is the measurement of HBV DNA in the blood; the polymerase chain reaction (PCR) is the most sensitive assay (Table 9.11).

Acute hepatitis B will resolve on its own in most symptomatic individuals and so management usually includes a high-carbohydrate diet and avoidance of hepatotoxins (e.g. alcohol). Antiviral therapy is not warranted.

HBV viral load increases in cirrhosis or hepatocellular carcinoma, and chronic HBV infection can be effectively treated with pegylated interferon-alpha 2b (PEG-IFN). Adefovir, entecavir, lamivudine, telbivudine, tenofovir and dipivoxil are also available. PEG-IFN is given for 4–6 months but can have several adverse reactions. Lamivudine is used for those who fail to respond to interferon and is usually better tolerated, but treatment for 1–3 years is usually needed and a variant mutant virus strain –YMDD – eventually emerges in 50% of treated patients.

Health clearance for HCPs is defined in the UK as *standard* or *additional*. Standard health clearance applies to all staff; additional health clearance is needed for anyone who undertakes exposure-prone procedures (EPPs). EPPs are defined as:

those invasive procedures where there is a risk that injury to the worker may result in the exposure of the patient's open tissues to the blood of the worker. These include procedures where the worker's gloved hands may be in contact with sharp instruments, needle tips or sharp tissues (e.g. spicules of bone or teeth) inside a patient's open body cavity, wound or confined anatomical space where the hands may not be completely visible at all times.

Additional health clearance also means being hepatitis B surface antigen-negative or, if positive, being e antigen-negative with a viral load of 103 genome equivalents/mL or less; and hepatitis C antibody-negative or, if positive, being negative for HCV RNA. There is also guidance for tuberculosis.

Prevention is best achieved by HBV vaccination and by avoiding contact with the virus (Box 9.4). Vaccination is recommended for all clinical students and staff, and is essential for anyone (trainee or qualified) who undertakes EPP – which includes most of dentistry – and for people working with high-risk groups, and those travelling to high-prevalence areas. Infection of infants born to HBV-infected mothers from contact with HBV can also be minimized by giving hepatitis B immunoglobulin (HBIg) and vaccine within 12 hours of birth.

The HBV vaccine is a recombinant vaccine of HBsAg. After vaccination, anti-HBs develops and confers 90% protection for many years and possibly for life, but may not protect against pre-core variants. HBV vaccination also protects indirectly against hepatitis D. Hepatitis B vaccine rarely causes any significant adverse effects.

After routine vaccination of most infants, children, adolescents or adults, post-vaccination testing for adequate antibody response is not necessary. For HCPs with normal immune status who have demonstrated an anti-HBs response following vaccination, booster doses of vaccine are not recommended; neither is periodic anti-HBs testing. Post-vaccination testing is recommended for persons who:

- are immunocompromised (e.g. haemodialysis patients)
- received the vaccine in the buttock
- are infants born to HBsAg-positive mothers
- are HCPs who have contact with blood
- are sex partners of persons with chronic HBV infection.

Post-vaccination testing in these groups should be completed 1–2 months after the third vaccine dose for results to be meaningful. A protective antibody response is 10 mIU/mL or more.

Combined hepatitis A and hepatitis B vaccine is available for some travellers, injecting drug users, promiscuous individuals who do not practise safe sex, and persons with clotting factor disorders who receive therapeutic blood products. It is indicated for vaccination of persons aged over 18 years in these groups. Hepatitis B vaccine is recommended for travellers to areas of high or intermediate hepatitis B endemicity, who plan to stay for more than 6 months and have frequent close contact with the local population.

Dental aspects

All dental professionals should be immunized against HBV. Drugs should be used with caution (see Tables 9.1 and 9.7). There may be a bleeding tendency if the platelet count is low (Ch. 8), or if the pro-thrombin time (and INR) is prolonged. Patients with normal platelet counts and normal prothrombin times (INR) can undergo dental intervention safely.

Although pure parotid saliva does not contain HBsAg, saliva collected from the oral cavity may contain HBV (presumably derived from serum via gingival exudate) and may be a source for non-parenteral transmission. However, the risk of transmission by this route appears to be low except where there is very close contact, as in families, children's nurseries or sexual contact. HBV can also be transmitted by human bites. Blood, plasma or serum can be infectious. As little as 0.0000001 mL of HBsAg-positive serum can transmit hepatitis B.

The main danger is from needlestick injuries; some 25% may transmit HBV infection. There is a higher risk for oral surgeons and periodontologists, and for those working with high-risk patients, probably because of needlestick injuries. However, if adequate precautions are taken, the dental surgery is no longer a significant source of transmission. In the past, HBsAg carriage was found in about 1% of dental practitioners and up to 20% of oral surgeons, who occasionally transmitted the infection to their patients. Now the risk appears to be low, since standard infection control precautions are taken and dental professionals have been immunized against HBV. Practitioners who are ill with hepatitis should stop dental practice until fully recovered. Testing for HBeAg may indicate those individuals likely to spread hepatitis B. HBeAg-positive dental surgeons and those who are HBeAg-negative but have more than 1000 HBV viral particles per millilitre of blood should discontinue practice involving exposure-prone procedures.

Needlestick injuries involving HBV can transmit the virus; post-exposure prophylaxis (PEP) with HBIg and/or hepatitis B vaccine series should be considered for occupational exposures after evaluation of the HBsAg status of the source and the vaccination and vaccine-response status of the exposed person within 24 hours of contact (Ch. 31).

Hepatitis C

General aspects

HCV infection was identified from what was formerly known as post-transfusion non-A non-B hepatitis (NANBH). HCV now ranks second only to alcoholism as a cause of liver disease in the developed world and is responsible for much sporadic viral hepatitis, particularly in intravenous drug abusers, among whom its prevalence is rising. Hepatitis C is increasing in the UK and many intravenous drug abusers are infected here too, most asymptomatically.

By contrast, transfusion-associated hepatitis C has declined, as blood is now routinely tested for HCV. The virus can also be transmitted between HCPs and patients. Persons at special risk for hepatitis C

include those who: have received blood from a donor who later tested positive for hepatitis C; have ever injected illegal drugs; have received a blood transfusion or solid organ transplant before about 1992; have received a blood product for clotting disorders produced before about 1987; have ever been on long-term renal dialysis; or have evidence of liver disease (e.g. persistently abnormal ALT levels).

Six major HCV genotypes (different genetic variations or strains) are recognized; genotype 1 accounts for most cases. HCV genotypes and subtypes are distributed differently across the world:

- Genotypes 1, 2 and 3 are found worldwide:
  - Subtype 1a is prevalent in North and South America, Europe and Australia.
  - Subtype 1b is common in North America and Europe, and is also found in parts of Asia.
- Genotype 4 is prevalent in the Middle East and Africa.
- Genotype 5 is prevalent in South Africa.
- Genotype 6 is prevalent in South-East Asia.

Some studies suggest that different types of HCV may be associated with different transmission routes. Subtype 3a appears to be prevalent among injection drug users and it is believed to have been introduced into North America and the UK with the widespread use of heroin in the 1960s. It has been suggested that genotype 1b is associated with a more severe disease progression than genotype 1a or 2. People with HCV genotype 3 are more likely to develop steatosis; it is believed that this genotype is an independent risk factor and may actually play a direct role in the development of steatosis.

Clinical features

Hepatitis C has a similar incubation period to hepatitis B (usually less than 60 but up to 150 days) but most HCV-infected persons develop no signs or symptoms. Clinical hepatitis C is also usually a less severe and shorter illness than hepatitis B (see Table 9.9), but a greater proportion (25–80%) of patients have persisting abnormal liver function tests, many develop chronic liver disease (up to 85%), and some develop liver cancer, or die (<3%). There are associations of HCV in some populations with sicca syndrome, lichen planus, lymphoma, cryoglobulinaemia and other extrahepatic manifestations.

About 15% of patients infected with HCV are co-infected with hepatitis G virus (HGV). Co-infection with HBV and SEN (see below) is also common.

General management

The initial test for HCV infection is serological testing for the hepatitis C antibody. Diagnosis is usually confirmed by measurement of serum levels of HCV RNA with use of the reverse-transcriptase PCR.

Acute HCV infection resolves spontaneously in 50% of patients; both interferon-alpha and PEG-IFN, with or without ribavirin, have been used with some success but can have significant adverse effects. A protease inhibitor (e.g. boceprevir or telaprevir) may also be given.

Genotype-1 patients require the longest treatment duration and have the lowest response rates. Treatment is with PEG-IFN plus ribavirin (PR) for 6–12 months. Testing for interleukin (IL)-28 polymorphisms could be used for the purposes of counselling patients, since a patient with the IL-28 CC genotype may require only 28 weeks of PR therapy instead of 48 weeks. Side-effects may include influenza-like symptoms, fatigue and bone marrow suppression. Boceprevir or telaprevir may be added to PR. Ribavirin causes anaemia as its main side-effect. Telaprevir is associated with a rash. Boceprevir may cause dysgeusia, neutropenia and anaemia; it is a reversible inhibitor of cytochrome P450 3A4, so all who receive boceprevir therapy require an assessment of drug–drug interactions.

There is as yet no vaccine against HCV. Hepatitis C prevention is shown in Box 9.4.

Dental aspects

HCV has been transmitted to patients and staff in health-care facilities. There has been a raised prevalence of HCV infection in some dental populations studied, and the virus has been found in saliva and infection has followed a human bite. HCV is transmitted in about 10% of needlestick injuries.

For HCV PEP, the HCV status of the source and of the exposed person should be determined; for health-care personnel exposed to an HCV-positive source, follow-up HCV testing should be performed to determine whether infection has developed. Immune globulin and antiviral agents (e.g. interferon with or without ribavirin) are not recommended for PEP of hepatitis C. However, early treatment of acute hepatitis C infection may prevent chronic hepatitis C infection (Ch. 31).

Staff infected with HCV should not perform exposure-prone procedures (see above, Ch. 31 and Appendix 9.2).

HCV may be associated with oral features – sicca syndrome, non-Hodgkin lymphoma and, in some populations (mainly patients originating from the Mediterranean basin or Japan), with lichen planus. Chronic HCV infection and sicca syndrome have an association with human leukocyte antigen (HLA)-DQB1*02.

Hepatitis D

General aspects

HDV (or delta agent) is an incomplete virus carried within the HBV particle and will only replicate in the presence of HBsAg. Therefore, there is no HDV without HBV infection. HDV spreads parenterally, mainly by shared hypodermic needles. Risk groups are as for HBV (see Box 9.3). HDV has been transmitted to patients and staff in health-care facilities.

HDV is endemic, especially in the Mediterranean littoral and among intravenous drug abusers, and is found worldwide. It is not endemic in northern Europe or the USA, but some haemophiliacs and others have acquired the infection and the prevalence is rising.

Clinical features

HDV infection may coincide with hepatitis B or may superinfect patients with chronic hepatitis B. Infection may produce a biphasic pattern with double rises in liver enzymes, and bilirubin. The incubation period of hepatitis D is unknown; 90% of infections are asymptomatic and HDV infection does not necessarily differ clinically from hepatitis B but can cause fulminant disease with a high mortality. About 70–80% of HBV carriers with HDV superinfection develop chronic liver disease with cirrhosis, compared with 15–30% with chronic HBV infection alone.

General management

Hepatitis D virus antigen indicates recent infection; delta antibody indicates chronic hepatitis or recovery. Drug treatment with interferon-alpha is effective. Vaccination against HBV protects indirectly against HDV.

Dental aspects

The same considerations apply as for hepatitis B.

Hepatitis E

HEV spreads mainly via the faecal–oral route and is responsible for large epidemics in India, South-East Asia, parts of the Commonwealth of Independent States (CIS; the old USSR) and Africa. HEV causes a disease similar to hepatitis A, but in pregnant women it has a high mortality rate (up to 40%).

Hepatitis E virus is not known to be transmitted during dentistry.

Hepatitis G

HGV may co-infect some patients infected with HCV or HBV. About 1.5% of healthy blood donors in the USA are infected with HGV and it is of high prevalence in intravenous drug users.

HGV infection, if it produces clinical hepatitis, tends to be less severe than hepatitis C but is followed by persistent infection in 15–30%. HGV appears to respond to interferon-alpha.

HGV is not known to be transmitted during dentistry. GB virus C is related to HGV.

Transfusion-transmitted virus (torque teno virus)

Transfusion-transmitted virus (TTV) has a single strand only of DNA and there is a high prevalence of chronic viraemia in apparently healthy people (up to nearly 100% in some countries). Like HGV, the pathogenicity of TTV has not been proven; it has not yet been aetiologically linked to any other disease and the virus is not known to be transmitted during dentistry.

SEN viruses

SEN is named after the initials of the patient from whom the virus was isolated. SEN V-D and SEN V-H are DNA viruses that are transmitted parenterally and can cause post-transfusion hepatitis. These viruses are otherwise of unknown pathogenicity and not known to be transmitted during dentistry.

LEPTOSPIROSIS

The bacteria *Leptospira icterohaemorrhagiae*, associated with rats, and *Leptospira hardjo*, found in cattle, can be transmitted to humans by contact with the urine of rats, foxes or cattle, usually via contaminated water or soil. Leptospirosis is an occupational hazard for people who work outdoors or with animals (e.g. farmers and vets), and for sewer workers, and is a recreational hazard for those who participate in water sports and for campers. There is usually an influenza-like illness with severe headaches. The severe form (Weil disease), which affects only about 10–15%, causes liver damage and jaundice, and has a death rate between 4% and 40%. It may respond to penicillin or tetracycline.

ALCOHOLIC HEPATITIS

Alcohol is the major and increasing cause of hepatitis in developed countries. It injures the liver by blocking the metabolism of protein, fats and carbohydrates, and causes fatty change (alcoholic steatosis); in response there is inflammation (alcoholic hepatitis), which is probably reversible initially. The amount of alcohol that can injure the liver varies greatly from person to person: in women, as few as 2–3 units per day may be responsible, and in men, as few as 3–4 units per day. Exposure to alcohol over long periods may cause liver fibrosis, which, in itself, is largely asymptomatic; as it progresses, however, it can turn into cirrhosis, where the fibrosis alters the architecture and impairs liver function. If cirrhosis progresses, the liver may fail.

NON-ALCOHOLIC STEATOHEPATITIS (NASH; MACROVESICULAR STEATOSIS; NON-ALCOHOLIC FATTY LIVER DISEASE, NAFLD)

Non-alcoholic fatty liver disease (NAFLD) is the most common chronic liver disease, strongly associated with obesity, the metabolic syndrome and type 2 diabetes. NASH is present in more than 25% of severely obese patients, 40% of whom have advanced fibrosis.

The histologic spectrum of NAFLD ranges from simple steatosis to non-alcoholic steatohepatitis (NASH), fibrosis and eventually cirrhosis. Patients with NASH and significant fibrosis seen on liver biopsy have an increased risk for liver-related morbidity and mortality compared to patients with simple steatosis. The only clinical evidence of hepatic steatosis and NASH may be mildly raised aminotransferase levels. Steatosis appears to have a benign course, whereas NASH can progress to cirrhosis.

Fatty infiltration of the liver can be identified by ultrasonography or computed tomography (CT).

Tests that can accurately predict the presence of advanced disease without the need for liver biopsy include those that predict NASH (such as markers of hepatocyte apoptosis, oxidative stress and inflammation) and those that predict fibrosis. Caspase-generated CK18 fragment levels can be measured in plasma using enzyme-linked immunosorbent assay (ELISA), and these levels have been found to be significantly higher in NASH patients than simple steatosis. Ferritin levels more than 1.5 times the upper limit of normal were associated with the diagnosis of NASH and advanced fibrosis.

Liver failure as a result of NASH is uncommon. Weight loss is the cornerstone of treatment in patients who are obese. Other treatments for NASH that are being studied include vitamin E and ursodiol.

DRUG-INDUCED HEPATITIS

Apart from alcohol, the main offender, many other drugs can cause hepatitis. These include halothane; some non-steroidal anti-inflammatory drugs (NSAIDs), antimicrobials, herbs and nutritional supplements; and paracetamol (acetaminophen) in overdose (Box 9.5). With some drugs, liver damage is a predictable dose-related effect, while with others the damage is unpredictable and may be immunologically mediated (Table 9.12).

Aspirin ingestion by children, during and after a viral illness (e.g. chickenpox, influenza or other respiratory tract illness), significantly increases the chance of developing Reye syndrome – liver damage with encephalopathy and abnormal accumulations of fat in the liver and other organs, along with a severe rise in intracranial pressure. Reye syndrome can follow several (1–14) days after aspirin use, usually in a viral infection, and generally progresses through two stages. The first includes persistent or continuous vomiting, severe tiredness, belligerence due to illness (moodiness), nausea and loss of energy. The second stage follows, with personality changes, bizarre mental and physical behaviour (confusion, restlessness and irrational behaviour), lethargy or inactivity, and sometimes coma and convulsions. There is a 90% chance of recovery for those diagnosed early but only 10%

are likely to recover if diagnosed late. Treatment is typically provided in an intensive care unit for monitoring of fluids, electrolytes, blood gases, intracranial pressure and nutrition. About 90% of cases of Reye syndrome develop in the first 15 years of life, so aspirin or other salicylates are contraindicated for children under 16, except for certain specific diseases. Many over-the-counter medications, including mouth ulcer preparations, may contain salicylates and these must be avoided. Paracetamol (acetaminophen) in moderate dosage is now the preferred analgesic and antipyretic for children below the age of 16.

Antimicrobials that may sometimes cause liver problems include tetracyclines, erythromycin and flucloxacillin. Tetracyclines in massive doses can cause liver damage, especially if there is impaired urinary excretion. Erythromycin estolate is potentially hepatotoxic but the effect is reversible when the drug is stopped (erythromycin stearate, however, is not hepatotoxic). Flucloxacillin can be cholestatic.

Box 9.5 *Hepatotoxic drugs, not including alcohol*

- Allopurinol
- Amiodarone
- Amitriptyline
- Atomoxetine
- Azathioprine
- Erythromycin estolate
- Flucloxacillin
- Halothane
- Ibuprofen
- Indometacin
- Isoniazid (INH)
- Ketoconazole
- Loratadine
- Methotrexate
- Methyldopa
- Minocycline
- Nifedipine
- Nitrofurantoin
- Oral contraceptives
- Paracetamol (acetaminophen)
- Phenytoin
- Pyrazinamide
- Rifampicin
- Sulphonamides
- Tetracyclines
- Valproic acid
- Zidovudine

Table 9.12 *Drug and chemically related liver damage*

Dose-related liver damage	Non-dose-related liver damage
Alcohol	Antithyroid drugs
Anabolic steroids	Erythromycin estolate
Isoniazid	Flucloxacillin
Ketoconazole	Halothane
Methyldopa	Nitrofurantoin
Methyltestosterone	Phenylbutazone, phenothiazines, vinyl chloride and carbon tetrachloride
Paracetamol (acetaminophen)	Phenytoin
Tetracyclines	Sulphonamides

Table 9.13 *Autoimmune hepatitis*

Clinical features	Type 1	Type 2	Type 3
Diagnostic autoantibodies	SMA	Anti-LKM	Soluble liver–kidney antigen
	ANA	P450 IID6	Cytokeratins 8 and 18
	Anti-actin	Synthetic core motif peptides 254–271	
Age mainly affected	Any	Children	Adults
Concurrent autoimmune disease (%)	41	34	58
IgG raised	+++	+	++
HLA associations	B8, DR3, DR4	B14, Dw3, C4AQO	Uncertain
Progression to cirrhosis (%)	45	82	75

ANA = antinuclear antibody; IID = ???; LKM = liver–kidney microsomal; SMA = smooth muscle antibody.

Halothane can cause hepatitis, which may follow a single exposure in 1 in 35 000 cases. Transient impairment of liver function appears after halothane as after other anaesthetics, but hepatitis is more likely when anaesthetics are given repeatedly at intervals of less than 3 months, in middle-aged females, and in the obese. The reaction may be some form of hypersensitivity, but the precise mechanism is uncertain and pre-existing liver disease does not appear to be contributory. There also appears to be a genetic susceptibility. Clinically, halothane hepatitis causes pyrexia developing after a week post-operatively. Malaise, anorexia and jaundice may then appear, and if jaundice is severe the prognosis is very poor. Unfortunately, there are no dependable criteria or laboratory tests to indicate when halothane is truly contraindicated. Serum antibodies reacting with halothane-altered liver membrane determinants have been reported in about 75% of patients but, as with antibodies to penicillin, few of these patients have a reaction on a further exposure. Halothane should never be given repeatedly, or within a period of 3 months, and never to any patient who has had malaise, pyrexia or jaundice after exposure to it. Fortunately, newer halogenated anaesthetic agents, such as enflurane, isoflurane, desflurane and sevoflurane, do not induce hepatitis in those who have had an episode of halothane hepatitis. In many hospitals, these agents have, despite their cost, replaced halothane, particularly to carry out several operations on the same patient at short intervals.

AUTOIMMUNE HEPATITIS

Autoimmune hepatitis (autoimmune liver disease; autoimmune chronic active hepatitis) is associated with various autoantibodies and the complement allele C4AQO and with HLA haplotypes B8, B14, DR3, DR4 and Dw3; it often progresses to cirrhosis. Several types of autoimmune hepatitis are recognized (Table 9.13). Multisystem manifestations are common, especially in young women, and can include acne, arthralgia, amenorrhoea, haemolytic anaemia, nephritis, pulmonary fibrosis, thyroiditis and ulcerative colitis.

Diagnosis of autoimmune hepatitis is based on the presence of elevated aminotransferase levels. More than 80% of patients with autoimmune hepatitis have hypergammaglobulinaemia, antibodies against smooth muscle, and liver–kidney microsomal antibodies. Autoimmune hepatitis is typically responsive to immunosuppressants.

FULMINANT HEPATIC FAILURE

Fulminant hepatic failure is a dangerous clinical syndrome characterized by rapid onset of hepatic encephalopathy and a marked decline in hepatic synthetic function within 28 days of the onset of symptoms, in those without a history of chronic liver disease. The aetiology of fulminant hepatic failure, when known, is mainly paracetamol (acetaminophen) overdose, other drug reactions, hepatitis B or hepatitis A.

Hepatic encephalopathy and severe coagulopathy are the hallmarks of fulminant hepatic failure. Severe coagulopathy often precedes evolution of hepatic encephalopathy to coma. As soon as the diagnosis is made, it is important to establish the cause. Certain aetiologies demand immediate specific treatment, including *N*-acetylcysteine for paracetamol (acetaminophen) poisoning, penicillin for *Amanita* mushroom poisoning, delivery of the infant in acute fatty liver of pregnancy, or zinc and trientine therapy for Wilson disease.

Overall survival is poor without liver transplantation, with a mortality of up to 97%. Patients should be admitted to the intensive care unit and transferred for liver transplantation – the only effective therapy.

CIRRHOSIS

General aspects

Cirrhosis is characterized by liver cell necrosis and inflammation, followed by replacement with fibrotic tissue and regenerating nodules of hepatocytes, and vascular derangement. Liver function deteriorates and the blood flow becomes obstructed.

Clinical features

Cirrhosis is a potentially fatal disorder. Obstruction to the portal circulation can lead to portal hypertension, oesophageal varices, gastrointestinal haemorrhage and the risk of vomiting of blood (haematemesis), which can be fatal. Thrombocytopenia from splenomegaly, and low blood clotting factor levels, leads to a bleeding tendency that can worsen the haemorrhage. Anaemia may also result. Portal obstruction can also lead to portal–systemic (hepatic) encephalopathy and tremor (liver flap or asterixis), due to failure to detoxify normal metabolites; this can be exacerbated by drugs, gastrointestinal haemorrhage or a high-protein diet and can lead to coma. Metabolism is disturbed, and sex-steroid accumulation can lead to gynaecomastia and testicular atrophy.

Spontaneous bacterial peritonitis is a potential and serious problem. Diabetes mellitus, peptic ulceration, renal dysfunction, gallstones, immune dysfunction and hepatoma are other potential complications.

The patient may develop (see Fig. 9.2): finger-clubbing, opaque nails (leukonychia), palmar erythema, asterixis, spider naevi (angiomata; Fig. 9.6), scratch marks, purpura, gynaecomastia, scant body hair, testicular atrophy, hepatomegaly, splenomegaly, distended abdominal

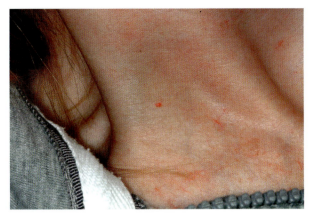

Fig 9.6 Spider naevi.

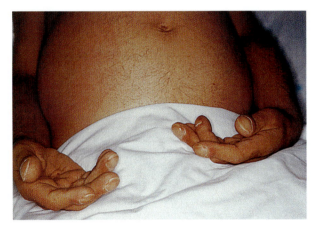

Fig. 9.7 Ascites and finger-clubbing in chronic liver disease.

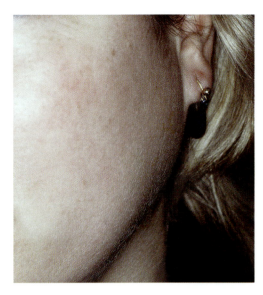

Fig. 9.8 Sialosis.

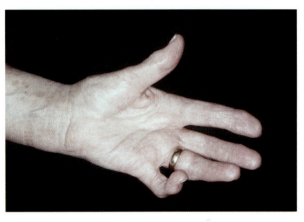

Fig. 9.9 Dupuytren contractures involve the fifth and fourth fingers in alcoholic liver disease. This may be also hereditary or have other causes.

veins in which flow is away from the umbilicus (caput medusae), ascites (fluid in the peritoneal cavity) (Fig. 9.7) and ankle oedema. Alcoholic cirrhosis may have associated parotid swelling (sialosis) (Fig. 9.8), Dupuytren contracture (Fig. 9.9), gastric ulceration or pancreatitis.

General management

The diagnosis depends on the history, physical examination, evaluation of liver function tests (see Table 9.2) and other studies. Liver enzymes, especially aminotransferases, are raised. Values of bilirubin and alkaline phosphatase are variable. Serological markers are common in autoimmune hepatitis and include IgG elevations, antinuclear antibody, smooth muscle (anti-actin) antibody, LE (lupus erythematosus) cells, rheumatoid factor, and antibodies directed against liver and kidney microsomes. CT, ultrasound or other imaging may be indicated. Liver biopsy is essential for definitive diagnosis.

Autoimmune hepatitis generally improves with treatment with corticosteroids, with or without azathioprine. Treatment for chronic HBV and HCV with interferon-alpha suppresses viral replication. Treatment of chronic HBV infection with lamivudine gives results comparable to interferon and is well tolerated, but treatment for 1–3 years is usually needed and a mutant strain of the virus often emerges. Treatment with adefovir dipivoxil is another choice. Chronic HCV is treated with a combination of ribavirin plus interferon-alpha or PEG-IFN.

Prognosis is highly variable and patients with chronic hepatitis often survive years or decades, but often hepatocellular failure, cirrhosis or both eventually follow. Liver transplantation is fairly successful for HCV-related hepatitis and long-term survival rates are relatively high.

Transplantation has not generally been effective for HBV end-stage liver disease because of aggressive disease recurrence in the graft, but treatment with lamivudine can now help ameliorate it.

In cirrhosis, laboratory tests for haemochromatosis or Wilson disease are specific but many others are non-specific. Serum albumin is often low but bilirubin, immunoglobulins, transaminases and alkaline phosphatase may be raised. Haematological abnormalities include a prolonged prothrombin time, thrombocytopenia, anaemia, macrocytosis and sometimes leukocytosis.

Treatments that can stop or delay further progression and complications include treatment of any viral cause, and interferon to inhibit activation of hepatic stellate cells and degradation of the collagenous matrix by metalloproteinases, activated by tissue inhibitor of metalloproteinases (TIMP). Adequate nutrition should be maintained and management is mainly directed towards prevention and treatment of complications. For example, for ascites and oedema, a low-sodium diet or the use of diuretics may help. For portal hypertension, beta-blockers may be needed. Varices are managed by ligation, beta-blockers and possibly transjugular intrahepatic portosystemic shunting. Encephalopathy can be managed with a low-protein diet supplemented with ornithine, aspartate, benzoate or phenylacetate. Lactulose plus neomycin may also be used.

The molecular absorbent recirculating system (MARS) removes water-soluble and protein-bound toxins that accumulate in liver failure, based on an albumin-filled circuit recirculating through a charcoal and colestyramine column.

Liver transplantation is necessary when complications cannot be controlled, or when the liver becomes so damaged that it ceases functioning.

Dental aspects

Patients can present serious bleeding problems if surgery is needed. Certain drugs may be contraindicated. There may be a risk from transmission of infection. Surgery is hazardous also because of possible HCV or HBV carriage, or infection, diabetes, anaemia, drug therapy, poor wound healing and a liability to peritonitis. The hepatologist should be consulted if surgery, GA or drug therapy is needed. A clotting screen and prothrombin time may be indicated. If the prothrombin time is prolonged, vitamin K1 10 mg parenterally (phytomenadione) should be given daily for several days preoperatively to improve haemostatic function. If there is an inadequate response, as shown by the prothrombin time, a transfusion of fresh blood or plasma may be required. Repeated gastrointestinal bleeding may cause anaemia (Ch. 8) or be fatal.

Routine dental treatment can usually be carried out without any particular problem, though alcoholism may influence treatment planning and procedures (Ch. 34).

Impaired drug detoxification and excretion mean that drug effects are not entirely predictable: age, gender, the type and severity of the liver disease, hypoalbuminaemia (depressed protein-binding of drugs) and the induction of hepatic drug-metabolizing enzymes by previous medication may influence outcomes of drug use. Especial care must be taken when considering the use of drugs, particularly some analgesics, antimicrobials and drugs exerting their effect on the central nervous system (CNS; see Table 9.7). Drugs that are hepatotoxic should obviously be avoided.

LA is safe given in normal doses, but prilocaine or articaine is preferred to lidocaine. Drugs liable to cause respiratory depression are dangerous and coma can be precipitated by sedatives, hypnotics or opioids. The doses of midazolam used for CS should thus be reduced. Inhalational sedation is preferable. Nitrous oxide with pethidine or phenoperidine appears to be suitable for GA but it is essential to avoid hypoxia; isoflurane or sevoflurane is preferable to halothane (see 'halothane hepatitis' earlier). Desflurane should be used in lower-than-normal doses. Suxamethonium is best avoided because of impaired cholinesterase activity.

Aspirin and most other NSAIDs, such as indometacin, should be avoided because of the risk of gastric haemorrhage in those with portal hypertension or peptic ulcers. Analgesia is best achieved with paracetamol (acetaminophen) or codeine used in lower-than-normal doses.

Antimicrobials that can usually be used safely in normal doses include penicillin, cefalexin, cefazolin and imipenem. Broad-spectrum antibiotics (at least in theory) should be avoided as they may further reduce vitamin K availability by destroying the gut flora.

If a jaundiced patient must undergo major surgery, aggressive treatment with intravenous fluids and diuresis with mannitol are indicated to avoid acute renal failure, which may complicate hepatic failure (hepatorenal syndrome; Ch. 12). There may also be considerations related to alcoholism (Ch. 34), autoimmune disease, hepatitis B, C or D antigen carriage or diabetes (Ch. 6).

Spontaneous bacterial peritonitis is a potential problem in cirrhosis with ascites. Though most infections are with normal gut aerobic bacteria or Gram-positive bacteria, invasive dental or oral surgical procedures may increase the risk and, since the mortality approaches 30%, antibiotic prophylaxis must be considered. Amoxicillin orally 2–3 g with metronidazole 1 hour preoperatively or intravenous imipenem is recommended.

Some patients have sialosis, or tooth erosion from gastric regurgitation. There is an association between liver cirrhosis and oral carcinoma.

PRIMARY BILIARY CIRRHOSIS

General aspects

Primary biliary cirrhosis (PBC) is an uncommon, progressive, autoimmune disorder with antibodies directed against mitochondrial pyruvate dehydrogenase complex, affecting small intrahepatic bile ducts; it is seen mainly in middle-aged women. PBC begins with non-suppurative destructive cholangitis and jaundice, and culminates in cirrhosis.

Clinical features

Patients with PBC may be asymptomatic for many years but, eventually, complaints of weakness, lethargy, weight loss, pale stools, dark urine, jaundice and pruritus emerge. Complications include xanthomas and skin pigmentation, or the complications of any chronic liver disease. Osteoporosis and connective tissue diseases, particularly systemic sclerosis (scleroderma) or Sjögren syndrome, may occur.

General management

PBC must be distinguished from other conditions with similar symptoms, such as *autoimmune hepatitis* or *primary sclerosing cholangitis*. The biochemical features of PBC resemble those of obstructive jaundice with raised serum alkaline phosphatase and elevated AST, ALT and GGT levels. Antibodies against mitochondria are found in about 90%. Approximately 50% have antinuclear antibodies, sometimes against proteins specific to nuclear components; the M2-IgG antimitochondrial antibody is the most specific test.

Antinuclear antibodies appear to be prognostic agents in PBC; *anti-glycoprotein-210 antibodies* and, to a lesser degree, *anti-p62 antibodies* correlate with progression toward end-stage liver failure. *Anticentromere antibodies* correlate with development of portal hypertension.

Abdominal ultrasound or a CT scan is usually performed to rule out blockage to the bile ducts. Previously, most suspected sufferers underwent a liver biopsy and – if uncertainty remained – endoscopic retrograde cholangiopancreatography (ERCP; an endoscopic investigation of the bile duct). Now most patients are diagnosed without invasive investigation since the combination of antimitochondrial antibodies and typical (cholestatic) liver function tests is considered diagnostic. Liver biopsy is still necessary to determine the stage of disease.

Medical treatment includes colestyramine to relieve pruritus, vitamins and calcium for osteoporosis prevention, and oral medium-chain triglycerides to improve nutrition. Ursodeoxycholic acid may help improve laboratory values but the effect on prognosis is unclear. Colchicine may play a role in inhibiting liver fibrosis and improves laboratory values but not signs or symptoms.

Orthotopic liver transplantation is highly successful for end-stage liver disease resulting from PBC.

Dental aspects

Patients with PBC may present similar management problems to those with other parenchymal liver diseases. Sjögren syndrome complicates 70% or more cases of PBC. Telangiectasias may be seen and oral lichen planus is an occasional complication. Penicillamine, once used for treatment, occasionally caused thrombocytopenia, polymyositis, pemphigus or myasthenia, and also caused lichenoid lesions, oral ulceration and loss of taste.

PRIMARY SCLEROSING CHOLANGITIS

Primary sclerosing cholangitis (PSC) is an autoimmune form of cholangitis that leads to accumulation of bile; this damages the liver, leading in turn to jaundice and liver failure.

LIVER CANCER

General aspects

Cancer of hepatocytes is termed hepatocellular carcinoma (HCC) or malignant hepatoma. Common in Africa, South-East Asia, Japan and some Mediterranean countries (areas of high endemicity for HBV and HCV), it is uncommon in the USA and UK – where metastatic cancer to the liver from the colon, lungs, breasts, uterus or other parts of the body is far more common.

Risk factors for HCC include male gender, old age, a positive family history, chronic HCV or HBV, oral contraceptive use and cirrhosis. Aflatoxin, a mould that forms on peanuts, corn and other nuts and grains, is an important cause in Asia and Africa.

Clinical features

Liver cancer in the early stages often causes no symptoms. Later manifestations may include wasting, jaundice, pain or swelling in the abdomen, anorexia and fever.

General management

High alpha-fetoprotein serum levels can be a feature of liver cancer. Ultrasound, isotope and MRI scans, and biopsy are often needed for diagnosis.

Treatment usually consists of surgical resection (partial hepatectomy) but the prognosis is invariably poor. Liver transplantation may be required.

Radiotherapy, chemotherapy and targeted therapy may be used. Image-guided radiation therapy (IGRT) and respiratory gating may reduce toxicity. Doxorubicin alone or in combination with cisplatin, 5-fluorouracil and interferon (PIAF) is a chemotherapeutic approach that has improved survival for some. For HCC, anti-angiogenic drugs are the most common targeted therapy (sorafenib). More information on treatment options may be found at: http://www.cancer.net/cancer-types/liver-cancer/treatment (accessed 30 September 2013).

Dental aspects

There appear to be no significant dental considerations other than those applying to other types of severe liver disease.

EXTRAHEPATIC BILIARY OBSTRUCTION

General aspects

The main causes of extrahepatic biliary obstruction are gallstones and carcinoma of the pancreas (Ch. 7). Gallstones are common with advancing age, particularly in females. Around 10–20% of adults have gallstones but most are symptomless. About 80% of the stones contain cholesterol, while others are bile-pigment stones. The aetiology of cholesterol stones is usually unclear but some patients with Crohn disease or those on clofibrate, oral contraceptives or oestrogens appear to be susceptible. Pigment gallstones may complicate chronic haemolytic anaemias (hereditary spherocytosis, thalassaemia or sickle cell anaemia).

Clinical features

Gallstones are often asymptomatic but passage of the stones into the bile ducts can precipitate pain because of biliary colic, acute cholecystitis or acute pancreatitis. Extrahepatic biliary obstruction causes jaundice, pruritus, dark urine and pale stools with impaired absorption of fats and of vitamin K.

General management

There is usually a rise in serum bilirubin esters, alkaline phosphatase, 5′-nucleotidase, GGT and transaminases. Diagnosis may be by ultrasound and ERCP. Lithotripsy and medical treatment with chenodeoxycholic acid or ursodeoxycholic acid have a place in the treatment of asymptomatic stones. Cholecystectomy is usually indicated if obstructive jaundice develops.

Dental aspects

The main danger in surgery is excessive bleeding resulting from vitamin K malabsorption. Surgical intervention should therefore be deferred wherever possible in the presence of jaundice until haemostatic function returns to normal. If surgery is essential, vitamin K1 should be given parenterally for several days in an attempt to correct the bleeding tendency (Ch. 8).

GA in a severely jaundiced patient can lead to renal failure (hepatorenal syndrome).

POSTOPERATIVE JAUNDICE

Postoperative jaundice is discussed in Chapter 3 and its causes are listed in Table 9.14.

Table 9.14 *Causes of postoperative jaundice*

Excessive bilirubin load	Hepatocellular disease	Others
Haemolysis due to haemolytic anaemia or incompatible transfusions	Gilbert syndrome	Bile duct damage
	Viral hepatitis	Obstructive jaundice
Resorption of blood from large haematoma	Halothane and other drug-induced hepatitis	Sepsis
		Shock
		Gallstone disease
		Pancreatitis

LIVER TRANSPLANTATION

General aspects

Liver transplantation is provided for treatment of end-stage liver disease, such as from biliary atresia, metabolic disease, cirrhosis or malignancy. Usually, the liver is obtained from a cadaveric or brain-dead donor. Fortunately, even pieces of liver, when transplanted, will grow into a normal size. *Deceased organ transplantation* involves transplanting a liver that has been removed from a person who recently died. In *living donor liver transplantation*, a section of liver is removed from a living donor and used for transplant. *Split donation transplantation* is when a liver is removed from a person who recently died and then split into two pieces, each piece then being transplanted into a different patient.

The 1-year survival after liver transplantation is around 80% and, of survivors, 90% survive 5 years and 85% for 10 years. Graft-versus-host disease can follow liver transplantation (Ch. 35).

Several extracorporeal bioartificial liver devices are also undergoing clinical evaluation.

General management

All liver transplant recipients require lifelong immunosuppression with agents such as corticosteroids and calcineurin inhibitors to prevent a T-cell, alloimmune rejection response. TNFα inhibitors and other biological therapies may play an important role in solid-organ transplantation.

Liver transplant recipients may be susceptible to infections with viruses and/or fungi and to recurrence of their original disease; they may develop recurrence of hepatitis B or C, alcoholic liver disease, one of the autoimmune hepatitides, or diabetes, kidney disease, post-transplant lymphoproliferative syndrome or malignant neoplasms (Ch. 35).

The severity of hepatitis recurrence varies from mild to development of progressive allograft failure. Hepatitis B immunoglobulin is available for the prevention of hepatitis B reinfection in liver transplant patients. HCV recurrence after transplantation is almost universal but the extent of the graft damage is variable. The survival in the short term is not significantly affected, but concerns exist regarding long-term recurrence because the rate of developing cirrhosis at 5 years can be as high as 8–25%. Type 2 diabetes is a common and potentially serious complication of a liver transplantation, affecting about 1 in 5 people.

More information on liver transplantation may be found at: http://www.nhs.uk/conditions/Liver-transplant/Pages/Introduction.aspx (accessed 30 September 2013).

Dental aspects

In addition to those discussed in Chapter 35, dental aspects include:

- liver failure (bleeding tendencies, impaired drug metabolism)

- retarded tooth eruption and discoloured and hypoplastic teeth in children needing liver transplants
- gingival swelling in patients on ciclosporin or some other drugs.

KEY WEBSITES

(Accessed 27 May 2013)
BMJ. <http://www.bmj.com/specialties/liver-disease>.
National Institutes of Health. <http://health.nih.gov/topic/LiverDiseasesGeneral>.

USEFUL WEBSITES

(Accessed 27 May 2013)
Macmillan. <http://www.macmillan.org.uk/Cancerinformation/Cancertypes/AtoZ.aspx>.
MedlinePlus. <http://www.nlm.nih.gov/medlineplus/hepatitis.html>.
NHS Choices. <http://www.nhs.uk/Conditions/Pages/hub.aspx>.
Wikipedia. Cirrhosis. <http://en.wikipedia.org/wiki/Cirrhosis>.
Wikipedia. Hepatitis. <http://en.wikipedia.org/wiki/Hepatitis>.

FURTHER READING

Aimetti, M., et al. 2008. Non-surgical periodontal treatment of cyclosporin A-induced gingival overgrowth: immunohistochemical results. Oral Dis. 14, 244.
Carrozzo, M., 2008. Oral diseases associated with hepatitis C virus infection. Part 1. Sialadenitis and salivary glands lymphoma. Oral Dis. 14, 123.
Ferreiro, M.C., et al. 2005. Transmission of hepatitis C virus by saliva? Oral Dis. 11, 230.
Golecka, M., et al. 2007. Influence of oral hygiene habits on prosthetic stomatitis complicated by mucosal infection after organ transplantation. Transplant Proc. 39, 2875.
Guggenheimer, J., et al. 2007. Dental health status of liver transplant candidates. Liver Transpl. 13, 280.
Kajiya, T., et al. 2008. Pyogenic liver abscess related to dental disease in an immunocompetent host. Intern Med 47, 675.
Lodi, G., et al. 2002. Infectious hepatitis C, hepatitis G, and TT virus: review and implications for dentists. Special Care Dent. 22, 53.
Lodi, G., et al. 2000. Hepatitis G virus-associated oral lichen planus; no influence from hepatitis G virus co-infection. J. Oral Pathol. Med. 29, 39.
Modi, A.A., Liang, T.J., 2008. Hepatitis C: a clinical review. Oral Dis. 14, 10.
Naudi, A.B., et al. 2008. A report of 2 cases of green pigmentation in the primary dentition associated with cholestasis caused by sepsis. J. Dent. Child (Chic) 75, 91.
Perry, J.L., et al. 2006. Infected health care workers and patient safety: a double standard. Am. J. Infect. Control 34, 313.
Redd, J.T, et al. 2007. Patient-to-patient transmission of hepatitis B virus associated with oral surgery. J. Infect. Dis. 195, 1311.
Rustemeyer, J., Bremerich, A., 2007. Necessity of surgical dental foci treatment prior to organ transplantation and heart valve replacement. Clin. Oral Invest. 11, 171.
Scully, C., Chaudhry, S., 2007. Aspects of human disease 15. Chronic liver disease. Dent. Update 43, 525.
Scully, C, Chaudhry, SI., 2007. Aspects of human disease. Dent. Update 34, 525.
Valerin, M.A., et al. 2007. Modified Child–Pugh score as a marker for postoperative bleeding from invasive dental procedures. Oral Surg. Oral Med. Oral Pathol. Oral Radiol. Endod. 104, 56.

APPENDIX 9.1 SYNDROMES WITH CONGENITAL HYPERBILIRUBINAEMIA

	Gilbert	Crigler–Najjar	Dubin–Johnson	Rotor
Prevalence	Common	Rare	Rare	Rare
Prognosis	Usually benign	May be fatal	Benign	Benign
Bilirubinaemia	Unconjugated	Unconjugated	Conjugated	Conjugated
Pigment in urine	–	–	+	+
Associated problems	–	Kernicterus	–	–
Comments	May become jaundiced after GA but no other clinical problems	Serious disease	No clinical problems Liver pigmented	Liver not pigmented

APPENDIX 9.2 HEALTH PROTECTION AGENCY GUIDANCE

UK ADVISORY PANEL FOR HEALTHCARE WORKERS INFECTED WITH BLOODBORNE VIRUSES (UKAP)

Information on UKAP is available in the Infections A-Z under the 'Blood-borne viruses and occupational exposure' tab at: http://www. hpa.org.uk/Topics/InfectiousDiseases/ (accessed 30 September 2013).

The panel is available for consultation:

- when advice is needed regarding restricting the practice of HCPs infected with blood-borne viruses
- when a lookback exercise may be needed as a result of exposure-prone procedures being undertaken on patients by an HCP infected with a blood-borne virus
- for general advice concerning the categorization of clinical procedures as exposure-prone.

The panel works within the framework of government guidance concerning HCPs and blood-borne viruses, and aims to interpret the guidance in relation to individual cases on a consistent basis.

UK DEPARTMENT OF HEALTH GUIDANCE

Hepatitis B infected healthcare workers and antiviral therapy (2007)

See http://www.dh.gov.uk/en/publicationsandstatistics/publications/publicationspolicyandguidance/dh_073164 (accessed 30 September 2013).

Health clearance for tuberculosis, hepatitis B, hepatitis C and HIV: new healthcare workers (2007)

See http://www.dh.gov.uk/en/publicationsandstatistics/publications/publicationspolicyandguidance/dh_073132 (accessed 30 September 2013).

Medical and dental students: health clearance for hepatitis B, hepatitis C, HIV and tuberculosis. Medical Schools Council (February 2008)

See http://www.medschools.ac.uk/Students/howtoapply/publications/Pages/BBV.aspx (accessed 30 September 2013).

Health service circular HSC 2000/020: hepatitis B infected health care workers

See http://www.dh.gov.uk/en/publicationsandstatistics/publications/publicationspolicyandguidance/dh_4008156 (accessed 30 September 2013).

Guidance extended the previous restrictions placed upon hepatitis B-infected HCPs. Both those who carry the e antigen (i.e. are HBeAg-positive) and those who are e-antigen–negative with a viral load

(hepatitis B virus [HBV] DNA level) that exceeds 10^3 genome equivalents per millilitre are restricted from performing exposure-prone procedures. The guidance names two dedicated laboratories in the UK where tests for HBV DNA are to be carried out using a specified assay and standardized controls.

Hepatitis B-infected HCPs who are HBeAg-negative and do not have an HBV DNA level exceeding 10^3 are not restricted from performing exposure-prone procedures but are subject to exposure-prone procedures.

Protecting health-care workers and patients from hepatitis B

The guidance recommends that carriers of the hepatitis B virus who are known to be e-antigen–positive must not carry out procedures where there is a risk that injury to themselves will result in their blood contaminating a patient's open tissues. Such procedures are termed 'exposure-prone procedures':

- Addendum to HSG(93)40: *Protecting health care workers and patients from hepatitis B* (April 2004)
- Addendum to HSG(93)40: *Protecting health care workers and patients from hepatitis B* (26 September 1996)
- *Protecting health care workers and patients from hepatitis B* (HSG[93]40)
- *Protecting health care workers and patients from hepatitis B* (*Olive Book*).

Health service circular HSC 2002/010: hepatitis C infected health care workers

Guidance recommends that HCPs known to be infected with hepatitis C and who are viraemic (i.e. HCV RNA-positive) should not perform exposure-prone procedures. The guidelines also recommend that HCPs intending to embark upon careers that rely upon the performance of exposure-prone procedures should be tested for hepatitis C (antibodies and, if positive, HCV RNA). This would mean prospective dental students before entry into dental schools. The guidelines are intended to apply to prospective students for undergraduate training, and not to those already qualified who are seeking postgraduate training. As in the HIV guidance, there is also a section about those at risk coming forward for testing for hepatitis C.

Guidance for clinical health care workers: protection against infection with blood-borne viruses (HSC 1998/063)

See http://www.dh.gov.uk/en/publicationsandstatistics/publications/publicationspolicyandguidance/dh_4002766 (accessed 30 September 2013). This booklet contains guidance on measures to protect clinical HCPs against occupational infection with blood-borne viruses. It is based on the recommendations of the Expert Advisory Group on AIDS and the Advisory Group on Hepatitis. It draws also on work done by the Advisory Committee on Dangerous Pathogens and the Microbiology Advisory Committee.

10 Mental health

Mental health problems include mental illness; medically unexplained symptoms (MUS – formerly termed psychogenic problems); dementia, discussed in Chapter 13; and learning impairment, discussed in Chapter 28. The brain is a highly complex organ, the functions of many areas remaining unclear (Fig. 10.1). The rapid and widespread effects of mental reactions and emotions can readily be seen from the vasodilatation with blushing seen in anger, anxiety or embarrassment (Fig. 10.2).

All systems of mental disorders and diagnosis stem from the work of Kraepelin, who claimed that certain groups of symptoms often occur together, thus allowing us to call them *diseases* or *syndromes*.

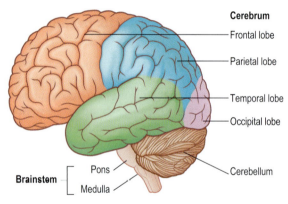

Fig. 10.1 Brain structure.

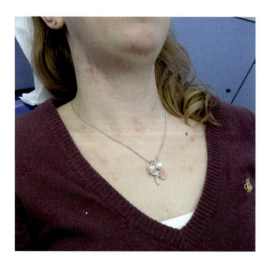

Fig. 10.2 Blushing – an almost immediate vasodilatation emanating from a mental reaction to anxiety, anger or embarrassment.

He regarded each mental illness as distinct, with its own origins, symptoms, course and outcomes, and identified two major groups:

- *Dementia praecox* (schizophrenia)
- *Manic-depressive psychosis*.

This helped to establish the organic nature of mental disorders and formed the basis of the *Diagnostic and Statistical Manual of Mental Disorders* (DSM), the official classification system of the American Psychiatric Association (APA), and the World Health Organization's *International Classification of Diseases* (ICD; see below). The Diagnostic and Statistical Manual of Mental Disorders (5th ed.; DSM–5; American Psychiatric Association [APA], 2013) is the most widely accepted up-to-date nomenclature used for the classification of mental disorders. Kraepelin's classification is also embodied in the Mental Health Act 1983, which contains three major categories of mental disturbances – mental illness, personality disorder and mental impairment.

Most disorders are caused by the interaction of:

- biological factors
- sociological factors
- psychological factors.

Genetics plays a role in shaping our personality and consequently our psychological status. The interactions of genetic and environmental factors are believed to cause a number of mental health problems ranging from autism (Ch. 28) to bipolar disorder.

Life stresses, such as bereavement and divorce, can play a significant role in mental health. Lifestyles can also influence mental health; brisk exercise can, by stimulating release of noradrenaline and endorphins, lift depression and create a sense of euphoria. Sunlight stimulates the pineal gland to release serotonin and melatonin, which influence mood. This is one reason why more people tend to be depressed during the darker winter months – seasonal affective disorder (SAD).

Although mental health and mental illness are related, they represent different psychological states.

Mental health is 'a state of well-being in which the individual realizes his or her own abilities, can cope with the normal stresses of life, can work productively and fruitfully, and is able to make a contribution to his or her community'. Indicators of mental health include the following:

- Emotional well-being – such as perceived life satisfaction, happiness, cheerfulness, peacefulness.
- Psychological well-being – such as self-acceptance, personal growth including openness to new experiences, optimism, hopefulness, purpose in life, control of one's environment, spirituality, self-direction and positive relationships.
- Social well-being: social acceptance, belief in the potential of people and society as a whole, personal self-worth and usefulness to society, sense of community. The social determinants of mental health include adequate housing, safe neighbourhoods, equitable jobs and wages, quality education, and equity in access to quality health care.

Good mental health is not just the absence of diagnosable mental health problems but is characterized by the ability to:

- learn
- feel, express and manage a range of positive and negative emotions
- form and maintain good relationships with others
- cope with and manage change and uncertainty.

Mental (psychiatric) illness is defined as 'collectively all diagnosable mental disorders' or 'health conditions that are characterized by alterations in thinking, mood, or behaviour (or some combination thereof) associated with distress and/or impaired functioning'.

Depression is the most common type of mental illness and it has been estimated that depression will soon be the second leading cause of disability throughout the world, trailing only ischaemic heart disease. Evidence has shown that mental disorders, especially depressive disorders, are strongly related to the occurrence, successful treatment and course of many chronic diseases, including diabetes, cancer, cardiovascular disease, asthma, obesity and many risk behaviours for chronic disease, such as physical inactivity, smoking, excessive drinking and insufficient sleep.

When people experience severe and/or enduring mental health problems, they are sometimes described as mentally ill but there is no universally agreed cut-off point at which behaviour becomes abnormal enough to be termed mental illness. In any event, the term can imply that all such problems are caused solely by medical or biological factors, whereas most seem to result from complex interactions of medical, biological, social and/or psychological factors.

Personality disorder is defined as 'an enduring pattern of inner experience and behaviours that deviates markedly from the expectation of the individual's culture, is pervasive and inflexible, has an onset in adolescence or early adulthood, is stable over time and leads to distress or impairment'.

Mental health problems traditionally have been classified as *organic* (identifiable brain disease) or *functional* (no obvious brain structural abnormality); or as *neuroses* or *psychoses*. The term 'neuroses' covers those symptoms that can be regarded as severe forms of 'normal' emotional experiences, such as depression, anxiety or panic; they are now more often called 'common mental health problems' and include anxiety (with insight retained), depression, phobias, and obsessive–compulsive and panic disorders. Psychoses are less common and manifest with symptoms that constitute a severe distortion of a person's perception of reality with loss of insight; they may include hallucinations such as seeing, hearing, smelling or feeling things that no one else can, and also severe and enduring mental health problems such as schizophrenia and bipolar affective disorder (manic depression).

Several diagnostic and classification frameworks have been developed to help identify mental health problems. As mentioned earlier, the two main ones are the ICD (the current one is version 10 – ICD-10) and the DSM (the latest is version 4 revised – DSM-IV-TR); these classify mental health problems in a series of families or categories (Box 10.1).

Therapies include psychotherapy and various psychoactive medications. Cognitive–behavioural therapy (CBT) is an increasingly used short-term, problem-focused psychosocial intervention. Evidence from randomised controlled trials and meta-analyses shows that CBT can be an effective intervention for depression, panic disorder, generalised anxiety and obsessive–compulsive disorder, and its usefulness in a growing range of other issues such as health anxiety/hypochondriasis, social phobia, schizophrenia and bipolar disorders. Most patients are

---

Box 10.1 *International Classification of Diseases (ICD) 1 F00–F99: mental and behavioural disorders*

1.1. (F00–F09) Organic, including symptomatic, mental disorders
1.2. (F10–F19) Mental and behavioural disorders due to psychoactive substance use
1.3. (F20–F29) Schizophrenia, schizotypal and delusional disorders
1.4. (F30–F39) Mood (affective) disorders
1.5. (F40–F48) Neurotic, stress-related and somatoform disorders
1.6. (F50–F59) Behavioural syndromes associated with physiological disturbances and physical factors
1.7. (F60–F69) Disorders of adult personality and behaviour
1.8. (F70–F79) Mental retardation
1.9. (F80–F89) Disorders of psychological development
1.10. (F90–F98) Behavioural and emotional disorders with onset usually occurring in childhood and adolescence
1.11. (F99) Unspecified mental disorder

---

cared for in the community, with rare recourse to 'sectioning' (admission to hospital against a patient's will). In the UK, under the Mental Health Act 1983, intended to help doctors manage patients with a mental disorder, patients can be sectioned or detained against their will and given treatment. The types of defined 'mental disorder' include 'severe mental impairment', 'psychopathic disorder' or 'mental illness'. Under the Act, patients can be sectioned if they are perceived to be a threat to themselves or others.

A patient can only be sectioned if an approved social worker or a close relative and two doctors believe it is necessary. One of these doctors is usually a psychiatrist, while the other knows the patient well, but in an emergency a single doctor's recommendation may be sufficient.

If a patient is sectioned as an emergency case, they may then be detained under section 4 of the Mental Health Act for up to 72 hours. If doctors believe that further assessment or treatment is necessary, then the patient can be detained under section 2 of the Act, meaning that they can be admitted to hospital and detained for up to 28 days to undergo a full psychiatric assessment. At the end of the 28-day period, if the medical recommendation is for the patient's stay in hospital to be extended, section 3 of the Act permits a further 6-month extension. A patient can be discharged from hospital at any time if doctors believe they are no longer a threat to themselves or anyone else.

LEGISLATION

Legislation and policy decisions affect individuals' rights and, in particular, their entitlement to health-care provision, including oral health care. Legislation in the UK has evolved significantly over recent years to protect the rights of the individual, and a summary is presented below.

MENTAL HEALTH ACTS 1983 AND 2007

This Act is primarily concerned with the care and treatment of people with a mental health problem that requires that they be detained or treated in the interests of their own health and safety or with a view to protecting other people. It is now 30 years old and new legislation was passed through parliament in the form of the Mental Health Act 2007.

Table 10.1 *Main parts and functions of the brain*

Main part of brain (see Fig. 10.1)		Neurological functions	Mental and other functions
Supratentorial	Cerebrum	Initiation of movement, coordination of movement, temperature, touch, vision, hearing	Higher functions, memory, judgment, ideas, reasoning, problem-solving, emotions, learning
			Skilful intellectual tasks (e.g. reading, writing, mathematical calculations)
			Limbic system contains several nuclei of grey matter around the brainstem; it commands certain behaviours necessary for survival, e.g. distinction between agreeable and disagreeable; affective functions are developed, e.g. inducing females to nurse and protect their toddlers, or inducing playful moods. Emotions and feelings, like anger, fright, passion, love, hate, joy and sadness, originate in the limbic system, which is also responsible for aspects of personal identity and important functions related to memory
	Brainstem, including mid-brain, pons and medulla	Movement of eyes and mouth, relaying sensory messages (i.e. heat, pain, loudness), hunger, respiration, consciousness, cardiac function, body temperature, involuntary muscle movements, sneezing, coughing, vomiting, swallowing	Self-preservation. Mechanisms of aggression and repetitive behaviour. Instinctive reactions of the so-called reflex arcs and the commands that allow some involuntary actions and control of visceral functions (cardiac, pulmonary, intestinal, etc.)
Infratentorial	Cerebellum	Coordination of voluntary muscle movements and maintenance of posture, balance, equilibrium	–

MENTAL CAPACITY ACT 2005

This Act is relevant to everyone involved in the care, treatment or support of people aged 16 years and over in England and Wales who lack capacity to make all or some decisions for themselves. It also applies to situations where a person may lack capacity to make a decision at a particular time due to illness, drugs or alcohol. Assessments of capacity should be time- and decision-specific.

The Act clarifies the terms 'mental capacity' and 'lack of mental capacity', and says that a person is unable to make a particular decision if they cannot do one or more of the following:

- Understand information given to them
- Retain that information for long enough to be able to make the decision
- Weigh up the information available to make the decision
- Communicate their decision; this could be done, for example, by talking, using sign language or even simple muscle movements, such as blinking an eye or squeezing a hand.

The new criminal offence of ill treatment or wilful neglect of people who lack capacity also came into force in 2007. Within the law, 'helping with personal hygiene' (including tooth-brushing) attracts protection from liability as long as the individual giving this assistance has complied with the Act by assessing a person's capacity and acting in their best interests. 'Best-interest' decisions made on behalf of people who lack capacity should place the fewest restrictions possible on their basic rights and freedoms.

Further changes within the Act include the introduction of *lasting powers of attorney* (LPA), which extend to health and welfare decisions. When a health professional has a significant concern relating to decisions about serious medical treatment taken under the authority of an LPA, the case can be referred for adjudication to the Court of Protection, which is ultimately responsible for the proper functioning of the legislation. The Act also created an *Office of the Public Guardian*, which has responsibility for the registration and supervision of both LPAs and court-appointed deputies. Furthermore, independent mental capacity advocates were introduced to support particularly vulnerable incapacitated adults – most often those who lack any other forms of external support – in making certain decisions.

DENTAL ASPECTS

Preventive dentistry is crucial in patients with mental health problems. The individual may neglect oral hygiene, dental appointments and instructions unless a caregiver or family member is also involved. Dental staff must use great tact, patience and a sympathetic, unpatronizing manner in handling patients with mental health problems. To avoid causing adverse drug interactions, special precautions should be taken when administering certain antibiotics, analgesics and sedatives. The treatment should be given in the morning, when cooperation tends to be best, with the usual caretakers present and in a familiar environment, and time must be allowed to explain every procedure before it is carried out. The patient should be treated while sitting upright in the dental chair or slightly reclined, to avoid aspiration and postural hypotension (Ch. 5).

Mental health is often affected by social, psychological, biological, genetic and environmental factors, as well as by changes in the brain neurotransmitters of the central nervous system (CNS) (Table 10.1).

Emotion is not a function of any specific brain area but of a circuit that involves interconnected basic structures: the hypothalamus, the anterior thalamic nucleus, the cingulate gyrus, the hippocampus, the prefrontal area, the parahippocampal gyrus and subcortical groupings like the amygdala, the medial thalamic nucleus, the septal area, the basal nuclei and a few brainstem formations (Table 10.2)

BIOLOGICAL ASPECTS

BRAIN NEUROTRANSMITTERS

Brain neurotransmitters include monoamines, acetylcholine (ACh), amino acids, gamma-aminobutyric acid (GABA), peptides, substance P and opioids (Table 10.3).

Monoamines include catecholamines (noradrenaline [norepinephrine], adrenaline [epinephrine] and dopamine), serotonin (5-hydroxytryptamine; 5-HT) and histamine. Noradrenaline is released by post-ganglionic neurons of the sympathetic branch of the autonomic nervous system. ACh mediates transmission at brain synapses involved in the acquisition of short-term memory. Amino acids such as glutamic

Table 10.2 *Main parts and functions of the brain involved with emotion and mood*

Brain area	Emotions/moods
Amygdala	Mediates and controls major affective activities like friendship, love and affection, expressions of mood and fear, rage and aggression
Cingulate gyrus	Coordinates smells and sights with pleasant memories of previous emotions and participates in the emotional reaction to pain and regulation of aggressive behaviour
Hippocampus	Responsible for long-term memory
Hypothalamus	Connects with other prosencephalic areas and the mesencephalus. Involved with several vegetative functions and some so-called motivated behaviours, like thermal regulations, sexuality, combativeness, hunger and thirst. Also plays a role in emotion, e.g. pleasure, rage, aversion and laughing
Nucleus accumbens	Responsible for pleasurable sensations, some of them similar to orgasm
Septal region	Associated with different kinds of pleasant sensations, mainly those related to sexual experiences. Anterior frontal lobe is important in the genesis and expression of affection, joy, sadness, hope or despair, as well as the capacity for concentration, problem-solving and abstraction
Thalamus	Associated with emotional reactivity due to connections with other limbic system structures. The medial dorsal nucleus connects with the frontal area and hypothalamus. The anterior nuclei connect with the mammillary bodies and, through them, via the fornix, with the hippocampus and cingulate gyrus

acid (Glu) are involved in transmission at excitatory synapses and are essential for long-term potentiation (LTP), a form of memory. GABA is released at inhibitory synapses to hyperpolarize the post-synaptic membrane, resulting in an inhibitory post-synaptic potential (IPSP). Peptides not only serve as brain neurotransmitters but some are also hormones; these include vasopressin (antidiuretic hormone; ADH), oxytocin, gonadotropin-releasing hormone (GnRH), angiotensin II and cholecystokinin (CCK). Other transmitters include substance P, which transmits pain impulses and opioids – a term used for all enkephalins, endorphins and morphine-like peptide chemicals, including dynorphin.

Enkephalins (from the Greek *kephale*, meaning head) are pentapeptides. One enkephalin, leu-enkephalin, terminates in a leucine; the other, met-enkephalin, terminates in a methionine. Enkephalins are released at synapses on neurons involved in transmitting pain signals to the brain and act as an intrinsic pain-suppressing system, hyperpolarizing the post-synaptic membrane and thus inhibiting pain signals.

Endorphins are small-chain peptides that activate opiate receptors, producing feelings of well-being, as well as tolerance to pain. These compounds are hundreds or even thousands of times more potent than morphine. Four groups of endorphins – alpha, beta, gamma and sigma – have been identified.

Dynorphins are other brain opioid peptides.

Factors that influence the production of enkephalins, endorphins and dynorphins include prolonged strenuous activity, transcutaneous electrical nerve stimulation (TENS), acupuncture and placebos. Enkephalins and endorphins bind to neuroreceptors in the brain to give relief from pain. This effect appears to be responsible for the so-called 'runner's high', the temporary loss of pain after severe injury, and the analgesic effects that acupuncture and chiropractic adjustments of the spine can offer.

Enkephalins are found especially in the thalamus and in parts of the spinal cord that transmit pain impulses, and in the adrenal medulla.

They act as analgesics and sedatives, and appear to affect mood and motivation. Blood levels rise after exercise and sexual activity, and may explain how a severely wounded person can continue to function. Endorphins may act to prevent the release of substance P, which may account for the sedating effects of endogenous endorphins and of opioids given therapeutically. Endorphins also have anti-ageing effects by removing superoxide, anti-stress activity, pain-relieving effects and memory-improving activity. Endorphins may link the emotional state of well-being and the health of the immune system.

Once any neurotransmitter has acted, it must be removed from the synaptic cleft, usually by reuptake or breakdown, to prepare the synapse for the arrival of the next action potential. All the neurotransmitters except ACh do this via reuptake. ACh is removed from the synapse by enzymatic breakdown by acetylcholinesterase into inactive fragments.

OTHER FACTORS THAT AFFECT MENTAL HEALTH

These include the following:

- *Antidepressant drugs* include monoamine oxidase inhibitors (MAOIs), which block the breakdown of monoamines, such as noradrenaline and serotonin. Selective serotonin reuptake inhibitors (SSRIs) block the reuptake of serotonin only, but tricyclic antidepressants (TCAs) interfere with noradrenaline and serotonin reuptake from synapses and thus enhance their action.
- *Amino acids*, such as tyrosine, phenylalanine, methionine, tryptophan and GABA, are essential for the production of neurotransmitters and are, therefore, natural antidepressants. Organic sulphur in the form of methylsulphonylmethane (MSM) is needed for their production and utilization. Dietary supplementation with MSM may improve alertness and elevate mood.
- *Hormones* act indirectly via control of blood sugar, calcium and sodium balance, and affect behaviour in general – anger, love, anxiety, panic attacks and agitation. Hypoglycaemia can cause agitation, depression and poor mental concentration. Hypothyroidism can cause impotence and depression. Hyperthyroidism can cause agitation, irritability and lack of sleep. Addison disease can cause severe depression, while those treated with high corticosteroid doses can become euphoric or have hallucinations and psychoses. Sex steroids such as testosterone clearly affect mood and behaviour. The mood swings associated with premenstrual stress and menopause may be reduced with natural progesterone cream derived from wild yam – all sex steroids were originally produced from wild (elephant foot) yam. Melatonin may affect depression.
- *Drugs that bind to the GABA receptor* to enhance the inhibitory effect of GABA in the CNS include sedatives such as phenobarbital, alcohol, and anxiolytics such as benzodiazepines.
- *Drugs such as chlorpromazine and haloperidol bind to dopamine receptors*, leading to greater synthesis of dopamine at the synapse and easing some of the symptoms of schizophrenia.
- *Naloxone binds to the opioid kappa receptor*, and blocks both enkephalin-degrading enzyme inhibitors (enkephalinase inhibitors) and kappa antagonists.

NEUROIMMUNOLOGICAL MECHANISMS

There appears to be a relationship between mental health and the immune system, which can be either overactive or suppressed, leading to associated diseases. There is growing evidence that such

Table 10.3 *Some neurotransmitters, with their functions and associated disorders*

Neurotransmitter	Functions	Associated disorders
Acetylcholine (ACh)	Alertness, memory	Alzheimer disease is associated with 90% loss of ACh in the forebrain and hippocampus
	Muscle tone, learning, primitive drives, emotions, release of vasopressin (involved in learning and regulation of urine output). ACh-releasing neurons in the pons are active in rapid eye movement (REM) sleep (dreaming)	
	Relation to sexual performance and arousal – helps control blood flow to genitals, heart rate and blood pressure during sexual intercourse	
Adrenaline (epinephrine)	Physiological expressions of fear and anxiety (fright, fight and flight)	Adrenaline in excess is seen in anxiety disorders
Dopamine	Feelings of bliss ('the pleasure chemical'). More dopamine in the frontal lobe lessens pain and increases pleasure	Parkinson disease is brought on when dopamine fails to reach the basal ganglia
	Regulation of information flow into the frontal lobe from other areas of brain	Relation to attention deficit hyperactivity disorder (ADHD)
	Effect on voluntary movement, learning, memory and emotion	Schizophrenia is associated with the inability of dopamine to reach the frontal lobe
		Excess dopamine in the limbic system and not enough in the cortex may produce paranoia or inhibit social interaction
		A shortage of dopamine in the frontal lobes may cause poor memory
		Cocaine, opiates and alcohol produce their effects in part via dopamine release
Endorphins and enkephalins	Involvement in pain reduction, pleasure (enhance release of dopamine) and hibernation, as well as a number of other behaviours	Opiates (natural and synthetic) bind to endorphin and enkephalin brain receptors and alter behaviour
	Endorphins block pain at receptor sites and facilitate the dopamine pathway that feeds into the frontal lobe, thereby replacing pain with pleasure	
	Also produced by the pituitary gland and released as hormones	
Gamma-aminobutyric acid (GABA)	Major inhibitory neurotransmitter lessening anxiety. Brain produces substances that enhance anxiety (beta-carbolines), as well as substances that lower anxiety (e.g. allopregnanolone). All modify GABA brain receptors to produce effects	Anxiolytic drugs, such as benzodiazepines, act by enhancing effects of GABA at synapses
Glutamate	The main brain excitatory neurotransmitter, with actions mediated at NMDA and AMPA receptors involved in memory formation	Involvement in a 'suicidal' response when the brain is damaged, as in stroke. Excess glutamate is neurotoxic and neurons are damaged by the excessive calcium that enters the cell due to glutamate-binding. Glutamate is produced excessively in amyotrophic lateral sclerosis
Neuropeptide Y/polypeptide YY (NPY/PPYY)	Effect on hypothalamus and stimulation of excessive food intake and fat storage	Link with anxiety and eating disorders
Noradrenaline (norepinephrine)	Stimulant to the body and mind. Causes some of the physiological expressions of fear and anxiety (fright, fight and flight response). Modulation of heart rate, blood pressure, learning, memory, waking, emotion	Most forms of depression are associated with a deficiency of noradrenaline
		High levels can cause aggression
		Stress in children can lead to permanently high levels of noradrenaline, creating the potential for violent behavior
		Raised levels of norepinephrine mixed with dopamine and phenylethylamine produce feelings of infatuation
Oxytocin	Raised levels give mothers an impulse to cuddle their newborns	High levels contribute to multiple orgasms in women
Phenylethylamine	In the limbic system gives feelings of bliss	Low levels in ADHD
	A natural ingredient in chocolate	
Serotonin (5-hydroxytryptamine, 5-HT)	The 'feel-good' hormone that enables relaxation and enjoyment of life	Most forms of depression are associated with a deficiency of serotonin at functionally important serotonergic receptors
	Synthesized from the amino acid l-tryptophan	
	Also a precursor for the pineal hormone melatonin, which regulates the body clock: sleep, appetite, sensory perception, temperature regulation, pain suppression and mood	
Substance P	A neurotransmitter that mediates pain; found throughout the pain pathway	–
	Release can be blocked by enkephalins and endorphins	

neuroimmunological mechanisms might influence immunological and inflammatory disorders and defence against infection. It has, for example, been suggested that stress might underlie some periodontal and other oral diseases. The major route identified for neuroimmunomodulation is via the neuroendocrine system.

In addition to recognizable neurotransmitters, the nervous system contains significant levels of cytokines and their receptors. Thus the possibility of a two-way exchange of information is clearly present. Immune cells possess a host of receptor profiles for modulatory substances and many of these are common to the nervous system. Two different pathways and effects of immediate stress can be demonstrated:

- The endocrine path, in which the CNS is central to the control of release of glucocorticosteroids such as cortisol, which have an immunosuppressive effect and temporary adverse effects on cognitive functions, such as learning and memory.
- The second, direct neural pathway to the adrenal medulla releases other transmitters, particularly catecholamines, which depress chemotaxis and phagocytosis, and beta-adrenergic agonists, which have general effects on white blood cells.

In severe long-term stress, natural opioids are released; the adrenals release met-enkephalin and the hypothalamus releases beta-endorphin, which leads to enhanced anti-tumour activity of natural killer (NK) cells and proliferative response of lymphocytes.

Inflammatory cytokines – interleukin (IL)-1b, IL-6 and tumour necrosis factor alpha (TNFα) – activate the hypothalamo–pituitary–adrenal (HPA) axis. IL-1 modulates brain catecholamine activity; depletion of central catecholamines potentiates severity of inflammation and also affects the release of corticotropin-releasing hormone (CRH) and adrenocorticotropic hormone (ACTH). IL-1, IL-6 and nitric oxide modulate brain serotonin activity, depletion of which enhances the inflammatory response.

Under stress conditions, if immune activity is not controlled, it may reach a state of activation in which host injury and tissue destruction can take place (autoimmunity).

ANXIETY AND STRESS

Anxiety disorders are characterized by excessive and unrealistic worry about everyday tasks or events, or may be specific to certain objects or rituals. Stress keeps people alert and ready to avoid danger, but when it persists, illness can result.

ANXIETY DISORDERS

Clinical features

Anxiety can cause several physical effects as a result of overwhelming autonomic activity. Sympathetic activity via the release of catecholamines causes apprehension, tachycardia, hyperventilation, hypertension, sweating, tremor and dilated pupils. Parasympathetic activity may lead to involuntary defecation and urinary incontinence. These changes may be recognized by features such as those listed in Table 10.4.

Pathological anxiety may be difficult to diagnose and requires careful consideration of an individual's personal history and presenting clinical features. A thorough history and perhaps psychiatric assessment may be appropriate, but underlying organic causes such as hyperthyroidism and mitral valve prolapse should be excluded first.

Anxiety can be classified into the following diagnostic categories:

- Panic disorder – discrete attacks with no external stimulus
- Phobias – discrete attacks with stimuli

Table 10.4 *Features suggesting anxiety*

Physiological	Behavioural	Cognitive
Child		
Pallor	Crying	Being scared
Increased pulse rate	Being uncooperative, restless or disruptive	Anxiety
Tension		Negative thoughts
Hyperventilation	Silence or sullenness	
Adult		
Dry mouth	Verbal abuse	Negative thoughts
	Excessive talking	
	Cancelling appointments, arriving late or not at all	

- Generalized anxiety disorder (GAD) – a generalized persistent state of anxiety
- Anxiety as a manifestation of other psychiatric disease such as depression.

General management

Treatment of anxiety and stress may require:

- appropriate management of any underlying organic disease
- lifestyle changes – to reduce stressors and avoid precipitating factors
- behavioural techniques
- pharmacotherapy (anxiolytics and beta-blockers)
- psychotherapy – this may be used to aid adjustment of lifestyle (supportive) or to explore patient conflicts and secondary gain (psychodynamic).

Psychotherapy involves talking with a mental health professional, such as a psychiatrist, psychologist, social worker or counsellor, to learn how to deal with problems. Cognitive behavioural therapy (CBT) and behavioural therapy are effective for several anxiety disorders, particularly panic disorder and social phobia. There are two components to CBT: the cognitive component helps to change thinking patterns that keep people from overcoming their fears, while the behavioural component seeks to change reactions to anxiety-provoking situations. Anxiety disorders may be addressed by exposure (to the object or event of concern) and response prevention – not permitting the compulsive behaviour, to help the individual learn that it is not needed. A key element of this component is exposure, in which people have to confront the things they fear. Behavioural therapy alone, without a strong cognitive component, has been used effectively to treat specific phobias. Here, persons are gradually exposed to the objects or situations that are feared. Often the therapist will accompany them to provide support and guidance. After treatment, the beneficial effects of CBT may last longer than those of medication for people with panic disorder; the same may be true for obsessive–compulsive disorder (OCD), post-traumatic stress disorder and social phobia.

Drugs can play a part in the treatment of some people with anxiety or phobias. Anti-anxiety medications (anxiolytics) either alter or inhibit the amount or action of a targeted neurotransmitter. Anxiolytics include benzodiazepines (BZPs – which enhance GABA inhibitory activity), serotonin selective reuptake inhibitors (SSRIs), and azapirones such as buspirone (which act on 5-HT [serotonin]1A receptor). Other drugs, like beta blockers, are used as anxiolytics since they can inhibit some of the physical manifestations, such as rapid heartbeat and sweating. BZPs relieve symptoms quickly with few side-effects, except often for some drowsiness. BZPs include clonazepam, which is used for social phobia and GAD; alprazolam, which is helpful for panic disorder and GAD; and lorazepam, which is also useful for panic disorder. BZPs should be prescribed for short periods of time because of development of tolerance (rising doses to achieve the same effect) and dependence. Panic disorder is an exception, for which BZPs may be used for 6 months to a year. Those who abuse drugs or alcohol are not usually good candidates for BZPs because they can become dependent. Withdrawal symptoms, and in certain instances rebound anxiety, can follow after stopping BZPs. They should not be given to children, the elderly, alcoholics (except to treat withdrawal), or pregnant or lactating women. Temazepam is particularly prone to becoming abused and is a controlled drug. Azapirones (AZPs) are used to treat a range of mental health problems, including anxiety disorders, depression and psychosis. Adverse effects may include drowsiness, dizziness, nausea, weakness, insomnia and lightheadedness.

Beta-blockers, such as propanolol, are helpful in certain anxiety disorders, particularly social phobia. Antidepressants can help to relieve anxiety.

Dental aspects

Anxiety can be generated by dental or medical appointments, even amongst normal patients, and is a perfectly natural reaction to an unpleasant experience. A total of 65% of patients report some level of fear of dental treatment. It is essential, therefore, not to dismiss patients who will not accept a proposed treatment as being 'phobic' or 'uncooperative', though a small number will require psychological or even psychiatric assessment and/or treatment. Younger patients have significantly more fear of treatment than older patients. Among fearful patients, changes in pulse rate (>10 beats/min) and blood pressure are detectable.

Quantification of anxiety levels can be achieved using a modified dental anxiety scale (see Box 2.2). Other scales and a range of techniques to manage such patients are outlined by Rafique et al. (2008).

Dental 'phobia' is more extreme than straightforward anxiety, and previous frightening dental experiences are often cited as the major factor in their development. Patients fear the noise and vibration of the drill (56%), the sight of the injection needle (47%) and sitting at the treatment chair (42%) especially. Effects include muscle tension (64%), faster heart beat (59%), accelerated breathing (37%), sweating (32%) and stomach cramps (28%). Patients with a true phobic neurosis about dental treatment are uncommon but, when seen, demand great patience. Phobic patients, who may genuinely want dental care but are unable to cooperate, are often unaware of their anxiety and, as a consequence, may be hostile in their responses or behaviour. Some individuals are difficult or even impossible to manage because of anxiety, phobia or personality disorders.

Patients who apply for treatment at a dental fear clinic are not just dentally anxious; they often show a wide range of other complaints. Persons with clinically significant fear tend to have poorer perceived dental health, a longer interval since their last dental appointment, a higher frequency of past fear behaviours, more physical symptoms during dental injections, and a higher percentage of symptoms of anxiety and depression. They may chatter incessantly, have a history of failed appointments, and appear tense and agitated ('white knuckle syndrome').

Dental treatment in anxiety states is usually straightforward. Early morning appointments, with pre-medication and no waiting, can help. The main aids are careful, painlessly performed dental procedures, psychological approaches, confident reassurance, patience and, sometimes, the use of pharmacological agents – for example, anxiolytics such as oral diazepam, supplemented if necessary with intravenous, transmucosal or inhalational sedation during dental treatment. General techniques to help overcome anxiety include relaxation techniques (e.g. deep breathing), distraction (e.g. watching TV), control strategies (e.g. 'put your hand up if you wish me to stop') and positive reinforcement (e.g. praise). Other measures include systematic desensitization, biofeedback, modelling and hypnosis, and may need support from a psychologist.

Symptoms such as agitation, slight tachycardia and dry mouth, mainly caused by sympathetic overactivity, are usually controllable by reassurance and possibly a very mild anxiolytic or sedative, such as a low dose of a beta-blocker or a short-acting (temazepam) or moderate-acting (lorazepam or diazepam) BZP, provided the patient is not pregnant and does not drive, operate dangerous machinery or make important decisions for the following 24 hours. Temazepam 10 mg orally on the night before and 1 hour before dental treatment can be used to supplement gentle sympathetic handling and reassurance of the anxious patient. Intravenous or intranasal sedation with midazolam, or relative analgesia using nitrous oxide and oxygen, is also useful. BZP metabolism is impaired by azole antifungals, and by macrolide antibiotics such as erythromycin and clarithromycin. Alcohol, antihistamines and barbiturates have additive sedative effects with BZPs. The analgesic dextropropoxyphene should be avoided in patients taking alprazolam, as it may cause toxicity.

Difficulties may also result from alcoholism or drug dependence, or drug treatment with major tranquillizers, MAOIs or TCAs. Oral manifestations, such as facial arthromyalgia, dry mouth, lip-chewing or bruxism, may be complaints in chronically anxious people. Cancer phobia is also an indication of an anxiety.

STRESS

General aspects

The brain areas involved in regulation of stress responses include the prefrontal cortex, amygdala, hippocampus and nucleus accumbens. Acute stress enhances immune function whereas chronic stress suppresses it.

Besides the hypothalamus and brainstem, which are essential for autonomic and neuroendocrine responses to stressors, higher cognitive areas of the brain play a key role in memory, anxiety and decision-making, and are targets of stress and stress hormones. The effects of glucocorticoids on the hippocampus and other brain regions are regulated by: corticosteroid-binding globulin (CBG), multiple drug resistance P-glycoprotein (MDRpG), and metabolism by 11-hydroxysteroid dehydrogenase type 1 (11-HSD-1). Four peptide/protein hormones – IGF-1, insulin, ghrelin and leptin – affect the hippocampus.

Different alleles of commonly occurring genes determine how individuals will respond to stress. For example, the serotonin transporter is associated with alcoholism, and individuals who have one allele are more likely to respond to stress by developing depression. Individuals with an allele of the monoamine oxidase A gene are more vulnerable to abuse in childhood and more likely to become abusers themselves and to show antisocial behaviours. Stress begins in and affects the brain, as well as the rest of the body. Acute stress responses promote adaptation and survival via neural, cardiovascular, autonomic, immune and metabolic responses. Chronic stress can promote and exacerbate pathophysiology through the same systems. The burden of chronic stress and accompanying changes in personal behaviours (smoking, eating too much, drinking, poor-quality sleep – otherwise referred to as 'lifestyle') is called allostatic overload. Brain regions such as the hippocampus, prefrontal cortex and amygdala respond to acute and chronic stress and show changes in morphology and chemistry that are largely reversible if the chronic stress lasts only for weeks. However, it is not clear whether prolonged stress for many months or years may have irreversible effects.

In obese individuals, the final common pathway of the stress response – the HPA axis – is altered, and concentrations of cortisol are raised in adipose tissue due to raised activity of 11β-HSD-1. Short sleep and decreased sleep quality are also associated with obesity. In addition, sleep curtailment induces HPA-axis alterations that, in turn, may negatively affect sleep.

CRH plays a central role in the regulation of the HPA axis. CRH action on ACTH release is potentiated by vasopressin, whereas oxytocin inhibits it. ACTH release results in the release of corticosteroids from the adrenals, which subsequently, through mineralocorticoid and glucocorticoid receptors, exert negative feedback on the hippocampus, the pituitary and the hypothalamus. The most important glucocorticoid in humans is cortisol. Vasopressin production is increased in depression. The suprachiasmatic nucleus, the biological clock of the brain, shows lower vasopressin production and a smaller circadian amplitude in depression, which may explain the associated sleep problems. The hypothalamo–pituitary–thyroid (HPT) axis is inhibited in depression. Although cortisol and CRH may well be causally involved in depression, there is no evidence for any major irreversible damage in the hippocampus in depression.

The stress response is mediated by the HPA system and reliant on activity of the CRH neurons in the hypothalamic paraventricular nucleus (PVN). The CRH neurons co-express vasopressin (ADH), which potentiates the CRH effects. CRH neurons regulate the adrenal innervation of the autonomic system and affect mood. Both centrally released CRH and increased levels of cortisol contribute to the features of depression. Depression is also a frequent side-effect of steroid treatment and is one of the symptoms of Cushing syndrome. The ADH neurons in the hypothalamic PVN and supraoptic nucleus are also activated in depression, which contributes to the increased release of ACTH from the pituitary. Increased levels of circulating ADH are also associated with the risk for suicide. The prevalence, incidence and morbidity risk for depression are higher in females than in males and fluctuations in sex hormone levels are considered to be involved.

Causes of stress

The causes of stress can be different for each person and individuals vary in their ways of coping.

Common causes of stress include:

- accidents
- confrontations
- crowds
- deadlines
- death of a loved one
- divorce
- examinations
- financial problems
- heavy traffic
- house-moving
- illness
- job change or loss
- legal problems
- marriage
- pregnancy
- retirement
- separation.

Clinical features of stress

Signs include the following:

- Emotional
  - Anger
  - Inability to concentrate
  - Mood swings
  - Sadness
  - Unproductive worry
- Physical
  - Chronic fatigue
  - Sweaty palms
  - Tremors
  - Weight changes
  - Headaches
- Mental/behavioural
  - Acting on impulse
  - Changing jobs frequently
  - Over-reacting
  - Using alcohol or drugs
  - Withdrawing from relationships.

Stress is a reaction caused by anything that requires adjustment to a change in the environment. The reactions can be physical, mental/behavioural and/or emotional. Emotional stress can release chemicals that provoke brain blood vessel changes, which in turn can trigger tension (stress) headaches. The sympathetic nervous system turns on the fight or flight response with adrenaline (epinephrine) release; the brain limbic system immediately responds. Cortisol secretion rises but other hormones shut down; growth, reproduction and the immune system are suppressed. Later, the tranquillizing parasympathetic nervous system activates to calm things down.

Tension headaches can be either episodic or chronic. Episodic tension headache is usually triggered by an isolated stressful situation or a build-up of stress; it can usually be treated by analgesics. Daily stress, such as from a high-pressure job, can lead to chronic tension headaches. Treatment for chronic tension headaches usually involves counselling, stress management and possibly anxiolytics or antidepressants.

Coping with stress

The key to coping with stress is identifying stressors, learning ways to reduce stress and managing stress. Coping is a process, not an event.

Helpful advice includes the following measures:

- Lower your expectations; accept that there are events beyond your control
- Ask others to help
- Take responsibility for the situation
- Problem-solve
- Be assertive rather than aggressive
- Maintain emotionally supportive relationships
- Maintain emotional composure
- Try to change the source of stress and distance yourself from it
- Learn to relax
- Eat and drink sensibly
- Maintain a healthy self-esteem
- Exercise regularly
- Avoid smoking or other bad habits.

Stress may play a greater role in health and disease than formerly supposed. Humans are sensitive to stressors (e.g. operations) and even visits for health care can activate the HPA system. Anxiety generated

Table 10.5 *Some possible effects of acute and chronic stress*

	Mild stress	Acute stress	Chronic stress
Central nervous system	Mood change	Improved concentration and clarity of thought	Anxiety, loss of sense of humour, depression, fatigue, headaches, migraines, tremor
Cardiovascular	Rise in pulse rate and blood pressure	Tachycardia, arrhythmias	Hypertension, chest pain, ischaemic heart disease
Respiratory	Raised respiratory rate	Hyperventilation	Cough, asthma
Mouth	Slight dryness	Dry mouth	Dry mouth, ulcers
Gastrointestinal	Raised bowel activity	Impaired digestion	Peptic ulceration, irritable bowel syndrome
Sexual	Male impotence, female irregular menstruation	Male impotence, female irregular menstruation	Male impotence, female amenorrhoea

by such ordeals as dental or medical appointments, or by public speaking, solo musical performances, examinations or interviews, is normal. Stress is also fairly common in dental students and staff. Work stressors may include examinations, fear of failure, difficulties with accommodation or study facilities, inadequate holidays or relaxation time, financial difficulties, criticism, and time and scheduling demands. Stress can lead to reactions affecting a wide range of functions (Table 10.5).

Fear, an emotion that deals with danger, causes an automatic, rapid protective response in many body systems, coordinated by the amygdala. Emotional memories stored in the central amygdala may play a role in disorders involving very distinct fears, such as phobias, while different parts may be involved in other forms of anxiety.

The hippocampus – an area of the brain critical to memory and emotion – is involved in intrusive memories and flashbacks typical of post-traumatic stress disorder, and results in raised levels of stress hormones – cortisol, adrenaline (epinephrine) and noradrenaline (norepinephrine).

Danger induces high levels of enkephalins and endorphins, natural opioids, which can temporarily mask pain, and in some anxiety states higher levels persist even after the danger has passed.

Cortisol is the major steroid hormone produced in the adrenal glands and is essential for the body to cope with stress. Cortisol levels exhibit a natural rise in the morning and fall at night. If this rhythm is disturbed, mineral balance, blood sugar control and stress responses are affected. Lack of cortisol can lead to fatigue, allergies and arthritis, while excess cortisol can have an even greater negative effect on the body. While short-term elevations of cortisol are important for dealing with the stress of life-threatening issues, illness and wound-healing, chronically elevated levels can result in tiredness, depression and accelerated ageing with hypertension, muscle loss, bone destruction, obesity and diabetes. Prolonged stress or prolonged exposure to glucocorticoids can also have adverse effects on the hippocampus to cause atrophy, and memory deficits such as have been demonstrated in Cushing syndrome, depression and post-traumatic stress disorder.

Dehydroepiandrosterone (DHEA), the most abundant steroid hormone in the body, appears to counter the effects of high levels of cortisol and improves the ability to cope with stress. Low levels of DHEA have been associated with impaired immunity, cardiovascular disease, Alzheimer disease, hypothyroidism and diabetes.

Anxious or stressed patients may require drugs to control the anxiety but they respond better to beta-blocking agents (such as propranolol) than to BZPs, and with less impairment of performance. Stress may lead to substance abuse (Ch. 34). Anxiety may be caused or aggravated by using caffeine or street drugs like amphetamines, LSD or ecstasy.

Stress in dental staff

Dentistry can be a stressful occupation for both the dentist and the ancillary staff. There appears to be a significant level of dissatisfaction amongst dental nurses and hygienists in general practice, in terms of working conditions, relations with other staff and management skills of the dentist.

Increasingly, dentists in general practice appear concerned about the business aspects of practice, and seem to experience more physical and mental ill-health compared with other health professionals. In contrast, community dentists may be more worried about clinical matters, such as treating medical emergencies or difficult patients.

POST-TRAUMATIC STRESS DISORDER (PTSD)

General aspects

Post-traumatic stress disorder is an anxiety state that can follow exposure to a terrifying event where victims can see danger, where life is threatened, or where they see other people dying or being injured. Traumatic events that can trigger PTSD include personal assaults, such as rape or mugging, disasters, accidents or military combat.

Many people with PTSD repeatedly re-experience the ordeal in the form of flashback episodes, memories, nightmares or frightening thoughts, or being 'on guard', especially when exposed to events or objects reminiscent of the trauma. Anniversaries of the event can also trigger symptoms. Most people with PTSD thus try to avoid any reminders or thoughts of the ordeal (avoidance and numbing).

Clinical features

Symptoms of PTSD typically begin within 3 months of the traumatic event but occasionally not until years later. Headaches, gastrointestinal complaints, dizziness, chest pain or discomfort elsewhere can be disabling. Emotional numbness and sleep disturbance, depression, anxiety, irritability, outbursts of anger and feelings of intense guilt are common.

Associated depression, alcohol or other substance abuse, or another anxiety disorder is also common.

General management

CBT, group therapy, eye movement desensitization and reprocessing (EMDR) and exposure therapy, in which patients gradually and repeatedly relive the frightening experiences under controlled conditions to help them work through the trauma, can be effective. Medications, particularly SSRIs, are frequently prescribed (TCAs are as effective), and help to ease associated symptoms of depression and anxiety and to promote sleep.

Dental aspects

Frightening though dentistry may be, it is not known to have precipitated PTSD. However, patients who are suffering from PTSD may present with a variety of unexplained pain problems.

GENERALIZED ANXIETY DISORDER (GAD)

General aspects

Generalized anxiety disorder differs from normal anxiety in that it is chronic and fills the day with exaggerated and unfounded worry and tension. GAD is twice as common in women as in men.

Clinical features

People with GAD are always anticipating disaster, often worrying excessively about health, money, family or work; they may have physical symptoms, such as fatigue, headaches, muscle tension, muscle aches, difficulty in swallowing, trembling, twitching, irritability, sweating and hot flushes, and trouble falling or staying asleep. Unlike individuals with other anxiety disorders, people with GAD do not characteristically avoid certain situations. GAD is often accompanied by other conditions associated with stress, such as irritable bowel syndrome. GAD may be accompanied by another anxiety disorder, depression or substance abuse.

General management

Generalized anxiety disorder is diagnosed when someone spends at least 6 months worrying excessively about everyday problems. GAD is commonly treated with CBT and BZPs such as clonazepam or alprazolam. Venlafaxine, a drug closely related to the SSRIs, is also useful. Buspirone, an azapirone, is also used: it must be taken consistently for at least 2 weeks to achieve effect, and possible adverse-effects include dizziness, headaches and nausea.

PANIC DISORDER

General aspects

Panic disorder is the term given to recurrent unpredictable attacks of severe anxiety with physical symptoms such as palpitations, chest pain, dyspnoea, paraesthesiae and sweating ('panic attacks'). There are associations with mitral valve prolapse in 50%.

Clinical features

Panic attacks can come at any time, even during sleep. In a panic attack, there are features of catecholamine release – the heart pounds and the patient may feel sweaty, weak, faint or dizzy. The hands may tingle or feel numb, and there may be nausea, chest pain, a sense of unreality or fear of impending doom.

Many or most of the symptoms may result from hyperventilation. An attack generally peaks within 10 minutes but some symptoms may last much longer. Many individuals suffer intense anxiety between episodes, worrying when and where the next attack will strike.

Panic disorder is often accompanied by other conditions such as depression, drug abuse or alcoholism, and may lead to a pattern of avoidance of places or situations where panic attacks have struck.

General management

Panic disorder is one of the most readily treatable disorders and usually responds to psychotherapy or medication with alprazolam or lorazepam. Fluoxetine or another SSRI is frequently prescribed but TCAs are as effective. Hyperventilation is effectively treated by rebreathing into a paper bag.

SOCIAL PHOBIA (SOCIAL ANXIETY DISORDER)

General aspects

Social phobia involves overwhelming anxiety and excessive self-consciousness in normal social situations, resulting in a persistent, intense and chronic fear of being watched and judged by others and being embarrassed or humiliated by one's own actions. Women and men are equally likely to develop social phobia, usually beginning in childhood or early adolescence.

Clinical features

Accompanying physical symptoms may include blushing, profuse sweating, trembling, nausea and difficulty in talking. Anxiety disorders and depression are common and substance abuse may develop.

General management

Social phobia can usually be treated successfully with psychotherapy or medications. Beta-blockers, such as propanolol or clonazepam, are helpful. Fluoxetine or other SSRIs are frequently prescribed but TCAs are as effective.

SPECIFIC PHOBIAS (PHOBIC NEUROSES)

General aspects

A phobia is a morbid fear or anxiety out of all proportion to the threat, an intense irrational fear of something that poses little or no actual danger. Twice as common in women as in men, phobias usually appear first during childhood or adolescence and tend to persist into adulthood.

Clinical features

Phobic neuroses differ from anxiety neuroses in that the phobic anxiety arises only in specific circumstances, whereas patients with anxiety neuroses are *generally* anxious. Claustrophobia (fear of closed spaces) is probably the most common phobic disorder. Magnetic resonance imaging (MRI) is sometimes impossible to carry out because of claustrophobia.

Some of the other more common specific phobias are centred around heights, tunnels, driving, water, flying, insects, dogs and injuries involving blood. When phobias are centred on threats such as flying, anaesthetics or dental treatment, normal life is possible if such threats are avoided. Phobias may also be a minor part of a more severe disorder, such as depression, obsessive neurosis, anxiety state, personality disorder or schizophrenia.

General management

Specific phobias are highly treatable with carefully targeted psychotherapy. Behaviour therapy aims at desensitization by slow and gradual exposure to the frightening situation. Implosion is a technique in which patients are asked to imagine a persistently frightening situation for 1 or 2 hours. Phobias can sometimes be controlled by anxiolytic drugs. Buspirone is particularly useful, since it lacks the psychomotor impairment, dependence and some other effects of BZP use. Antidepressants, especially TCAs, are used if there is a significant depressive component.

PERSONALITY DISORDERS

In mental health, the word 'personality' refers to the collection of characteristics or traits that makes each of us an individual, including the ways that we think, feel and behave.

Personality may develop in a way that makes it difficult for us to live with ourselves and/or other people – traits or disorders usually noticeable from childhood or early teens. Personality disorders are chronic abnormalities of character or maladjustment to life that shade into neuroses or psychoses and may make it difficult to make or keep relationships, get on with friends and family or with people at work, keep out of trouble or control feelings or behaviour. However, insight is retained and most patients manage to pursue a relatively normal life. Personality disorders are shown in Table 10.6.

Causes include upbringing (neglect, physical or sexual abuse, violence in the family, parents who drink too much alcohol), early problems (childhood severe aggression, disobedience and temper tantrums) or brain problems (these remain to be defined). Personality disorders may be aggravated by drugs or alcohol, interpersonal conflicts, financial problems or other mental health problems.

People with personality disorders are often made unhappy by poor relationships or frequent conflicts, and severe antisocial personality disorders can lead to criminal behaviour. Dangerous and severe personality disorders are the subject of a recent review of the Mental Health Act; these patients may be detained under the Act, regardless of the absence of treatable disease.

Handling patients with personality disorders requires enormous patience and tolerance, and the exercise of tact and skills. These skills only come with appreciation of the existence of these disorders and with experience, but are difficult to acquire. Even with such skills, little progress may still be possible. Antipsychotics or antidepressant or mood-stabilizing drug therapy may be helpful.

BORDERLINE PERSONALITY DISORDER (BPD)

General aspects

Borderline personality disorder is characterized by pervasive instability of mood, interpersonal relationships, self-image and behaviour. It frequently disrupts family and work, long-term planning and the individual's sense of self-identity. BPD affects 2% of adults, mostly young women.

Brain imaging studies in BPD show that individual differences in the ability to activate regions of the prefrontal cerebral cortex thought to be involved in inhibitory activity predict the ability to suppress negative emotion.

Clinical features

A person with BPD may experience intense bouts of anger, depression and anxiety that may last only hours, or at most a day, while a person with depression or bipolar disorder (see below) typically endures the same types of mood for weeks. Bouts of BPD may be associated with episodes of impulsive aggression, self-injury, and drug or alcohol

Table 10.6 *Types of personality disorder*

Personality disorder	Features
Cluster A	Paranoid
Paranoid	Suspicious, distrustful, litigious, lacking humour, blaming others
	Feeling that other people are being unpleasant (even when evidence shows this is false), sensitive to rejection, tending to hold grudges
Schizoid	Socially distant, detached, secretive, isolated, lacking friends
	Emotionally 'cold', disliking contact with other people, preferring own company; having a rich fantasy world
Schizotypal	Odd, eccentric, having difficulties with thinking, lacking emotion or appropriate emotional reactions, seeing or hearing strange things, related to schizophrenia
Cluster B	Emotional and impulsive
Antisocial or dissocial	Impulsive, aggressive, manipulative, selfish, callous, disloyal, in conflict with everyone and everything, not caring about the feelings of others, easily frustrated
	Tending to be aggressive, committing crimes, finding it difficult to make intimate relationships, not feeling guilty or learning from unpleasant experiences
Borderline	Impulsive, self-destructive, unstable, finding it hard to control emotions
	Feeling bad about self, often self-harming, feeling 'empty', making relationships quickly but easily losing them, possibly feeling paranoid or depressed
	When stressed, possibly hearing noises or voices
Histrionic	Emotional, dramatic, theatrical, immature, manipulative, attention-seeking, having shallow interpersonal relationships, over-dramatizing events, self-centred
	Showing strong emotions that change quickly and do not last long
	Can be suggestible, worrying a lot about appearance, craving new things and excitement, can be seductive
Narcissistic	Boastful, egotistical, 'superiority complex', strong sense of own self-importance
	Dreaming of unlimited success, power and intellectual brilliance, craving attention but showing few warm feelings in return, exploiting others, asking for favours but not returning them
Cluster C	Anxious
Avoidant	Shy, timid, 'inferiority complex', very anxious and tense, worrying a lot
	Feeling insecure and inferior, having to be liked and accepted
	Extremely sensitive to criticism
Dependent	Dependent, submissive, clinging, passive, relying on others to make decisions for them, finding it hard to cope with daily chores, feeling hopeless and incompetent
	Easily feeling abandoned by others
Obsessive–compulsive (anankastic)	Perfectionist, rigid, controlling, chronically worried about standards and self-image; unable to relax, often depressed
	Cautious, preoccupied with detail, worrying about doing the wrong thing, finding it hard to adapt; often having high moral standards
	Judgmental; sensitive to criticism; possibly having obsessional thoughts and images (although not as bad as in obsessive–compulsive disorder)

abuse. People with BPD may exhibit other impulsive behaviours, such as excessive spending, binge eating or risky sex. Distortions in cognition and sense of self can lead to frequent changes in long-term goals, career plans, jobs, friendships, gender identity and values.

BPD is often associated with other psychiatric problems, particularly bipolar disorder, depression, anxiety disorders, substance abuse and other personality disorders. Thus BPD often causes highly unstable patterns of social relationships.

General management

Dialectical behaviour therapy, developed specifically to treat BPD, involves four primary modes of treatment: individual therapy, group skills training, telephone contact and therapist consultation. Antidepressants and antipsychotic drugs may also be used.

Dental aspects

Persons with personality disorders may make unreliable patients. They are unlikely to have any conscience about missing appointments or to pay much attention to oral health-care instructions. Treatment plans may be argued about or frankly refused. Payment may be withheld and litigation threatened.

Dental staff may also have personality disorders and find themselves in conflict with others, including colleagues – often to the dental staff's disadvantage, and may find it difficult not to antagonize patients and colleagues.

OBSESSIVE–COMPULSIVE DISORDER (OCD)

General aspects

Obsessional personality traits are common, especially amongst dental and medical personnel, and are often salutary. Many healthy people have features of obsessive–compulsive disorder with secondary ritualistic behaviours, such as checking that the door is locked several times before or after leaving the house. In true OCD, the urge to do or think certain things repeatedly can dominate life unhelpfully, with obsessive activities consuming at least 14 hours a day and causing significant disruption of normal life. For example, one dental surgeon felt compelled to telephone his patients late at night because he was obsessed with the notion that, having prepared the cavity, he might have forgotten to place the restoration. The basal ganglia and striatum appear to be involved in OCD. OCD strikes males slightly more commonly and usually starts in childhood, adolescence or early adulthood.

OCD is the fourth most common mental disorder, affecting 1–2% of the population, and it appears to be increasing.

Clinical features

OCD is comprised of thoughts (obsessions) that create anxiety, and things the patient does to reduce the anxiety (compulsions). Obsessional patients are often intelligent, many are unmarried and many have a pre-morbid state, such as an uncertain and vacillating – or alternatively, a stubborn, rigid, morose and irritable – personality. Obsessional thoughts are those that come repeatedly into consciousness against the patient's will; they are usually unpleasant but always recognized as the patient's own thoughts. Typical obsessions are the repeated checking, questioning of decisions, hoarding, counting, religious compulsions, the fear of harm or harming, or the fear of dirtiness or contamination. This may manifest with repeated hand-washing, for example (Fig. 10.3).

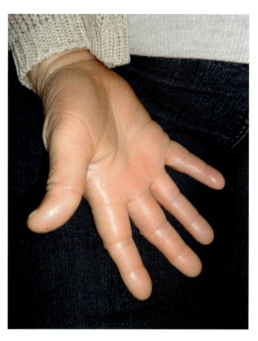

Fig. 10.3 Effects of repeated hand-washing in obsessive–compulsive disorder.

However, the thoughts are not accepted by the patient as harmless or inevitable, and an internal struggle against them leads to secondary ritualistic thought or behaviour patterns (compulsions). The compulsions may include rituals, checking, avoidance, hoarding and reassurance. A prominent example was the millionaire Howard Hughes, who was so severely affected that he eventually ended up sitting naked in the middle of his hotel room, obsessed with concerns about 'contamination' and with six aides 'cleaning' him.

The obsessional thoughts may also in turn generate depression or other anxiety disorders, and some people with OCD also have eating disorders. Obsessional features can also be associated with disorders such as depression, schizophrenia or, rarely, organic brain disease.

The course of OCD is variable. Symptoms may come and go, may ease over time or can grow progressively worse.

General management

Treatment is often difficult, though OCD may respond to psychotherapy or to medication with antidepressants, especially SSRIs, clomipramine and the TCAs, which are useful when there is also depression. The BZPs may be useful when anxiety is predominant.

Dental aspects

It is questionable whether true obsessions often become centred on the mouth but they may, for example, result in compulsive tooth-brushing or excessive use of antiseptic mouthwashes. Occasional patients become obsessed with the possibility of infections or cancer in the mouth (as, for example, one man who was obsessed with the idea that his Fordyce spots were thrush) and refuse to be reassured. Some individuals become obsessed with the notion that they have oral malodour.

CHILDHOOD DISORDERS

These include attention-deficit/hyperactivity disorder, conduct disorder (the antisocial personality disorder of childhood) and oppositional defiant disorder (not only in children).

ATTENTION-DEFICIT/HYPERACTIVITY DISORDER (ADHD)

This is a disorder that interferes with the ability to persist in a task and to exercise age-appropriate inhibition. ADHD is usually diagnosed in childhood, but the condition can continue into the adult years. It manifests with a failure to listen to instructions, inability to organize oneself, fidgeting with hands and feet, talking too much, leaving projects and work unfinished, and having trouble paying attention to and responding to details.

ADHD types include:

- a predominantly inattentive subtype
- a predominantly hyperactive–impulsive subtype
- a combined subtype.

General aspects

Mischievous children are not abnormal. Overactivity or hyperactivity applies to gross misbehavior, such as reckless escapes from parents while on public transport. Hyperactive children always seem to be in motion and seem unable to curb their immediate reactions or think before they act. Although parents not infrequently describe their badly behaved child as 'overactive', the term should be limited to those who demonstrate gross behavioural abnormalities, including uncontrolled activity, impulsiveness, impaired concentration, motor restlessness and extreme fidgeting. These activities are seen particularly when orderliness is required – for example, in the dental waiting room or surgery. Deficit in attention and motor control and perception may be a variant.

Once called *hyperkinesis* or *minimal brain dysfunction*, ADHD is characterized by inattention and hyperactivity and/or impulsivity, which are excessive, long-term and pervasive. It is one of the most common of childhood mental disorders, affecting 3–5% of children; it is twice as common in boys as in girls and often continues into adolescence and adulthood.

Commonly associated disorders may include:

- oppositional defiant disorders – these affect nearly half of all children with ADHD, who overreact or lash out when they resent anything
- developmental language disorders
- motor and coordination difficulties
- specific learning disabilities
- Tourette syndrome.

Overactivity can be caused by minor head injuries, undetectable brain damage or refined sugar and food additives. It is also caused by factors affecting the parents, the child or the child–parent relationship, or by external factors (Table 10.7).

Table 10.7 *Causes of hyperactivity in a child*

Child	Parental	External
Hyperkinetic syndrome	Child–parent relationship	Institutionalization
Brain damage		Excessive demands at school
Low intelligence	Rejection or overprotection	
Tartrazine sensitivity	Inconsistent discipline	
Anxiety states	Lack of parental love	
Drug abuse	Marital disharmony	
	Depression	

Clinical features

To make a diagnosis of ADHD, the abnormal behaviours listed above must be severe, appear before the age of 7 years, and continue for at least 6 months. Signs of inattention include becoming easily distracted by irrelevant sights and sounds, failing to pay attention to details and making careless mistakes, rarely following instructions carefully and completely, or losing or forgetting things such as toys, pencils, books and tools needed for a task.

Signs of hyperactivity and impulsivity include feeling restless, often fidgeting with hands or feet, squirming, running, climbing or leaving a seat, in situations where sitting or quiet behaviour is expected, blurting out answers before hearing the whole question, and having difficulty waiting in a queue or for a turn.

General management

Behavioural therapy, emotional counselling and practical support, including structured classroom management and tutoring, are required for the child, along with parent education. Sedatives and tranquillizers should be avoided, as they may impair learning ability or cause paradoxical reactions – such as aggressive behaviour. Stimulants surprisingly seem to be the most effective treatment in both children and adults, and treatment may include methylphenidate (Ritalin), atomoxetine and dexamfetamine (dextroamphetamine; Dexedrine); in the USA, Adderall – a 'cocktail' of four different amphetamine salts – is also available. The non-stimulant antihypertensive agent guanfacine may also have a role.

Dental aspects

- Overactive children can often be almost impossible to manage in the dental surgery and frequently succeed in frustrating all concerned.
- 'Tell–show–do' may be of value.
- Tranquillizers such as diazepam should be avoided, as they usually exacerbate rather than depress overactivity.
- Dental treatment may not be possible without conscious sedation (CS) or general anaesthesia (GA). Such patients are, therefore, often referred to hospital for dental care. The drug treatment may create resistance to CS. Local anaesthesia (LA) containing adrenaline (epinephrine) may interact with atomoxetine to increase blood pressure.

SOMATIZATION DISORDERS

General aspects

Many people suffer inner anxieties and some are prone to turn these into symptoms; these individuals are termed 'somatizers'. They typically develop inappropriate health-seeking behaviours, with multiple consultations and investigations, and use of many conventional and alternative therapies, and may accumulate huge medical records ('fat folder syndrome'). *Somatic disorders* are those that are thought to be initiated or aggravated by psychological factors and that persist for over 2 years. Typical examples are unexplained breathlessness, chest pain, fatigue, dizziness, paraesthesiae or chronic facial pain. Allergies, migraine, anorexia nervosa, psychogenic vomiting and, sometimes, obesity may also have a psychogenic basis. In addition, psychological factors may contribute to factitious injuries.

Psoriasis from head to inbetween toes
Perpetual scream in left ear
Spasmodic pressure above left ear
Constant ulcers in mouth and on tongue
Asthma, bronchitis, severe bouts of indigestion
Sore mouth due to grinding of bottom right molar
Severe pain under crutch after any exertion
Constant irritation around back passage
Spasmodic bleeding piles

Medicines taken internally
Predisalone
Ventolin
Asilone suspension
Bronchipax

Fig. 10.4 Note as presented by a patient. Such histories vary in length, detail and imagination, and sometimes suggest that the patient is disturbed (*maladie du petit papier*).

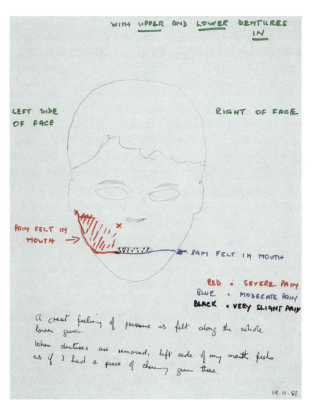

Fig. 10.5 Drawing produced by a patient.

Features that may suggest that symptoms are related to somatization, but not necessarily depressive, may include any of the following:

- *Absence of organic cause or physical signs.* The affected area typically appears normal and if, for example, a putatively diseased tooth is extracted, symptoms are unaffected. The symptoms cause real enough suffering to the patient and this must be acknowledged while emotional factors are explored.
- *Persistence of symptoms for very long periods, sometimes for years.* Clearly, after such periods any organic cause would have become apparent.
- *Bizarre symptoms.* The may include 'drawing' or 'gripping' sensations or apparently exaggerated 'unbearable' pain in spite of normal physical health or often sleep.
- *Vague localization of symptoms.* The distribution of pain, for example, may not follow an anatomical pattern, and the patient may be unable to put a finger precisely upon the painful area.
- *Unrecognizable stimuli.* Symptoms are usually not provoked by recognizable stimuli such as hot or cold foods, or mastication.
- *Multiple physical disorders.* Patients may have several chronic physical complaints at the same time.

In contrast to patients with severe organic disease, who typically reach for medication, many patients with chronic pain make little attempt to seek relief from them. After a brief trial, drugs are frequently said to be totally ineffective.

Patients' personality and manner are highly variable. Some appear obviously neurotic but few are overtly depressed. Indeed, the organic symptoms can be regarded as more acceptable substitutes ('depressive equivalents') for more typical manifestations of depression. These varied clinical pictures are discussed more fully below.

Sometimes the patients bring notes (Fig. 10.4) or drawings (Fig. 10.5) to illustrate their problems. These may reflect genuine disease, or may indicate the emotional nature of the complaint(s) (*la maladie du petit papier*). However, increasingly, informed patients who have no mental health problems bring notes or computer printouts to consultations.

In some patients, the response to antidepressant drugs is dramatic, with relief of symptoms and striking general improvement in mood, sometimes before the drug has had time to produce a true antidepressant effect. However, effective dosage varies widely and, in the case of TCAs, the response is generally related to the plasma levels achieved. Thus doses may sometimes have to be very high before an effect is evident.

Many patients go from specialist to specialist (doctor-shopping) over the course of years, with negative results from innumerable investigations or no response to any form of treatment. Indeed, the patient persistently refuses to accept advice or reassurance, and may even seem to take a sort of perverse pride in the resistance of the pain to the challenge of medical science.

Conflict between patient and carer is not uncommon, and patients may believe they are not receiving proper care.

Chronic physical symptoms can generally be regarded as a plea for help or attention. This occasionally becomes distressingly apparent in a patient who, at the start, appears well-balanced and self-controlled – even occasionally joking about symptoms – but after a little while is crying uncontrollably. At the other extreme, many patients reject the possibility of mental illness and aggressively assert that 'It's not my nerves' (even if no such suggestion has been made) and typically also reject the idea of psychiatric help, however obliquely and sympathetically suggested.

Examples of these varied clinical pictures therefore include the following:

- The patient may be overtly depressed and cries readily or is obviously having difficulty in restraining tears. Alternatively, initial self-control is followed by unrestrained crying.
- The patient may complain (in effect) of depression by saying that the pain or other symptom makes them miserable.
- Some, when allowed to discuss their symptoms, relate them to 'stress' or trouble with the family or at work.
- A few are already taking, or have taken, antidepressant drugs but the symptoms have not been controlled.
- A few have associated bizarre (delusional) symptoms, such as 'powder' or 'slime' coming out of the painful area, as mentioned earlier.
- A few, given the chance of a sympathetic hearing, gratefully expand on their problems and welcome the suggestion of help.

■ The most difficult and relatively common group is the 'rejectors', who will not accept the idea of mental disturbance, refuse to have the possibility investigated and are unwilling to accept that any drugs (which they equate with drugs of dependence) may be helpful.

It should not need to be emphasized that, where psychological problems are suspected, discussion with the patient must be conducted patiently, gently and sympathetically. Surprisingly, this may perhaps be the first opportunity that patients have had to unburden themselves. Listening, tolerance, empathy and compassion are required. Unfortunately, some doctors are at least as intolerant of such 'neurotic' patients as some members of the public. This is not to suggest that the dentist should attempt to be an amateur psychiatrist but an effort must be made understand the nature of the symptoms. It is probably unnecessary to enquire into full details of family relationships or broken homes. If a patient is depressed, the cause is often as much the patient's susceptibility to depression as the so-called life situation. In any case, improvement in the life situation is unlikely to be feasible, and it is only too common for those so affected to be unable to overcome their difficulties without help from drugs or other sources. It is important to stress to the patient that we now understand that damage to the periphery, perhaps from unnecessary dental treatment, causes wind-up and central sensitization so that the brain becomes hypervigilant. Such an explanation allows both doctor and patient to understand how the pain changes and moves around; the problem is not some localized pathology but a disorder of pain signalling requiring both pharmacological and cognitive help.

The key feature is the fact that the presenting complaint cannot be explained by any known medical condition and there appears to be unconscious/involuntary symptom production; these are sometimes termed medically unexplained symptoms (MUS).

Careful investigation is therefore essential to exclude possible organic causes; however, the dentist must be careful not to over-investigate the patient, as this has been shown to make problems more difficult to treat. It is important to achieve a shared understanding and management plan. Try diaries to record the problems; avoid manipulation by the patient; and minimize involvement of other health-care professionals ('doctor-shopping').

The concurrence of emotional and physical disease is one of the most common problems in medicine that require a mature clinical understanding.

Types of disorder previously termed 'psychosomatic' include those shown in Box 10.2.

SOMATIZATION DISORDER

This consists of complaints of multiple unexplained symptoms, which rarely remit completely but are presented in colourful, exaggerated terms.

Box 10.2 *Types of somatization disorder*

- Somatization disorder
- Hypochondriasis
- Conversion disorder
- Somatoform pain disorder
- Body dysmorphic syndrome
- Malingering
- Factitious disorders
- Hysterical states

Patients are rarely men but rather are inconsistent historians with depressed mood and anxiety symptoms. Diagnostic criteria include:

■ four pain symptoms, *plus*
■ two gastrointestinal symptoms, *plus*
■ one sexual/reproductive symptom, *plus*
■ one pseudoneurological symptom
■ if within a medical condition, excessive symptoms
■ absence of laboratory abnormalities
■ symptoms that cannot be intentionally feigned or produced.

HYPOCHONDRIASIS

Health anxiety (hypochondriasis) is obsessive worrying about health, often to the point where it causes great distress and affects the ability to function properly. Some people with health anxiety have unexplained physical symptoms, e.g. chest pain, abdominal pain, facial pain or headaches, which they assume are a sign of disease despite reassurance. Hypochondriasis neurosis (health anxiety) is a morbid preoccupation with physical symptoms or bodily functions, in which minute details are related incessantly; there is excessive preoccupation with fear of disease or a strong belief in having disease due to false interpretation of a trivial symptom. The condition may be graphically described as 'illness as a way of life'. Minor degrees of hypochondriasis are common, especially among older people, particularly (and quite understandably) if they are living alone. Features include:

■ presentation of the medical history in excessive detail
■ absence of organic disease or physiological disturbance
■ unwarranted fears or ideas persisting despite reassurances
■ clinically significant distress
■ complaints not restricted to appearance or delusional intensity
■ negative physical examination and laboratory results.

General management

Organic disease should always be excluded, as should depression and schizophrenia. Most patients with hypochondriasis are depressed and some are deluded.

Reassurance, CBT and supportive care are then needed, and antidepressant drugs may be helpful. Unnecessary interventions must also be avoided.

Dental aspects

The common oral symptoms are dry or burning mouth, disturbed taste and oral or facial pain.

Other syndromes related to dentistry include the so-called but unproven chronic candidosis ('candidiasis') syndromes and mercury allergy syndrome.

CONVERSION DISORDER ('HYSTERIA')

In conversion disorder, the patient complains of isolated symptoms that appear to be motivated by the desire to achieve a gain of some sort and have no physical cause (e.g. blindness, deafness, stocking anaesthesia and features that do not conform to known anatomical pathways or physiological mechanisms).

Diagnostic criteria include:

■ symptoms preceded by stress
■ no neurological, medical, substance abuse or cultural explanation
■ severe distress
■ absent or insufficient significant laboratory findings.

Nevertheless, in 10–50% of these patients, a physical disease process will ultimately become apparent.

SOMATIZATION PAIN DISORDER (BRIQUET SYNDROME)

Somatization disorder is characterized by physical symptoms that mimic disease or injury, for which there is no identifiable physical cause, but that are not the result of conscious malingering or factitious disorders (Ch. 13).

BODY DYSMORPHIC DISORDER (BDD; DYSMORPHOPHOBIA)

In BDD, the affected person is excessively concerned and preoccupied by a perceived defect in their physical features, causing psychological distress that impairs occupational and/or social functioning, sometimes to the point of depression, anxiety or social withdrawal. BDD affects men and women equally, with the onset of symptoms generally in adolescence or early adulthood. BDD is characterized by an unusually exaggerated degree of worry or concern about a specific part of the face or body, rather than the general size or shape of the body. The most common area of focus is the face (size, shape or lack of symmetry).

BDD is distinguished from anorexia nervosa and bulimia nervosa, as those patients are generally preoccupied with their overall weight and body shape. About 50% of patients with BDD, however, also meet the criteria for a delusional disorder, which is characterized by beliefs that are not based in reality. The defect in BDD exists only in the eyes of the beholder, and others can rarely agree that anything is defective. Thus the patient may adopt compulsive behaviour, which can include:

- compulsive checking in mirrors, windows and other reflective surfaces
- attempts to camouflage the imagined defect
- excessive grooming
- compulsive skin-touching
- reassurance-seeking
- compulsive information-seeking
- obsession with cosmetic procedures, such as orthognathic or plastic surgery, with few satisfactory results for the patient; with the number of elective cosmetic dentistry procedures being performed, the dentists may be the first health-care provider to notice BDD.

Patients with BDD may well be unrealistically dissatisfied with results of treatments and procedures, or unable to verbalize expectations. BDD has a high rate of comorbidity, most commonly with major depression, social phobia or OCD. BDD patients can also be self-destructive, and may even perform surgery on themselves (e.g. sawing down teeth or removing facial scars with sandpaper) and attempt or complete suicide. There is a completed suicide rate double that of major depression and so BDD is a major risk factor for suicide. CBT and SSRIs are indicated.

MALINGERING

Malingering is the deliberate simulation or exaggeration of symptoms for obvious and understandable gain. The gain can be monetary (e.g. compensation or incapacity benefit), or to avoid work or other unpleasant tasks (e.g. service in the armed forces) or criminal prosecution. True malingering is rare. Diagnosis can be difficult but a key is whether the symptoms persist when the patients believe they are not being watched.

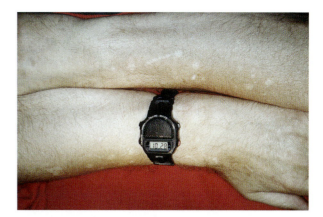

Fig. 10.6 Self-induced burns from cigarettes as an attention-seeking device.

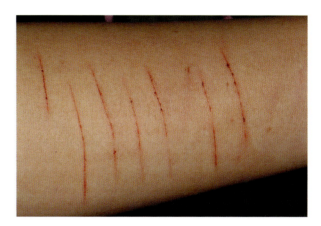

Fig. 10.7 Self -harm.

FACTITIOUS INJURIES

Factitious (self-induced) disorders are distinguished from somatoform disorders by the voluntary production of symptoms, and distinguished from malingering by the lack of external incentive. Physical or psychological symptoms are intentionally produced to assume a sick role. They are more common in men than women, and seen most frequently in health-care professionals (HCPs), who intentionally produce signs of medical and/or mental disorders.

Serious and deliberate self-inflicted lesions in the mouth are considerably less common than on the skin. This may be due to an underlying need or desire for attention, and oral lesions are insufficiently obvious.

Factitious disorders are not uncommon in depressed patients and in those with schizophrenia and learning disability. Examples include self-induced cigarette burns (Fig. 10.6) or cuts (Fig. 10.7). Rare causes of self-injury also include any cause of sensory loss or pain insensitivity, such as the Riley–Day syndrome, Lesch–Nyhan syndrome (Ch. 23) and Gilles de la Tourette syndrome – multiple tics and coprolalia (involuntary uttering of obscenities).

Clinical features

Minor, subconsciously self-induced oral lesions are common, the classic examples being bruxism and cheek-biting (morsicatio buccarum) and exfoliative cheilitis ('tic de lèvres'; Fig. 10.8). Other lesions may be accidentally self-inflicted when the oral mucosa is anaesthetized, after a local anaesthetic, surgery or damage to the trigeminal nerve.

The most commonly reported type of self-inflicted oral injury has been so-called self-extraction of teeth. Soft-tissue lesions can also be produced, typically by picking at the gingivae with the fingernails. In

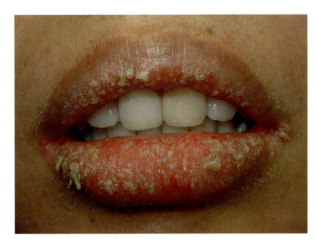

Fig. 10.8 Exfoliative cheilitis.

adults, injuries may be produced by use of the pointed end of a nail file, often also at the gingival margins.

Other types of injury include the application of caustic substances to the lips or injuries from attempts at suicide.

General management

Self-inflicted lesions should be suspected when they do not correspond with those of any recognized disease; are of bizarre configuration with sharp outlines; are found in an otherwise healthy patient; are in sites accessible only to the patient; or if the patient shows signs that suggest emotional disturbance, is under stress, is known to be under psychiatric treatment, or has a learning impairment.

Few patients will admit to injuring themselves. More frequently, the diagnosis can be confirmed only by discreet observation after admission of the patient to hospital. However, even when seen to cause the injuries, the patient may still deny having made them. Once the diagnosis has been made, the family doctor or specialist psychiatrist should see the patient.

HYSTERICAL STATES

Hysterical personality disorders, neuroses and acute psychoses are recognized.

Hysterical neuroses

Hysterical neuroses mainly affect females – sometimes those working in medical or paramedical occupations – as conversion neurosis or as a dissociative state. Hysterical conversion neurosis is characterized by physical complaints that have no demonstrable organic basis, such as pain, anaesthesia, dysphagia, fainting, fits, paralysis or tremor, but frequently result in patients submitting to repeated operations; there may, as a result, be multiple scars (see 'Munchausen syndrome'). Dissociative states are characterized by disturbances of consciousness or identity (but no physical symptoms) in the absence of demonstrable organic disease. Amnesia, states of fugue (when the patient wanders aimlessly away), or (rarely) multiple personalities are examples.

It is often difficult to establish that the patient is gaining something by the illness, although in compensation neurosis the nature of the potential gain is easily recognized.

Dental aspects

Patients who aggressively insist on their symptoms and demand surgery for undetectable lesions are fortunately rare.

Munchausen syndrome

Munchausen syndrome is a disorder in which patients go to considerable length to fabricate histories and simulate symptoms without an external incentive (compare malingering) but apparently for the sake of undergoing operations. This may be done repeatedly, even occasionally by assuming false names and travelling to many hospitals scattered about the country. Patients are often intelligent and resourceful. Common complaints are of acute abdominal pain; fever; haematuria; or infected wounds. Ultimately, the patient may become extensively scarred and develop complications from the repeated operations.

Munchausen syndrome-by-proxy is the term given to a parent or other carer who invents symptoms in, and demands unnecessary medical or surgical treatment for, a child.

Treatment is difficult and often fails; the main aims should be to avoid unnecessary drug use (especially opiates) and surgery.

Compensation neurosis

Compensation neurosis usually follows an accident (especially a head injury) or operation, and is characterized by paralysis, chronic pain (often headache) or other symptoms of obscure origin and of no obvious organic cause. Men and women are equally susceptible, there is no previous history, and the lack of insight is less convincing than in hysteria.

Settlement of the claim for compensation typically results in rapid disappearance of the symptoms.

SELF-HARM

Self-harm (SH) or deliberate self-harm (DSH) includes self-injury (SI) and self-poisoning, and is defined as the intentional, direct injuring of body tissue. Discrete from most body art such as piercings/tattoos, SH is most common in adolescence and young adulthood, usually first appearing between the ages of 12 and 24.

The most common form of SH is skin-cutting but there is a wide range of behaviours including, but not limited to, burning, scratching, banging or hitting body parts, interfering with wound healing, hair-pulling (trichotillomania) and ingestion of objects (pica) or toxic substances. It is not intended to be suicidal but that might result.

Connotations include:

- neurotic – nail-biting, picking, extreme hair removal and unnecessary cosmetic surgery
- religious – self-flagellation and other forms
- cultural – such as the Shi'ite ritual of self-flagellation, Mayan self-cutting/piercing
- psychotic – eye or ear removal, genital self-mutilation, autocastration and extreme amputation
- organic brain diseases – repetitive head-banging, hand-biting, finger-fracturing or eye removal.

SH is classed as a borderline personality disturbance or a coping mechanism which provides temporary relief of intense feelings such as anxiety, depression, stress, emotional numbness or a sense of failure. Munchausen syndrome, war avoidance behaviour and attention-seeking may be involved. DSH is especially prevalent in prison populations.

SH may also feature in:

- genetic disorders: e.g. Lesch–Nyhan syndrome
- mental issues: bipolar disorder, schizophrenia, depression
- substance abuse or withdrawal.

Box 10.3 *Some possible behavioural reactions to organic disease*

- Denial
- Anger
- Frustration
- Aggression
- Anxiety
- Fear
- Withdrawal
- Apathy
- Dependency
- Depression

Care plans should be multidisciplinary and developed collaboratively with the person who self-harms and, provided the person agrees, with their family, carers or significant others. Psychological, pharmacological and psychosocial interventions may be needed (see http://www.nice.org.uk/newsroom/pressreleases/LongerTermManagementOfSelfHarmGuidance.jsp).

PSYCHIATRIC DISORDERS

Psychiatric disorders are common; perhaps one-third of the population suffer at some time during their life. These disorders are often under-diagnosed, and what may appear simply to be unusual behaviour may actually be a manifestation. Psychiatric illnesses cause significant incapacity but, equally, organic illness can cause major behavioural changes and sometimes precipitate psychiatric disease (Box 10.3). Mental disorders underlie many complaints and extend the recovery time from many others.

Mental disorders frequently coexist with diverse other illnesses. Depression, for example, may be associated with a high prevalence (around 65%) of common chronic medical conditions, such as hypertension, coronary artery disease, diabetes, arthritis and chronic lung disorders. About 15% of people with a mental disorder also indulge in substance abuse.

Diagnostic criteria for the most common mental disorders are outlined in DSM-IV (American Psychiatric Association, 1994; revised 2000; Table 10.8 and Box 10.4). The most significant psychiatric disorders are shown in Table 10.9.

Dental aspects

Mental disorders can significantly influence oral health care, not least because of behavioural disorders or interpersonal difficulties. Patients with mental disease may be unable to cooperate. Drug misuse may explain abnormal behaviour in some patients:

- Compliance with appointments or treatment is often poor.
- There may be difficulties in gaining informed consent to treatment.
- There may also be oral neglect with a high prevalence of caries and periodontal disease, difficulties coping with dental prostheses, and self-induced lesions or other oral symptoms caused by the psychiatric illness or its treatment.
- Some of the more severely ill or neglected patients with mental disorders are at high risk from diseases of deprivation and lifestyle, such as tuberculosis.
- Drugs such as antidepressants, phenothiazines, lithium or barbiturates can cause xerostomia or other orofacial disorders, or otherwise influence dental care.

Table 10.8 *Classification of psychosocial health*

Axis	Description
I	Clinical disorders (see Box 10.4)
II	Personality disorders
III	General medical conditions
IV	Psychosocial and environmental problems
V	Global assessment of functioning

Box 10.4 *Axis I*

- Disorders first diagnosed in infancy
- Delirium, dementia, and amnestic and other cognitive disorders
- Mental disorders caused by a general medical condition
- Substance-related disorders
- Schizophrenia and other psychotic disorders
- Mood disorders
- Anxiety disorders
- Somatoform disorders
- Factitious disorders
- Dissociative disorders
- Sexual and gender identity disorders
- Eating disorders
- Sleep disorders
- Psychological factors affecting medical conditions
- Impulse control disorders not classified elsewhere
- Adjustment disorders
- Other conditions that may be the focus of medical attention

Table 10.9 *The most common mental disorders*

Condition	Anxiety disorders	Depression	Schizophrenia
Prevalence (approximate)	1 in 10 people	1 in 10 people	1 in 100 people

MOOD DISORDERS

Depression

General aspects

Depression is more than just a 'bad day'; diagnostic criteria established by the APA dictate that five or more symptoms must be present for a continuous period of at least 2 weeks. Depression is characterized by depressed or sad mood, diminished interest in activities that used to be pleasurable, weight gain or loss, psychomotor agitation or retardation, fatigue, inappropriate guilt and difficulties concentrating, as well as recurrent thoughts of death.

Major depression frequently goes unrecognized and untreated, and may foster tragic consequences, such as suicide and impaired interpersonal relationships at work and at home. The use of medications and/or specific psychotherapeutic techniques has proven effective in the treatment of major depression.

Dysthymia, a depressive disorder characterized by low-grade mood impairment of at least 2 years that commonly has an initial presentation in childhood or young adulthood, has been likened to a less severe major depression, but one more likely to assume a chronic course.

Depression is a common emotion which all of us experience at some time. It becomes a disorder of emotion when it is characterized by a persistent lowering of mood and negative patterns of thinking, and may impact significantly on an individual's quality of life. Depression is also often a feature of a medical problem but is sometimes so severe and enduring that it becomes an illness in itself.

Depression as an illness, involves mood and thoughts, and affects the way persons eat and sleep, feel about themselves and think about things. Although depression alone may be seen (unipolar disorder), about 1 in 10 people who suffer from serious depression will also have periods when they are too happy and overactive (bipolar disorder – which used to be called manic depression).

The lifetime risk for depression is approximately 10%, with rates being doubled in women; hormonal factors may contribute, particularly menstrual cycle changes, pregnancy, miscarriage, the postpartum period, pre-menopause and the menopause. Depression may be genetic and can often run in families; onset may be at any stage from childhood onwards. Episodes can be triggered by adverse life events, such as a serious loss, difficult relationships, financial problems or any stressful (unwelcome or even desired) change in life patterns.

Some cases are precipitated by serious medical illnesses such as stroke, heart attack, cancer, Parkinson disease, hormonal disorders, or illnesses that are long and uncomfortable or painful, such as arthritis or bronchitis. Some people become depressed after viral infections like influenza or glandular fever.

The main effects of depression appear to relate to changes in hypothalamic centres that govern food intake, libido and circadian rhythms; various hormones, particularly serotonin, dopamine and noradrenaline (norepinephrine), are implicated and hypercortisolism is common. Antidepressants increase concentrations of these chemicals at brain nerve endings and so seem to boost the function of those parts of the brain that use serotonin and noradrenaline.

The danger in depression is of suicide; death from suicide in men is four times that of women, though more women attempt it.

In addition to being a chronic disease in its own right, depression appears to be associated with behaviours linked to other chronic diseases:

- *Smoking.* Depression is a risk factor for smoking, with nicotine stimulating receptors in the brain that may improve mood in certain types of depression; furthermore, depression may impede smoking cessation efforts.
- *Alcohol consumption.* Early onset of drinking is associated with a range of problematic outcomes, including depressive symptoms.
- *Physical inactivity.* Physical inactivity and obesity are modifiable risk factors for depression.
- *Sleep disturbance.* Depression appears to be associated with poor sleep.

Clinical features

Features of major depression (Box 10.5) include: a persistently sad, anxious or 'empty' mood; feelings of hopelessness and pessimism; of guilt, worthlessness and helplessness; loss of interest or pleasure in hobbies and activities that were once enjoyed, including sex; lack of energy, fatigue and a feeling of being 'slowed down'; difficulty concentrating, remembering, and making decisions; insomnia, early-morning awakening or oversleeping; appetite and/or weight loss, or overeating/weight gain; and restlessness and irritability. A depressive episode is diagnosed if five or more of the following symptoms last most of the day, nearly every day, for a period of 2 weeks or longer:

- feeling unhappy most of the time (but may feel a little better in the evenings)
- loss of interest in life and inability to enjoy anything

Box 10.5 *Features of depression*

- Sadness
- Hopelessness
- Pessimism
- Lack of pleasure
- Irritability
- Fatigue
- Sleep disturbance
- Loss of libido and appetite

- finding it harder to make decisions
- inability to cope with things that the patient used to be able to deal with
- feeling utterly tired
- feeling restless and agitated
- loss of appetite and weight (some people find they do the reverse and put on weight)
- taking 1–2 hours to get off to sleep, and then waking up earlier than usual
- loss of interest in sex
- loss of self-confidence
- feeling useless, inadequate and hopeless
- avoidance of other people
- feeling irritable
- feeling worse at a particular time each day, usually in the morning
- thoughts of suicide.

Patients may exhibit: lack of energy, fatigue, reduced concentration, insomnia, early-morning awakening, oversleeping, loss of appetite and weight loss or gain. Depression may also manifest as chronic pain; 50% of patients who are depressed have pain as their presenting complaint. Chronic pain or other persistent bodily symptoms that are not caused by physical illness or injury are common.

Men are less likely to admit to depression and doctors are less likely to suspect it. It is often masked in men by manifesting, not as feeling hopeless and helpless, but as being irritable, angry and discouraged. Alternatively, depression may be suppressed by alcohol or drugs, or by the socially acceptable habit of working excessively long hours.

There may be thoughts of death or suicide, and suicide attempts. Warning signs include: talking about feeling suicidal or wanting to die; feeling hopeless, that nothing will ever change or get better; feeling helpless, that nothing the patient does makes any difference; feeling a burden to family and friends; abusing alcohol or drugs; putting affairs in order (e.g. organizing finances or giving away possessions to prepare for death); writing a suicide note; and putting themselves in harm's way, or in situations where there is a danger of being killed. Risks for suicide appear to be higher earlier in the course of the illness.

Dysthymic disorder is a chronic, less intense form of depression but may progress to major depression. It involves long-term, chronic symptoms that do not disable patients, but keep them from functioning well or from feeling happy. Many dysthymics also experience major depressive episodes at some time.

Seasonal affective disorder (SAD) is a chronic cyclical form of depression that appears as daylight hours shorten and is related to melatonin and serotonin production. Its features also include winter somnolence and a craving for carbohydrates. Light therapy may be beneficial.

Involutional melancholia is characterized by severe anxiety and hypochondriasis, beginning in later life and mainly affecting women.

Bipolar disorder is the term given to depression alternating with mania, which may amount to a psychosis. The various mood states in bipolar disorder may be regarded as a spectrum with severe depression at one end and mania at the other. Bipolar I disorder consists of alternating depression and mania; bipolar II disorder is alternating depression with hypomania; while mixed bipolar disorder is when depression and mania occur concurrently – usually as aggression plus depression.

General management

Diagnosis of depression is dependent upon identifying:

- a persistent lowering of mood
- alterations of biological function (as outlined above)
- altered thought content – patients have negative pessimistic thoughts about themselves, the world and the future (Beck cognitive triad).

It is important to remember that depressed patients often present with other symptoms, such as pain, and questionnaires to screen for thought and biological disturbances are therefore useful diagnostically.

Anyone thinking about committing suicide needs immediate attention, preferably from a psychiatrist. Important measures, if there is an attempt, are calling a doctor or emergency services to seek immediate help; ensuring that the suicidal person is not left alone; and denying access to medications, weapons or other items that could be used for self-harm.

Treatment of depression is by psychotherapy and medication. (Fig. 10.9) Psychotherapy involves talking with a mental health professional, such as a psychiatrist, psychologist, social worker or counsellor, to learn how to deal with problems.

The majority of patients with depression can be managed in the primary health-care setting by using the following measures:

- Appropriate risk assessment for suicide, self-neglect and danger to others. Psychiatric referral is needed if suicide risk is high or the depression is severe and unresponsive to initial treatment. Following the recent review of the Mental Health Act 2008 in the UK, all doctors are required to be able to judge a patient's capacity to make decisions; psychiatrists are further required to assess dangerousness.
- Psychological techniques (cognitive behavioural and supportive therapy).
- Pharmacotherapy (Tables 10.10 and 10.17).
- Electroconvulsive therapy (ECT) for very severe cases, where significant physical retardation or delusions (fixed unshakeable false beliefs) are present.

Antidepressants

Antidepressant drugs raise brain levels of serotonin and noradrenaline (norepinephrine). None of them is perfect and all suffer from at least one of the following drawbacks:

- Delayed onset of action from 7 to 28 days – although some improvements may be seen in the first few weeks, most antidepressant medications must be taken regularly for 3–4 weeks (in some cases, as many as 8 weeks) before the full therapeutic effect starts
- Anticholinergic effects
- Sedation
- Agitation
- Cardiotoxicity
- Weight gain.

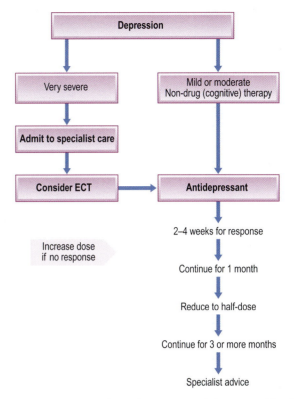

Fig. 10.9 Depression, CBT, tricyclic antidepressants and electroconvulsive therapy (ECT).

Table 10.10 *Classification of antidepressants[a] (see Table 10.16)*

Class	Examples
Tricyclic antidepressant (TCA)	Amitriptyline
Serotonin noradrenaline (norepinephrine) reuptake inhibitor (SNRI)	Venlafaxine
Selective serotonin reuptake inhibitor (SSRI)	Fluoxetine
Noradrenaline (norepinephrine) reuptake inhibitor (NRI)	Reboxetine
Noradrenaline (norepinephrine) and specific serotonergic agonist	Mirtazapine
Serotonin reuptake inhibitor (SRI)	Nefazodone
Reversible inhibitor of monoamine oxidase A (RIMA)	Moclobemide
Monoamine oxidase inhibitor (MAOI)	Phenelzine

[a]See Table 10.16.

Table 10.11 *Monoamine oxidase inhibitors (MAOIs)*

MAOI	Special comments (see text about food reactions)
Isocarboxazid	Contraindicated in liver or cardiovascular disease
Phenelzine	Contraindicated in liver or cardiovascular disease
Tranylcypromine	The most dangerous MAOI
Moclobemide	Less reactive with foods or drugs

Patients often are tempted to stop medication too soon but they should continue for at least 4–9 months to prevent recurrence.

Monoamine oxidase inhibitors (MAOIs) These were the first effective antidepressants but are now rarely prescribed because of their adverse effects (Table 10.11). Dry mouth and hypotension are common side-effects of MAOIs. The most serious adverse effects of the earlier and non-selective irreversible MAOIs, such as phenelzine, isoniazid and tranylcypromine, are drug or food interactions.

Table 10.12 *Monoamine oxidase inhibitors: possible adverse effects and interactions*

Possible adverse effects	Possible interactions
Hyposalivation	Hypertensive reactions with noradrenaline (norepinephrine), ephedrine or phenylephrine, or with tyramine-containing foods
Hypotension	
Anorexia	
Nausea	Adrenaline (epinephrine) can be used safely
Constipation	Enhanced action of respiratory depressants such as general anaesthetic agents, sedatives, antihistamines, opioids
Sexual dysfunction	
	Risk of seizures with tramadol

Table 10.13 *Some possible adverse effects and interactions of tricyclic antidepressants*

	Possible adverse reactions	Possible interactions
Cardiovascular	Arrhythmias	Hypertensive reaction with noradrenaline (norepinephrine)
	Cardiotoxicity	
	Postural hypotension	
	Tachycardias	
Neurological	Agitation	Potentiation of CNS depressants
	Ataxia	
	Dizziness	Risk of seizures with tramadol
	Drowsiness	
	Insomnia	
	Seizures	
	Tremor	
Liver	Jaundice	
Blood	Leukopenia	
Others	Blurred vision	
	Constipation	
	Dry mouth	
	Nausea	
	Sexual dysfunction	
	Urinary retention	

Hypertensive crises have resulted from interaction of these MAOIs with foods containing tyramine, particularly cheese, and also with yeast products, chocolate, bananas, broad beans, some red wines and beer, pickled herring or caviar. However, the frequency of such reactions has been greatly overestimated. Selective MAOIs, such as selegiline, used mainly in parkinsonism rather than depression, can also provoke similar reactions contrary to earlier beliefs. Interactions of MAOIs with pethidine and other opioids are the most dangerous reactions and have sometimes been fatal (Table 10.12). Interactions with TCAs are also dangerous. Ephedrine and similar drugs, which are often present in nasal decongestants or cold remedies, may cause severe hypertension.

The most commonly used MAOIs are phenelzine and isocarboxazid; phenelzine, for example, is helpful for people with panic disorder and social phobia.

Tricyclic antidepressants (TCAs) These are probably the most effective antidepressants, which have stood the test of time, despite their undesirable adverse effects (Table 10.13); they are useful when there is associated anxiety. Their most common adverse effects, and ways to deal with some of them, are:

- dry mouth – it is helpful to drink sips of water, chew sugarless gum and clean teeth daily
- constipation – bran, prunes, fruit and vegetables should be in the diet
- bladder difficulties – emptying the bladder may be troublesome and the urine stream may be weak
- sexual difficulties – sexual function may deteriorate
- blurred vision
- dizziness – rising from the bed or chair slowly is helpful
- drowsiness as a daytime problem (see Table 10.13) – the more sedating antidepressants are generally taken at bedtime to help sleep and minimize daytime drowsiness. A person feeling drowsy or sedated should not drive or operate dangerous equipment.

The onset of action of TCAs is slow and they may take 4 weeks to exert their full effect. The action is dose-dependent and lack of effect is often the result of failure to achieve adequate plasma levels. TCAs are contraindicated in patients with cardiac disorders (recent myocardial infarct, arrhythmias, heart block, cardiac failure), epilepsy, liver dysfunction, blood dyscrasias, glaucoma and urinary obstruction (e.g. prostatic hypertrophy). They should only be given after a full blood count and liver function tests; if the patient is over 45, an ECG is also indicated. TCAs should not be given within 2 weeks of the use of MAOIs.

The most commonly used TCAs are amitriptyline, dosulepin and imipramine. Sedation is a common side-effect, particularly with amitriptyline, but this may be an advantage if the patient is agitated

Table 10.14 *Tricyclic and related antidepressants*

Drug	Special comments[a]
Tricyclic antidepressant (TCA)	
Amitriptyline	More cardiotoxic, sedative and antimuscarinic than many TCAs; caution with general anaesthesia
Amoxapine	May cause tardive dyskinesia
Clomipramine	Possibly low sedative activity
Dosulepin	Sedative
Doxepin	Sedative; fewer cardiac effects
Imipramine	Less sedative than most but more antimuscarinic and cardiac effects
Lofepramine	Avoid in renal or hepatic disease
Nortriptyline	Possibly low antimuscarinic effects
Trimipramine	Photosensitive rashes
Related drugs	
Maprotiline	Less antimuscarinic but more epileptogenic than TCAs
Mianserin	Possible hepatic and haematological reactions
Trazodone	Fewer antimuscarinic and cardiac effects

[a]Up to 4 weeks are required before symptom control can be expected. Reduced doses should be used in the elderly. Arrhythmias and heart block may be seen, as well as drowsiness, dry mouth, urinary retention and constipation (antimuscarinic actions). Contraindicated after myocardial infarction. Cardiotoxic in overdose.

(Table 10.14). Side-effects of the TCAs are more serious in older people. Various other TCAs have particular advantages: imipramine, for example, is mildly stimulating and clomipramine appears to be useful where there are obsessional or phobic problems. Lofepramine has fewer antimuscarinic effects than some others and is less dangerous in overdose. Doxepin (similar to imipramine) is the drug of choice if there is cardiovascular disease. Clomipramine is the only tricyclic prescribed for OCD, while imipramine may be given for panic disorder and GAD.

Selective serotonin reuptake inhibitors (SSRIs) These are newer antidepressants, and have the advantage over older antidepressants of less severe antimuscarinic activity, weight gain or cardiac conduction effects. SSRIs do not interact with alcohol and are thus often preferred by both patients and practitioners; however, gastrointestinal effects are common.

Adverse effects of SSRIs include anorexia, nausea, anxiety, diarrhea, sexual dysfunction, and rarely mania, paranoia or extrapyramidal features (Table 10.15). Fluoxetine (Prozac) has been hailed as a valuable antidepressant (makes you feel 'better than well'!), but in the USA has allegedly been associated with aggressive behaviour, including murders. More recently, the same allegations have been made against paroxetine.

SSRIs may interact with TCAs or neuroleptics to cause a rise in plasma concentration and exaggerated effects of these drugs. SSRIs may interact with MAOIs, TCAs, carbamazepine or lithium to produce the serotonin syndrome (see Table 10.15), which comprises CNS irritability, hyper-reflexia and myoclonus, and is occasionally fatal. SSRIs should not therefore be used with TCAs or within 2 weeks of MAOIs. They are also contraindicated in epilepsy, cardiac disease, diabetes, glaucoma, bleeding tendencies, pregnancy, liver or renal disease.

They may have other adverse effects:

- Arrhythmias if the patient is using terfenadine
- Headache

- Nausea
- Nervousness and insomnia (trouble falling asleep or waking often during the night) – dosage reductions or time will usually resolve these complaints
- Agitation
- Dry mouth.

SSRIs such as fluoxetine or sertraline are commonly prescribed for panic disorder, OCD, PTSD and social phobia, and may be preferred for anxiety disorders. SSRIs can inhibit cytochrome P450 enzymes and thus impair the metabolism of BZPs, carbamazepine, codeine and erythromycin.

Newer antidepressants These include agomelatine, a melatonin receptor agonist; ketamine-like N-methyl-D-aspartate receptor (NMDA) antagonists; and vortioxetine - a SSRI variant which has antagonistic properties at 5-HT3A and 5-HT7 receptors, partial agonistic properties at 5-HT1B receptors, agonistic properties at 5-HT1A receptors, and potent inhibition of the serotonin reuptake transporter.

Summary of antidepressants (see Appendix 10.1) The SSRIs and other newer antidepressants (Table 10.16) that affect neurotransmitters, such as dopamine or noradrenaline (norepinephrine), generally have fewer adverse effects than TCAs, and both SSRIs and TCAs are safer overall than MAOIs, which can interact, even fatally, with some foods and drugs. Other agents used in severe depression may include some antipsychotics such as quetiapine and aripiprazole.

Herbal therapy

St John's wort (*Hypericum perforatum*) has been shown to be effective in mild depression but it may interact with SSRIs to produce the serotonin syndrome. It also stimulates cytochrome P450, and thus impairs the activity of drugs such as chemotherapeutic drugs (e.g. irinotecan, the vinca alkaloids, etoposide, teniposide, anthracycline, paclitaxel, docetaxel and tamoxifen), ciclosporin, digoxin, warfarin, indinavir (a protease inhibitor used in human immunodeficiency virus [HIV] infection), oral contraceptives, opioids and general anaesthetic agents.

Table 10.15 *Selective serotonin reuptake inhibitors: possible adverse effects and drug interactions*

Possible adverse effects	Possible interactions	
	Drug	Effect
Xerostomia	Carbamazepine	Serotonin syndrome
Arrhythmias	Lithium	Serotonin syndrome
Gastrointestinal upsets	Monoamine oxidase inhibitors	Serotonin syndrome
	Terfenadine	Arrhythmias
	Tramadol	Risk of seizures
	Tricyclics	Serotonin syndrome

Table 10.16 *Antidepressants and their actions*[a]

Class	Abbreviation	Actions	Examples
Monoamine oxidase inhibitors	MAOIs	Inhibit monoamine oxidase A (MAO-A)	Moclobemide
Noradrenergic and specific serotonergic antidepressants	NASSAs	Block noradrenaline (norepinephrine), 5HT2 and 5HT3 reuptake	Mirtazapine
Noradrenaline (norepinephrine) reuptake inhibitors	NRIs	Block noradrenaline (norepinephrine) reuptake	Reboxetine
Selective serotonin reuptake inhibitors	SSRIs	Block 5HT (serotonin) reuptake	Citalopram
			Fluoxetine
			Fluvoxamine
			Paroxetine
			Sertraline
Serotonin noradrenaline (norepinephrine) reuptake inhibitors	SNRIs	Block noradrenaline (norepinephrine) and 5HT reuptake	Duloxetine
			Venlafaxine
Serotonin reuptake inhibitors	SRIs	5HT antagonists	Nefazodone
Tricyclic antidepressants	TCAs	Block noradrenaline (norepinephrine) and 5HT reuptake	Amitriptyline
			Clomipramine
			Dosulepin
			Doxepin
			Lofepramine
			Nortriptyline
			Protriptyline

[a]See Table 10.10. For adverse effects, see Tables 10.11–10.15.

Electroconvulsive therapy (ECT)

ECT is sometimes given for severe depression, where drugs have been ineffective or where there is a strong risk of suicide. A muscle relaxant is given before treatment, which is delivered under GA. Electrodes are placed at precise locations on the head to deliver electrical impulses. The stimulation causes a brief seizure. The patient does not consciously experience the electrical stimulus. Amnesia is the main side-effect.

Dental aspects of depression

The features aiding recognition of depression have been suggested above. Dental staff should be alert to this possibility, particularly where the patient appears withdrawn, difficult or aggressive, or where there are oral complaints of the types described earlier. Great tact, patience and a sympathetic, friendly manner are needed. Dental treatment is preferably deferred until depression is under control but preventive programmes should be instituted at an early stage.

In patients taking TCAs, adrenaline (epinephrine) in local anaesthetics has not been shown clinically to cause hypertension (despite statements to the contrary). However, severe hypertension has resulted from high concentrations of noradrenaline (norepinephrine) in local anaesthetics, whether or not the patient was receiving antidepressants. Noradrenaline has no advantages as a vasoconstrictor and noradrenaline preparations have been withdrawn.

Paracetamol (acetaminophen) can inhibit the metabolism of TCAs, and atropinics are potentiated by TCAs.

Patients on MAOIs are at risk from GA, since prolonged respiratory depression may result. Any CNS depressant, especially opioids and phenothiazines, given to patients on MAOIs (or within 21 days of their withdrawal) may precipitate coma. Pethidine is particularly dangerous.

Indirectly acting sympathomimetic agents, such as ephedrine or cocaine, can interact with MAOIs to cause hypertension, and must therefore not be used. There is no evidence of any danger to patients on MAOIs from adrenaline (epinephrine) in LA solutions.

Tricyclics and MAOIs can cause postural hypotension. Dental patients using these drugs should not be stood immediately upright if they have been recumbent during treatment and the chair should be brought upright slowly.

Some depressed patients resort to drug misuse, and this must be considered (Ch. 34).

BZPs, carbamazepine, codeine and erythromycin may be potentiated by SSRIs.

The most common oral complaint of depressed patients under treatment is that of a dry mouth, especially as a result of the use of TCAs, MAOIs or lithium. This may even predispose to oral candidosis and accelerated caries. Taste sensation may also be disturbed and patients tend to eat more sugar. The effect of xerostomia can occasionally result in ascending suppurative parotitis. The most effective treatment is to change the antidepressant to another that has little anticholinergic activity. If this is not acceptable, the dry mouth should be managed as in Sjögren syndrome (Ch. 16). Smoking, and other drugs that may add to the xerostomia, such as antihistamines, hyoscine (scopolamine) or other atropine-like drugs, or SSRIs, should therefore be avoided. Both MAOIs and TCAs have also been reported occasionally to cause facial dyskinesias, and prolonged use of flupentixol can lead to intractable tardive dyskinesia.

Bodily complaints, often related to the mouth, are common in depression and the dental surgeon should appreciate the possibility of a psychological basis for such oral disorders. Depression is associated especially with the following painful disorders of the orofacial region:

- Chronic facial pain
- Burning mouth or sore tongue (oral dysaesthesia)
- Occasionally temporomandibular pain dysfunction syndrome
- Other oral complaints, which may be delusional and include: discharges (of fluid, slime or powder coming into the mouth) dry mouth or sialorrhoea despite normal salivary flow spots or lumps halitosis disturbed taste sensation.

Depression may also accompany: other mental diseases, such as schizophrenia; viral infections (e.g. influenza, hepatitis or infectious mononucleosis); drugs (particularly reserpine, methyldopa, fenfluramine and corticosteroids) or their withdrawal (e.g. of amphetamines, BZPs or antidepressants); and serious medical disorders such as parkinsonism, stroke, myocardial infarction, malignant diseases or endocrinopathies, like diabetes.

Chronic fatigue syndrome (myalgic encephalitis/encephalomyopathy [ME])

General aspects

Chronic fatigue syndrome (CFS) is not a mental disorder but the cause is still unclear. It is a disorder characterized by lack of energy, tiredness, muscle and joint pains after minimal effort, emotional lability, poor concentration and memory, and often other symptoms. This clinical picture was described in 1867 and termed 'neurasthenia'. CFS is under-diagnosed in more than 80% of the people who have it; at the same time, it is often misdiagnosed as depression.

CFS often begins after an infection such as influenza or infectious mononucleosis, or after a period of high stress. Since the symptoms may resemble those of the recovery phase of a viral infection, the complaint is termed 'post-viral fatigue syndrome', but claims for Epstein–Barr virus, herpes virus 6 and Coxsackie B having a causative role have not been substantiated. Parvovirus has been implicated in some patients. Xenotropic murine leukaemia virus-related virus (XMRV), a human retrovirus apparently first identified in tissue samples from prostate cancer, was also reported to have been detected in two-thirds of patients with CFS. However, evidence of XMRV in these conditions was controversial and the suggested links have since been disproved.

Genetic, immunological, infectious, metabolic and neurological aetiologies have been suggested to explain CFS. Several mechanisms have been proposed, such as excessive oxidative stress following exertion, immune imbalance characterized by decreased natural killer cell and macrophage activity, immunoglobulin G subclass deficiencies (IgG1, IgG3), and decreased serum concentrations of complement component. Autoantibodies have also been suggested as a possible factor; recent studies indicate that antiserotonin, anti-microtubule-associated protein 2 and antimuscarinic cholinergic receptor 1 antibodies may play a role. It has been demonstrated that impairment in vasoactive neuropeptide metabolism may explain the symptoms of CFS. Genes for haematological disease and function, immunological disease and function, cancer, cell death, immune response and infection have altered expression. Increases in elastase activity and protein kinase and ribonuclease (RNase) L enzymes support the clinical importance of these immune dysfunctions in CFS.

Clinical features

Unlike most post-viral symptoms, which usually abate in a few days or weeks, CFS symptoms, particularly fatigue, either persist or fluctuate, frequently for more than 6 months. CFS also has eight other possible primary symptoms, which include: loss of memory or concentration, sore throat, painful and mildly enlarged lymph nodes in the neck or axilla, myalgia, polyarthralgia without swelling or redness, headache of a new type, pattern or severity, sleep disturbance; or extreme exhaustion after normal exercise or exertion. A person meets the diagnostic criteria of CFS when unexplained fatigue persists for 6 months or more with at least 4 of the above 8 primary symptoms are also present.

Similar features may be seen in infection with:

- Epstein–Barr virus
- human herpesvirus 6
- enterovirus
- rubella
- *Candida albicans*
- bornaviruses
- mycoplasma
- Ross River virus
- *Coxiella burnetti*
- human retroviruses, such as HIV or XMRV.

CFS is a post-infective condition in approximately 10–12% of cases.

Neurally mediated hypotension (NMH) or postural orthostatic tachycardia syndrome (POTS) have been incriminated in some CFS patients.

General management

Tests showing any disorders of muscle function or any other organic lesion have not been substantiated. By contrast, those with organic neuromuscular diseases do not have the mental symptoms characteristic of CFS.

Management of CFS aims to relieve symptoms by using gradual but steady exercise and treatment of symptoms. CFS may respond to antidepressant drugs.

Dental aspects

Unexpectedly, perhaps, atypical (idiopathic) facial pain has not been reported as a feature of CFS. The only oral symptom reported has been dry mouth.

PSYCHOSES

Psychotic disorders are serious conditions characterized by dysregulation of thought processes, in which insight is often lacking (Table 10.17). In particular, schizophrenia has hallmark symptoms of delusions (false, strongly held beliefs not influenced by logical reasoning or explained by a person's usual cultural concepts) and hallucinations (hearing and/or seeing sensory information which is not actually present and is not apparent to others). Typically, psychotic disorders are treated with antipsychotic medications and psychosocial interventions.

Bipolar disorder

Bipolar disorder (formerly known as 'manic–depressive psychosis') is a major mood disorder in which the individual most commonly experiences episodes of depression and episodes of mania (a clearly elevated, unrestrained or irritable mood that may manifest in an exaggerated assessment of self-importance or grandiosity, sleeplessness, racing thoughts, pressured speech, and the tendency to engage in activities

Table 10.17 *Main psychoses: features*

Bipolar disorder (manic depression)	Mainly severe depression but there may be manic episodes for weeks, months or years
Schizophrenia	Severe disorder of thought, behaviour and affect, with hallucinations, delusions and illusions
Korsakoff syndrome	Recent amnesia and confabulation
Brief psychotic disorder	Short, non-recurrent psychosis
Delusional disorder	One or more fixed beliefs
Shared psychotic disorder	'Folie à deux' – a delusional disorder shared by two people

Table 10.18 *Bipolar disorders*

Terminology	Comments
Bipolar I	At least one high, or manic episode, lasting longer than 1 week. Some people with bipolar I will have only manic episodes, although most will also have periods of depression
	Untreated, manic episodes generally last 3–6 months
	Depressive episodes last rather longer – 6–12 months without treatment
Bipolar II	More than one episode of severe depression but only mild manic episodes – 'hypomania'
Cyclothymia	Mood swings not as severe as in full bipolar disorder but can be longer. May develop into full bipolar disorder
Rapid cycling	More than four mood swings in a 12-month period

that appear pleasurable but have a high potential for adverse consequences). Medications and psychotherapy are effective treatments of bipolar disorder.

Mu-opioids (endorphins), CRH, noradrenaline (norepinephrine), dopamine and serotonin appear to be altered in depression.

General aspects

Bipolar disorder is characterized by cycling mood changes of severe highs (mania) and lows (depression). Hypomania with major depression is termed bipolar I disorder (Table 10.18). Sometimes the mood switches are dramatic and rapid, but most often they are gradual.

About 1 in every 100 adults has bipolar disorder. Men and women are affected equally. It usually starts in late adolescence or early adulthood. It is unusual for it to start after the age of 40. However, symptoms may sometimes start during childhood, or alternatively in later in life, when they may indicate organic disease: for example, a neoplasm or an effect of drugs such as corticosteroids, alcohol or another drug of dependence.

When in the manic cycle, the person may be overactive and overtalkative, and have excessive energy. In the depressed cycle, any or all of the symptoms of a depressive disorder are prominent.

Mania

Mania, left untreated, may worsen to a psychotic state. It is characterized by:

- abnormal or excessive elation, 'high', excessively euphoric mood
- unusual irritability
- less need for sleep
- grandiose notions and unrealistic beliefs in abilities and powers

- excessive talking
- racing thoughts, jumping from one idea to another ('butterfly mind')
- distractibility
- excessive sexual desire
- greatly increased energy and provocative, intrusive or aggressive behaviour
- poor judgment
- inappropriate social behaviour
- spending sprees
- abuse of drugs, particularly cocaine, alcohol and sleeping medications
- denial that anything is wrong.

A manic episode is diagnosed if elevated mood comes with three or more of the other symptoms for most of the day, nearly every day, for 1 week or longer.

Mania often affects thinking, judgment and social behaviour in ways that can cause serious problems and embarrassment. The individual in a manic phase may feel elated and full of grand schemes that might range from unwise business decisions to romantic sprees. Frequently, therefore, the family rather than the patient feel the ill-effects and complain accordingly.

A mild to moderate level of mania is called hypomania and it may be enjoyed by the patient; it may even be associated with good functioning and enhanced productivity. Thus, even when family and friends learn to recognize the mood swings as possible bipolar disorder, the person may deny that anything is wrong. Alternation between mild mania and depression is termed cyclothymia.

Sometimes, severe episodes of mania or depression include psychotic symptoms, such as hallucinations and delusions. Psychotic symptoms in bipolar disorder tend to reflect the extreme mood state at the time. For example, delusions of grandiosity, such as believing one is the president or has special powers or wealth, may be experienced during mania. Delusions of guilt or worthlessness, such as believing that one is ruined and penniless or has committed some terrible crime, may appear during depression. People with bipolar disorder who have these symptoms are sometimes incorrectly diagnosed as having schizophrenia.

General management of mania

CBT may be effective. Psychoeducation involves teaching people with bipolar disorder about the illness and its treatment, and how to recognize signs of relapse so that early intervention can be instituted before a full-blown episode. Lithium, carbamazepine and valproate are the main mood-stabilizing drugs. 'Atypical' antipsychotic medications (such as olanzapine) may help.

Lithium can have several adverse effects. It affects thyroid function and the ECG, and can produce nephrogenic diabetes insipidus. It is also a teratogen. It must only be used where blood levels can be monitored, as overdose can cause tremor, ataxia, convulsions and renal damage. Patients with cardiovascular, renal or thyroid disorders are at risk. Side-effects include thirst, dry mouth and nausea. Povidone–iodine is contraindicated.

Carbamazepine has fewer adverse effects than lithium and is given when the latter is not tolerated. An important adverse effect is ataxia.

Valproate may lead to adverse effects. It depresses platelet numbers and function to produce a bleeding tendency. Valproate may lead to adverse hormone changes in teenage girls and polycystic ovary syndrome in women who start taking the medication before age 20, so

Table 10.19 *Potential drug interactions with lithium*

Drug interacting with lithium	Consequences
Carbamazepine	Lithium toxicity
Diazepam	Hypothermia
Droperidol and other neuroleptics	Facial dyskinesias
Non-steroidal anti-inflammatory drugs (NSAIDs)	Lithium toxicity
Metronidazole	Lithium toxicity
Phenytoin	Lithium toxicity
Selective serotonin reuptake inhibitors (SSRIs)	Serotonin syndrome
Suxamethonium and other muscle relaxants	Prolonged muscle relaxation
Tetracyclines	Lithium toxicity

young female patients who are prescribed valproate should be monitored carefully by a physician. NSAIDs, erythromycin and BZPs are also contraindicated.

Newer anticonvulsant medications, including lamotrigine, gabapentin and topiramate, are being studied for their effect in stabilizing mood. Atypical antipsychotic medications, including clozapine, olanzapine, risperidone and ziprasidone, are also possible treatments.

If insomnia is a problem, a high-potency BZP, such as clonazepam or lorazepam, may help. These medications may be habit-forming and should be prescribed in the short term only; therefore other types of sedative medication, such as zolpidem, are sometimes used instead.

Treatments of unproven worth in mania include St John's wort (*Hypericum perforatum*) and omega-3 fatty acids found in fish oil.

Dental aspects

An excited manic patient can be difficult to manage and treatment may have to be delayed until after stabilization. Lithium treatment should be monitored by regular assay of plasma levels. Arrhythmias may be precipitated, particularly during GA. Lithium can interact with many drugs, and it may be advisable to stop lithium treatment 2–3 days before GA (Table 10.19).

Most NSAIDs and metronidazole should be avoided, as they can induce toxicity, but aspirin, paracetamol (acetaminophen) and codeine are safe to use.

Manic–depressive patients may be treated with lithium and also antidepressant drugs – with oral side-effects such as xerostomia.

Schizophrenia

The term 'schizophrenia' covers a number of chronic conditions of complex aetiology that are characterized by dopamine overactivity in the mesolimbic pathways of the brain. It is a disabling condition and has a lifetime prevalence of approximately 1%, although in recent years prevalence figures are falling for reasons that are not clear.

There is a significant genetic component in the aetiology, probably related to chromosomes 13 and 6. Schizophrenia appears to be due to some imbalance of the complex interrelated chemical systems of the brain, involving dopamine and glutamate; many studies have found abnormalities in brain structure, and suggest it may be a developmental disorder leading to neurons forming inappropriate connections during fetal development. Marijuana use may precipitate schizophrenia and abuse of phencyclidine (PCP), crack cocaine, LSD and amphetamines can cause a similar picture (Ch. 34). There is a high prevalence in the socially deprived and in penal institutions. It may also be common in some people of African heritage.

Clinical features

Acute schizophrenia typically presents in young individuals with positive symptoms (hallucinations, delusions and thought disorder). The person generally lacks insight and concern is initially raised by a friend or relative. Acute schizophrenia may develop in previously normal individuals, is often precipitated by organic disorders or external stress, and affective symptoms such as depression may be associated. Chronic schizophrenia is more common and characterized by inappropriate affect (mood), disordered thought processes, delusions and hallucinations. Some patients are strikingly paranoid, while others have mainly motor symptoms (catatonia), a bizarre mixture of emotional, behavioural and thought disturbances, or neuroses. Chronic schizophrenia may present insidiously with negative symptoms (apathy, loss of affect and social withdrawal) and thus be misdiagnosed.

Intelligence is unimpaired and insight may even be retained. Occasionally, as a result, patients may be aware that their behaviour is bizarre and even realize the consternation that such behaviour creates in others.

Mood, thoughts and behaviour are disorganized and appear irrational and exaggerated. Disorders of perception (hallucinations) and thought (delusions) are common. Disintegration of the individual's personality results in social isolation and withdrawal. Some patients are strikingly paranoid whilst others exhibit motor impairment (catatonia) or a mixture of emotional, behavioural and thought disturbances (hebephrenia). Thoughts and behaviour can be totally inappropriate and incomprehensible.

The first signs of schizophrenia often appear as confusing, or even shocking, changes in behaviour. Schizophrenics frequently suffer terrifying symptoms, such as hearing internal voices not heard by others, or believing that other people are reading their minds, controlling their thoughts or plotting to harm them. Such symptoms may leave them fearful and withdrawn.

Schizophrenics often suffer a severely impaired emotional expressiveness – a 'blunted' or 'flat' affect. Signs of normal emotion are diminished or missing, the voice monotonous and facial expressions mask-like; the person may appear apathetic. Schizophrenics may withdraw socially, avoiding contact with others; when forced to interact, they may have nothing to say ('impoverished thought').

Disordered thinking is common. Schizophrenics may not be able to sort out what is relevant and what is not relevant to a situation. Thoughts may come and go rapidly. The patient may not be able to concentrate on one thought for very long and may be easily distracted and unable to focus attention. Schizophrenic thought disorder causes loss of cohesion between logical thought sequences, with thoughts becoming disorganized and fragmented. Speech and behaviour can be so disorganized as to be incomprehensible or frightening to others. Speech may include non-existent words (neologisms) or be inconsequential ('word salad'). There may be disruption of the stream of speech (thought-blocking), which can make conversation very difficult.

If people cannot make sense of what an individual with schizophrenia is saying, they are likely to become uncomfortable and tend to leave that person alone, and this, together with inappropriate affect and withdrawal from social contact, leads to isolation. Motivation can thus be greatly weakened, as can interest in or enjoyment of life. In some severe cases, a person can spend entire days doing nothing at all, even neglecting basic hygiene. These problems with emotional expression and motivation may

be extremely troubling to family members and friends, but are symptoms of schizophrenia, not character flaws or personal weaknesses.

Hallucinations and delusions have no connection to an appropriate source and can involve any sensory form – auditory, visual, tactile, gustatory and olfactory. However, hearing voices that other people do not hear is the most common type of hallucination. Such voices may describe the patient's activities, carry on a conversation, warn of impending dangers or even issue orders. Schizophrenics live in a world distorted by hallucinations and delusions, and may feel frightened, anxious and confused; they may behave very differently at various times. Sometimes they may seem distant, detached or preoccupied, and may even sit as rigidly as a stone, not moving for hours or uttering a sound. At other times they may move about constantly – always occupied, appearing wide awake and alert. The bizarre nature of the disorder may be made obvious when they shout back at the unheard voices.

Delusions, on the other hand, describe a sensory stimulus that is present but is incorrectly interpreted by the individual. As we have seen, delusions are false personal beliefs not subject to reason or contradictory evidence, and are not explained by a person's usual cultural concepts. Delusions may take on different themes. For example, patients suffering from paranoid-type symptoms – roughly one-third of schizophrenics – often have delusions that they, or a member of the family or someone close to them, are the focus of persecution. Alternatively, they may have false and irrational beliefs that they are being cheated, harassed, poisoned or conspired against. Delusions of grandeur, in which the individual believes that he or she is a famous or important figure, are common. The best-known schizophrenic delusion, in the past, was that of being Napoleon! Sometimes the delusions are quite bizarre: for instance, believing that a neighbour is controlling their behaviour with magnetic waves; that people on television are directing special messages to them, or that their thoughts are being broadcast aloud to others. Murderous attacks on others are sometimes ordered by the illusory inner voices.

Paranoia is a projection of the patient's internal disturbance, which, as a consequence, is believed to be the result of the hostility of others, such as neighbours, secret agents or foreign powers, who may be projecting mysterious rays to achieve their malign objectives, for example.

Catatonia, with abnormalities of movement, posture and speech, negativism, echolalia, mannerisms and stereotypia, may also be a feature.

General management

Diagnosis is not easy at times, since even normal individuals may feel, think or act in ways that resemble schizophrenia. At the same time, people with schizophrenia do not always act abnormally. Indeed, some people with the illness can appear completely normal and be perfectly responsible, even while they experience hallucinations or delusions. An individual's behaviour may change over time, seeming close to normal when appropriate treatment is being received, but becoming bizarre when medication is stopped.

The diagnosis should thus only be made by an experienced psychiatrist. The diagnostic criteria for schizophrenia vary but include the recognition of Schneider's first-rank symptoms:

- Auditory hallucinations – thought echo or voices talking about the patient in the third person
- Passivity – the feeling of being controlled by external forces
- Thought insertion or withdrawal
- Thought broadcasting
- Delusions
- Hallucinations.

Some people with symptoms of schizophrenia exhibit prolonged extremes of elated or depressed mood, mimicking a manic–depressive (or bipolar) disorder or major depressive disorder. When such symptoms cannot be clearly categorized, a diagnosis of 'schizoaffective disorder' is sometimes made.

It is important to rule out other illnesses, as sometimes similar symptoms are due to undetected underlying medical conditions or drug abuse; for this reason, a medical history should be taken and a physical examination and laboratory tests should be done to rule out other possible causes.

Coping with the symptoms of schizophrenia can be especially difficult for family members who remember how involved or vivacious a person was before they became ill.

Treatment of schizophrenia includes:

- early active intervention before the illness becomes chronic
- assessment of the risk a patient poses to themselves or others (individuals may require acute psychiatric admission under the Mental Health Act ["sectioning"])
- family therapy
- CBT
- long-term psychotherapy and antipsychotic drug therapy (Table 10.20)
- supportive therapy via community psychiatric services.

A person with schizophrenia can be more sensitive to stress, so it is best to avoid arguments and keep calm.

Treatment with individual psychotherapy is of questionable value. Rehabilitation, family education and self-help groups can help. Treatment usually includes drugs, which can be the older (typical) antipsychotics that work by reducing brain dopamine but can cause side-effects, such as stiffness and shakiness, feeling slow, restlessness, sexual difficulties and unwanted movements, mainly of the mouth and tongue. Some of these antipsychotic medications, including haloperidol, fluphenazine, perphenazine and others, are available in long-acting injectable forms that eliminate the need to take pills every day. The newer (atypical) antipsychotics are less likely to produce unwanted movements but can cause weight gain, diabetes, tiredness and sexual problems (see Table 10.20).

Antipsychotic medications alter the dopamine/cholinergic balance in the basal ganglia so that extrapyramidal and anticholinergic effects are common and can be disabling. All may variably produce weight gain, extrapyramidal side effects, prolactin increase, prolonged QT interval (Ch. 5) and sedation. The long-term side-effects of antipsychotic drugs, especially drowsiness, hypotension, xerostomia, interference with temperature regulation and extrapyramidal symptoms, may pose particularly serious problems. Extrapyramidal features from medication are most common with the piperazine phenothiazines, butyrophenones and depot preparations, and include:

- dystonia and dyskinesia (abnormal movements)
- akathisia (restlessness)
- Parkinsonism; anti-parkinsonian drugs, such as benzatropine or orphenadrine, are required to control extrapyramidal symptoms, which sometimes develop after only a few doses. L-dopa is contraindicated.

Maintenance therapy is conveniently carried out with long-acting preparations such as fluphenazine or flupentixol, but these can cause intractable tardive dyskinesia. Phenothiazines can also cause the neuroleptic malignant syndrome, dose-related impaired temperature regulation, obstructive jaundice, leukopenia or ECG changes.

Most schizophrenic patients need and show substantial improvement with antipsychotic drugs but there have been sudden deaths in asthmatics. Some people have only one such psychotic episode; others have many episodes during a lifetime but lead relatively normal lives during the interim periods; but those with 'chronic' schizophrenia, or a continuous or recurring pattern of illness, typically require long-term treatment. Schizophrenia can be remarkably disturbing for patients and for those in contact with them; hospitalization may therefore be necessary in severe cases. Overall, about 10% remain hospitalized and a further 30% remain seriously handicapped.

ECT may be given if there is a poor response to medication or if there is catatonia.

Tardive dyskinesia Tardive dyskinesia (TD) is characterized by involuntary movements, most often involving the mouth, lips and tongue, and sometimes the trunk or other parts of the body, such as arms and legs. It affects about 15–20% of patients who have been receiving phenothiazines for many years, but sometimes only for short periods. The symptoms of TD are usually mild so that the patient may be unaware of the movements. TD does not respond to withdrawal of the causative drug or to any other medication.

Table 10.20 *Important drugs used to treat schizophrenia*

Class	Examples	Features
Phenothiazines		
Phenothiazines with pronounced sedative effects, but moderate antimuscarinic and extrapyramidal effects	Chlorpromazine, promazine	If there is considerable anxiety or hyperactivity, chlorpromazine is most commonly used but parenteral fluphenazine enanthate or decanoate, pipotiazine palmitate and zuclopenthixol decanoate by biweekly injection overcome compliance difficulties
Phenothiazines with low extrapyramidal effects, and moderate sedative and antimuscarinic effects	Pericyazine, pipotiazine, thioridazine	Fewer extrapyramidal effects than other phenothiazines
		Thioridazine may be cardiotoxic
Piperazine phenothiazines, with low sedative and antimuscarinic activity	Fluphenazine, perphenazine, prochlorperazine, trifluoperazine	May be given if no sedation is needed, but may have pronounced extrapyramidal effects and may worsen depression
Butyrophenones	Benperidol, droperidol, haloperidol	Useful mainly for violent patients
Thioxanthines	Flupentixol, zuclopenthixol	Extrapyramidal effects common
Atypical antipsychotics	Clozapine, amisulpride, olanzapine, quetiapine, risperidone, sertindole, zotepine	All apart from clozapine are first-line treatment for newly diagnosed schizophrenia. Clozapine is used for resistant cases; it does not cause tardive dyskinesia but has significant antimuscarinic effects and can cause agranulocytosis
		All can cause long QT syndrome
Diphenylbutylpiperidines	Fluspirilene, pimozide	Danger of sudden unexplained, probably cardiac, death

Neuroleptic malignant syndrome Neuroleptic malignant syndrome (NMS) is a rare but potentially life-threatening drug-induced disorder associated with the use of antipsychotic medications. It is characterized by disturbances in mental status, hyperpyrexia, and disturbed autonomic and extrapyramidal functions. Laboratory findings include leukocytosis, raised creatine phosphokinase and metabolic acidosis. Treatment of NMS consists primarily of early recognition, discontinuation of triggering drugs, management of fluid balance, cooling, and monitoring for complications. Use of dopamine agonists or dantrolene, or both, should be considered and may be indicated in more severe, prolonged or refractory cases.

Dental aspects

Mild schizophrenic features (which are often unrecognized) include loss of social contact, flatness of mood or inappropriate social behaviour, which may appear at first as mere tactlessness or stupidity. Thus the patient, when asked to sit down in the surgery, may sit in the operator's rather than the dental chair. Attempts at communication are met by a response that indicates a failure to get through or are interrupted by totally irrelevant remarks. Such patients may have delusional oral symptoms, the treatment of which is beyond the expertise of dental staff, and then psychiatric help must be sought.

Phenothiazines can cause adrenaline (epinephrine) reversal in patients given a LA; there is vasodilatation instead of the anticipated vasoconstriction because of the alpha-adrenergic blocking activity of phenothiazines. Any practical importance of this in relation to LA is unclear:

- Conscious sedation is safe.
- With tramadol, there is a risk of seizures.
- Haloperidol and phenothiazines may cause orthostatic hypotension. Patients should be raised slowly and carefully assisted from the dental chair.
- Haloperidol and droperidol reportedly block the vasoconstrictor activity of adrenaline (epinephrine).
- GA, especially with intravenous barbiturates, can lead to severe hypotension and should therefore be avoided if possible.
- The long-term use of neuroleptics can lead to xerostomia (with susceptibility to candidosis and caries, and, occasionally, ascending parotitis), oral pigmentation and severe extrapyramidal symptoms.
- Muscular rigidity or tonic spasms (facial dyskinesias), frequently involving the bulbar or neck muscles, with subsequent difficulties in speech or swallowing. Alternatively, there may be uncontrollable facial grimacing (orofacial dystonia), which may start after only a few doses. This may be controlled by stopping the neuroleptic and giving anti-parkinsonian antimuscarinic drugs.
- Haloperidol and clozapine can cause hypersalivation.

Korsakoff psychosis

Korsakoff psychosis is characterized by amnesia for recent events, impaired ability to learn new facts and fabricated descriptions of recent events (confabulation). Nevertheless the patient is alert, responsible and behaves in an otherwise normal manner.

The disease results from a symmetrical lesion in the periaqueductal area, thalamus, mammillary bodies and cerebellar vermis; chronic alcoholism associated with thiamine deficiency is an important cause, though

Table 10.21 *Some drug-induced mental states*

Mental State	Drugs sometimes responsible	
	Used in medicine mainly	Used in dentistry too
Confusion	Antihypertensives	Benzodiazepines
	Antihistamines	
	Tricyclic antidepressants	
Aggressive behaviour	Dopa derivatives	Benzodiazepines (in children)
Nightmares or hallucinations	Some antihypertensives	Pentazocine or ketamine
Mania	L-dopa	Corticosteroids
Depression	Antihypertensives	Pentazocine
	Contraceptive pill	Corticosteroids
Delirium	Antihypertensives	Procaine penicillin
	Antitubercular drugs	Sulphonamides
	Anticonvulsants	
	Oral hypoglycaemics	
Paranoia	Antihypertensives	Ephedrine
	Anticonvulsants	Corticosteroids
	Amphetamines	

relatively few alcoholics develop the syndrome. Other possible causes include cerebrovascular disease, tumours or degenerative disorders.

Other psychoses

Psychoses can complicate various endocrine disturbances, the puerperium, or the use of drugs such as alcohol, amphetamine, cannabis or psychotomimetics (Table 10.21).

SYSTEMIC DISEASE CAUSING MENTAL DISORDERS

Many endocrine diseases can be complicated by mental disturbances, as may alcoholism, drug abuse or drug treatment. Major trauma, surgery or severe life-threatening disease can also frequently cause emotional reactions, such as anxiety or depression, or conditions such as compensation neurosis.

KEY WEBSITES

(Accessed 27 May 2013)
BMJ. <http://www.bmj.com/specialties/psychiatry>
Centers for Disease Control and Prevention. <http://www.cdc.gov/mentalhealth/mental-health-inf.htm>
General Medical Council. Consent: patients and doctors making decisions together 2008. General Medical Council 51. <http://www.gmc-uk.org/guidance/ethical_guidance/consent_guidance/index.asp>
Mental Capacity Act 2005. s2(1) Department of Constitutional Affairs. <http://www.legislation.gov.uk/ukpga/2005/9/contents>
National Institute of Mental Health. <http://www.nimh.nih.gov/index.shtml>

USEFUL WEBSITES

(Accessed 27 May 2013)
Anxiety UK. <http://www.anxietyuk.org.uk>
CCBT Ltd. <http://www.ccbt.co.uk>
David Baldwin's Trauma Information Pages. <http://www.trauma-pages.com/>
Depression Alliance. <http://www.depressionalliance.org/>
John F. Abess MD. <http://www.abess.com/glossary.html>
National Institute for Health and Care Excellence (NICE). <http://www.nice.org.uk/guidance/index.jsp>

NICE clinical guideline 26. Post-traumatic stress disorder: the management of PTSD in adults and children in primary and secondary care. <http://www.nice.org.uk/Guidance/CG26>

Royal College of Psychiatrists. <http://www.rcpsych.ac.uk/>

Samaritans. <http://www.samaritans.org>

FURTHER READING

Abrahamsson, K.H., et al. 2000. Psychosocial aspects of dental and general fears in dental phobic patients. Acta Odontol. Scand. 58, 37.

Adshead, G., 2000. Psychological therapies for post-traumatic stress disorder. Br. J. Psychiatr. 177, 144.

American Psychiatric Association, 2013. Diagnostic and statistical manual of mental disorders, fifth ed. American Psychiatric Publishing, Arlington, VA.

Barskey, A.J., 2001. The patient with hypochondriasis. N. Engl. J. Med. 345, 1395.

Bassi, N., et al. 2008. Chronic fatigue syndrome: characteristics and possible causes for its pathogenesis. Isr. Med. Assoc. J. 10, 79.

Bateman, A., Tyrer, P., 2004. Psychological treatment for personality disorders. Adv. Psychiatr. Treat. 10, 378.

Bateman, A., Tyrer, P., 2004. Services for personality disorder: organisation for inclusion. Adv. Psychiatr. Treat. 10, 425.

Blenkiron, P., 2001. Treatment of obsessive compulsive disorder (review). Cont. Prof. Dev. Bull. Psychiatr. 2, 68–72.

British Medical Association and Law Society, 2004. Assessment of mental capacity: guidance for doctors and lawyers. BMJ, London.

Coid, J., 2003. Epidemiology, public health and the problem of personality disorder. Br. J. Psychiatr. 182 (Suppl 44), s3–s10.

Coid, J., et al. 2006. Prevalence and correlates of personality disorder in Great Britain. Br. J. Psychiatr. 188, 423–431.

Foa, E. (Ed.), 2000. Effective treatments for PTSD: guidelines from the International Society of Traumatic Stress Studies. Guilford Press, New York

Freeman, R., 2000. The psychology of dental patient care: a common sense approach. BDJ Books, Basingstoke.

Friedlander, A.H., Norman, D.C., 2002. Late-life depression: psychopathology, medical interventions and dental implications. Oral Surg. 94, 404.

Geddes, J., 2003. Bipolar disorder. Evid. Based Ment. Health. 6, 101.

Glaros, A.G., 2000–01. Emotional factors in temporomandibular joint disorders. J. Indiana Dent. Assoc. 79 (4), 20.

Goodwin, G.M., 2003. Evidence-based guidelines for treating bipolar disorder: recommendations from the British Association for Psychopharmacology. J. Psychopharmacol. 17, 149.

Griffith, J.P., Zarrouf, F.A., 2008. A systematic review of chronic fatigue syndrome: don't assume it's depression. Prim. Care Companion J. Clin. Psychiatr. 10, 120.

Hagglin, C., et al. 2001. Dental anxiety in relation to mental health and personality factors: a longitudinal study of middle-aged and elderly women. Eur. J. Oral Sci. 109, 27.

Hill, J., 2003. Early identification of individuals at risk for antisocial personality disorder. Br. J. Psychiatr. 182 (Suppl 44), s11.

Hull, A.M., et al. 2002. Survivors of the Piper Alpha oil platform disaster: long-term follow-up study. Br. J. Psychiatr. 181, 433.

Humphris, G.M., et al. 2000. Further evidence for the reliability and validity of the Modified Dental Anxiety Scale. Int. Dent. J. 50, 367.

Kendell, R., 2002. The distinction between personality disorder and mental illness. Br. J. Psychiatr. 180, 110.

Kerr, J.R., et al. 2008. Gene expression subtypes in patients with chronic fatigue syndrome/myalgic encephalomyelitis. J. Infect. Dis. 197, 1171.

Lab, D., et al. 2008. Treating post-traumatic stress disorder in the 'real world': evaluation of a specialist trauma service and adaptations to standard treatment approaches. Psychiatr. Bull. 32, 8.

Locker, D., et al. 2001. Psychological disorder, conditioning experiences, and the onset of dental anxiety in early adulthood. J. Dent. Res. 80, 1588.

McEwen, B.S., 2008. Central effects of stress hormones in health and disease: understanding the protective and damaging effects of stress and stress mediators. Eur. J. Pharmacol. 583 (2–3), 174. Epub 2008 Jan 30

Mellor, A., 2007. Management of the anxious patient: what treatments are available? Dent. Update 34, 108.

Morriss, R., 2004. The early warning symptom intervention for patients with bipolar affective disorder. Adv. Psychiatr. Treat. 10, 18.

National Institute for Health and Clinical Excellence (NICE), 2005. Core interventions in the treatment of obsessive-compulsive disorder and body dysmorphic disorder *Clinical guidelines 31* (Quick reference guide). NICE, London.

NICE clinical guideline 28, 2005. The treatment of depression in children and young people. NICE, London.

NICE clinical guideline 38, 2006. Bipolar disorder: the management of bipolar disorder in adults, children and adolescents, in primary and secondary care. National Collaborating Centre for Mental Health, London.

Rafique, S., et al. 2008. Management of the petrified dental patient. Dent. Update 35, 196. 201, 204 *passim*.

Rey, J.M., Tennant, C.C., 2002. Cannabis and mental health. BMJ 325, 1183.

Scully, C., et al. 2007. Special care in dentistry: handbook of oral healthcare. Churchill Livingstone, Edinburgh.

Scully, C., Chaudhry, S., 2008. Aspects of human disease 21. Anxiety, stress and depression. Dent. Update 35, 213.

Scully, C., Chaudhry, S., 2008. Aspects of human disease 22. Schizophrenia. Dent. Update 35, 285.

Seishima, M., et al. 2008. Chronic fatigue syndrome after human parvovirus B19 infection without persistent viremia. Dermatology 216, 341.

Talis, F., 1992. Understanding obsessions and compulsions: a self-help manual. Sheldon Press, London.

Tate, P., 2007. The doctor's communication handbook. Radcliffe Publishing, Oxford.

Tyrer, P. (Ed.), 2002. Personality disorders, psychiatry 2002. Medicine Publishing Company, Oxford

Tyrer, P., Bateman, A., 2004. Drug treatment for personality disorders. Adv. Psychiatr. Treat. 10, 389.

Tyrer, P., et al. 2007. Critical developments in the assessment of personality disorder. Br. J. Psychiatr. 190 (Suppl 49), s51.

Understanding NICE guidance: *information for people with OCD or body dysmorphic disorder, their families and carers, and the public.* Printed copies from NHS response line; downloadable from: <http://www.nice.org.uk/guidance/index.jsp?action=byID&o=10976> [accessed 30 11.13].

US Department of Health and Human Services, 1999. Mental health: a report of the Surgeon General. National Institute of Mental Health, Rockville, MD.

Veale, D, Willson, R., 2009. Overcoming obsessive-compulsive disorder: a self-help book using cognitive-behavioural techniques. Constable & Robinson, London.

Yehuda, R (Ed.), 2002. Treating trauma: survivors with PTSD. American Publishing, Washington, DC

APPENDIX 10.1 WORLD HEALTH ORGANIZATION'S NOMENCLATURE FOR ANTIDEPRESSANTS, WITH EXAMPLES

NON-SELECTIVE MONOAMINE REUPTAKE INHIBITORS

- Tricyclic antidepressants: imipramine, amitriptyline*, clomipramine, lofepramine, amoxapine
- Noradrenaline reuptake inhibitors: desipramine, nortriptyline, maprotiline

SELECTIVE SEROTONIN REUPTAKE INHIBITORS

- Fluoxetine*, fluvoxamine, zimelidine, paroxetine, sertraline, citalopram, escitalopram

MONOAMINE OXIDASE INHIBITORS (NON-SELECTIVE)

- Phenelzine, tranylcypromine, isocarboxazid

MONOAMINE OXIDASE A INHIBITORS

- Moclobemide, toloxatone

OTHER ANTIDEPRESSANTS

- Serotonin noradrenaline reuptake inhibitors: venlafaxine, duloxetine
- Noradrenaline dopamine reuptake inhibitors: nomifensine, buproprion
- Noradrenaline and selective serotonin antagonists: mirtazapine
- Serotonin antagonist and reuptake inhibitor: trazadone
- Melatonin receptor agonist with 5-HT2C receptor antagonist properties: agomelatine
- Serotonin partial agonist: gepirone

*Listed in the WHO's list of essential medicines for use in depressive disorders; adapted from Hatcher S, and Arroll B. BMJ *2012; 344 doi: http://dx.doi.org/10.1136/bmj.d8300.*

SKIN DISEASES

The common and more important skin diseases only are discussed here.

ACNE

General aspects

Acne is a common skin disorder in which hair follicles become blocked with oil and hypertrophied epithelium; it is characterized by clogged pores and pimples. More than 4 out of 5 people, particularly adolescent males, develop acne. Several factors – including hormones, bacteria, medications such as corticosteroids, heredity and stress – play a role. Many adult women experience mild to moderate acne due to hormonal changes associated with menstrual cycles, starting or stopping oral contraceptives, or pregnancy.

Clinical features

Pimples appear as hair follicles and become plugged with oil and dead skin cells, causing the follicle wall to bulge and produce a 'whitehead'. If the pore stays open and traps dirt, the plug surface oxidises and darkens, causing a 'blackhead'. Blockages and inflammation deep inside hair follicles can produce scarring and cysts. Acne is rarely serious but it often causes emotional distress.

General management

Effective lotions generally contain benzoyl peroxide or azelaic acid. Topical erythromycin and clindamycin are effective treatments for inflamed lesions. Systemic acne treatment should start with antimicrobials (tetracyclines or erythromycin). Options for scarring cystic acne or acne that fails to respond to other treatments are, in women, cyproterone acetate or isotretinoin (vitamin A analogue, only prescribable by consultant dermatologists). For men, only isotretinoin is available. Oral contraceptives, including a combination of norgestimate and ethinylestradiol, can improve acne in women. Maternal use of vitamin A congeners must be avoided since birth defects similar to those in Di George syndrome can result – the *fetal isotretinoin syndrome*.

Dermabrasion (removing the top skin layers with a rapidly rotating wire brush) may help more severe scarring. Laser resurfacing can achieve the same effect.

CANCER

General aspects

The three major types of skin cancer, all on the increase, are (see also Ch. 22):

- basal cell carcinoma (BCC; rodent ulcer; Fig. 11.1)
- squamous cell carcinoma (SCC; Fig. 11.2)
- melanoma.

All are on the increase; nearly half of all men over 65 years will develop a skin cancer. Risk factors are shown in Box 11.1.

Clinical features and general management

Skin cancer develops mainly on areas of sun-exposed skin: the scalp, face, lips, ears, neck, chest, arms and hands, and on the legs in women. BCC is superficial and highly treatable, especially if found early. It appears as a pearly or waxy lump on the face, ears or neck, or a flat,

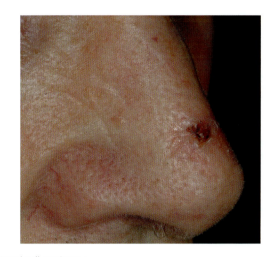

Fig. 11.1 Basal cell carcinoma.

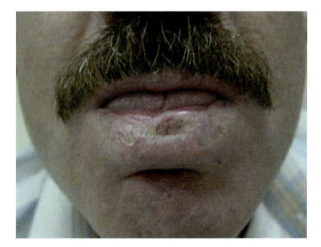

Fig. 11.2 Squamous cell carcinoma.

flesh-coloured or brown scar-like lesion on the chest or back, typically in persons after middle age, but responds to excision. In Gorlin syndrome, BCC can start to form in childhood.

SCC is superficial, slow-growing and highly treatable, especially if found early. It presents as a firm, red nodule on the face, lip, ears, neck, hands or arms, or a flat lesion with a scaly, crusted surface on the face, ears, neck, hands or arms. It usually responds to wide excision.

Melanoma has the greatest potential to spread and may be fatal. It typically appears as: a large brownish spot with darker speckles, anywhere; a simple mole anywhere that changes in colour or size or consistency, or that bleeds or exhibits new growth; a small lesion with an irregular border and red, white, blue or blue–black spots on the trunk or limbs; shiny, firm, dome-shaped nodules anywhere; dark lesions on palms, soles, tips of fingers and toes, or on mucous membranes; or a red flat lesion (amelanotic melanoma). Malignant melanomas can also form in the retina or, rarely, even in areas protected from sunlight such as the mouth.

Treatment of melanoma is usually excision, and if the tumour is superficial (Breslow depth <1.5 mm) the prognosis is excellent at 90% 5-year survival. The prognosis of malignant melanoma is usually poor as a consequence of late diagnosis and rapid spread: survival averages only 2 years.

Dental aspects

Dentists are a risk group for skin cancers (from excess vacational sun exposure!).

ECZEMA

General aspects

Eczema is a term describing a range of persistent skin conditions that include dryness and recurring rashes characterized by redness, itching, crusting, flaking, blistering, cracking, oozing or bleeding.

Clinical features

Common types of eczema include the following:

- *Atopic eczema* is believed to have a hereditary component (often runs in families whose members also have asthma and/or hay fever). It is particularly noticeable on face and scalp, neck, inside of elbows, behind knees and buttocks.

- *Contact dermatitis* is irritant (resulting from direct reaction to a solvent) or allergic.
- *Seborrhoeic dermatitis* causes dry or greasy scaling of scalp and eyebrows, scaly pimples and red patches.

General management

Patch-testing, raised serum immunoglobulin E (IgE), eosinophilia, radioallergosorbent test (RAST) or paper radioimmunosorbent test (PRIST; Ch. 17) may be diagnostically helpful. There is no known cure. Treatments, which aim to control symptoms, reduce inflammation and relieve itching, include topical emollients, corticosteroids, or calcineurin inhibitors. Ciclosporin, azathioprine or methotrexate may rarely be needed.

PSORIASIS

General aspects

Psoriasis is a common chronic skin disease characterized by scaling and inflammation. It has a strong genetic background with human leukocyte antigen (HLA)-Cw6 and HLA-DR7. T cells trigger inflammation, and excessive skin cell reproduction underlies the pathogenesis. There are sometimes associations with stress and alcoholism.

Clinical features

Psoriasis causes thick pruritic erythematous plaques covered with silvery scales (Fig. 11.3), predominantly on scalp, elbows and knees, lower back, face, palms, and soles of feet, and 'ice-pick' pitting or onycholysis of fingernails and toenails (Fig. 11.4). About 15% have joint inflammation (psoriatic arthropathy).

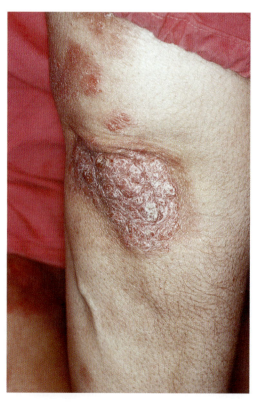

Fig. 11.3 Psoriasis. Silvery flaky rash on the elbows.

General management

Treatment of psoriasis initially is with topical agents – corticosteroids, vitamin D3, vitamin A analogues (retinoids), coal tar or dithranol (anthralin). Failing this, light (phototherapy) is used. Sunlight often helps but more controlled artificial light treatment may be used in mild psoriasis (ultraviolet B phototherapy), or psoralen and ultraviolet A (PUVA) therapy in more severe or extensive psoriasis.

Severe cases of psoriasis may need systemic treatment with methotrexate, ciclosporin or retinoids.

Dental aspects

Local anaesthesia (LA) is safe. Conscious sedation (CS) can be given if required.

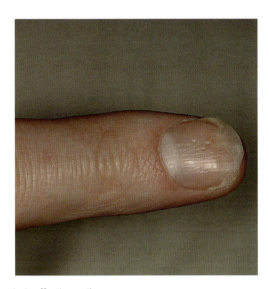

Fig. 11.4 Psoriasis affecting nails.

Oral lesions, such as white or reddish mucosal plaques, are rare. There may be a higher prevalence of erythema migrans and fissured tongue, particularly in pustular psoriasis. The temporomandibular joint is involved in up to 60% of patients with psoriatic arthropathy.

Oral complications of the treatment of psoriasis, such as gingival swelling from ciclosporin, or ulceration from methotrexate, may be seen.

ACQUIRED MUCOCUTANEOUS DISORDERS

Several mucocutaneous diseases can involve the mouth or may influence dental treatment. The most common is lichen planus. The most serious are pemphigus (which is potentially fatal), erythema multiforme and mucous membrane pemphigoid (which may involve other mucosae). Oral lesions herald some mucocutaneous diseases or may be the main manifestation. Immunostaining can often help the diagnosis (Table 11.1).

Many of the mucocutaneous diseases are treated with corticosteroids (topically or systemically), which may, if used for prolonged periods, cause adrenocortical suppression (Ch. 6).

LICHEN PLANUS

General aspects

Lichen planus (LP) is a common skin and mucosal disease. The immunopathogenesis includes a dense T-lymphocyte infiltrate, to an unidentified provoking antigen.

Lesions clinically and histologically similar or identical to LP (lichenoid lesions) can be related to dental restorations, particularly amalgam and drugs, especially to non-steroidal anti-inflammatory drugs (NSAIDs), gold, antimalarials and beta-blockers. Reported associations of oral LP with diabetes mellitus and hypertension have not been confirmed, and the so-called Grinspan syndrome of LP, diabetes mellitus and hypertension is probably related to drug treatment.

Table 11.1 *Immunostaining in skin and oral mucosal diseases*

Disease	Direct immunofluorescence	Epithelial location	Indirect immunofluorescence	Type of antibody[a]	Main epithelial antigen
Pemphigus vulgaris	Yes	Intercellular	Yes	IgG	Desmoglein
Paraneoplastic pemphigus	Yes	Intercellular[b]	Yes	IgG	Desmoplakin
IgA pemphigus	Yes	Intercellular	Yes	IgA	?Desmocollin
Bullous pemphigoid	Yes	Basement membrane area	Yes	IgG	BP1
Mucous membrane pemphigoid	Yes	Basement membrane area	Rarely	IgG	BP2
Angina bullosa haemorrhagica	No	–	No	–	–
Dermatitis herpetiformis	Yes	Basement membrane area	No	IgA	Transglutaminase
Linear IgA disease	Yes	Basement membrane area	No	IgA	Laminin
Systemic lupus erythematosus	Yes	Basement membrane area	Yes	ANA	NR
Chronic discoid lupus erythematosus	Yes	Basement membrane area	No	ANA	NR
Lichen planus	Often	Basement membrane area	No	(Usually fibrin)	?
Chronic ulcerative stomatitis	Yes	Basal cell layer	No	IgG/ANA	?

ANA = antinuclear antibody; BP = bullous pemphigoid; Ig = immunoglobulin; NR = not relevant.
[a]Usually with complement deposits.
[b]Transitional epithelium.

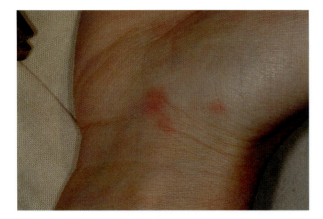

Fig. 11.5 Lichen planus rash.

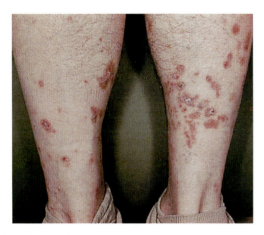

Fig. 11.6 Lichen planus rash.

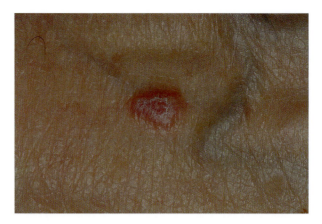

Fig. 11.7 Wickham striae in lichen planus.

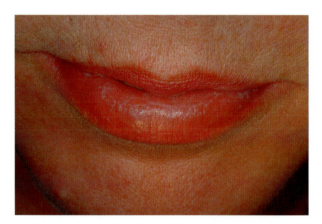

Fig. 11.8 Lichen planus on lips.

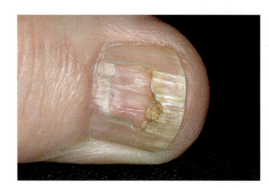

Fig. 11.9 Lichen planus affecting nails.

Similar lesions may be reactions to chemicals, such as photographic developing solutions, graft-versus-host disease (Ch. 35), chronic liver disease and virus infections – hepatitis C or human immunodeficiency virus (HIV).

Approximately 1% of cases of oral LP may develop malignant change after 10 years.

Clinical features

Skin lesions are usually small polygonal purplish or violaceous itchy papules, particularly affecting the flexor surfaces of the wrist (Fig. 11.5), and also elsewhere such as the shins (Fig. 11.6) or periumbilically, but rarely, if ever, on the face. Examination with a lens may show a fine lacy white network of striae (Wickham striae) on these papules (Fig. 11.7). Mouth and genital lesions in LP include white striae, papules, plaques, or red atrophic areas or erosions (Fig. 11.8). The nails or hair may be affected (Fig. 11.9).

General management

A drug history should be taken in order to exclude possible reactions. If there is any doubt about the diagnosis, a biopsy is needed, particularly to differentiate LP from lupus erythematosus, chronic ulcerative stomatitis or keratoses. Topical corticosteroids or tacrolimus can be useful to control symptomatic LP, especially severe erosive lesions. Aloe vera reportedly gives effective symptomatic relief.

Exceptionally severe LP sometimes responds only to systemic corticosteroids. Other drugs, such as vitamin A analogues (etretinate), dapsone, ciclosporin or alefacept, are used only rarely.

Dental aspects

Oral lesions in LP can persist for years, although the skin lesions frequently resolve within a few months. Oral lesions characteristically are bilateral and sometimes strikingly symmetrical; they affect particularly the posterior buccal mucosa but may also involve the tongue, gingivae or other sites. Gingival lesions are usually atrophic and red ('desquamative gingivitis').

Replacement of amalgam with non-metallic alternatives may sometimes cause lesions to resolve, but relapse is possible. LA is safe. CS can be given if required.

PEMPHIGUS

Pemphigus is a potentially fatal autoimmune reaction against proteins, usually within the stratified squamous epithelium; it is characterized

Table 11.2 *Pemphigus variants*

Pemphigus variant	Desmosomal antigens	Serum antibodies	Oral lesions	Comments
Pemphigus vulgaris localized to mucosae (mucosal)	Desmoglein 3	IgG	Common	Fatal
Pemphigus vulgaris also involving skin/other mucosae (mucocutaneous)	Desmoglein 3 Desmoglein 1	IgG	Common	Fatal
Pemphigus vegetans	Desmoglein 1	IgG	Uncommon	Variant of vulgaris
Pemphigus foliaceus	Desmoglein 1	IgG	Uncommon	–
Pemphigus erythematosus	Desmoglein 1	IgG	Uncommon	Variant of foliaceus
Drug-induced pemphigus	Desmoglein 3	IgG	Common	–
Paraneoplastic pemphigus	Desmoplakin 1 Desmoplakin 2	IgG or IgA	Common	Rare. Associated with lymphoproliferative disorders
IgA pemphigus	Desmocollin 1 Desmocollin 2 Desmoglein 3	IgA	Common	Rare

by widespread formation of skin vesicles and bullae. The mouth is frequently the first site of attack. Variants include those listed in Table 11.2.

Pemphigus vulgaris

General aspects

Pemphigus vulgaris is an uncommon disease, which mainly affects middle-aged women. Pemphigus may occasionally be associated with other autoimmune diseases, such as lupus erythematosus, inflammatory bowel disease, or thymoma and myasthenia gravis. Rarely, it is induced by a drug such as rifampicin, penicillamine or captopril. The main immunological finding is circulating antibodies to desmogleins of intercellular attachments (desmosomes) of epithelial cells of stratified squamous epithelia. These IgG antibodies, and complement components, are deposited (and can also be localized by immunostaining) around the epithelial cells, and result in loss of adherence of the cells to one another (acantholysis). Pemphigus is characterized by widespread formation of intraepithelial vesicles and bullae.

Clinical features

Pemphigus vulgaris is characterized by thin-roofed vesicles or bullae, followed by ulceration (Fig. 11.10). It frequently appears in the mouth first. Stroking the skin or mucosa with a finger may induce vesicle formation in an apparently unaffected area or cause a bulla to extend (Nikolsky sign). If untreated, pemphigus vulgaris is usually fatal, as a result of extensive skin and mucosal damage leading to fluid and electrolyte loss, and often infection.

General management

Rapid and precise diagnosis of pemphigus vulgaris is essential since acute cases need immediate immunosuppressive treatment. Diagnosis is confirmed by biopsy. The specimen should be halved to enable both light and immunofluorescent microscopy to be carried out. Light microscopy on a paraffin section is usually distinctive and shows suprabasal cleft formation and intraepithelial vesicles containing free-floating acantholytic cells. Immunofluorescence examination shows IgG and C3 deposits intercellularly. It can be carried out by the direct method using fluorescein-conjugated anti-human IgG and anti-complement (C3) sera

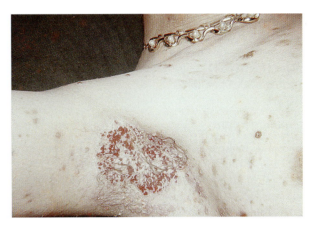

Fig. 11.10 Pemphigus.

on the frozen specimen or on exfoliated cells. In the indirect method, the patient's serum is incubated with normal animal mucosa, which is then labelled with fluorescein-conjugated antihuman globulin (see Table 11.1). Antibodies to desmoglein 1 may be found in pemphigus vulgaris with cutaneous lesions, or in pemphigus foliaceus; antibodies to desmoglein 3 may herald oral involvement in pemphigus vulgaris.

The usual treatment of pemphigus vulgaris is with high doses of systemic corticosteroids plus a steroid-sparing agent such as azathioprine. Gold may sometimes be used. Cyclophosphamide, methotrexate or mycophenolate mofetil also appear to be effective. With current methods of treatment, the mortality may be reduced to about 8% but is often a complication of immunosuppressive treatment. Long-term remission has been reported but many require prolonged therapy.

Dental aspects

LA and CS can be given as required. Orofacial manifestations are as described above. However, blisters are so fragile as rarely to be seen intact in the mouth. They leave painful erosions.

Mucous membrane pemphigoid

General aspects

Mucous membrane pemphigoid is a group of subepithelial immune blistering diseases with autoantibodies directed to different epithelial basement membrane proteins. Oral pemphigoid-like lesions have occasionally been reported in association with internal cancers or the use of certain drugs, such as penicillamine. Autoantibodies against basement membrane proteins cause loss of attachment of the epithelium to the connective tissue and blister formation. The common variant of mucous membrane pemphigoid has antibodies against bullous pemphigoid antigen 2 (BP2) but the types that mainly affect the mouth have antibodies against integrin or epiligrin. Serum autoantibodies are demonstrable by conventional techniques in relatively few patients.

Clinical features

Mucous membrane pemphigoid predominantly affects women between 50 and 70 years of age. Intact vesicles or bullae are frequently visible. Sometimes the blisters fill with blood and then must be distinguished from generalized or localized oral purpura. The gingivae may be particularly affected and pemphigoid is an important cause of so-called 'desquamative gingivitis'. Progress is typically indolent and lesions may remain restricted to one site, such as the mouth, for several years or possibly never develop elsewhere, depending on the type.

Scarring after healing of the bullae is a serious complication in sites such as the eyes, larynx, oesophagus or genitalia. Ocular involvement is the most common dangerous manifestation since it can impair or destroy sight (Fig. 11.11). Laryngeal or oesophageal stenosis secondary to scarring is also possible.

General management

The diagnosis of pemphigoid must be confirmed by biopsy. The section should be halved and a frozen section tested for localization of immunoglobulins or complement components along the basement membrane (see Table 11.1). It may be difficult otherwise to differentiate pemphigoid from other mucosal blistering diseases. Paraffin sections show separation of the epithelium from the underlying connective tissue, which is infiltrated by inflammatory cells, often with many eosinophils. Localization of immunoglobulins (IgG) along the line of the epithelial basement membrane can be shown in fewer than 50% but complement components may be demonstrable in about 80%. If there is any suspicion of ocular involvement, referral to an ophthalmologist is essential. The danger of ocular involvement is regarded as an indication for giving systemic corticosteroids. Other lesions can often be adequately controlled by potent topical corticosteroids. Dapsone or systemic corticosteroids may be needed for more severe cases.

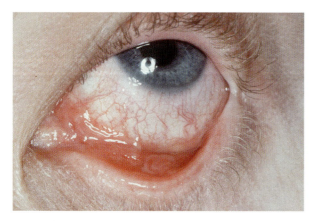

Fig. 11.11 Pemphigoid affecting conjunctiva.

Dental aspects

LA is safe and CS can be given if required. Orofacial manifestations are as described above.

BULLOUS PEMPHIGOID

Bullous pemphigoid is essentially a skin disease that rarely affects the mouth but histologically or immunologically does not appear to differ from mucous membrane pemphigoid. There are associations with diabetes or psoriasis.

DERMATITIS HERPETIFORMIS

Dermatitis herpetiformis is an uncommon chronic skin disease related to coeliac disease.

Clinical features

Dermatitis herpetiformis usually affects males past middle age, and causes an itchy papulovesicular eruption, usually on the extensor surfaces of the upper limbs and trunk. It leaves pigmented areas on healing. The coeliac disease is milder than in isolated coeliac disease. There may be associations with thyroid disease, gastric achlorhydria, pernicious anaemia and lymphoma.

General management

Diagnosis of dermatitis herpetiformis is by demonstrating deposits of IgA in the papillae at the epithelial basement membrane zone (BMZ), with papillary tip microabscesses and a subepithelial split. The biopsy should be from uninvolved skin. Anti-endomysial and anti-transglutaminase antibodies may be detectable. Serum immune complexes are often detectable but decline if the patient is put on a gluten-free diet, which may be of considerable benefit (Ch. 7). Patients are usually treated with dapsone, sulfapyridine or sulfamethoxypyridazine.

Dental aspects

Indometacin may exacerbate the condition and should be avoided. Oral lesions are usually innocuous but may be erythematous, vesicular, purpuric or sometimes erosive. They may be confused with pemphigoid. Coeliac-type enamel defects may rarely occur.

Drug reactions may be seen. Dapsone rarely causes a lichenoid eruption; sulfapyridine or other sulphonamides may cause erythema multiforme.

LINEAR IGA DISEASE

General aspects

Linear IgA disease (LAD) is a rare variant of dermatitis herpetiformis, in which the IgA deposits are linear at the BMZ but coeliac disease is absent. LAD may occasionally be induced by vancomycin.

Clinical features

Similar oral manifestations to dermatitis herpetiformis may be seen and LAD is most likely to be confused with pemphigoid. A variant seen in childhood is termed chronic bullous dermatosis of childhood. There may be an association with lymphoma.

General management

The diagnosis and treatment are as for dermatitis herpetiformis but a gluten-free diet is not required.

Dental aspects

Oral lesions are clinically indistinguishable from those in dermatitis herpetiformis.

ERYTHEMA MULTIFORME

General aspects

Erythema multiforme primarily affects young males and is characterized by recurrent mucosal and/or cutaneous lesions, including virtually any type of rash. The aetiology is uncertain but it may be an immune complex disorder in which the antigens can be various microorganisms or drugs (Table 11.3). Herpes simplex may be involved in most cases limited to the mouth.

Severe cases with multiple mucosal involvement and fever are termed toxic epidermal necrolysis (TEN), or Stevens–Johnson syndrome. TEN is the term often used when there is very extensive skin detachment and involvement of mucosae, and the condition is drug-induced. It has up to 40% mortality. Stevens–Johnson syndrome is a less severe form than TEN, also affecting several sites.

Clinical features

Skin, and ocular, genital or oral mucous membranes, may be involved together or in isolation. The typical skin lesion is the target or iris lesion (Figs. 11.12 and 11.13), in which there are concentric erythematous rings affecting particularly the hands and feet. Vesicles or bullae may also be seen. Typical oral features are grossly swollen, crusted and blood-stained lips, and widespread superficial oral ulceration with ill-defined margins (Fig. 11.14).

General management

When typical mucosal lesions are associated with dermal lesions, the diagnosis can usually be made largely on clinical grounds. Diagnosis can be difficult when the disease is limited to mucosae. Other suggestive features are recent use of drugs (particularly sulphonamides) or recent infections, particularly by herpes simplex or *Mycoplasma pneumoniae*. Biopsy can be useful to exclude other more serious diseases, such as early-onset pemphigus. An ophthalmological opinion should be obtained if the conjunctivae are involved. Oral lesions can be symptomatically managed with topical corticosteroids, chlorhexidine or lidocaine gel to ease the pain. Healing usually takes 10–14 days.

Severe erythema multiforme and TEN may necessitate hospital admission, as feeding may be difficult; systemic corticosteroids are frequently given but may not provide anything more than symptomatic relief. Aciclovir is indicated for prophylaxis of recurrent erythema multiforme, since herpes simplex virus (HSV) is often involved.

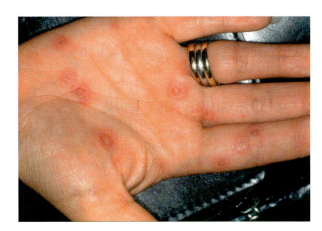

Fig. 11.12 Erythematous rings in erythema multiforme.

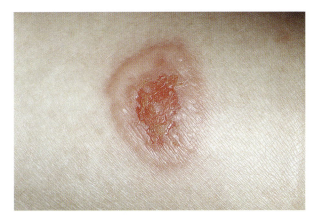

Fig. 11.13 Erythema multiforme target lesion.

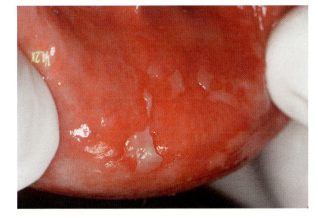

Fig. 11.14 Erythema multiforme on lips.

Table 11.3 *Erythema multiforme: possible causes*

Microorganisms	Drugs[b]	Others
Herpes simplex virus[a]	Barbiturates	Internal malignancy
Mycoplasma	Carbamazepine	Irradiation
	Chlorpropamide	Pregnancy
	Codeine	
	Hydantoins	
	Penicillins	
	Phenylbutazone	
	Salicylates	
	Sulphonamides	
	Tetracyclines	
	Thiazides	

[a]Most common cause of recurrent erythema multiforme.
[b]Most drugs have at some time been implicated in erythema multiforme.

- Lichen planus
- Pemphigoid
- Chronic ulcerative stomatitis
- Dermatitis herpetiformis
- Linear IgA disease
- Pemphigus
- Erythema multiforme
- Pyostomatitis vegetans

Orals
- Aphthous-like stomatitis

Ocular
- Uveitis and hypopyon
- Retinal vasculitis
- Optic atrophy
- Blindness

Genital
- Ulcers

Cutaneous
- Pustules
- Erythema nodosum

Joints
- Arthralgia (large joints)

Vascular
- Aneurysms
- Thromboses of vena cava

Renal
- Proteinuria
- Haematuria

Neuropsychiatric
- Syndromes resembling multiple sclerosis
- Syndromes resembling pseudobulbar palsy
- Benign intracranial hypertension
- Brainstem lesions
- Depression

Dental aspects

LA is safe. CS can be given if required. Orofacial manifestations are as described above.

DESQUAMATIVE GINGIVITIS

Desquamative gingivitis is the term given to the clinical description of chronically red and occasionally sore gingivae. It is caused mainly by pemphigoid or lichen planus, and sometimes by other mucocutaneous disorders (Box 11.2).

BEHÇET DISEASE

General aspects

Behçet disease is a clinical triad of oral and genital ulceration, and uveitis, tending particularly to strike people with 'Silk Road' bloodlines, especially those from Turkey and Japan. Behçet disease mainly affects young adult males, and there is an association with HLA-B5 and HLA-B51(B5101). Features such as arthralgia and leukocytoclastic vasculitis suggest an immune complex-mediated basis. The immunological changes seen mimic those in patients with recurrent aphthous stomatitis (RAS), with various T-lymphocyte abnormalities (especially T-suppressor cell dysfunction), changes in serum complement, and increased polymorphonuclear leukocyte motility. There is also evidence that mononuclear cells may initiate antibody-dependent cellular cytotoxicity to oral epithelial cells, and evidence of disturbance of natural killer cell activity.

Clinical features

Behçet disease is a multisystem disease with a wide variety of manifestations. Oral ulceration is the most constant feature and is indistinguishable from the common types of aphthous-like stomatitis. Ocular and genital lesions are common, as are rashes, arthritis, thrombophlebitis, cardiovascular disease and central nervous system (CNS) involvement (Box 11.3).

MAGIC syndrome (*m*outh *a*nd *g*enital ulcers and *i*nterstitial *c*hondritis) is a recognized variant of Behçet disease.

General management

A clinical diagnosis of Behçet disease is usually made on the presence of any two of the oral, genital and ocular features, but similar oral ulceration may also develop in other diseases that have multisystem involvement and these must be excluded when making the diagnosis. Behçet disease must enter into the differential diagnosis of recurrent

aphthae but the diagnosis may be difficult to confirm for the reasons given earlier. Oral and genital ulceration may also result from folate deficiency, when other features characteristic of Behçet syndrome are lacking. Recurrent oral, ocular and genital lesions may also be seen in erythema multiforme and sometimes in ulcerative colitis and other conditions. The primary features of Behçet disease are as follows:

- Recurrent oral ulceration (painful aphthous-like ulcers, testing negative for herpes) in almost 100% of patients *plus*
- Any two of the following four:
  Recurrent genital ulcerations
  Eye inflammation (uveitis or retinal vasculitis)
  Skin lesions (erythema nodosum, pseudofolliculitis, papulopustular lesions or acneiform nodules)
  A positive pathergy test (a skin-prick test using a sterile needle and sterile saline solution).

However, UK or US patients rarely test positive, even during disease activity. Behcet disease international criteria were revised in 2013.

Other manifestations that may be useful in diagnosis but are not considered part of the international Behçet criteria, include:

- subcutaneous thrombophlebitis, deep vein thrombosis
- epididymitis, arterial occlusion and/or aneurysm
- CNS involvement (including difficulties in movement or speech, or memory loss)
- severe headaches with stiff neck, joint pain or non-destructive arthritis

- gastrointestinal tract involvement (bloating, cramping, diarrhoea, bloody stools)
- renal involvement
- pulmonary vascular inflammation and pleuritis.

Reliable diagnostic tests for Behçet disease are not available but there are many immunological findings including: circulating autoanti-bodies (e.g. against intermediate filaments, cardiolipin and neutrophil cytoplasm); circulating immune complexes and abnormal levels of complement; immunoglobulins and complement deposition within and around blood vessel walls; and a depressed T-helper (CD4): T-suppressor (CD8) ratio. Behçet disease is thus diagnosed mainly on clinical grounds alone, though findings of HLA-B5101 and pathergy are supportive, as are antibodies to cardiolipin and neutrophil cyto-plasm. Activity of the disease may be assessed by serum levels of acute-phase proteins or antibodies to intermediate filaments, both raised in active Behçet disease.

Medical and ophthalmological opinions should be obtained since ocular involvement often culminates in impaired sight.

Available treatments include mainly colchicine, systemic corticos-teroids, azathioprine, interferon alpha, mycophenolate mofetil and thalidomide. However, the multiplicity of other medications, including levamisole, cyclophosphamide, dapsone and ciclosporin or chloram-bucil, confirms their overall low level of success. Anti-tumour necrosis factor (TNF) biological therapies and rituximab have been used with some success.

Dental aspects

Oral lesions can be managed symptomatically like common aph-thae. Topical tetracycline mouthwash is the topical drug of choice for controlling the ulcers. Topical corticosteroids and LA may help. Colchicine may be of value and thalidomide may be the most effective treatment for otherwise intractable oral ulceration.

SWEET SYNDROME

Sweet syndrome, or acute neutrophilic dermatosis, is rare but consists of persistent high fever, raised erythrocyte sedimentation rate and neutrophilia, and a rash. Some cases are associated with malignancy (especially acute myeloid leukaemia), and some have followed infec-tions – especially upper respiratory tract infections.

The rash consists of dull red skin nodules or plaques on the neck and forearms especially; these may become pustular. Sweet syndrome may also include oral ulceration, conjunctivitis, episcleritis and arthralgia. Treatment is with systemic corticosteroids.

GENETIC MUCOCUTANEOUS DISORDERS

ECTODERMAL DYSPLASIA

The ectodermal dysplasias (EDs) are a family of hereditary diseases that involve defects in two or more tissues derived from ectoderm – skin, hair, teeth, nails and sweat glands. Oral manifestations of the EDs are associated with the teeth. Alterations in tooth development can include hypodontia, anodontia and conically shaped teeth.

General aspects

ED is a relatively common genodermatosis characterized by hypoplasia or agenesis of many skin appendages. There are many variants. The skin is fragile and nails may be defective. The teeth and salivary glands may also be defective or fail to form. Sweat glands may also fail to form and heat control is then disrupted (hypohidrotic ectodermal dysplasia).

Clinical features

There may be frontal bossing and a depressed nasal bridge. The hair is fine, blond and scanty (hypotrichosis), especially in the tonsural region, and the eyelashes and eyebrows may be absent. If the teeth are absent, there may be a prematurely senile (nutcracker) profile with protuberant lips.

Dental aspects

ED rarely causes management problems, apart from those related to its oral manifestations. LA is safe, as is CS. General anaesthesia (GA), as with other dental patients, must be given in hospital. Especial care is indicated in intubation in hypohidrotic forms. Teeth are often few in number (hypodontia or oligodontia), and those present may be of simple conical form. The enamel is thin. Either the deciduous or the permanent dentition, or in extreme cases both, may fail to form (anodontia), causing hypoplasia of the jaws. Salivary glands may also fail to form, which causes xerostomia. Preventive dental care is therefore particularly important.

EPIDERMOLYSIS BULLOSA

General aspects

Epidermolysis bullosa is an uncommon bullous disease affecting mainly skin and mucosae. There are several forms that show different patterns of inheritance and vary greatly in severity. The severe form appears soon after birth; milder forms may not become evident until adolescence or later (Table 11.4).

An acquired form, with antibodies against collagen VII, is also recognized.

Clinical features

Vesicles and bullae form in response to mild or insignificant trauma and may lead to disabling scarring.

General management

Corticosteroids may help prevent blister formation and some success has been claimed for vitamin E and phenytoin.

Dental aspects

Early dietary advice and preventive dental care is overwhelmingly important, since even 'normal' toothbrushing can cause ulceration. Adequate oral hygiene is difficult to achieve, and dental diseases such as caries and periodontal disease are common. Oral scarring and severe microstomia may restrict access. Blistering, erosions and aggravation of scarring following dental treatment (however carefully carried out) may possibly be reduced by applying KY jelly or silicone oil to the mucosa. A short preoperative course of corticosteroids an hour before treatment, and again on the following day, then tapering the dose off over the next 3 days may possibly help.

Intramuscular injections can cause sloughing and adhesive tapes easily traumatize the epidermis and thus should be avoided. Antimicrobials to cover surgery may possibly be helpful.

Table 11.4 *The main types of epidermolysis bullosa*

Type	Onset	Main site of lesions[a]	Oral mucosal lesions	Dental defects	Nail defects	Scarring	Inheritance
I. Non-scarring types							
Simplex[b]	Neonatal onwards	Hands, feet and elbows	Rarely	No	No	No	AD
Letalis[c]	Birth	Widespread	Yes[d]	Yes	Severe	No	AR
II. Scarring types							
Dermolytic dominant (dystrophic)[e]	Childhood	Extremities	Uncommon	No	Yes	Yes. Soft scars	AD
Dermolytic recessive (polydysplastic)[f]	Birth or infancy	Widespread	Yes. Severe, mutilating	No	Destruction	Mutilating[g]	AR

AD = autosomal dominant; AR = autosomal recessive.
[a]Usually also any site of trauma.
[b]May improve by puberty; commonest type.
[c]Usually fatal in neonatal period or childhood; also known as Herlitz disease.
[d]Vermilion border of lips spared: lesions are perioral and perinasal. May be corneal lesions.
[e]A cemental defect has been reported, but destruction and loss of teeth from caries and periodontal care is a typical result of inability to brush the teeth.
[f]Rare and fatal.
[g]Typically leads to destruction of hands and feet. Oesophageal stricture may lead to aspiration into airway.

GA should be avoided where possible. Bullae may form on the face or in the airway if intubation is attempted. If intubation must be used, the face should be protected with petroleum jelly gauze and the route should be oral rather than nasal. Iron deficiency anaemia is common and may need correction before GA (Ch. 8). Intravenous ketamine has proved a useful anaesthetic in these patients. Atropinics are often needed to control excessive salivation.

Rarely, squamous cell carcinoma can complicate the oral lesions. Rare cases are associated with poikiloderma congenitale and may present with early-onset periodontitis or desquamative gingivitis.

MULTIPLE BASAL CELL NAEVI SYNDROME (GORLIN–GOLTZ SYNDROME)

General aspects

The multiple basal cell naevi syndrome consists of multiple basal cell carcinomas of early onset, keratocystic odontogenic tumours, anomalies of the vertebrae and ribs, and many other abnormalities. It is an autosomal dominant trait with poor penetrance.

Clinical features

Skin lesions appear in childhood or adolescence. Multiple naevoid basal cell carcinomas over the nose, eyelids, cheeks and elsewhere are often an early sign (Fig. 11.15).

There is frontal and temporoparietal bossing, a broad nasal root, prominent supraorbital ridges and a degree of mandibular prognathism. Multiple jaw cysts develop. Short fourth metacarpals are common. There may also be pitting of the palms or soles.

Many other problems may be associated, including learning impairment or cerebral tumours. Pseudohypoparathyroidism has been described in some patients and there is also a slightly greater incidence of diabetes mellitus. Cardiac lesions may be present and cerebral tumours can be fatal.

General management

Radiography may reveal bifid ribs, vertebral defects with kyphoscoliosis and calcification of the falx cerebri.

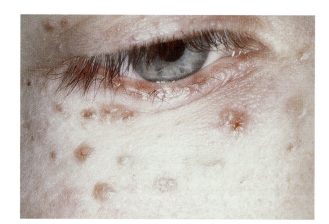

Fig. 11.15 Basal carcinomas in multiple basal cell naevi (Gorlin–Goltz) syndrome.

Dental aspects

LA is safe. CS can be given. GA must be given in hospital for treatment of the jaw cysts.

GARDNER SYNDROME (FAMILIAL ADENOMATOUS POLYPOSIS COLI)

General aspects

Gardner syndrome is the association of multiple osteomas, skin fibromas and epidermoid cysts, and pigmented ocular fundus lesions with colonic polyposis.

It is an autosomal dominant trait of variable penetrance.

Clinical features

Multiple osteomas characteristically involve the jaws, facial skeleton or frontal bone, and appear in adolescence. Fibromas, desmoid tumours, epidermoid cysts or lipomas affect any site. Multiple colonic polyps invariably undergo malignant change. Thyroid, adrenal and biliary carcinomas may also develop.

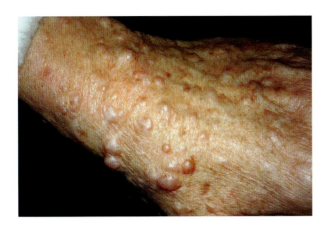

Fig. 11.16 Neurofibromatosis.

General management

Colonic resection is usually required. Desmoid tumours often arise in the abdominal wall scar.

Dental aspects

LA is safe. CS can be given if required. Multiple osteomas, particularly on the alveolar margins, should suggest the presence of Gardner syndrome. Compound odontomas and dental anomalies may be associated.

COWDEN SYNDROME

This is an autosomal dominant condition of multiple hamartomas, with a predisposition to carcinomas of the breast, thyroid or colon. Skin and mucosal papules precede the onset of malignant disease. Other lesions include keratoses on the palms and soles, and sometimes learning impairment.

Oral mucosal papillomatosis may suggest the diagnosis. When associated with cerebellar hypertrophy, the syndrome is known as Cowden–L'Hermitte syndrome.

PHAKOMATOSES

The phakomatoses (neurodermatoses) are hereditary hamartomatous autosomal dominant disorders affecting the skin and nervous system. They include neurofibromatosis, tuberous sclerosis and Sturge–Weber syndrome. Sporadic cases are not uncommon. The fourth member of this group, cerebroretinal angiomatosis, is not discussed here.

Neurofibromatosis type I (von Recklinghausen disease)

General aspects

Neurofibromatosis type I is a simple autosomal dominant condition in which there are multiple neurofibromas or, less often, neurilemmomas.

Clinical features

Neurofibromas sometimes form in vast numbers (Fig. 11.16). These may be disfiguring but are often asymptomatic unless pressure effects develop: for example, on the spinal nerve roots with compression of the spinal cord. Patches of skin hyperpigmentation (café-au-lait spots)

are common. Sarcomatous change may develop in about 10% of severely affected patients. There is also a greater frequency of cerebral gliomas.

Complications may include learning impairment and epilepsy in a minority. Multiple neuroendocrine adenoma syndrome may be associated (Ch. 6).

Dental aspects

LA can be given safely. CS can be given if required. GA must, as always, be given in hospital.

Oral mucosal neurofibromas are uncommon and more typically associated with endocrine disorders (multiple endocrine adenoma [MEA] type III; Ch. 6).

Neurofibromatosis type II is characterized by bilateral acoustic neuromas, which can cause deafness and any of the symptoms of cerebellopontine angle lesions, but the skin lesions of type I are lacking.

Tuberous sclerosis (Bourneville disease; epiloia)

General aspects

Tuberous sclerosis is characterized by adenoma sebaceum and leaf-shaped depigmented naevi of the skin, epilepsy and sometimes learning disability.

It is a simple autosomal dominant trait linked to chromosome 9 or 16.

Clinical features

The skin adenoma sebaceum are angiofibromas typically distributed in a butterfly pattern across the cheeks, nasolabial folds, bridge of the nose, forehead and chin. Epilepsy, learning impairment and cardiac or renal involvement, or endocrinopathies, particularly diabetes mellitus, may be features.

Dental aspects

Dental management may be complicated by cardiac or renal involvement, or diabetes mellitus, in addition to epilepsy and sometimes learning impairment. LA with or without CS can be given, unless there is severe cardiac or renal involvement. GA must, as always, be given in hospital.

The facial 'adenomas' may be conspicuous and suggest the diagnosis. Oral lesions include hyperplastic gingivitis and pit-shaped dental defects in both dentitions.

Sturge–Weber syndrome

General aspects

Sturge–Weber syndrome (encephalotrigeminal angiomatosis) is characterized by an angiomatous defect (hamartoma), which is usually on the upper part of the face and also within the skull.

Clinical features

The angioma is often large, usually sited in the upper part of the face, and may appear to occupy the area of a division of the trigeminal nerve, extending into the mouth. The occipital lobe of the brain is usually involved, but the parietal and frontal lobes may be affected if the lower face is involved by the angioma.

Clinically, there are often convulsions, hemiplegia and learning impairment.

Dental aspects

Dental surgery in the area affected by the haemangioma may be complicated by profuse haemorrhage and should therefore only be attempted in hospital. When the vascular naevus involves the face, it usually extends to the underlying oral mucosa and gingivae, which are red and sometimes hyperplastic, and also to the alveolar bone.

LA is safe. CS can usually be given if required.

PSEUDOXANTHOMA ELASTICUM

Pseudoxanthoma elasticum is a rare autosomal recessive disorder of connective tissue characterized by yellow papular or reticular skin lesions, visual impairment and cardiovascular abnormalities. The skin is hyperextensible and there may be blue sclerae and loose-jointedness. Abnormalities in the eyes include streaks beneath the retina (angioid streaks) and often haemorrhages and scarring.

Cardiovascular involvement includes calcification of elastic tissue in vessel walls, leading to poor blood flow, which in turn causes ischaemic heart disease and intermittent claudication. Hypertension is common. Some patients have a normal lifespan but others succumb to haemorrhage, cardiac disease or cerebrovascular accidents. Some individuals develop hypothyroidism; others bleed from the upper gastrointestinal tract, uterus, or renal or respiratory tracts.

Dental management may be complicated particularly by cardiovascular disease.

Lesions may be seen around the face and mouth, and there may be nodules in the lips or rarely in the mouth.

ORAL MUCOSAL DISORDERS

Mouth ulcers are generally caused by local factors but some are recurrent aphthae; others are due to malignant disease (Ch. 22), drugs or systemic disease (diseases of blood, infections, gastrointestinal disease or skin diseases; Chs 7, 8 and 21).

RECURRENT APHTHAE (RECURRENT APHTHOUS STOMATITIS)

General aspects

Recurrent aphthae (recurrent aphthous stomatitis; RAS) typically appear as round or ovoid ulcers, with onset usually in childhood or adolescence, and recurrences at intervals. RAS is common and may affect up to 25% of the population. The cause is usually unclear and most patients are otherwise healthy, but there are occasional associations with a familial basis, no tobacco use, menstrual cycle, haematinic deficiency (iron, folate or vitamin B_{12}), trauma, stress and particular foods.

Aphthous-like ulcers may be seen in relation to a number of conditions (Box 11.4).

Box 11.4 *Aphthous-like ulcers: related conditions*

- Autoinflammatory syndromes such as periodic fever, aphthous stomatitis, pharyngitis and cervical adenitis (PFAPA)
- *Behçet syndrome*, when there is usually genital ulceration, uveitis and other lesions
- *Coeliac or Crohn disease*, or other intestinal diseases, notably ulcerative colitis
- *Drugs* (e.g. cytotoxics, mammalian target of rapamycin [mTOR] inhibitors, NSAIDS, nicorandil) or defective immunity (e.g. HIV infection: major aphthae may be the presenting feature) or cyclic neutropenia: typically (but rarely) causes recurrent infections, fever, malaise and enlarged cervical lymph nodes. Oral ulceration may appear at 21-day intervals, coincident with the falls in circulating neutrophils, and may be the main manifestation of the disease. In others, severe periodontal disease may develop

---

Table 11.5 *Clinical variants of aphthae*

Minor aphthae	Major aphthae	Herpetiform aphthae
Common	Uncommon	Uncommon
Usually round or ovoid discrete ulcers	Usually round or ovoid discrete ulcers	Ulcers initially 1–3 mm across but later coalesce to form ragged ulcers
Not on attached gingiva or hard palate and rarely on dorsum of tongue	Ulcers may be 1 to several cm in diameter	Ulcers form in crops of 10–100 with widespread erythema
Most are 2–4 mm in diameter	Persist for months before healing with scarring	
Heal within 10 days without scarring		

Clinical features

The onset is usually in childhood or adolescence. Ulcers are typically round or ovoid, and recur at intervals. Three different clinical patterns are recognized (Table 11.5).

General management

In addition to a careful history, patients with aphthous-like ulcers should be screened haematologically, particularly if the history suggests a systemic disorder or if the ulcers develop or worsen in middle age or later. A full screen includes haemoglobin and blood indices, serum ferritin (or iron and iron-binding capacity), vitamin B_{12} levels, corrected whole blood or red cell folate levels, and transglutaminase and anti-endomysial antibodies (to exclude coeliac disease). There are no useful laboratory diagnostic tests for RAS. Systemic conditions, such as Behçet disease and HIV infection, should be excluded if the history is suggestive.

There is no specific or reliably effective treatment; topical corticosteroids are often used. For severe or intractable RAS, systemic corticosteroids or other immunosuppressants may be given, but overall thalidomide appears to be most effective. In patients with HIV infection, aphthous-like ulcers may respond to antiretroviral therapy (ART), granulocyte–macrophage colony-stimulating factor or thalidomide. Anti-TNF biological therapies may be successful in severe aphthae.

PERIODIC FEVER, APHTHOUS STOMATITIS, PHARYNGITIS AND CERVICAL ADENITIS (PFAPA)

See Chapter 19.

CHRONIC ULCERATIVE STOMATITIS

General aspects

Chronic ulcerative stomatitis (CUS) is a rare disease with an appearance similar to erosive lichen planus, which mainly affects the oral mucosa. CUS is associated with unusual antinuclear antibodies reacting exclusively with squamous epithelia (squamous epithelium-specific antinuclear antibodies; SES-ANA). Sera from CUS patients bind a keratinocyte protein, KET, which is closely related to the *p53* tumour suppressor gene. The *KET* gene is expressed exclusively in epithelia and thymus, and thus may play a role in keratinocyte cell-cycle control. This might explain the specificity of SES-ANA for keratinocytes. However, the antibodies persist after clearance of mucosal lesions, are fixed *in vivo* and also in uninvolved skin and other mucosa, and may appear in patients without CUS. Thus their pathogenic potential remains to be established.

Clinical features

CUS mainly affects older females. The clinical appearances are similar to erosive lichen planus (see earlier) and it seems likely that many cases of CUS have been misdiagnosed clinically as lichen planus.

General management

Antimalarials are highly effective initially. Relapses usually respond only to combined therapy with chloroquine and small doses of corticosteroids.

INFLAMMATORY DENTAL DISEASE: RELATIONSHIP WITH SYSTEMIC DISEASE

Increasing evidence supports, but does not prove, an association between periodontal infection and various systemic diseases, especially with atherosclerotic cardiovascular disease or its sequelae, and possibly other conditions. The possible mechanisms behind these associations ultimately include increased systemic inflammation due to periodontal diseases and/or dissemination of bacteria and direct damage on endothelium and other target organs. There is some evidence supporting links with pre-eclampsia, pre-term and low-birthweight babies, endometriosis, ischaemic heart disease, cerebrovascular disease, aspiration pneumonia, diabetes mellitus, metabolic syndrome, chronic kidney disease, osteoporosis, Alzheimer disease, pancreatic cancer, kidney cancer, haematological cancers and even oral cancer. It is possible that endodontic infections have similar associations, as chronic inflammatory lesions following carious lesions could both trigger a systemic inflammatory state as well as induce short-lived bacteraemias (for this vast topic, see Chapple and Hamburger, 2006).

ORAL CANCER

See Chapter 22.

SALIVARY NEOPLASMS

See Chapter 14.

KEY WEBSITES

(Accessed 27 May 2013)
BMJ. <http://www.bmj.com/specialties/dermatology>
National Institutes of Health: National Institute of Arthritis and Musculoskeletal and Skin Diseases. <http://www.niams.nih.gov/health_info/pemphigus/>
National Institutes of Health: Office of Rare Diseases Research. <http://rarediseases.info.nih.gov/GARD/Condition/7352/Pemphigus.aspx>
NHS Choices:
  Behçet disease. <http://www.nhs.uk/conditions/Behcets-disease/Pages/introduction.aspx>
  Lichen planus. <http://www.nhs.uk/conditions/Lichen-planus/Pages/Introduction.aspx>
  Pemphigus vulgaris. <http://www.nhs.uk/Conditions/pemphigus-vulgaris/Pages/Definition.aspx>

USEFUL WEBSITES

(Accessed 27 May 2013)
American Academy of Dermatology. <http://www.aad.org/skin-conditions/dermatology-a-to-z/lichen-planus>
International Pemphigus & Pemphigoid Foundation. <http://www.pemphigus.org/living-with-pp/understanding-pp/>
MedlinePlus. <http://www.nlm.nih.gov/medlineplus/oralcancer.html>

FURTHER READING

Amagai, M., 2009. The molecular logic of pemphigus and impetigo: the desmoglein story. Vet. Dermatol. 20, 308.
Aoki, T., et al. 2000. Beneficial effects of interferon-alpha in a case with Behçet's disease. Intern. Med. 39, 667.
Avangco, L., Rogers 3rd, R.S., 2003. Oral manifestations of erythema multiforme. Dermatol. Clin. 21 (1), 195.
Bagan, J., et al. 2005. Mucous membrane pemphigoid. Oral Dis. 11, 197.
Baioni, C.S., et al. 2008. Analysis of the association of polymorphism in the osteoprotegerin gene with susceptibility to chronic kidney disease and periodontitis. J. Periodontal. Res. 43, 578.
Bez, C., et al. 2001. Lack of association between hepatotropic transfusion transmitted virus infection and oral lichen planus in British and Italian populations. Br. J. Dermatol. 145, 990.
Black, M., et al. 2005. Pemphigus. Oral Dis. 11, 119.
Calabrese, L., Fleischer, A.B., 2000. Thalidomide: current and potential clinical applications. Am. J. Med. 108, 487.
Challacombe, S.J., et al. 2001. Immunodiagnosis of pemphigus and mucous membrane pemphigoid. Acta Odontol. Scand. 59, 226.
Chapple, I.L., Hamburger, J., 2006. Periodontal medicine: a window on the body. Quintessence, New Malden.
Chen, M.C., et al. 2008. The incidence and risk of second primary cancers in patients with nasopharyngeal carcinoma: a population-based study in Taiwan over a 25-year period (1979–2003). Ann. Oncol. 19, 1180.
Choonhakarn, C., et al. 2008. The efficacy of aloe vera gel in the treatment of oral lichen planus: a randomized controlled trial. Br. J. Dermatol. 158, 573.
Cirillo, N., et al. 2012. Urban legends series: pemphigus vulgaris. Oral Dis. 18 (5), 442.
Cote, B., et al. 1995. Clinicopathologic correlation in erythema multiforme and Stevens–Johnson syndrome. Arch. Dermatol. 131 (11), 1268.
Farthing, P., et al. 2005. Erythema multiforme. Oral Dis. 11, 261.
Femiano, F., et al. 2002. Pemphigus vulgaris with oral involvement: evaluation of two different systemic corticosteroid therapeutic protocols. J. Eur. Acad. Dermatol. Venereol. 16, 353.
Franek, E., et al. 2006. Chronic periodontitis in hemodialysis patients with chronic kidney disease is associated with elevated serum C-reactive protein concentration and greater intima-media thickness of the carotid artery. J. Nephrol. 19, 346.
Gonzalez-Moles, M.A., et al. 2008. Oral lichen planus: controversies surrounding malignant transformation. Oral Dis. 14 (3), 229. doi: 10.1111/j.1601-0825.2008.01441.x. Epub 2008 Feb 22.
Hatemi, G., Seyahi, E., Fresko, I., Hamuryudan, V., 2012 May-Jun;30. Behçet's syndrome: a critical digest of the recent literature. Clin. Exp. Rheumatol. (3 Suppl 72), S80–S89. Epub 2012 Sep 25. Review. PubMed PMID: 23009740.
Herranz, P., et al. 2000. Successful treatment of aphthous ulcerations in AIDS patients using topical granulocyte–macrophage colony-stimulating factor. Br. J. Dermatol. 142, 171.

International Team for the Revision of the International Criteria for Behçet's Disease (ITR-ICBD), Davatchi, F., Assaad-Khalil, S., Calamia, K.T., Crook, J.E., Sadeghi-Abdollahi, B., et al., 2013 Feb 26. The International criteria for Behçet's disease (ICBD): a collaborative study of 27 countries on the sensitivity and specificity of the new criteria. J. Eur. Acad. Dermatol. Venereol. 10.1111/jdv.12107. [Epub ahead of print] PubMed PMID: 23441863.

Koga, H., et al. 2012. Five Japanese cases of antidesmoglein 1 antibody-positive and antidesmoglein 3 antibody-negative pemphigus with oral lesions. Br. J. Dermatol. 166, 976.

Lodi, G., et al. 2000. Hepatitis G virus-associated oral lichen planus: no influence from hepatitis G virus co-infection. J. Oral Pathol. Med. 29, 39.

Porter, S.R., et al. 2000. Recurrent aphthous stomatitis. Clin. Dermatol. 18, 569.

Porter S.R., Scully C. Aphthous ulcers: recurrent. Clin Evid 2000; 5:606/2001; 6:1037/2002; 7:1232; Clin. Evid. Concise. 2002; 7:234.

Scully, C., 2001. The mouth in dermatological disorders. Practitioner 245, 942.

Scully, C., Bagan, J.V., 2008. Oral mucosal diseases: erythema multiforme. Br. J. Oral Maxillofac. Surg. 46, 90. 2007 Sep 1 [Epub ahead of print].

Scully, C., et al. 1999. Update on mucous membrane pemphigoid (an immune mediated sub-epithelial blistering disease): a heterogeneous entity. Oral Surg. Oral Med. Oral Pathol. 88, 56.

Scully, C., Carrozzo, M., 2008. Oral mucosal diseases: lichen planus. Br. J. Oral Maxillofac. Surg. 46, 15. Epub 2007 Sep 5.

Scully, C, Challacombe, S.J., 2002. Pemphigus vulgaris: update on etiopathogenesis, oral manifestations and management. Crit. Rev. Oral Biol. Med. 13, 397.

Scully, C., et al. 2000. Management of oral lichen planus. Am. J. Clin. Dermatol. 1, 287.

Scully C., et al. 2002. Aphthous ulcerations. Diagnosis and treatment of oral lesions. Dermatol. Ther. (ed. C. Camisa), 15.185.

Scully, C., Lo Muzio, L., 2008. Oral mucosal diseases: pemphigoid. Br. J. Oral Maxillofac. Surg. 46, 358. Epub 2007 Sep 4.

Scully, C., Mignogna, M., 2008. Oral mucosal diseases: pemphigus. Br. J. Oral Maxillofac. Surg. 46, 272. Epub 2007 Sep 17.

Scully, C., Porter, S., 2008. Oral mucosal diseases: recurrent aphthous stomatitis. Br. J. Oral Maxillofac. Surg. 46, 198. Epub 2007 Sep 11.

Shotts, R., Scully, C., 2002. How to identify and deal with tongue problems. Pulse 62, 73.

Williams, P.M., Conklin, R.J., 2005. Erythema multiforme: a review and contrast from Stevens–Johnson syndrome/toxic epidermal necrolysis. Dent. Clin. N. Am. 49, 67.

APPENDIX 11.1 CONGENITAL ORAL AND INTESTINAL DISORDERS

Syndrome	Cutaneous and other extraintestinal features	Gastrointestinal lesions
Cowden syndrome	Skin nodules Breast malignancy	Polyps
Gardner syndrome (familial adenomatous polyposis coli)	Osteomas of jaws (especially mandible), epidermal cysts, sebaceous cysts, lipomas, fibroma, dental anomalies	Colon polyps, adenocarcinomas, biliary neoplasia
Multiple endocrine adenoma (MEA) III	Ch. 6	Mucosal neuromas
Peutz–Jeghers syndrome	Pigmented macules of mouth, lips and digits Risk of neoplasia	Small intestine polyps and carcinoma rarely
Tylosis	Hyperkeratosis of palms and soles	Oral leukoplakia Oesophageal carcinoma

The kidneys (nephrons) have many functions, especially fluid and electrolyte balance, waste removal, acid–base balance, vitamin D metabolism and stimulation of erythrocyte production. The kidney makes urine by filtering small molecules and ions from the blood and then reclaiming useful materials such as glucose (Fig. 12.1). The nephron consists of a Bowman's capsule, glomerulus (a capillary network within Bowman's capsule), proximal convoluted tubule, loop of Henle, and distal convoluted and collecting tubules (Table 12.1).

The kidneys constantly pass urine through the ureters to the bladder; it is stored in the bladder to be passed from time to time via the urethra (Fig. 12.2). Nearly a quarter of the blood volume perfuses the kidneys each minute. The glomerular filtration rate (GFR) can be calculated from creatinine clearance, inulin clearance, or clearance of isotopes, such as ^{125}I-iothalamate, ^{51}Cr-EDTA (ethylenediamine tetra-acetic acid) or ^{99m}Tc-DPTA (diethylenetriamine penta-acetic acid), or plasma creatinine levels; it is increasingly expressed as an estimate calculated by using the Modification of Diet in Renal Disease (MDRD) study equation, which takes into account patient age, gender and serum creatinine level. In health, the GFR is around 120 mL/min per 1.73 m^2 for women and 130 mL/min per 1.73 m^2 for men. In population terms, this declines by 1–2 mL/min per year over the age of 20 years. The kidneys also act in the excretion of drugs and hormones, and as endocrine organs for the synthesis of hydroxycholecalciferol (active vitamin D), erythropoietin, renin and prostaglandins, and as target organs for parathyroid hormone and aldosterone.

Renal failure can come on suddenly (acute renal failure; ARF), as after surgery or severe injuries, or when renal blood vessels become obstructed, but more usually develops slowly (chronic renal failure, CRF; chronic kidney disease, CKD). Renal failure results in fluid retention, acidosis, accumulation of metabolites and drugs, damage to platelets (leading to a bleeding tendency), hypertension, anaemia and endocrine effects.

ACUTE RENAL FAILURE

Acute renal failure can be caused by pre-renal, renal or post-renal factors:

- *Pre-renal factors* (55%) include: hypotension (haemorrhage or severe burns), renal thrombosis, sepsis, dehydration, heat stroke or drugs, e.g. non-steroidal anti-inflammatory drugs (NSAIDs), fluroquinolones, androgen-deprivation therapy and angiotensin-converting enzyme inhibitors (ACEIs). Clarithromycin given to patients on antihypertensive calcium-channel blockers may cause acute kidney injury, hypotension, and even death.
- *Renal factors* (15%) include: interstitial nephritis; toxic acute tubular necrosis; complicated surgery or trauma (myoglobin blocks tubular function); drugs – contrast dyes used in arteriography, antibiotics (especially streptomycin, gentamicin or amphotericin), aspirin and other NSAIDs, paracetamol (acetaminophen) overdose; toxins (betel, heavy metals, solvents); multiple organ failure, in which the heart, lungs, liver, brain and kidneys totally or partially shut down (most often the result of major trauma or sepsis); the haemolytic–uraemic syndrome, which is caused in children by *Escherichia coli* O157:H7 (which expresses verotoxin – also called Shiga toxin) and in adults by HIV, antiphospholipid syndrome, post-partum renal failure, malignant hypertension, scleroderma or cancer chemotherapy.
- *Post-renal factors* include: obstructed urine flow.

ARF is a medical emergency, which may lead to confusion, seizures and coma. Management is often by dialysis.

CHRONIC KIDNEY DISEASE (CKD; CHRONIC RENAL DISEASE)

General aspects

Chronic kidney disease is defined as kidney damage, or a reduction in the GFR, for 3 or more months. All individuals with a GFR of less than 90 mL/min per 1.73 m^2 for 3 months are classified as having CKD, if there is also proteinuria or haematuria. They are at increased risk of loss of kidney function and development of cardiovascular disease (Table 12.2).

Historically, CKD has been classified according to the part of the renal anatomy involved, as follows:

- *Vascular*, which includes disease of large vessels (e.g. bilateral renal artery stenosis) or small vessels (e.g. ischaemic nephropathy, haemolytic–uraemic syndrome, vasculitis)
- *Glomerular*, a diverse group subclassified into disease that is primary (e.g. focal segmental glomerulosclerosis, immunoglobulin A [IgA] nephritis) or secondary (e.g. diabetic nephropathy, lupus nephritis)
- *Tubulointerstitial*, which includes polycystic kidney disease, drug- and toxin-induced chronic tubulointerstitial nephritis and reflux nephropathy
- *Obstructive*, as with renal or bladder stones and prostate diseases.

CKD is said to be present when damaged kidneys perform their functions less well, causing waste substances such as urea to accumulate and leading to other issues. CKD is not a specific disease. The most common causes (75% of all adult cases) are diabetes, hypertension and glomerulonephritis. Renal diseases (e.g. chronic glomerulonephritis, polycystic renal disease, renal artery stenosis), systemic diseases (lupus erythematosus, myeloma, amyloid), poisoning (e.g. lead or betel) and drugs (e.g. long-term use of aspirin or other NSAIDs, or large amounts of paracetamol [acetaminophen]) are other causes.

CKD is more common among women than men. In men, it is 50% more likely than in women to progress to renal failure. It is seen in 35% of people aged 20 years or older with diabetes, and 20% of people aged 20 years or older with hypertension. Since diabetes and hypertension are both common in people of South Asian and of African heritage, such individuals have a high prevalence of CKD.

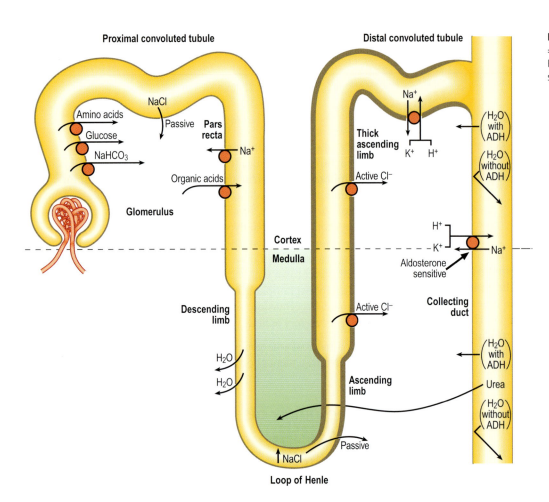

Fig. 12.1 Diagram of renal tubular structure. ADH = antidiuretic hormone; Cl⁻, chloride; H_2O = water; H^+, hydrogen; K^+, potassium; Na^+ = sodium; NaCl = sodium chloride; $NaHCO_3$ = bicarbonate.

Table 12.1 *The kidney: constituents and functions*

Proximal convoluted tubule	Loop of Henle	Distal convoluted tubule	Collecting tubule
Actively reabsorbs glucose, amino acids, uric acid and inorganic salts	Water continues to leave by osmosis	More Na^+ is reclaimed by active transport, and still more water follows by osmosis	Final adjustment of body Na^+ and water content
Active transport out of Na^+ controlled by angiotensin II			Surplus or waste ions and molecules flow out as urine
Active transport of phosphate (PO_4^{3-}) suppressed by parathyroid hormone			
Water follows by osmosis			

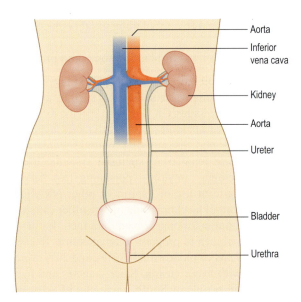

Fig. 12.2 Genitourinary anatomy.

Other risk factors include cardiovascular disease, obesity, hypercholesterolaemia and a family history of CKD. Inadequately controlled diabetes and hypertension increase the risk of progression of CKD to kidney failure. Repeated kidney injury (e.g. infections, drugs or toxins injurious to the kidney) can also contribute to progression to kidney failure, especially in older people. CKD is usually irreversible and progressive and can lead to end-stage renal disease (ESRD; renal failure), through five stages defined by the National Kidney Foundation (see Table 12.2). CKD can be compensated by structural and functional hypertrophy of surviving nephrons, to a point at which around 50% of renal function remains, when chronic renal insufficiency ensues. This inevitably progresses to ESRD.

Clinical features

People with early CKD often have no symptoms; at this point, only a blood test to estimate kidney function and a urine test to assess kidney damage will help the diagnosis. Only when kidney function has fallen to less than 25% of normal do nocturia and anorexia appear, and

Table 12.2 *Stages of chronic kidney disease*

Stages[a]	Renal health	GFR mL/min/1.73 m^2	Features
–	Normal	130	–
1	Diminished renal reserve (early CKD)	>90	Abnormalities in blood or urine tests or imaging studies but few overt symptoms
2	Mild CKD (azotaemia)	60–89	Abnormalities in blood or urine tests or imaging studies
3	Moderately severe	30–59	Abnormalities in blood or urine tests or imaging studies
4	Severe CKD	15–29	Uraemic symptoms
5	End-stage renal failure (ESRF), also called end-stage renal disease (ESRD), chronic kidney failure (CKF) or chronic kidney disease (CKD)	<15	Life-threatening and requires some form of renal replacement therapy

[a]Stages are based on estimated glomerular filtration rate (eGFR): National Kidney Foundation. *Am J Kidney Dis* 2002; 39(2 Suppl 1):S1.

Table 12.3 *Laboratory features of chronic kidney disease*

Urea	Creatinine	Potassium	Phosphate	Calcium	Haemoglobin
Raised	Raised	Normal or Raised	Raised	Low	Low

serum levels of nitrogenous compounds (urea) become raised (azotaemia or uraemia). Later, problems such as cardiovascular disease (heart attacks, heart failure, heart rhythm disturbances and strokes), anaemia and bone disease cause clinical features.

Leading causes of ESRD are diabetes and hypertension. Less common causes include glomerulonephritis, hereditary kidney disease, and malignancies such as myeloma.

Premature death from both cardiovascular disease and from all causes is higher in adults with CKD compared to adults without CKD.

CKD can be associated with fluid overload, sodium and potassium imbalances, bone and mineral disorders, and anaemia. Advanced CKD causes significant impairment of all renal functions, affects virtually all body systems, and causes changes in urea and electrolytes and other blood constituents (Table 12.3; Fig. 12.3). CKD can manifest in a range of clinical features (Table 12.4). Purpura and a bleeding tendency may appear from abnormal platelet production (a consequence of diminished thrombopoietin production); diminished platelet factor 3 (thromboxane), which impairs conversion of prothrombin to thrombin; raised prostacyclin (prostaglandin I), leading to vasodilatation and poor platelet aggregation; and defective von Willebrand factor. Hypertension is common. Anaemia is frequently found and is caused by toxic suppression of the bone marrow, lack of renal production of erythropoietin and/or iron deficiency, from blood loss in the gut. A tendency to infection arises because of defective phagocyte function, which results from reduced interleukin-2 (IL-2) and increases in pro-inflammatory cytokines (IL-1, IL-6, tumour necrosis factor [TNF]).

Renal osteodystrophy is common; phosphate retention leads to depression of plasma calcium levels and subsequently raised parathyroid activity (secondary hyperparathyroidism). There is also deficiency of renal production of 1,25-dihydroxycholecalciferol (vitamin D$_3$) and calcium absorption is thereby impaired. Parathyroid hyperplasia may eventually become adenomatous and irreversible (tertiary hyperparathyroidism).

General management

CKD is diagnosed by clinical history and presentation, and by rising plasma urea (in the USA, blood urea nitrogen; BUN) and creatinine levels and a falling GFR, which is increasingly expressed as an estimate (eGFR; calculated by using the Modification of Diet in Renal Disease [MDRD] equation, which takes into account patient age, gender and serum creatinine level). There is also a correction that can be applied for those of Afro-Caribbean background.

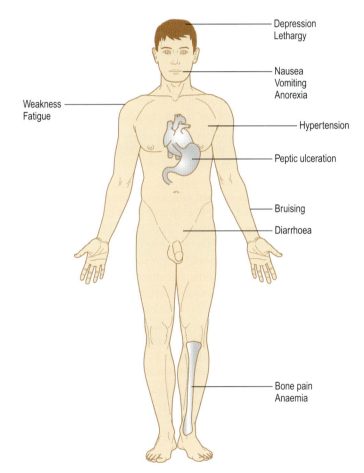

Fig. 12.3 Chronic kidney disease.

The decline in eGFR can be plotted over time, allowing accurate prognosis (such as timing of requirement for dialysis, creation of arteriovenous fistulae, etc.). It also allows for demonstration of effects of therapy, the most important of which is control of blood pressure – by using ACEIs and angiotensin II blockers (ARBs). Underlying causes of CKD should be treated where possible and any stress, infection or urinary tract obstruction should be dealt with, as this may precipitate symptoms. The treatment goal is to slow down or halt the progression of CKD to stage 5, measured by a falling eGFR and rising plasma urea and rising creatinine levels, and aimed at reducing cardiovascular risk, which is the main cause of mortality. A normal diet (low-protein diets are now rarely

Table 12.4 *Clinical features of chronic kidney disease*

Blood and immune	Cardiovascular	Gastrointestinal	Neuromuscular	Metabolic and endocrine	Skin
Bleeding	Hypertension	Anorexia	Weakness and lassitude	Nocturia and polyuria	Pruritus
Anaemia	Congestive cardiac failure	Nausea and vomiting	Drowsiness leading to coma	Thirst	Bruising
Lymphopenia	Pericarditis	Hiccoughs	Headaches, confusion	Glycosuria	Hyperpigmentation
Liability to infections	Cardiomyopathy	Peptic ulcer and gastrointestinal bleeding	Disturbances of vision	Raised urea, creatinine, lipids and uric acid	Infections
	Atheroma, peripheral vascular disease		Sensory disturbances	Electrolyte disturbances	
			Tremor	Secondary hyperparathyroidism	
				Renal osteodystrophy	
				Impotence, amenorrhoea, infertility	

advocated); potassium restriction; and salt or water control are used. As cardiovascular risk is high in patients with low GFR, management includes statins, aspirin, smoking cessation and other measures (Ch. 5).

Symptoms and complications, such as hiccough, vomiting, fits and calcium loss, are treated. Iron stores are replenished using iron and epoietin (recombinant erythropoietin) or darbepoietin, which has a longer half-life. Calcium carbonate, vitamin D$_3$ or its synthetic analogue, a low-phosphate diet or intravenous clodronate help inhibit bone resorption. Cinacalcet, which reduces parathyroid hormone, may be used. Parathyroidectomy may be necessary in cases of tertiary hyperparathyroidism (Ch. 6). A bisphosphonate may be needed for the management of renal osteodystrophy.

Drug therapy requires certain cautions. Dosages of drugs cleared renally, such as penicillins, cephalosporins and erythromycin, should be reduced based on renal function (Table 12.5). The least nephrotoxic agents should be used (NSAIDs or tetracyclines should be avoided), and alternative medications should be prescribed if necessary to avoid potential drug interactions. Clinicians should be aware of drugs with active metabolites that can exaggerate pharmacological effects in patients with CKD. Patients with CKD should also be asked about over-the-counter and herbal medicine use.

CKD can be treated through medication and lifestyle changes to slow disease progression, and to prevent or delay the onset of kidney failure. However, the only treatment options for kidney failure/ESRD are dialysis or a renal transplant. When the patient reaches stage 5 CKD (end-stage renal failure; ESRF), renal replacement therapy is required – dialysis or transplantation.

Dialysis

There are two primary types of dialysis – peritoneal dialysis and haemodialysis.

Peritoneal dialysis (PD) works on the principle that the peritoneal membrane can act as a natural semi-permeable membrane. Dialysis fluid is instilled via a catheter (often a Tenckhoff catheter) placed near the umbilicus, into the abdominal cavity (Fig. 12.4) or tunnelled under the skin from near the sternum (called a pre-sternal catheter). PD has advantages since it is relatively easy to learn, fluid balance is usually easier than on haemodialysis, it is usually done at home and it is relatively easy to travel with (e.g. dialysis solution bags can be transported); though less efficient than haemodialysis, it is as beneficial overall, since it is performed more frequently. Continuous ambulatory peritoneal dialysis (CAPD) has around 4–5 manual changes daily, while with continuous cyclic peritoneal dialysis (CCPD) a machine does the exchanges at night. Intermittent peritoneal dialysis (IPD) uses the same type of machine as CCPD; if done overnight, it is called nocturnal intermittent peritoneal dialysis (NIPD). Control of infection is of paramount importance. PD carries the risk of peritonitis (as well as fluid leaks into the tissues and hernias). Infections of the PD catheter's exit site or 'tunnel', however, are less serious.

Haemodialysis (HD) is used to remove metabolites (e.g. urea, potassium) and excess water, by exposing the patient's blood across a semi-permeable membrane to a hypotonic solution to allow the diffusion and osmosis of solutes and fluid from the body. The dialysis solution has levels of minerals like potassium and calcium that are similar to their natural concentration in healthy blood. For another solute, bicarbonate, the dialysis solution level is set slightly higher than that in normal blood, to encourage diffusion of bicarbonate into the body and thus to neutralize the metabolic acidosis often present. HD is often carried out at home or as an outpatient. Optimal effects are from 5–7 dialysis sessions of 6–8 hours each per week, but most patients have two or three 3–6-hourly sessions per week. An arteriovenous fistula is usually created surgically above the wrist to facilitate the introduction of infusion lines (Fig. 12.5); alternatively, a Gortex or polytetrafluoroethylene (PTFE) graft is placed, or an indwelling tunnelled cuffed catheter used. The patient is heparinized during dialysis to keep both the infusion lines and the dialysis machine tubing patent and the patient's blood is passed through an extracorporeal circulation (Fig. 12.6).

Dialysis can totally rehabilitate up to 20% of patients but cannot prevent all complications, and is itself associated with some adverse effects (collectively referred to as dialysis 'hangover' or 'washout'). These features are caused by removing fluid too rapidly or to excess, and may include:

- Hypotension
- Cramps
- Febrile reactions
- Arrhythmias
- Haemolysis
- Hypoxaemia.

Other and longer-term adverse effects include worsened ischaemic heart disease, cardiac valve calcification (especially affecting the aortic valve), dialysis-related amyloidosis and neuropathies. Cardiovascular disease and infection are the leading causes of death. In addition, haemodialysis may mechanically damage platelets – creating an additional bleeding tendency.

HD grafts and catheters may be at risk of infection, and bacterial endocarditis, osteomyelitis, blood-borne virus infections (mainly hepatitis or HIV) and tuberculosis were common in the past. Patients who

Table 12.5 *Drug modification in patients with chronic kidney disease*[a]

	Usually safe (no dosage change usually required)	Fairly safe (dosage change only in severe CKD)	Less safe (dosage reduction indicated[b] even in mild CKD)	Avoid (best avoided in any patient with CKD)
Anaesthetics	Lidocaine	Prilocaine, articaine	–	–
Analgesics	Paracetamol (acetaminophen)	Codeine	Aspirin NSAIDs	Dextropropoxyphene opioids Meperidine, morphine Pethidine Tramadol
Antimicrobials	Azithromycin Cloxacillin Doxycycline Flucloxacillin Fucidin Minocycline Rifampicin	Ampicillin Amoxicillin Benzylpenicillin Clindamycin Co-trimoxazole Erythromycin Ketoconazole Lincomycin Metronidazole Phenoxymethyl penicillin	Aciclovir[c] Cephalosporins[d] Ciprofloxacin Fluconazole Levofloxacin Ofloxacin Vancomycin	Aminoglycosides Carbenicillin Cefadroxil Cefalexin Cefixime Cefalotin Gentamicin Imipenem/cilastatin Itraconazole Sulphonamides Tetracyclines[e] Valaciclovir
Anticonvulsants			Carbamazepine Gabapentin Lamotrigine	
Sedatives	Diazepam Midazolam			

[a]Many other drugs unlikely to be used in oral health care may be contraindicated; check the formulary. Gadolinium-containing contrast agents are contraindicated as they may cause nephrogenic system fibrosis. Clarithromycin should not be prescribed for patients already taking antihypertensive calcium-channel blockers.
[b]Severe CKD – glomerular filtration rate (GFR) < 10 mL/min; moderately severe CKD – GFR < 25 mL/min; mild CKD – GFR < 50 mL/min.
[c]Systemic aciclovir.
[d]Except cephaloridine and cefalotin, which are contraindicated.
[e]Except doxycycline and minocycline.

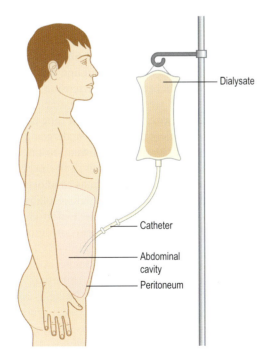

Fig. 12.4 Peritoneal dialysis.

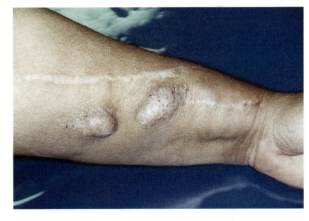

Fig. 12.5 Arteriovenous anastomosis (shunt) for haemodialysis.

undergo haemodialysis still have a higher risk of infection, due to the following:

- Frequent use of catheters or insertion of needles
- Compromised immunity
- Frequent hospital stays and surgery.

In order to take some basic steps to prevent infections in HD patients, staff should:

- clean hands before and after every patient contact
- wear gloves and other personal protective equipment (PPE) for all patient care
- promote vascular access safety
- promote fistula use
- improve catheter care
- remove catheters
- separate clean areas from contaminated areas
- use medication vials safely
- clean and disinfect the dialysis station between patients
- perform safe handling of dialysers.

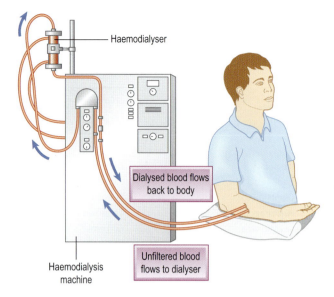

- Haemodialyser
- Dialysed blood flows back to body
- Unfiltered blood flows to dialyser
- Haemodialysis machine

Fig. 12.6 Haemodialysis.

Haemofiltration

In haemofiltration, the blood is pumped through a 'haemofilter', as in dialysis; rather than a dialysate being used, however, a pressure gradient is applied. Water thus moves across the very permeable membrane rapidly, facilitating removal of metabolites, especially those with large molecular weights that are cleared less well by haemodialysis. The salts and water lost from the blood during haemofiltration are replaced with a 'substitution fluid' infused into the extracorporeal circuit during the treatment.

Haemodiafiltration combines haemodialysis and haemofiltration in one process.

Renal transplantation

See below.

Dental aspects of chronic kidney disease

In CKD there is a correlation between tooth loss and the proportion of patients with low protein and calorie intake. Oral disease is common, especially periodontitis, and preventive measures may be lacking. Oral hygiene measures are important. The haematologist should first be consulted about the bleeding tendency; dental treatment is usually best carried out on the day after dialysis, when there has been maximal benefit from the dialysis and the effect of the heparin has abated. Careful haemostasis should be ensured if surgical procedures are necessary (Ch. 8). Should bleeding be prolonged, desmopressin (DDAVP) may provide haemostasis for up to 4 hours. If this fails, cryoprecipitate may be effective; it has a peak effect at 4–12 hours and lasts up to 36 hours. Conjugated oestrogens may aid haemostasis; the effect takes 2–5 days to develop but persists for 30 days.

Infections are poorly controlled by the patient with CKD, especially if immunosuppressed, and may spread locally as well as giving rise to septicaemia. They also accelerate tissue catabolism, causing clinical deterioration, and there is some evidence that periodontitis can perpetuate inflammation in CKD. Tuberculosis is also more frequent, but is usually extrapulmonary and therefore does not constitute a risk to dental staff. Infections can be difficult to recognize, as signs of inflammation are masked. Haemodialysis predisposes to blood-borne viral infections, such as hepatitis viruses. Odontogenic infections should be treated vigorously (see Table 12.5). Erythromycin, particularly when prescribed to patients with CKD, has been associated with reversible hearing loss. Flucloxacillin and fucidin can be given in standard dosage. Patients with CKD receiving doxycycline, azithromycin, sparfloxacin, trovafloxacin, and grepafloxacin require no alteration of dosage. Tetracyclines can worsen nitrogen

retention and acidosis, and are best avoided, though doxycycline or minocycline may be given. Benzylpenicillin has significant potassium content and may be neurotoxic; penicillins (other than phenoxymethyl penicillin and flucloxacillin) and metronidazole should be given in lower doses, since high serum levels can be toxic to the central nervous system.

Vascular access infections are usually caused by skin organisms such as *Staphylococcus aureus* and only rarely by oral microorganisms; thus patients with most arteriovenous fistulas are not considered at risk from infection during dental treatment and not considered to require antimicrobial prophylaxis. Patients with indwelling intraperitoneal catheters are also not considered to need antimicrobial prophylaxis. Before having dental extractions, scaling or periodontal surgery, patients with CKD may be considered for antimicrobial prophylaxis, especially those with renal transplants (Ch. 35), those with polycystic kidneys (who may also have mitral valve prolapse), those on PD, or those on HD with prosthetic bridge grafts of PTFE or tunnelled cuffed catheters. One regimen is to give 400 mg teicoplanin intravenously during dialysis, which gives cover for at least a day.

Drugs excreted mainly by the kidney may have undesirably enhanced or prolonged activity if doses are not lowered, depending on the degree of renal failure, the dialysis schedule or the presence of a transplant. Except in an emergency, such drugs should be prescribed only after consultation with the renal physician. Drugs that are directly nephrotoxic must be avoided (see Table 12.5). Aspirin (often a 75 mg dose will already be being given as prophylaxis against cardiovascular disease) and other NSAIDs should be avoided, since they aggravate gastrointestinal irritation and bleeding associated with CKD. Their excretion may also be delayed and they may be nephrotoxic, especially in the older patient or where there is renal damage or cardiac failure. Some patients have peptic ulceration – a further contraindication to aspirin. Even cyclo-oxygenase (COX)-2 inhibitors may be nephrotoxic and are best avoided. Use of NSAIDs is linked to a risk for ARF, nephrotic syndrome with interstitial nephritis, and CKD. Sodium excretion is reduced and can lead to peripheral oedema, elevated blood pressure and exacerbation of heart failure. Antihypertensive effects of beta-blockers, ACEIs or ARBs can be decreased. Short-term NSAID use is well tolerated if the patient is well hydrated and has good renal function and no heart failure, diabetes or hypertension. Serum creatinine should be checked every 2–4 weeks in early treatment.

Antihistamines or drugs with antimuscarinic side-effects may cause dry mouth or urinary retention. In patients undergoing haemodialysis, there may be: difficulties in chewing, swallowing, tasting and speaking; increased risk of oral disease, including lesions of the mucosa, gingiva and tongue; bacterial and fungal infections, such as candidiasis, dental caries and periodontal disease; interdialytic weight gain resulting from increased fluid intake; and a reduction in quality of life. Unfortunately, there is no effective treatment for hyposalivation in patients on chronic haemodialysis. Uraemic stomatitis is now a rare complication of CKD (Fig. 12.7).

Systemic fluorides should not be given because of doubt about fluoride excretion by damaged kidneys, but they can usually be used safely as a topical treatment for caries prophylaxis. Antacids containing magnesium salts should not be given, as there may be magnesium retention. Antacids containing calcium or aluminium bases may impair absorption of penicillin V and sulphonamides. Colestyramine, sometimes used in CKD, may also interfere with the absorption of penicillins.

Consideration must also be given to the effect on dental care of underlying diseases, such as hypertension (Ch. 5), diabetes (Ch. 6), systemic lupus erythematosus (Ch. 16), polyarteritis nodosa (Ch. 5), myelomatosis (Ch. 8) and amyloidosis (Ch. 8), or complications such as peptic ulceration (Ch. 7). Major surgical procedures may be complicated by hyperkalaemia as a result of tissue damage, acidaemia and blood transfusion, which predisposes to arrhythmias and may cause

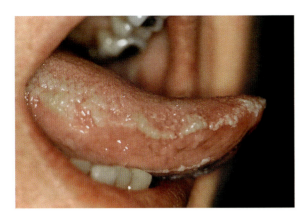

Fig. 12.7 Uraemic stomatitis in chronic kidney disease.

cardiac arrest. Dialysis is deferred postoperatively if possible, since heparinization is required.

Local anaesthesia (LA) is safe unless there is a severe bleeding tendency. For conscious sedation (CS), relative analgesia is preferred, since the veins of the forearms and the saphenous veins are lifelines for patients on regular haemodialysis. If it is necessary to give intravenous sedation or to take blood, other veins, such as those at or above the elbow, should be used because of the risk of consequent fistula infection or thrombophlebitis. Never put a cannula into the arteriovenous fistula arm. Midazolam is preferable to diazepam because of the lower risk of thrombophlebitis.

General anaesthesia (GA) is contraindicated if the haemoglobin is below 10 g/dL. Patients are also highly sensitive to the myocardial depressant effects of anaesthetic agents, and may develop hypotension at moderate levels of anaesthesia. Myocardial depression and cardiac arrhythmias are especially likely in those with poorly controlled metabolic acidosis and hyperkalaemia. Enflurane is metabolized to potentially nephrotoxic organic fluoride ions and therefore should be avoided if other nephrotoxic agents are used concurrently. Isoflurane and sevoflurane are probably safer. Induction with thiopental followed by very light GA with nitrous oxide is generally the technique of choice.

Although data are conflicting, most studies show that dental health of CKD patients is comparable with that of controls but there is more periodontal disease. Secondary hyperparathyroidism does not have an appreciable effect on periodontal indices and radiographic bone height. Osseous lesions include loss of the lamina dura, osteoporosis and osteolytic areas (renal osteodystrophy). Secondary hyperparathyroidism may lead to giant cell lesions. There may be abnormal bone repair after extractions, with socket sclerosis. Patients with renal disease should therefore be screened carefully for bone disease before implant placement. Dry mouth, halitosis and a metallic taste, and insidious oral bleeding and purpura can also be conspicuous. The salivary glands may swell, salivary flow is reduced, and there are protein and electrolyte changes, and calculus accumulation. In children with CKD, jaw growth is usually retarded and tooth eruption may be delayed. There may be malocclusion and enamel hypoplasia with brownish discolouration, but tetracycline staining of the teeth should no longer be seen. A lower caries rate and less periodontal disease have been reported in children with CKD. A variety of mucosal lesions may be seen. The oral mucosa may be pale because of anaemia and there may be oral ulceration.

THE NEPHROTIC SYNDROME

General aspects

The nephrotic syndrome is a non-specific condition in which glomerular damage (usually because of minimal change disease, diabetic nephropathy or systemic lupus erythematosus) leads to massive proteinuria with hypoalbuminaemia and oedema.

Clinical features

Oedema affects especially the face, genitals and lower limbs, and there are transudates in serous cavities (especially the peritoneal cavity – ascites). Loss of immunoglobulins (especially IgG) in the urine predisposes to infections with encapsulated bacteria such as *Haemophilus influenzae* and *Streptococcus pneumoniae*. Loss of antithrombin III, with raised factor VIII, fibrinogen and other clotting factors, leads to hypercoagulability – predisposing to thromboses. Loss of cholecalciferol-binding protein leads to vitamin D deficiency, secondary hyperparathyroidism and bone disease. In response to albumin loss, the liver synthesizes more of its proteins and levels of large proteins (such as alpha$_2$-macroglobulin and lipoproteins) increase. Patients also develop hypercholesterolaemia and become susceptible to atheroma and ischaemic heart disease.

General management

Treatment aims to reduce proteinuria, control infections and prevent thromboembolism, and to remove or treat the basic cause of nephrosis. Many of the considerations in the management of the patient with CKD are also applicable to the nephrotic patient. Corticosteroids, a low-salt but high-protein diet, warfarin and prophylactic antimicrobials may be given.

Dental aspects

Long-term corticosteroid therapy is the main problem (Ch. 6). Prophylactic antimicrobials may be indicated for procedures likely to cause a bacteraemia. Cardiovascular and haematological disorders and anticoagulation may complicate care (Ch. 8).

RENAL STONES (NEPHROLITHIASIS)

Renal stones (calculi) are not uncommon and may cause symptoms of renal colic or secondary renal damage; 90% can be seen on radiography. Systemic disease is rarely identified as underlying renal stones, but they may complicate gout, hyperparathyroidism, hyperoxaluria, cystinosis or renal tubular acidosis. A recent outbreak in China was related to melamine contamination of milk. There is no known predisposition to salivary calculi or dental calculus formation in patients who develop renal stones. An enamel-renal syndrome of amelogenesis imperfecta and nephrocalcinosis, and the amelogenesis imperfecta-gingival fibromatosis syndrome have both been associated with mutations in FAM20A. Renal calculi are treated by lithotripsy or surgical removal.

RENAL CANCER

Most kidney cancers (90%) are adenocarcinomas – renal cell cancers. Transitional cell cancer is rare. It is rare for people under 40 to have renal cancer, but the rare Wilms tumour (nephroblastoma) affects very young children. Renal cancer affects more men than women. Risk factors are shown in Box 12.1.

Clinical features

Renal cancer may be symptomless but blood in the urine is the most common feature. There can be pain or a lump in the area of the kidney, or persistent fevers, night sweats, tiredness and weight loss.

General management

Diagnosis is confirmed by cystoscopy, ultrasound, computed tomography/magnetic resonance imaging, intravenous urography and biopsy. The main treatment is surgery, usually nephrectomy. Other treatments may include biological treatments (interferon-alpha or the IL-2 analogue aldesleukin) or targeted treatments (the multikinase inhibitors sorafenib or sunitinib, or bevacizumab or temsirolimus]. Occasionally, radiotherapy or chemotherapy is used, or hormones.

Dental aspects

Renal cancer occasionally metastasizes to the jaws or mouth.

RENAL TRANSPLANTATION

Transplantation is now recommended for patients with ESRD who are medically suitable, since a successful transplant offers enhanced quality and duration of life, and is more effective (medically and economically) than chronic dialysis. Transplantation is the renal replacement modality of choice for child patients and for patients with diabetic nephropathy.

Outcomes are improved by 'pre-emptive' live donor transplantation – using a kidney from an unaffected relative and performing the transplant before the patient needs to have dialysis. Transplants can be from cadaveric or living donors. Graft survival is as high as 90% at 1 year and about 70% survival at 5 years, while overall mortality is less than 5%. The transplanted kidney is usually sited in the right iliac fossa of the abdomen.

All kidney transplant recipients require lifelong immunosuppression to prevent a T-cell alloimmune rejection response. Immunosuppressive regimens vary among transplantation centers but most often include a calcineurin inhibitor (CNI) and an adjuvant agent, with or without corticosteroids. The most common maintenance immunosuppressive agents include:

- CNIs (ciclosporin and tacrolimus)
- co-stimulation blockers (belatacept)
- mammalian target of rapamycin (mTOR) inhibitors (sirolimus and everolimus)
- antiproliferatives (azathioprine and mycophenolic acid derivatives)
- corticosteroids.

Alemtuzumab, basiliximab or daclizumab is increasingly used, with a CNI. Systemic complications of transplantation include transplant rejection, increased risk of atheroma and ischaemic heart disease, ciclosporin-induced nephropathy and immunosuppression-induced infection or malignancy (Ch. 35).

Dental aspects of renal transplantation

See also above and Chapter 35.

Any oral sign of infection must be examined immediately and treated aggressively in an immunosuppressed transplant recipient. There should be careful observation to detect any malignant complications. Drug-induced gingival overgrowth (DIGO) is commonly caused by ciclosporin or nifedipine. Oral ulceration may be caused by sirolimus and everolimus. Dental pulp narrowing has been noted – apparently a corticosteroid effect.

Consideration should also be given to haematological abnormalities, such as anaemia and platelet–haemostatic dysfunction; viral hepatitis B and C; and cardiovascular disorders such as hypertension, atherosclerotic heart disease with myocardial infarction, congestive heart failure, and left ventricular hypertrophy. Bone and joint disease is common because of low calcium levels, high phosphorus concentrations and elevated serum parathyroid hormone.

LA is safe unless there is a severe bleeding tendency. For CS, relative analgesia is preferred. If it is necessary to give intravenous sedation, midazolam is preferable to diazepam because of the lower risk of thrombophlebitis.

KEY WEBSITES

(Accessed 27 May 2013)
BMJ. <http://www.bmj.com/specialties/renal-medicine>.
MedlinePlus. <http://www.nlm.nih.gov/medlineplus/ency/article/002289.htm>.
National Institutes of Health: National Kidney Disease Education Program. <http://www.nkdep.nih.gov/learn/are-you-at-risk.shtml>.

USEFUL WEBSITES

(Accessed 27 May 2013)
Macmillan. <http://www.macmillan.org.uk/Cancerinformation/Cancertypes/Kidney/Kidneycancer.aspx>.
National Institutes of Health: National Cancer Institute. <http://www.cancer.gov/>.
National Institutes of Health: National Institute of Diabetes and Digestive and Kidney Diseases. <http://kidney.niddk.nih.gov/>.
National Kidney Federation. <http://www.kidney.org.uk/>.
Scottish Intercollegiate Guidelines Network. <http://www.sign.ac.uk/guidelines/fulltext/103/index.html>.
University of Iowa Hospitals & Clinics. <http://www.uihealthcare.org/Adam/?/HIE + Multimedia/0/200000>.

FURTHER READING

Bansal, N., Hsu, C.Y., 2008. Long-term outcomes of patients with chronic kidney disease. Nat. Clin. Pract. Nephrol. 4, 532.
Bayraktar, G., et al. 2004. Evaluation of salivary parameters and dental status in adult hemodialysis patients. Clin. Nephrol. 62, 380.
Bayraktar, G., et al. 2007. Dental and periodontal findings in hemodialysis patients. Oral Dis. 13, 393.
Bayraktar, G., et al. 2008. Evaluation of periodontal parameters in patients undergoing peritoneal dialysis or hemodialysis. Oral Dis. 14, 185.
Chou, C.Y., et al. 2008. Association between betel-nut chewing and chronic kidney disease in men. Public Health Nutr. 23, 1.
Craig, R.G., 2008. Interactions between chronic renal disease and periodontal disease. Oral Dis. 14, 1.
Crawford, P.W., Lerma, E.V., 2008. Treatment options for end stage renal disease. Prim. Care 35, 407.
Cunha, F.L., et al. 2007. Oral health of a Brazilian population on renal dialysis. Spec. Care Dentist. 27, 227.
Frankenthal, S., et al. 2002. The effect of secondary hyperparathyroidism and hemodialysis therapy on alveolar bone and periodontium. J. Clin. Periodontol. 29, 479.
Kerr, A.R., 2001. Update on renal disease for the dental practitioner. Oral Surg. 92, 9.
Kotano, P., 2008. Chronic inflammation in dialysis patients – periodontal disease, the new kid on the block. Oral Dis. 14, 8.
Lee, R.A., Gabardi, S., 2012. Current trends in immunosuppressive therapies for renal transplant recipients. Am. J. Health Syst. Pharm. 69 (22), 1961. doi: 10.2146/ajhp110624. PubMed PMID: 23135563.
Moghaddam, S.M., et al. 2008. Hepatitis C and renal transplantation: a review on historical aspects and current issues. Rev. Med. Virol. 18, 375.
Munar, M.Y., Singh, H., 2007. Guidelines for drug dosing regimens in chronic kidney disease. Am. Fam. Physician. 75, 1487.

The central nervous system (CNS) consists of the brain and spinal cord. The brain is the chief regulator of neuroendocrine, autonomic and immune systems, as well as behaviour. The brain contains the cerebral motor and sensory cortices essential for life, and other areas have specialized functions (Tables 10.1, 13.1 and 13.2; Figs 10.1, 13.1 and 13.2). Brain damage can lead to motor and/or sensory defects, variable disability, or even to loss of consciousness and/or death.

The CNS controls the peripheral nervous system (PNS), which consists of the somatic (SNS) and (ANS) autonomic nervous systems, and extends to the limbs and organs (Fig. 13.3). The SNS is under conscious control and is responsible for receiving external stimuli and for coordinating movement. The ANS consists of the sympathetic, parasympathetic and enteric nervous systems. The sympathetic system responds to danger or stress by release of adrenaline (epinephrine) – increasing anxiety, cardiac rate and output, and other physiological changes. The parasympathetic system is responsible for slowing the

Table 13.1 *Functions of main parts of the brain*

Part of brain	Known functions
Cerebral lobe	
Frontal	Higher mental functions, such as motivation, planning, social behaviour and speech production
Occipital	Visual processing and visual cortex
Parietal	Integration of sensory information from various parts of the body, knowledge of numbers and their relations, manipulation of objects, processing of information relating to the sense of touch, visuospatial processing
Temporal	Auditory perception, such as hearing and language, interpretation of visual stimuli, aiding recognition of long-term memory
Lower brain	
Basal ganglia	Voluntary motor control, procedural learning relating to routine behaviours or 'habits' such as eye movements, cognitive emotional functions
Cerebellum	Motor control, coordination, precision, accurate timing, attention, language, fear and pleasure responses
Brainstem	Basic functions, including regulation of heart rate, breathing, sleeping, eating and central nervous system – pivotal in maintaining consciousness. Main motor and sensory innervation to face, mouth and neck via cranial nerves. Nerve connections of motor and sensory systems from the brain to the rest of the body pass through the brainstem

Table 13.2 *Location of the main functions in the cerebral cortex*

Frontal lobe	Pre-central gyrus	Post-central gyrus	Superior temporal lobe	Occipital lobe
Olfactory	Motor	Sensory (somatosensory)	Hearing	Vision
Language (on dominant side) and speech (Broca's area)			Word comprehension (Wernicke's area)	

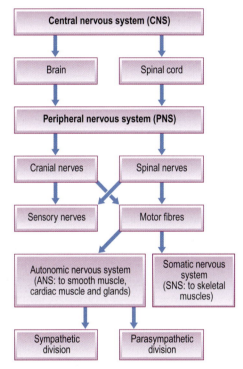

Fig. 13.1 Nervous system.

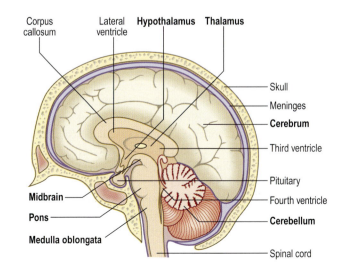

Fig. 13.2 Brain.

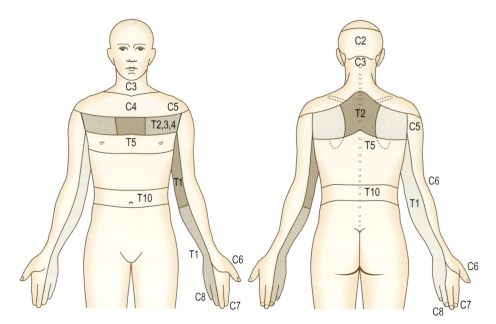

Fig. 13.3 Cervical and thoracic dermatomes.

heart, dilating blood vessels, and stimulating digestive and genito-urinary systems. The enteric nervous system controls digestion in the gastrointestinal tract.

The core components of the nervous system are neurons. Action potentials travel down the neuronal axon to open calcium (Ca^{2+}) channels in the plasma membrane, triggering the exocytosis of vesicles containing neurotransmitters, which affect a receiving cell. The main neurotransmitters are acetylcholine (ACh) and noradrenaline (norepinephrine), but there are many others (see Tables 13.1 and 10.3).

ACh at excitatory synapses depolarizes the post-synaptic membrane, causing an excitatory post-synaptic potential and an action potential in the post-synaptic cell. ACh is released at the terminals of all motor neurons activating skeletal muscle, all pre-ganglionic neurons of the ANS and post-ganglionic neurons of the parasympathetic system. ACh also mediates transmission at brain synapses involved in acquisition of short-term memory.

Amino acids such as glutamic acid are involved in CNS transmission at excitatory synapses and are essential for long-term potentiation, a form of memory. Gamma-aminobutyric acid (GABA) at inhibitory synapses hyperpolarizes the post-synaptic membrane, causing an inhibitory post-synaptic potential.

NEUROLOGICAL DISEASE

Patients whose symptoms have a neurological basis are relatively common. Dental professionals may well be involved in the care of these people, especially of those with the most important brain disorders, such as cerebral palsy, epilepsy, cerebrovascular accidents (CVAs; strokes) and facial palsy. The most common neurological complaints are shown in Box 13.1. The role of stress is discussed in Chapter 10.

Orofacial pain is common and may have a neurological cause. Patients with head or maxillofacial injuries may have brain damage with impaired ocular movements or pupil reactions and loss of the sense of smell (anosmia). Dental professionals should therefore be able to examine and recognize gross neurological abnormalities, and especially problems involving the cranial nerves – particularly the trigeminal, facial, glossopharyngeal, vagal and hypoglossal nerves.

Box 13.1 *The 12 most common neurological complaints*

- Cerebrovascular accidents
- Compressive neuropathies (e.g. carpal tunnel syndrome)
- Diabetic neuropathy
- Epilepsy
- Headaches
- Meningitis
- Multiple sclerosis
- Parkinsonism
- Tremors
- Trigeminal neuralgia
- Tumours
- Zoster

NEUROLOGICAL EVALUATION

The nervous system may need to be evaluated, as in Table 13.3. Mental status can be assessed using a standard screening test, such as the Mini-Mental State Examination (MMSE) or Folstein test (simple questions and problems in a number of areas: the time and place of the test, repeating lists of words, arithmetic, language use and comprehension, and basic motor skills). Testing can also be achieved as shown in Table 13.4.

If cognitive functions seem unaffected, there is no related complaint, and the patient appears, behaves and supplies a history normally, formal cognitive evaluation is not required.

HEADACHES AND OROFACIAL PAIN

Pain is broadly divided into nociceptive pain and neuropathic pain.

Nociceptive pain is caused by actual or potential damage to tissues (e.g. trauma, cut, burn). Nerve endings become activated or damaged by the injury, with pain that tends to be sharp or aching and is often

Table 13.3 *Neurological evaluation*

Aspects	Details	Assessment
Speech	Dysarthria may be detected	
Mental state or higher mental function	See Table 13.4	
Level of consciousness	See Ch. 24	Glasgow Coma Scale is widely used
Cognition	See Table 13.4	
Sensory system	Sensory nerves carry information from the body to the brain about such things as touch, pain, heat, cold, vibration, position of body parts, and shape of objects	Test using a pin and a blunt object to see if the patient can distinguish. Test ability to feel light touch, heat and vibration. Test position sense – move finger or toe up or down and ask the person to describe its position without looking. Dermatomes are shown in Figure 13.3
Motor system	Muscle weakness or paralysis may indicate damage to the muscle, motor nerve or synapse, brain or spinal cord	Assess muscle size change (increased size or wasting/atrophy); involuntary movements or twitching; strength; and tone changes – increase (spasticity, rigidity) or decrease (flaccidity)
	A reflex is an automatic response to a stimulus. Those most commonly tested are the knee jerk, and elbow, ankle and plantar reflexes. The knee jerk tests the pathway consisting of the sensory nerve to the spinal cord, the spinal cord connections, and the motor nerves back to the muscle	The plantar reflex, tested by firmly stroking the outer border of the sole of foot with an object that causes minor discomfort, normally causes toes to curl downward; if the big toe goes upward and other toes spread out, this suggests a brain or spinal cord lesion (except in infants <6 months)
		The extent of brain injury in a comatose person is tested by noting whether pupils constrict when light is shined on them (pupillary light reflex). Facial sensation and movement are determined by whether eyes blink when the cornea is touched (corneal reflex)
Cerebrum and cerebellum	Gait, coordination and balance testing require integration of signals from sensory and motor nerves by brain and spinal cord	Gait is tested by asking the patient to walk in a straight line, placing one foot in front of the other; walk on heels and then on toes; and then hop on each foot
		Coordination is tested by asking the patient to use the forefinger to reach out and touch an object, and then their own nose, and then to repeat actions rapidly and then with the eyes closed
		Balance is assessed by the Romberg test: the patient stands still, with feet together and eyes closed. In health, balance should be retained
Autonomic nervous system (ANS)	–	Test by determining whether blood pressure changes when the person lies, sits or stands (orthostatic hypotension), or if there is a reduction or absence of sweating
Cranial nerves	See Table 13.12	

Table 13.4 *Testing mental status*

Test	Test indicates
Give today's date	Orientation in time, place and person
State the place where you are	
Name specific people	
Name the last three Prime Ministers	Knowledge
Describe an event that happened yesterday	Recent memory
Describe events from schooldays	Remote memory
Interpret a proverb (e.g. 'There's many a slip between cup and lip')	Abstract thinking
Do simple arithmetic	Ability to calculate numbers
Repeat a short list of objects	Attention
Recall the short list of objects after 5 minutes	Immediate recall
Describe feelings and opinions about your illness	Insight
Explain how you feel today	Mood
Comb your hair	Ability to perform action
Name simple objects and body parts	Ability to use language
Identify, without seeing them, small objects held in the hand, and discriminate between being touched in two places	Ability of brain to process and interpret complex information from the hand
Follow simple command involving different body parts on different sides (such as 'put your right thumb in your left ear and stick out your tongue')	Language comprehension
Draw a clock, cube or house	Ability to understand spatial relationships

eased by traditional analgesics such as paracetamol (acetaminophen), non-steroidal anti-inflammatory drugs (NSAIDs) and opioids.

Neuropathic pain (neuralgia) is a pain arising from nerve signal problems and is often persistent, with features such as burning, stabbing, aching or electric shock-like qualities. Neuropathic pain may be experienced in:

- alcoholism
- burning mouth syndrome
- cancer
- chemotherapy pain
- diabetic neuropathy
- human immunodeficiency virus (HIV) infection
- idiopathic (atypical) facial pain
- multiple sclerosis
- phantom pain (follows surgery)
- post-herpetic neuralgia (follows zoster)
- trigeminal neuralgia.

Related to these pains there may also be phenomena including:

- *Allodynia* – Pain starts, or worsens, with a touch or stimulus that would not normally cause pain.
- *Hyperalgesia* – Severe pain is experienced from a stimulus or touch that would normally cause slight discomfort only.
- *Paraesthesia* – Unpleasant or painful feelings are experienced, even when there is no stimulus.

Neuropathic pain is less likely than nociceptive pain to be eased by traditional analgesics but is often improved by:

- antidepressants
- antiepileptics
- capsaicin
- physical treatments (physiotherapy, acupuncture, nerve blocks and transcutaneous electrical nerve stimulation [TENS])
- psychological treatments (stress management, counselling, cognitive behavioural therapy and pain management programmes).

Pain receptors can be stimulated by stress, muscular tension, dilated blood vessels and other triggers. Headache and orofacial pain are the most common neurological complaints; they are often chronic and are mainly caused by local disease, vascular disease, referred pain, neurological disorders or psychogenic disorders (Table 13.5 and Box 13.2). Headaches can also occasionally herald serious brain disorders, such as tumour, infection or bleeding (Box 13.3). Features suggesting serious or life-threatening headaches are shown in Box 13.4.

Some headaches have quite specific and less serious precipitating factors (Table 13.6); foods such as alcohol, caffeine, chocolate, cheeses and nuts can cause headaches in some people and may trigger migraine. About 50% of patients seen in headache clinics are thought to suffer from muscle contraction (tension) headaches, which appear to involve the tightening or tensing of facial and neck muscles because of stress (see Ch. 10 and below). Virtually *all* types of headache are influenced, at least to some extent, by stress, emotional factors and individual personalities.

Table 13.5 *Causes of headache and orofacial pain*

Cause	Diseases
Local	Dental or oral disease
	Infections or tumours of paranasal sinuses and nasopharynx
	Ocular or aural lesions
	Neck lesions
Vascular	Migraine
	Migrainous neuralgia
	Idiopathic stabbing headache
	Chronic paroxysmal hemicranias
	Temporal arteritis
Neurological	Trigeminal neuralgia
	Glossopharyngeal neuralgia
	Herpetic neuralgia
	Raeder neuralgia
	Intracranial disease: pontine infarction, cerebellopontine angle tumours, middle cranial fossa lesions, cavernous sinus thrombosis, Bell palsy
Psychogenic	Tension headaches
	Oral dysaesthesia
	Idiopathic (atypical) facial pain
	Temporomandibular pain–dysfunction syndrome
Other	Trauma
	Raised intracranial pressure
	Diseases of the skull
	Meningeal irritation
	Drugs (e.g. vinca alkaloids, nitrites, dapsone, some analgesics)
	Referred pain (e.g. heart or chest)
	Medical diseases (e.g. severe hypertension)

Box 13.2 *International Headache Society (IHS) classification of headache*

1. Migraine
    1.1. Migraine without aura
    1.2. Migraine with aura
    1.3. Ophthalmoplegic migraine
    1.4. Retinal migraine
    1.5. Childhood periodic syndromes that may be precursors to or associated with migraine
    1.6. Complications of migraine
    1.7. Migrainous disorder not fulfilling above criteria
2. Tension-type headache
    2.1. Episodic tension-type headache
    2.2. Chronic tension-type headache
    2.3. Tension-type headache not fulfilling above criteria
3. Cluster headache and chronic paroxysmal hemicrania
    3.1. Cluster headache
    3.2. Chronic paroxysmal hemicrania
    3.3. Cluster headache-like disorder not fulfilling above criteria
4. Miscellaneous headaches not associated with structural lesion
    4.1. Idiopathic stabbing headache
    4.2. External compression headache
    4.3. Cold stimulus headache
    4.4. Benign cough headache
    4.5. Benign exertional headache
    4.6. Headache associated with sexual activity
5. Headache associated with head trauma
    5.1. Acute post-traumatic headache
    5.2. Chronic post-traumatic headache
6. Headache associated with vascular disorders
    6.1. Acute ischaemic cerebrovascular disorder
    6.2. Intracranial haematoma
    6.3. Subarachnoid haemorrhage
    6.4. Unruptured vascular malformation
    6.5. Arteritis
    6.6. Carotid or vertebral artery pain
    6.7. Venous thrombosis
    6.8. Arterial hypertension
    6.9. Headache associated with other vascular disorder
7. Headache associated with non-vascular intracranial disorder
    7.1. High cerebrospinal fluid (CSF) pressure
    7.2. Low CSF pressure
    7.3. Intracranial infection
    7.4. Intracranial sarcoidosis and other non-infectious inflammatory diseases
    7.5. Headache related to intrathecal injections
    7.6. Intracranial neoplasm
    7.7. Headache associated with other intracranial disorder
8. Headache associated with substances or their withdrawal
    8.1. Headache induced by acute substance use or exposure
    8.2. Headache induced by chronic substance use or exposure
    8.3. Headache from substance withdrawal (acute use)
    8.4. Headache from substance withdrawal (chronic use)
    8.5. Headache associated with substances but with uncertain mechanism
9. Headache associated with non-cephalic infection
    9.1. Viral infection
    9.2. Bacterial infection
    9.3. Headache related to other infection
10. Headache associated with metabolic disorder
    10.1. Hypoxia
    10.2. Hypercapnia

10.3. Mixed hypoxia and hypercapnia

10.4. Hypoglycaemia

10.5. Dialysis

10.6. Headache related to other metabolic abnormality

11. Headache or facial pain associated with disorder of cranium, neck, eyes, ears, nose, sinuses, teeth, mouth, or other facial or cranial structures

11.1. Cranial bone

11.2. Neck

11.3. Eyes

11.4. Ears

11.5. Nose and sinuses

11.6. Teeth, jaws and related structures

11.7. Temporomandibular joint disease

12. Cranial neuralgias, nerve trunk pain and deafferentation pain

12.1. Persistent (in contrast to tic-like) pain of cranial nerve origin

12.2. Trigeminal neuralgia

12.3. Glossopharyngeal neuralgia

12.4. Nervus intermedius neuralgia

12.5. Superior laryngeal neuralgia

12.6. Occipital neuralgia

12.7. Central causes of head and facial pain other than tic douloureux

12.8. Facial pain not fulfilling criteria in groups 11 or 12

13. Headache not classifiable

Box 13.3 *Serious causes of headache*

- Acute glaucoma
- Acute hypertension
- Acute lesions affecting the carotid vessels
- Brain tumours
- Giant cell arteritis
- Meningitis
- Subarachnoid haemorrhage
- Subdural or epidural haemorrhage

Box 13.4 *Indicators of seriousness in headache*

- Abrupt, severe 'thunderclap' or bilateral headache
- Confusion, loss of consciousness, convulsions, fever, stiff neck, rash, mental confusion, seizures, diplopia, weakness, numbness, pain in the eye or ear, or dysarthria
- Disruption of normal life
- Follows a recent sore throat or respiratory infection
- New headache pain after age 55
- Persistence in a person who was previously headache-free
- Preceded by head trauma
- Recurrence in children
- Severity of headache
- Worsening after coughing, exertion, straining or a sudden movement

---

Table 13.6 *Some less serious causes of headache*

Conditions	Causes
Chinese restaurant syndrome	Monosodium glutamate
Hangover headache	Acetaldehyde
Hot dog headache	Nitrites/nitrates
Post-coital headache	Intercourse
Vitamin A-induced headache	Vitamin A

LOCAL CAUSES OF OROFACIAL PAIN

The mouth

Oral causes of facial pain (e.g. pulpitis, apical periodontitis, periodontal abscesses, pericoronitis and various intraosseous lesions) are common and are discussed in other texts.

The sinuses and nasopharynx

Sinusitis causes localized pain. In acute maxillary or frontal sinusitis, local pain and tenderness (but not swelling), with radio-opacity of the affected sinuses, usually follow a cold (Ch. 14).

Tumours of sinuses or nasopharynx can also cause facial pain. These are rare, usually carcinomas, and involve trigeminal nerve branches; they may cause pain simulating pain–dysfunction syndrome. They can remain undetected until late in their course.

Eagle syndrome, due to calcification of the stylohyoid ligament, may be a rare cause of pain on chewing, swallowing or turning the head. The elongated styloid process may be visualized radiographically, and palpation of it in the wall of the pharynx causes intense pain. The stylohyoid process can be shortened surgically, but regrowth and relapse are common.

The eyes

Glaucoma (raised intraocular pressure) may cause pain in and around the orbit. Disorders of refraction can cause frontal headaches. Retrobulbar neuritis (e.g. in multiple sclerosis) can cause pain in and around the orbit.

The ears

Pharyngeal or middle ear disease may cause headaches. Oral disease can rarely cause pain referred to the ear; the classic picture is that of the older man with tongue cancer whose complaint is earache.

The neck

Cervical vertebral disease occasionally causes headache or pain referred to the face and may aggravate tension headaches. Nerve block with local anaesthesia (LA) may temporarily relieve this pain. Carotidynia is unilateral pain arising from the cervical carotid artery that radiates to the ipsilateral face and ear, and sometimes to the head; it is associated with carotid artery tenderness and overlying soft tissue swelling, and is responsive to corticosteroids.

VASCULAR CAUSES OF FACIAL PAIN

Vasomotor states are responsible for certain headaches; either widening or narrowing of extracranial and intracranial arteries may produce pain. Both vasodilatation and neurogenic inflammation are under the influence of serotonin (5-hydroxytryptamine; 5HT); the $5HT_{1B}$ receptor controls vasodilatation, whereas $5HT_{1D}$ regulates neurogenic inflammation.

Serotonin agonists, such as ergotamine and triptans, can prevent neurogenic inflammation.

Migraine

Further information on migraine may be found at: http://www.disabled-world.com/health/neurology/migraine/ (accessed 30 September 2013).

General aspects

Migraine is a recurrent headache combined with autonomic disturbances, affecting over 14% of women and 7% of men. The prodrome is usually accompanied by diminished cerebral blood flow, possibly the result of a neuronal trigger mechanism in the trigeminovascular nucleus, but the headache itself is usually associated with increased cerebral and extracranial blood flow, possibly caused by serotonin adsorbed to blood vessel walls, since platelet serotonin rises before a migraine headache. This may cause the trigeminal nerve to release neuropeptides; the combination of serotonin and bradykinin may cause blood vessels to become dilated and inflamed.

Clinical features

Migraine triggers can include:

- weather, season, altitude, or time zone changes
- drugs (e.g. cimetidine, fenfluramine, nifedipine and theophylline)
- low blood sugar
- mealtime changes, skipped meals or fasting
- intense physical exertion, including sexual activity
- tobacco
- lack of sleep
- bright lights, loud noises or strong odours
- menstrual cycle hormone changes
- stress, anxiety, or relaxation after stress
- alcohol (often red wine)
- caffeine (excess or withdrawal)
- nitrates, such as in hot dogs and lunch meats
- monosodium glutamate (MSG), a flavour enhancer in fast foods, broths, seasonings and spices
- tyramine, such as in aged cheeses, soy products, broad (fava) beans, hard sausages, smoked fish and Chianti wine. The highest levels of tyramine are in aged cheeses, spoiled meats, aged and cured meats, Marmite®, sauerkraut, fermented soybean products, broad bean pods and draft (tap) beer, but there is little or no tyramine in non-alcoholic beverages, breads, fats, cottage cheese, ricotta, cream cheese, soft farmer's cheese, mozzarella cheese, processed cheese slices, sour cream, yogurt, milk, eggs, tomatoes, fresh meat, poultry, fish, shellfish and soy milk (Table 13.7; see also http://www.headaches.org/pdf/Diet.pdf, accessed 30 September 2013).
- aspartame
- botulinum toxin A (Botox) injections.

Large quantities of nuts (peanuts, coconuts and brazil nuts) may trigger hypertensive reactions and headaches, but not via tyramine.

The fact that migraine attacks are more frequent at weekends, for example, should not be interpreted as excluding stress, as there is no doubt that some find the company and demands of their families more stressful than their work. Going away on holiday (Freud's *Reisefieber* – 'travel fever') is also highly stressful for many.

Several types of migraine are recognized (Table 13.8); migraine without aura is the most frequent – presenting with unilateral headache – but migraine with aura is the most readily recognizable.

Classical migraine presents with an aura (warning symptoms), which may last about 15 minutes and consists of visual, sensory, motor or speech disturbances. Visual phenomena are typically of zigzag flickering light (fortification spectra) or other transient visual defects. Sensory phenomena include paraesthesia or anaesthesia – usually of the contralateral upper limb, or face and mouth. Motor symptoms are mainly weakness – again, of the contralateral upper limb. Obvious vascular phenomena may be

Table 13.7 *Tyramine in foods*

Tyramine-containing	Low in tyramine	Not usually tyramine-containing
All draft (tap) beer and ale, Chianti, port, sherry, vermouth, red wine, white wine	Domestic bottled beers	Non-alcoholic beverages
Most aged cheeses	Cream cheese and cottage cheese	Normal cheese of the type typically used on bread and pizza
Banana skin, figs, grapes, oranges, pineapples, plums, prunes, raisins, overripe avocados	Avocados – provided not overripe	Chocolate
		Tomatoes
		Processed cheese
Broad (fava) beans, aubergine (eggplant)		Fresh liver, meat, poultry, fish and shellfish
Processed foods; Marmite®, Vegemite®, sauerkraut and shrimp paste		Soy milk
Processed meats, cured or pickled meats, and meat by-products and broths. Game birds and wild animals if hung; old liver and meat		
All soy products: soya beans, soy sauce, tofu, miso and teriyaki sauce		

Table 13.8 *Migraine variants*

Type/subtype	Clinical features
Migraine	
Status	Intense pain that usually lasts longer than 72h
Abdominal	Abdominal pain without a gastrointestinal cause (lasts up to 72h), nausea, vomiting, and flushing or paleness. Children who have abdominal migraine often develop typical migraine as they age
Headache-free	Aura without headache
Migraine without aura	Tiredness or mood changes the day before the headache, which may be on one or both sides of head. Nausea, vomiting and also sensitivity to light
Classic	Unilateral headache preceded by an aura (a neurological phenomenon) experienced 10–30min before the headache. Most auras are visual (bright shimmering lights around objects or at the edges of the field of vision or zigzag lines, castles, wavy images, or hallucinations). Other patients have temporary vision loss. Non-visual auras include motor weakness, speech or language abnormalities, dizziness, vertigo, and tingling or numbness of face, tongue or extremities
Hemiplegic	Often familial; hemiparesis may outlast headache by several days; may rarely cause facial palsy
Ophthalmoplegic	Affects children (boys) mainly. As headache progresses, eyelid droops and eye movements become paralysed. Ptosis may persist for days or weeks
Vertebrobasilar	Affects adolescent girls mainly. Aura associated with ataxia, vertigo, diplopia; headache usually occipital; there may be loss of consciousness at the onset
Complicated	Any form of migraine complicated by residual neurological defect after attack
Migrainous neuralgia	
Classic	Pain typically around the eye, often with visible effects of vasodilatation
Facial migraine	Affects lower face (lower-half migraine or carotidynia). Episodes may occur several times weekly and last a few minutes to hours. Deep, dull, aching and sometimes piercing pain in the jaw or neck. There is usually tenderness and swelling over the carotid artery

associated and range from facial flushing and oedema on the affected side to temporary hemiplegia. Unilateral headache (hemicrania), which is usually severe, often becomes throbbing and generalized, may be associated with facial pallor, and can last for hours or days. Photophobia and sometimes phonophobia, nausea and sometimes vomiting may be seen. The number, frequency, intensity and duration of migraine attacks vary widely, but they tend to diminish in frequency and intensity with increasing age.

General management

The diagnosis of migraine is clinical. Spontaneous remissions are not uncommon and migraine tends to improve during pregnancy. Management is usually with drugs and avoidance of precipitating factors but there is also a significant placebo factor.

In acute attacks, patients usually prefer to lie in a quiet, dark room. Analgesics such as aspirin, paracetamol (acetaminophen) or ibuprofen can be effective. Intranasal lidocaine can give early relief within 5 minutes in over half of those suffering from migraine, but the pain returns after about an hour in half of the responders. Triptans (serotonin ($5HT_1$) receptor agonists), such as sumatriptan, are effective in up to 80% if given within 1 hour; possible adverse effects include nausea, dizziness, muscle weakness and, rarely, stroke or myocardial infarction. Sumatriptan may cause coronary spasm and angina, or permanent neurological damage if given in hemiplegic migraine or with ergotamine. Triptans are contraindicated for patients taking monoamine oxidase inhibitors (MAOIs).

If triptans are ineffective, ergotamine given orally may abort an attack but, in many cases, absorption by mouth is too slow to be effective and a better alternative is to use it by inhalation from a Medihaler. Even so, ergotamine must not be used within 6 hours of sumatriptan. The maximum permissible dose of ergotamine is 4 mg in 24 hours; this must not be exceeded and treatment must not be repeated at intervals of less than 4 days. Ergotamine can cause peripheral vasospasm and gangrene, abdominal pain, nausea and vomiting. It can also be given with caffeine, or as a suppository, which overcomes the problem of poor absorption if the patient is vomiting.

Oral antiemetics, such as metoclopramide, domperidone or buclizine, should be given early to overcome the autonomic dysfunction preventing gastric emptying. In severe cases of vomiting, an antiemetic such as metoclopramide or prochlorperazine by suppository may also be required.

If attacks of migraine are more frequent than two a month, the treatment of choice is prophylaxis with propranolol or another beta-blocker, but sometimes a serotonin antagonist (pizotifen or cyproheptadine) or amitriptyline is used. Pizotifen can cause drowsiness and should be used with caution in renal disease, pregnancy, glaucoma or urinary retention. Low-dose aspirin may reduce attacks by 20%, probably by blocking prostaglandin production in response to stimulation of a 5HT (serotonin) receptor. Calcium-channel blockers, such as verapamil or nifedipine, may be useful alternatives. Methysergide may help but has dangerous toxic effects (retroperitoneal fibrosis, and fibrosis of heart valves and pleura) and is therefore given only for refractory cases under specialist supervision. The Transcranial Magnetic Stimulator (TMS) is FDA approved for use in mibraine in people who have no epilepsy and have no metals in the head, neck, or upper body that are attracted by a magnet, or an active implanted medical device such as a pacemaker or deep brain stimulator.

Dental aspects

Dental procedures, such as tooth extraction, amalgam removal or the use of occlusal splints, are of no proven value in the management of true migraine.

Trigeminal autonomic cephalgias

The trigeminal autonomic cephalgias (TACs) include migrainous neuralgia and short-lasting unilateral neuralgia with conjunctival injection and tearing (SUNCT).

Migrainous neuralgia (periodic migrainous neuralgia, cluster headaches, Horton neuralgia, superficial petrosal neuralgia, histamine cephalgia, Sluder headaches)

General aspects
Migrainous neuralgia is less common than migraine. It is a pain in the head and face, defined by the International Headache Society (HIS) as:

> *unilateral excruciatingly severe attacks of pain principally in the ocular, frontal and temporal areas, recurring in separate bouts with daily or almost daily attacks for weeks or months, usually with ipsilateral lacrimation, conjunctival injection, photophobia and nasal stuffiness and/or rhinorrhoea.*

Males are mainly affected and attacks often begin in middle age.
Occasionally, pain mimicking migrainous neuralgia is caused by organic disease, such as ocular disorders or lesions of the trigeminal nerve, brainstem or middle cranial fossa near the midline, including the cavernous sinus, circle of Willis or pituitary. Presentation is then often atypical.

Clinical features
Attacks of migrainous neuralgia are sometimes precipitated by the factors shown in Box 13.5. Typical features are the onset of severe pain at night (classically at around 2.00 a.m.), and clustering of attacks at the same time, for several weeks. Migrainous neuralgia causes unilateral pain usually localized around the maxillary premolars, eye, forehead, cheek and temple (Table 13.9). Pain may occasionally be occipital, cervical or scapular. Episodes, which commence and often terminate suddenly, last less than 1 hour (often 30–45 minutes), and may recur from 1 to 8 times daily. Autonomic features include flushing and/or sweating on the affected side of the face and features such as lacrimation, conjunctival injection and nasal congestion, sometimes with Horner syndrome.

General management
Migrainous neuralgia should be differentiated from migraine and other headaches (see Table 13.9). Diagnosis is clinical but, as similar symptoms may be related to tumours around the cavernous sinus and craniospinal junction, a scan (computed tomography/magnetic

---

Box 13.5 *Precipitants of migrainous neuralgia*

- Alcohol
- Cocaine
- Exercise
- High altitude
- Histamine
- Hot baths
- Hypoxaemia
- Nitroglycerin

Table 13.9 *Differentiation of headaches and orofacial pain of different cause*

Factor	Temporomandibular joint (TMJ) pain–dysfunction	Psychogenic	Idiopathic trigeminal neuralgia	Migraine	Migrainous neuralgia
Age (years)	20–30	35–60	50+	Any	30+
Sex	F > M	F > M	F > M	F > M	M > F
Site	Temple, ear, jaws, teeth Usually unilateral	Diffuse, deep, sometimes across midline	Mandible or maxilla Unilateral	Any	Retro-orbital Unilateral
Associated features	Click in TMJ, trismus	Life events, back pain, etc. Stress, fatigue	± Trigger area	± Photophobia Nausea Vomiting	Nasal stuffiness, lacrimation
Character	Dull, continuous	Dull, boring, continuous	Lancinating	Throbbing	Throbbing
Duration of episode	Weeks to years	Weeks to years	Brief (seconds)	Hours (or usually days)	Minutes to hours, Early mornings, may be daily for a few days

resonance imaging [CT/MRI]) is indicated. Precipitants should be avoided and oxygen inhalations help (pain relief from these is sometimes regarded as diagnostic). Other therapies include ipsilaterally applied intranasal lidocaine; triptans (usually sumatriptan), when there is neither hypertension nor coronary artery disease – zolmitriptan, rizatriptan, eletriptan or naratriptan are also available; ergotamine; butorphanol tartrate nasal spray; capsaicin; and pizotifen. Preventive medications include ergotamine, propranolol, amitriptyline, cyproheptadine, diltiazem, lithium carbonate, prednisolone (prednisone) and verapamil. Neurosurgery may be required for those with intractable cluster headaches.

Dental aspects
Migrainous neuralgia must be distinguished from dental pain by the characteristic history and confirmation of the absence of a dental cause.

Short-lasting unilateral neuralgia with conjunctival injection and tearing (SUNCT)

This syndrome is a form of TAC seen mainly in males above 50 years, who have short-lasting unilateral attacks of intermittent, moderate to severe, burning, piercing or throbbing daytime pain, usually unilaterally, around the eye or temple; these last 5 seconds to 5 minutes per episode and are accompanied by autonomic disturbances, such as conjunctival injection, lacrimation, nasal stuffiness, rhinorrhoea and subclinical forehead sweating. Systolic blood pressure may rise during the attacks. Movement of the neck may trigger these headaches. SUNCT is therefore similar to migrainous neuralgia but may occur in the daytime. SUNCT is generally non-responsive to analgesics. Trigeminal injections of glycerol may provide temporary relief in some severe cases. Corticosteroids and antiepileptics (e.g. gabapentin, lamotrigine or carbamazepine) may help relieve some symptoms.

Idiopathic stabbing headache (ice-pick pains)

Idiopathic stabbing headache is pain confined to the head and exclusively or predominantly felt unilaterally in the distribution of the first division of the trigeminal nerve (orbit, temple and parietal area), mostly in the orbital region. It often recurs in the same place, but may move to other places on the same side of the head or, less commonly, to the opposite side. Pain forms a single stab or a series of stabs; each stab lasts for seconds only and episodes recur at irregular intervals of hours to days.

Diagnosis depends upon the exclusion of structural changes at the site of pain and in the distribution of the affected cranial nerve. Indometacin may relieve idiopathic stabbing headache.

Chronic paroxysmal hemicrania

Chronic paroxysmal hemicrania is similar to migrainous neuralgia, but only sometimes comes at night and is rarely triggered by alcohol. In 20% it follows head injury or whiplash injury, and invariably responds well to indometacin.

Cranial arteritis (temporal or giant cell arteritis)
General aspects

Cranial arteritis is an immunologically mediated vasculitis closely related to polymyalgia rheumatica, causing inflammation of the walls of medium-sized arteries with prominent giant cells, and obliteration of the vessel lumen. Women are predominantly affected, usually after the age of 55.

Clinical features

The most common complaint is severe unilateral, mainly temporal, throbbing headache. Associated features may be malaise, proximal muscle stiffness, weight loss and fever. The superficial temporal artery is typically prominent, tortuous and tender.

The most severe complication of cranial arteritis is ischaemia of the optic nerve, causing blindness in up to 30%. Hemiplegia or myocardial infarction is also possible. Pain on mastication (misnamed jaw claudication) is seen in about 20% of cases and occasionally there is limited mouth opening.

General management

Cranial arteritis should be suspected in an older patient who suddenly experiences headache associated with a warm, tender scalp vessel. There is no diagnostic serological test but erythrocyte sedimentation rate (ESR) is usually greatly raised. Serum levels of interleukin (IL)-6 and alkaline phosphatase may also be raised. Temporal artery biopsy is the one confirmatory diagnostic measure and even this may be negative, as lesions are patchily distributed.

As soon as the diagnosis is made it is obligatory to give systemic corticosteroids (60 mg prednisolone [prednisone] daily, reducing as the

ESR returns to normal) because of the risk of eye involvement. The clinical response is rapid.

Dental aspects

Ischaemic pain in the muscles of mastication can cause severe discomfort when eating and has been reported in 20% of patients. A rare manifestation is ischaemic necrosis and gangrene of the tongue or lip.

NEUROLOGICAL CAUSES OF FACIAL PAIN

Sensory innervation of the face and scalp is carried by the trigeminal nerve. Lesions of the trigeminal at any stage from its nuclei along its course from the pons can cause facial pain or sensory loss, sometimes with serious implications. Pain may be amenable to treatment with pregabalin, gabapentin or carbamazepine.

Idiopathic trigeminal neuralgia

General aspects

Trigeminal neuralgia (TN) has been described by the IHS as 'a painful, unilateral affliction of the face, characterized by brief electric-shock, lightning-like (lancinating) pains limited to the distribution of one or more divisions of the trigeminal nerve'. TN usually afflicts patients over the age of 50. The incidence is less than 0.2% in those under 40 years but rises to 25% in those over 70.

About 15% of cases have structural causes; about 5% are produced by posterior fossa tumours (meningiomas, acoustic neurinomas or carcinomas) that are not suspected before operation and a slightly smaller percentage have multiple sclerosis.

The cause of *idiopathic* TN is unclear but may be demyelination triggered by a tortuous arteriosclerotic blood vessel in the posterior cranial fossa that presses on the trigeminal (the disease predominantly affects older people, many of whom have hypertension or arteriosclerosis).

Clinical features

The pain of TN has the following characteristics:

- It is confined to the trigeminal area of one side, usually the maxillary or mandibular division, or occasionally both. Infraorbital or lower lip/lower jaw pain is common, and supraorbital pain uncommon.
- It is severe and sharply stabbing (lancinating), of only a few seconds' duration, but paroxysms may follow in quick succession. Typically, the pain is remarkably severe and a patient seen crying with pain during an attack is not easily forgotten.
- Triggers are mild stimuli, which, applied to trigger zones within the trigeminal area, typically provoke an attack, and include:
  shaving
  stroking or touching the face
  eating
  drinking a hot or cold liquid
  brushing teeth
  talking
  putting on cosmetics
  encountering a cold breeze
  walking into an air-conditioned room.

Idiopathic TN is likely when there is an intact corneal reflex, no abnormal neurological signs, no objective sensory loss in the area and no other defined neurological deficit.

Secondary TN is more likely if the patient's pain started when younger than 40 years, if there is predominant forehead and/or orbit pain (i.e. first division of the trigeminal nerve), if the pain is bilateral, if there are abnormal trigeminal reflexes, or if there are physical signs such as facial sensory or motor impairment. The latter can result from posterior cerebral fossa lesions, particularly tumours or aneurysms (the combination of neuralgia with hemifacial spasm also suggests a posterior cranial fossa lesion), multiple sclerosis, brainstem ischaemia or infarction in cerebrovascular disease, neurosyphilis or other lesions.

Atypical TN is a syndrome that overlaps TN and trigeminal neuropathy, and affects up to 5% after facial surgery or significant trauma, and up to 1% after the removal of impacted teeth. It includes unusual symptoms, such as more continuous rather than lightning attacks of pain, or triggering by warmth rather than cold, and may result from lesions or injuries of the trigeminal nerve root distal to the root entry zone but with even greater compression than found in the idiopathic form of TN. Attacks consist of constant pain that episodically intensifies and produces both lancinating triggered pain and a baseline, constant, dull and throbbing discomfort.

General management

The diagnosis is clinical. Organic disease must be excluded by neurological examination to confirm normal corneal reflexes, sensory appreciation, and masseter muscle bulk and strength. Loss of the corneal reflex excludes the diagnosis of idiopathic TN, unless a previous trigeminal nerve section procedure has been performed. The other main differential diagnoses are glossopharyngeal neuralgia (the two can coexist), idiopathic facial pain, Raeder paratrigeminal syndrome and Frey syndrome.

Investigations, required especially if there are any neurological features, may include skull radiographs, MRI or CT brain scans, and occasionally cerebrospinal fluid (CSF) examination or neurophysiological tests (e.g. trigeminal evoked potentials and corneal reflex latency). Many now advocate MRI as routine.

A few patients with mild symptoms recover spontaneously but most require treatment. This is initially with anticonvulsants, particularly carbamazepine, which change GABA levels in the central pain-inhibiting systems. Spontaneous remissions of a month or two are relatively common and may make the assessment of treatment difficult. Carbamazepine is indicated first, if only because its use may constitute a therapeutic challenge to the correct diagnosis. If, for example, a patient presumed to have TN does not respond to carbamazepine in 24–48 hours, then the physician may wish to reconsider the initial diagnosis. Carbamazepine is not an analgesic and, if given when an attack starts, will not relieve the pain. If used prophylactically, it may control up to 90% of cases over the first few months, but this falls to about 25% by 1 year.

Carbamazepine absorption is slow, and its antineuralgic activity depends on its metabolites; it must therefore be given continuously for long periods until symptoms are controlled or adverse effects become excessive. Though about 80% obtain pain relief within 24 hours, about 20 days are required before the full effect is noted. Carbamazepine can cause severe ataxia but the many other possible toxic effects are uncommon. Ataxia and drowsiness are dose-related, may interfere with driving and can be dose-limiting.

Some Asians metabolize carbamazepine poorly and can thus suffer from overdose or other adverse events, so they should be screened for the human leukocyte antigen (HLA). The HLA-B*1502 allele has been shown to be strongly correlated with carbamazepine-induced Stevens–Johnson syndrome and toxic epidermal necrolysis (SJS–TEN) in Han Chinese and other Asian populations but not in European populations. The presence of HLA-A*3101 allele is associated with carbamazepine-induced hypersensitivity among people of northern European ancestry. Carbamazepine is contraindicated in pregnancy and porphyria, and should be used with caution in persons with hepatic, renal, cardiac (especially atrioventricular conduction defects) or bone marrow disease. Monitoring of blood carbamazepine levels and, for adverse reactions, regular assessment of blood pressure, blood urea and electrolytes, liver function, platelet and white cell counts is helpful. Carbamazepine may predispose to liver damage from paracetamol (acetaminophen) and may interfere with the effectiveness of the contraceptive pill, though most patients are beyond the age of concern in that respect. Drugs such as erythromycin, cimetidine and isoniazid can raise serum carbamazepine levels.

Should carbamazepine in maximum dosage fail to control neuralgia, oxcarbazine, gabapentin, baclofen and lamotrigine are second choices. Additional therapeutic agents that may be added or may replace carbamazepine include phenytoin, tizanidine, topical capsaicin, and valproate.

Surgery may be indicated if medical therapy fails (25–50% of patients eventually fail to respond to drugs) or adverse effects are intolerable. Surgery (surgical division, cryosurgery, injections of alcohol or phenol) to the trigeminal nerve branches involved is usually carried out under open operation under LA. Cryosurgery can bring pain relief without permanent anaesthesia. However, the benefit of all peripheral nerve procedures may only be temporary, with relapse common within 2 years. If these treatments fail, intracranial neurosurgery is available. All destructive surgical procedures result in a sensory deficit in up to 20% of patients; relapse is common beyond 2 years and the more peripheral the procedure, the greater the risk of recurrence. Although all the surgical procedures are inherently supported by low-level evidence, the results in thousands of patients indicate that surgical treatments for TN are efficacious and acceptably safe. Percutaneous Gasserian lesions can be safely performed in older people but often cause facial numbness. Microvascular decompression provides the longest-lasting pain relief but involves some risk of major neurological complications. Gamma-knife surgery is the least invasive and safest procedure but pain relief may take 1 month to develop.

Percutaneous radiofrequency trigeminal (retrogasserian) rhizotomy (PRTR) is the most widely used technique and is minimally invasive, involving the insertion of a needle, but has morbidity and some mortality. Trigeminal-innervated muscle weakness is a significant early side-effect and anaesthesia also results, causing danger of damage to the cornea.

Percutaneous trigeminal ganglion compression (rhizotomy) is minimally invasive and uses a Fogarty balloon. This may be effective. Over 50% of patients have mild to moderate postoperative numbness but this does not affect the cornea; 16% have ipsilateral masseter/pterygoid weakness. The overall recurrence rate is 26% but 60% of patients are pain-free 8 years after surgery.

Microvascular decompression (MVD) is an invasive procedure performed via a suboccipital craniotomy. This may be effective but occasionally results in damage to the VII or VIII cranial nerves and also carries a small risk of mortality.

Gamma knife radiosurgery (GKR) is non-invasive. It involves delivering high doses of radiation to the trigeminal nerve root without any need for injection or skin incision. It can be successful in eliminating pain in up to 80% but pain recurs in more than half the cases.

Neurosurgical techniques can occasionally be followed by continuous facial pain (anaesthesia dolorosa) that responds very poorly to treatment.

Dental aspects

Patients may be reluctant to brush their teeth or attend for dental treatment.

Glossopharyngeal (vagoglossopharyngeal) neuralgia

Glossopharyngeal neuralgia is rare and usually idiopathic, possibly caused by an abnormal intracranial blood vessel, as in trigeminal neuralgia. The pain is similar to that of TN (rarely, the two coexist), but affects the throat, especially the tonsillar region, and is typically triggered by swallowing or coughing. Pain may also be felt in the ipsilateral ear (vago-Collet–Sicard syndrome) and this may simulate neuralgia of the nervus intermedius (Hunt neuralgia). There are no sensory or motor defects but, in 10%, there is associated bradycardia and fall in blood pressure, sometimes with syncope, especially when the neuralgia is secondary to a throat tumour. During longer attacks, asystole may occur and long, severe attacks may be marked by protracted cardiac arrest, absence of pulse, pallor, mental confusion, syncope or convulsions.

The mechanism usually proposed has been spillover of impulses from the glossopharyngeal nerve via the tractus solitarius to the dorsal motor nucleus of the vagus nerve, resulting in reflex bradycardia, heart block or asystole.

Unlike TN, glossopharyngeal neuralgia rarely appears to be associated with intracranial tumours and even more rarely with multiple sclerosis. Tumours in the posterior cranial fossa or jugular foramen (jugular foramen syndrome) can rarely cause similar pain, together with lesions of the vagus (X) and accessory (XI) nerves (Appendix 13.1). Hoarseness, dysphagia, palatal deviation to the intact side, anaesthesia of the posterior pharyngeal wall, and weakness of the sternomastoid and upper trapezius are then seen.

A 10% cocaine or other anaesthetic throat spray will cause temporary pain relief and is diagnostic. Therapy is as for TN, but carbamazepine is usually less effective and gabapentin is probably better. If drugs fail to give adequate relief, neurosurgery is indicated but is more difficult than for TN and has a higher morbidity and mortality.

Raeder paratrigeminal neuralgia

Raeder paratrigeminal neuralgia is severe, persistent pain in and around the eye, with associated Horner syndrome; it is often caused by a lesion at the skull base that requires neurological attention.

Herpetic and post-herpetic facial neuralgia

Herpes zoster (shingles) is often preceded, usually accompanied and sometimes followed by neuralgia in up to 70% of cases. It mainly affects older people, but antivirals may help prevent it (Ch. 21).

Post-herpetic neuralgia is defined as pain persisting a month after the eruption of zoster, causing continuous burning pain, worse with movement and thermal change, and sometimes sensory changes in the affected area. Treatment is difficult, and pain may be so intolerable that suicide can become a risk. However, spontaneous improvement may sometimes follow after about 18 months.

NSAIDs are generally ineffective but topical lidocaine or capsaicin cream may help. Tricyclic antidepressants, particularly desipramine or amitriptyline, may relieve the pain better than valproate or carbamazepine. TENS or neurosurgery may sometimes help.

Pontine infarction

Pontine ischaemia may be due to bilateral ventral pontine infarction. Lateral medullary infarction may cause a similar but unilateral effect. Burning orofacial pain may be an early symptom.

Bilateral ventral pontine infarction causes the syndrome of quadriplegia and lower cranial nerve palsies but preservation of movement of the upper eyelids and vertical gaze (termed the 'locked-in syndrome' because the patient, though able to understand what is being said and what is happening, is imprisoned by an inability to speak or move anything apart from the eyes; see later). The prognosis is poor.

Cerebellopontine angle tumours

Lesions in the posterior cranial fossa (e.g. cerebellopontine angle tumours) can cause facial pain associated with an absent corneal reflex (V nerve), deafness, tinnitus and vertigo (from involvement of the VIII nerve), facial palsy (VII nerve involvement), ataxia, intention tremor and nystagmus (cerebellar involvement), and spasticity of the leg (pyramidal tract involvement). Acoustic neuromas and meningiomas are usually operable.

Middle cranial fossa lesions

Middle cranial fossa lesions can involve the V and VI nerves, and also cause lateral rectus palsy. Carotid aneurysms, especially those in the cavernous sinus, or cavernous sinus thrombosis may also cause facial pain and associated cranial nerve lesions (III, IV and VI nerves; see Fig. 6.3).

Cavernous sinus thrombosis

Cavernous sinus thrombosis is a life-threatening complication that may rarely result from infection spreading back through the emissary veins from the maxillary or nasal region, or upper teeth, or from infected thrombi in the anterior facial vein or less commonly the pterygoid plexus. Infection can reach the cavernous sinus via either the ophthalmic veins or the foramen ovale.

Clinically, cavernous sinus thrombosis causes gross eyelid oedema, ipsilateral pulsatile exophthalmos, cyanosis due to venous obstruction, rigors and high swinging pyrexia. The superior orbital fissure syndrome (proptosis, fixed dilated pupil and limitation of eye movements) rapidly develops.

There is a mortality of up to 50%, and a further 50% of those that survive are likely to lose the sight of one or both eyes. Vigorous and early use of anticoagulants, antibiotics, drainage and elimination of infection are essential.

Bell palsy

Bell (facial) palsy is preceded or accompanied by pain in the region of the ear, spreading down the jaw in about half the cases. However, the appearance of the typical facial paralysis leaves little doubt as to the diagnosis (see below).

Facial pain caused by extracranial lesions

Branches of the trigeminal nerve may be affected by inflammatory, traumatic or neoplastic lesions causing pain or sensory loss in their distribution.

PSYCHOGENIC CAUSES OF HEADACHE OR OROFACIAL PAIN

See Chapter 10. This type of pain may need treatment with antidepressant agents, particularly selective serotonin reuptake inhibitors (SSRIs) and serotonin–noradrenaline (norepinephrine) reuptake inhibitors (SNRIs).

Tension headaches

Tension headaches are common, especially in young adults, and particularly in emotionally tense, aggressive, frustrated and anxious individuals. They may be caused by sustained contraction of the head and neck muscles and vasoconstriction of nutrient arterioles. Patients are frequently adamant that they suffer from migraine and sometimes the two conditions do coexist. The possibility of associated depression should also be considered.

Clinical features

The pain must be experienced on more than 15 days monthly to be classified as tension headache. It affects the frontal, occipital or temporal muscles, and is felt as a constant ache or band-like pressure, of mild or moderate intensity, bilateral in location, and lasting from 30 minutes to 7 days. The pain onset often is associated with emotional conflict but does not worsen with routine physical activity. Nausea is absent, but photophobia or phonophobia may be present. Pain can often be elicited by palpation of the trapezius or pericranial muscles; it is often worse in the evening and at night but does not waken the patient.

General management

Hypertension and hyperthyroidism should be excluded, as must drug-associated headaches (e.g. analgesics, antihistamines, anticonvulsants, ergotamine, steroids and antibiotics). The pain may be treated by rest, simple analgesics, or combination drugs with biofeedback, and particularly with counselling. Reassurance may be effective and may be bolstered by a short course of diazepam, which is both an anxiolytic and a muscle relaxant. Failing this, amitriptyline is usually effective. Even acupuncture may offer relief.

Oral dysaesthesias

A complaint of a burning tongue or mouth is the common type of oral dysaesthesia. Dry mouth, disturbed taste sensations and delusions of halitosis are other dysaesthesias. These are often manifestations of monosymptomatic hypochondriasis, somatization pain disorder or a depressive neurosis. There is sometimes cancer phobia, or anxiety about the possibility, for example, of venereal disease or human immunodeficiency virus (HIV) infection.

Burning mouth syndrome (glossopyrosis; glossodynia)

General aspects

Burning mouth 'syndrome' (BMS) is a common chronic complaint seen especially in middle-aged or elderly females. Organic causes of burning mouth include:

- glossitis
- erythema migrans (geographic tongue)

- candidosis
- lichen planus
- dry mouth
- drugs (such as angiotensin-converting enzyme inhibitors [ACEIs] or proton pump inhibitors [PPIs])
- habits and denture difficulties
- diabetes.

Burning mouth syndrome is the term usually used when symptoms persist in the absence of identifiable organic aetiological factors. Many of these cases appear related to psychogenic factors such as cancer phobia, depression or anxiety. Sometimes, factors such as restricted tongue space from poor denture construction, or parafunction, such as tongue-thrusting, may be at play. Denture allergy is rarely responsible. Systemic disorders, such as a haematological deficiency state or hypothyroidism, are found in some (Table 13.10).

Clinical features
A burning sensation starts after waking and grows in intensity during the day. It may sometimes be relieved by chewing or drinking. By contrast, pain caused by organic lesions is typically made worse by eating.

BMS most frequently affects the tongue but may also involve the palate or, less commonly, the lips or lower alveolus. There are often multiple oral and/or other psychogenic related complaints, such as dry mouth, a bad taste in the mouth, headaches, chronic back pain, irritable bowel syndrome or dysmenorrhoea.

Patients are often high users of health-care services; there have often already been multiple consultations and attempts at treatment. There are no clinically detectable signs of mucosal disease and no tenderness or swelling of the tongue or affected areas; there is a total lack of objective signs and all investigations are negative. Patients use analgesics only uncommonly.

Three types have been described on the basis of the pattern of symptoms of burning sensation (Table 13.11).

General management
Laboratory screening may be indicated to rule out anaemia and vitamin or iron deficiency (blood tests), diabetes (blood and urine analyses), hyposalivation (salivary flow rates) and candidosis (smear). Pontine infarction should be excluded (see above).

Table 13.10 *Organic causes of burning mouth*

Examples	Comments/examples
Local causes	
Candidosis	Sometimes associated with hyposalivation
Denture problems	–
Erythema migrans (geographical tongue)	–
Lichen planus	–
Systemic causes	
Deficiency	B vitamins, especially B$_{12}$
	Folate
	Iron
Diabetes	–
Drugs	–
Dry mouth	–
Psychogenic	Anxiety states
	Cancer phobia
	Depression
	Hypochondriasis

Few patients with BMS have spontaneous remission and thus treatment is indicated, including attention to any local factors such as dentures, psychogenic assessment and occasionally psychiatric care, but many refuse this. Psychological screening using, for example, the hospital anxiety and depression (HAD) scale may be helpful. Treatment may include topical agents such as capsaicin or clonazepam, alpha lipoic acid, or antidepressants such as amitriptyline, dosulepin, doxepin, fluoxetine or trazodone.

Idiopathic facial pain (atypical or psychogenic facial pain)
General aspects

The IHS defines this as 'facial pain not fulfilling other criteria' or:

persistent facial pain that does not have the characteristics of the cranial neuralgias and is not associated with physical signs or demonstrable organic causes. It is present daily and persists for most or all of the day. It is confined at onset to a limited area on one side of the face and may spread to the upper and lower jaws or other areas of the face or neck. It is deep and poorly localized. The pain is not associated with sensory loss or other physical signs. Laboratory investigations including radiographs of face and jaws do not demonstrate relevant abnormalities.

A few patients with similar symptomatology eventually prove to have organic disorders, such as an adenocystic carcinoma that has invaded perineurally, but in others it may be a somatization pain disorder (Ch. 10).

Clinical features

Pain is continuous, often of a dull boring or burning type; it generally has an ill-defined location but involves the maxilla particularly. The pain may waken the patient in the early morning and has no obvious precipitating factors, although it may be attributed to dental disease or treatment; it is rarely relieved completely by analgesics. There are often multiple oral and/or other psychogenic related complaints. There have often been multiple consultations and treatment attempts.

General management

Idiopathic facial pain is a clinical diagnosis reached by careful examination of the mouth, perioral structures and cranial nerves. Imaging with CT or MRI to exclude organic disease is important.

Cognitive therapy is indicated but, since many of these patients have already rejected the idea of mental illness, it may be difficult to persuade them of the need for this type of help. Sometimes it is helpful to make it clear that depression both is common and is an illness like

Table 13.11 *Types of burning mouth syndrome*

Type	Symptom pattern	Frequency	Other features
1	No symptoms on waking but increasing during the day	–	Unremitting
2	Symptoms on waking and through the day	Most common	Unremitting
3	No regular pattern of symptoms	Least common	May remit

any other; as with other disorders, it can also cause physical symptoms. Sometimes the pain may appear as a hysterical conversion neurosis and many patients have obsessional personality traits.

Antidepressants that can be useful include amitriptyline, dosulepin, nortriptyline and fluoxetine.

Idiopathic odontalgia is a variant characterized by the complaint of severe throbbing pain in one or several teeth, which are hypersensitive to any stimulus. Extractions typically lead to transference of the symptoms to adjacent teeth.

Temporomandibular pain–dysfunction syndrome (facial pain–dysfunction, myofascial pain–dysfunction, TMJ pain–dysfunction or facial arthromyalgia)

General aspects

Temporomandibular joint (TMJ) pain–dysfunction is a common problem, predominantly affecting young women. The TMJ shows no pathology, in contrast to internal derangement of the TMJ, which may also lead to pain. The cause is unclear but there have been many hypotheses, ranging from trauma to malocclusion and even psychogenic factors.

Some occupations or hobbies, such as scuba diving, may predispose to abnormal habits and TMJ pain–dysfunction.

There may be a greater frequency of migraine, rhinitis, peptic ulcer and irritable bowel syndrome associated, leading some to believe that depression may be contributory. A psychiatric basis for the syndrome is, however, controversial, but it may be seen particularly in ambitious, obsessional personalities, in anxiety states or in agitated depression.

Clinical features

There is typically dull pain, usually in front of the TMJ; the pain tends to radiate over the masseter and temporalis muscles and sometimes occipitally or cervically. Tenderness in the masticatory muscles, including the pterygoids, is characteristic.

There may be an audible click or palpable crepitus in the joint, the mandible often deviates towards the affected side on opening and there may be restricted mouth opening, or 'locking'. There is sometimes faceting on the teeth, ridging of the tongue margins and buccal mucosa at the occlusal line, and sometimes signs of lip-chewing if patients frequently grind or clench their teeth or develop various (parafunctional) habits, such as pencil chewing.

General management

Radiography shows no significant abnormality but, nevertheless, organic disease must be excluded. In any case, symptoms eventually resolve spontaneously. Degenerative joint disease is not usually a consequence. Treatment consists of reassurance. A bite-raising appliance to provide a free, sliding occlusion may help. Mild anxiolytics, such as diazepam, which is also a muscle relaxant, may help but should only be given for a limited period and may need to be supplemented with analgesics or peri-articular injection of benzocaine. If there is real evidence of depression, tricyclic antidepressants may be more useful.

Dental aspects

Limited mouth-opening may interfere with dental treatment. Attrition may require special restorative care. Dental treatment may be blamed for the onset of symptoms.

OTHER CAUSES OF HEADACHE AND OROFACIAL PAIN

See Table 13.5. Orofacial pain may be referred from the chest, particularly in ischaemic heart disease but occasionally in lung cancer. Headache can be a feature of many systemic diseases, such as any fever, hypertension, chronic obstructive airways disease or some endocrinopathies, and head injuries.

Head injuries

Headaches after head injuries, though common, do not normally persist. If they do, neurological advice must be sought to exclude intracranial haemorrhage. In the absence of neurological complications, persistent post-traumatic headaches may be due to compensation neurosis (Ch. 10).

Raised intracranial pressure

Raised intracranial pressure is one of the most serious but also the least common cause of headache. It is a dangerous condition, usually related to space-occupying lesions such as intracranial haemorrhage, abscess or tumours; it is occasionally drug-induced (e.g. by tetracyclines) and may be caused by malignant hypertension. The headache is severe and often worse on waking, but improves during the day. Nausea and vomiting are common and the headache is aggravated by straining, coughing, sneezing or lying down. Neurological attention is essential.

Skull disease

Headache is occasionally the presenting feature of diseases of the skull, such as bony metastases or Paget disease (Ch. 16).

Meningeal irritation

Meningeal irritation, seen in meningitis or subarachnoid haemorrhage, provokes severe headache with nausea, vomiting, neck pain or stiffness (inability to kiss the knees) or pain on raising the straightened legs (Kernig sign). Urgent neurological attention is needed.

New daily persistent headache

Epstein–Barr virus appears to be associated with these headaches in young adults; they recur daily but resolve spontaneously within a year.

Drugs

Facial pain may occasionally be induced by drugs (e.g. nitrites, vinca alkaloids, phenothiazines or even analgesics). Daily or near-daily analgesic use can perpetuate the headache process. Analgesia rebound headache (medication overuse headache, or MOH) mimics tension-type or migraine-like headaches and is usually associated with products containing caffeine or butalbital (a barbiturate often combined with other medications, such as paracetamol [acetaminophen], codeine or aspirin). To avoid MOH, simple analgesics should not be used for more than 15 days per month, while those such as ergots, triptans, opioids and barbiturates should not be taken on more than 10 days per month. Usually, when analgesics are discontinued, MOH may worsen for several days and the sufferer may have nausea or vomiting, but then begins to improve spontaneously.

GENERAL MANAGEMENT OF HEADACHE AND OROFACIAL PAIN

Features of pain that need to be ascertained are previous episodes, duration, onset, site, nature, duration, moderating factors, referral and severity. Patients with headache should be evaluated initially by history supplemented by physical examination, including examination of the cranium, sinuses, ears and eyes, and mental and neurological status. Some differentiating features are shown in Table 13.9.

Investigations may need to include a full blood picture, basic blood chemistry and possibly endocrinological examination, as well as urinalysis, imaging (CT or MRI) and sometimes lumbar puncture, electroencephalography (EEG), electrocardiography (ECG) or arteriography.

CRANIAL NERVE LESIONS

Cranial nerves can be damaged by trauma, infections, tumours, drugs or chronic diseases (e.g. diabetes, connective tissue diseases, leukaemia, sarcoidosis, midline granulomas, Behçet disease or demyelinating diseases; Table 13.12).

Table 13.12 *Cranial nerves: main features, causes of lesions and testing*

Number	Name	Main functions	How to test the nerve	Main lesion features	Main causes
I	Olfactory	Olfaction	With an odorous substances	Anosmia or hyposmia	Trauma
					Infection
					Neoplasm
II	Optic	Vision	Vision chart. Ask patient to stare at your face from about 30 cm away and (with both eyes open and with each eye shut in turn) report if any part of your face is missing	Visual defect or blindness	Trauma
					Infection
					Neoplasm
					Cerebrovascular accident (CVA)
					Multiple sclerosis
III	Oculomotor	Most eye muscles	'Follow the moving finger' in a 'rugby post' configuration	Ptosis	Diabetes
				Dilated pupil	Trauma
				Diplopia	
				Eye points 'down and out'	
IV	Trochlear	Superior oblique eye muscle	Look down at the tip of the nose	Diplopia	Trauma
				Unable to look down when looking medially	
V	Trigeminal	Facial sensation, muscles of mastication	Touch the face, clench the teeth	Anaesthesia or hypo-aesthesia	Trauma
					Infection
					Neoplasm
					Multiple sclerosis
					Connective tissue disease
VI	Abducens	Lateral rectus eye muscle	Look to each side	Diplopia	Trauma
				Unable to look laterally to the affected side	Neoplasm
					CVA
					Raised intracranial pressure
VII	Facial	Facial expression, taste	Smile, raise the eyebrows	Facial palsy	Trauma
			Test taste for sugar and salt		Infection
					Neoplasm
					CVA
					Multiple sclerosis
					Connective tissue disease
VIII	Auditory/ vestibular	Hearing and balance	Tuning fork	Impaired hearing or balance	Trauma
					Infection
					Neoplasm
					CVA
					Bone disease
IX	Glossopharyngeal	Pharynx sensation	Test gag reflex	Impaired gag reflex	Trauma
					Neoplasm
X	Vagus	Pharynx and larynx muscles, parasympathetic	Check for hoarseness, open wide and say 'Ah'	Voice changes	Trauma
				Impaired gag reflex	Neoplasm
					CVA
XI	Accessory	Sternomastoid and trapezius	Test turning the head or shrugging shoulders	Weakness	CVA
					Trauma
					Infection (poliomyelitis)
XII	Hypoglossal	Tongue muscles	Protrude tongue	Tongue deviation to affected side, and sometimes wasting	Trauma
					Neoplasm

History and full neurological and physical examinations are essential aspects of assessment, including that of people with cranial nerve lesions. Investigations that may be useful include: blood tests (full blood count, electrolytes, liver, kidney or endocrine function tests); CSF examination – lumbar puncture; electrophysiological studies (EEG); and imaging (plain radiography, CT, MRI and positron emission tomography [PET]) – allows cerebral functional studies and opened the way for advances, such as single-photon emission computed tomography (SPECT).

OLFACTORY NERVE (CRANIAL NERVE I)

The olfactory nerve permits the smelling of odours. Unilateral anosmia is often unnoticed but bilateral anosmia causes loss of ability to smell odours; in practice, the patient may complain of loss of taste rather than of smell. Anosmia is common in upper respiratory infections and after head injuries, as the nerves may be torn as they pass through the cribriform plate; this is experienced especially in Le Fort III fractures of the middle third of the facial skeleton. Olfactory neuroblastoma is a rare tumour linked tentatively to dental staff. An olfactory lesion is confirmed by inability to smell substances, such as orange, soap, coffee, cloves or peppermint oil. Each nostril is tested separately. Ammoniacal solutions must not be used, as they stimulate the trigeminal rather than the olfactory nerve.

OPTIC NERVE (CRANIAL NERVE II)

The optic nerve is central to vision (Fig. 13.4) and can be damaged by trauma, glaucoma, raised intracranial pressure, neoplasms, radiation, toxins or drugs, resulting in impaired vision. Visual ability is tested by asking the person to read an eye chart. Peripheral vision is tested by asking the person to detect objects or movement from the corners of the eyes.

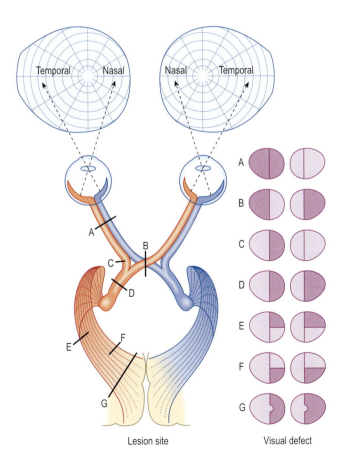

Lesion site   Visual defect

Fig. 13.4 Optic nerve lesions, site of lesion and resultant visual defects.

The ability to detect light is tested in a darkened room by shining a bright light (as from a torch) into each pupil.

OCULOMOTOR NERVE (CRANIAL NERVE III)

Extraocular (orbital) muscles are complex but responsible for moving the globe. The medial rectus (supplied by the third nerve) moves the eye medially (adducts). The adducted eye is depressed by the superior oblique muscle (fourth nerve) and elevated by the inferior oblique (third nerve). The lateral rectus (sixth nerve) abducts the eye. The abducted eye is depressed by the inferior rectus (third nerve) and elevated by the superior rectus (third nerve).

The oculomotor nerve thus supplies most of the orbital muscles (not the lateral rectus and superior oblique), as well as the ciliary muscle, the constrictor of the pupil, and the muscle that raises the upper eyelid. Disruption of the third nerve can be caused by extracranial causes (trauma, arteriosclerosis, diabetes, orbital apex disease, cavernous sinus disease, aneurysm of the posterior communicating artery) or supratentorial (raised intracranial pressure with uncal herniation). Disruption of the third nerve causes the following:

- Paralysis of internal, upward and downward movement of the eye. Lateral movement is retained
- Double vision (diplopia) and a divergent squint with the affected eye pointing downwards and laterally – 'down and out' in all directions except when looking towards the affected side
- Ptosis (drooping upper eyelid)
- A dilated pupil, which fails to constrict on accommodation or when light is shone either on to the affected eye (negative direct light reaction) or into the unaffected eye (negative consensual light reaction), i.e. a fixed pupil.

The upper eyelid is checked for drooping (ptosis). The pupils' response to light is checked by shining a bright light (as from a torch) into each pupil in a darkened room. The ability to move each eye up, down and inward is tested by asking the person to follow a target moved by the examiner.

TROCHLEAR NERVE (CRANIAL NERVE IV)

The trochlear nerve supplies only the superior oblique muscle, which moves the eye downwards and medially towards the nose. Damage may be caused by vascular disease, diabetes, cavernous sinus syndrome, trauma or orbital apex syndrome. A trochlear lesion is characterized by:

- the head tilted away from the affected side
- diplopia, maximal on looking downwards and inwards, and causing difficulty descending stairs or reading
- normal pupils.

The ability to move each eye down and inward is tested by asking the person to follow a target moved by the examiner. There is often damage to the third and fourth nerves as well.

TRIGEMINAL NERVE (CRANIAL NERVE V)

The trigeminal (= three twins) nerve supplies sensation over the face (apart from the angle of the jaw), scalp (back to a line drawn across the vertex, between the ears) and most of the mucosae of the oral cavity, conjunctivae, nose, tympanic membrane and paranasal sinuses (Fig. 13.5). Taste fibres from the anterior two-thirds of tongue are carried in the trigeminal nerve. The motor division of the trigeminal nerve supplies the muscles of mastication. Secretomotor fibres to submandibular and sublingual salivary glands and lacrimal glands are

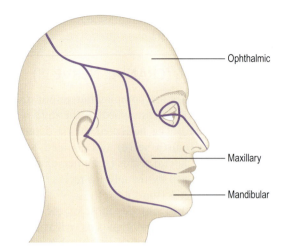

Fig. 13.5 Distribution of sensory divisions of the trigeminal nerve.

Table 13.13 *Causes of sensory loss in the trigeminal area*

Source	Type	Main causes
Intracranial		
Congenital	Syringobulbia	–
Acquired	Inflammatory	Multiple sclerosis
		Neurosyphilis
		Sarcoidosis
		Tuberculosis
		Connective tissue disease
		HIV/AIDS
	Neoplastic	Cerebral tumours
	Vascular	Cerebrovascular disease
		Aneurysms
	Drugs	Stilbamidine
	Occupational	Trilene (dry cleaning)
	Idiopathic	Benign trigeminal neuropathy
		Paget disease
Extracranial		
Acquired	Trauma	To infraorbital, inferior dental, lingual or mental nerves or middle cranial fossa fracture
	Inflammatory	Osteomyelitis
	Neoplastic	Carcinoma of antrum or nasopharynx
		Oral carcinoma
		Metastatic tumours
		Leukaemic deposits

also carried in trigeminal branches. Damage to the trigeminal can be extracranial (trauma [e.g. surgical, fractures], bone disease, drugs, multiple sclerosis, diabetes or tumours) or intracranial (trauma [e.g. surgical, fractures], inflammatory [infections, sarcoidosis, connective tissue disorders], tumours, cerebrovascular disease, syringobulbia, diabetes, bone disease, drugs or multiple sclerosis).

Trigeminal sensory loss (Table 13.13)

Normal facial sensation, mediated by the trigeminal, is important to protect the skin, mucosae and especially the cornea from damage. Loss of facial sensory awareness, which can be caused by lesions of a sensory branch of the trigeminal nerve or the central connections,

may be completely lost (*anaesthesia*) or partially lost (*hypoaesthesia*). *Paraesthesia* does not mean loss of sensation; rather it means abnormal sensation, often 'pins and needles' or similar discomfort.

Extracranial causes of facial sensory loss are most common and include damage to the trigeminal from trauma, which is the usual cause – especially by inferior alveolar local analgesic injections, fractures or surgery (particularly lower third molar removal, osteotomies or jaw resections), mainly after orthognathic or cancer surgery. Rarely, endodontics or implants may be responsible. Ipsilateral lower labial hypoaesthesia or anaesthesia usually results. The lingual nerve may be damaged, especially during removal of lower third molars, and particularly when the lingual split technique is used. Ipsilateral lingual hypoaesthesia or anaesthesia usually results. Occasionally, the mental foramen is close beneath a lower denture and there is anaesthesia of the lower lip on the affected side, as a result of pressure from the denture. Damage to branches of the maxillary division may be caused by the following:

- Trauma – usually middle-third facial fractures
- Bone disease – osteomyelitis in the mandible may affect the inferior alveolar nerve to cause labial anaesthesia. Paget disease is a rare cause of sensory loss
- Malignant disease – oral carcinomas may invade the jaws to cause anaesthesia. Jaw metastases or malignant disease in the bone marrow may damage the nerve supply. Tumours such as carcinoma of the maxillary antrum may cause ipsilateral upper labial hypoaesthesia or anaesthesia. Nasopharyngeal carcinomas may invade the pharyngeal wall to infiltrate the mandibular division of the trigeminal nerve, causing pain, sensory loss and, by occluding the Eustachian tube, deafness (Trotter syndrome). Tumours around the skull base may also involve the trigeminal nerve. Numbness that spreads is a possible indicator of malignancy
- Neuropathies – multiple sclerosis, diabetes, sarcoidosis, toxin
- Drug-induced – e.g. mefloquine; infections – e.g. HIV, herpes simplex virus (HSV), syphilis, Lyme disease, leprosy; amyloidosis; or sickle cell disease.

Intracranial lesions affecting the trigeminal or connections are uncommon but serious, and include inflammatory disorders (multiple sclerosis, sarcoidosis, connective tissue disorders), infections (e.g. HIV, HSV, syphilis, leprosy), neoplasms (tumours around the Gasserian ganglion or posterior cranial fossa may involve the trigeminal nerve; numbness that spreads is a possible indicator of malignancy), syringobulbia or drugs.

Since other cranial nerves are anatomically close, there may be neurological deficits associated with intracranial causes of facial sensory loss. In posterior cranial fossa lesions, for example, there may be cerebellar features such as ataxia. In middle cranial fossa lesions, there may be associated neurological deficits affecting cranial nerve VI and thus mediolateral eye movements.

Benign trigeminal neuropathy is a transient sensory loss in one or more divisions of the trigeminal nerve that seldom occurs until the second decade or affects the corneal reflex. The aetiology is unknown, though some patients prove to have connective tissue disorder. *Psychogenic causes of facial sensory loss* include hysteria, and particularly hyperventilation syndrome. Facial sensation is mediated through the trigeminal nerve but the skin over the angle of the mandible is supplied by cervical nerves.

Trigeminal neuropathy or post-traumatic trigeminal neuropathy may develop after irreparable damage to the trigeminal nerve, most commonly after destructive procedures, such as rhizotomies used for treatment of trigeminal neuralgia, but also after craniofacial trauma (road traffic accidents), or dental or sinus trauma (e.g. Caldwell–Luc procedures).

Other causes of neuropathic pain can be metabolic (diabetes), inflammatory, infective (post-herpetic neuralgias), neoplastic and, rarely, after local analgesic injections.

Hypoaesthesia or anaesthesia may become associated with abnormal sensations or pain, related to excessive firing of pain-mediating nerve cells (phantom or deafferentation pain), which can start immediately or days to years later. Neuropathic pain may be burning, stabbing, stinging or like an electric shock. Trigeminal neuropathic pain often presents as a constant, unilateral, often mild facial pain with prominent sensory loss; it is spontaneous and unremitting. In the most extreme form (anaesthesia dolorosa), there is continuous severe pain in areas of complete numbness.

Analgesics are rarely effective. The first-line treatment is with a tricyclic antidepressant, such as amitriptyline; gabapentin is the best alternative. Topical capsaicin, which appears to deplete substance P, may also be effective. Trigeminal nerve stimulation procedures may offer relief. More invasive procedures, such as brain surface (pre-motor cortex) stimulation or tractotomy, may be needed.

The blink reflex is tested by touching the cornea of the eye with a wisp of cotton wool. Facial sensation is assessed using a pin and a wisp of cotton wool. Strength and movement of muscles that control the jaw are tested by asking the person to clench the teeth and open the jaw against resistance.

Damage to a sensory branch of the trigeminal causes hypoaesthesia in its area of distribution, initially resulting in a diminishing skin response to pinprick and, later, complete anaesthesia. Lesions involving the ophthalmic division cause corneal anaesthesia: gently touching the cornea with a wisp of cotton wool (which the patient must not see), twisted to a point (corneal reflex), normally causes a blink, but not if the cornea is anaesthetic or the facial nerve is damaged.

It is important, with patients complaining of facial anaesthesia, to test all areas but particularly the corneal reflex, and the reaction to pinprick over the angle of the mandible. If, however, the patient complains of complete facial or hemifacial anaesthesia but the corneal reflex is retained or there is anaesthesia over the angle of the mandible, the symptoms are probably functional rather than organic.

Damage to taste can be tested with sweet, salt, sour or bitter substances carefully applied to the dorsum of the tongue.

Trigeminal motor neuropathy

Trigeminal motor neuropathy may occasionally be seen in isolation – possibly related to a viral infection. Trigeminal motor neuropathy is more frequently associated with trigeminal sensory neuropathy or due to lesions affecting the motor division of the trigeminal nerve when there are usually other cranial nerve deficits, sometimes caused by an intracranial tumour. Weakness may develop, sometimes with masseter and temporalis wasting. Damage to the motor part of the trigeminal can be difficult to establish; it is usually asymptomatic if unilateral but the jaw may deviate towards the affected side on opening. It is easier to detect motor weakness by asking the patient to open the jaw against resistance, rather than by trying to test the strength of closure.

ABDUCENS NERVE (CRANIAL NERVE VI)

The abducens nerve supplies only the lateral rectus muscle. Damage to this nerve may be caused by vascular disease, cavernous sinus syndrome, trauma, orbital apex syndrome or raised intracranial pressure. Lesions can be surprisingly disabling, presenting with (Fig. 13.6):

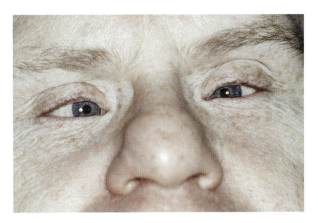

Fig. 13.6 Lesions of the abducens nerve. With the patient looking directly ahead, the affected left eye deviates medially as its lateral rectus muscle is functionless.

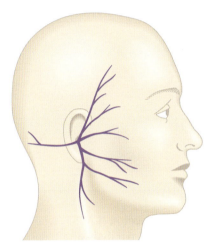

Fig. 13.7 Motor branches of the facial nerve to muscles of facial expression.

- paralysis of abduction of the eye
- deviation of the affected eye towards the nose, and convergent squint – the diplopia is maximal on looking laterally towards the affected side
- normal pupils.

The ability to move each eye outward beyond the midline is tested by asking the person to look to the side.

FACIAL NERVE (CRANIAL NERVE VII)

The facial nerve is the motor supply to the muscles of facial expression (Fig. 13.7), but it also carries taste sensation from the anterior two-thirds of the tongue (via the chorda tympani), secretomotor fibres to the submandibular and sublingual salivary glands and lacrimal glands, and branches to the stapedius muscle.

Causes of damage to the facial nerve include, especially, stroke, trauma and infection; these and other causes are shown in Table 13.14.

The motor neurons supplying the lower face receive upper motor neurons (UMNs) from the contralateral motor cortex, whereas the neurons to the upper face receive bilateral UMN innervation. Thus a UMN lesion (e.g. stroke) causes unilateral facial palsy with some sparing of the frontalis and orbicularis oculi muscles (because of the bilateral cortical representation) and, although voluntary facial movements are impaired, the face may still move with emotional responses (e.g. laughing). Paresis of the ipsilateral arm (monoparesis) or of the arm and leg (hemiparesis), or dysphasia, may also be associated because of more extensive cerebrocortical damage.

Table 13.14 *Localization of site of lesion in, and causes of, unilateral facial palsy*

Muscles paralysed	Lacrimation	Hyperacusis	Sense of taste	Other features	Probable site of lesion	Type of lesion
Lower face	N	–	N	Emotional movement retained ± monoparesis or hemiparesis ± aphasia	Upper motor neuron (UMN)	Stroke Brain tumour Trauma HIV infection
All facial muscles	↓	+	↓	± VIth nerve damage	Lower motor neuron (LMN) Facial nucleus	Multiple sclerosis
				± VIIIth nerve damage	Between nucleus and geniculate ganglion	Fractured base of skull Posterior cranial fossa tumours Sarcoidosis
	N	±	N or ↓	–	Between geniculate ganglion and stylomastoid canal	Otitis media Cholesteatoma
		–	N	–	In stylomastoid canal or extracranially	Bell palsy Trauma Local analgesia (e.g. misplaced inferior dental block) Parotid malignant neoplasm Guillain–Barré syndrome Herpes simplex virus Lyme disease HIV infection Granulomatous disorders
Isolated facial muscles	N	–	N	–	Branch of facial nerve extracranially	Trauma Local analgesia

N = normal.

In contrast, lower motor neuron (LMN) facial palsy (e.g. Bell palsy) is characterized by unilateral paralysis of all muscles of facial expression – for both voluntary and emotional responses.

In facial palsy, the forehead is unfurrowed; the patient is unable to close the eye on that side and attempted closure causes the eye to roll upwards (Bell sign). Lacrimation is diminished in a seventh nerve lesion but, because of the weakness, tears tend to overflow on to the cheek (epiphora), the nasolabial fold is obliterated, and the corner of the mouth droops and saliva may dribble from it and cause angular stomatitis. On the affected side, food collects in the vestibule and plaque accumulates on teeth. Other defects, such as loss of taste or hyperacusis, may be associated.

Facial weakness is demonstrated by asking patients to smile, close their eyes against resistance, raise the eyebrows, whistle or raise the lips to show their teeth. The Schirmer test, carried out by gently placing a strip of filter paper on the lower conjunctival sac and comparing the wetting of the paper with that on the other side, may show reduced lacrimation. Taste is tested by applying sugar, salt, sour lemon juice or vinegar, and bitter substances (aspirin, quinine or aloes) on the tongue and asking the patient to identify each one.

Bell palsy

Bell palsy is facial paralysis for which no local or systemic cause can be identified, though it is now recognized to be a lower motor neuron palsy and mainly due to infection with herpes simplex virus. There appears to be inflammation of the facial nerve in the stylomastoid canal, sometimes with demyelination.

Similar features may occasionally be seen after other herpes virus infections (e.g. varicella zoster virus [VZV], cytomegalovirus [CMV] and Epstein–Barr virus [EBV]), influenza viruses, retroviruses (e.g. HIV and human lymphotropic virus-1 [HTLV-1]), and other infections

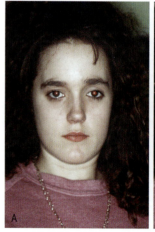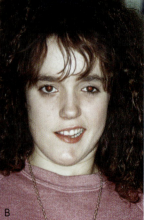

Fig. 13.8 Bell palsy. The right side of the face is completely paralysed (A), as demonstrated when the patient tries to smile (B).

such as Lyme disease (*Borrelia burgdorferi*). There are occasional associations with hypertension, lymphoma, Melkersson–Rosenthal syndrome, Crohn disease, orofacial granulomatosis, sarcoidosis, connective tissue disorders, acoustic neuroma, Guillain–Barré syndrome, multiple sclerosis and a variety of other disorders (see Table 13.14). Bell palsy is more common in pregnancy, diabetes, influenza, a cold or another respiratory illness.

Clinical features

There is acute unilateral facial paralysis (with no other paralyses) over a few hours, maximal within 48 hours (Fig. 13.8). Pain in the region of the ear or in the jaw may precede the paralysis by a day or two. Occasionally, hyperacusis (oversensitivity to sound due to loss of function of the nerve to stapedius) or loss of taste (chorda tympani) on the anterior tongue, or changes in salivation/lacrimation are associated (see Table 13.14). Patients may complain of facial numbness but sensation is intact on testing.

General management

LMN palsy must be distinguished from UMN palsy (Table 13.15) and the degree of palsy assessed (Table 13.16).

Electromyography (EMG) can confirm nerve damage and its severity. If paralysis is progressive, imaging of the internal acoustic canal, cerebellopontine angle and mastoid may be needed to exclude an organic lesion. Most patients with Bell palsy, however, are otherwise healthy, present no management difficulties and totally recover spontaneously within weeks. Nevertheless, active treatment is indicated and includes anti-inflammatory medication (a short course of prednisolone [prednisone] may result in 80–90% complete recovery, compared with about 50–60% in the absence of such treatment); antiviral medication (aciclovir or famciclovir); and facial massage (may help prevent permanent contractures of the paralysed muscles during the acute phase; the cornea should be protected with an eye pad). Patients offered antivirals should be counselled that a benefit from antivirals has not been fully established; if there is a benefit, it is likely to be only modest.

Where paralysis is complete, only 50% recover completely within 1 week but another 25% recover over 2 weeks or so. Few who have not recovered by 2 weeks will do so. Favourable prognostic signs are incomplete paralysis in the first week and persistence of the stapedial reflex, measured by electroneurography. Bad prognostic signs are hyperacusis, severe taste impairment and/or diminished lacrimation or salivation, especially in older, diabetic or hypertensive patients. Although many patients recover spontaneously, the after-effects in the remaining 10–20% can be severe and distressing, when surgical decompression of the nerve in the stylomastoid canal may be attempted. If paralysis persists and function remains incomplete, the palpebral fissure may narrow, the nasolabial fold deepens and facial spasm may develop. Rare complications, apparently caused by anomalous regeneration of the facial nerve, include irregular or anomalous lacrimation (crocodile tears) when the facial muscles are used – for example, during eating, retraction of the commissure when the eye is closed, or hemifacial spasm.

Dental aspects

In chronic palsy, construction of a splint to support the angle of the mouth may improve aesthetics to some degree, as may a facial graft or other manœuvres such as facial–hypoglossal nerve anastomosis, but results are not always entirely satisfactory.

Ramsay–Hunt syndrome

Severe facial paralysis with vesicles in the ipsilateral pharynx and external auditory canal (Ramsay–Hunt syndrome) may be due to varicella zoster virus (VZV) of the facial nerve geniculate ganglion.

Bilateral facial paralysis

Bilateral facial paralysis is rare but may result from acute idiopathic polyneuritis (Guillain–Barré syndrome, Ch. 37), sarcoidosis (Heerfordt syndrome, Ch. 37), arachnoiditis or posterior cranial fossa tumours.

Other causes of facial weakness

An apparent facial palsy may be caused by myasthenia gravis, some myopathies or Romberg syndrome.

Table 13.15 *Differentiation of upper motor neuron (UMN) from lower motor neuron (LMN) lesions of the facial nerve*

Action	UMN lesion	LMN lesion
Emotional movements of the face	Retained	Lost
Blink reflex	Retained	Lost
Ability to wrinkle forehead	Retained	Lost
Drooling from commissure	Uncommon	Common
Lacrimation, taste and hearing	Unaffected	May be affected
Tongue protrusion	Normal	Deviates to unaffected side

Table 13.16 *Facial palsy severity score*

House and Brackmann grades	Facial function	Features	Dysfunction and outcomes
I	Normal	–	–
II	Incomplete paralysis	Slight weakness. The patients may have a slight synkinesis	Mild dysfunction
		Normal symmetry and tone at rest	Good outcomes
		Forehead motion is moderate to good, complete eye closure is achieved with minimal effort but slight mouth asymmetry	
III	Incomplete paralysis	An obvious but not disfiguring difference between the sides. A noticeable but not severe synkinesis, contracture or hemifacial spasm	Moderate dysfunction
		Normal symmetry and tone at rest	
		Forehead movement is slight to moderate, complete eye closure is achieved with effort, and a slightly weak mouth movement is noted	
IV	Incomplete paralysis	An obvious weakness and/or disfiguring asymmetry	Moderate dysfunction
		Symmetry and tone normal at rest	
		No forehead motion. Eye closure is incomplete and an asymmetric mouth is noted	
V	Incomplete facial paralysis	Only a barely perceptible motion	Severe dysfunction
		Asymmetry at rest	
		No forehead motion	
		Eye closure is incomplete and mouth movement is only slight	
VI	Complete facial paralysis	Gross asymmetry	Severe dysfunction
		Total palsy: no movement	

VESTIBULOCOCHLEAR (OR AUDITORY) NERVE (CRANIAL NERVE VIII)

This nerve has two components, the vestibular (concerned with appreciation of the movements and position of the head) and the cochlear (hearing).

Damage to the auditory nerve can be caused by loud noise (explosions, music or occupations where loud sounds are produced), ageing, infections of inner ear and brain, drugs (e.g. aminoglycosides), trauma, stroke or multiple sclerosis. Damage to the vestibular component may be caused by infections (vestibular neuritis and labyrinthitis).

Lesions of the auditory nerve may cause loss of hearing, vertigo or ringing in the ears (tinnitus). An otological opinion should be obtained, as special tests are needed for diagnosis. Hearing is tested with a tuning fork or with headphones that play tones of different frequencies (pitches) and loudness (audiometry). Balance is tested by asking the person to walk a straight line.

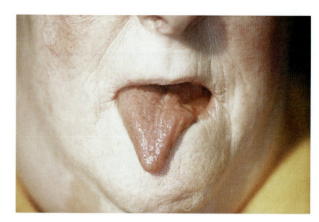

Fig. 13.9 Lesion of hypoglossal nerve with wasting of the left side of the tongue (lower motor neuron lesion).

GLOSSOPHARYNGEAL NERVE (CRANIAL NERVE IX)

The glossopharyngeal nerve supplies the posterior third of the tongue and the pharynx; it carries taste sensation from the posterior third of the tongue, motor supply to the stylopharyngeus and secretomotor fibres to the parotid. The glossopharyngeal can be damaged by infections, trauma, tumours or surgery in the cerebellopontine angle, pharynx or parapharyngeal space, and lesions are usually associated with lesions of vagus, accessory and hypoglossal nerves (bulbar palsy). They typically cause impaired pharyngeal sensation, so that the gag reflex may be weakened. Bulbar palsy is the term given to weakness or paralysis of muscles supplied by the medulla (tongue, pharynx, larynx, sternomastoid and upper trapezius; cranial nerves IX–XII inclusive). Acute bulbar palsy can be caused by poliomyelitis or diphtheria, chronic progressive bulbar palsy by tumours or aneurysms of the posterior cranial fossa or nasopharynx, or strokes. Various other syndromes, some of which are rare, are tabulated in Appendix 13.1. Because the ninth and tenth cranial nerves control similar functions, they are tested together. The person is asked to swallow, and to say 'aah' (to check movement of the palate and uvula); the back of the throat may be touched with a tongue blade, which evokes the gag reflex in healthy people. The person is asked to speak to determine whether the voice sounds nasal.

VAGUS NERVE (CRANIAL NERVE X)

The vagus has a wide parasympathetic distribution to the thoracic and upper abdominal viscera and the motor supply to some soft palate, pharyngeal and laryngeal muscles. The vagus can be damaged particularly by trauma, including neck surgery, and in particular carotid artery or thyroid surgery. Lesions of one vagus are rare in isolation but can cause impaired gag reflex, hoarse voice and bovine cough; if the patient is asked to say 'aah', the soft palate moves towards the unaffected side.

ACCESSORY NERVE (CRANIAL NERVE XI)

The accessory nerve provides the motor supply to sternomastoid and trapezius muscles. It can be damaged iatrogenically, surgically in neck resections or occasionally in lymph node biopsy or excision. Accessory nerve lesions are often associated with damage to the ninth and tenth nerves and cause ipsilateral sternomastoid weakness (on turning the head away from the affected side) and weakness of the trapezius on shrugging the shoulders. There may be an asymmetric neckline, a drooping shoulder, weakness of forward elevation of the shoulder, and a winged scapula – exaggerated on arm abduction.

Testing this nerve is also useful in differentiating patients with genuine palsies from those with functional complaints since, in an accessory nerve lesion, there is weakness on turning the head away from the affected side but those shamming paralysis often simulate weakness when turning the head towards the 'affected' side.

HYPOGLOSSAL NERVE (CRANIAL NERVE XII)

The hypoglossal nerve is the motor supply to the tongue muscles and may be damaged in its intracranial or extracranial course. A tumour or bone disease at the skull base, stroke, infection of the brainstem, an injury to the neck – such as during endarterectomy, or amyotrophic lateral sclerosis can damage the nerve. Intracranial lesions typically cause bulbar palsy (see later). Disease in the condylar canals, such as Paget disease or bone tumours, and peripheral lesions, such as glomus jugulare, carotid body or other tumours, trauma or radiation damage, can cause an isolated hypoglossal nerve deficit. In a UMN lesion the tongue is spastic but not wasted; in an LMN lesion there is wasting and fibrillation of the affected side (Fig. 13.9).

Hypoglossal lesions cause dysarthria (difficulty in speaking), particularly for lingual sounds, and deviation of the tongue towards the affected side on protrusion.

DISORDERS OF TASTE

The complex process of tasting begins when molecules stimulate special sensory (gustatory or taste) cells in the nose, mouth or throat. Another chemosensory mechanism, the common chemical sense, contributes to appreciation of food flavour, especially to sensations like the sting of ammonia, the coolness of menthol and the irritation of chilli peppers.

Humans can commonly identify at least five different taste sensations: sweet, sour, bitter, salty and umami (the taste elicited by glutamate, found in chicken broth, meat extracts and some cheeses). Flavours are recognized largely through the sense of smell. Taste buds are present on the tongue mainly, but also on the soft palate, uvula, epiglottis, pharynx, larynx and oesophagus. Taste perception can be tested with salt (sodium chloride), sweet (saccharin), acidic (citrus) and bitter (quinine) or by electrogustometry. Disorders of taste (dysgeusia) are fairly common and have a wide range of causes (Table 13.17), similar to those causing halitosis.

Table 13.17 *Causes of taste loss or change*

Cause	Examples
Ageing	–
Local causes	Hyposalivation
	Irradiation of the oral cavity or salivary glands
Drugs	Acetazolamide
	Albuterol
	Amiloride
	Angiotensin-converting enzyme inhibitors (ACEIs)
	Anticholinergics
	Antidepressants
	Antihistamines
	Antihypertensives
	Aspirin
	Azelastine
	Captopril
	Carbimazole
	Chlorhexidine
	Clarithromycin
	Clofibrate
	Cytotoxic agents
	Dorzolamide
	Eszopiclone
	Etoposide
	Gold
	Griseofulvin
	Imipramine
	L-dopa
	Lithium
	Metformin
	Metronidazole
	Penicillamine
	Phenindione
	Protease inhibitors
	Salbutamol (albuterol)
	Terbinafine
	Topiramate
	Zopiclone
Neurological disorders	Alzheimer disease
	Bell palsy
	Carotid dissection
	Encephalitis
	Facial palsy
	Head trauma
	Multiple sclerosis
	Nerve damage (chorda tympani, facial, glossopharyngeal, lingual)
	Parkinson disease
	Posterior cranial fossa disorders
	Riley–Day syndrome
	Temporal lobe epilepsy
Nutritional defects	Cancer
	Vitamin B deficiency
	Zinc deficiency
Endocrinopathies	Addison disease
	Cushing syndrome
	Diabetes
	Hypopituitarism
	Hypothyroidism
Metabolic disorders	Chronic renal failure
	Hepatic disease
Viral infections	Various

Perceived loss of taste usually reflects a smell loss, which is often confused with a taste loss. The sense of taste can also be temporarily disturbed by the use of chemicals such as chlorhexidine.

Rarely, there is complete lack of perception to taste sweet, sour, bitter, salty and umami (ageusia). More commonly, testing may demonstrate a weakened ability to taste (hypogeusia). In other disorders of the chemical senses, the system may misread and/or distort an odour, a taste or a flavour. The most common taste complaint is that of phantom taste perceptions. Alternatively, a person may detect a foul taste from a substance that is normally pleasant-tasting.

Loss of taste can be due to medical disorders, or anaesthesia of the nerves involved, particularly surgery with lingual nerve damage (e.g. resections or third molar extraction); damage to the chorda tympani (from middle ear surgery, herpes zoster oticus, otitis media, mastoiditis or cholesteatoma); upper respiratory infections; head injury; radiation therapy; diabetes; hypertension; malnutrition; chemicals such as insecticides; some drugs (gymnemic acid abolishes the perception of sweet tastes while amiloride abolishes salt perception); or degenerative neurological diseases (Parkinson disease, Alzheimer disease and Korsakoff psychosis).

CEREBROVASCULAR ACCIDENTS, STROKES AND TRANSIENT ISCHAEMIC ATTACKS

General aspects

Blood enters the brain from the two carotid and two vertebral arteries, which branch to supply each specific area of brain. If blood flow from these arteries is interrupted for more than a few seconds, brain cells can die, causing infarction and damage, and resulting in loss of function – a stroke or cerebrovascular accident (CVA) – the syndrome of rapidly developing clinical signs and symptoms of focal and, at times, global disturbance of cerebral function lasting more than 24 hours (or death within that time).

Strokes are a common cause of death (the third leading cause of death, accounting for 1 out of every 15 deaths in the developed world) and disability, especially in older people. The high mortality relates not only to the acute brain damage but also to complications (thrombosis and infection, especially respiratory). A stroke may be preceded by a transient ischaemic attack (TIA), which, by definition, is characterized by a focal neurological deficit that lasts less than 60 minutes and resolves completely within 24 hours. Patients who have had a TIA are at high risk of a stroke and require prompt evaluation. A reversible ischaemic neurological deficit (RIND) is similar but persists for more than 24 hours; again, it is a predictor of a stroke.

The most common cause of CVA is carotid or intracerebral artery atheroma, in which plaque rupture results in arterial occlusion or thrombosis. An embolism from the left side of the heart (a potential complication of atrial fibrillation) may also obstruct cerebral blood flow, and intracerebral or subarachnoid haemorrhages account for the other 20% of strokes. TIAs are typically embolic and cause focal cerebral and neurological deficits. Risk factors for CVA include increasing age, hypertension, atrial fibrillation, ischaemic or valvular heart disease, preceding CVA, diabetes, hypercholesterolaemia, smoking, alcohol, obesity, hyperviscosity syndromes, and prothrombotic and haemorrhagic states. Emboli may also reach the cerebral vessels from fibrillating atria. Rarely, CVAs are secondary to carotid stenosis or dissection; cocaine use; fibromuscular dysplasia; or syphilis. Prevention involves controlling risk factors and taking more exercise.

Clinical features

The clinical manifestations vary according to the duration, severity and pattern of cerebral ischaemia. Typical features include sudden visual deterioration (monocular or homonymous), speech disturbance (expressive or receptive dysphasia) and hemiplegia (loss of voluntary movement of the opposite side of the body to the cerebral lesion). Most patients who sustain an ischaemic or haemorrhagic stoke remain conscious but, if the ischaemia, oedema or haemorrhage is extensive, raised intracranial pressure may impair consciousness – progressing to coma and/or death. Approximately 45% of people with a stroke die within a month; 50% of those who survive 6 months may survive another 7 years. Of survivors, 40% have mild disability, 40% require special care, 10% recover completely and 10% require long-term hospitalization. Prognosis is better in young patients and if there is incomplete paralysis of a limb, no loss of consciousness at onset or later, and no confusion.

Transient ischaemic attacks are typically embolic and may cause focal cerebral deficits such as facial numbness, hemiplegia or dysarthria; about 30% progress to stroke. *Reversible ischaemic neurological deficit* is similar to TIA but persists for more than 24 hours.

Stroke-in-evolution is when such a cerebral deficit persists and worsens. Common symptoms include changes in vision, speech and comprehension, weakness, vertigo, loss of sensation in part of the body, or changes in conscious level.

Typical features of *full stroke* (Table 13.18) include: sudden unconsciousness, often going on to coma or death; hemiplegia (loss of voluntary movement of the opposite side of the body to the brain lesion); changes in speech (slurred, thick, difficult speech or inability to speak – aphasia), often with loss of the ability to write (both the result of a left-sided brain lesion); and visual loss or deterioration, especially in one eye. Other symptoms depend on the area of brain affected, the extent of damage and the cause, but may include numbness, paraesthesia or other sensation changes, or problems with recognizing or identifying sensory stimuli (agnosia), resulting in 'neglect' of one side of the body; difficulty in understanding speech, reading or writing; vertigo; swallowing difficulties; personality or emotional changes, including depression or apathy; loss of bladder or bowel control; and cognitive decline, dementia, ease of distraction, impaired judgment and limited attention.

The four main types of stroke (Table 13.19) are as follows:

- *Cerebral arterial thrombosis*, the most common cause, follows atherosclerosis; it tends to be the least rapid in development and has lowish acute mortality (30%).
- *Intracerebral haemorrhage* mainly affects individuals past middle age and is the most lethal type, with a mortality of 80%. Bleeding into the brain destroys and tears apart the tissue and acts as an expanding lesion, distorting the brain and causing gross cerebral oedema. Predisposing factors are hypertension and atherosclerosis.
- *Subarachnoid haemorrhage* accounts for only about 10% of strokes, originates from a ruptured congenital aneurysm (berry aneurysm) on the arterial circle of Willis (more common in polycystic kidney disease, Ehlers–Danlos syndrome, fibromuscular dysplasia with renal artery stenosis, polyarteritis nodosa and coarctation of the aorta). Hypertension, atherosclerosis, trauma, cocaine or amphetamine abuse, and acute physical or emotional stress may be contributory. Clinically, subarachnoid haemorrhage is characterized by sudden, excruciatingly severe headache, which is quickly followed by coma; unlike other types of stroke, localizing signs, such as hemiplegia, are typically absent. In some cases, slow aneurysm leakage causes headache or minor neurological dysfunction preceding the acute attack. The prognosis is poor: about 30% of patients die from the initial haemorrhage and only 50% survive.
- *Cerebral embolism* is relatively uncommon and usually originates from a fibrillating atrium or intracardiac thrombosis secondary to a myocardial infarct, and rarely from endocarditis or a thrombosed prosthetic heart valve. Embolic strokes are *not* associated with activity levels, can occur at any time, and typically are dramatically sudden and may affect a younger person.

General management

Diagnosis of a CVA is essentially clinical, based upon a history and clinical features. Specific neurological, motor and sensory deficits often correspond closely to the location of the brain damage. Neck stiffness, Brudzinski sign (flexing the neck causes the patient to flex knees and hips) and Kernig sign (flexing the hip 90° and straightening the knee causes pain) become positive in subarachnoid haemorrhage. Examination may also show changes in vision or visual fields, abnormal eye movements, muscle weakness, impaired sensation and other changes. A 'bruit' may be heard over the carotid arteries in the neck.

Table 13.18 *Disability following stroke*[a]

	Right-sided brain lesion	Left-sided brain lesion
Side paralysed	Left	Right
Other deficits	Thought, perception	Language, speech
Other problems	Memory	Memory
	Problems with performing tasks and using mirrors	Problems with organization

[a]See Table 13.19.

Table 13.19 *Clinical features of different types of stroke*

	Haemorrhage		Thrombosis	Embolism
	Intracerebral	Subarachnoid		
Prodrome	–	±	Transient ischaemic attacks (TIAs)	–
Onset	Rapid	Rapid	Gradual	Sudden
First symptom	Headache	Intense headache	Ill-defined	Headache
Progression	Hemiplegia and aphasia	Coma	Gradual and intermittent	Immediate
Underlying diseases	Hypertension	Aneurysm	Hypertension	Atrial fibrillation, etc.
	Atherosclerosis		Atherosclerosis	
Prognosis	High mortality	High mortality	From minimal dysfunction to death in a week	80% recur

There may be signs of atrial fibrillation. It is also important to assess risk factors, including co-morbid medical conditions. MRI or CT may localize the site and assess the degree of cerebral damage. However, MRI is not always possible and CT may be normal in the early stages of ischaemic stroke or in patients with minor symptoms. Cardiac investigations (ECG and echocardiogram) help in arrhythmias and valvular heart disease. Carotid duplex scans assess carotid artery stenosis and arterial blood flow to the brain.

Cerebral arteriography can identify a source of haemorrhage. Brainstem evoked response audiometry and clotting, thrombophilia and vasculitic screens may help. Blood biomarkers of stroke, such as S-100b (a marker of astrocytic activation), B-type neurotrophic growth factor, von Willebrand factor, matrix metalloproteinase-9 and monocyte chemotactic protein-1, have yet to be proved superior to conventional investigations.

Virtually all stroke victims or those with developing stroke should be admitted early to hospital for assessment and management, the goal being to prevent a stroke or to prevent its spread, and to maximize the patient's ability to function. The time of the stroke, progression and conscious level (using the Glasgow Coma Scale; Ch. 24) should be recorded. Early treatment in a dedicated stroke unit lowers mortality and morbidity. Supportive care includes protection of the airway with appropriate ventilatory support; speech and language assessment; keeping the patient nil by mouth if swallowing is impaired, and placing a nasogastric tube to reduce the risk of an aspiration pneumonia; pressure-sensitive nursing to avoid the development of bed sores; urinary catheterization and incontinence pads if urethral and anal sphincteric reflexes are impaired; physiotherapy to reduce muscle wasting and disuse atrophy; and occupational therapy for long-term rehabilitation. The airway must be protected during the acute phase and, for virtually all strokes, hospitalization is required, possibly including intensive care, life support and oxygen.

It is essential to establish the type of stroke since patients under good care have mortality reduced by 25% and recurrence by a similar amount. The degree of disability can be assessed according to one of several scales (e.g. the Barthel Index, Glasgow Outcome Scale, Hunt and Hess Classification of Subarachnoid Hemorrhage, Modified Rankin Scale or NIH Stroke Scale). Anticoagulation may be useful if it is certain that the stroke is thrombotic or embolic. Alteplase is recommended for ischaemic stroke. Recombinant tissue plasminogen activator (RTPA) lyses clots and potentially restores blood flow to the affected area to prevent further cell death and permanent damage, but there are strict criteria because of the risk of serious bleeding for those who can receive it. The most important is that the stroke victim be evaluated and treated by a specialized stroke team within 3 hours of onset of symptoms. Aspirin and other antiplatelet drugs are also used to prevent non-haemorrhagic strokes.

Antihypertensive medication is frequently indicated. Control of atrial fibrillation is needed to prevent recurrent strokes. Analgesics are required to control severe headache. Nimodipine (a calcium antagonist) helps reduce intracranial vasospasm.

Surgical treatment may include emergency neurosurgery or interventional neuroradiology to clip or glue a leaking aneurysm, or evacuate a large intracerebral bleed. Carotid endarterectomy facilitates removal of atheroma to improve blood flow to the cerebral arteries.

Precautions must be taken in the later care of the comatose patient, to prevent pressure sores and sometimes urinary catheterization or bladder/bowel control programmes are needed to control incontinence. If the person has swallowing difficulties, nutrients and fluids may be given through an intravenous line or via a nasogastric or gastrostomy tube. Longer-term care involves rehabilitation, based on the symptoms, and prevention of future strokes. Recovery is possible as other areas of the brain take over functioning for the damaged areas. Depression and other symptoms should be treated. People should stay active within their physical limitations but safety must be considered, since some stroke victims appear to have no awareness of their surroundings on the affected side. Friends and family members should repeatedly reinforce important cues, like name, age, date, time and where they live, to help reduce disorientation. Communication may require pictures, demonstration, verbal cues or other strategies, depending on the type and extent of language deficit. In-home care, nursing homes, adult day care or convalescent homes may be needed to provide a safe environment, control aggressive or agitated behaviour, and meet physiological needs. Visiting nurses or aides, volunteer services, homemakers, adult protective services and other community resources may be helpful. Speech therapy, occupational therapy, physical therapy, positioning, range-of-motion exercises, and other therapies may prevent complications and promote maximum recovery of function. Legal action may make it easier to make ethical decisions regarding the care of the person with organic brain syndromes such as stroke.

For TIAs or RIND, aspirin reduces the chance of progression to full stroke. Antihypertensive medication is frequently indicated. Otherwise, the investigations are as above for stroke.

Dental aspects

Many patients with a stroke initially suffer confusion and emotional lability; therefore, encouragement is an extremely important motivating factor. Access, mobility and communication may be impaired in many, since they may have cognitive and visual defects, as well as dysarthria, aphasia, confusion, memory loss, and emotional distress and depression. Support with preventive care is critical; oral hygiene tends to deteriorate on the paralysed side, and impaired manual dexterity may interfere with tooth-brushing. Use of an electric toothbrush or adapted holders may help.

Dentists should defer elective and invasive dental care for 3–6 months. It is important to communicate clearly with the patient by not wearing a mask, by facing the patient and by speaking slowly and clearly, using language that is not complex. Short treatment sessions in mid-morning are desirable for these patients, who are best treated in the upright position, with extra care taken to prevent foreign bodies from entering the pharynx. The practitioner needs to monitor blood pressure and anticoagulation status before beginning any dental treatment.

Dental management modifications in a patient with a stroke may also include consideration of problems relating to loss of protective reflexes, such as swallowing and gag reflexes in brainstem lesions. Patients are best treated sitting upright and extra care must be taken to avoid foreign bodies entering the pharynx. Good suction must be at hand.

Subarachnoid or cerebral haemorrhage can be precipitated by acute hypertension and, in the past, has resulted from the use of noradrenaline (norepinephrine) in LA. Cerebral haemorrhage can also stem from hypertension caused by interactions of MAOIs with other drugs, particularly pethidine (meperidine). Opioids are best avoided in strokes, as they may cause severe hypotension and these and benzodiazepines may cause respiratory depression. It is thus important to have short stress-free treatment sessions in mid-morning and to monitor blood pressure; use the minimal amount of adrenaline (epinephrine) in LA; avoid the use of adrenaline-containing gingival retraction cords; and possibly avoid electronic dental analgesia.

Multidisciplinary care is required for modifications related to anticoagulation, hypertension, cardiovascular disease, diabetes mellitus or old age.

After a stroke, patients may have unilateral (UMN) facial palsy. Oral hygiene tends to deteriorate on the paralysed side and impaired manual dexterity may interfere with tooth-brushing. An electric toothbrush may help. Oropharyngeal dysphagia post-stroke in around 50% of patients makes a significant contribution to morbidity and mortality, since it predisposes to respiratory infection, malnutrition and weight loss.

Strokes are a possible cause of sudden loss of consciousness in the dental surgery and should be recognizable, especially by the sudden loss of consciousness and, usually, signs of one-sided paralysis as already described. Protection of the airway and a call for an ambulance are the only useful immediate measures (Ch. 1).

Calcified atherosclerotic plaques may sometimes be detected on dental panoramic radiographs.

LOCKED-IN SYNDROME

Locked-in syndrome is a condition in which a patient is aware and awake, but cannot move or communicate due to complete paralysis of nearly all voluntary muscles. It is usually due to a brainstem lesion, such as a stroke, trauma, infection or tumour, but higher centres remain intact. Some patients can move certain facial muscles, most often some extraocular eye muscles. There is a 90% early mortality. Of survivors, most do not regain motor control but assistive computer interface technologies may help patients to communicate.

MOVEMENT DISORDERS

Muscles may move without the person meaning them to. For example, tiny muscle twitches (fasciculations) may indicate nerve damage to that muscle. Other possible involuntary movements are rhythmic movements of a body part (tremor), twitches (tics), sudden flinging of a limb (hemiballismus), quick fidgety movements (chorea) or snake-like writhing (athetosis), all of which suggest motor incoordination due to basal ganglia disease. Muscle tone that is evenly increased (rigidity) may be due to Parkinson disease. Muscle tone is severely reduced (flaccid) immediately and temporarily after a spinal cord injury produces paralysis. Muscle tone that is uneven and suddenly increased (spasticity) may be due to a stroke or spinal cord injury.

One of the most common involuntary movements is a tremor, which may have many causes – essential tremor, Parkinson disease, Huntington chorea and cerebellar disease (Table 13.20).

PARKINSON DISEASE (PD; PARALYSIS AGITANS)

General aspects

Parkinson disease (PD) is a common but serious brain disorder that causes trembling, muscle rigidity, difficulty in walking, and problems with balance and coordination; its prevalence increases with age. PD affects mainly the basal ganglia with degeneration of the substantia nigra pigmented cells that normally release dopamine – the neurotransmitter that travels between the substantia nigra and corpus striatum, which enables muscles to make smooth controlled movements. Profound depletion of nigrostriatal dopamine results in disequilibrium of the extrapyramidal motor circuits and development of parkinsonism (i.e. tremor, bradykinesia and rigidity).

PD usually affects people over the age of 50. Most cases are idiopathic and people who have an affected first-degree relative are at three times greater risk of developing it themselves. *PINK1* mutations tend to be diagnosed as the early-onset autosomal recessive form of PD. Parkinsonism may also be caused by cerebrovascular disease, head injury (particularly in boxers), drugs (particularly phenothiazines and butyrophenones [dopamine receptor blockers], valproate, metoclopramide and prochlorperazine), and (rarely) encephalitis lethargica (von Economo disease). Severe parkinsonism has followed the use of an illicitly manufactured opioid (methyl phenyl tetrahydropyridine, MPTP) and this led to the suggestion that many cases of apparently idiopathic disease are due to environmental toxins, such as pesticides, herbicides, manganese, heavy metals or carbon monoxide. PD is more common in people who are engaged in farming, live in rural areas or drink well water. Lower oestrogen levels may also raise the risk of PD; menopausal women who receive little or no hormone replacement therapy (HRT) and those who have had hysterectomies may be at higher risk, while menopausal women using HRT appear to have a decreased risk.

Clinical features

The earliest features of PD can be as subtle as an arm that does not swing when walking, a mild tremor in the fingers, or soft or mumbling speech that is difficult to understand. The primary features are:

- tremor, or trembling in hands, arms, legs, jaw and face
- rigidity, or stiffness of limbs and trunk
- bradykinesia, or slowness of movement
- postural instability, or impaired balance and coordination.

Early symptoms of PD are subtle and often occur gradually. PD is chronic and progressive and, as the disease follows its course, the tremor may begin to interfere with daily activities. As features become more pronounced, patients may have difficulty walking, talking or completing other simple tasks. Other features may include depression

Table 13.20 *Motor abnormalities: terms, features and main causes*

Disorder	Features	Main causes
Akathisia	Restlessness	Neuroleptic drugs
Akinesia	Lack of movement	Parkinsonism
Athetosis	Dystonia of limbs	Athetoid cerebral palsy
Chorea	Continual flow of jerky movements	Huntington and Sydenham chorea (rheumatic fever)
Clonus	Rhythmic contractions	Upper motor neuron (UMN) lesions
Dyskinesia	Involuntary chewing or grinding	Phenothiazines
Dystonia	Sustained spasms causing abnormal posture	Phenothiazines
Fasciculation	Spontaneous contractions of muscle fibres	Lower motor neuron (LMN) lesions
Hemiballismus	Chorea affecting half of the body	Subthalamic lesion
Rigidity	Limbs resist passive movement	Parkinsonism
Spasticity	Excess tone in arm flexors, leg extensors	Cerebral palsy; UMN lesion
Tremor	Rhythmic movements of a part at rest	Parkinsonism, anxiety, drugs, thyrotoxicosis, benign, or brain lesion. Worse with anxiety; better with alcohol, benzodiazepines or beta-blockers
	On intention to move	Cerebellar disease

and other emotional changes; difficulty in swallowing, chewing and speaking; urinary problems; constipation; skin problems; and sleep disruption (Box 13.6 and Fig. 13.10).

Many people with PD develop voices that become monotonous and very soft, a special problem for older adults because the voice may not be audible to a partner with poor hearing. Even the functioning of the digestive tract may slow down, causing difficulties with swallowing, digestion and elimination, and constipation is often a major problem. PD may cause either urinary incontinence or urine retention, and anticholinergic drugs used to treat the disease make it hard to urinate. Bradykinesia may progress to akinesia and total rigidity.

Complications of PD may include subtle psychiatric disorders, deformities of the hands and feet, ocular abnormalities, urinary and gastrointestinal disturbances, and autonomic dysfunction (which may cause mild postural hypotension, disordered respiratory control and hypersalivation that, with the movement defect, may result in drooling). The face in PD is often expressionless and there is a loss of the blink reflex as a response to gentle tapping of the bridge of the nose. Oculogyric crises may be seen in drug-induced or post-encephalitic disease.

General management

There are no diagnostic tests for PD.

Supportive care is required. Treatment aims to enhance brain dopamine – but treatment with dopamine itself is impossible, since it fails to cross the blood–brain barrier. Drug treatment with dopaminergic agents aims to increase dopamine by increasing L-dopa; by inhibiting dopamine breakdown; or by using agonists of dopamine (Table 13.21) hopefully with minimal adverse effects such as confusion; may interfere with driving; may cause fibrotic reactions (lungs, heart, retroperitoneal); and may cause impulse control disorders (e.g. gambling, hypersexuality, or binge eating). Symptom relief may be possible with L-dopa combined with carbidopa – which delays the conversion of L-dopa into dopamine until it reaches the brain. Bradykinesia and rigidity respond best, while tremor may be only marginally reduced. Monoamine oxidase inhibitors such as rasagiline or seligiline enhance L-dopa activities (see below). Dopaminergic drugs may cause daytime sleepiness.

Other drugs, such as bromocriptine, pramipexole and ropinirole, mimic dopamine. Anticholinergics (antimuscarinic drugs) reduce tremor and rigidity, and they (or catechol-*O*-methyl transferase [COMT] inhibitors such as entacapone or tolcapone) may be given together with L-dopa in severe cases.

Box 13.6 *Features of parkinsonism*

- Tremor – mainly affecting the hands (pill-rolling) and arms, and worst at rest. Tremors also may develop in the head, lips or feet
- Rigidity – the arms are flexed and held stiffly at the sides. Limb movement has a so-called cog-wheel rigidity
- Abnormal posture – the neck and shoulders are rigid, causing a stooping posture
- Restlessness (akathisia) – typical
- Slowness (bradykinesia) – slowness in the initiation and execution of movements and poverty of spontaneous movements. The patient may be slow at starting to walk but then runs forwards (festinant gait) or shuffles with slow short steps. Speech may be affected

---

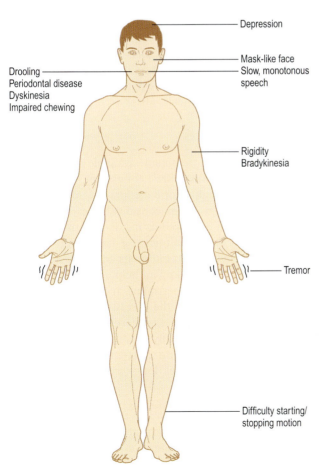

Fig. 13.10 Parkinsonism.

Depression

Mask-like face
Slow, monotonous speech

Drooling
Periodontal disease
Dyskinesia
Impaired chewing

Rigidity
Bradykinesia

Tremor

Difficulty starting/
stopping motion

Table 13.21 *Drug treatment in Parkinson disease*

Drug examples	Action	Comments
L-dopa (levodopa); usually given with inhibitor of degradative enzyme dopa decarboxylase, e.g. carbidopa (co-careldopa) or benserazide (co-beneldopa)	Replaces dopamine	L-dopa is converted into dopamine in the brain and may improve akinesia and imbalance. Adverse effects include involuntary movements (dyskinesia), nausea, arrhythmias, liver dysfunction, depression, psychoses and hallucinations. L-dopa is contraindicated in glaucoma
Bromocriptine Pergolide Lysuride Ropinirole Cabergoline Pramipexole Apomorphine (injection)	Dopamine agonists	Useful when L-dopa cannot be tolerated, but can cause hypotension or serious neuropsychiatric adverse effects, and pulmonary, retroperitoneal and pericardial fibrosis
Amantadine	Acts like a dopamine agonist	An antiviral
Monoamine oxidase B (MAO-B) inhibitor (selegiline)	Inhibits MAO-B and thus dopamine breakdown	Toxic reactions have occurred in some patients who took selegiline with the narcotic pethidine (meperidine)
Catechol-*O*-methyl transferase (COMT) inhibitors	Block the liver enzyme that breaks down dopamine and dopa	Tolcapone has been linked to liver damage and liver failure. Entacapone may help manage fluctuations in the response to L-dopa in people with Parkinson disease
Trihexyphenidyl/benzhexol Benzatropine Orphenadrine Procyclidine	Anticholinergics (block acetylcholine)	Effective at reducing tremor at rest

Propargylamine MAOIs demonstrate antioxidant and antiapoptotic activity. The physiological role of MAO is to catalyse the biotransformation of a variety of arylalkylamine neurotransmitters, such as dopamine, adrenaline (epinephrine), noradrenaline (norepinephrine) and serotonin, as well as to detoxify biogenic amines, such as tyramine. MAO-B found within glial cells is the predominant isoform responsible for breakdown of dopamine to 3,4-dihydroxyphenylacetic acid and homovanillic acid (HVA), as well as deamination of alpha-phenylethylamine, an endogenous amine that stimulates the release of dopamine and inhibits its neuronal reuptake. Selective inhibition of MAO-B increases synaptosomal dopamine concentrations. Therefore, selective inhibition of brain MAO-B is pharmacologically desirable for treating PD. Rasagiline potently and completely inhibits MAO-B and increases basal synaptosomal levels of striatal dopamine. Rasagiline mesylate (*N*-propargyl-1[R]-aminoindan) is a second-generation, selective and irreversible inhibitor of MAO-B, and is therefore used along with L-dopa for patients with advanced PD or as a single-drug treatment for early PD.

An antiviral, amantadine, also appears to reduce symptoms. Adenosine A(2A) receptor antagonists may prove useful in the future. Rotigotine, a non-ergoline dopamine agonist is available as a transdermal preparation.

Deep brain stimulation (DBS), which involves implanting a brain stimulator, similar to a heart pacemaker, within the subthalamic nucleus, may reduce tremors, slowness of movements and gait problems, as well as the need for L-dopa and related drugs; this in turn decreases the dyskinesias that are a common adverse effect of L-dopa. The device can also be placed in the thalamus for tremor control or the globus pallidus to produce effects similar to pallidotomy. Neurosurgery may reduce tremor but carries a number of risks, including slurred speech, disabling weakness and vision problems, especially when performed bilaterally. Thalamotomy, the destruction of small amounts of tissue in the thalamus, is useful to reduce tremor. Pallidotomy, use of an electric current to destroy a small amount of tissue in the pallidum (globus pallidus), may improve tremors, rigidity and slowed movement but benefits do not always persist.

Experimentally, brain grafts of fetal substantia nigral tissue have been given but their value is as yet unclear; one large study reported that as many as 15% of recipients developed severe dyskinesias as a result of *excess* dopamine.

Dental aspects

It is essential in patients with PD not to let the blankness of expression and apparent unresponsiveness be mistaken for lack of reaction or intelligence. Sympathetic handling is particularly important, as anxiety increases tremor, which may affect the tongue and/or lips. Patients should be raised upright only cautiously and carefully assisted out of the dental chair, since parkinsonism, L-dopa and some other agents may cause hypotension. The movements, drooling and head positioning associated with PD can make the use of sharp and rotating instruments hazardous and may compromise restorative care. L-dopa in combination with a dopa-decarboxylase inhibitor may interact with adrenaline (epinephrine) to cause tachycardia, arrhythmias and hypertension. Adrenaline may interact with COMT inhibitors (tolcapone, entacapone) to cause tachycardia, arrhythmias and hypertension; therefore, LA without adrenaline should be used in these patients. Erythromycin and other macrolides may increase levels of bromocriptine or cabergoline. Pergolide may rarely induce cardiac valvulopathy; pramipexole may cause sudden onset of sleepiness. It is important not to stop anti-Parkinsonian medication, since this might precipitate the neuroleptic malignant syndrome (Ch. 10).

Conscious sedation (CS) should be safe. Pethidine (meperidine) should be avoided in patients receiving selegiline or other MAOIs,

since a serious interaction is possible. Selegiline differs from other MAOIs in that it should not cause acute hypertensive episodes when it is used with most other drugs.

Drooling of saliva may be troublesome; injection of botulinum toxoid into salivary glands significantly decreases saliva production, which may be beneficial. Orofacial involuntary movements (dyskinesia), such as 'flycatcher tongue' and lip-pursing, are side-effects of L-dopa and bromocriptine, and may make the use of rotating dental instruments more hazardous.

L-dopa may cause taste disturbances and reddish saliva. Antimuscarinic drugs may produce dry mouth.

Drills and ultrasonic scalers are safe to use in a patient with a DBS pacemaker but check that it is still switched on after treatment.

HUNTINGTON CHOREA

General aspects

Huntington chorea is an autosomal dominant condition related to a gene on chromosome 4 and the protein huntingtin. It is due to atrophy of the caudate nucleus of the basal ganglia and characterized by involuntary movements (chorea), emotional disturbances and progressive dementia; currently, it is incurable.

Clinical features

The name *chorea* comes from the Greek for 'dance' and refers to the characteristic and incessant quick, jerky and involuntary movements.

Signs and symptoms usually appear in early to middle age (30–50 years) and may include: involuntary jerky movements of fingers, feet, arms, neck, trunk and face; hesitant, halting or slurred speech; clumsiness or poor balance; wide, prancing gait; personality changes (moodiness, paranoia); and deterioration in cognitive function (memory, attention, decision-making).

Progress of disease is slow, often leading to difficulty walking so that patients become chair-bound. Life is often ended by intercurrent infection, or sometimes suicide, since patients are usually aware of the family history and poor prognosis.

General management

There is no satisfactory treatment available to stop or reverse Huntington disease and thus genetic counselling, though available, is not always taken up. A high-calorie diet may be advised, as the involuntary movements can burn up considerable calories. Medications may help. Some signs and symptoms may be controlled by neuroleptics (e.g. clonazepam). Antipsychotics (e.g. haloperidol and clozapine) help control movements, violent outbursts and hallucinations. Speech therapy can be valuable. Lithium can help control extreme emotions and mood swings. Fluoxetine, sertraline and nortriptyline can assist in the control of depression and the obsessive–compulsive rituals that some people with Huntington disease develop. Most individuals who have Huntington disease eventually become physically and mentally disabled, and therefore may require short-term psychiatric hospitalization and, as the disease progresses, long-term nursing care.

Dental aspects

Patients can often understand what they are being told but may be unable to respond; this can give a false impression of the degree of dementia.

There may be darting movements of the head and tongue that subside somewhat if physical control is applied. The chorea can make operative dentistry or the construction and wearing of prostheses difficult or nigh impossible; general anaesthesia (GA) or CS may then help but especial care must be taken to protect the airway at all times. Oral hygiene may be impaired through reduced manual dexterity, and a predilection to caries and periodontal disease is worsened by medications that cause xerostomia or by a high-calorie diet unless thought is given to avoiding cariogenicity. Orofacial trauma may occur.

NEURAL TUBE DEFECTS (SPINA BIFIDA)

See Chapter 28.

POLIOMYELITIS

General aspects

Anterior poliomyelitis (polio) is an enteroviral infection, spread faeco-orally, that may damage the lower motor neurons and sometimes motor cranial nerves. Rare in the developed world since the introduction of an effective vaccine, it is still common in developing countries; it appears in the developed world in some immigrants or where vaccine uptake is poor.

Clinical features

Typically causing wasting and paralysis of a lower limb, polio may affect other areas, including the medulla oblongata, when it can cause bulbar palsy and respiratory paralysis.

General management

Patients with respiratory paralysis must be artificially ventilated (on an 'iron lung') permanently.

Dental aspects

Patients with bulbar palsy or a high-level spinal lesion may also have impaired gag and cough reflexes, and thus their airway must be carefully protected. Good suction must be used. Patients with quadriplegia may benefit from the dentist constructing a mouthstick or bitestick appliance with which they can perform manual functions or operate a computer, telephone and other means of communication. Those with paraplegia require care similar to persons with spina bifida (see Ch. 28).

SPINAL CORD DAMAGE AND PARAPLEGIA

See Chapter 28.

ABNORMAL FACIAL MOVEMENTS

Dystonias

Dystonias are a group of uncommon basal ganglia diseases characterized by abnormal movements associated with muscle spasm, and are focal or generalized. An example of focal dystonia is torticollis. Most dystonias are primary (a neurological disorder cannot be identified). Those that result from defined organic diseases affecting the brain are known as secondary dystonias.

Oromandibular dystonia refers to recurrent spasmodic episodes of lip movement, tongue protrusion and retraction, and jaw clenching or opening. This may be associated with blepharospasm, and respiratory muscles and speech may be impaired. Over one-third of patients may suffer from depression. Treatment is difficult but benzodiazepines may be helpful.

Acute oromandibular dystonia (drug-induced parkinsonism) can appear within a short time (hours or days) of starting treatment with neuroleptics, such as phenothiazines and butyrophenones. It may resolve after withdrawal of the drug or be improved with antimuscarinics such as benzatropine. However, it is made worse by L-dopa, which can itself also cause involuntary spasmodic movements if the dose is too great.

Torticollis

Torticollis (from the Latin *torti* – twisted – and *collis* – neck) refers to the neck being held in a twisted or bent position. It can be congenital or acquired.

Infants born with torticollis appear healthy at delivery, but over days to weeks develop soft-tissue swelling over an injured sternocleidomastoid due to birth trauma or intrauterine malpositioning. This mass, which may be confused with a branchial cleft cyst, regresses and leaves a fibrous band in place of the muscle, causing contracture of the neck.

Acquired torticollis or idiopathic spasmodic torticollis is a focal dystonia known as acute wry-neck; it is the type most frequently encountered and develops overnight in young and middle-aged adults. Symptoms usually resolve spontaneously within 2 weeks with use of heat, massage, supportive cervical collar, muscle relaxants and analgesics. Torticollis may be associated with other forms of focal dystonia, such as blepharospasm, writer's cramp, spasmodic dysphonia or orobuccal dystonia.

Dyskinesias

Dyskinesias are abnormal movements of the tongue or facial muscles, sometimes with abnormal jaw movements, bruxism or dysphagia.

Common dyskinesias are involuntary tongue protrusion and retraction, and facial grimacing. Tardive dyskinesia is usually a late (hence tardive) complication of long-term treatment with neuroleptics. It is somewhat similar to oromandibular dystonia. It rarely responds to withdrawal of the offending drug, is usually made worse by giving antimuscarinics, and may be resistant to treatment.

Facial tics

Most facial tics are benign spasms (habit spasms) and usually affect children. Common tics are blinking, grimacing, shaking the head, clearing the throat, coughing or shrugging. Emotion or fatigue intensifies tics but the natural history is of spontaneous remission. If the tic is persistent, haloperidol may be helpful.

Gilles de la Tourette syndrome

This includes tics and compulsive behavioural rituals, sometimes with coprolalia (utterance of obscenities).

Hemifacial spasm and blepharospasm

Hemifacial spasm (clonic facial spasm) mainly affects adults, particularly older people, with a spasm that involves especially the angle of mouth or the eyelid and worsens towards evening. Many cases of hemifacial spasm are idiopathic, but some herald a cerebellopontine angle lesion or other lesion and some follow facial palsy. Occasionally, facial paralysis or trigeminal neuralgia follows.

Blepharospasm is a spasm of both eyelids that may be seen in the elderly, either in isolation or with hemifacial spasm.

Local injections of botulinum toxin into the affected muscles may give relief for up to 3 months but must be given with extreme care, as there is a hazard of corneal exposure and glaucoma.

Facial myokymia

Facial myokymia is a rare but serious condition in which there are continuous fine, worm-like contractions of one or more facial muscles, especially the perioral or periorbital muscles. It must be distinguished from facial hemispasm, facial tics or blepharospasm (which involves several muscles synchronously), and from benign fasciculation and myokymia of the lower eyelid, which are quite innocuous.

Facial myokymia starts suddenly, lasts for variable periods and is unaffected by voluntary movements; it is frequently associated with multiple sclerosis, brainstem or posterior cranial fossa tumours, or other neurological disorders. Neurological assessment is crucial.

Myoclonus

Myoclonus refers to a quick, abnormal, involuntary muscle jerk, that usually comes infrequently or many times a minute. In severe cases, it can distort movement and limit the ability to walk, talk and eat. Jerking leg movements while the person is at rest used to be called myoclonus, but they are now referred to as periodic leg movements (restless legs syndrome). Myoclonus can be normal if it only affects persons as they fall asleep (hypnic jerks). However, it can also be a sign of drug adverse effects (e.g. amitriptyline); metabolic disorders, such as hepatic or renal failure or hyponatraemia; or CNS disorders, such as infection, viral encephalitis or Creutzfeldt–Jakob disease, brain damage (trauma or stroke), multiple sclerosis, epilepsy, Parkinson disease or Alzheimer disease.

Treatment of myoclonus is usually with anticonvulsants.

BOTULINUM TOXIN

Botulinum toxins are increasingly used, especially in cosmetic surgery, but they are neurotoxins and severe, life-threatening, respiratory muscle problems and death have occasionally occurred when the toxin has spread through the body.

Botulinum toxin type A (Botox [Allergan]: BTX; Dysport (Ipsen); Xeomin [Merz Pharma]) is one of seven distinct neurotoxins produced by *Clostridium botulinum*. It has high specificity and potency, and *small* doses of purified, sterilized toxin may be injected to block the release of acetylcholine and thus temporarily paralyse muscles. It is widely used to paralyse facial muscles to improve the appearance of moderate to severe frown lines between the eyebrows (glabellar lines) or other wrinkles for up to 120 days.

Botulinum toxin type A has been used for an extensive range of conditions but there is most evidence that it can be useful to treat blepharospasm, hemifacial spasm and cervical dystonia. It also acts on cholinergic synapses in the autonomic nervous system, and injection into salivary glands significantly decreases saliva production, which may be beneficial for patients with sialorrhoea, such as in Parkinson disease or amyotrophic lateral sclerosis. There are no randomized controlled trials of botulinum toxoid in a range of applications (orofacial pain syndromes, cluster headache, chronic paroxysmal hemicrania, trigeminal neuralgia) and only a few small-sized trials in others (cervicogenic headache, chronic neck pain, temporomandibular disorders).

Botox should be injected no more frequently than once every 3 months and the lowest effective dose should be used. Botulinum toxin type A is contraindicated for use in pregnancy and neuromuscular disorders. Air travel should be avoided for 72 hours, as a decrease in pressure may affect distribution of the toxin. The most common adverse events following injection of Botox are generally temporary but can last several months, and include headache, respiratory infection, an influenza syndrome, blepharoptosis (droopy eyelids) and nausea. In less than 3%, adverse reactions may include pain in the face, redness at the injection site and muscle weakness. Botulinum toxin type A has occasionally caused severe, life-threatening breathing problems and death. These symptoms occurred as soon as one day and as late as several weeks after botulinum toxin type A injections were given.

Botulinum toxin type B (BoNTB; Myobloc) acts at a slightly different site from toxin A, and is used to treat cervical dystonia. It may cause severe xerostomia and many of the adverse effects seen with botulinum toxin type A. Botulinum toxin type B has occasionally caused severe, life-threatening breathing problems and death as soon as one day and as late as several weeks after injections were given.

DEMYELINATING AND DEGENERATIVE DISEASES

MULTIPLE (DISSEMINATED) SCLEROSIS

General aspects

Multiple sclerosis (MS) is the most common demyelinating disease of young adults, especially women. There is a high prevalence in northern Europe and North America, and there may be a familial predisposition. MS is thought to be an autoimmune disease in genetically susceptible individuals, perhaps of viral aetiology, and possibly due to human herpes virus 6 (HHV-6), with autoantibodies directed against myelin sheath proteins. Vitamin D is possibly associated with some protection against MS and reduced relapse risk in certain patients. It is a chronic relapsing disorder, characterized by the formation of 'plaques' (areas of demyelination) throughout the CNS. Inflammation of and damage to the myelin sheath with multiple areas of scarring (sclerosis) impair muscle coordination, visual sensation and other nerve signals.

Clinical features

The hallmark of MS is a series of neurological deficits, distributed in time and space, that are not explained by any other causes. Up to 35% of cases are subclinical. Clinical features depend on the area of the CNS affected and may include fatigue, dizziness, numbness, weakness or paralysis in a limb, brief pain, tingling or electric-shock sensations, tremor, lack of coordination or unsteady gait, visual disturbances causing diplopia or a moving field of vision and pain on eye movement (optic neuritis), urinary incontinence, constipation and sexual dysfunction, or cognitive changes (memory loss and impaired concentration). Nystagmus, ataxia, jerky (scanning) speech, tremors and loss of muscular coordination develop as a result of cerebellar involvement. Occasionally, mental changes, such as forgetfulness or confusion, occur. MS varies in severity and speed of evolution, ranging from a mild illness to one that results in permanent disability (Table 13.22). As the disease progresses, muscle spasms, vision loss, problems with bladder, bowel or sexual function, and paralysis may develop and,

Table 13.22 *Multiple sclerosis (MS) subtypes*

Subtype	Frequency	Features
Relapsing–remitting	80%+	Short acute attacks about once each year
Primary progressive	10%	Progressive deterioration from outset
Secondary progressive	Uncommon	Progressive deterioration in patients with relapsing–remitting MS, after approximately 10 years
Progressive–relapsing	Rare	Relapses in patients with primary progressive MS

ultimately, there can be widespread paralysis, loss of sphincter control and urinary incontinence.

General management

Diagnosis is assisted by MRI to identify demyelinating disease (T2-weighted MRI shows demyelinating plaques and gadolinium-enhancing lesions); delayed visual evoked response potentials (VEPs) and CSF examination may demonstrate a slightly raised white cell count, increased protein concentration and oligoclonal bands indicating intrathecal immunoglobulin synthesis.

Management requires a multidisciplinary team. Symptomatic care may include physical and occupational therapy, counselling and drugs.

There is no specific reliably effective treatment for MS, but acute episodes may be ameliorated by disease-modifying agents (DMAs) beta-interferons (interferon-beta-1b and beta-1a) and glatiramer – an immunomodulator that shifts pro-inflammatory T-helper 1 (Th1) cells to regulatory Th2 cells that suppress the inflammatory response. Neither interferon nor glatiramer is recommended by the National Institute for Health and Care Excellence (NICE) for the treatment of MS in England and Wales. Other potent anti-inflammatory agents like natalizumab (a monoclonal antibody that inhibits leukocyte migration in the CNS) and alemtuzumab are increasingly used, particularly in patients with breakthrough disease activity. Mitoxantrone – a topoisomerase inhibitor – may help in severe attacks. Dimethyl fumarate (Tecfidera) is approved for use in adults with relapsing forms of MS. Intravenous immunoglobulin has a positive effect in relapsing and advanced MS. Corticosteroids promote remission in acute episodes but do not influence long-term prognosis. Low-dose methotrexate is also used. Oral fumarate appears to reduce disease activity significantly in relapsing–remitting MS. Experimental approaches include plasma exchange. Muscle relaxants (baclofen, tizanidine, dantrolene and benzodiazepine) may reduce pain from spastic muscle paralysis. Antidepressants (e.g. fluoxetine), the antiviral amantadine or modafinil (a medication used for narcolepsy) may reduce fatigue.

Dental aspects

There are no specific oral manifestations of MS but this diagnosis should always be considered in a young patient presenting with trigeminal neuralgia, particularly if bilateral, or if there have been other neurological disturbances, or if the pain lasts minutes or hours. It may respond to carbamazepine. Other presentations may include cerebellar tremor; abnormal speech; abnormal perioral sensation, such as extreme hypersensitivity or anaesthesia; or facial palsy, myokymia or hemispasm. Atropinics used in the treatment of bladder dysfunction may cause dry mouth, as may tizanidine. Glatiramer may cause facial oedema.

Dental preventive care and treatment are important since oral hygiene may be poor. Limited mobility and psychological disorders may interfere with routine dental treatment. Patients with severe MS are best not treated fully supine, as respiration may be embarrassed. Treatment is best carried out under LA if possible. Nitrous oxide is probably best avoided since it may theoretically cause demyelination. Some patients are on corticosteroids, with attendant complications (Ch. 6).

GUILLAIN–BARRÉ SYNDROME (INFECTIVE OR IDIOPATHIC POLYNEURITIS)

General aspects

Guillain–Barré syndrome (GBS) appears to be an immunologically mediated disorder mainly of peripheral nerves, which may follow bacterial infections (campylobacteriosis, from eating undercooked food, especially poultry); viral infections (approximately two-thirds of people affected by GBS have had an infection, such as sore throat, diarrhoea, cold or influenza, or EBV or CMV infection, up to 4 weeks before the onset); or operations (5–10% of all cases). GBS occasionally follows vaccinations (within 1.5–5 weeks of vaccination).

Clinical features

GBS is a serious neurological disorder characterized by subacute onset of progressive, symmetrical weakness in the arms and legs. There is loss of reflexes, and there may be sensory abnormalities, respiratory paralysis and involvement of the cranial nerves. There is a low mortality, and 20% of hospitalized patients can suffer prolonged disability. GBS can be devastating because of its sudden onset; signs and symptoms usually appear rapidly over the course of a single day, and may include weakness, paraesthesia or loss of sensation in legs and feet, or in arms or upper body, with hypoaesthesia, paraesthesia or moderate pain throughout the body. Difficulty with breathing, eye and facial movement, speaking, chewing or swallowing, and paralysis of legs and arms, may follow. There may be bradycardia, hypotension and difficulty with bladder or intestinal control. Generally, GBS progresses quickly, with most patients experiencing the most profound weakness in the legs, arms, chest and other areas within 3 weeks. In some cases, GBS may progress very rapidly with complete paralysis of legs, arms and respiration over a few hours. Recovery may take as little as a few weeks or as long as a few years, and up to 30% have some residual weakness after 3 years.

Miller Fisher syndrome is a rare variant of GBS, characterized by ataxia, ophthalmoplegia and areflexia.

General management

Diagnosis is confirmed by lumbar puncture and EMG. Hospitalization is required and treatment approaches include plasmapheresis, intravenous immunoglobulin and physiotherapy.

MOTOR NEURON DISEASE

General aspects

Motor neuron disease (MND) comprises a group of uncommon fatal neurodegenerative diseases affecting males, especially in old age, and causing damage to motor neurons (especially anterior horn cells;

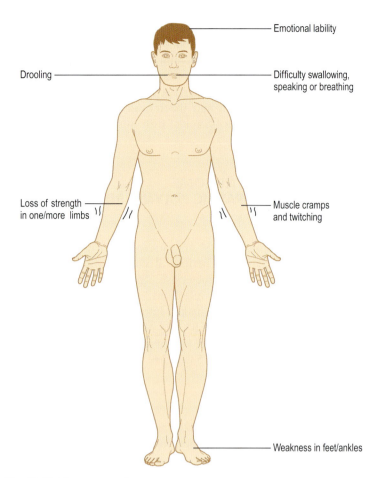

Emotional lability

Drooling

Difficulty swallowing, speaking or breathing

Loss of strength in one/more limbs

Muscle cramps and twitching

Weakness in feet/ankles

Fig. 13.11 Motor neuron disease.

Fig. 13.11). The aetiology is unclear but may be viral; 90% of cases of the most common type are sporadic, while a few others are due to a defect in the gene for superoxide dismutase, which normally protects against free radical damage.

Clinical features

There are three subtypes of MND:

Amyotrophic lateral sclerosis (ALS) is the most common subtype and has an intermediate prognosis. It affects oligodendrocytes and motor neurones in the anterior horn and pyramidal tract, and begins in the hands, feet and limbs, but is rapidly progressive and spreads to the trunk. UMN and LMN damage cause hand wasting and weakness, and leg spasticity. Early signs and symptoms include cramps and twitching in arms, shoulders and tongue (the hypoglossal nerve may be affected); slow loss of strength and coordination in one or more limbs; and weakness in feet and ankles, resulting in a stiff and clumsy gait and in foot-dragging. ALS eventually affects bulbar functions such as chewing, swallowing, speaking and breathing but, even in the late stages, sensory, bowel, bladder and cognitive functions are spared. Involvement of the brainstem may lead to pseudobulbar palsy – bulbar palsy with emotional lability (involuntary weeping or laughing). When muscles in the diaphragm and chest wall fail, individuals lose the ability to breathe without ventilatory support. Riluzole (an antiglutamate) prolongs life by 2–3 months but does not relieve symptoms. Other drugs are available to help individuals with spasticity, pain, panic attacks and depression. Physiotherapy, occupational therapy and rehabilitation may help, as may forms of mechanical ventilation (respirators). ALS is relentless, with respiratory paralysis and death supervening within 5 years.

Progressive bulbar palsy affects brainstem anterior horn cells and thus cranial nerve motor neurons arising in the medulla (IX–XII inclusive). It has the worse prognosis, and is characterized by wasting, weakness and fasciculation of the muscles of the pharynx, tongue, palate, sternomastoid and trapezius.

Progressive muscular atrophy has the best MND prognosis, affecting the anterior horn below the foramen magnum and causing LMN lesions with wasting and weakness starting in small muscles of the hands and spreading proximally.

General management

Diagnosis is clinical, based on the history and findings of muscle fasciculation, weakness, wasting, spastic dysarthria and exaggerated reflexes. Nerve conduction studies and EMG are confirmatory. Riluzole may slow the progress of ALS. Physical and occupational therapy, speech therapy, nutritional support and, eventually, breathing assistance are needed and can be remarkably successful (as in the case of Prof Stephen Hawking). Morphine or pethidine (meperidine) is frequently needed for terminal care.

Dental aspects

Oral hygiene may be impaired, as in other conditions with disability. Weakness or paralysis in the neck and head can lead to dysphagia and drooling. Protection of the airway may also be impaired. Botulinum toxoid injection into salivary glands significantly decreases saliva production.

SYRINGOMYELIA

General aspects

Syringomyelia is cavitation of the spinal cord, of unknown aetiology, causing disruption of pain and temperature neurons of the anterior commissure. *Syringobulbia* is the term used if it affects the brainstem (usually the medulla).

Clinical features

Symptoms begin in adolescence or adult life and progress erratically. Syringomyelia leads to segmental loss of pain and temperature but preservation of touch senses, causing painless ulcers, injuries or burns and deranged (Charcot) joints. Damage to sympathetic neurons in the intermediolateral column of the spinal cord can cause Horner syndrome. Later, the pyramidal tracts may be involved, causing leg spasticity. Kyphoscoliosis develops at an early stage.

Syringobulbia may also cause facial or oral sensory changes or paralyses, but medullary damage rarely affects the respiratory or cardiovascular centres significantly.

General management

There is no effective treatment. Patients should be protected from injuries, especially from heat.

Dental aspects

Syringobulbia can cause facial sensory loss with unilateral palatal and vocal cord palsies, nystagmus, weakness and atrophy of the tongue, dysphagia and dysarthria.

PATIENTS WITH RESPIRATORY PARALYSIS

Spinal cord trauma, infarction, haemorrhage, myelitis, tumours or poliomyelitis may cause severe and permanent disablement, but the type of disability depends largely on the level and extent of the lesion within the spinal cord. High-level lesions can be fatal, or cause respiratory paralysis and quadriplegia. Lower-level lesions may cause paraplegia and many of the problems that afflict persons with spina bifida (Ch. 28).

ORGANIC BRAIN DISORDERS

Damage to focal areas of brain from trauma, stroke, tumours or infections may lead to a range of defined neurological defects (Table 13.23) and epilepsy, whilst damage that is more gross may also cause coma or death.

More diffuse cortical damage can lead to acute or chronic organic brain disease (dementia) and widespread brain dysfunction. *Acute organic brain disease* can have many causes (Table 13.24). Characterized by disorientation, anxiety, fear, hallucinations, delusions and impaired consciousness, patients with acute organic brain disease must be handled carefully with tact and reassurance, and may need sedation and psychiatric help (Ch. 10).

Chronic organic brain disease (dementia) is more common than acute, and probably affects 1% of those aged 60 years, doubling every 5 years thereafter so that, by age 85 years, up to 50% are affected. Dementia is not a feature of old age *per se* but has many causes; almost two-thirds is Alzheimer disease and one-quarter is multi-infarct (vascular) dementia (Table 13.25).

Everyone has occasional lapses in memory, especially with advancing age, and it is often quite normal to forget the names of people whom you rarely see, but it is not a normal part of ageing to forget the names of familiar people and objects.

Dementia is an acquired progressive loss of cognitive functions, intellectual and social abilities, severe enough to interfere with daily functioning, and characterized by amnesia (especially for recent events), inability to concentrate, disorientation in time, place or person, and intellectual impairment (including loss of normal social awareness; Box 13.7). Other less specific symptoms include mood changes or paranoia. Anxiety, fear, hallucinations and delusions can be features.

Dementia is often accompanied by disruptive behaviour, and may be mimicked by acute organic brain disease, confusional states, drug-induced disorders and psychiatric disease.

Informed consent is a fraught issue in patients with dementia. They themselves are rarely able to give informed consent and, in many countries, relatives and staff have no legal right to give such consent on the patient's behalf. If a person is not capable of giving or refusing consent, and has not validly refused such care in advance, treatment may still be given lawfully if it is deemed to be in the patient's best interests. However, this should happen only after full consideration of its potential benefits and unwanted effects, and consultation with the carer(s), relatives and other people close to the patient.

DEMENTIA

Dementia may be caused by systemic disorders such as metabolic syndrome, in which the combination of high blood pressure, high cholesterol, and diabetes causes confusion and memory loss, or by Alzheimer disease.

Table 13.23 *Defects resulting from brain cortex damage*

Area damaged	Examples of resulting defects
Frontal	Anosmia, abnormal affect, difficulty in motivation/planning, aphasia, perseveration, personality changes
Occipital	Cortical blindness, homonymous hemianopia, visual agnosia, impaired visual perception
Parietal	Astereognosis (failure to recognize common objects by feel), disorders of learned movements such as writing
Temporal	Memory impairment, cortical deafness, auditory agnosia, impaired musical perception

Table 13.24 *Possible causes of acute organic brain disorders*

Causes	Mental complications that may result
Chemicals	Various
Drugs	Various
Endocrine disease	
Acromegaly	Emotional lability
Addison disease	Apathy, mild recent amnesia
Corticosteroid therapy	Euphoria
Cushing syndrome and disease	Euphoria or depression, psychoses with delusions or hallucinations
Hypoglycaemia (in treated diabetes mellitus)	Confusion, dementia
Hypothyroidism	Impaired concentration, amnesia, depression, paranoia, acute confusion
Hyperparathyroidism with hypercalcaemia	Apathy, depression
Thyrotoxicosis	Anxiety and agitation, depression
Infections	See text
Trauma	Ch. 24
Tumours	See text

Table 13.25 *Causes of dementia*

Common causes	Uncommon causes
Alcoholism	Brain-occupying lesion
Alzheimer disease	Chronic traumatic encephalopathy
Hydrocephalus	Creutzfeldt–Jakob disease
Lewy body dementia	HIV infection/AIDS
Multi-infarct dementia	Hypothyroidism
Tumours	Huntington chorea
	Pick disease (frontal lobar atrophy)
	Syphilis
	Vitamin B_{12} deficiency
	Wernicke–Korsakoff syndrome

Box 13.7 *Diagnostic features of dementia*

Development of multiple cognitive defects	Cognitive disturbances	Language (aphasia)
Memory impairment		Motor activities (apraxia)
		Recognition (agnosia)
		Planning
		Organizing

Alzheimer disease (Alzheimer dementia)

General aspects

Alzheimer disease (AD) is the most common form of dementia. It may affect 10–15% of those over 65, 20% of those over 80 years of age and nearly half of those aged 85 and older. AD involves parts of the brain that control thought, memory and language, and can seriously affect a person's ability to carry out daily activities.

It seems likely that a combination of factors is responsible:

- *Age* – This is a major factor.
- *Gender* – Women are more likely to develop AD, even allowing for their longer life expectancy.
- *Head injury* – Severe head injury or whiplash, or trauma over an extended period (e.g. boxing), increases the risk.
- *Lifestyle* – Smoking, hypertension, low folate and high blood cholesterol increase the risk. Aluminium or mercury appears not to be causal. Evidence for physical, mental and social activities as protective factors against AD is growing.
- *Genetic* – Abnormalities on chromosome 1, 14 or 21 account for a small number of cases of early-onset dementia. Down syndrome is also caused by an abnormality of chromosome 21 and, as these individuals age, 50% will show the physical brain changes and behavioural symptoms of AD. A gene on chromosome 19 that controls apolipoprotein E4 has been implicated in later-onset AD. The genes involved in AD (*ApoE4*, *TREM2* or *Fad*) seem responsible for a common pathogenic pathway centred around cellular trafficking, maturation and abnormal processing of beta-amyloid precursor protein (β-APP), and the subsequent generation, aggregation and intracellular deposition of toxic beta-amyloid (Aβ: Aβ 1–42) peptides.

The three major pathological hallmarks of AD are:

- *amyloid plaques* – These are made of beta-amyloid peptide and other fragments
- *neurofibrillary tangles* (NFTs) – Damage to tau proteins in neurons causes malfunction and loss of microtubule stabilization, and neuronal atrophy
- *loss of connections between neurons responsible for memory and learning* – Neurons die throughout the brain, and affected regions atrophy.

The brain degenerates, with reduced neurotransmitter levels, creating signalling problems and a progressive decline in memory and mental abilities. Similar brain changes can be seen in Down syndrome; both have a defect on chromosome 21, where the *APP* gene is located. Mutations in this *APP* gene, or the pre-senilins PS-1 or PS-2, or inheritance of the ApoE allele, are responsible for some cases of AD.

Clinical features

AD may manifest with slight memory loss and confusion, and an inability to perform previously simple tasks, but eventually leads to decreasing cognitive skills and severe, irreversible mental impairment that destroys a person's ability to remember, reason, learn and imagine (Box 13.8). Initially, people with AD experience memory loss and confusion, which may be mistaken for age-related memory changes ('senior moments'). However, there are gradual behavioural and personality changes, a decline in cognitive abilities such as decision-making and language skills, and problems recognizing family and friends. AD ultimately leads to a severe loss of mental function. In most people with AD, features include:

Box 13.8 *Changes in cognition (mental ability) in Alzheimer disease*

- Dementia (dysfunction of multiple cognitive functions)
- Difficulty performing common motor skills, such as combing one's hair, despite normal strength (apraxia)
- Difficulty in understanding or using language to speak or write (aphasia)
- Failing memory
- Inability to recognize familiar objects (agnosia)
- Inability to perform simple arithmetic (acalculia)
- Inability to sustain concentration when performing a task
- Inability to distinguish right from left
- Poor visual–spatial comprehension (e.g. getting lost driving in a familiar area)

- memory loss – one of the most common signs is forgetting recently learned information
- challenges in planning or solving problems, such as ability to develop and follow a plan or work with numbers
- difficulty completing familiar daily tasks
- confusion about time or place
- trouble understanding visual images and spatial relationships, such as difficulty reading, judging distance and determining colour or contrast
- trouble following or joining a conversation
- misplacing things and losing the ability to retrace steps
- decreased or poor judgment
- withdrawal from work or social activities
- changes in mood and personality, such as becoming confused, suspicious, depressed, fearful or anxious
- features of anxiety and depression – these may also be present, often contributing to social difficulties and self-neglect.

In advanced dementia, individuals may be disoriented in time, place and person. The ability to recognize family or friends, or carry out the simplest, once-routine tasks that require sequential steps, such as combing the hair or tooth-brushing, decreases. There are also general deteriorations in motor skills and difficulties with abstract thinking, decision-making and finding the right word. People with AD may initially have trouble balancing their cheque book, a problem that progresses to trouble understanding and recognizing numbers. Eventually, reading and writing are also affected and inability to solve everyday problems, such as knowing what to do if food on the stove is burning, makes independent living impossible. Ultimately, there can be disorientation and grossly inappropriate or bizarre behaviour, in which loss of a sense of time and dates, personality changes, delusions, mood swings or depression, and disordered behaviour of many kinds may be associated. Patients may express distrust in others, show increased stubbornness and withdraw socially. Restlessness is also a common sign and eventually patients may even wander from home.

General management

No definitive test is available. The diagnosis depends on evidence of a progressive decline in cognitive function in the absence of focal neurological deficits and the exclusion of other organic disease, such as hypothyroidism and vitamin B_{12} deficiency. Investigations include full blood count, renal and liver profiles, serum vitamin B_{12} and folate levels, syphilis serology, infection screen and MRI. Additional diagnostic studies included serial neurocognitive testing, NeuroSPECT, ApoE genotyping, and a CSF assay of tau and beta-amyloid. AD differs from multi-infarct dementia, as shown in Table 13.26.

Table 13.26 *Comparison of Alzheimer disease and multi-infarct dementia*

	Alzheimer disease	Multi-infarct dementia
Gender	F > M	M > F
Age at onset	70–90 years	60–80 years
Aetiopathogenesis	? Possibly environmental/familial	Transient ischaemic attack (TIA) or stroke
Hypertension and ischaemic heart disease	±	+ + +
Onset	Slow, progressive deterioration	Acute and stepwise deterioration
Main symptoms	Cognitive loss	Emotional disturbance
Cognitive loss	Global	Patchy
Insight	Lost	Preserved
Personality	Lost	Preserved
Focal signs	±	+ + +

Medications used to treat AD, to assist individuals carry out activities of daily living by maintaining thinking, memory or speaking skills, and which can also help some of the associated behavioural and personality disturbances, include drugs that stabilize acetylcholine levels (donepezil, rivastigmine, galantamine) and an antagonist of glutamate, a neurotransmitter present at abnormally high levels in AD (memantine). Oestrogens, NSAIDs, and antioxidants such as vitamin E may improve cognition. Ginkgo biloba may improve memory. An unexpected benefit of statins (inhibitors of 3-hydroxy-3-methyl-glutaryl-CoA [HMG-CoA]) has been their effect on enzymes that generate Aβ peptides. Glutamatergic agonist and Aβ-peptide immunization, however, have had little impact. Methylene blue is an innovation and looks promising in early clinical trials. Sedatives and antidepressants may help manage associated anxiety and depression.

Patients with dementia should be managed in the community if possible, although a detailed assessment by a psychogeriatrician is often needed. People with AD are individuals with their own likes and dislikes, struggling to make sense of a world they can no longer fully understand. It is essential to treat them with respect and dignity, using good verbal and non-verbal communication:

- Engage their attention. Eliminate distractions, such as traffic noise or other people's conversations. Make eye contact. Be relaxed and calm.
- Gently hold their hand or put your arm around their shoulder to comfort them.
- Give verbal cues: 'I'm your dentist,' rather than the more challenging 'Do you remember who I am?' Use simple short sentences. Ask questions one at a time in such a way that they can answer 'yes' or 'no'. Repeat or rephrase your words if they do not understand.
- Listen carefully to what the person says. If you have to interpret their meaning, check that you have guessed correctly.
- Never speak down to someone with dementia, or speak across them as if they were not there. Even if you get no response, include them in your conversations.
- Reassure them constantly. Use gentle humour to form a bond between you.

Once you know them, it may be appropriate to call them by their first name, which they will recall long after they have forgotten their surname.

Nothing is worse than delivering treatment that the patient neither understands nor appreciates, and struggles to avoid. Treatment planning should be realistic and patient-centred, aiming to maintain quality of life. When the many complex issues are evaluated, there are essentially four choices:

- Comprehensive routine care, including aesthetic and prosthodontic treatments
- Monitoring and maintaining the existing dentition by restoring new cavities and implementing prevention
- Emergency care only, relieving pain and infection, and implementing prevention if possible
- No dental treatment at all because of poor general health or inability to cooperate.

As AD progresses, the person must be constantly reassessed, and individualized care plans revised to take into account physical and cognitive changes.

Treatment may involve management of concurrent problems, which may make dementia worse (e.g. respiratory or urinary tract infections); social services (supportive interventions for both patients and carers – long-term residential or nursing home care may become necessary); and drugs.

In advanced AD, the inability of patients to care for themselves leads to: difficulty eating, incontinence and health problems, such as pneumonia and other infections; urinary incontinence, which may require catheterization and raises the risk of infections; and falls and their complications. Prolonged immobilization, which may be necessary to recover from injuries related to a fall, raises the risk of deep vein thrombosis and pulmonary embolism.

Dental aspects

Up to 75% of patients with AD require dental attention but the chief problems are behavioural. It is crucial to anticipate future decline in oral hygiene. Carers must be involved. Attention to diet, oral hygiene and preventive care are important but after a time may no longer be practicable. Dental treatment should be planned with the knowledge that the patient may sooner or later become unmanageable for treatment under LA. In the early stages, dental appointments and instructions are forgotten. Later, there is progressive neglect of oral health as a result of forgetting the need, or even how, to brush the teeth or clean dentures. Dentures are also frequently lost or broken, or cannot be tolerated. Deterioration of dental care, together with hyposalivation, can lead to destruction of the dentition by caries and periodontal disease, and increase the problems of management because of difficulty in eating and halitosis. Periodontitis has even been suggested as an aetiological factor in AD. Injuries are also common in demented patients. Drugs, such as phenothiazines used to manage behavioural problems, may aggravate xerostomia and may cause dyskinesias. Loss of taste is common. Salivary substitutes may give some symptomatic relief.

Treatment should, as far as possible, be carried out in the morning, when cooperation tends to be best, and with the usual carers present in a familiar environment; care is needed to explain every procedure before it is carried out and to avoid discomfort. Time-consuming and complex treatments should be avoided.

Access can be a serious handicap. Preoperative sedation with a short-acting benzodiazepine or haloperidol may be required.

Frontotemporal dementia (Pick's disease)

Frontotemporal dementia (FTD) is a progressive dementia, which is typically associated with shrinking of the frontal and temporal anterior lobes of the brain. The current designation of the syndrome groups together Pick's disease, primary progressive aphasia and semantic dementia as FTD. Some doctors propose adding corticobasal degeneration and progressive supranuclear palsy to frontotemporal dementia and calling the group Pick complex.

Symptoms of FTD fall into two groups: changes in behaviour or problems with language. The first type features behaviour that can be either impulsive (disinhibited) or bored and listless (apathetic) and includes:

- inappropriate social behaviour
- lack of social tact
- lack of empathy
- distractibility
- loss of insight into the behaviours of oneself and others
- an increased interest in sex
- changes in food preferences
- agitation or, conversely, blunted emotions
- neglect of personal hygiene
- repetitive or compulsive behaviour
- decreased energy and motivation.

The second type primarily features symptoms of language disturbance, including difficulty making or understanding speech, often in conjunction with symptoms of the behavioural type of FTD. Spatial skills and memory remain intact.

BRAIN TUMOURS

Brain (cerebral) tumours are second only to cerebrovascular lesions as a cause of neurological disease. Most are metastatic from carcinomas of the lung, breast, gastrointestinal tract and kidney, but primary cerebral tumours are also usually malignant. A possible relationship between brain tumours and dental radiography has been reported but not as yet confirmed. Intracranial lymphomas are a well-recognized feature of HIV disease and are rising in prevalence. In children, brain tumours account for approximately 2% of all cancer deaths but are second only to leukaemia as a cause of death.

Epileptiform fits developing for the first time in an adult are strongly suggestive of a cerebral tumour. Typical features of a tumour are localizing signs dependent on the site (e.g. convulsions or paralysis), and signs of raised intracranial pressure (headache, vomiting, papilloedema, lapsing consciousness, rising blood pressure and slowing pulse). Cerebral tumours, even those that are histologically benign, have a poor prognosis if not amenable to surgery.

Acoustic neuroma (neurofibroma)

Acoustic neuroma is usually a benign tumour that arises from the neural axon or sheath of the vestibular part of cranial nerve VIII, where it leaves the brainstem in the posterior cranial fossa. Bilateral acoustic neuromas are characteristic of neurofibromatosis type II (Fig. 13.12). Clinically, this causes tinnitus (ringing in the ears), deafness and rotational vertigo (a sensation of spinning), and then post-auricular pain, disturbance of balance, facial twitching or weakness and paraesthesia; as the trigeminal, facial, glossopharyngeal and vagus nerves become stretched over the tumour, there is difficulty in speaking and swallowing – a highly characteristic picture. The neuroma can be completely removed surgically in about 60% of cases.

Meningioma

Ionizing radiation is a risk factor for meningioma, the most common primary brain tumour. An increased risk of meningioma is associated

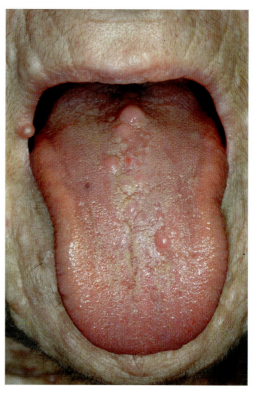

Fig. 13.12 Neurofibromatosis.

with bitewing examination on a yearly or more frequent basis, and was also linked to Panorex films® taken at a young age or on a yearly or more frequent basis. Exposure to some dental X-rays performed in the past, when radiation exposure was greater than in the current era, appears to be associated with an increased risk of intracranial meningioma.

The American Dental Association's statement on the use of dental radiographs (American Dental Association 2006) highlights the need for dentists to examine the risk/benefit ratio associated with the use of dental X-rays and confirms that there is little evidence to support the use of dental X-rays to search for occult disease in asymptomatic patients or to obtain routine dental X-rays from all patients at preset intervals.

Pituitary tumours

Adenomas are the most common pituitary tumours. Their endocrine effects dominate the clinical picture (Ch. 6) but they may compress the gland and cause hypopituitarism, or produce signs common to other cerebral tumours.

The craniopharyngioma arises from Rathke's pouch, an upgrowth from the primitive stomatodeum, may resemble an ameloblastoma or calcifying odontogenic cyst microscopically. Most manifest in childhood with headache, vomiting, papilloedema and visual defects. Short stature, delayed sexual development and diabetes insipidus may be associated. Suprasellar calcification may be seen, especially on CT.

Pituitary tumours can be removed, often through a trans-sphenoidal approach.

CENTRAL NERVOUS SYSTEM INFECTIONS

Meningitis

Meningitis is infection of the membranes (meninges) that surround the brain and spinal cord, and has a number of possible causes and

Table 13.27 *Causes and sequelae of meningitis*

Causes		Comments
Infective		
Viral	Enteroviruses: Coxsackie viruses, ECHO viruses and mumps	Thousands of cases occur each year, mostly affecting babies and children. Most common; usually self-limited to 10 days or less and a mild disease. Although most recover fully, some remain with serious and debilitating after-effects. Specific treatment rarely available
Bacterial	Neisseria meningitidis (meningococcus)	Most cases in babies and young children. Uncommon. Around 7% die and 15% left with severe disability. Meningococcal disease describes meningitis and septicaemia, which can occur alone or more commonly together. Treat urgently with antimicrobials (benzyl penicillin or cefotaxime)
	Streptococcus pneumoniae (pneumococcus)	Most cases in babies and young children under 18 months of age. Increasingly important in adult life, particularly in those with impaired resistance (e.g. alcoholism or sickle cell disease). A life-threatening infection; 20% die and 25% are left with severe and disabling after-effects. Treat with intravenous ceftriaxone or cefotaxime (often penicillin-resistant), or if cause is unclear. Vaccine is available
	Haemophilus influenzae	Usually in babies and children under the age of 4. Hib vaccine significantly reduced cases. Treat with cefotaxime
	Listeria monocytogenes	Treat with amoxicillin plus gentamicin
	Mycobacterium tuberculosis	Usually originates from lungs but in about 2% is haematogenous. Develops slowly. Difficult to diagnose and treat
	Group B streptococcus (Streptococcus agalactiae) and Escherichia coli	The most common causes in newborn babies. Risks higher for premature babies. Fatality rates as high as 20%
	Staphylococcus aureus	May complicate neurosurgical procedures
	Listeria monocytogenes	Associated with malnutrition and alcoholism
Fungal	Cryptococcus neoformans, Candida albicans	Rare. Typically seen in immunocompromised people. Often develop slowly. Difficult to diagnose and treat
Non-infective		
Physical injury		–
Cancer		
Drugs		
Systemic lupus erythematosus		

sequelae (Table 13.27; see also Ch. 21). Viral meningitis is usually fairly inconsequential and self-limiting. However, high fever, severe and persistent headache, stiff neck, nausea and vomiting may appear suddenly and require prompt medical attention since some forms of meningitis, notably bacterial, are potentially fatal.

Bacterial (suppurative) meningitis

General aspects

A number of bacteria may cause meningitis, notably *Neisseria meningitidis* (meningococcus), *Streptococcus pneumoniae* (pneumococcus)

and *Haemophilus influenzae* B (Hib; see Table 13.27). *N. meningitidis* (12 serotypes are known) is carried in the nasopharynx and sometimes causes meningitis epidemics, mainly in children or adolescents. Most cases are caused by serogroups A, B and C, less commonly by serogroups W-135 and Y. Recent outbreaks have been caused by groups B and C. Group B, type 15 meningococcus, in particular, causes a severe form of the disease. Spread of bacteria to the meninges is by the bloodstream or occasionally results from a maxillofacial fracture involving the ethmoid cribriform plate (Ch. 24).

Clinical features

Meningitis is characterized by severe headache, nausea or vomiting, pain and stiffness of the neck, drowsiness, photophobia, fever, stupor or coma and, occasionally, convulsions. A purpuric rash is characteristic of meningococcal septicaemia, which, as a result of bleeding into the adrenal cortex, can go on to adrenocortical failure with vasomotor collapse, shock and death (Waterhouse–Friderichsen syndrome).

General management

Diagnosis is confirmed with a Gram-stained smear, culturing and examining for meningococci by the polymerase chain reaction (PCR) from throat, lumbar puncture (CSF) specimen and blood. Antibiotic treatment should start immediately, even before microbiology results are available. If treatment is prompt, the overall mortality is low, but about 20% suffer permanent neurological damage (e.g. cranial neuropathies – blindness, deafness or palsies, epilepsy or learning impairment).

Patients with middle third maxillofacial injuries should be given prophylactic antimicrobials because of the danger of meningitis (Ch. 24). Family contacts of patients with contagious meningitis require chemoprophylaxis with rifampicin or ciprofloxacin. ACWY Vax is a meningitis quadrivalent vaccine that contains inactivated polysaccharide extracts of meningococci types A, C, W-135 and Y.

Brain abscess

General aspects

Brain abscesses usually arise secondary to middle ear, sinus or pulmonary infections, head trauma or infective endocarditis. Bacteria from periodontal pockets, particularly anaerobes, or periapical periodontitis are also a recognized focus for cerebral abscess; inhalation of a tooth fragment or materials used in dentistry can cause a lung abscess, which can metastasize to the brain with serious consequences. Patients with congenital heart disease, particularly those with right-to-left shunts, and those with hereditary haemorrhagic telangiectasia are also at risk of brain abscess.

In immunocompetent persons, frontal lobe abscesses often result from sinusitis and contain a heavy growth of *Streptococcus milleri*. Sphenoidal sinusitis is notorious in this respect and can be difficult to diagnose. Post-traumatic or postoperative brain abscesses are often related to *Staphylococcus aureus*.

Temporal lobe abscesses frequently arise from middle ear mixed bacterial infections, with large numbers of anaerobes. In immunocompromised persons, brain abscesses may also be fungal (mainly *Candida*, *Aspergillus* or *Cryptococcus*) or protozoal (*Toxoplasma*).

Clinical features

Cerebral abscess causes signs and symptoms similar to those of other space-occupying lesions of the brain (i.e. headache, nausea, vomiting, diminished level of consciousness, hypertension, bradycardia and respiratory changes).

General management

CT and MRI are valuable in the diagnosis. Treatment is by immediate high doses of antibiotics (usually penicillin or metronidazole, or both), followed, where necessary, by aspiration or drainage. The mortality is still between 10% and 20%.

Encephalitis

Encephalitis (inflammation of the brain) is usually caused by viral infection. Symptoms include sudden fever, headache, vomiting, photophobia (abnormal visual sensitivity to light), stiff neck and back, confusion, drowsiness, clumsiness, unsteady gait and irritability.

Some cases are mild, short and relatively benign, and patients recover fully; others are severe, and permanent impairment or death is possible. The acute phase of encephalitis may last for 1–2 weeks, with gradual or sudden resolution of fever and neurological symptoms. Neurological symptoms may require many months before full recovery. No specific treatment is available unless infection is caused by herpes simplex virus.

Herpetic simplex encephalitis

Herpetic simplex encephalitis is rare, although still the most frequent cause of encephalitis in temperate climates. Evidence as to whether it is a primary or reactivation infection is conflicting. Clinical effects are highly variable, ranging from early symptoms, such as disorientation, personality changes, hallucinations and ataxia (which can be mistaken for drunkenness or psychosis) to stupor, fits, paralyses and sensory loss. Coma is often pre-terminal.

Herpetic simplex encephalitis has often been fatal, particularly because confirmation of the diagnosis has had to be by brain biopsy, but the prognosis has improved greatly as a result of treatment with aciclovir and related antiviral drugs, which are frequently given on suspicion. The incidence of neurological damage among survivors has also declined.

Neurosyphilis

See Chapter 32.

HIV-associated neurological disease

See Chapter 21.

Prion disease (transmissible spongiform encephalopathies)

Transmissible spongiform encephalopathies (TSEs) are a group of fatal degenerative brain diseases (encephalopathies) characterized by the appearance of microscopic vacuoles in the brain grey matter, giving a sponge-like (spongiform) appearance. TSEs were originally termed slow virus infections – though no virus has ever been associated and current evidence points to the specific association with an abnormal form of a host-encoded protein termed a prion (proteinaceous infectious particle).

Prions are composed of a cell-surface glycoprotein PrP, and accumulation in the brain of a protease-resistant isoform (PrP^{sc}) is the common mechanism of pathogenesis of TSEs. PrP^{sc} is remarkably resistant to inactivation by sterilization methods, and this presents significant infection control problems when patients with TSEs undergo health interventions.

All TSEs have prolonged incubation periods of months to years, gradually leading to death over months or years, with varying amounts of PrP^{sc} accumulating in the CNS.

There are several animal TSEs, including bovine spongiform encephalitis (BSE; also known as 'mad cow disease') in cattle, and scrapie in sheep and goats. The classic example of a human TSE is Creutzfeldt–Jakob disease (CJD). Incubation periods in humans, after peripheral or oral exposure, range from at least 4 years to 40 years, with a mean of 10–15 years.

Infectivity in TSEs is highest in brain tissue but is also present in some peripheral tissues; it is not found in most body fluids, including saliva. Animal studies show prions in the trigeminal nerve, tooth pulp, gingiva and salivary glands, and the potential for prion transmission via the dental route. Prions do not evoke a protective immune response or detectable diagnostic antibodies. Nevertheless, attempts at vaccine production are under way.

Human TSE types are inherited, acquired or sporadic (Table 13.28), but are frequently referred to collectively as CJD. The acquired forms include kuru, and iatrogenic and variant CJD. Overall, CJD affects approximately 1 per 1 000 000 of the population per annum across the world.

Creutzfeldt–Jakob disease (CJD)

Creutzfeldt-Jakob disease is a rare illness and is one of a group of diseases called prion diseases, which affect humans and animals. Prion diseases exist in different forms, all of which are progressive, currently untreatable and ultimately fatal. Their name arises because they are associated with an alteration in a naturally occurring protein: the prion protein.

CJD was first described in 1920. The commonest form is called sporadic CJD and occurs worldwide, causing around 1 death per million population per year. A new form of CJD (variant CJD; see below), linked to BSE in cattle, was identified in 1996. There are also inherited forms of human prion disease associated with mutations of the prion protein gene (*PRNP*) and cases caused by infection via medical or surgical treatments (iatrogenic CJD).

Sporadic CJD (sCJD) accounts for about 85% of all cases of CJD. The underlying cause is unknown but the disease commonly develops in middle to late life as a rapidly progressive multifocal dementia. Up to a third of patients have non-specific prodromal symptoms, such as insomnia, fatigue, depression, weight loss, headache, malaise and pain. Over weeks there is rapid progression to akinetic mutism, with mental deterioration, myoclonus, extrapyramidal and pyramidal signs,

Table 13.28 *Types of Creutzfeldt–Jakob disease (CJD)*

Type	Abbreviation	Source
Sporadic	sCJD	–
Familial	fCJD	Autosomal dominant
Kuru	–	Ritualistic cannibalism
Iatrogenic	iCJD	Contaminated surgical instruments; dura mater grafts or pituitary hormones
Variant; sometimes termed new-variant CJD	vCJD; nvCJD	Consumption of material infected with bovine spongiform encephalopathy (BSE)

cerebellar ataxia and cortical blindness. The EEG shows characteristic changes.

Familial CJD (fCJD), which accounts for around 10% of cases, includes rare autosomal dominant disorders that manifest in early to middle adult life. *Fatal familial insomnia* is characterized by progressive insomnia, dysautonomia, disruption of circadian rhythms, motor dysfunction and deterioration in cognition. *Gerstmann–Straussler–Scheinker syndrome* is distinct, with many PrP^sc^-positive plaques throughout the brain.

Kuru, first described in the 1950s, was endemic among the Fore ethnic group in the eastern highlands of Papua New Guinea and spread by cannibalism. Most cases were in children and women, who ritually consumed brains from deceased relatives. Typically, there was progressive cerebellar ataxia but, unlike in CJD, dementia was not common.

Iatrogenic CJD (iCJD) can be transmitted mainly by exposure to cadaver-derived growth hormone, pituitary gonadotropins, dura mater homografting, corneal grafts or inadequately sterilized neurosurgical equipment. There is no evidence to suggest that any patients who have received dura mater allografts for the management of maxillofacial defects have developed iCJD. Concerns exist about the theoretical risk of the use of non-human animal-derived graft materials and heterologous human graft materials in oral or periodontal surgery.

Variably protease-sensitive prionopathy (VPSPr) is a relatively newly described (in 2008) human prion disease of unknown aetiology. Its precise relationship with other prion diseases is uncertain but no mutations have been found in the *PRNP* coding sequence and the patients have no (known) risk factors for iatrogenic CJD. The reported cases have clinicopathological profiles and protein biochemical characteristics that differ from those seen in variant or sporadic CJD. The clinical features are not yet fully characterized but the reported cases have been middle-aged to elderly with relatively longer disease durations than for sporadic CJD.

Variant Creutzfeldt–Jakob disease (vCJD)

General aspects

BSE was first recognized in UK cattle in 1986, and it was eventually established that the infective agent was spread by the use of meat and bonemeal in cattle food. Then, in 1990, TSE appeared in domestic cats in the UK, suggesting that TSE was transmitted in pet foods and that the causative agent was by no means species-specific. In 1996, a variant of sporadic CJD (variant or vCJD) was first observed in humans in the UK, and linked with the consumption of infected bovine offal. Pathological examination of the CNS revealed plaques of PrP^sc^ and a specific genetic predisposition, with all vCJD patients analysed being homozygous for methionine at codon 129 of the *PrP* gene. CNS, posterior orbit and (unusually for prion diseases) lymphoreticular tissue are, in descending order of risk, the tissues most likely to be infective. Transfusions of blood or blood derivatives can also transmit the prion; plasma products were banned in the UK in 1998 and all donor blood has been leukodepleted since 1999. To avoid the possibility of transmission via infected brain tissue, recipients of human growth hormone were excluded from blood donation in 1989, and recipients of other human-derived pituitary hormones have been excluded since 1993. There may also be other potential but unproven sources of infection, such as products from cell lines grown in the presence of fetal bovine serum, some vaccines, and bovine products such as collagen.

Clinical features

Persons with vCJD have prominent early psychiatric symptoms (severe depression and behavioural manifestations), together with paraesthesias and dysaesthesias, followed by dementia, cerebellar and other neurological signs, myoclonus or other involuntary movements and, finally, akinetic mutism.

General management

The clinical course of vCJD is much longer than that of sCJD and affected patients do not have the same typical EEG changes. Tests and investigations that can contribute to a diagnosis include MRI, which shows characteristic bilateral symmetrical high signals in the thalamic pulvinar nuclei ('the pulvinar sign'). Other investigations include blood tests for the genetic mutations, EEG, psychometric tests, and CSF analyses to show a rise in the specific CSF proteins 14-3-3 and to exclude other infections. Tonsillar biopsy may help confirm a diagnosis of CJD.

There is no effective treatment for vCJD or other prion diseases. *In vitro*, some success has been achieved with mepacrine (quinacrine) and chlorpromazine.

Dental aspects

Conventional dental treatment has no proven association with transmission of any form of CJD. However, PrP^sc^ is remarkably resistant to inactivation with heat, most disinfectants, and ionizing, ultraviolet and microwave radiations. Concentrated bleach does appear to achieve inactivation and 20 000 ppm available chlorine of sodium hypochlorite for 1 hour or 2M sodium hydroxide for 1 hour are considered effective (Box 13.9), as is an enzyme (prionzyme).

Effective cleaning to remove adherent tissue, coupled with autoclaving, significantly reduces infectivity levels on contaminated instruments if a non-porous load steam sterilizer is used at 134–137°C for a single cycle of 18 minutes or six successive cycles of 3 minutes each.

For management purposes, it is useful to divide patients with TSEs into three main groups, as follows:

- Confirmed cases of CJD – all instruments used for invasive procedures should be destroyed after use.
- Suspected cases of CJD (patients who present with a clinical history that is suggestive of CJD but a confirmed diagnosis is unavailable) – the instruments used for invasive procedures should be quarantined pending a confirmation of diagnosis.
- Cases 'at risk' of CJD who are clinically well, including those 'at risk' by virtue of an inheritable defect in the prion protein gene producing fCJD, and those who have been exposed to infectious material through the use of human cadaveric derived pituitary hormones, and dural and corneal homografts (iatrogenic CJD) – most guidelines recommend that surgical instruments used to operate on 'high-risk ' tissues (CNS, spinal cord and eye) in patients 'at risk' of CJD should be disposed of by incineration. For interventions such as routine dental treatment, which do not involve 'high-risk' tissues, some national guidelines recommend the use of stringent instrument decontamination.

Dental health care staff infected or potentially infected with prion disease should not practise invasive clinical procedures in view of the risk of motor and cognitive dysfunction.

Box 13.9 *Recommended methods of inactivation of human and transmissible spongiform encephalopathy (TSE) agents*

- 20 000 ppm available chlorine of sodium hypochlorite for 1 h
- 2M sodium hydroxide for 1 h
- Non-porous load steam sterilizer 134–137°C for a single cycle of 18 min, or six successive cycles of 3 min each

Orofacial manifestations of human TSEs comprise dysphagia and dysarthia (due to pseudobulbar palsy); in vCJD patients, there may be orofacial dysaesthesia or paraesthesia or abnormal taste sensation.

BRAIN DAMAGE

Trauma, hypoxia, infections and hypoglycaemia are the main causes of brain damage.

Traumatic brain injury (TBI)

TBI can occur when the head suddenly and violently hits an object, or when an object penetrates the skull and enters the brain. Consequences can be mild, moderate or severe, depending on the extent of brain damage.

A person with a mild TBI may remain conscious or may experience a loss of consciousness for a few seconds or minutes. Other symptoms may include headache, confusion, light-headedness, dizziness, blurred vision or tired eyes, tinnitus, a bad taste in the mouth, fatigue or lethargy, a change in sleep patterns, behavioural or mood changes, and trouble with memory, concentration, attention or thinking.

A person with a moderate or severe TBI may show the same symptoms but also have a headache that increases or does not resolve, repeated vomiting or nausea, convulsions or seizures, an inability to awaken from sleep, dilatation of one or both pupils, slurred speech, weakness or numbness in the extremities, loss of coordination, and increased confusion, restlessness or agitation.

Patients with moderate or severe TBI should receive urgent medical attention to prevent further injury by ensuring proper oxygen supply to the brain, maintaining adequate blood flow and controlling blood pressure. Patients with mild to moderate injuries may receive skull and neck imaging (usually CT) to check for fractures or spinal instability.

Disabilities resulting from a TBI depend upon the severity of the injury, the location of the injury, and the age and general health of the individual; they can include problems with cognition (thinking, memory and reasoning), sensory processing (sight, hearing, touch, taste and smell), communication (expression and understanding), and behaviour or mental health (depression, anxiety, personality changes, aggression, acting out and social inappropriateness). More serious head injuries may result in stupor – an unresponsive state but one in which an individual can be aroused briefly by a strong stimulus, such as sharp pain; coma – a state in which an individual is totally unconscious, unresponsive, unaware and unarousable; vegetative state – in which an individual is unconscious and unaware of their surroundings but continues to have a sleep–wake cycle and periods of alertness; and a persistent vegetative state (PVS; see below) – in which an individual stays in a vegetative state for more than a month. Approximately half of severely head-injured patients will need surgery to remove or repair haematomas or contusions.

Cerebral palsy

See Chapter 28.

Hypoxic encephalopathy

Acute cerebral hypoxia is particularly important, as it can readily cause brain damage. Some patients can die and others suffer damage leading, depending on the age, duration and degree of hypoxia, to cerebral palsy, epilepsy or a persistent vegetative state.

Hypoxia can follow head injuries, airway obstruction, severe hypotension (e.g. cardiac arrest, shock syndrome, severe bradycardia, stroke) or impaired oxygenation (e.g. respiratory failure or the situation during GA, when the anaesthetic agent can depress respiration but there may also be partial, often unnoticed, respiratory obstruction). Cerebral hypoxia can remain unrecognized if the patient is already unconscious.

Cerebral hypoxia causes loss of consciousness in less than a minute but, if the blood circulation and oxygenation are restored within about 3 minutes, recovery should be complete. Hypoxia for longer than about 3 minutes causes brain damage and coma, with dilated pupils unresponsive to light, inert or rigid limbs, unresponsiveness to all stimuli, abolition of brainstem reflexes and, ultimately, no electrical activity on EEG (brain death). *The most vigilant supervision of all patients with head injuries, and other patients undergoing or recovering from GA or sedation, is, therefore, essential.* Special care must be taken to ensure that the patient is breathing effectively, that oxygen supplies are adequate and maintained, and that no hypoxia, however slight, develops.

Persistent vegetative state

'Persistent vegetative state' (PVS) is a term that describes the condition of patients with severe brain damage. Patients with PVS have no cerebral cortical function (they are unconscious and unaware), but exhibit irregular circadian sleep–wake cycles with either full or partial hypothalamic and brainstem autonomic functions, and persisting reflexes. PET scan studies have shown metabolic activity to be decreased by approximately 50% in the cerebral cortex and cerebellum of patients in PVS.

Patients in a PVS may be aroused by certain stimuli, opening their eyes if they are closed, changing their facial expressions, or even moving their limbs, and they may grind their teeth, swallow, smile, shed tears, grunt, moan or scream without reason. They may move their eyes, but this is merely reflexive and does not indicate awareness if they neither fixate on a visual object nor track a moving target with their eyes. Nevertheless, despite no evidence of awareness, their heads and eyes can follow a moving object or move towards a loud sound.

PVS is considered permanent when a diagnosis of irreversibility can be established, based on the fact that the chances of the patient regaining consciousness are exceedingly small.

Patients with PVS need close medical and nursing support, similar to that for stroke victims, including attention to oral health.

EPILEPSY

General aspects

Epilepsy, or seizure disorder, refers to a tendency to recurrent seizures. A seizure (fit) is a convulsion or transient disturbance in consciousness, caused by abnormal cerebral cortical electrical activity. Different causes prevail at different ages (Table 13.29). Disturbances of nerve cell activity produce symptoms that vary, depending on which part (and how much) of the brain is affected. Seizures may produce changes in awareness or sensation, involuntary movements, or other changes in

Table 13.29 *Causes of fits at different ages of onset*

Age at onset	More common causes
Young child	Birth trauma, fevers, metabolic disease, congenital disease or idiopathic
Adolescent	Idiopathic or traumatic
Young adult	Traumatic, neoplastic, idiopathic, alcoholism or barbiturate abuse, acquired immune deficiency syndrome (AIDS)
Middle-aged	Neoplastic, traumatic, cerebrovascular disease, AIDS or drug abuse
Older	Cerebrovascular disease or neoplasm

behaviour. In general, seizures do not indicate epilepsy but may only occur as a result of a temporary medical condition, such as a high fever, hypoglycaemia, alcohol or drug use or withdrawal, or following brain injury.

Typically, a seizure lasts from a few seconds to a few minutes. There are many seizure types but they fall into two main groups:

- *Primary generalized seizures* – seizures begin with widespread involvement of both sides of the brain.
- *Partial seizures* – seizures begin with involvement of a smaller, localized area of the brain, though in some the disturbance spreads within seconds or minutes to involve widespread areas of the brain (secondary generalized seizure).

Some people have an absence seizure, a type of primary generalized seizure called petit mal – rapid blinking or a few seconds of staring into space, and this may be hardly noticeable to others. In contrast, a person having a complex partial seizure may appear confused or dazed and unable to respond to questions for up to a few minutes. Finally, a person having a generalized tonic–clonic seizure, often called grand mal, may cry out, lose consciousness, fall to the ground, and have rigidity and muscle jerks for up to a few minutes, with an extended period of confusion and fatigue afterward.

In nearly two-thirds of the cases of epilepsy, a specific underlying cause is not identified but some known conditions and events that may lead to epilepsy are:

- oxygen deprivation
- brain infections (e.g. meningitis, encephalitis, cysticercosis or brain abscess)
- traumatic brain injury or head injury
- stroke
- other neurological diseases (e.g. Alzheimer disease)
- brain tumours
- certain genetic disorders.

Epilepsy is a predisposition for *recurrent* seizures; it affects approximately 1% of the adult population and may reflect underlying brain pathology (injury, tumours or infections). A total of 10% of the population suffer at least one seizure in their lifetime, but mainly in childhood when it may be caused by febrile convulsions. Epilepsy is more prevalent in the young and in the mentally or physically impaired. Most cases begin between the ages of 5 and 20 years.

Epilepsy is occasionally secondary (symptomatic epilepsy) to cerebral hypoxia; metabolic disturbances (hypoglycaemia or hyperglycaemia) and drugs (alcohol, amphetamines, anticonvulsants, barbiturates, benzodiazepines, cocaine and opioids) may predispose to epilepsy. Many cases, however, have no detectable structural or metabolic cause and are known as idiopathic – when there is likely to be a positive family history and a genetic predisposition (Box 13.10).

Many seizures in epileptic people have no clear trigger but, in some instances, food and sleep deprivation, hormonal changes (e.g. pregnancy or menstruation), concurrent illness, metabolic disturbances, sensory stimuli (flashing lights, sounds and touch – even, very rarely, an electric toothbrush), and prescribed or illicit drugs (alcohol, chlorpromazine, enflurane, flumazenil, fluoxetine, ketamine, methohexitone, tramadol, tricyclic antidepressants) or their withdrawal may be implicated.

Clinical features

The International League Against Epilepsy (ILAE) Classification of Epileptic Seizures 1981 and 1989 are the two systems in use. ILAE 1981 classifies seizures as:

Box 13.10 *Causes of epilepsy*

- Metabolic abnormalities
  - Diabetes mellitus or hypoglycaemia
  - Electrolyte imbalances
  - Renal failure
  - Nutritional deficiencies
  - Inborn errors of metabolism, e.g. phenylketonuria (PKU)
  - Use of, intoxication from or withdrawal from alcohol
  - Use of, intoxication from or withdrawal from illicit drugs, especially cocaine and amphetamines; also anticonvulsants, barbiturates, benzodiazepines, ecstasy, opioids
- Brain trauma
  - May affect any age, highest incidence in young adults
  - Most likely if the brain membranes are damaged
  - Seizures usually begin within 2 years of injury
  - Early seizures (within 2 weeks of injury) do not necessarily indicate that chronic seizures (epilepsy) will develop
- Brain tumours and other space-occupying brain lesions (such as haematomas)
  - May affect any age, more common after age 30
  - Partial (focal) seizures most common initially
  - May progress to generalized tonic–clonic seizures
- Cerebrovascular disease
  - Most common cause of seizures after age 60
- Degenerative disorders (senile dementia, Alzheimer disease or similar organic brain syndromes)
  - Mostly affect older people
- Drugs
- Infections, which may affect all ages
  - Meningitis
  - Encephalitis
  - Brain abscess
  - Acute severe systemic infections
  - Chronic infections (e.g. neurosyphilis)
  - HIV/AIDS or other immune disorders

- partial (seizures involving only part of the brain)
- generalized (seizures involving both sides of the brain)
- unclassifiable.

A problem presented by this simple classification is that the same patient may have more than one type of seizure, either together or in sequence. ILAE 1989 is meant to supplement the 1981 classification and describes epilepsies as:

- localization-related (involving one or more distinct parts of the brain)
- generalized (involving both sides of the brain at the same time)
- undetermined whether localized or generalized
- special syndromes (Table 13.30).

In addition to seizures, there may be other features, such as headache, changes in mood or energy level, confusion and memory loss.

The main types of epilepsy are generalized seizures (grand mal [tonic–clonic]), when consciousness is typically lost, and partial seizures, which include simple seizures during which the person remains alert, along with abnormal movements or sensations. Generalized seizures are the most dramatic but partial seizures are the most common.

Generalized: grand mal (tonic–clonic) epilepsy

Grand mal epilepsy usually begins in childhood, or sometimes at about puberty. There is a warning (aura), followed by loss of consciousness, tonic and clonic convulsions, then, finally, a variably

Table 13.30 *Classification and features of generalized and focal/partial epilepsy*

Type	Subtype	Clinical features
Generalized seizures	Tonic–clonic (grand mal)	Loss of consciousness, tonic phase, clonic phase, tongue-biting, incontinence
		Seizure lasts <5 min
	Absence seizure (petit mal)	Brief period of unresponsiveness
		Duration of absences <30 s
Partial seizures	Simple (Jacksonian epilepsy)	No impairment of consciousness
		Motor, sensory and autonomic features
	Complex (temporal lobe epilepsy)	Impaired consciousness
		Automatic repetitive acts

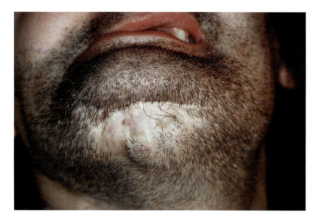

Fig. 13.13 Results of trauma in a person with epilepsy.

prolonged recovery. The aura may consist of a mood change, irritability, brief hallucination or headache. The attack then begins suddenly, with total body tonic spasm and loss of consciousness. The sufferer falls to the ground and is in danger of injury. Initially, the face becomes pale and the pupils dilate, the head and spine are thrown into extension (opisthotonos), and glottic and respiratory muscle spasm may cause an initial brief cry and cyanosis. There may also be incontinence and biting of the tongue or lips. The tonic phase passes, after less than a minute, into the clonic phase, when there are repetitive jerking movements of trunk, limbs, tongue and lips. Salivation is profuse with bruxism, sometimes tongue-biting and, occasionally, vomiting. There may be urinary or faecal incontinence, and autonomic phenomena such as tachycardia, hypertension and flushing. Clonus is followed by a state of flaccid semi-coma for a further 10–15 minutes. Confusion and headaches are common afterwards and the patient may sleep for up to 12 hours or more before full recovery. The attack may occasionally be followed by a transient residual paralysis (Todd palsy) or by automatic or aggressive behaviour. This full sequence is not always completed.

Complications of major convulsions can be trauma (Fig. 13.13), respiratory embarrassment or brain damage; seizures may progress to *status epilepticus* but most end without mishap. A major fit is so dramatic that it seems to be of longer duration than is in fact the case, but if it lasts more than 5 minutes (by the clock) or starts again after apparently ceasing, the patient must be regarded as being in status epilepticus, which is particularly dangerous – the mortality rate can be up to 20%. Brain damage may result from cerebral hypoxia, when tonic and clonic phases alternate repeatedly without consciousness being regained and there can also be inhalation of vomit and saliva. *Status*

epilepticus is a medical emergency because it causes severe hypoxia, and is potentially fatal.

Partial seizures

Petit mal seizures come most often during childhood and are characterized by minimal or no movements (except for eye-blinking) and an apparently blank stare, with a brief sudden loss of awareness or of conscious activity that may last only seconds. Seizures may recur many times and may involve learning difficulties (the child is often thought to be daydreaming). Most patients who have petit mal also have grand mal attacks.

Simple partial (focal) seizures can be motor, sensory or behavioural, typically remain confined to one area, and include muscle contractions of a specific body part – focal motor epilepsy, which may take the form of clonic movements of a limb or group of muscles, usually in the face, arm or leg, though the clonus may spread (march) to adjacent muscles on the same side of the body (Jacksonian epilepsy). There are abnormal sensations; sometimes nausea, sweating, skin flushing and dilated pupils; and sometimes other focal (localized) symptoms.

Partial complex seizures, or temporal lobe epilepsy (psychomotor epilepsy), are characterized by automatism (automatic performance of complex behaviours), such as lip-smacking and chewing movements, or facial grimacing; recalled or inappropriate emotions; changes in personality or alertness; sometimes disorientation, confusion and amnesia, or loss of consciousness; and sometimes olfactory (smell) or gustatory (taste) hallucinations or impairments.

General management of epilepsy

Having a single seizure as the result of a high fever (febrile seizure) or head injury does not necessarily mean that a person has epilepsy. Only when individuals have had two or more seizures are they considered to have epilepsy, and the diagnosis requires careful review.

Disorders that may show features resembling seizures include transient ischaemic attacks, rage or panic attacks, and any disorder that causes loss of consciousness, tremors or tics. Witness accounts are invaluable. A physical examination, including a detailed neurological component, is indicated to confirm the diagnosis; it may show focal neurological deficits but often is normal. CT and MRI are used to screen for cerebral pathology. An EEG records brain electrical activity and may aid in the diagnosis, usually confirming the seizures and possibly, in some cases, indicating the location of a lesion. It displays 3-Hz spike-and-wave activity in primary generalized absence seizures. However, a normal EEG does not completely rule out a seizure disorder. Tests for the cause may also include a full blood picture, blood glucose, liver function tests, renal function tests, inflammatory markers (erythrocyte sedimentation rate [ESR], C-reactive protein [CRP]), and CSF analysis to exclude infection.

Management of a seizure is outlined in Ch 1. Management of epilepsy includes patient education; identification and avoidance of precipitating or trigger factors; treatment of any identifiable predisposing pathology or disease; and prophylactic anticonvulsants. Antiepileptic drugs (AEDs) are the treatment modality used for most people (Table 13.31) and are of two broad groups – GABA or receptor potentiators, and neuronal inhibitors. Therapy is typically started with a single drug, raising doses until the disorder is controlled. A second-line drug is then substituted and some 50% will eventually be able to relinquish medication. However, most patients with major epilepsy having more than one attack in a year need to be maintained on AEDs.

A second drug should only be given *additionally* if a single agent in maximal dosage fails to control fits or causes undesirable toxic effects. Plasma levels may sometimes need to be monitored, particularly with phenytoin, where small changes in dosage can cause disproportionately large changes in plasma levels and toxic effects. Since treatment

Table 13.31 *AED treatment of epilepsy*

Type of epilepsy	Drugs	Adverse effects[a]
Tonic–clonic seizure	Carbamazepine	Skin rashes
	Phenytoin	Blood dyscrasias
	Sodium valproate	Liver impairment
	Gabapentin	
Absence seizure	Sodium valproate	Sleep disturbance
	Ethosuximide	
Partial seizures	Carbamazepine	As above
	Sodium valproate	

[a]Sodium valproate is best avoided in women of childbearing age because of significant risk (5–7%) of fetal malformation. Phenytoin and carbamazepine may also be teratogenic.

Box 13.11 *Possible adverse effects of phenytoin apart from teratogenicity*

- In large doses, nystagmus, ataxia and, possibly, cerebellar damage
- Gingival swelling, thickening of the facial features, hypertrichosis
- Folic acid deficiency and, occasionally, megaloblastic anaemia
- Enhanced catabolism of vitamin D, causing osteomalacia, usually subclinical
- Lymphadenopathy with lymphoma-like changes histologically
- Slightly enhanced risk of lymphoma
- Allergy – rashes, erythema multiforme or lupus erythematosus-like reactions

Table 13.32 *Drugs used in dentistry that can increase anticonvulsant activity, leading to overdose*

Drug	Comment
Aspirin	Can increase the bleeding tendency induced by valproate
Azole antifungals	Can interfere with phenytoin
	Can increase the bleeding tendency induced by valproate
	Can interfere with carbamazepine
Metronidazole	Can interfere with phenytoin
	Can increase the bleeding tendency induced by valproate
Non-steroidal anti-inflammatory drugs (NSAIDs)	Can increase the bleeding tendency induced by valproate
Propoxyphene	Can interfere with carbamazepine

Table 13.33 *Drugs used in dentistry whose activity can be altered by AEDs*

Drug	Comment
Paracetamol (acetaminophen)	Hepatotoxicity may be increased by anticonvulsants
Doxycycline	Metabolism may be increased by carbamazepine

of major epilepsy is often lifelong, adverse effects can be a problem (Box 13.11).

Patients with epilepsy who are drowsy from medication should not operate unguarded machinery or drive. Epileptics may not drive a motor vehicle until they have been seizure-free for more than 1 year, or over a 3-year period have only had sleep attacks.

AEDs may interact with other drugs (Tables 13.32 and 13.33); some interfere with the oral contraceptives. Traditional AEDs in pregnancy, particularly phenytoin, are potentially teratogenic but there is a greater risk to the fetus from uncontrolled epilepsy. Phenytoin (Epanutin), carbamazepine (Tegretol) and sodium valproate (Epilim) are all known to be teratogenic and can cause fetal anticonvulsant syndrome (FACS), which affects up to 10% of babies born to women taking anticonvulsants during pregnancy. Folic acid can reduce the risk of some of the congenital problems seen. Anomalies reported in FACS include spina bifida, cleft palate, and heart, kidney and limb malformations. The children also usually have distinctive facial features (prominent forehead, broad flattened nasal bridge, thin upper lip, medial deficiency of the eyebrows and infraorbital grooves); these may be particularly apparent in pre-school children but change, becoming more normal as the children mature. Anticonvulsant medication is also a risk factor for the development of an autistic spectrum disorder.

Valproate depresses platelet numbers and function to produce a bleeding tendency. Valproate may lead to adverse hormone changes in teenage girls and polycystic ovary syndrome in women who start taking the medication before age 20, so young female patients taking it should be monitored carefully by a physician. NSAIDs, erythromycin and benzodiazepines are also contraindicated.

Newer-generation AEDs which are not teratogenic, include:

- Gabapentin
- Lamotrigine
- Levetiracetam
- Oxcarbazepine
- Topiramate.

Antiepileptic drugs should be continued during breast-feeding. Drug treatment should follow the same principles as for non-pregnant patients but plasma levels need to be monitored, as they may fall during the later stages.

The uses and adverse effects of anticonvulsant drugs are summarized in Appendix 13.2.

With certain types of partial epilepsy, especially when seizures consistently arise from a single area of brain (the 'seizure focus') such as the temporal lobe, surgical removal of that focus may be effective in stopping seizures or making them amenable to medical control.

Other supplemental treatments that are sometimes beneficial include a ketogenic diet (a high-fat, low-carbohydrate diet with restricted calories) and vagus nerve stimulation therapy (VNST). VNST involves the use of an implantable electronic device in the neck to stimulate the vagus nerve intermittently. Little is understood about how vagal nerve stimulation modulates seizure control but about 50% of patients experience a 40% or greater reduction in seizure frequency and severity. Adverse effects may include intermittent decrease in respiratory flow during sleep and up to one-third of patients develop mild obstructive sleep apnoea post treatment. Thus screening for obstructive sleep apnoea (OSA) in patients undergoing a VNST implant is important. VNST may also cause stimulation of the superior and recurrent laryngeal nerves and problems ranging from alteration of voice, coughing, pharyngitis and throat pain, and hoarseness (common) to laryngeal muscle spasm and upper airway obstruction (rare). Transcutaneous vagus nerve stimulation (t-VNS) permits vagal stimulation without surgical intervention (Lisowska and Daly 2012).

Dental aspects

Dental treatment should be carried out in a good phase of epilepsy, when attacks are infrequent. Various factors can precipitate attacks (Box 13.12).

Those who have infrequent seizures or who depend on others (such as those with a learning impairment) may fail to take regular medication and thus be poorly controlled. When dental treatment is being carried out in a known epileptic, a strong mouth prop should be kept in position and the oral cavity kept as free as possible of debris. As much apparatus as possible should be kept away from the area around the patient. Drugs can be epileptogenic or interfere with anticonvulsants, or can themselves be changed by anticonvulsant therapy and may, therefore, be contraindicated (see Tables 13.32 and 13.33; Box 13.13).

In the past, particularly, gingival swelling due to phenytoin required treatment by gingival surgery. Carbamazepine or gabapentin obviates this problem.

Aspirin, azoles and metronidazole can interfere with phenytoin. Propoxyphene and erythromycin can interfere with carbamazepine.

Large doses of lidocaine given intravenously for severe arrhythmias may occasionally cause convulsions. An overenthusiastic casualty officer may therefore blame a dental LA for causing a fit. There is no evidence that this can happen, especially as intravenous lidocaine has also been advocated for the control of status epilepticus.

CS in epilepsy should be safe. Stress reduction should reduce the chance of a fit. Benzodiazepines are anti-epileptogenic, but occasionally fits have been recorded in epileptics undergoing intravenous sedation with midazolam. Flumazenil, however, can be epileptogenic. Nitrous oxide can increase the CNS depression in patients on anticonvulsants. It is probably best to avoid electronic dental analgesia.

Temporal lobe (psychomotor) epilepsy, in particular, is associated with paranoid and schizophrenic features. Antisocial and psychopathic behaviour may then make dental management difficult.

Acrylic is probably better used for prostheses than porcelain, as it is more resilient.

Convulsions may have craniofacial sequelae, especially lacerations, haematomas and fractures. Trauma frequently results from a grand mal attack when the patient falls unconscious or from the muscle spasm, and a range of injuries can result, e.g. fractures of the vertebrae or limbs; dislocations; periorbital subcutaneous haematomas in the absence of facial fractures; injuries to the face from falling (lacerations, haematomas, fractures of the facial skeleton); fractures, devitalization, subluxation or loss of teeth (a chest radiograph may be required); TMJ subluxation; or lacerations or scarring of the tongue, lips or buccal mucosa.

FEBRILE CONVULSIONS (FEBRILE SEIZURES)

Febrile convulsions are more common than epilepsy, usually affect children and result from a rise in body temperature commonly caused by infection; they are seen in about 4% of infants or small children, the child typically losing consciousness and shaking. The seizures characteristically last only last a minute or two; some can be as brief as a few seconds. Risk factors include young age (below 15 months), frequent fevers, and immediate family members who have a history of febrile seizures.

Children who develop high fevers (above 38°C) should therefore be put in a cool environment, bathed with tepid water and given paracetamol (acetaminophen) elixir (*not* aspirin). Children under 18 months should be admitted to hospital since the fit may be due to meningitis. Severe febrile convulsions can cause brain damage and about 3% of children with febrile convulsions go on in later life to develop epilepsy; most do not.

There is no evidence that short febrile seizures cause brain damage – most are harmless and warrant no treatment. However, children who have cerebral palsy, delayed development or other neurological abnormalities, or who have febrile seizures that are lengthy or affect only one part of the body, may have an increased risk of developing epilepsy.

PERIPHERAL NEUROPATHIES

Mononeuropathies are commonly caused by nerve compression (e.g. carpal tunnel syndrome) or by vascular disease. Polyneuropathies have a wide range of causes, as seen in Box 13.14.

AUTONOMIC DYSFUNCTION

Many disorders can be associated with autonomic dysfunction, most importantly ageing, alcoholism, amyloidosis, diabetes, familial dysautonomia, liver failure, parkinsonism, porphyria and renal failure. Autonomic dysfunction manifests with: abnormal sweating (sometimes gustatory sweating), bladder dysfunction, dry mouth and eyes, gastrointestinal dysfunction, impotence and orthostatic (postural) hypotension. Autonomic dysfunction may also underlie sialosis.

Patients with autonomic dysfunction are sensitive to any agent causing hypotension, such as those used in GA, and to being raised quickly from the supine position. Some have mitral valve prolapse.

HORNER SYNDROME

Horner syndrome comprises unilateral:

- miosis (constricted pupil), unreactive to mydriatics
- ptosis (drooping eyelid)
- loss of sweating of the face
- apparent enophthalmos (because of ptosis).

Horner syndrome is usually caused by post-ganglionic interruption of sympathetic nerve fibres, or interruption at the cervical sympathetic trunk or in the spinal cord or brainstem. It may result, for example, from surgery or trauma to the neck, or bronchogenic or metastatic breast carcinoma infiltrating the sympathetic supply from the superior cervical sympathetic ganglion.

CHOLINERGIC DYSAUTONOMIA

Post-ganglionic cholinergic autonomic dysfunction may be autoimmune, characterized by impaired lacrimation and salivation, mydriasis, decreased gastrointestinal motility, bladder atony, sweating and taste disturbance.

RILEY–DAY SYNDROME (FAMILIAL DYSAUTONOMIA)

Familial dysautonomia, a rare autosomal recessive disorder found almost exclusively in Ashkenazi Jews, is characterized by selective damage to the sensory, motor and autonomic peripheral nervous system.

The main features are depressed pain sensation and impaired regulation of temperature and blood pressure. Aspiration pneumonias and episodes of acute abdominal pain are common.

Orthostatic hypotension can occur, so patients should be raised upright only cautiously. The other most important dental aspect is self-mutilation of hard and/or soft tissues. Splints may be used to protect the soft tissues.

Hypersalivation may be seen, the lingual fungiform papillae and taste sensation are diminished, and oral hygiene may be poor.

DISORDERS OF NEUROMUSCULAR TRANSMISSION

MYASTHENIA GRAVIS

See Chapter 16.

SLEEP

Sleep affects daily functioning and physical and mental health. Sleep and wakefulness are controlled by neurotransmitters; brainstem serotonin (5-hydroxytryptamine; 5HT) and noradrenaline (norepinephrine) keep parts of the brain active during wakefulness, while other neurons at the base of the brain begin signalling during sleep and 'switch off' signals that maintain wakefulness. Adenosine accumulates throughout waking hours, causing drowsiness, but gradually breaks down during sleep.

Sleep passes through stages 1, 2, 3, 4 and rapid eye movement (*REM*) sleep; then the cycle starts all over again with stage 1. A complete sleep cycle takes 90–110 minutes on average, the first REM period usually occurring about 70–90 minutes after falling asleep. It manifests with more rapid, irregular and shallow breathing, rapidly jerking eyes, temporary paralysis of limb muscles and increase in heart rate; blood pressure rises and males can develop erections. REM sleep stimulates the brain regions used in learning, which may be important for normal brain development; this would explain why infants spend much more time in REM sleep than adults.

In stage 1, light sleep, the person can be awakened easily, the eyes move slowly and muscle activity slows. In stage 2 sleep, eye movements stop and brain electrical activity subsides, with occasional bursts of rapid waves called *sleep spindles.* In stage 3, extremely slow brain waves called *delta waves* begin to appear, interspersed with smaller, faster waves. By stage 4, the brain produces delta waves almost exclusively. Stages 3 and 4 are called *deep sleep* and this is typified by lack of eye movement and muscle activity; people awakened during deep sleep do not adjust immediately and often feel disoriented for several minutes after they wake up. Some children experience bed-wetting, night terrors or sleepwalking during deep sleep. Deep sleep coincides with growth hormone release in children and young adults, and increased production and reduced breakdown of proteins. Activity in parts of the brain that control emotions, decision-making processes and social interactions is drastically reduced during deep sleep, suggesting that this type of sleep may help people maintain optimal emotional and social functioning while awake.

The first sleep cycles each night contain relatively short REM periods and long periods of deep sleep; as the night progresses, REM sleep periods lengthen while deep sleep decreases so that, by morning, most people spend nearly all their sleep time in stages 1, 2 and REM.

Circadian (from the Latin for 'around a day') rhythms are regular changes in mental and physical characteristics that occur in the course of a day; they are usually controlled by the body's biological 'clock' – the hypothalamic suprachiasmatic nucleus (SCN). The SCN receives information about the amount of light or darkness, and connects with the pineal gland, which produces melatonin. Tryptophan is converted to serotonin and finally to the hormone melatonin (N-acetyl-5-methoxytryptamine). The less light there is, the more melatonin is released, and nocturnal melatonin secretion may be involved in physiological sleep onset. At sunset, light cessation triggers the pineal to begin releasing melatonin and this rises, peaking around 2.00 a.m. (3.00 a.m. for the elderly), after which it steadily declines to minimal levels by morning. Melatonin regulates many neuroendocrine functions. The SCN has melatonin receptors, and melatonin may have a direct action on the SCN to influence circadian rhythms. The SCN also governs functions synchronized with the sleep–wake cycle, including temperature, hormone secretion, urine production and changes in blood pressure.

SLEEP DISORDERS

The amount of sleep each person needs depends on many factors, including age. Children generally require about 12 hours a day, teenagers need about 9 hours and most adults 7–8 hours. Women in the first 3 months of pregnancy often need more. The amount of sleep needed also increases if a person has been deprived of sleep previously – a dangerous situation when operating machinery or driving. Too little sleep causes drowsiness and inability to concentrate, impaired memory and physical performance, and reduced ability to carry out calculations. If it continues, hallucinations and mood swings may develop. Reduced sleep duration is associated with increased body mass and obesity; sleep restriction to 4 hours of sleep per night increases blood pressure, decreases parasympathetic tone, increases evening cortisol and insulin levels, and promotes increased appetite, possibly through the elevation of ghrelin, a pro-appetitive hormone, along with decreased levels of leptin. Moreover, proinflammatory cytokine levels are increased with sleep deprivation, along with decreased performance in tests of psychomotor vigilance, and this has been reported to result from a modest sleep restriction.

Foods can change neurotransmitters and affect sleep, as can drugs (e.g. alcohol, amphetamines, antidepressants, caffeine, cocaine, decongestants, dopaminergic drugs, ecstasy, hypnotics, pramipexole, sedatives, statins and valproate). Antidepressants may suppress REM sleep. Heavy smokers often sleep lightly, have reduced amounts of REM sleep and tend to wake after 3–4 hours due to nicotine withdrawal.

The ability to thermoregulate is lost during REM, so abnormally hot or cold environmental temperatures can disrupt sleep.

Sleep and sleep-related problems play a role in a large number of disorders (Table 13.34).

Insomnia

The best measure of the amount of sleep needed is how a person feels, if they awaken feeling refreshed, they are getting enough sleep. Insomnia can affect almost everyone occasionally because of stress, jet lag, diet or many other factors, and insomnia tends to increase with age. It affects about 40% of women, 30% of men and over 50% of older people. Insomnia is a key symptom of depression and often the major disabling symptom of an underlying medical disorder (Table 13.35).

Insomnia can be a chronic and persistent difficulty in either:

- falling asleep (initial insomnia)
- remaining asleep through the night (middle insomnia)
- waking up too early (terminal insomnia).

Insomnia almost always affects well-being and job performance the next day. Those who have insomnia frequently or for extended periods of time can develop even more serious sleep deficits.

Mild insomnia often can be prevented or cured by practising good sleep hygiene habits (Box 13.15). For short-term insomnia, hypnotics may help. Counselling may be valuable for psychological disorders that lead to insomnia; antidepressants such as amitriptyline or trazodone can often be helpful. Antihistamines and long-acting or high-dose sedatives can increase daytime drowsiness, making the problem worse over time, not better.

Jet lag

Jet lag is the result of long-distance travel east/west, crossing time zones at a rapid rate, and consists of symptoms such as sleep disturbance, loss of appetite, reduced psychomotor efficiency and general malaise. Circadian rhythms need about 1 day to adapt for each time zone crossed; people adapt more easily after a flight westward because there is a longer day. Melatonin will almost certainly have a role in the treatment but the exact dose regime still requires to be worked out. Benzodiazepines are the current treatments; they appear to suppress melatonin secretion.

Delayed sleep phase syndrome

This is the condition when people are only able to fall asleep late into the night or early in the morning. It is quite common among adolescents.

Somnambulism (sleepwalking)

This disorder falls under the parasomnia group – undesirable motor, verbal or experiential events that occur during sleep. Sleepwalking occurs most commonly in middle childhood and pre-adolescence, with a peak incidence around puberty. There are no specific diagnostic tests. Reassurance usually suffices. Parents may need to lock windows and

Table 13.34 *Effects of disease on sleep*

Disorder	Sleep-related problems
Depression	Often causes early morning wakening. Extreme sleep deprivation can lead to a seemingly psychotic state of paranoia and hallucinations in otherwise healthy people and disrupted sleep can trigger episodes of mania (agitation and hyperactivity) in people with manic depression
Epilepsy	Rapid eye movement (REM) sleep seems to help prevent seizures, while deep sleep may promote the spread of these seizures. Sleep deprivation may trigger seizures
Infectious diseases	Cytokines are powerfully sleep-inducing
Pain	Hospital routines may disrupt sleep, and patients who are unable to sleep also notice pain more
Sleep apnoea	Ch. 15
Stroke and asthma	Attacks tend to occur more frequently during the night and early morning, perhaps due to changes in hormones and heart rate

Table 13.35 *Causes of insomnia*[a]

Causes	Detail
Disrupted waking hours	Jet lag, shift work, wake–sleep pattern disturbances, excessive sleep during day
Disturbance of sleep	Bed or bedroom not conducive to sleep, noise, interference with sleep by diseases, including prostate hypertrophy (men), cystitis (women), chronic obstructive pulmonary disease, arthritis, heartburn and cardiorespiratory problems
Drugs	Nicotine, alcohol, caffeine, food or stimulants at bedtime, medications or illicit 'street drugs' (e.g. excessive thyroxine, amphetamines, caffeine-containing beverages, cocaine, ephedrine, phenylpropanolamine, theophylline), withdrawal of medications (such as sedatives or hypnotics), alcoholism or abrupt alcohol cessation
Endocrine	Hyperthyroidism
Light exposure	Inadequate bright-light exposure during waking hours
Others	Ageing, restless legs syndrome (see later)
Psychological factors	Depression, grief, anxiety, stress, exhilaration or excitement, excessive physical or intellectual stimulation at bedtime

[a]See also Table 13.35.

Box 13.15 *Sleep hygiene*[a]

- Having a routine
- Going to the toilet before retiring
- Taking a warm bath
- Going to sleep at a reasonable time
- Ensuring that the bed is comfortable, warm and in a quiet place
- Avoiding stimulants

[a]See http://umm.edu/programs/sleep/patients/sleep-hygiene (accessed 26 May 2013).

doors, remove obstacles and add alarms (if necessary) to decrease the likelihood of injury. Benzodiazepines or tricyclic antidepressants may be useful if necessary.

Seasonal affective disorder (SAD; winter depression)

This is depression occurring in the winter months, associated with hypersomnia, weight gain and carbohydrate craving. Environmental magnetic fields have diminished strength during the winter months and there may be desynchronization of the circadian rhythm. SAD improves with bright-light treatment, or melatonin.

Narcolepsy

Narcolepsy is a disorder of sleep regulation that manifests with 'sleep attacks' lasting from several seconds to more than 30 minutes, at various times, even after a normal night's sleep. Narcolepsy is usually hereditary, linked to HLA-DR2 and the hypocretin receptor 2 gene, but is occasionally caused by brain damage from a head injury or neurological disease. People with narcolepsy also may experience cataplexy (sudden onset of falling or collapse), hallucinations whilst falling asleep, temporary paralysis on awakening and disrupted night-time sleep. Nearly 50% of patients develop a personality or major affective disorder.

Restless legs syndrome

This is one of the most common sleep disorders, especially among older people. A familial disorder causing unpleasant crawling, prickling or tingling sensations in legs and feet and an urge to move them for relief, it may sometimes be linked to anaemia, pregnancy or diabetes. Many restless legs syndrome (RLS) patients also have a disorder known as *periodic limb movement disorder* (PLMD), which causes repetitive jerking movements of the limbs, especially the legs. These movements occur every 20–40 seconds and cause severely fragmented sleep. RLS and PLMD often can be relieved by drugs that affect dopamine.

Snoring

Snoring is caused by the vibration of the uvula and soft palate during breathing whilst asleep. It is at the lower end of a spectrum of sleep-disordered breathing (SDB), which may be related to weak activity of tongue, palate and pharynx muscles. SDB has simple snoring at its minimal level, then upper airways resistance syndrome (UARS) and, finally, obstructive sleep apnoea syndrome (OSAS; Ch. 15). SDB has been associated with insulin resistance and glucose intolerance, and is frequently found in people with type 2 diabetes.

At least 30% of adults snore, more as age increases. Snorers tend to have a higher body mass index and snoring is usually due to nasal or pharyngeal obstruction or weakness. Snoring is usually a minor problem, but complications may include interpersonal difficulties from annoyance to others, mouth-breathing and dryness, headache and daytime tiredness. Almost all treatments for snoring are based on ensuring upper airway patency. Advice includes sleeping on the side, losing weight and stopping smoking. Rarely, single-dose injection snoreplasty with sodium tetradecyl sulfate or surgery (or radiofrequency uvulopalatopharyngoplasty or laser-assisted palatoplasty) is indicated.

Central sleep apnoea is a disorder that may occur particularly in people who have life-threatening brainstem problems, since control of breathing is located there. The condition may be associated with:

- cervical spine disorders:
  arthritis
  surgery
  radiation
- CNS conditions:
  bulbar poliomyelitis
  brainstem stroke or encephalitis
  Parkinson's disease
  primary hypoventilation syndrome
- use of narcotics.

REPETITIVE MOTION DISORDERS (OVERUSE SYNDROME)

Repetitive motion disorders (RMDs) are muscular conditions that result from repeated motions performed in the course of normal work or daily activities. RMDs most commonly affect the upper limbs (hands, wrists, elbows and shoulders), but can also be seen in the neck, back, hips, knees, feet, legs and ankles. RMDs include carpal tunnel syndrome, bursitis, tendonitis, epicondylitis, ganglion cyst, tenosynovitis and trigger finger.

RMDs are characterized by pain, tingling, numbness, swelling or redness of the affected area, and loss of flexibility and strength.

Treatment for RMDs usually includes reducing or stopping the causative motions. Applying ice to the affected area and analgesics, NSAIDs and steroids can reduce pain and swelling. Splints may relieve pressure on the muscles and nerves. Physical therapy may help. In rare cases only, surgery may be required.

KEY WEBSITES

(Accessed 27 May 2013)
BMJ. <http://www.bmj.com/specialties/neurology>.
National Institutes of Health: National Institute of Neurological Disorders and Stroke. <http://www.ninds.nih.gov/disorders/disorder_index.htm>.

USEFUL WEBSITES

(Accessed 27 May 2013)
American Epilepsy Society. <http://www.aesnet.org/>.
Brain & Spine Foundation. <http://www.brainandspine.org.uk>.
British Sleep Society. <http://www.sleepsociety.org.uk/>.
Epilepsy Action. <http://www.epilepsy.org.uk/>.
Facial Neuralgia Resources. http://facial-neuralgia.org.
IMigraine.net. http://imigraine.net.
Meningitis Now. <http://www.meningitis-trust.org/>.
Multiple Sclerosis Society. <http://www.mssociety.org.uk/>.
National CJD Research & Surveillance Unit. <http://www.cjd.ed.ac.uk>.
Stroke Association. <http://www.stroke.org.uk/>.

FURTHER READING

Al-Jassim, A.H., Lesser, T.H., 2008. Single dose injection snoreplasty: investigation or treatment? J. Laryngol. Otol. 122, 1190.
American Dental Association Council on Scientific Affairs, 2006. The use of dental radiographs: update and recommendations. J. Am. Dent. Assoc. 137, 1304.
Bacigaluppi, M., Hermann, D.M., 2008. New targets of neuroprotection in ischemic stroke. Sci. World J. 8, 698.

Bakheit, A.M., 2006. The possible adverse effects of intramuscular botulinum toxin injections and their management. Curr. Drug. Saf. 1, 271.

Blanchet, P.J., et al. 2005. Oral dyskinesia; a clinical overview. Int. J. Prosthodont. 18, 10.

Boyle, C.A., et al. 2008. Providing dental care for patients with Huntington's disease. Dent. Update 35, 333.

Chemaly, D., et al. 2000. Oral and maxillofacial manifestations of multiple sclerosis. J. Can. Dent. Assoc. 66, 600.

Claus, E.B., et al. 2012. Dental X-rays and risk of meningioma. Cancer 118 (18), 4530.

Combarros, O., et al. 2000. Hemiageusia from an ipsilateral multiple sclerosis plaque at the midpontine tegmentum. J. Neurol. Neurosurg. Psychiatry 68, 796.

Costa, M.M., et al. 2008. Prevalence of dental trauma in patients with cerebral palsy. Spec. Care Dentist. 28, 61.

Cruccu, G., et al. 2008. AAN-EFNS guidelines on trigeminal neuralgia management. Eur. J. Neurol. 15, 1013.

Dave, S.J., 2008. Pilocarpine for the treatment of refractory dry mouth (xerostomia) associated with botulinum toxin type B. Am. J. Phys. Med. Rehabil. 87, 684.

Fedok, F.G., 2008. Advances in minimally invasive facial rejuvenation. Curr. Opin. Otolaryngol. Head Neck Surg. 16, 359.

Fiske, J., Boyle, C., 2002. Epilepsy and oral care. Dent. Update 29, 180.

Frenkel, H., 2004. Alzheimer's disease and oral care. Dent. Update 31, 273.

Gronseth, G.S., Paduga, R., 2012. Evidence-based guideline update: steroids and antivirals for Bell palsy. Report of the Guideline Development Subcommittee of the American Academy of Neurology. Neurology 79, 1.

Hankey, G.J., 2008. Review: statins prevent stroke and reduce mortality. Evid. Based Med. 13, 113.

Haytac, M.C., et al. 2008. Epileptic seizures triggered by the use of a powered toothbrush. Seizure 17, 288.

Holland, J.N., Weiner, G.M., 2004. Recent developments in Bell's palsy. Br. Med. J. 329, 553.

Hupp, W.S., 2001. Seizure disorders. Oral Surg. 92, 593.

Jacobsen, P.L., Eden, O., 2008. Epilepsy and the dental management of the epileptic patient. J. Contemp. Dent. Pract. 9, 54.

Jagoda, A., Chan, Y.F., 2008. Transient ischemic attack overview: defining the challenges for improving outcomes. Ann. Emerg. Med. 52, S3.

Kang, Y.K., et al. 2000. Pure trigeminal motor neuropathy: a case report. Arch. Phys. Med. Rehabil. 81, 995.

Katsara, M., et al. 2008. Towards immunotherapeutic drugs and vaccines against multiple sclerosis. Acta Biochim. Biophys. Sin. (Shanghai) 40, 636.

Kocaelli, H., et al. 2002. Alzheimer's disease and dental management. Oral Surg. 93, 521.

Kumazawa, R., et al. 2008. Mutation analysis of the PINK1 gene in 391 patients with Parkinson disease. Arch. Neurol. 65, 802.

Lamonte, M.P., 2008. Ensuring emergency medicine performance standards for stroke and transient ischemic attack care. Emerg. Med. Clin. North Am. 26, 703.

Lisowska, P., Daly, B., 2012. Vagus nerve stimulation therapy (VNST) in epilepsy – implications for dental practice. Br. Dent. J. 212 (2), 69.

Lobbezoo, F., Naeije, M., 2007. Dental implications of some common movement disorders. Arch. Oral Biol. 52, 395.

Lumley, J.S.P., 2004. Creutzfeld–Jakob disease (CJD) in surgical practice. Ann. R. Coll. Surg. Eng. 86, 86.

McCormack, M., et al. 2011. HLA-A*3101 and carbamazepine-induced hypersensitivity reactions in Europeans. N. Engl. J. Med. 364 (12), 1134.

Meeks, S.L., et al. 2000. Calculation of cranial nerve complication probability for acoustic neuroma radiosurgery. Int. J. Radiat. Oncol. Biol. Phys. 47 (3), 597.

Moore, P., Naumann, M., 2003. Handbook of botulinum treatment, 2nd ed. Blackwell, Oxford.

Penarrocha, M., et al. 2001. Acyclovir treatment in 2 patients with benign trigeminal sensory neuropathy. J. Oral Maxillofac. Surg. 59, 453.

Penarrocha, M., et al. 2007. Trigeminal neuropathy. Oral Dis. 13, 141.

Ramagopal, M., et al. 2008. Obstructive sleep apnea and history of asthma in snoring children. Sleep Breath. 12, 381.

Schulte-Mattler, W.J., 2008. Use of botulinum toxin a in adult neurological disorders: efficacy, tolerability and safety. CNS Drugs 22, 725.

Scully, C., Chaudhry, S., 2008. Aspects of human disease 23. Cerebrovascular accident (CVA). Dent. Update 35, 357.

Scully, C., Chaudhry, S., 2008. Aspects of human disease 24. Dementia. Dent. Update 35, 428.

Scully, C., Chaudhry, S., 2008. Aspects of human disease 25. Epilepsy. Dent. Update 35, 501.

Scully, C., Chaudhry, S., 2008. Aspects of human disease 26. Multiple sclerosis. Dent. Update 35, 581.

Scully, C., Chaudhry, S., 2008. Aspects of human disease 27. Migraine. Dent. Update 35, 645.

Scully, C., Diz Dios, P., 2000. Oral dyskinesias and palsies. In: Alio Sanz, J.J. (Ed.), Rapport XV congress of international association of disability and oral health. Aula Medica, Madrid, pp. 306.

Scully, C., Shotts, R., 2001. The mouth in neurological disorders. Practitioner 245, 539.

Shaw, J.E., et al. 2008. Sleep-disordered breathing and type 2 diabetes: a report from the International Diabetes Federation Taskforce on Epidemiology and Prevention. Diabetes Res. Clin. Pract. 81, 2.

Simola, N., et al. 2008. Adenosine A2A receptor antagonists and Parkinson's disease: state of the art and future directions. Curr. Pharm. Des. 14, 1475.

Smith, A.J., et al. 2003. Prions and the oral cavity. J. Dent. Res. 82, 769.

Stone, C.A., O'Leary, N., 2008. Systematic review of the effectiveness of botulinum toxin or radiotherapy for sialorrhea in patients with amyotrophic lateral sclerosis. J. Pain Symptom Manage. 37, 246.

Sullivan, F.M., et al. 2007. Early treatment with prednisolone or acyclovir in Bell's palsy. N. Engl. J. Med. 357, 1598.

Suryadevara, A.C., 2008. Update on perioral cosmetic enhancement. Curr. Opin. Otolaryngol. Head Neck Surg. 16, 347.

Swope, D., Barbano, R., 2008. Treatment recommendations and practical applications of botulinum toxin treatment of cervical dystonia. Neurol. Clin. 26 (Suppl. 1), 54.

Toulouse, A., Sullivan, A.M., 2008. Progress in Parkinson's disease: where do we stand? Prog. Neurobiol. 85, 376.

Vorkas, C.K., et al. 2008. Epilepsy and dental procedures: a review. N Y State Dent. J. 74, 39.

Voss, N.F., et al. 2000. Meningiomas of the cerebellopontine angle. Surg. Neurol. 53, 439.

Welsby, P.D., 2004. The 12, 24, or is it 26 cranial nerves? Postgrad. Med. J. 80, 602.

Xue, M., et al. 2008. Autism spectrum disorders: concurrent clinical disorders. J. Child Neurol. 23, 6.

Zivadinov, R., et al. 2008. Mechanisms of action of disease-modifying agents and brain volume changes in multiple sclerosis. Neurology 71, 136.

APPENDIX 13.1 CRANIAL NERVE SYNDROMES

Syndrome	Cranial nerves involved	Site of lesion	Other features
Avellis	X	Medulla	Hemiplegia
			Horner syndrome
Benedikt	III	Midbrain	Cerebellar ataxia
			Tremor
			Hemiplegia
Cerebellopontine angle	V, VII, VIII, sometimes IX	Posterior cranial fossa	Cerebellar ataxia
Claude	III	Midbrain	Cerebellar ataxia
			Tremor
Collet–Sicard	IX, X, XI, XII	Retroparotid space	Paralysed palate, pharynx, tongue
Foix	III, IV, V (ophthalmic), VI	Cavernous sinus	Proptosis
Gradenigo	V, VI	Petrous temporal	Pain
Jackson	X, XII	Medulla	Hemiplegia
			Horner syndrome
Jacob	II, III, IV, V, VI	Middle cranial fossa	–
Millard–Gubler	VII, VI	Pons	Hemiplegia
Moebius	VI, VII	Pons	Lack of facial expression
Nothnagel	III	Midbrain	Cerebellar ataxia
Parinaud	III, IV, VI	Midbrain	Abnormal eye movements with pupil dysfunction
Sphenoid fissure (superior orbital fissure)	III, IV, V (ophthalmic), VI, sometimes II	Superior orbital fissure	Proptosis
Vernet	IX, X, XI	Jugular foramen	Paralysed soft palate, pharynx and vocal cords
		Nasopharynx	
Villaret	IX, X, XI, XII	Retroparotid space	Horner syndrome
Wallenberg (posterior inferior cerebellar artery [PICA]; lateral medullary)	V, IX, X, XI	Medulla	Ipsilateral cerebellar ataxia and Horner syndrome, loss of pain and temperature sense on face, and paralysis of palate/pharynx/larynx
			Contralateral loss of pain and temperature sense elsewhere
			Vertigo, nystagmus
Weber	III	Midbrain	Hemiplegia

APPENDIX 13.2 ANTICONVULSANT DRUGS: USES AND ADVERSE EFFECTS

Drug	Use	Systemic adverse effects	Oral adverse effects
Carbamazepine	Temporal lobe epilepsy (TLE)	Ataxia	Dry mouth
	Grand mal (GM)	Drowsiness	Dyskinesias
		Leukopenia	Erythema multiforme
		Lupoid syndrome	
		Syndrome of inappropriate antidiuretic hormone secretion (SIADH; Ch. 6)	
Valproate	GM	Bleeding diathesis	Purpura
	Petit mal (PM)	Drowsiness	
Phenytoin	GM	Cerebellar damage	Cervical lymphadenopathy, dental anomalies
	TLE	Hirsutism	Erythema multiforme
		Hyperglycaemia	Gingival swelling
		Nephrotic syndrome	Lupoid syndrome or ulcers
Ethosuximide	PM	Eosinophilia	–
		Lupoid syndrome	
		Renal damage	
Primidone	GM	Ataxia	Megaloblastic anaemia causing ulcers
	TLE	Drowsiness	
	PM	Oculomotor palsy	
Gabapentin	GM	Dizziness	Dry mouth
	PM	Drowsiness	
Topiramate	GM	Allergic reactions	Dry mouth, oedema
	PM	Various others	

APPENDIX 13.3 PERIPHERAL NEUROPATHIES

Hereditary

- Charcot–Marie–Tooth disease
- Dejerine–Sottas disease
- Refsum disease

Acquired

- Infective
  - Diphtheria
  - Guillain–Barré syndrome
  - Herpes zoster
  - Human immunodeficiency virus (HIV)
  - Human T-lymphotropic virus 1 (HTLV-1)
  - Leprosy
  - Lyme disease

- Neoplasms
  - Various
- Trauma
- Metabolic
  - Diabetes mellitus
  - Vitamin deficiencies, especially B_{12}
- Toxic
  - Alcohol
  - Gold
  - Heavy metals
  - Nitrous oxide abuse
- Idiopathic
  - Bell palsy

The upper respiratory tract (URT) includes the nose, paranasal sinus, pharynx and larynx but the salivary glands and oral cavity are closely adjacent. Otorhinolaryngology specialists (ear, nose and throat; ENT) deal mainly with the nose, paranasal sinus, pharynx and larynx, and often employ binocular microscopy (Fig. 14.1) and nasendoscopy. Salivary disorders are discussed mainly in this chapter, as well as Chapters 18 and 22, oral disorders in Chapters 11 and 22. The URT may become damaged by pollutants such as smoke, soot, dust and chemicals, or infected with microorganisms from the inspired air. Pain from sinus or aural problems may radiate or be referred to the mouth; equally, oral problems may cause pain in the sinus or ear.

UPPER RESPIRATORY TRACT INFECTIONS (URTI)

A wide variety of respiratory pathogens may cause a single clinical syndrome and, *vice versa*, any one pathogen may cause a range of clinical diseases. Most URTI are viral.

The URT is also colonized by normal bacterial flora, which rarely cause disease, but may under certain circumstances cause upper or lower respiratory tract (LRT) or even systemic or transmissible infections. For example, the normal nasal bacterial flora may include *Staphylococcus aureus*, *S. epidermidis* and aerobic corynebacteria ('diphtheroids'). Some people carry meticillin-resistant *S. aureus* (MRSA) in their nose, which can cause disease (Ch. 21). Bacterial infection caused by a foreign body introduced into the nose of a child (e.g. a small toy) is a well-recognized cause of halitosis, as are tonsillitis and sinusitis. The nasopharyngeal bacterial flora may include non-encapsulated or non-virulent strains of *Streptococcus pneumoniae*, *Neisseria meningitidis* and *Haemophilus influenzae*, which may cause meningitis. Pharyngitis can be caused by group A streptococci (and can rarely lead to rheumatic fever and occasionally rheumatic carditis; Ch. 5) or can be caused by Epstein–Barr virus (Ch. 21).

VIRAL UPPER RESPIRATORY TRACT INFECTIONS

Viruses frequently evade URT defences to produce infections; children have up to eight UTRIs per year, and adolescents up to four. Viral URTIs are highly infectious in the early stages and most are contracted by shaking the hands of infected persons or by touching things that they have touched (and then touching the nose, mouth or conjunctivae; Table 14.1); infection may also be spread via sneezes. The incubation periods rarely exceed 14 days. The incubation times of the common agents are:

- rhinoviruses, 1–5 days
- influenza and parainfluenza viruses, 1–4 days
- respiratory syncytial virus (RSV), 7 days
- Epstein–Barr virus (EBV), 4–6 weeks.

The three main clinical patterns of URTI are the common cold syndrome (coryza), pharyngitis and tonsillitis, and laryngotracheitis.
Other URTIs are discussed in Chapter 21.

The common cold syndrome

General aspects

The common cold is caused not by a single organism but usually by rhinoviruses; it can, however, be caused by more than 200 different viruses (Table 14.2), particularly by respiratory syncytial virus (RSV), coronaviruses, and para-influenza and influenza viruses).

Clinical features

Sneezing, mucus overproduction with nasal obstruction, nasopharyngeal soreness and mild systemic upset are common. Bacterial infection may supervene and cause sinusitis or middle ear infection (otitis media), but serious complications are rare in otherwise healthy patients.

General management

Only symptomatic treatment is available.

Dental aspects

Elective dental care is best deferred. General anaesthesia (GA) should be avoided since there is often some respiratory obstruction and

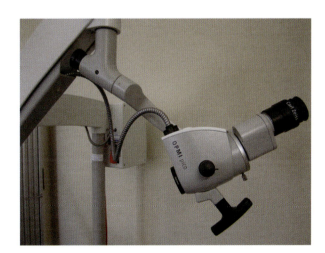

Fig. 14.1 Microscope.

Table 14.1 *The main respiratory viruses*

Viral respiratory pathogens	Presumed viral respiratory disease
Adenoviruses	Coronaviruses
Influenza viruses	Coxsackie viruses
Para-influenza virus	Cytomegalovirus
Respiratory syncytial virus	ECHO viruses
Rhinoviruses	Epstein–Barr virus
	Herpes simplex viruses
	Severe acute respiratory syndrome (SARS)

Table 14.2 *Upper respiratory tract infections and their main causes*

Condition	Micro-organisms
Common cold	Coronavirus
	Coxsackie viruses
	ECHO viruses
	Para-influenza virus
	Respiratory syncytial virus
	Rhinoviruses
Pharyngitis	Adenoviruses
	Coxsackie viruses
	ECHO viruses
	Epstein–Barr virus
	Beta-haemolytic streptococci
	Influenza viruses
	Candida
Tonsillitis	Adenoviruses
	Beta-haemolytic streptococci
	Enteroviruses
	Epstein–Barr virus
	Herpes simplex virus
	Influenza viruses
	Para-influenza viruses
Influenza	Influenza viruses
Sinusitis	*Streptococcus pneumoniae*
	Streptococcus milleri
	Haemophilus influenzae
	Moraxella catarrhalis
	Aspergillus
	Mucorales

Box 14.1 *Factors predisposing to sinusitis*

- Diving – water may be forced into the nose and sinuses
- Barotrauma in air flight, conversely
- Foreign body in nose or sinus
- Peri-apical infection of upper posterior teeth
- Oro-antral fistula
- Prolonged endotracheal intubation and mechanical ventilation
- Rhinitis – vasomotor or allergic
- Viral upper respiratory tract infection

infection can spread to the lungs. If a GA is unavoidable, it is best to intubate with a cuffed tube, so that nasal secretions do not enter the larynx. Antimicrobials may be indicated for prophylaxis. Xylitol chewing gum has been shown to reduce the risk of otitis media, presumably by inhibiting pneumococcal superinfection.

Pharyngitis and tonsillitis

General aspects

Most cases of pharyngitis and tonsillitis are caused by viruses (see Table 14.2), some by streptococci.

Clinical features

The throat is sore, with pain on swallowing (dysphagia) and sometimes fever and conjunctivitis. Enlargement of the tonsils with an infected exudate from the crypts, together with cervical lymphadenopathy, is characteristic of tonsillitis. Prominent submucosal aggregates of lymphoid tissue may be evident in those with pharyngitis. Complications are rare but may include peritonsillar abscess (quinsy), otitis media and, rarely, scarlet fever, acute glomerulonephritis or rheumatic fever.

General management

Infectious mononucleosis (glandular fever) or, rarely, diphtheria may need to be considered in the differential diagnosis.

Tonsillitis caused by bacterial infection is best treated with benzyl or phenoxymethyl penicillin, or, if the patient is allergic, by erythromycin

or a cephalosporin. Ampicillin and amoxicillin should be avoided, as they tend to cause rashes, especially if the sore throat is misdiagnosed as a streptococcal sore throat but is due to glandular fever.

Pharyngitis is not often treated with antimicrobials, as there is no evidence that they accelerate resolution or reduce complications; an increasing body of opinion advises simple analgesics.

Dental aspects

Elective dental care is best deferred. GA should be avoided since there is often a degree of respiratory obstruction and infection may spread to the lungs.

Laryngotracheitis

General aspects

Various microbes may be involved, such as respiratory syncytial virus (RSV), particularly in children.

Clinical features

Hoarseness, loss of voice and persistent cough are common. In children, partial laryngeal obstruction may cause noisy inspiration (stridor or croup) and is potentially dangerous.

General management

Symptomatic treatment only is available but ribavirin or palivizumab may be appropriate in RSV infection in infants who may otherwise subsequently develop bronchiolitis.

Dental aspects

Dental treatment should be deferred until after recovery. GA must be avoided, as it may exacerbate progression of infection to the lungs. Antimicrobials may be indicated for prophylaxis.

BACTERIAL RESPIRATORY TRACT INFECTIONS

Sinusitis

General aspects

Infection of the paranasal air sinuses (maxillary most commonly, but also ethmoid, sphenoid and frontal) is usually bacterial. It may be preceded by viral or other factors (Box 14.1).

Table 14.3 *Paranasal sinusitis*

Sinus	Location of pain	Other features
Maxillary	Cheek and/or upper teeth, worsened by biting	Tenderness over antra
Frontal	Over frontal sinuses	Tenderness of sides of nose
Ethmoidal	Between eyes	Anosmia, eyelid swelling
Sphenoidal	Ear, neck, and top or centre of head	–

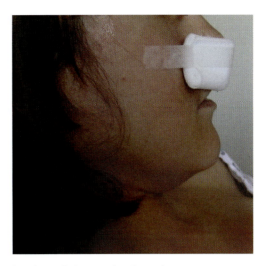

Fig. 14.2 Nasal pack, used after nasal and antral surgery.

Clinical features

Headache on wakening is typical, with pain worse on tilting the head or lying down; there is also nasal obstruction with mucopurulent nasal discharge (Table 14.3).

General management

Diagnosis is from the history, plus tenderness over the sinus, dullness on transillumination, and radio-opacity or a fluid level on plain X-rays of the sinuses (sinus opacity may be due to mucosal thickening rather than infection, but a fluid level is highly suggestive of infection). Antral opacities in children can be difficult to evaluate since they are seen in up to 50% of healthy children under the age of 6 years. Computed tomography (CT) is now the standard care. Ultrasonography may be helpful. However, the gold standard for diagnosis remains sinus puncture and aspiration.

Sinusitis is classified as acute, chronic or recurrent.

In *acute sinusitis*, the bacteria most commonly incriminated are *Streptococcus pneumoniae* and *Haemophilus influenzae*. Infection resolves spontaneously in about 50%, but analgesics are often indicated and antibiotics may be required if symptoms persist or there is a purulent discharge. Treatment is drainage using vasoconstrictor nasal drops, such as ephedrine or xylometazoline. Inhalations of warm, moist air, with benzoin, menthol or eucalyptus, may give symptomatic relief. In adults, a course of antimicrobials for longer than 7 days is indicated, using amoxicillin, ampicillin or co-amoxiclav (erythromycin or azithromycin, if penicillin-allergic), or a tetracycline, such as doxycycline, or clarithromycin. In children, high-dose amoxicillin, cefuroxime or co-amoxiclav is recommended especially if the child has received antibiotics during the 4–6 weeks prior to the infection.

Chronic sinusitis involves anaerobes, especially *Porphyromonas* (Bacteroides), and half are beta-lactamase producers. It may follow acute sinusitis, especially where there are local abnormalities, allergic rhinitis, or impaired defence mechanisms such as cystic fibrosis or human immunodeficiency virus (HIV) disease. Gram-positive cocci and bacilli, as well as Gram-negative bacilli, may also be found – especially in HIV/acquired immunodeficiency syndrome (AIDS) patients and those on prolonged endotracheal intubation. *Pseudomonas aeruginosa* (up to 5% of cases are caused by *Pseudomonas*, especially in cystic fibrosis), *Acinetobacter baumannii* and Enterobacteriaceae are also implicated. In immunocompromised persons, fungi may also be involved, including *Mucor*, *Aspergillus* or other species. Chronic sinusitis responds better to drainage by functional endoscopic surgical techniques (Fig. 14.2), plus antimicrobials, such as metronidazole with amoxicillin, erythromycin, clarithromycin or a cephalosporin.

Recurrent sinusitis should be treated with drainage, plus antimicrobials, and investigation to determine whether there is any underlying cause.

Dental aspects

Dental treatment should be deferred until after recovery. GA should be avoided, since there is often some respiratory obstruction and infection can spread to the lungs. Inhalational sedation may be impeded if the nasal airway is obstructed

Mycoses may infect the sinuses in immunocompromised persons (Ch. 20).

Otitis media

General aspects

Otitis media is a common middle-ear infection in children; 3 out of 4 experience it by the age of 3 years. Otitis media usually follows a viral URTI, often followed by bacterial superinfection. The most common bacterial pathogen is *Streptococcus pneumoniae*, followed by non-typeable *Haemophilus influenzae* and *Moraxella catarrhalis*.

The most important predisposing factor is Eustachian tube (ET) dysfunction but immune defects and palatal dysfunction, such as cleft palate or submucous cleft, occasionally contribute. Interference with the ET mucosa by inflammatory oedema, adenoidal hypertrophy, negative intratympanic pressure or, rarely, a tumour facilitates direct extension of infections from the nasopharynx to the middle ear. Oesophageal contents regurgitated into the nasopharynx can enter the middle ear through the ET if it is patulous.

Clinical features

When the ears are infected, the ET becomes inflamed and swollen, the mucociliary pathways from the middle ear to the nasopharynx become paralysed or dysfunctional, and fluid is trapped inside the middle-ear cleft. The adenoids can also become infected and can block the openings of the ET, trapping air and fluid.

Acute otitis media is very painful, and is worse when the child is lying down. If the infection is not controlled, the eardrum ruptures and pus escapes through the perforation – otorrhoea – when there is an immediate decrease in pain. It may become evident that the child has diminished hearing in that ear. If ET dysfunction merely prevents the normal drainage of the middle-ear cleft, with or without previous acute infection, a condition referred to as otitis media with effusion or 'glue ear' becomes established. This also affects the hearing but is painless. In either case, temporary speech and language problems may become evident as a result of the hearing loss, but usually resolve spontaneously with time. Complications that are rare but can be serious include mastoiditis, meningitis, brain abscess, lateral sinus thrombosis, otitic hydrocephalus, facial palsy, cholesteatoma and tympanosclerosis.

General management

Medical treatment includes antibiotics (usually penicillin) and decongestants and/or antihistamines together with analgesia. If fluids from otitis media stay in the ear for several months, drainage by surgery, usually myringotomy (incision of the ear drum) and grommets (small drainage tubes placed in the incision), may be recommended. Adenoidectomy may also be indicated.

MALIGNANT NEOPLASMS

Most head and neck cancers are squamous cell carcinomas; other tumour types include lymphoepithelioma, spindle cell carcinoma, verrucous cancer, undifferentiated carcinoma, Kaposi sarcoma and lymphoma. Use of computer guided surgery seems likely to improve outcomes, especially in patients whose anatomy has been altered.

MAXILLARY ANTRAL CARCINOMA

General aspects

Antral carcinoma is a rare neoplasm of unknown aetiology, seen mainly in older people.

Clinical features

From the outset, antral carcinoma presents with severe maxillary pain. As the tumour increases in size, the effects of expansion and infiltration of adjacent tissues also become apparent. There is intraoral alveolar swelling; ulceration of the palate or buccal sulcus; swelling of the cheek; unilateral nasal obstruction, often associated with a blood-stained discharge; obstruction of the nasolacrimal duct with consequent epiphora; hypoaesthesia or anaesthesia of the cheek in the infraorbital nerve distribution; proptosis and ophthalmoplegia consequent on invasion of the orbit; and trismus from infiltration of the muscles of mastication.

General management

Combinations of surgery and radiochemotherapy are usually required. Further details can be found in standard textbooks of otorhinolaryngology or maxillofacial surgery.

NEOPLASMS OF THE PHARYNX

Cancer can develop in the nasopharynx (see below and Ch. 22), oropharynx (consisting of the base of tongue, the tonsillar region, soft palate and back of the oral cavity) or the hypopharynx. Patients with pharyngeal cancer are at greater risk of cancer elsewhere in the upper aerodigestive tract.

Factors that increase the risk of pharyngeal cancers include smoking (both tobacco and marijuana) or chewing tobacco; alcohol use; leukoplakia; human papillomavirus (oropharyngeal carcinoma); Epstein–Barr virus (nasopharyngeal carcinoma); anaemia (Paterson–Brown-Kelly syndrome); radiation; and immune defects.

Pharyngeal cancer is treated by one, or a combination, of radiotherapy, chemotherapy or surgery.

NASOPHARYNGEAL CARCINOMA

General aspects

Nasopharyngeal carcinoma is a rare neoplasm that may be associated with Epstein–Barr virus and dietary nitrosamines; it is especially common amongst the southern Chinese, some Inuit races and people in parts of North Africa, such as Tunisia. A similar tumour, undifferentiated carcinoma with lymphoid stroma, is one of the most common salivary gland cancers in Inuits and southern Chinese.

Clinical features

Nasopharyngeal carcinoma often remains asymptomatic for some time, as it rarely obstructs the nasopharynx. The ways in which it presents include:

- isolated cervical lymph node enlargement
- unilateral conductive deafness (from obstruction of the Eustachian tube)
- abducens nerve palsy
- soft palate elevation and immobility
- ipsilateral pain, sometimes with anaesthesia, in the distribution of the major divisions of the trigeminal nerve, e.g. over the eye (ophthalmic division), tongue, lower teeth and lower lip (mandibular division)
- a combination of the above – known as *Trotter's triad.*

General management

Treatment is usually by radiotherapy.

LARYNGEAL CARCINOMA

Laryngeal cancer is found in the glottis, supraglottis or subglottis. It is most common in males, patients of both sexes over the age of 55 who smoke or drink alcohol, are infected with human papillomavirus or have immune defects. Risk factors may also include genetics (people of African descent are more likely than whites to be affected); a personal history of head and neck cancer; exposure to asbestos, sulphuric acid mist or nickel; or a diet low in vitamin A.

Clinical features

Symptoms and signs may include hoarseness, persistent sore throat, dysphagia, pain referred to the ear when swallowing, haemoptysis and cervical lymphadenopathy.

General management

Laryngoscopy, computed tomography (CT) and biopsy are required to confirm the diagnosis. Laryngeal cancer is treated by one, or a combination, of radiotherapy, chemotherapy or surgery. Laser surgery may be used for very early cancers of the larynx. A cordectomy removes the vocal cord. A supraglottic laryngectomy takes out only the supraglottis. A partial or hemi-laryngectomy removes only part of the larynx. A total laryngectomy removes the entire larynx and commits the patient to a permanent tracheostomy. Despite loss of part or all of the vocal apparatus, most patients are able to communicate by speech with or without further surgical procedures and electronic voice aids.

- Epstein–Barr virus infection
  - At least in Asian patients and Inuits
- Occupation
  - Rubber manufacturing
  - Plumbing industry
  - Woodworking
  - Hairdressing
  - Asbestos exposure
- Smoking
  - At least for Warthin tumour
- Other malignant disease
  - Breast cancer
  - Nasopharyngeal carcinoma
  - Thyroid cancer
- X-ray repair cross-complementing group 1 (XRCC1) single-nucleotide polymorphisms
- Radiation exposure, as in:
  - sun exposure
  - ionizing radiation exposure
  - survivors of atomic explosions in Japan (mucoepidermoid carcinomas and Warthin tumour)
  - survivors of childhood malignancies treated with radiation and chemotherapy
  - iodine-131 in the treatment of thyroid disease
  - radiotherapy to the head and neck
  - radiographs of the head and neck

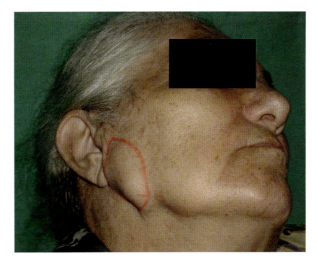

Fig. 14.3 Salivary gland neoplasms are mainly in the parotid gland.

ORAL AND OROPHARYNGEAL CARCINOMA

See Chapter 22.

SALIVARY NEOPLASMS

General aspects

A wide range of different neoplasms can affect the salivary glands but most are uncommon; they are epithelial neoplasms, which present as unilateral swelling of the parotid and are benign. Most salivary gland neoplasms are seen in older people. There is a female predisposition.

Neoplasms in the major salivary glands (parotid, submandibular) are most commonly pleomorphic adenomas but others are usually monomorphic adenomas (such as adenolymphomas), mucoepidermoid tumours or acinic cell tumours. Neoplasms in the minor salivary glands are most commonly pleomorphic adenomas but carcinomas, particularly adenoid cystic carcinomas, account for about 50%.

Salivary gland tumours are more common in certain geographical locations. Inuits, for example, have an increased prevalence. The aetiology is unknown but there are various associations (Box 14.2). A suggested association of parotid tumours with mobile phone use is controversial.

Apart from the above epithelial neoplasms, the next most common salivary neoplasms are lymphomas. Sjögren syndrome is recognized as predisposing to lymphomas, which have arisen in up to 6% of patients over 10 years in some studies.

Clinical features

Salivary gland swelling is the main clinical feature of a neoplasm (Fig. 14.3). A long history of gradual gland enlargement suggests a benign process, while pain, facial palsy, rapid growth and change in growth pattern are ominous and suggest carcinoma.

General management

On clinical examination, a mass is usually palpable. In the case of the parotid, this will often be in the retromandibular region but is sometimes pre-tragal. Tumours confined to the deep lobe of the parotid present like other parapharyngeal tumours with medial displacement of the palate, tonsil and pharyngeal wall. A few malignant neoplasms may be small and almost impalpable, and present with pain only. Magnetic resonance imaging (MRI) is particularly helpful for diagnosing parotid and submandibular tumours. CT is often degraded in this region by amalgam artefacts. Ultrasonography has utility in determining whether a mass is in the tail of the parotid or posterior pole of the submandibular gland. Regardless of the image appearances, the precise diagnosis can only be firmly established by histological examination of either the operative specimen or, increasingly frequently, by fine-needle aspiration biopsy.

The treatment of choice for salivary gland neoplasms is surgical excision. Most salivary gland neoplasms are relatively radioresistant. Chemotherapy is used only on a very limited basis and as an adjunct in the treatment of some malignant salivary gland neoplasms, such as adenocarcinoma or adenoid cystic carcinoma.

LYMPHOMAS

See Chapter 8.

ORO-ANTRAL FISTULA

Oro-antral fistula is discussed in surgical textbooks. Palatal perforations can be caused by trauma, malignant neoplasms or the use of cocaine.

OBSTRUCTIVE SLEEP APNOEA SYNDROME

General aspects

Obstructive sleep apnoea syndrome (OSAS) is characterized by periods of prolonged apnoea during sleep. Patients with OSAS snore extremely loudly, often termed 'heroic snoring'!

The cause is airway obstruction, usually in the region of the oropharynx; enlarged tonsils, nasal septum deformity, narrow dental arches and abnormalities in the larynx may contribute. Enlarged tonsils or tongue (macroglossia) are uncommon causes. Alcohol or other sedatives inducing muscle relaxation can aggravate the situation.

As the patient relaxes in the early phase of sleep, the tongue falls back into the oropharynx and causes obstruction. OSAS is the extreme end of a spectrum of sleep-disordered breathing (SDB), which may be related to weak activity of muscles in (or obstruction to) the tongue, palate and pharynx. SDB has as its minimal level simple snoring, then upper airways resistance syndrome (UARS) and, finally, OSAS, in which there are periods of apnoea during sleep; each period lasts for up to a minute and episodes range from the occasional one to hundreds per night, waking the patient. Sleep is lost and patients with significant OSAS have daytime sleepiness that often culminates in road traffic accidents, an increased risk of acute cardiopulmonary complications and stroke.

Oronasal obstruction in weak senile patients results from blockage of the nose and lack of teeth or dentures, causing the mouth to become overclosed. It may cause a dangerous degree of dyspnoea and cyanosis, even when the person is awake. Hypoxia, thus caused, may contribute to the death of these vulnerable patients.

Clinical features

Partial upper airways obstruction during sleep in anyone can cause snoring that is not OSAS. People with OSAS are characteristically obese middle-aged men. In OSAS, snoring is far more severe and, because there is apnoea, arterial oxygen saturation falls, and cardiac arrhythmias and stroke may develop, particularly in obese middle-aged men. In even more severe cases, pulmonary hypertension and right ventricular failure result. There is also a raised mortality rate from road traffic and other accidents, since affected patients are constantly drowsy.

General management

Severity of OSAS is scored by an apnoea/hypopnoea index calculated from the combined number of episodes per night (less than 20 is mild, 20–40 is moderate and more than 40 is classed as severe). Tiredness can be scored on the Epworth scale (Table 14.4); a score of 10 or more is considered 'sleepy', while 18 or more is 'very sleepy'. Diagnosis is assisted by polysomnography and measurement of arterial blood oxygen.

Treatment includes obesity reduction and nasal continuous positive airways pressure (CPAP). Other measures include various appliances (sometimes termed non-sleep apnoea dental orthotics [NADOs], e.g. *Silent Nite, Klearway, NAPA, Snore aid, Herbst, Silencer*), orthognathic surgery (maxillary–mandibular and hyoid advancement; MMA), or uvulopalatopharyngoplasty (UPPP), adenoidectomy, tonsillectomy or even tracheostomy.

UPPP using scalpel surgery or lasers has been the standard treatment for OSAS, but is often overprescribed and its efficacy is under review.

Dental aspects

Dental appliances that hold the mandible forward are claimed to be as effective as surgical measures and should certainly be tried initially. However, where the obstruction is predominantly hypopharyngeal, surgical advancement of the facial skeleton and hyoid (MMA) may effectively

Table 14.4 *Score sheet for Epworth daytime sleepiness scale*

Situation	Chance of dozing or sleeping[a]
Sitting and reading	Total = Epworth score
Watching TV	
Sitting inactive in a public place	
Being a passenger in a motor vehicle for an hour or more	
Lying down in the afternoon	
Sitting and talking to someone	
Sitting quietly after lunch (no alcohol)	
Stopped for a few minutes in traffic while driving	

[a]0 = would *never* doze or sleep; 1 = *slight* chance of dozing or sleeping; 2 = *moderate* chance of dozing or sleeping; 3 = *high* chance of dozing or sleeping.

expand the airway. When there is both oropharyngeal and hypopharyngeal obstruction, UPPP may need to be combined with MMA.

Nasal obstruction may also have to be relieved, but staged maxillofacial surgery to assess the degree of improvement may relieve nocturnal hypoxia, snoring and daytime sleepiness.

FREY SYNDROME (GUSTATORY SWEATING)

General and clinical aspects

Parotidectomy or trauma to the parotid region is sometimes followed by sweating and flushing of the pre-auricular skin on that side, in response to stimulation of salivation. Similar conditions may follow surgery to other salivary glands.

Gustatory sweating is due to the joining of the damaged postganglionic parasympathetic nerve fibres with the sympathetic nerve endings, so that sweating and flushing occur rather than salivation.

General management

Antiperspirants, such as 20% aluminium chloride hexahydrate, may be effective in controlling the sweating.

DEVELOPMENTAL DISORDERS

By the third week after fertilization, the first of four paired swellings – the branchial arches – at the sides of the head end of the embryo have formed, as well as three germ layers (ectoderm, endoderm and mesoderm). Some craniofacial anomalies result from branchial arch defects and others from the germ layers.

Genes that orchestrate the development of craniofacial structures also direct the development of brain, limbs and some internal organs, such as the heart, lungs and liver. If affected very early in gestation, there may be widespread and devastating consequences. Craniofacial birth defects are rare but fortunately may be ameliorated by surgery, dental care, psychological counselling, and rehabilitation.

CRANIOFACIAL ANOMALIES CAUSED BY BRANCHIAL ARCH DEFECTS

The primary palate forms by merging of the two medial nasal prominences, which arise from the frontonasal process. The primary palate

Table 14.5 *Main genes involved in cleft palate development*

Defects	Genes implicated
Defects in growth of the palatal shelves	Homeobox-containing transcription factor *MSX1*
	Paired-related genes *Pax-1, 3, 6, 7* and *9*
	Dlx transcription factors
	Activin A
	LIM homeobox genes
Elevation of palatal shelves	*Gli* transcription factors
	Jagged 1, 2
	BMP7/BMPreceptor1B
	Hox genes
Impairment of the midline epithelial seam, adhesion, dispersion	*Tgfβ3*
	Transforming growth factor (*TGF*)
Epithelio-mesenchymal transition	Fibroblast growth factor (*FGF*)
	Twist transcription factor
Cell deficiency (proliferation, differentiation, migration defects)	*SHH* (Sonic Hedgehog)
	Endothelin-1 (*Et-1*)

Drugs most commonly implicated

- Alcohol
- Anticonvulsants
- Cocaine
- Fluconazole
- Heroin
- Phenytoin
- Retinoids
- Tobacco
- Topiramate

Drugs occasionally implicated

- Antihypertensives
- Corticosteroids
- Cytotoxic agents
- Thalidomide

Box 14.4 *Genes implicated in non-syndromic cleft palate*

- Transforming growth factor (*TGF*)
- Retinoic acid receptor alpha (*RARA*)
- Long arm of chromosome 2 (2q32)
- Chromosome 4
- Short arm of chromosome 6 (*Et-1* gene 6p24)

will fuse laterally with the maxillary processes of the first branchial arch during the sixth and seventh weeks, forming the upper lip. The palate contains the maxillary incisor teeth.

Secondary palate development involves bilateral palatal shelves arising from the maxillary processes in 6.5-week human embryos, which eventually make contact above the tongue. The palatal shelves adhere with each other over the space of about 10 days to form the midline epithelial seam. The epithelial seam disperses to allow merging of the mesenchyme to form fused palatal shelves, by the 10th week of gestation. The midpalatal seam often disappears incompletely, leaving epithelial rests or remnants (Epstein's pearls) in the midline. Impaired formation of the secondary palate results in cleft palate (CP), usually quickly recognized after birth, especially when associated with a cleft lip (CL). A submucous cleft can be more difficult to diagnose.

Pathogenesis of cleft palate

The development of the face and the upper lip takes place during the fifth to ninth week of pregnancy. Clefts of the lip with or without cleft palate, and cleft palate alone, result from the failure of the first branchial arches to complete fusion processes; they are the most common of all craniofacial anomalies. The male-to-female ratio of cleft lip/palate (CLP) is 2:1; the ratio for CP alone is just the reverse, 1:2.

Failed fusion of the palatal shelves can be caused by different gene defects (Table 14.5), culminating in:

- a problem in the formation of the midline epithelial seam
- small size of the palatal processes
- unsynchronized timing of the elevation or growth of the palatal shelves with the growth of surrounding structures such as the cranial base
- a small mandible preventing the downward relocation of the tongue, which mechanically may prevent palatal fusion.

CP as an isolated malformation behaves as an entity distinct from CL with or without CP. It has an incidence of 0.5 per 1000 births. The risk of recurrence in subsequent children is about 2% if one child has it, 6% if one parent has it, and 15% if one parent and one child have it.

Non-syndromic cleft palate

Not all cases of clefting are inherited; a number of teratogens (environmental agents that can cause birth defects) have been implicated, as well as defects in essential nutrients. Environmental factors present during the first trimester of pregnancy, and which may generate CP, include maternal URTI in the first trimester, smoking (especially when the mother has glutathione-S-transferase theta 1 [GSTT1] – null variants), obesity, diabetes, stress or exposure to the agents shown in Box 14.3. Paternal smoking has also been implicated.

CLP is more prevalent in the lower socioeconomic classes. The teratogens incriminated include isotretinoin, used to treat acne, which causes birth defects such as brain malformations, learning disability and heart problems, as well as facial abnormalities. Thalidomide given to pregnant mothers was, and anticonvulsants (phenytoin, valproic acid, lamotrigine, carbamazepine) and corticosteroids may be, associated with an increased incidence. Phenytoin may act via an effect causing fetal arrhythmias and hypoxia. Systemic corticosteroids have been reported to increase the risk (this is controversial) and there are also concerns about possible effects from topical steroids used in the first trimester. There has been suspicion of aspirin and diazepam as possible causes but there is no real evidence. Folic acid given periconceptually may lower the risk but the evidence is weak.

Inheritance of non-syndromic CP is multigenic, with a number of genes implicated (Box 14.4).

Clefting can occur independently or as part of a larger syndrome that may include the heart and other organs. Affected infants have facial deformity and may have difficulty with feeding, breathing, speaking and swallowing; they are susceptible to respiratory infections.

General aspects

The primary palate or pre-maxilla includes that portion of the alveolar ridge containing the four incisors. The secondary palate forms the remaining hard palate and all the soft palate. Orofacial clefts result from an embryopathy in which there is failure of the frontonasal process and/or fusion of the palatal shelves. In the submucous CP, the palatal shelves may fail to join, but the overlying mucous membranes are intact and the muscle attachments of the soft palate are abnormal, causing velopharyngeal insufficiency. Bifid uvula may signify a submucous CP.

CP is the fourth most common birth defect, affecting approximately 1 in 700–1000 live births. There are also racial differences, with a high incidence in South-East Asians and a low incidence in Afro-Caribbean races. The common clefts are cleft lip with or without cleft palate (CL ± P) and CP only. The total incidence of facial clefting is between 2 and 3 per 1000 live births. A number of these do not develop as full-term fetuses. Facial clefts are associated with a syndrome in up to 15–60% of cases and are then termed syndromic clefts (see below). More than 400 syndromes may include a facial cleft as one manifestation, and CLP may be associated with many congenital syndromes.

The cause of non-syndromic cleft lip with or without cleft palate (NSCLP) is unclear but there is still a strong genetic component; there may be a family history of clefts and typically the same type of cleft is seen in affected members. In monozygotic twins, there is nearly 40% concordance. No single gene defect appears responsible, however. Several loci have been identified. Candidate genes in CLP include transforming growth factor alpha (*TGF*), poliovirus receptor-like 1 (*PVRL1*), retinoic acid receptor alpha (*RARA*), T-box transcription factor-22 (*TBX22*), specific isoforms of glutamic acid decarboxylase (*GAD*), interferon regulatory factor 6 (*IRF6*), *MSX1* (formerly *homeobox 7* – encodes a member of the muscle segment *homeobox* gene family) and fibroblast growth factor (*FGF*) (see Table 14.5).

Clinical features

Clefts have a major impact from birth from both aesthetic and functional viewpoints, since the neonate with a CP is unable to suckle. Later, speech development is also impaired. A person may have a CL, CP, or both.

A unilateral CL occurs on one side of the upper lip. A bilateral CL occurs on both sides of the upper lip. In its most severe form, the cleft may extend through the nose base.

CP may be incomplete, involving only the uvula and the muscular soft palate (velum). A complete CP extends the entire length of the palate. CP can be unilateral or bilateral. There may also be feeding difficulties and associated congenital defects such as dental, hearing and speech defects.

General management

Health-care providers that frequently participate in a multidisciplinary CP team include: audiologists; maxillofacial, ear, nose and throat, and plastic surgeons; geneticists; neurosurgeons; nurses; dentists (paediatric dentist/orthodontist/prosthodontist); paediatricians; social workers/psychologists; and speech and language pathologists.

A high percentage of patients with CP develop otitis media with effusion. Up to 20% have additional abnormalities that can affect management in various ways (Fig. 14.4). Systemic disorders are more frequent in patients with CP than in those with CL alone, and include especially skeletal, cardiac, renal and central nervous system defects.

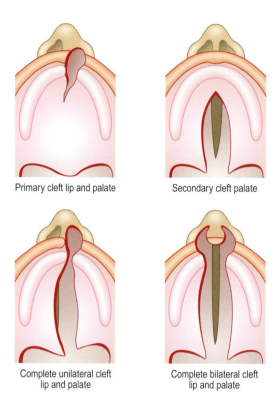

Primary cleft lip and palate
Secondary cleft palate
Complete unilateral cleft lip and palate
Complete bilateral cleft lip and palate

Fig. 14.4 Cleft palate.

Newborn to 12 months

Treatment of the airway takes priority and may be managed with positioning but, in severe cases, may need tracheostomy. There can be significant difficulties in management of the airway for anaesthesia in children under the age of 5 years, particularly in young infants and in those with feeding difficulties, bilateral clefts and/or retrognathia. Patients with mandibular dysostoses and those requiring midface advancement (Le Fort II osteotomy) have the greatest problems. Difficulties are common in Pierre Robin, Treacher Collins and Goldenhar syndromes, and the cervical spine may be problematic in Klippel–Feil syndrome. The laryngeal mask has been recommended as a guide to fibreoptic endoscopic intubation. Aesthetics is a major issue for parents (Fig. 14.5). One of the problems for the child is feeding; a Rosti bottle with Gummi teat often helps.

The timing of the initial CLP repair is controversial. In general, when the lip alone is cleft, initial cosmetic repair is carried out at about 3–6 months of age, though earlier operations are becoming popular. Many repair CLP within the first few days of life since, after repair, the appearance is dramatically improved, feeding difficulties are significantly minimized and speech develops better. If the palatal defect is too wide, it can be repaired 3 months later to allow for sufficient palatal growth. In any event, CP is now usually repaired before the child speaks, between 6 and 18 months, and typically at 6–12 months of age.

Years 1 to 18

Age 1–5 years is when it is important to have good hearing and normal appearance to avoid low self-esteem and help speech develop. These children need a hearing assessment; if hearing is impaired, ear ventilation tubes (grommets) may be indicated.

Age 5–13 years is when the orthodontist can help correct malocclusion, and alveolar bone grafting may be needed. Speech, if poor despite the best efforts on the part of the child and the speech pathologist, may be corrected with pharyngoplasty.

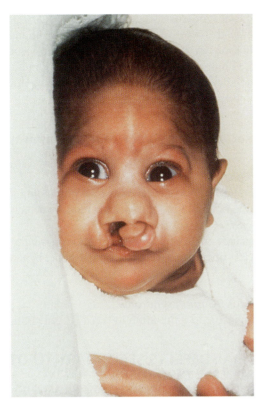

Fig. 14.5 Cleft lip.

Age 13–18 years is the time for final adjustments. Fine-tuning, such as scar revisions, rhinoplasty and orthognathic surgery, is carried out to enable the child's appearance and speech to be restored to as near normal as possible.

Dental aspects

Palatal ulcers seen in neonates with CLP appear to result from trauma from the tongue and resolve if a palatal plate is fitted. Dental abnormalities include malocclusion (almost 100%), hypodontia (50%), hypoplasia (30%) and supernumerary teeth (20%). Children may have a higher prevalence of caries in both primary and permanent dentitions, and significantly more gingivitis, especially in the maxillary anterior region. Adult CLP patients may have poorer oral hygiene and more gingivitis. Prevention and continuity of care are essential and a high rate of success can be achieved.

Submucous cleft palate can be recognized by a notched posterior nasal spine, a translucent zone in the midline of the soft palate and a bifid uvula, but not all these features are necessarily present and a bifid uvula may be seen in isolation. About 1 in 1200 births is affected and feeding difficulties, speech defects and middle-ear infections may develop in 90% of affected children. Adenoidectomy is contraindicated, as it may reveal latent velopharyngeal insufficiency. A minority have other issues such as Loeys–Dietz syndrome (similar to Marfan syndrome), where there is a risk of arterial aneurysm and rupture.

Syndromic cleft palate

Current molecular epidemiology investigations have examined both syndromic and non-syndromic (isolated) cleft lip/palate and cleft palate. Linkage studies have identified a number of candidate genes, including *MSX1*, *RAR*, an X-linked locus, and the genes for TGF beta-3 and TGF alpha.

Van der Woude and Waardenberg syndromes are associated with CL, with or without CP. Common syndromes with CP include Apert, Stickler and Treacher Collins syndromes. CLP may also be seen in velocardiofacial, Pierre Robin and KlippelαFeil syndromes and in various chromosome anomalies (Down syndrome, Edwards syndrome; Appendix 14.1).

A small subgroup of patients have CLP with median facial dysplasia and cerebrofacial malformations, while others have laryngotracheal oesophageal clefts (Opitz–Frias or G syndrome) or cranial asymmetry (Opitz or B syndrome).

One of the common syndromic forms of CLP, the van der Woude syndrome, is caused by an autosomal dominant form of inheritance at a locus on chromosome 1.

Other examples include:

- branchial arch syndromes
- craniosynostoses
- diseases associated with mutations in the Sonic Hedgehog pathway (*SHH*).

Branchial arch syndromes

Pierre Robin syndrome
Deficient development of the mandibular portion derived from the first branchial arch results in micrognathia, with the tongue set back and possibly obstructing the airway. CP may be another consequence. The infant is also at risk of cor pulmonale.

Treacher Collins syndrome (mandibulofacial dysostosis)
Treacher Collins syndrome has an autosomal dominant inheritance and is associated with mutation of the *Treacle* gene (5q32-q33.1), which encodes a phosphorylated nucleolar trafficking protein. First branchial arch structures are deficient, and all derivative craniofacial components are affected. Treacher Collins syndrome manifests with cleft palate; downward-sloping eyelids; partial absence of lower eyelashes; depressed cheekbones; a large, fish-like mouth; deformed ears with conductive deafness; a small, receding chin and lower jaw; a highly arched or cleft palate; and severe dental malocclusion. These defects result from defective cranial neural crest cell differentiation, migration and proliferation.

The underdeveloped facial structures can contribute to airway blockage and repeated upper respiratory infections, and maldevelopment of the ears leads to a conductive deafness.

DiGeorge syndrome, velocardiofacial syndrome (Shprintzen syndrome, CATCH 22)
General aspects. Velocardiofacial syndrome (VCFS; from the Latin *velum* – palate, *cardia* – heart, and *facies* – to do with the face) is a genetic disorder involving chromosome 22 (a deletion at 22q11). Its features include *c*ardiac defects, *a*bnormal facies, *t*hymic hypoplasia, *c*left palate and *h*ypocalcaemia – hence it is termed 'CATCH 22'. It affects approximately 5–8% of children born with CP. There is a characteristic facial appearance, minor learning problems and speech and feeding difficulties, and heart defects. It is inherited in only about 10–15% and, usually, neither parent has the syndrome or carries the defective gene.

Also known as Shprintzen syndrome, craniofacial syndrome or conotruncal anomaly unusual face syndrome, at least 30 different defects have been associated with the 22q11 deletion of VCFS. DiGeorge syndrome is similar (Ch. 20).

- Cleft palate, usually of the soft palate
- Heart disease
- Facies (elongated face, almond-shaped eyes, wide nose, small ears)
- Learning difficulties
- Eye defects
- Otitis media
- Hypoparathyroidism
- Immune defects
- Weak muscles
- Short height
- Curvature of the spine (scoliosis)
- Tapered fingers

Clinical features. There is great variation in the features (Box 14.5), although none of these problems occurs in all cases.

Dental aspects. There may be difficulties associated with CLP, cardiac disease and immune defects.

Maldevelopment of the fourth branchial arch and the third and fourth pharyngeal pouches leads to deficiencies affecting the thymus, parathyroid glands and the great vessels. Facial features include a squared-off nasal tip, small mouth and widely spaced eyes. Similar facial features, along with heart defects, are seen in the velocardiofacial syndrome. Both syndromes are associated with deletions on the long arm of chromosome 22 (22q11).

The thymic defect severely compromises cellular immunity. Inadequate or missing parathyroid glands cause severe hypocalcaemia and seizures. The great vessel abnormalities lead to compromised circulation.

Features include:

- cardiac abnormality
- abnormal facies
- T-cell deficit due to thymic hypoplasia
- cleft palate
- hypocalcaemia due to hypoparathyroidism.

Craniosynostoses

The premature fusion of certain skull bones (craniosynostosis) prevents normal skull growth, affects the shape of the head and face, and puts pressure on the developing brain. It is seen in Crouzon, Apert, Saethre–Chotzen and Pfeiffer syndromes and in Boston-type craniosynostosis (Ch. 37).

Crouzon syndrome

Crouzon syndrome is a rare genetic disorder characterized by abnormal skull growth with wide-set, bulging eyes (hypertelorism; proptosis) and visual problems caused by shallow eye sockets; eyes that do not point in the same direction (strabismus); a beaked nose; and an underdeveloped maxilla. In addition, there may be cleft lip and palate, dental problems and hearing loss, which is sometimes accompanied by narrow ear canals. People with Crouzon syndrome are usually of normal intelligence.

Mutations in the fibroblast growth factor receptor 2 (*FGFR2*) gene cause Crouzon syndrome.

Apert craniofacial synostosis

Apert craniofacial synostosis is an autosomal dominant disorder, caused by mutations in the chromosome 10q26 gene encoding *FGFR2*. CP is associated more significantly with the *S252W* mutation.

Features include craniosynostosis, facial dysmorphology, hand and feet defects, and learning impairment.

Diseases associated with Sonic Hedgehog pathway (SHH) mutations

Holoprosencephaly

Holoprosencephaly affects neural crest cells populating the frontonasal mass and the forebrain, with associated midface defects. Some cases are caused by *SHH* mutations.

Features include wide phenotypic variation, a single central incisor, median cleft lip and palate, absent nasal bone, hypertelorism and cyclopia.

Basal cell naevus ('Gorlin') syndrome

This condition is due to a mutation in the *PTC* gene (Ch. 37).

CRANIOFACIAL DEFECTS SECONDARY TO OTHER DEVELOPMENTAL DISORDERS

Craniofacial defects may be secondary to a more generalized structural or biochemical defect.

Osteogenesis imperfecta

See Chapter 16.

Waardenburg syndrome

See Chapter 37.

Cleidocranial dysplasia

The inheritance of a regulatory gene defect in cleidocranial dysplasia leads to features that include delayed tooth eruption, supernumerary teeth, altered or missing collarbones, short stature, and possible failure of cranial suture closure. The exact mechanism of the associated gene, *CBFA1*, located on chromosome 6, has not been determined but appears to be essential for bone development.

KEY WEBSITES

(Accessed 27 May 2012)
American Academy of Otolaryngology – Head and Neck Surgery. <http://www.entnet.org/healthinformation/>
BMJ. <http://www.bmj.com/specialties/otolaryngology-ent>

USEFUL WEBSITES

(Accessed 27 May 2012)
American Academy of Allergy, Asthma & Immunology. <http://www.aaaai.org/home.aspx>
Bandolier. <http://www.medicine.ox.ac.uk/bandolier/booth/booths/ent.html>
ENT UK. <http://www.entuk.org/publications/>
Genetics Home Reference. ghr.nlm.nih.gov/
National Institutes of Health: National Institute of Allergy and Infectious Diseases. <http://www.niaid.nih.gov/topics/Pages/default.aspx>
NHS Direct Wales. <http://www.nhsdirect.wales.nhs.uk/encyclopaedia/c/article/cleftlipandpalate/>

FURTHER READING

Avila, J.R., et al. 2006. PVRL1 variants contribute to non-syndromic cleft lip and palate in multiple populations. Am. J. Med. Genet. A 140, 2562.

Azarbayjani, F., Danielsson, B.R., 2001. Phenytoin-induced cleft palate: evidence for embryonic cardiac bradyarrhythmia due to inhibition of delayed rectifier K+ channels resulting in hypoxia-reoxygenation damage. Teratology 63, 152.

Azarbayjani, F., Danielsson, B.R., 2002. Embryonic arrhythmia by inhibition of HERG channels: a common hypoxia-related teratogenic mechanism for antiepileptic drugs? Epilepsia 43, 457.

Bettega, G., et al. 2000. Obstructive sleep apnea syndrome. Am. J. Respir. Crit. Care Med. 162, 641.

Bille, C., et al. 2007. Oral clefts and life style factors – a case-cohort study based on prospective Danish data. Eur. J. Epidemiol. 22, 173.

Bloch, K.E., et al. 2000. A randomised, controlled crossover trial of two oral appliances for sleep apnea treatment. Am. J. Respir. Crit. Care Med. 162, 246.

Boscolo-Rizzo, P., et al. 2008. Long-term quality of life after total laryngectomy and postoperative radiotherapy versus concurrent chemoradiotherapy for laryngeal preservation. Laryngoscope 118, 300.

Boysen, T., et al. 2008. The Inuit cancer pattern – the influence of migration. Int. J. Cancer 122, 2568.

Carinci, F., et al. 2003. Recent developments in orofacial cleft genetics. J. Craniofac. Surg. 14, 130.

Carinci, F., et al. 2005. Non-syndromic orofacial clefts in Southern Italy: pattern analysis according to gender, history of maternal smoking, folic acid intake and familial diabetes. J. Craniomaxillofac. Surg. 33, 91.

Carmichael, S.L., et al. 2007. Maternal stressful life events and risks of birth defects. Epidemiology 18, 356.

Cedergren, M., Källén, B., 2005. Maternal obesity and the risk for orofacial clefts in the offspring. Cleft Palate Craniofac. J. 42, 367.

Chevrier, C., et al. 2008. Genetic susceptibilities in the association between maternal exposure to tobacco smoke and the risk of nonsyndromic oral cleft. Am. J. Med. Genet. A 146A, 2396.

Clark, J.D., et al. 2003. Socioeconomic status and orofacial clefts in Scotland, 1989 to 1998. Cleft Palate Craniofac. J. 40, 481.

Cohen, M., et al. 2007. Isolated uvulitis. Ear Nose Throat J. 86 (462), 464.

Cohen, M., et al. 2008. Palatal perforation from cocaine abuse. Ear Nose Throat J. 87, 262.

de la Chaux, R., et al. 2007. [Snoring: therapeutic options.]. MMW Fortschr. Med. 149, 33.

Deacon, S., 2005. Maternal smoking during pregnancy is associated with a higher risk of non-syndromic orofacial clefts in infants. Evid. Based Dent. 6, 43.

Edwards, M.J., et al. 2003. Case-control study of cleft lip or palate after maternal use of topical corticosteroids during pregnancy. Am. J. Med. Genet. A 120A, 459.

Eng, C.Y., et al. 2007. A comparison of the incidence of facial palsy following parotidectomy performed by ENT and non-ENT surgeons. J. Laryngol. Otol. 121, 40.

Eppley, B.L., et al. 2005. The spectrum of orofacial clefting. Plast. Reconstr. Surg. 115, 101e.

Eros, E., et al. 2002. A population-based case-control teratologic study of nitrazepam, medazepam, tofisopam, alprazolum and clonazepam treatment during pregnancy. Eur. J. Obstet. Gynecol. Reprod. Biol. 101, 147.

Fallin, M.D., et al. 2003. Family-based analysis of MSX1 haplotypes for association with oral clefts. Genet. Epidemiol. 25, 168.

Gilgen-Anner, Y., et al. 2007. Iodide mumps after contrast media imaging: a rare adverse effect to iodine. Ann. Allergy Asthma Immunol. 99, 93.

Grewal, J., et al. 2008. Maternal periconceptional smoking and alcohol consumption and risk for select congenital anomalies. Birth Defects Res. A Clin. Mol. Teratol. 82, 519.

Hardell, L., et al. 2004. No association between the use of cellular or cordless telephones and salivary gland tumours. Occup. Environ. Med. 61, 675.

Hart, T.C., et al. The impact of molecular genetics on oral health paradigms. Crit. Rev. Oral Biol. Med. 11, 26.

Holmes, L.B., et al. 2008. Increased frequency of isolated cleft palate in infants exposed to lamotrigine during pregnancy. Neurology 70, 2152.

Honein, M.A., et al. 2007. Maternal smoking and environmental tobacco smoke exposure and the risk of orofacial clefts. Epidemiology 18, 226.

Hughes, J.P., et al. How we do it: changes in thyroid and salivary gland surgery since 1989: who's doing it and what are they doing? Clin. Otolaryngol. 2006; 31:443.

Johnson, J.T., et al. 2008. Reduction of snoring with a plasma-mediated radiofrequency-based ablation (Coblation) device. Ear Nose Throat J. 87, 40.

Källén, B., Otterblad Olausson, P., 2007. Use of anti-asthmatic drugs during pregnancy. 3. Congenital malformations in the infants. Eur. J. Clin. Pharmacol. 63, 383.

Kim, D.S., et al. 2007. Dental otalgia. J. Laryngol. Otol. 121, 1129.

Koch, M., et al. 2008. [Diagnostic and interventional sialoscopy in obstructive diseases of the salivary glands.]. HNO 56, 139.

Kouwen, H.B., DeJonckere, P.H., 2007. Prevalence of OME is reduced in young children using chewing gum. Ear Hear 28, 451.

Kozer, E., et al. 2002. Aspirin consumption during the first trimester of pregnancy and congenital anomalies: a meta-analysis. Am. J. Obstet. Gynecol. 187, 1623.

Krapels, I.P., et al. 2006. Periconceptional health and lifestyle factors of both parents affect the risk of live-born children with orofacial clefts. Birth Defects Res. A Clin. Mol. Teratol. 76, 613.

Lie, R.T., et al. 2008. Maternal smoking and oral clefts: the role of detoxification pathway genes. Epidemiology 19, 606.

Little, J., et al. 2004. Tobacco smoking and oral clefts: a meta-analysis. Bull. World Health Organ. 82, 213.

Lönn, S., et al. 2006. Mobile phone use and risk of parotid gland tumor. Am. J. Epidemiol. 164, 637.

Manrique, D., et al. 2007. Drooling: analysis and evaluation of 31 children who underwent bilateral submandibular gland excision and parotid duct ligation. Braz. J. Otorhinolaryngol. 73, 40.

Matalon, S., et al. 2002. The teratogenic effect of carbamazepine: a meta-analysis of 1255 exposures. Reprod. Toxicol. 16, 9.

Mueller, D.T., Callanan, V.P., 2007. Congenital malformations of the oral cavity. Otolaryngol. Clin. North Am. 40, 141. vii

Nahlieli, O., et al. 2008. Endoscopic treatment of salivary gland injuries due to facial rejuvenation procedures. Laryngoscope 118, 763.

Nørgård, B., et al. 2005. Aspirin use during early pregnancy and the risk of congenital abnormalities: a population-based case-control study. Am. J. Obstet. Gynecol. 192, 922.

Pavelec, V., Polenik, P., 2006. Use of Er,Cr:YSGG versus standard lasers in laser assisted uvulopalatoplasty for treatment of snoring. Laryngoscope 116, 1512.

Perez-Aytes, A., et al. 2008. In utero exposure to mycophenolate mofetil: a characteristic phenotype? Am. J. Med. Genet. A 146A, 1.

Puhó, E.H., et al. 2007. Drug treatment during pregnancy and isolated orofacial clefts in Hungary. Cleft Palate Craniofac. J. 44, 194.

Puraviappan, P., et al. 2007. Efficacy of relocation of submandibular duct in cerebral palsy patients with drooling. Asian J. Surg. 30, 209.

Ramirez, D., et al. 2007. Maternal smoking during early pregnancy, GSTP1 and EPHX1 variants, and risk of isolated orofacial clefts. Cleft Palate Craniofac. J. 44, 366.

Ricciardiello, F., et al. 2006. Otorhinolaryngology-related tuberculosis. Acta Otorhinolaryngol. Ital. 26, 38.

Rubino, C., et al. 2003. Second primary malignancies in thyroid cancer patients. Br. J. Cancer 89, 1638.

Sadetzki, S., et al. 2008. Cellular phone use and risk of benign and malignant parotid gland tumors – a nationwide case-control study. Am. J. Epidemiol. 167, 457.

Sadetzki, S., et al. 2008. Smoking and risk of parotid gland tumors: a nationwide case-control study. Cancer 112, 1974. Erratum in Cancer 2008; 113:662.

Sandow, P.L., et al. 2006. Taste loss and recovery following radiation therapy. J. Dent. Res. 85, 608.

Sandy, J.R., 2003. Molecular, clinical and political approaches to the problem of cleft lip and palate. J. R. Coll. Surg. Edinb. Irel. 1, 9.

Schüz, J., et al. 2006. Cellular telephone use and cancer risk: update of a nationwide Danish cohort. J. Natl. Cancer Inst. 98, 1707.

Shaw, G.M., et al. 2005. Endothelial nitric oxide synthase (NOS3) genetic variants, maternal smoking, vitamin use, and risk of human orofacial clefts. Am. J. Epidemiol. 162, 1207.

Shi, M., et al. 2007. Orofacial cleft risk is increased with maternal smoking and specific detoxification-gene variants. Am. J. Hum. Genet. 80, 76.

Shi, M., et al. 2008. Review on genetic variants and maternal smoking in the etiology of oral clefts and other birth defects. Birth Defects Res. C Embryo. Today 84, 16.

Smith, S.D., 2007. Oral appliances in the treatment of obstructive sleep apnea. Atlas Oral Maxillofac. Surg. Clin. North Am. 15, 193.

Sorrenti, G., et al. 2006. One-phase management of severe obstructive sleep apnea: tongue base reduction with hyoepiglottoplasty plus uvulopalatopharyngoplasty. Otolaryngol. Head Neck Surg. 135, 906.

Vieira, A.R., 2008. Unraveling human cleft lip and palate research. J. Dent. Res. 87, 119.

Webster, W.S., et al. 2006. The relationship between cleft lip, maxillary hypoplasia, hypoxia and phenytoin. Curr. Pharm. Des. 12, 1431.

Wikner, B.N., et al. 2007. Use of benzodiazepines and benzodiazepine receptor agonists during pregnancy: neonatal outcome and congenital malformations. Pharmacoepidemiol. Drug. Saf. 16, 1203.

Wilcox, A.J., et al. 2007. Folic acid supplements and risk of facial clefts: national population based case-control study. BMJ 334, 464.

Wong, F.K., Hagg, U., 2004. An update on the aetiology of orofacial clefts. Hong Kong Med. J. 10, 331.

Yazdy, M.M., et al. 2007. Reduction in orofacial clefts following folic acid fortification of the U.S. grain supply. Birth Defects Res. A Clin. Mol. Teratol. 79, 16.

Zeiger, J.S., et al. 2005. Oral clefts, maternal smoking, and TGFA: a meta-analysis of gene-environment interaction. Cleft Palate Craniofac. J. 42, 58.

APPENDIX 14.1 SYNDROMES THAT MAY INCLUDE CLEFT LIP/PALATE

- Apert syndrome
- Basal cell carcinoma naevoid syndrome
- Carpenter syndrome
- Cleidocranial dysplasia
- Craniosynostosis
- Crouzon syndrome
- Down syndrome
- Edwards syndrome
- Freeman–Sheldon syndrome
- Goldenhar syndrome
- Hallermann–Streiff syndrome
- Hemifacial microsomia
- Hydrocephalus
- Klippel–Feil syndrome
- Microtia
- Miller syndrome

- Moebius syndrome
- Nager syndrome
- Nasal encephalocoeles
- Neurofibromatosis
- Orbital hypertelorism
- Parry–Romberg syndrome
- Pfeiffer syndrome
- Pierre Robin sequence
- Saethre–Chotzen syndrome
- Shprintzen syndrome
- Stickler syndrome
- Treacher Collins syndrome
- van der Woude syndrome
- Velocardiofacial syndrome
- Waardenburg syndrome

Respiratory medicine 15

The respiratory tract consists of the upper respiratory tract (URT – nose, paranasal sinuses, pharynx and larynx; discussed in Ch. 14) and the lower respiratory tract (LRT): the respiratory airways (trachea, bronchi and bronchioles) and lungs (respiratory bronchioles, alveolar ducts, alveolar sacs and alveoli), discussed in this chapter.

Protective mechanisms in the respiratory tracts include a mucociliary lining. Particles or pathogens are trapped in the mucus and driven by ciliary action (the ciliary elevator) to the pharynx. Mucociliary transport declines with age but any effect on clinical infection has not been proved. Lymphoid tissues of the Waldeyer ring (adenoids, palatine and lingual tonsils) are important in developing an immune response to pathogens. However, the best respiratory defence mechanism is the cough reflex, the components of which include cough receptors, afferent nerves, the cough centre, and efferent nerves and effector muscles. Impairment of any of these – as may be seen in older patients or those with conditions associated with lowered consciousness (e.g. sedative use and neurological disease) – can weaken protection. Dysphagia or impaired oesophageal motility may exacerbate the tendency to aspirate foreign material. The alveolar defence mechanisms include macrophages, immunocytes, surfactant, phospholipids, immunoglobulin G (IgG), IgE, secretory IgA, complement components and factor B; many immune defects manifest with recurrent respiratory infections.

Lung function is vital to gas exchange – the blood absorbs oxygen and releases carbon dioxide. Normal gas exchange requires adequate alveolar ventilation, normal ventilation/blood flow relationships and adequate alveolar–capillary membrane surface area. Breathing (ventilation) depends on respiratory drive, which reacts to the respiratory load. This process requires work and results in gas exchange.

Oxygen is transported in combination with haemoglobin in erythrocytes and a small amount dissolved in plasma. The oxyhaemoglobin dissociation curve is sigmoidal; once the oxygen saturation falls below 95%, the amount of O_2 transported to the tissues and brain falls rapidly. High temperatures, acidosis, raised CO_2 and raised 2,3-diphosphoglycerate (2,3-DPG) levels encourage oxygen offloading, whereas fetal haemoglobin and carboxyhaemoglobin have the contrary effect. Chronic hypoxaemia (e.g. at high altitudes) stimulates release of erythropoietin from the kidneys, with a rise in red cell production, and raised 2,3-DPG. Athletes have abused erythropoietin to gain competitive advantage (Ch. 33).

LOWER RESPIRATORY DISEASE

The most common LRT disorders are asthma and chronic obstructive pulmonary disease (COPD).

General aspects

Respiratory disorders are common, and are often caused or aggravated by tobacco smoking. They may significantly affect general anaesthesia (GA) and conscious sedation (CS), since they are often a contraindication to use of benzodiazepines, opioids, GA agents and other respiratory depressants.

Clinical features

Impaired gas exchange leads to laboured breathing and can cause significant incapacity. Features include cough, sputum production, wheeze, dyspnoea, chest pain, cyanosis, finger-clubbing (Fig. 15.1), use of accessory muscles of respiration with indrawing of the intercostal spaces (hyperinflation), and abnormalities in chest shape, movements, respiratory rate and breath sounds.

Cough may be a feature of any respiratory problem but, if chronic, may herald serious disease – for example, COPD, cancer or infection such as tuberculosis. Mucoid or mucopurulent sputum is often a feature (Fig. 15.2); purulent sputum indicates acute bronchitis, bronchiectasis or lung abscess. Blood (haemoptysis) or blood-stained sputum, though common in acute infections (especially in pre-existing COPD), bronchiectasis and pulmonary embolism, may herald an even more serious condition – for example, possibly one due to carcinoma or tuberculosis. Wheezing is caused by airways obstruction and is a typical sign of asthma or COPD. Breathlessness (dyspnoea) is distressing, and may be caused by respiratory or cardiovascular disease, or by anaemia, and is particularly ominous if it persists at rest.

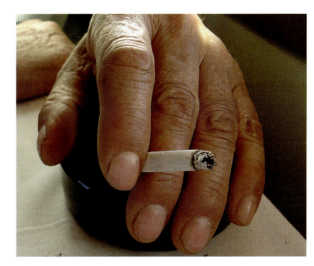

Fig. 15.1 Tobacco smoker with clubbing in lung cancer.

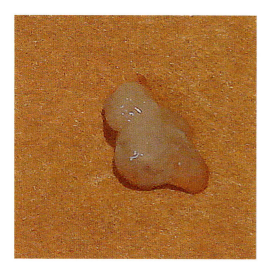

Fig. 15.2 Mucoid sputum from chronic obstructive pulmonary disease.

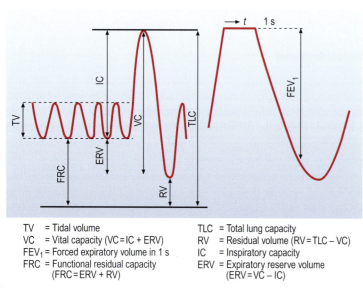

TV = Tidal volume	TLC = Total lung capacity
VC = Vital capacity (VC = IC + ERV)	RV = Residual volume (RV = TLC – VC)
FEV₁ = Forced expiratory volume in 1 s	IC = Inspiratory capacity
FRC = Functional residual capacity (FRC = ERV + RV)	ERV = Expiratory reserve volume (ERV = VC – IC)

Fig. 15.3 Spirometry.

Excessive resistive load, such as in asthma, COPD and cystic fibrosis, impairs airflow. Elastic load increases because of, for example, interstitial fibrosis, muscle paralysis and obesity.

General management

Diagnosis of respiratory disorders is from the clinical features supported by imaging (especially chest radiography). Spiral computed tomography (CT) can now scan the lungs in a quick 20–30-second breath-hold and therefore, instead of producing a stack of individual CT slices, which may be misaligned due to patient movement or breathing in between slices, provides high-resolution three-dimensional images.

Respiratory function tests can measure individual components of the respiratory process. *Spirometry* is the basic screening test for assessing mechanical load problems, the quantification involving determination of the vital capacity (VC) – slow vital capacity (SVC) and/or forced vital capacity (FVC) – and the speed of maximal expiratory flow (MEF; Fig. 15.3). In health, about 75% of a normal-sized VC is expelled in 1 second (FEV_1). The peak flow meter, which measures the peak expiratory flow rate (PEFR; the earliest portion of forced

Table 15.1 *Adult values for PaO_2 and oxygen saturation[a]*

	PaO_2 (kPa)	SaO_2 (%)
Normal (range)	13 (≥10.7)	97 (95–100)
Hypoxaemia	<10.7	<95
Mild hypoxaemia	8–10.5	90–94
Moderate hypoxaemia	5.3–7.9	75–89
Severe hypoxaemia	<5.3	<75

[a]From Williams AJ. Assessing and interpreting arterial blood gases and acid–base balance. BMJ 1998; 317:1213. http://www.bmj.com/cgi/content/full/317/7167/1213 (accessed 30 September 2013).

expiration), is a simple measure of airflow obstruction, when the FEV_1 is a much smaller fraction of the VC. In lung restriction, the diminished VC can be mostly expelled in about 1 second. Serial measurements (e.g. in asthma) provide valuable information about disease progress. The reversibility of airways obstruction is usually assessed by spirometry before and after use of a bronchodilator agent.

Arterial blood gas analysis yields considerable information about gas exchange efficiency. Arterial hypoxaemia in adults is defined as PaO_2 below 10.7 kPa breathing room air, although it is not usually treated as clinically important unless below 8 kPa, when oxygen saturation will be 90% or less (Table 15.1).

Arterial carbon dioxide tension ($PaCO_2$) is used as an inversely proportional index of 'effective' alveolar ventilation. Hence, a high $PaCO_2$ is taken to indicate poor alveolar ventilation. Alveolar hypoventilation (raised $PaCO_2$) with a normal pH probably represents a primary ventilatory change present long enough for renal mechanisms to compensate, as in chronic ventilatory failure. Ventilation/blood flow relationships are most simply assessed by considering the size of the difference between the amounts of oxygen and carbon dioxide in the blood and in the air; the differences are small if the lungs are working efficiently. Disparity between ventilation/blood flow ratios results in abnormally wide differences – and then alveolar–arterial PO_2 and arterial–alveolar PCO_2 gradients will be abnormal.

Alveolar capillary surface area is assessed by measuring the uptake of carbon monoxide – usually abnormal in diffuse interstitial inflammatory and fibrotic processes and in emphysema.

Assessing bronchial reactivity and the exercise response can help evaluate breathlessness. Simple exercise testing provides information about overall fitness and the appropriateness of cardiorespiratory responses. Radionuclide lung scanning, blood gas analysis and sputum cytology or culture are sometimes needed in addition.

Management can include oxygen administration by mask or nasal cannula (Figs 15.4 and 15.5).

Dental aspects

LRT disorders can cause significant incapacity and are often a contraindication to GA, and even to CS.

ASTHMA

General aspects

Asthma is common, affecting 2–5% of the overall population; it is on the increase, particularly in childhood, with a frequency of up to 20% in some high-income countries. Asthma usually begins in childhood or early adult life; about half the patients with asthma develop it before age 10 years.

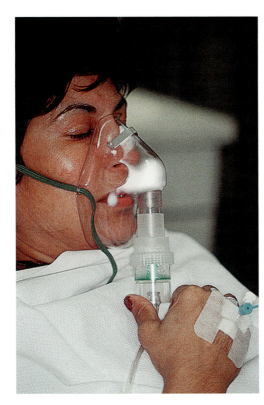

Fig. 15.4 Oxygen by mask in a patient with severe bronchospasm.

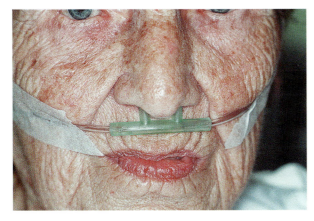

Fig. 15.5 Nasal catheter.

Bronchial hyper-reactivity causes reversible airway obstruction from smooth muscle constriction (bronchospasm), mucosal oedema and mucus hypersecretion. There are two main types, extrinsic (allergic) and intrinsic asthma (Table 15.2).

Extrinsic (allergic) asthma, the main childhood type, may be precipitated by allergens in animal dander, feathers or hair, drugs (e.g. non-steroidal anti-inflammatory drugs [NSAIDs] and some antibiotics), food (e.g. eggs, fish, fruit, milk, nuts), house dust (mite allergens) or moulds. Patients frequently have or develop other allergic diseases, such as eczema, hay fever and drug sensitivities. Extrinsic asthma is associated with IgE overproduction on allergen exposure, and release of mast cell mediators (histamine, leukotrienes, prostaglandins, bradykinin and platelet activating factor), which cause bronchospasm and oedema. About 75% of asthmatic children lose their asthma or improve by adulthood.

Intrinsic asthma is usually of adult onset and not allergic, but appears rather to be related to mast cell instability and

Table 15.2 *Types of asthma*

	Extrinsic asthma	Intrinsic asthma
Frequency	Most common	Least common
Aetiopathogenesis	Allergens causing IgE-mediated mast cell degranulation	Mast cell instability and airway hyper-responsivity
Association with atopy	+	–
Typical age of onset	Child	Adult

airway hyper-responsivity. Triggers include emotional stress, gastro-oesophageal reflux or vagally mediated responses.

Either type of asthma can be triggered by: infections (especially viral, mycoplasmal or fungal); irritating fumes (e.g. traffic or cigarette smoke); exercise (possibly due to cold air); weather changes; emotional stress; foods (e.g. nuts, shellfish, strawberries or milk) or additives (such as tartrazine); and drugs (e.g. aspirin and other NSAIDs, beta-blockers and angiotensin-converting enzyme inhibitors [ACEIs]).

Clinical features

In well-controlled patients with asthma, clinical features may be absent. During an asthmatic episode, symptoms may include dyspnoea, cough and paroxysmal expiratory wheeziness with laboured expiration. The frequency and severity of attacks vary widely between individuals (Table 15.3). Patients may become distressed, anxious and tachycardic, have reduced chest expansion and be using accessory respiratory muscles to increase their ventilatory effort. Nasal polyps are common, especially in aspirin-sensitive asthmatics. Children with asthma initially suffer from repeated 'colds' with cough, malaise and fever, often at night.

Asthma is typically diagnosed when the patient has more than one of the following – wheeze, cough, difficulty breathing and chest tightness – particularly if these are frequent and recurrent; are worse at night and in the early morning; occur in response to, or are worse after, exercise or other triggers, such as exposure to pets, cold or damp air, or with emotions or laughter; or occur without an association with colds. There is often:

- a personal history of atopic disorder
- a family history of atopic disorder and/or asthma
- widespread wheeze, heard on chest auscultation
- a history of improvement in symptoms or lung function in response to adequate therapy.

A prolonged asthmatic attack, which is refractory to treatment, may lead to life-threatening *status asthmaticus* (persisting for more than 24 hours). Failure of the patient to complete a sentence, indrawing of the intercostal muscles, a rapid pulse, a silent chest and signs of exhaustion are suggestive of impending respiratory arrest.

General management

Diagnosis of asthma is from the clinical history and presentation, based on recognizing a characteristic pattern of episodic symptoms in the absence of an alternative explanation. Investigations include a chest radiograph (to exclude other diagnoses, such as a pneumothorax), spirometry (serial PEFR), skin tests and blood examination (usually eosinophilia, raised total IgE and specific IgE antibody concentrations, which may help identify allergens). Occasionally, a histamine or methacholine challenge is used if the diagnosis is unclear.

Table 15.3 *Severity of asthma*

Severity of asthma	Symptom duration	Attack frequency per week	Other comments	Typical therapy
Mild	<1 h	<2	Attacks follow exercise or exposure to trigger	Beta-agonist as required
Moderate	Days	>2	Activity restricted	Beta-agonist plus steroid
Severe	Persistent	Persistent	Audible wheezing. Tachypnoea. Activity and sleep severely restricted	Beta agonist plus steroid plus theophylline

Table 15.4 *Medical management of asthma*[a]

Drug group	Examples	Comments
Beta-agonists	Selective β_2-agonists or stimulants (e.g. salbutamol). Others include:	Safest and most effective bronchodilators for routine control of asthma
		Relax bronchial smooth muscle with little cardiac effect
	Terbutaline, fenoterol, rimiterol	Act for 3–6 h
	Pirbuterol, reproterol, tulobuterol	Act for at least 12 h
	Bambuterol, salmeterol, formoterol	
Antimuscarinic bronchodilators	Ipratropium or oxitropium bromide	Useful particularly for those with asthma associated with bronchitis
		Act for up to 8 h
		Contraindicated in glaucoma and prostatic disease
Methylxanthines	Theophylline preparations (oral sustained release)	Prolonged action and useful for controlling nocturnal asthma
Corticosteroids	Corticosteroid (beclometasone, betamethasone valerate, budesonide or fluticasone) aerosol inhalations	Effective inhaled along with a bronchodilator but must be taken regularly
		High-dose corticosteroid inhalants can cause some adrenal suppression
Mast cell stabilizers	Sodium cromoglicate or nedocromil	Occasionally used as inhalants for prophylaxis, mainly in children, but some fail to respond
Leukotriene receptor antagonists	Montelukast, zafirlukast	May impair liver function and increase INR
5-Lipoxygenase inhibitor (impairs leukotriene release)	Zileuton	Given orally
		Effective when used alone or with inhaled steroids but may precipitate, and should not be used in Churg–Strauss syndrome, where deterioration and cardiac complications may be seen
Recombinant humanized monoclonal anti-immunoglobulin E (IgE) antibody	Omalizumab	Safe, effective treatment for allergic asthma

[a]In addition to oxygen.

In children with an intermediate probability of asthma, who can perform spirometry and have evidence of airways obstruction, assess the change in FEV_1 or PEFR in response to an inhaled bronchodilator (reversibility) and/or the response to a trial of treatment for a specified period; if there is significant reversibility, or if a treatment trial is beneficial, a diagnosis of asthma is probable.

Management includes patient education, smoking cessation advice, avoidance of identifiable irritants and allergens, and use of drugs. Home use of peak flow meters allows patients to monitor progress and detect any deterioration that may require urgent modification of treatment. Treatment should be based on the amount by which peak flow is reduced (a PEFR diary should be kept).

Drugs used for asthma management (Table 15.4) include oxygen, short-acting β_2 agonists (SABAs; such as salbutamol), corticosteroids, leukotriene receptor antagonists and omalizumab (a recombinant humanized monoclonal anti-IgE antibody that reduces the antigen-specific IgE).

Inhaled long-acting β_2 agonists (LABAs) may be needed (Fig. 15.6). Deaths from asthma are usually a result of failure to recognize deterioration or reluctance to use corticosteroids.

Other factors that have been studied include:

- **air pollution** – There is an association between air pollution and aggravation of existing asthma
- **allergen avoidance** – There is no consistent evidence of benefit
- **breast-feeding** – There is evidence of a protective effect in relation to early asthma
- **electrolytes** – There is no consistent evidence of benefit
- **fish oils and fatty acid** – There is no consistent evidence of benefit
- **house dust mites** – Measures to reduce the numbers of house dust mites do not affect asthma severity
- **immunotherapy** – Allergen-specific immunotherapy is beneficial in allergic asthma
- **microbial exposure** – There is insufficient evidence to indicate that the use of probiotics in pregnancy reduces the incidence of childhood asthma
- **modified milk formulae** – There is no consistent evidence of benefit

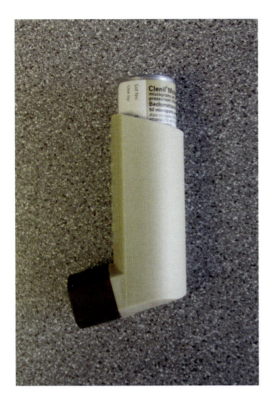

Fig. 15.6 Inhaler.

Box 15.1 *Agents that may precipitate asthmatic attack*
• Acrylic monomer
• Aspirin and other NSAIDs
• Barbiturates
• Beta-blockers
• Colophony
• Cyanoacrylates
• Histamine-releasing agents
• Mefenamic acid
• Opioids
• Pancuronium
• Pentazocine
• Suxamethonium
• Tubocurarine

Table 15.5 *Management complications from anti-asthmatic drugs*

Anti-asthmatic drug	Possible complications
β_2-agonists	Dry mouth
Corticosteroids	Steroid complications and adrenal crisis. Corticosteroid inhalers occasionally causes oral or pharyngeal thrush and, rarely, angina bullosa haemorrhagica
Ipratropium bromide	Dry mouth
Leukotriene antagonists	Bleeding tendency (and prolonged INR) because of impaired liver metabolism
Theophylline	Levels increased by epinephrine, erythromycin, clindamycin, azithromycin, clarithromycin or ciprofloxacin

- **nutritional supplementation** – There is limited, variable-quality evidence on the potential preventative effect of fish oil, selenium and vitamin E intake during pregnancy
- **pets** – There are no controlled trials on the benefits of removing pets from the home
- **tobacco** – Exposure to cigarette smoke adversely affects quality of life, lung function, need for rescue medications and long-term control with inhaled steroids. There is an association between maternal smoking and an increased risk of infant wheeze
- **weight reduction** – There is an association between increasing body mass index and symptoms of asthma.

Dental aspects

Elective dental care should be deferred in severe asthmatics until they are in a better phase; this can be advised by the patient's general practitioner.

Asthmatic patients should be asked to bring their usual medication with them when coming for dental treatment. Local anaesthesia (LA) is best used; occasional patients may react to the sulphites present as preservatives in vasoconstrictor-containing LA, so it may be better, where possible, to avoid solutions containing vasoconstrictor. Adrenaline (epinephrine) may theoretically enhance the risk of arrhythmias with beta-agonists and is contraindicated in patients using theophylline, as it may precipitate arrhythmias.

Relative analgesia with nitrous oxide and oxygen is preferable to intravenous sedation and gives more immediate control. Sedatives in general are better avoided as, in an acute asthmatic attack, even benzodiazepines can precipitate respiratory failure.

GA is best avoided, as it may be complicated by hypoxia and hypercapnia, which can cause pulmonary oedema even if cardiac function is normal, and cardiac failure if there is cardiac disease. The risk of postoperative lung collapse or pneumothorax is also increased. Halothane or, better, enflurane, isoflurane, desflurane and sevoflurane are the preferred anaesthetics, but ketamine may be useful in children.

Allergy to penicillin may be more frequent in asthmatics. Drugs to be avoided, since they may precipitate an asthmatic attack (see later), include those listed in Box 15.1.

Acute asthmatic attacks may also occasionally be precipitated by anxiety; it is important to attempt to lessen fear of dental treatment by gentle handling and reassurance. Even routine dental treatment can trigger a clinically significant decline in lung function in approximately 15% of asthmatics. Acute asthmatic attacks are usually self-limiting or respond to the patient's usual medication, such as a beta-agonist inhaler, but status asthmaticus is a potentially fatal emergency (Ch. 1). There may be complications caused by the anti-asthmatic drugs (Table 15.5).

Gastro-oesophageal reflux is not uncommon, with occasional tooth erosion. Periodontal inflammation is greater in asthmatics than in those without respiratory disease. Persons using steroid inhalers may develop oropharyngeal candidosis or, occasionally, angina bullosa haemorrhagica.

Guidelines on the management of asthma may be found at: http://www.sign.ac.uk/guidelines/fulltext/101/index.html, http://www.nice.org.uk/guidance/qualitystandards/indevelopment/Asthma.jsp and http://www.brit-thoracic.org.uk/Portals/0/Guidelines/AsthmaGuidelines/qrg101%202011.pdf (all accessed 30 September 2013).

Box 15.2 *Features of Churg–Strauss syndrome*

- Asthma
- Eosinophilia >10%
- Extravascular eosinophils
- Mono- or polyneuropathy
- Pulmonary infiltrates (non-fixed)
- Paranasal sinus abnormality

CHURG–STRAUSS SYNDROME (ALLERGIC GRANULOMATOSIS OR ANGIITIS)

General aspects

Churg–Strauss syndrome (CSS) is a rare, potentially fatal, systemic vasculitis similar to polyarteritis nodosa (PAN), characterized by severe asthma-like attacks with peripheral eosinophilia, and intravascular and extravascular granuloma formation with eosinophil infiltration and skin lesions in 70%. Cardiopulmonary involvement is the main cause of death.

Clinical features

CSS is diagnosed if at least 4 of the 6 criteria listed in Box 15.2 are positive.

General management

The 5-year survival of untreated CSS is 25%. Combination treatment with cyclophosphamide and prednisolone (prednisone) provides a 5-year survival of 50%.

Dental aspects

Management problems relating to patients with CSS may include respiratory impairment and corticosteroid treatment (Ch. 6).

CHRONIC OBSTRUCTIVE PULMONARY DISEASE (COPD)

General aspects

Chronic obstructive pulmonary disease (COPD; chronic obstructive airways disease, COAD) is a common, chronic, slowly progressive, irreversible disease (most frequently a combination of chronic bronchitis and emphysema), characterized by breathlessness and wheeze (airways obstruction), cough and sputum. *Chronic bronchitis* is defined as the excessive production of mucus and persistent cough with sputum production, daily for more than 3 months in a year over more than 2 consecutive years. It leads to production of excessive, viscous mucus, which is ineffectively cleared from the airway, obstructs and stagnates, and becomes infected, usually with *Streptococcus pneumoniae*, *Moraxella catarrhalis* and *Haemophilus influenzae*. Patchy areas of alveolar collapse can result. *Emphysema* is dilatation of air spaces distal to the terminal bronchioles with destruction of alveoli, reducing the alveolar surface area available for respiratory exchange. COPD is now the preferred term for conditions with airflow obstruction because of a combination of airway and parenchymal damage; patients were previously diagnosed as having chronic bronchitis or emphysema.

Table 15.6 *Clinical features differentiating COPD and asthma*

	COPD	Asthma
Smoker or ex-smoker	Nearly all	Possibly
Symptoms under age 35	Rare	Often
Chronic productive cough	Common	Uncommon
Breathlessness	Persistent and progressive	Variable
Night-time waking with breathlessness and/or wheeze	Uncommon	Common
Significant diurnal or day-to-day variability of symptoms	Uncommon	Common

Table 15.7 *Additional investigations in suspected COPD*

Investigation	Comments
Alpha$_1$-antitrypsin	If COPD has an early onset, or there is a minimal smoking history or positive family history
CT scan of thorax	To investigate symptoms that seem disproportionate to spirometric impairment
	To investigate chest radiograph abnormalities
	To assess suitability for GA and surgery
Echocardiogram	To assess cardiac status, if cor pulmonale is present
Electrocardiogram	To assess cardiac status, if cor pulmonale is present
Peak flow measurements (serial domiciliary)	To exclude asthma, if any diagnostic doubt
Pulse oximetry	To assess need for oxygen therapy, if cyanosis or cor pulmonale is present, or if FEV$_1$ is <50% predicted
Sputum culture	To identify organisms, if sputum is persistently present and purulent
Transfer factor for carbon monoxide (T_LCO)	To investigate symptoms that seem disproportionate to spirometric impairment

COPD is characterized by airflow obstruction – defined as an FEV_1/FVC ratio reduced to less than 0.7. If FEV_1 is 80% or more, a diagnosis of COPD should only be made if there are respiratory symptoms (e.g. dyspnoea or cough). The airflow obstruction is not fully reversible, does not change significantly over months, and is usually progressive in the long term.

The most important causes of COPD include cigarette smoking, environmental pollution, dusts, chemicals or occupational exposures to various substances. Exposure to smoke from home cooking or heating fuels may contribute. Deficiency of the antiproteolytic enzyme alpha1-antitrypsin is a rare cause of emphysema.

Clinical features

There is often significant airflow obstruction before the person is aware of it and so COPD typically remains undiagnosed until patients are in their fifties. Differentiation from asthma is important (Table 15.6).

A diagnosis of COPD should be considered in patients over the age of 35 who have a risk factor (e.g. smoking) and exertional breathlessness, chronic cough, regular sputum production, frequent winter 'bronchitis' or wheeze. Clinical judgment is based on history, physical examination, confirmation of airflow obstruction using spirometry (post-bronchodilator spirometry) and assessment of the severity of dyspnoea (Tables 15.7 and 15.8).

COPD is characterized by breathlessness and wheeze (airways obstruction), cough and an early morning mucoid sputum production.

Table 15.8 *MRC dyspnoea scale*

Grade	Degree of breathlessness related to activities
1	Not troubled by breathlessness except on strenuous exercise
2	Short of breath when hurrying or walking up a slight hill
3	Walks slower than contemporaries on level ground because of breathlessness, or has to stop for breath when walking at own pace
4	Stops for breath after walking about 100 metres or after a few minutes on level ground
5	Too breathless to leave the house, or breathless when dressing or undressing

Adapted from Fletcher CM, et al. The significance of respiratory symptoms and the diagnosis of chronic bronchitis in a working population. Br Med J 1959; 2:257.

Table 15.9 *Comparison of chronic bronchitis and emphysema*

	Chronic bronchitis	Emphysema
Cough	Chronic	Minimal
Sputum	Copious and mucoid	Minimal
Infections	Common	Uncommon
Dyspnoea	Mild	Severe
PO_2	Low	Low
PCO_2	Raised	Normal
Forced expiratory volume (FEV)	Low	Low
Clinical appearance	Blue bloater	Pink puffer

Progressive dyspnoea, low oxygen saturation, carbon dioxide accumulation (hypercapnia) and metabolic acidosis mean that patients may ultimately become dyspnoeic at rest ('respiratory cripples'), especially when recumbent (orthopnoea), and eventually develop respiratory failure, pulmonary hypertension, right ventricular hypertrophy and right-sided heart failure (cor pulmonale).

Two clinical patterns of COPD are recognized:

- '*Pink puffers*' – patients with emphysema who manage to maintain normal blood gases by hyperventilation, and are always breathless but not cyanosed; rather they are pink from vasodilatation
- '*Blue bloaters*' – patients with chronic bronchitis who lose their CO_2 drive, fail to maintain adequate ventilation and become both hypercapnic and hypoxic with central cyanosis, cor pulmonale and oedema (for these patients, the respiratory drive is from the low PO_2 and thus oxygen administration is contraindicated) (Table 15.9).

General management

The diagnosis of COPD is based upon clinical history and presentation. Investigations include a chest radiograph (which may show hyperinflated lung fields with loss of vascular markings); arterial blood gases (which should be measured if pulse oximetry shows oxygen saturation less than 92%); spirometry; and lung function tests. FEV1 is reduced in all cases (FEV_1 of less than 40% signifies severe COPD) and the flow–volume curve shows a typical pattern, with reduced flow rates at mid- and lower-lung volumes. A ratio of FEV_1:FVC of less than 70% confirms airways obstruction.

Patients with COPD and their family should be educated about the disease, and about required lifestyle changes and medication.

Non-drug therapy includes: stopping smoking (nicotine replacement therapy or bupropion may help); exercise by pulmonary rehabilitation – of proven benefit; weight loss (improves exercise tolerance); and vaccination (pneumococcal and influenza vaccines). Drug therapy includes short-acting bronchodilators (anticholinergic drugs [ipratropium bromide]) and β_2 agonists (salbutamol) to treat the reversible component of airway disease; corticosteroids (inhaled or systemic); and antibiotics (amoxicillin, trimethoprim or tetracycline). Mucolytics, such as carbocisteine, reduce acute exacerbations by almost one-third. Long-term oxygen therapy (LTOT) reduces mortality.

People with stable COPD who remain breathless or have exacerbations, despite using short-acting bronchodilators, should be offered the following as maintenance therapy:

- If FEV_1 is 50% of predicted or more: use either a long-acting β_2 agonist (LABA) or long-acting muscarinic antagonist (LAMA).
- If FEV_1 is less than 50% predicted: either a LABA with an inhaled corticosteroid (ICS) in a combination inhaler, or a LAMA.

Offer a LAMA in addition to a LABA plus ICS to people with COPD who remain breathless or have exacerbations, despite taking LABA plus ICS, irrespective of their FEV_1.

Provide pulmonary rehabilitation for all who need it; non-invasive ventilation (NIV) is the treatment of choice for persistent hypercapnic ventilatory failure during exacerbations not responding to medical therapy. The frequency of exacerbations should be reduced by appropriate use of inhaled corticosteroids and bronchodilators, and vaccinations.

Inhaled therapy

Bronchodilators (short-acting β_2 agonists [SABA] and short-acting muscarinic antagonists [SAMA]) should be the initial empirical treatment for the relief of breathlessness and exercise limitation. ICS have potential adverse effects (including non-fatal pneumonia) in people with COPD. Offer a once-daily LAMA in preference to four-times-daily SAMA to people with stable COPD who remain breathless or have exacerbations, despite using short-acting bronchodilators as required, and in whom a decision has been made to commence regular maintenance bronchodilator therapy with a muscarinic antagonist (see above).

Most patients – whatever their age – are able to acquire and maintain an adequate inhaler technique. Bronchodilators are usually best administered using a hand-held inhaler device (including a spacer device if appropriate).

Patients with distressing or disabling dyspnoea, despite maximal therapy using inhalers, should be considered for nebulizer therapy. They should be offered a choice between a face mask and a mouthpiece to administer their nebulized therapy, unless the drug specifically requires a mouthpiece (for example, anticholinergic drugs).

Oral therapy

Some patients with advanced COPD may require maintenance oral corticosteroids when these cannot be withdrawn following an exacerbation. These individuals should be monitored for the development of osteoporosis and given appropriate prophylaxis.

Theophylline should only be used after a trial of SABA and LABA, and only to those who are unable to use inhaled therapy, as there is a need to monitor plasma levels and interactions. The dose of theophylline prescribed should be reduced at the time of an exacerbation if macrolide or fluoroquinolone antibiotics (or other drugs known to interact) are given. There is insufficient evidence to recommend prophylactic antibiotic therapy in the management of stable COPD. Mucolytic drug therapy should be considered in patients with a chronic cough productive of sputum.

Combined inhaled and oral therapy
If patients remain symptomatic on monotherapy, their treatment should be intensified by combining therapies from different drug classes, such as:

- β_2 agonist and theophylline
- anticholinergic and theophylline.

Oxygen
Long-term oxygen therapy (LTOT). Inappropriate oxygen therapy in people with COPD may depress respiration. LTOT is indicated in patients with COPD who have a PaO_2 of less than 7.3 kPa when stable, or a PaO_2 greater than 7.3 kPa and less than 8 kPa when stable, and one of: secondary polycythaemia, nocturnal hypoxaemia (oxygen saturation of arterial blood [SaO_2] of less than 90% for more than 30% of the time), peripheral oedema or pulmonary hypertension.

To reap the benefits of LTOT, patients should breathe supplemental oxygen for at least 15 hours per day. To ensure that all those eligible for LTOT are identified, pulse oximetry should be available in all healthcare settings. The assessment of patients for LTOT should comprise the measurement of arterial blood gases on two occasions at least 3 weeks apart in patients who have a confident diagnosis of COPD, who are receiving optimum medical management and whose COPD is stable.

Patients should be warned about the risks of fire and explosion and told not to smoke when using oxygen.

Ambulatory oxygen therapy. Ambulatory oxygen therapy should be considered in patients on LTOT who wish to continue oxygen therapy outside the home, and who have exercise desaturation, are shown to have an improvement in exercise capacity and/or dyspnoea with oxygen, and are motivated to use oxygen.

Non-invasive ventilation (NIV). Adequately treated patients with chronic hypercapnic respiratory failure who have required assisted ventilation during an exacerbation, or who are hypercapnic or acidotic on LTOT, should be referred to a specialist centre for consideration of long-term NIV. Advanced emphysema is occasionally treated with surgery – excision of large acquired bullae or, rarely, lung transplantation.

Dental aspects
Patients with COPD who need dental care can be classified as follows:

- Patients at low risk – experience dyspnoea on effort but have normal blood gas levels. These patients can receive all dental treatment with minor modifications.
- Patients at moderate risk – experience dyspnoea on effort, are chronically treated with bronchodilators or recently with corticosteroids, and PaO_2 lowered. A medical consultation is advised to determine the level of control of the disease before any dental treatment.
- Patients at high risk – have symptomatic COPD that may be end-stage and poorly responsive to treatment. With these patients, a medical consultation is essential before any dental treatment is carried out.

Patients with COPD are best treated in an upright position at mid-morning or early afternoon, since they may become increasingly dyspnoeic if laid supine. It may be difficult to use a rubber dam, as some patients are mouth-breathers and not able to tolerate the additional obstruction. LA is preferred for dental treatment, but bilateral mandibular or palatal injections should be avoided. Patients with COPD should be given relative analgesia only if absolutely necessary, and only in hospital after full preoperative assessment. CS with diazepam and midazolam should not be used, as benzodiazepines are respiratory depressants. Patients should be given GA only if absolutely necessary, and intravenous barbiturates are contraindicated. Secretions reduce airway patency and, if lightly anaesthetized, the patient may cough and contaminate other areas of the lung.

Postoperative respiratory complications are more prevalent in patients with pre-existing lung diseases, especially after prolonged operations and if there has been no preoperative preparation. The most important single factor in preoperative care is cessation of smoking for at least 1 week preoperatively. Respiratory infections must also be eradicated; sputum should first be sent for culture and sensitivity, but antimicrobials such as amoxicillin should be started without awaiting results.

The medical management of COPD should be optimized prior to surgery. The ultimate clinical decision about whether or not to proceed with surgery should rest with a consultant anaesthetist and consultant surgeon, taking account of co-morbidities, functional status of the patient and necessity for the surgery.

Composite assessment tools, such as the American Society of Anesthesiologists (ASA) scoring system, and not just lung function, are the best criteria for the assessment of patients with COPD before surgery. Those taking corticosteroids should be treated with appropriate precautions (Ch. 6). Interactions of theophylline with other drugs, such as adrenaline (epinephrine), erythromycin, clindamycin, azithromycin, clarithromycin or ciprofloxacin, may result in dangerously high levels of theophylline. Ipratropium can cause dry mouth.

Guidelines for the management of COPD may be found at: http://publications.nice.org.uk/chronic-obstructive-pulmonary-disease-cg101 (accessed 30 September 2013).

INFECTIONS

General aspects
Respiratory viruses usually spread by touch or airborne transmission and the very small particles (2–0.2 micrometres) can avoid the upper respiratory tract defences and the mucociliary elevator to reach the lung alveoli. A range of viruses can cause lower respiratory tract infections (LRTIs; Table 15.10). Some viruses (e.g. influenza and respiratory syncytial) can spread from the upper to the lower respiratory tract via infection of the respiratory epithelium and can lead to bacterial superinfection and pneumonitis (pneumonia). Mycoplasmal (atypical) pneumonia and tuberculosis (TB) may be direct infections. Epidemics of a potentially fatal severe acute respiratory syndrome (SARS) have been caused by a coronavirus that originated in China and spread worldwide; H5N1 bird influenza also arose as an epidemic; and a similar epidemic, but of swine influenza (H1N1), emanated from Mexico (see later).

Bacterial infections, such as pneumonia or lung abscess, can also result from material aspirated into the lungs, and are usually unilateral. Those who aspirate more than others have, as a result, more frequent LRTI and this is seen in alcohol and other drug abusers, as well as comatose patients. Exogenous penetration and contamination

Table 15.10 *Lower respiratory tract infections and their main causes*[a]

Condition	Microorganisms
Laryngo-tracheo-bronchitis (croup)	Influenza viruses
	Mycoplasma pneumonia
	Para-influenza viruses
	Respiratory syncytial virus
Acute bronchiolitis	Human metapneumovirus (HMPV)
	Influenza viruses
	Respiratory syncytial virus
Acute bronchitis	Adenovirus
	Bordetella pertussis
	Chlamydia pneumoniae (Taiwan acute respiratory [TWAR] agent)
	Coronaviruses
	Coxsackie virus
	Haemophilus influenzae (non-typeable)
	Herpes simplex virus
	Influenza viruses
	Moraxella catarrhalis
	Mycoplasma pneumonia
	Para-influenza virus
	Respiratory syncytial virus
	Rhinovirus
Acute pneumonitis (pneumonia)	*Escherichia coli*
	Haemophilus influenza
	Klebsiella species
	Pseudomonas aeruginosa
	Severe acute respiratory syndrome-associated coronavirus (SARS-CoV)
	Streptococcus pneumoniae (pneumococcus)

[a]The most frequent are shown in bold.

Table 15.11 *Causes of pneumonia*

Infective route	Microorganisms
Inhalation	*Streptococcus pneumoniae, Streptococcus pyogenes*
	Mycobacteria, *Legionella, Coxiella burnetii* (Q fever)
	Influenza, measles virus, adenovirus
	Coccidioides, Histoplasma, Cryptococcus
Aspiration	Anaerobes, *Streptococcus pneumoniae, Staphylococcus aureus, Haemophilus influenzae*, Gram-negative bacilli
Haematogenous spread	*Staphylococcus aureus*, Gram-negative bacilli (*Pseudomonas aeruginosa*)
	Candida
	Strongyloides, Ascaris
Contiguous spread	Anaerobes, Gram-negative bacilli
	Entamoeba histolytica
Reactivation	Mycobacteria
	Cytomegalovirus
	Coccidioides, Histoplasma, Blastomyces
	Toxoplasma, Strongyloides, Pneumocystis jiroveci (P. carinii)

General management

Antimicrobial therapy is indicated, particularly for pneumonia. Antivirals have not been highly effective. Oxygen may be needed. Pneumococcal vaccine is indicated for older people.

Dental aspects

The majority of LRTIs are severe illnesses, and are contraindications to all but emergency dental treatment. GA is hazardous and absolutely contraindicated. Dental treatment should be deferred until recovery, or be limited to pain relief.

INFLUENZA ('FLU)

Influenza is mainly a community-based infection transmitted in households and communities. Health-care-associated influenza infections can arise in any health-care setting, most commonly when influenza is also circulating in the community.

General aspects

Influenza is a contagious disease caused by influenza virus types A, B or C. Type A has two main subtypes (H1N1 and H3N2); it causes most of the widespread influenza epidemics and can occasionally be fatal. Type B viruses generally cause regional outbreaks of moderate severity, and type C viruses are of minor significance.

A person can spread influenza starting 1 day before they feel sick and for another 3–7 days after symptoms start. Influenza can be prevented or ameliorated by vaccination each autumn; this is especially indicated for older people and those with cardiorespiratory disease.

Clinical features

Influenza attacks virtually the whole respiratory tract; symptoms appear suddenly after 1–4 days and include fever, sore throat, nasal congestion, headache, tiredness, dry cough and muscle pains (myalgia).

of the lung can result from trauma (e.g. a stab wound or road traffic accident) or surgery. *Entamoeba histolytica* can occasionally cause pneumonia – by direct extension from an amoebic liver abscess (Table 15.11). Patients with endocarditis, or septic pelvic or jugular thrombophlebitis, may experience LRTI acquired haematogenously and then it is often bilateral.

Immunocompromised persons (e.g. those with human immunodeficiency virus/acquired immune deficiency syndrome [HIV/AIDS] and transplant recipients) and people with bronchiectasis or cystic fibrosis are also susceptible to respiratory infections by a range of opportunistic microbes. *Pneumocystis jiroveci* (*P. carinii*), for example, is a common cause of potentially fatal pneumonia in immunocompromised patients – especially those with HIV/AIDS (Chs 20 and 21).

Clinical features

Clinical features of LRTI vary according to the part of the respiratory tract mainly affected:

- *Bronchiolitis* causes rapid respiration, wheezing, fever and dyspnoea – but is restricted mainly to infants.
- *Bronchitis* causes cough, wheezing and sometimes dyspnoea.
- *Pneumonia* causes cough, fever, rapid respiration, breathlessness, chest pain, dyspnoea and shivering.

Most people recover in 1–2 weeks but infection can be life-threatening, mainly because primary influenzal viral pneumonia can lead to secondary bacterial pneumonia or can exacerbate underlying conditions (e.g. pulmonary or cardiac disease). The old and very young, and those with chronic disorders, are more likely to suffer complications, such as pneumonia, bronchitis, sinusitis or otitis media. Influenza has also been followed by depression, encephalopathy, myocarditis, myositis, pericarditis, Reye syndrome and transverse myelitis.

General management

Rest, maintenance of fluid intake, analgesics, antipyretics, and avoidance of alcohol and tobacco help relieve symptoms. Aspirin must *never* be given to children under the age of 16 years who have 'flu-like symptoms, and particularly fever, as this can cause Reye syndrome.

Zanamivir (an antiviral that works against influenza types A and B) can shorten the symptoms by approximately 1 day, if treatment is started during the first 2 days of illness. Other antiviral drugs include amantadine, oseltamivir and rimantadine; they may be helpful but their use is restricted mainly to immunocompromised persons, since they can cause adverse effects.

Dental aspects

Influenza can be a severe contagious illness so all but emergency dental treatment should be deferred until recovery. GA is hazardous and absolutely contraindicated.

Bird 'flu

Influenza type A subtype H5N1 can cause an illness known as 'avian influenza' or 'bird 'flu' in birds, humans and many other animal species. HPAI A(H5N1) – 'highly pathogenic avian influenza virus of type A of subtype H5N1' – is the causative agent and is enzootic in many bird populations, especially in South-East Asia. It has spread globally and resulted in the deaths of over 100 people and the slaughter of millions of chickens. A vaccine that could provide protection (Prepandrix) has been cleared for use in the European Union. H5N7 is a more recent emergent infection, similar in many respects.

Swine 'flu

Swine influenza is common in pigs in the midwestern United States, Mexico, Canada, South America, Europe (including the UK, Sweden and Italy), Kenya, China, Taiwan, Japan and other parts of eastern Asia. Transmission of swine influenza virus from pigs to humans is not common, but can produce symptoms similar to those of influenza. A 2009 outbreak in humans ('swine 'flu') was due to an apparently new strain of H1N1 arising from a reassortment produced from strains of human, avian and swine viruses. It can pass from human to human. Antiviral agents such as oseltamivir may help. Vaccines are now available.

SEVERE ACUTE RESPIRATORY SYNDROME (SARS)

General aspects

An outbreak of a life-threatening febrile respiratory infection appeared in 2003, originating from Guangdong, China, and was named severe acute respiratory syndrome (SARS). Caused by a newly recognized coronavirus (SARS-associated coronavirus, SARS-CoV), SARS spread via close contact to many countries across the world. According to the World Health Organization, 8437 people worldwide became sick with SARS during the course of the first recognized outbreak and 813 died.

Clinical features

The incubation period of 2–7 days is followed by a high fever (above 38.0°C), malaise, headache and myalgia. Some people also experience mild upper respiratory symptoms and, after 2–7 days, lower respiratory signs – a dry cough and dyspnoea, potentially progressing to hypoxaemia. SARS can cause a pneumonia with a mortality approaching 10%, particularly in older or immunocompromised people.

General management

Artificial ventilation has been needed in 10–20% of cases. Antiviral agents, such as oseltamivir or ribavirin, may help. Inactivated vaccines, virally and bacterially vectored vaccines, recombinant protein and DNA vaccines, as well as attenuated vaccines, are under development.

Dental aspects

SARS is a severe illness, and all but emergency dental treatment should be deferred until recovery. GA is hazardous and absolutely contraindicated. For all contact with suspect SARS patients, careful hand hygiene is important, including hand-washing with soap and water; if hands are not visibly soiled, alcohol-based handrubs may be used as an alternative to hand-washing. If a suspected SARS patient is admitted to hospital, infection control personnel should be notified immediately. Infection control measures (www.cdc.gov/ncidod/hip/isolat/isolat.htm; accessed 30 September 2013) should include standard precautions (e.g. hand hygiene): health-care personnel should wear eye protection for all patient contact; contact precautions (e.g. gown and gloves for contact with the patient or their environment); and airborne precautions (e.g. an isolation room with negative pressure relative to the surrounding area and use of an N-95 filtering disposable respirator for persons entering the room).

BACTERIAL PNEUMONIA

General aspects

Pneumonia is classed as 'primary' if it occurs in a previously healthy individual, and is usually lobar; it is called 'secondary' if it follows some other disorder, such as previous viral respiratory infections, aspiration of foreign material, lung disease (bronchiectasis or carcinoma), depressed immunity (e.g. alcoholism or immunosuppression), or aspiration of oral bacteria (Table 15.12). It is usually bronchopneumonia.

Community-acquired pneumonia is often associated with *Streptococcus pneumoniae* or *Haemophilus influenzae* but Enterobacteriaceae, such as *Klebsiella* species, *Escherichia coli* and *Pseudomonas aeruginosa*, are especially likely in the very old and infirm (Table 15.13). Poor oral hygiene and periodontal disease may promote oropharyngeal bacterial colonization. Early on, hospital-acquired pneumonia is often associated with *Strep. pneumoniae* or *H. influenzae*. In late hospital-acquired pneumonia, polymicrobial infections or meticillin-resistant *Staphylococcus aureus* (MRSA) are particular hazards.

Clinical features

Pneumonia causes cough, fever, rapid respiration, breathlessness, chest pain, dyspnoea and shivering. Complications can include lung abscess or empyema (pus in pleural cavity).

Table 15.12 *Factors predisposing to pneumonia*

Exogenous	Endogenous
Viral respiratory infections, particularly influenza	Old age Immobility
Suppression of the cough reflex Aspiration of foreign material	Respiratory depression or chest injury
Mortality in patients in intensive care units (ventilator-associated pneumonia; VAP) – can range from 20% to 50%	Neurological disorders permitting aspiration of foreign material
	Underlying pulmonary disease, such as carcinoma or emphysema
Prolonged endotracheal intubation (increases risk by up to 20-fold)	Alcoholism
	Immunodeficiency (especially HIV/AIDS)
	Pneumocystis jiroveci (*carinii*) pneumonia – Chs 20 and 21

Table 15.14 *Differentiation of Legionnaire's disease from Pontiac fever*

	Legionnaire's disease	Pontiac fever
Isolation of bacterium	+	–
Incubation period	2–14 days	24–48 h
Percentage of persons who, when exposed to the source of an outbreak, become ill	<5%	>90%
Clinical features	Pneumonia: cough, fever, chest pain	'Flu-like illness (fever, chills, malaise) without pneumonia
Radiographic pneumonia	+	–
Case-fatality rate (%)	5–80	~0

Table 15.13 *Main causes of bacterial pneumonia*

Pathogen	Comments
Chlamydia pneumoniae	Seen in persons in institutions
Chlamydia psittaci	Seen after contact with psittacine birds (parrots, etc.)
Coxiella burnetii	Seen after contact with farm animals
Gram-negative anaerobes	Seen after aspiration
Haemophilus influenzae	Seen at extremes of life
Klebsiella pneumoniae	Seen in the elderly and debilitated, and in nursing homes
Legionella pneumoniae	Seen after exposure to water aerosols
Mycoplasma pneumoniae	Epidemics every 4 years
Staphylococcus aureus	Follows influenza
Streptococcus pneumoniae	Most common pathogen

General management

It is important to avoid alcohol and tobacco, but use analgesics and antipyretics to relieve the symptoms. Broad-spectrum antimicrobials given promptly and empirically usually include a macrolide (azithromycin, clarithromycin or erythromycin), quinolone (moxifloxacin, gatifloxacin or levofloxacin), or doxycycline for outpatients. For inpatients, cefuroxime or ceftriaxone plus a macrolide is used.

Prophylaxis includes immunization against influenza and pneumococci.

Dental aspects

Pneumonia is a severe illness and all but emergency dental treatment should be deferred until recovery. GA is hazardous and absolutely contraindicated.

Ventilator-associated pneumonia (VAP) is discussed later.

LEGIONELLOSIS

General aspects

Legionellosis is a bacterial respiratory infection caused by one of the family Legionellaceae, Gram-negative aerobic bacilli, ubiquitous in water and soil but particularly preferring warm aquatic environments. The term Legionnaire's disease was coined as a result of an outbreak of the previously unrecognized respiratory disease in an American Legion meeting in Philadelphia in 1976, but it is now recognized worldwide, many infections being contracted during travel abroad, particularly to Spain, Turkey and some other Mediterranean areas.

Legionella bacteria can be found in natural freshwater environments, usually in insufficient numbers to cause disease. *Legionella* grow best in warm water, as in hot tubs, cooling towers, hot water tanks, large plumbing systems, or the air-conditioning systems of large buildings. Though there are over 30 Legionellaceae, most infections are caused by *Legionella pneumophila*. Disease is contracted by inhalation of contaminated mist or vapour, mainly (approximately 46%) through aerosolization of infected water in air-conditioning systems, hot-water systems, humidifiers, nebulizers, showers and spa pools. Outbreaks have mostly been linked to aerosol sources in the community, cruise ships and hotels, with the most likely sources being whirlpool spas, air-conditioning units in large buildings, potable (drinking) water systems, and water used for bathing. Risk factors include:

- exposure to:
  recent travel with an overnight stay outside of the home (outbreaks of travel-associated legionellosis are infrequently identified but more than 20% of cases are thought to be associated with recent travel)
  whirlpool spas
  recent repairs or maintenance work on domestic plumbing
- systemic ill-health:
  alcohol use
  chronic kidney disease
  diabetes
  immune defects
  liver disease
  malignancy
  smoking.

Illness mainly affects males over 45, smokers, heavy drinkers, older people and the immunocompromised. Also vulnerable are travellers, especially middle-aged and older tourists, and conference or business groups, possibly because of tiredness or age. Many young people have been exposed to infection and become seropositive, but remained healthy.

There is no evidence of person-to-person transmission of legionellosis.

Clinical features

Legionellosis manifests as one of two clinical syndromes (Table 15.14). *Legionnaire's disease* is typically a lobular type of pneumonia, which

Table 15.15 *Sensitivity and specificity of Legionella diagnostic tests*

Test	Sensitivity (%)	Specificity (%)
Culture	80	100
Urine antigen	70	100
Paired serology[a]	70–80	>90
Direct fluorescent antibody stain	25–75	95

[a]A single antibody titre of any level is not diagnostic of legionellosis.

can be fatal but is fortunately rare; infection can range from discrete patches of inflammation and consolidation to involvement of whole lobes. *Pontiac fever* is milder and usually subsides rapidly, often without treatment.

People who should be tested for Legionnaire's disease include those with pneumonia in the following groups:

- Hospitalized patients with enigmatic pneumonia
- Patients who require care in an intensive care unit
- Compromised hosts
- Individuals who contract disease in the setting of a legionellosis outbreak
- Those who fail to respond to a beta-lactam or cephalosporin
- Patients who have travelled away from home within the preceding 2 weeks.

Because *Legionella* is commonly found in the environment, clinical isolates are necessary to interpret the findings of an environmental investigation. Diagnosis can be by rapid urine molecular testing for *L. pneumophila* antigen, and culture of respiratory secretions on selective media. Sensitivity and specificity of the diagnostic tests are shown in Table 15.15.

General management

Pontiac fever is a self-limited illness; most cases recover within 1 week and few benefit from antibiotic treatment. Overall mortality in Legionnaire's disease may be as high as 10%, and over 25% in older people and up to 80% in the immunocompromised. Erythromycin is standard treatment; cephalosporin is an alternative.

Dental aspects

Legionella species are present in roughly two-thirds of potable water samples collected from domestic and institutional taps and drinking fountains, and from a similar percentage of dental units, but water from these dental units often has higher bacterial concentrations (Ch. 31). There are reports of *Legionella* infections in dental unit water lines, and antibodies and occasionally frank infection demonstrated in dental staff; at least one patient appears to have contracted and died from infection emanating from a dental practice.

Prevention is crucial, involving (Ch. 31):

- continuous circulation water systems
- independent water reservoirs
- flushing lines
- regular disinfection of waterlines, handpieces and power scalers
- waterline filters
- regular water quality testing.

Further information on infection control measures is available at: http://www.legionellacontrol.com/legionella-control-association.htm (accessed 30 September 2013).

TUBERCULOSIS (TB)

General aspects

Tuberculosis (TB), an infection caused by mycobacteria, affects approximately one-third of the world's population (1.5 billion people); it is a major global health problem, some 2 million people dying from it annually. TB disproportionately affects the poorest persons in both high-income and developing countries. In high-income countries, most human TB arises from *Mycobacterium tuberculosis*, transmitted from person to person through the air. TB usually affects the lungs initially (pulmonary TB) but can also involve brain, kidneys, spine and other parts. From Victorian times to about the Second World War, *Mycobacterium bovis* infection from infected cows' milk (bovine or bTB) was a major cause of morbidity and mortality; it was clinically and pathologically indistinguishable from infection caused by *M. tuberculosis*. Cattle-testing and a slaughter programme became compulsory in 1950 and, by the 1980s, the incidence of TB in cattle had been substantially reduced. Tuberculosis from *M. bovis* in cows' milk was virtually eliminated in high-income countries by the tuberculin testing of cattle and pasteurization of milk. In the developing world, many cattle still have TB, and bTB is still seen. bTB has also increased in high-income countries over the last two decades and an infection rate of up to 38% in badgers – and transmission to cattle – may explain this.

TB is not spread by touch or by drinking glasses, dishes, sheets or clothing. It is usually transmitted by infected sputum, typically from close contacts such as family members, but is unlikely to be transmitted between normal social contacts. TB can present an occupational risk to health-care professionals, including dental staff. One outbreak of drug-resistant TB in New York involved at least 357 patients, most of whom contracted TB in one of 11 hospitals; nearly 90% of the patients were also HIV-positive, and most were young males of Hispanic or African heritage. TB has been transmitted between passengers during long-haul airline flights. The risk of transmitting TB though air circulation is now low because the high-efficiency particulate air (HEPA) filters on newer commercial aircraft are of the same type as those used in hospital respiratory isolation rooms; indeed, the number of times air is cleaned each hour exceeds the recommendation for hospital isolation rooms.

Sub-Saharan Africa has the highest rates of active TB per capita, driven primarily by the HIV epidemic. The absolute number of cases is highest in Asia, with India and China having the greatest burden of disease globally. In the USA and most Western European countries, the majority of cases occur in foreign-born residents and recent immigrants from countries in which tuberculosis is endemic. Immunocompromised people – such as diabetics and severely immunodeficient patients, like those with HIV/AIDS (about 30% of South Africans with HIV/AIDS also have TB) – and patients in prisons or institutions are at risk. TB also mainly affects medically neglected persons, such as vagrants, alcoholics, intravenous drug abusers or older homeless people. The main groups at increased risk for infection therefore include people who are resource-poor or immunoincompetent, especially:

- alcoholics
- older people
- people with cancer, diabetes mellitus, HIV/AIDS or liver disease
- people taking immunosuppressive or biological agents
- young children.

TB in developing countries is particularly widespread and is increasing, the highest rises in incidence being in South-East Asia, sub-Saharan Africa and Eastern Europe. In high-income countries,

Table 15.16 *Tuberculosis: differentiation of latent and active infections*

	Latent	Active
Mycobacteria present	+	+
Mycobacteria active	–	+
Contagious	–	+
Symptoms	–	+
Mantoux test	+	+
Chest radiograph	Normal	Abnormal
Sputum culture	–	+

Box 15.3 *Conditions in which tuberculosis may become activated*

- Alcohol abuse
- Cancer
- Chronic kidney disease
- Diabetes
- Drug abuse
- Gastric bypass/gastrectomy
- HIV
- Immunosuppression
- Leukaemia
- Recent infection
- Silicosis
- Young age at infection

the incidence is also rising, probably because of worsening social deprivation, homelessness, immigration, HIV infection and intravenous drug abuse. It is now as common in London as in the developing world, and is seen especially in immigrants, such as those from the Indian subcontinent, Africa and South Asia. This increase appears to be a result of the development of TB disease in individuals who may have been infected for some time and of new infections acquired in the UK, or as a result of travel to other countries where TB is common. London accounted for the highest proportion of cases in the UK in 2011 (39%), followed by the West Midlands region (11%); 74% of these were born outside the UK and mainly originated from South Asia and sub-Saharan Africa. In 2011, there was a rise in the number of TB cases compared to 2010, as well as an increase in drug resistance.

More information on TB, including statistics, can be found at: http://www.hpa.org.uk/Publications/InfectiousDiseases/Tuberculosis/ and http://www.tbfacts.org/tb-statistics.html (both accessed 30 September 2013).

Clinical features

Initial infection with TB is usually subclinical. About 10% of those infected develop overt disease; of these, half will manifest within 5 years (primary TB), while the remainder will develop post-primary disease. Inhaled mycobacteria may cause subpleural lesions (primary lesion) and lesions in the regional lymph nodes (primary complex). Body defences usually localize the mycobacteria, though these remain viable; infected persons are not obviously ill and are unlikely to know they are infected (latent; Table 15.16). Latent TB infection (LTBI) usually becomes active only after many years, if body defences become weakened (Box 15.3). However, active TB can develop shortly after mycobacteria enter the body, if body defences are impaired such as in ageing, drug or alcohol abuse, or HIV/AIDS. Also, in massive infections, acute active TB can result, typically causing a chronic productive cough, haemoptysis, weight loss, night sweats and fever. Erythema nodosum may be associated. Extrapulmonary TB is less common; it may appear as glandular involvement in the neck or elsewhere, and is less infectious than pulmonary TB. Lymph node TB may lead to lymphadenopathy, caseation of the nodes and pressure symptoms – for example, on the bronchi.

Post-primary TB follows reactivation of an old primary pulmonary lesion and results in features ranging from a chronic fibrotic lesion to fulminating tuberculous pneumonia. The pulmonary lesions may extend and lead to a pleural effusion. Reactivation or progression of primary TB may also result in widespread haematogenous dissemination of mycobacteria – 'miliary TB'. Multiple lesions may involve the central nervous system, bones, joints, and cardiovascular, gastrointestinal and genitourinary systems.

Clinical presentation in TB is thus variable, depending on the extent of spread and the organs involved. As it frequently passes unrecognized for so long, the mortality is high.

Similar illnesses to TB may also be caused by atypical (non-tuberculous) mycobacteria, such as *M. avium* complex (MAC; see below).

General management

The diagnosis of TB is suggested by the history and confirmed by physical examination, a massively raised erythrocyte sedimentation rate (ESR), positive tuberculin skin tests (TSTs; Mantoux or Heaf test for a delayed hypersensitivity reaction to protein from *M. tuberculosis* [purified protein derivative; PPD]) and chest imaging. Hypersensitivity develops with 2–8 weeks of infection and can be detected by conversion of the TST from negative to positive, but TSTs are neither 100% sensitive nor specific. A positive Mantoux reaction indicates previous immunization (BCG; bacille Calmette–Guérin – live attenuated *M. bovis*) or current infection – not necessarily disease. Chest radiography may show scarring and hilar lymphadenopathy. Computed tomography (CT) may show areas of calcification or highlight a tuberculous abscess. Smears and culture of sputum, blood, laryngeal swabs, bronchoalveolar lavage, gastric aspirates or pleural fluid may be tested for mycobacteria.

Polymerase chain reaction (PCR) techniques have greatly accelerated the diagnosis and speciation, though Ziehl–Neelsen, auramine or rhodamine microbial stains are still used. The mycobacteria growth indicator tube (MGIT) system gives results as early as 3–14 days. Blood assay for *M. tuberculosis* (BAMT) may be positive by interferon-gamma release assay (IGRA). Some 15% of people over 65 years have a positive IGRA. The IGRA can be used in place of (but not in addition to) TST. IGRAs measure the immune reactivity to *M. tuberculosis*. White blood cells from most persons that have been infected with *M. tuberculosis* will release interferon-gamma (IFN-γ) when mixed with *M. tuberculosis* antigens. A positive test result suggests that *M. tuberculosis* infection is likely; a negative result suggests that infection is unlikely.

Latent infection (LTBI) can be diagnosed with either a tuberculin skin test or an IGRA (more specific). IGRA gives a result within 24 hours and should be used biological therapy is given, such as for rheumatoid arthritis or inflammatory bowel disease. Prior BCG vaccination does not cause a false-positive IGRA test result. More information on the IGRA is available at: http://www.cdc.gov/tb/publications/factsheets/testing/igra.htm (accessed 30 September 2013).

Active TB is diagnosed by sputum microscopy and culture in liquid medium with subsequent drug-susceptibility testing. Nucleic acid

Table 15.17 *Antitubercular therapy*

Drug	Use	Main adverse effects
Ethambutol[a]	Initial therapy[b]	Ocular damage
Isoniazid	Initial therapy[b]	Peripheral neuropathy
	Continuation therapy[c]	Hepatotoxicity
Pyrazinamide	Initial therapy[b]	Hepatotoxicity
Rifampicin	Initial therapy[b]	Enhanced liver P450 drug-metabolizing enzymes
	Continuation therapy[c]	Red urine and saliva
		Bullous lesions
		Hepatotoxicity
		Nephrotoxicity
Streptomycin[a]	Initial therapy[b]	Vestibular nerve damage
		Circumoral paraesthesiae

[a]Increasing resistance.
[b]Initial therapy, usually = isoniazid + rifampicin + pyrazinamide or ethambutol for 2 months.
[c]Continuation therapy = isoniazid + rifampicin for 4 months.

amplification tests, imaging, and histopathological examination of biopsy samples help. IGRA and TSTs have no role in the diagnosis of active disease. A molecular diagnostic test now available in some high-income countries (Xpert MTB/RIF assay) detects *M. tuberculosis* complex within 2 hours, with a higher assay sensitivity than that of smear microscopy.

People who should be tested for TB include those who have symptoms, those who have had close day-to-day contact with active TB disease (family member, friend or co-worker), those who have HIV infection or AIDs, those with lowered immunity, those who are required to for employment or school, and those about to be treated with biological agents.

The top priority of TB control programmes is to identify and give complete treatment to all patients with active disease. TB is a notifiable disease and contact tracing is an important aspect of limiting spread. Treatment with antibiotics is indicated for people who are sick with TB, those infected but not sick, and those who are close contacts of infectious TB cases. Treatment for 'symptomatic sputum-positive' patients, which should be instituted as soon as possible, is combination chemotherapy, usually isoniazid plus rifampicin plus pyrazinamide or ethambutol for 2 months, with continuation of daily isoniazid and rifampicin for a further 4 months. Treatment for 'asymptomatic' patients who are believed to have been infected by contacts, but are not unwell, includes isoniazid for 6 months or isoniazid and rifampicin for 3 months. Rifapentine is a long-acting rifampicin used once weekly. Fluoroquinolones (moxifloxacin) may also act against TB. There may be resistance to one or more than one antibiotic.

Currently, given the potential risk of drug-resistant TB being present, treatment is usually started with isoniazid, rifampicin, pyrazinamide and ethambutol (or a quinolone such as gatifloxacin or moxifloxacin) for 2 months, then isoniazid and rifampicin for 4 months.

All antituberculous drugs (Table 15.17) have potentially serious adverse effects and require careful monitoring. If patient compliance is considered to be poor, directly observed therapy (DOT), where drugs are dispensed by and taken in the presence of a health-care professional, may be indicated. New drugs are on the horizon.

Immunization using BCG is advocated for schoolchildren, high-risk individuals and health-care professionals – although its efficacy has been questioned. New vaccines are in development.

Chemoprophylaxis with isoniazid and rifampicin is indicated in a number of situations (Box 15.4).

Box 15.4 *Indications for tuberculosis (TB) chemoprophylaxis*

- Previous inadequate treatment of TB
- Close contact with persons actively infected with TB
- Conversion of the tuberculin test within the past 2 years
- Biological therapy being considered
- A positive tuberculin test in the following groups:
  - Immunocompromised persons (diabetes, renal failure, cancer, HIV infection)
  - Persons under 35 years, or intravenous drug users
  - A foreign-born person who has migrated from a region of high prevalence within the previous 2 years

Drug-resistant TB (DR-TB)

TB can become resistant to the drugs used to treat it particularly when the drugs are misused or mismanaged. This may occur, for example, when:

- drugs are unavailable or of poor quality
- patients fail to complete the full treatment course
- health-care providers prescribe the wrong drugs, doses or length of treatment.

DR-TB is more common in people who:

- fail to take their TB drugs regularly or fail to take a complete course
- have recurrence of TB disease
- come from areas where DR-TB is common
- have spent time with someone who has DR-TB
- work in hospitals or health-care settings where DR-TB patients are seen.

More than 60% of DR-TB patients are in China, India, the Russian Federation, Pakistan and South Africa.

Multidrug-resistant TB (MDR-TB)

In some developing countries, approximately 10% of cases are multiple antibiotic-resistant; this is termed multidrug-resistant tuberculosis (MDR-TB); in the UK, only a small minority currently fall into this category but the number of cases is increasing. MDR-TB is defined as resistance to rifampicin and isoniazid; it may be atypical in presentation and the infection disseminates. More than 4% of people with TB worldwide have MDR-TB, and Eastern Europe has a high prevalence. MDR-TB is seen mainly in people with HIV/AIDS and in HIV/AIDS and in Africans. Bedaquiline, is a new anti-tubercular agent - the first active agent against tuberculosis to be registered since 1963.

Extensively drug-resistant TB (XDR-TB)

Extensively drug-resistant tuberculosis (XDR-TB) is a rare type of MDR-TB, not only resistant to isoniazid and rifampin, but also to any fluoroquinolone and at least one of three injectable second-line drugs (i.e. amikacin, kanamycin, or capreomycin). XDR-TB is of special concern for immunocompromised people (e.g. with HIV/AIDS), who are more likely to develop TB, and have a higher risk of death if they do develop it. XDR-TB is most often encountered in people from Eastern Europe, Russia and Africa. It has been transmitted in health-care facilities and is now seen worldwide. It is essentially untreatable, though capreomycin has been used effectively to treat MDR-TB in HIV-positive individuals.

Totally drug-resistant TB (TDR-TB or XXDR-TB)

Totally drug-resistant TB was reported initially in 2007–2009 in India, Iran and Italy; it is spreading, despite denials, and is most disquieting.

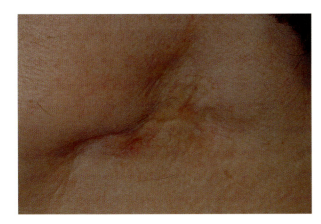

Fig. 15.7 Neck scarring from tuberculous lymphadenitis.

Table 15.18 *Dental management of patients with known or suspected tuberculosis (TB)*

History of TB	Potential infectivity	Comment
Active sputum-positive TB	High	Urgent dental treatment only; use special infection control precautions.
Recent history of TB and sputum known to be positive for TB	High	Defer elective dental care until TB treatment complete
Past history of TB	Refer to physician; needs confirmation	Use special infection control precautions for emergency dental care
No history of TB but signs or symptoms suggestive		Defer elective dental care until medical advice received
No history of TB but positive tuberculin test		

Dental aspects

Chronic ulcers, usually on the tongue dorsum, are the main oral manifestation of TB. They result from coughing of infected sputum from pulmonary TB, including in HIV-infected persons with TB, but are rare and such cases (usually middle-aged males) may result from neglect of symptoms or default from treatment. Occasionally, the diagnosis is made from biopsy of an ulcer after granulomas are seen microscopically. Acid-fast bacilli are rarely seen in oral biopsies, even with the help of special stains, so unfixed material should also be sent for culture if possible. Tuberculous cervical lymphadenopathy is the next most common form of the infection and is particularly common among those from South Asia. Most TB lymphadenitis is painless, with several enlarged, matted nodes, but systemic symptoms are present only in a minority and only about 15% have pulmonary manifestations on radiography (Fig. 15.7). Diagnosis relies on tuberculin testing, which can be positive in both tuberculous and non-tuberculous mycobacterial cervical lymphadenitis. Any person with lymphadenopathy and recent conversion from a negative to positive tuberculin test should be suspected of having mycobacterial infection, and this should prompt biopsy (e.g. fine-needle aspiration biopsy) for culture or histological confirmation. PCR will improve diagnosis, as culture must wait 4–8 weeks for a result. Oral complications of antitubercular therapy are rare, but rifabutin and rifampicin can cause red saliva.

Pulmonary TB is of high infectivity, as shown by cases of tuberculous infection of extraction sockets and cervical lymphadenitis in 15 patients treated by an infected member of staff at a dental clinic. Dental staff who themselves were HIV-positive, working in a dental clinic for HIV-infected persons in New York, have died from TB contracted occupationally. Transmission of MDR-TB between two dental workers may have occurred in an HIV dental clinic. Infection control is thus important, so staff with TB are usually precluded from their occupation until treated.

Management of a patient with TB depends upon the level of potential infectivity (Table 15.18). Patients with open pulmonary TB are contagious, and dental treatment is thus best deferred until the infection has been treated. Treatment with appropriate drugs for 2 weeks drastically reduces the infectivity of patients with pulmonary TB. If patients with open pulmonary TB must be given dental treatment, special precautions should be used to prevent the release of mycobacteria into the air, to remove any that are present and to stop their inhalation by other persons. Reduction of splatter and aerosols, by minimizing coughing and avoiding ultrasonic instruments, and use of a rubber dam, are important. Improved ventilation, ultraviolet germicidal light, new masks and personal respirators, and other personal protective devices,

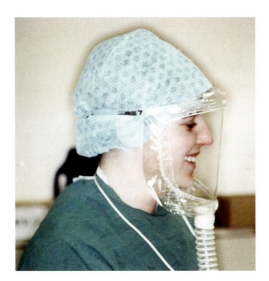

Fig. 15.8 Respirator.

such as HEPA filters, are indicated (Fig. 15.8). Mycobacteria are very resistant to disinfectants, so that heat sterilization must be used.

LA is safe and satisfactory. Relative analgesia is contraindicated because of the risk of contamination of the apparatus. GA is also contraindicated for dental treatment because of the risk of contamination of the anaesthetic apparatus and because of impaired pulmonary function. Aminoglycosides, such as streptomycin, enhance the activity of some neuromuscular blocking drugs and in large doses may alone cause a myasthenic syndrome. Possible drug interactions are shown in Table 15.19.

Other factors, such as alcoholism or intravenous drug use (Ch. 34), hepatitis (Ch. 9) or HIV disease (Ch. 20), may also influence dental management.

ATYPICAL MYCOBACTERIA (NON-TUBERCULOUS MYCOBACTERIA, NTM; MYCOBACTERIA OTHER THAN TUBERCULOSIS; MOTT)

General aspects

Mycobacteria other than tuberculosis (MOTT) are widely distributed in water, soil, animals and humans, and rarely cause disease. Severe MOTT infections have been seen, however, in individuals predisposed because of defects in the interleukin-12 (IL-12) and interferon-gamma (IFN-gamma) pathways.

Mycobacterium abscessus, a bacterium found in water, soil and dust, has been known to contaminate medications and products, including

Table 15.19 *Possible drug interactions in tuberculosis (TB)*

Drug	May cause interactions with
Paracetamol (acetaminophen)	Isoniazid
Azole antifungals	Rifampicin
Benzodiazepines	
Clarithromycin	
Diazepam	
Paracetamol (acetaminophen)	
Aspirin	Amikacin, capreomycin, kanamycin or streptomycin

Box 15.5 *Mycobacteria other than tuberculosis*

- *Mycobacterium abscessus*
- *M. avium*
- *M. chelonae*
- *M. fortuitum*
- *M. intracellulare* (*M. avium–intracellulare* complex; MAC)
- *M. kansasii*
- *M. marinum*
- *M. scrofulaceum*
- *M. ulcerans*
- *M. xenopi*

medical devices. Health-care-associated *M. abscessus* can cause a variety of infections, usually of the skin, but it can also cause lung infections in persons with various chronic lung diseases and is increasingly recognized as an opportunistic pathogen in *cystic fibrosis* (CF) patients.

Person-to-person transmission of atypical mycobacteria is *not* important in acquisition of infection, except for skin infections. On rare occasions, MOTT skin infections have followed tattooing with contaminated tattoo inks. Many people become infected with and harbour MOTT in their respiratory secretions without any symptoms or evidence of disease. Individuals with respiratory disease from MOTT do *not* readily infect others and, therefore, do not need to be isolated. MOTT are generally not infectious to others.

Infection with *M. abscessus* is usually caused by injections of contaminated substances or by invasive medical procedures employing contaminated equipment or material. Infection can also occur after accidental injury where the wound is contaminated by soil. There is very little risk of transmission from person to person.

Clinical features

Atypical mycobacteria include *M. avium, M. intracellulare* (MAC) species and others (Box 15.5). *Mycobacterium avium* complex (comprising *M. avium* and *M. intracellulare*; MAC) can cause several different syndromes:

- In children, MAC most commonly cause cervical lymphadenitis.
- In non-immunocompromised adults, pulmonary disease is a result of infection with MAC.
- In immunocompromised adults, disseminated MAC infections may arise. An immune defect, underlying illness or tissue damage may result in disseminated MAC infection.

MAC complex, *M. scrofulaceum* and *M. kansasii* are possible causes of tuberculous cervical lymphadenitis. MAC may also infect the lungs (similar to TB), skin or lymph nodes. Lung disease is also caused occasionally by *M. kansasii*, mainly in middle-aged and older persons

with underlying chronic lung conditions. *M. fortuitum* and *M. chelonae* may cause skin and wound infections and abscesses, frequently associated with trauma or surgery. *M. marinum* may cause 'swimming pool granuloma', a nodular lesion that may ulcerate, usually on an extremity. *M. ulcerans* may produce chronic ulcerative skin lesions, usually of an extremity. *M. abscessus* skin infections present with swollen and/or painful areas that are usually red, warm and tender to the touch, and which can also develop into boils or pustules. Other features of *M. abscessus* infection are fever, chills, muscle aches and malaise.

General management and dental aspects

Cervical lymphadenitis due to MAC, *M. scrofulaceum* and *M. kansasii* may affect otherwise healthy young children, most commonly preschool females who have unilateral cervical lymphadenopathy, typically in the submandibular or jugulodigastric nodes, and they may form a 'cold abscess'. MOTT is the usual cause in children under 12 years but TB is more common in older patients. Absence of fever or tuberculosis, a positive tuberculin test and failed response to conventional antimicrobials are highly suggestive of MOTT, but definitive diagnosis is by smear, culture or PCR of biopsy material obtained by fine-needle aspiration or removal of nodes.

Treatment is based on results of laboratory testing, which should identify the appropriate antibiotic. Preventive treatment of close contacts of persons with disease caused by MOTT is *not* needed. Most MOTT are resistant to standard antitubercular medication and, though it is possible that clarithromycin or clofazimine may have some effect, excision of affected nodes is the usual recommended therapy.

Water from dental units may contain MOTT species; mycobacterial proliferation in biofilms may explain the extent of this contamination (Ch. 31).

ASPIRATION SYNDROMES

Aspiration syndromes are conditions in which foreign substances are inhaled into the lungs and which can have consequences ranging from asphyxia to infection and lung abscess. Dental restorations or fragments of teeth, plaque, gastric contents and other materials may be aspirated, especially if material enters the pharynx, and particularly if the cough reflex is impaired for any reason.

Most commonly, aspiration syndromes involve oral or gastric contents associated with gastro-oesophageal reflux disease (GORD), swallowing dysfunction (Ch. 7), neurological disorders and structural abnormalities, such as a pharyngeal pouch. Cricopharyngeal dysfunction involves cricopharyngeal muscle spasm or achalasia of the superior oesophageal sphincter, and can be seen in infants who have a normal sucking reflex but have incoordination during swallowing, possibly secondary to delayed development or cerebral palsy. Anatomical disorders, such as cleft palate, pharyngeal pouch, oesophageal atresia, tracheo-oesophageal fistula, duodenal obstruction or malrotation, and motility disorders, such as achalasia, may have an aspiration risk. Infirm older patients are also at risk of aspiration, especially if they are bed-bound or have neurological disorders. Isolated superior laryngeal nerve damage, vocal cord paralysis, cerebral palsy, muscular dystrophy and Riley–Day syndrome (familial dysautonomia) are all associated with increased risk of aspiration.

VENTILATOR-ASSOCIATED PNEUMONIA (VAP)

Ventilator-associated pneumonia (VAP), as defined by the Centers for Disease Control and Prevention (CDC), is present when the chest radiograph shows new or progressive infiltrate, consolidation, cavitation or pleural effusion in conjunction with either new onset of purulent sputum or change in character of sputum, and an organism isolated from blood, or the isolation of an aetiological agent from a specimen obtained via suction aspiration through an endotracheal or tracheostomy tube.

The major route for acquiring endemic VAP is oropharyngeal colonization by endogenous flora or by exogenously acquired pathogens from intensive care units. VAP is the most commonly reported healthcare-acquired infection in patients receiving mechanical ventilation, with prevalence rates consistently in the 10–20% range. Mortality rates in VAP are at least double those in patients without VAP, ranging from 24% to 85% when the infection is caused by a multidrug-resistant Gram-negative pathogen.

The Healthcare Infection Control Practices Advisory Committee of the CDC has developed guidelines for the prevention of VAP. These include strategies aimed at preventing aspiration of contaminated oral or gastric material (e.g. raising the head of the bed and draining subglottic secretions), and interventions to alter bacterial colonization of stomach (e.g. stress ulcer prophylaxis and selective digestive decontamination) and mouth. Oral hygiene, suctioning and the provision of moisture to lips and oral mucosa, plus tooth-brushing, may be important in prevention of VAP. There are also strategies for managing ventilator circuits (e.g. replacement of ventilator circuits, use of closed rather than open suction, and use of heat moisture exchange as opposed to heated circuit technology).

LUNG ABSCESS

General aspects

Lung abscess is a localized infection leading to cavitation and necrosis. While some cases result from aspiration of foreign material, most develop from pneumonia caused by infection with *Staph. aureus* or *Klebsiella pneumoniae*. Bronchial obstruction by carcinoma is another important cause.

Clinical features

Symptoms resemble those of suppurative pneumonia. There is a risk of infection spreading locally or leading, via septicaemia, to a brain abscess.

General management

Diagnosis rests mainly on the chest radiograph, which may sometimes show cavitation or a fluid level. Antimicrobial chemotherapy, postural drainage and relief by bronchoscopy of any obstruction are indicated.

Dental aspects

A well-recognized cause of lung abscess is inhalation of a tooth or fragment, a restoration or rarely, an endodontic instrument. When undertaking endodontics or cementing restorations, such as inlays or crowns, a rubber dam or other protective device should always be used to avoid the danger of inhalation.

Lung abscesses may also result from aspiration of oral bacteria, particularly anaerobes, especially in infirm older patients or those who are intubated.

The other main dangers in dentistry are with GA, particularly if an inadequate throat pack has been used. Patients who inhale tooth fragments or dental instruments must have chest radiographs (lateral and postero-anterior) and, if necessary, bronchoscopy.

Table 15.20 *Sarcoidosis: possible clinical findings*

Type	Finding
Dermatological	Erythema nodosum, infiltrates around eyes and nose (lupus pernio)
Hepatic	Asymptomatic hepatomegaly, sarcoid liver disease
Lymph nodes	Lymphadenopathy (rarely lymphoma)
Musculoskeletal	Arthralgia, effusions, cyst-like radiolucent areas
Neurological	Cranial or peripheral neuropathies
Oral/para-oral	Salivary gland or gingival swelling
Ocular	Acute uveitis, cataracts, glaucoma
Pulmonary	Hilar lymphadenopathy; widespread infiltration
Renal	Nephrocalcinosis, renal calculi
Spleen	Splenomegaly
Systemic symptoms	Fever, weight loss, fatigue

LOEFFLER SYNDROME

Loeffler syndrome appears to be an allergic reaction, usually to the parasitic worm *Ascaris lumbricoides*, or drugs such as sulphonamides. It manifests with pulmonary infiltrates (and abnormal chest radiograph) and eosinophilia (eosinophilic pneumonia). The disease usually clears spontaneously.

SARCOIDOSIS

General aspects

Sarcoidosis, so named because skin lesions resembled a sarcoma, is a multisystem granulomatous disorder, seen most commonly in young adult females in northern Europe, especially in people of African heritage. The aetiology is unclear but *Propionibacterium acnes* and *P. granulosum* have been implicated and associations have been reported with exposure to inorganic particles, insecticides, moulds and occupations such as firefighting and metal-working. Serum samples contain antibodies directed against *Mycobacterium tuberculosis* antigens. Sarcoidosis is associated with HLA-DRB1 and DQB1, and a butyrophilin-like 2 (*BTNL2*) gene on chromosome 6. T-helper 1 (Th1) cells release IL-2 and IFN-γ, and augment macrophage tumour necrosis factor alpha (TNF-α) release. CD25 regulatory T cells cause a limited impairment of cell-mediated immune responses (partial anergy) but no obvious special susceptibility to infection.

Clinical features

Sarcoidosis affects the thorax in 90%, but has protean manifestations and can involve virtually any tissue (Table 15.20). Sarcoid most typically causes Löfgren syndrome (fever, bilateral hilar lymphadenopathy, arthralgia and erythema nodosum, especially around the ankles; Figs 15.9 and 15.10).

Other common presentations may include pulmonary infiltration and impaired respiratory efficiency, with cough and dyspnoea in severe cases, or acute uveitis, which can progress to blindness. Susceptibility to lymphomas has been suggested but not confirmed.

General management

Because of its vague and protean manifestations, sarcoidosis is underdiagnosed. In the presence of suggestive clinical features, helpful

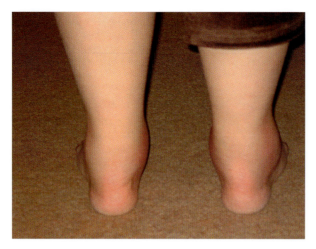

Fig. 15.9 Sarcoid causing ankle swelling in Löfgren syndrome.

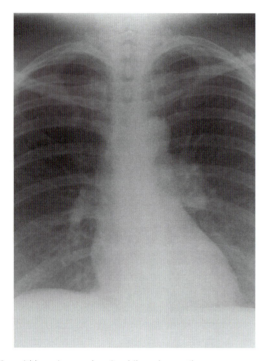

Fig. 15.10 Sarcoid lung image showing hilar adenopathy.

Table 15.21 *Sarcoidosis: laboratory findings*

Type	Finding
Histological	Non-caseating tubercle-like granulomas
Immunological	Anergy (partial)
	Negative response to tuberculin and some other common antigens on skin testing
	Lymphopenia; low numbers of T cells
	Raised serum levels of immunoglobulins
Biochemical	Hypercalcaemia
	Raised serum levels of lysozyme, serum angiotensin-converting enzyme (SACE) and adenosine deaminase

Half the patients with sarcoidosis remit within 3 years and about 66% remit by 10 years. Patients with only minor symptoms usually need no treatment but corticosteroids, sometimes with azathioprine, methotrexate, tetracyclines, hydroxychloroquine, infliximab or etanercept, are given if there is active organ disease (ocular disease, progressive lung disease, hypercalcaemia or cerebral involvement).

Dental aspects

Biopsy of the minor salivary glands frequently shows non-caseating granulomas and association with other features of sarcoidosis, particularly hilar lymphadenopathy. This is an important diagnostic finding that may obviate more invasive procedures. Sarcoidosis can involve any of the oral tissues but has a predilection for salivary glands. Asymptomatic swelling of the parotid glands or cervical nodes, and less frequently the lips, may accompany systemic disease. Superficial or deep-seated red submucosal nodules may develop intraorally and on the lips. Non-tender, well-circumscribed, brownish-red or violaceous nodules with superficial ulceration have also been reported. The oral and lip lesions may occasionally precede systemic involvement.

There is enlargement of the major salivary glands in about 6% of cases; some have xerostomia, and the association of salivary and lacrimal gland enlargement with fever and uveitis is known as uveoparotid fever (Heerfordt syndrome). Salivary swelling may also be seen without other features of Heerfordt syndrome. The salivary gland swellings usually resolve on treatment of sarcoidosis but this may take up to 3 years.

Facial palsy and other cranial neuropathies may be seen. There is also an association with Sjögren syndrome, when SS-A and SS-B serum autoantibodies are found. Rarely there is an association of thyroiditis with Addison disease, Sjögren syndrome and sarcoidosis (TASS syndrome). There is a group of patients who have histological features of sarcoid in one or more sites in the mouth, such as the gingivae, but no systemic manifestations. A few of these patients may ultimately develop other more or less systematized disease but the majority probably have isolated lesions. Such cases, where no exogenous cause for the granulomatous reaction can be found, are regarded as having 'sarcoid-like' reactions (orofacial granulomatosis) and treatment is unnecessary. However, patients should be kept under observation for as long as possible.

Management of patients with systemic sarcoidosis may include consideration of respiratory impairment, uveitis and visual impairment, renal disease, jaundice or corticosteroid treatment.

LA is safe and satisfactory. CS is contraindicated if there is any respiratory impairment. GA should only be given in hospital.

investigations include: chest radiography (enlarged hilar lymph nodes); raised serum angiotensin-converting enzyme (SACE; Table 15.21) in acute disease (this is insensitive, non-specific and a poor guide to therapy); positive gallium-67 citrate or gadolinium or positron emission tomography (PET) scans; labial salivary gland or transbronchial biopsy (for histological evidence of non-caseating epithelioid cell granulomas) – except in Löfgren syndrome, which is a classical clinical diagnosis. ^{18}F-deoxyglucose PET is helpful in identifying sites for biopsy.

Non-specific findings may include mild anaemia, leukopenia, eosinophilia, hypergammaglobulinaemia, raised ESR and low serum albumin. Hypercalcaemia is common because of extrarenal production of active vitamin D and can result in renal damage. Alkaline phosphatase, 5'-nucleotidase, lysozyme and adenosine deaminase levels are raised in hepatic sarcoidosis. Evidence of impaired delayed hypersensitivity reactions to some antigens may be useful. Kveim skin tests are not now used.

LUNG CANCER

General aspects

Lung cancer is the most common cancer in high-income countries in males and most frequently affects adult urban cigarette-smokers. Bronchogenic carcinoma accounts for 95% of all primary lung cancer and has also become increasingly common in women (because of increased tobacco use), to the extent that the mortality rate for the two sexes has become almost equal. Metastases from cancers elsewhere are also frequently found in the lungs.

Clinical features

Recurrent cough, haemoptysis, dyspnoea, chest pain and recurrent chest infections are the predominant features. Local infiltration may cause pleural effusion, lesions of the cervical sympathetic chain (Horner syndrome), brachial neuritis, recurrent laryngeal nerve palsy or obstruction of the superior vena cava with facial cyanosis and oedema (superior vena cava syndrome).

There are many non-metastatic extrapulmonary effects of bronchogenic (or other) carcinomas – for example, weight loss, anorexia, finger-clubbing, neuromyopathies, thromboses (thrombophlebitis migrans), muscle weakness, various skin manifestations and ectopic hormone production (of antidiuretic hormone, adrenocorticotropic hormone, parathyroid hormone and thyroid-stimulating hormone).

Metastases from bronchogenic cancer are common and typically form in the brain (which may manifest with headache, epilepsy, hemiplegia or visual disturbances), liver (hepatomegaly, jaundice or ascites) or bone (pain, swelling or pathological fracture).

General management

The diagnosis is based on history and physical examination, supported by radiography, CT and magnetic resonance imaging (MRI), sputum cytology, bronchoscopy and biopsy. Spiral CT appears to detect tumours at an early stage.

The overall 5-year survival rate is only 8%. Radiotherapy is the most common treatment. Only some 25% of patients are suitable for surgery but, even then, the 5-year survival is only about 25%. Chemotherapy has been disappointing, except in small-cell carcinomas.

Dental aspects

Dental treatment under LA should be uncomplicated. CS should preferably be avoided. GA is a matter for specialist management in hospital, as patients often have impaired respiratory function, especially after lobectomy or pneumonectomy. This, along with any muscle weakness (myasthenic syndrome, Eaton–Lambert syndrome) that can make the patient unduly sensitive to the action of muscle relaxants, makes GA hazardous.

Oral cancer may be associated with lung cancer, and *vice versa*, or develop at a later stage (Ch. 22). Such synchronous or metachronous primary tumours must always be ruled out.

Metastases can occasionally affect the orofacial region and cause enlargement of the lower cervical lymph nodes, epulis-like soft-tissue swellings or labial hypoaesthesia or paraesthesia in the jaw. Soft palate pigmentation is a rare early oral manifestation.

Lung cancer is a fairly common cause of death in dental technicians, but it is unknown whether this is due to smoking alone or to dust inhalation.

CYSTIC FIBROSIS (CF; FIBROCYSTIC DISEASE; MUCOVISCIDOSIS)

General aspects

Cystic fibrosis (CF) is one of the most common fatal hereditary disorders. Inherited as an autosomal recessive trait, with an incidence of about 1 in 2000 births, it is the most common inherited error of metabolism and is seen mainly in people of European descent. The gene responsible is on chromosome 7q. CF is caused by defects in the cystic fibrosis transmembrane conductance regulator (CFTR), a protein that appears to be part of a cyclic adenosine monophosphate (cAMP)-regulated chloride channel, regulating Cl^- and Na^+ transport across epithelial membranes, and ion channels and intracellular fluid flow in sweat, digestive and mucus glands.

The basic defect in CF is abnormal chloride ion transport across the cell membrane of nearly all exocrine glands. The blockage of salt and water movement into and out of cells results in the cells that line the lungs, pancreas and other organs producing abnormally thick, sticky mucus that can obstruct the airways and various glands, especially in the respiratory tract and pancreas. Involved glands (lungs, pancreas, intestinal glands, intrahepatic bile ducts, gallbladder, submaxillary and sweat glands) may become obstructed by this viscid or solid eosinophilic material.

Clinical features

Recurrent respiratory infections result in a persistent productive cough and bronchiectasis, with the lungs becoming infected with a variety of organisms including *Staph. aureus*, *Haemophilus influenzae*, *Pseudomonas aeruginosa*, *Strep. pneumoniae*, *Burkholderia cepacia*, and sometimes mycoses or mycobacteria. *Mycobacterium abscessus* is a non-tuberculous mycobacterium increasingly recognized as an opportunistic pathogen in CF patients. Viral infections, such as measles, can have severe sequelae.

Pancreatic duct obstruction leads to pancreatic insufficiency, with malabsorption and bulky, frequent, foul-smelling, fatty stools. Gallstones, diabetes, cirrhosis and pancreatitis may result. Sinusitis is very common.

Growth is frequently stunted. The mutations can also cause congenital bilateral absence of the vas deferens, so fertility is impaired in most males with CF. In women, fertility may be impaired by viscid cervical secretions, but many women have carried pregnancies to term.

General management

Most patients have a high concentration of sodium in their sweat (also reflected in the saliva); a sweat test showing sodium and chloride values of more than 60 mmol/L is considered positive, between 40 and 60 mmol/L equivocal, and less than 40 mmol/L negative.

Physiotherapy and postural drainage are crucially important. Clearance of sputum is helped by water aerosols and bronchodilators (terbutaline or salbutamol), but mucolytics such as carbocisteine, methyl cysteine and dornase alfa are of questionable effectiveness. Treatment with ivacaftor, a CFTR potentiator, improves chloride transport through the ion channel.

Amoxicillin and flucloxacillin are effective prophylactic antimicrobials and may be given by aerosol. Vaccination against measles, whooping cough and influenza is important. A low fat intake, adequate vitamins and oral pancreatic enzyme replacement (pancreatin) are also necessary.

Double-lung or heart–lung transplantation may eventually become necessary.

Dental aspects

Sinusitis is very common; most CF patients have recurrent sinusitis and nasal polyps. The major salivary glands may enlarge and hyposalivation sometimes occurs. The low-fat, high-carbohydrate diet and dry mouth may predispose to caries. Enamel hypoplasia and black stain may be seen, and both dental development and eruption are delayed. Tetracycline staining of the teeth was common but should rarely be seen now. Pancreatin may cause oral ulceration if held in the mouth.

LA is satisfactory but CS is usually contraindicated because of poor respiratory function. GA is contraindicated if respiratory function is poor. Lung disease, such as bronchiectasis, liver disease and diabetes, may complicate treatment.

BRONCHIECTASIS

General aspects

Bronchiectasis is dilatation and distortion of the bronchi. Causes include:

- Congenital defects, which should be considered in all patients include cystic fibrosis, Kartagener syndrome, alpha-1-antitrypsin deficiency, collagen defects (e.g. Marfan syndrome)
- Immunodeficiencies
- Postinfection
- Gastric aspiration
- Bronchial obstruction
- Autoimmune diseases, e.g. Sjögren's syndrome
- Asthma
- Inflammatory bowel disease

There is no identifiable underlying cause in about 50% of adults and 25% of children.

The damaged and dilated bronchi lose their ciliated epithelium and therefore mucus tends to pool, causing recurrent LRTIs, typically with *Strep. pneumoniae*, *Haemophilus influenzae* or *Pseudomonas aeruginosa*.

Clinical features

Overproduction of sputum, which is purulent during exacerbations, a cough (especially during exercise or when lying down) and finger-clubbing are typical features, with recurrent episodes of bronchitis, pneumonia and pleurisy. Haemoptysis is not uncommon. In advanced bronchiectasis, chest pain, dyspnoea, cyanosis and respiratory failure may develop. Complications may include cerebral abscess and amyloid disease.

General management

Chest radiography and pulmonary function tests are required. High-resolution CT (HRCT) is useful. Postural drainage is important. Antimicrobials, such as amoxicillin, cephalosporins or ciprofloxacin, are given for acute exacerbations and for long-term maintenance treatment.

Dental aspects

GA should be avoided where possible and is contraindicated in acute phases.

OCCUPATIONAL LUNG DISEASE (PNEUMOCONIOSES)

General aspects

Workers exposed to airborne particles may develop pulmonary disease (pneumoconiosis), which ranges from benign (e.g. siderosis) to malignant, as in mesothelioma from asbestosis (see Appendix 15.1), but any pneumoconiosis can cause significant incapacity.

Dental aspects

GA may be contraindicated; the physician should be contacted before treatment.

Berylliosis may be a hazard in some dental technical laboratories, when lung cancer is more frequent.

POSTOPERATIVE RESPIRATORY COMPLICATIONS

Respiratory complications following surgical operations under GA include segmental or lobar pulmonary collapse and infection. They are more common after abdominal surgery or if there is pre-existent respiratory disease or smoking (see also Ch. 3), and can be significantly reduced by smoking cessation, preoperative physiotherapy and bronchodilators, such as salbutamol.

If postoperative pulmonary infection develops, sputum should be sent for culture, and physiotherapy and antibiotics should be given. The common microbial causes are *Strep. pneumoniae* and *Haemophilus influenza*; in this case, suitable antibiotics include amoxicillin and erythromycin. Hospital infections may include other microorganisms, such as MRSA, *Klebsiella*, *Pseudomonas* and other Gram-negative bacteria.

Inhalation (aspiration) of gastric contents can cause pulmonary oedema and may be fatal (Mendelson syndrome); it is most likely if a GA is given to a patient who has a stomach that is not empty, has a hiatus hernia or is in the last trimester of pregnancy. Prevention is by ensuring the stomach is empty preoperatively; if it is not, an anaesthetist should pass an endotracheal tube. Antacids or an H2-receptor blocker, such as cimetidine or ranitidine, may be given by mouth preoperatively to lower gastric acidity.

If gastric contents are aspirated, the pharynx and larynx must be carefully sucked out. Systemic corticosteroids have been recommended but probably do not reduce the mortality.

RESPIRATORY DISTRESS SYNDROMES

Respiratory distress in premature infants may be caused by immaturity of surfactant-producing cells, when the alveoli fail to expand fully; this necessitates endotracheal intubation for many weeks. It may, in turn, result in midface hypoplasia, palatal grooving or clefting, or defects in the primary dentition. The same oral effects may be seen with prolonged use of orogastric feeding tubes. The degree to which subsequent growth corrects these deformations is currently unknown, though the palatal grooves typically regress by the age of 2 years. Using soft endotracheal tubes does not obviate this problem and, at present, the best means of avoiding palatal grooving appears to be the use of an intraoral acrylic plate to stabilize the tube and protect the palate.

Acute respiratory distress syndrome (ARDS) is a sequel to several types of pulmonary injury and some infections, including those with oral viridans streptococci.

LUNG TRANSPLANTATION

General aspects

Patients with end-stage pulmonary disease are considered for potential transplantation, usually using a lung from a brain-dead organ donor. A combination of ciclosporin, azathioprine and glucocorticoids is usually given for lifelong immunosuppression to prevent a T-cell, alloimmune rejection response.

Inhaled nitric oxide modulates pulmonary vascular tone via smooth muscle relaxation and can improve ventilation/perfusion matching and oxygenation in diseased lungs. Early graft failure following lung transplantation has been described by various investigators as reimplantation oedema, reperfusion oedema, primary graft failure or allograft dysfunction. Pathologically, this entity is diffuse alveolar damage.

Dental aspects

See also Chapter 35.

A meticulous pre-surgery oral assessment is required and dental treatment must be undertaken with particular attention to establishing optimal oral hygiene and eradicating sources of potential infection. Dental treatment should be completed before surgery. For 6 months after surgery, elective dental care is best deferred. If surgical treatment is needed during that period, antibiotic prophylaxis is probably warranted.

HEART AND LUNG TRANSPLANTATION

General aspects

Cardiopulmonary transplantation (heart and lung transplantation) is the simultaneous surgical replacement of the heart and lungs in patients with end-stage cardiac and pulmonary disease, with organs from a cadaveric donor.

General management

All transplant recipients require lifelong immunosuppression to prevent a T-cell, alloimmune rejection response.

Dental aspects

See also Chapter 35.

A meticulous pre-surgery oral assessment is required and dental treatment must be undertaken with particular attention to establishing optimal oral hygiene and eradicating sources of potential infection. Dental treatment should be completed before surgery. For 6 months after surgery, elective dental care is best deferred. If surgical treatment is needed during that period, antibiotic prophylaxis is probably warranted.

KEY WEBSITES

(Accessed 27 May 2013)
BMJ. <http://www.bmj.com/specialties/respiratory-medicine>

Centers for Disease Control and Prevention. <http://www.cdc.gov/ncird/overview/websites.html>
National Institutes of Health. <http://health.nih.gov/topic/RespiratoryDiseasesGeneral>

USEFUL WEBSITES

(Accessed 27 May 2013)
American Academy of Allergy, Asthma & Immunology. <http://www.aaaai.org/home.aspx>.
ERS e-Learning Resources. <http://www.ers-education.org/pages/default.aspx>.
Medic8.com. <http://www.medic8.com/lung-disorders>.
National Institutes of Health: National Institute of Allergy and Infectious Diseases. <http://www.niaid.nih.gov/topics/Pages/default.aspx>.

FURTHER READING

Bettega, G., et al. 2000. Obstructive sleep apnea syndrome. Am. J. Respir. Crit. Care Med. 162, 641.

Bloch, K.E., et al. 2000. A randomised, controlled crossover trial of two oral appliances for sleep apnea treatment. Am. J. Respir. Crit. Care Med. 162, 246.

Centers for Disease Control and Prevention, 2004. Healthcare Infection Control Practices Advisory Committee Guideline for the prevention of healthcare-associated pneumonia. Centers for Disease Control and Prevention, Atlanta.

Fields, L.B., 2008. Oral care intervention to reduce incidence of ventilator-associated pneumonia in the neurologic intensive care unit. J. Neurosci. Nurs. 40 (5), 291. PubMed PMID: 18856250

Flanders, S.A., et al. 2006. Nosocomial pneumonia: state of the science. Am. J. Infect. Control 34, 84.

Gandhi, N.R., et al. 2006. Extensively drug-resistant tuberculosis as a cause of death in patients co-infected with tuberculosis and HIV in a rural area of South Africa. Lancet 368, 1575.

Garcia, R., 2005. A review of the possible role of oral and dental colonization on the occurrence of health care-associated pneumonia: underappreciated risk and a call for interventions. Am. J. Infect. Control 33, 527.

Garcia, R., et al. 2009. Reducing ventilator-associated pneumonia through advanced oral-dental care: a 48-month study. Am. J. Crit. Care 18 (6), 523. Epub 2009 Jul 27. PubMed PMID: 19635805.

Garner, J.S., et al. 1996. CDC definitions for nosocomial infections. In: Olmsted, RN (Ed.), APIC infection control and applied epidemiology: principles and practice. Mosby, St Louis p. A-1.

Hutchins, K., et al. 2009 Sepp. Ventilator-associated pneumonia and oral care: a successful quality improvement project. Am. J. Infect. Control 37 (7), 590. PubMed PMID: 19716460.

Iannuzi, M.C., et al. 2007. Sarcoidosis. N. Engl. J. Med. 357, 2153.

Jensen, P.A., et al. 2005. Guidelines for preventing the transmission of *Mycobacterium tuberculosis* in health-care settings. MMWR 54 RR-17

Maartens, G., Wilkinson, R.J., 2007. Tuberculosis. Lancet 370, 2030.

Pobo, A., et al. 2009. A randomized trial of dental brushing for preventing ventilator-associated pneumonia. Chest 136 (2), 433. Epub 2009 May 29. PubMed PMID: 19482956.

Ricci, M.L., et al. 2012. Pneumonia associated with a dental unit waterline. Lancet 379 (9816), 684.

Rinaggio, J., 2003. Tuberculosis. Dent. Clin. N. Am. 47, 449.

Safdar, N., et al. 2005. The pathogenesis of ventilator-associated pneumonia: its relevance to developing effective strategies for prevention. Respir. Care 50, 725.

Scully, C., 2009. Aspects of human disease 32. Lung cancer. Dent. Update 36, 253.

Scully, C., Chaudhry, S., 2007. Aspects of human disease 8. Asthma. Dent. Update 34, 61.

Scully, C., Chaudhry, S., 2007. Aspects of human disease 9. Chronic obstructive pulmonary disease (COPD). Dent. Update 34, 125.

Scully, C., Chaudhry, S., 2009. Aspects of human disease 31. Tuberculosis. Dent. Update 36, 189.

Senol, G., et al. 2007. In vitro antibacterial activities of oral care products against ventilator-associated pneumonia pathogens. Am. J. Infect. Control 35, 531.

Sona, C.S., et al. 2009. The impact of a simple, low-cost oral care protocol on ventilator-associated pneumonia rates in a surgical intensive care unit. J. Intensive Care Med. 24 (1), 54. PubMed PMID: 19017665.

Tsai, H.H., et al. 2008. Intermittent suction of oral secretions before each positional change may reduce ventilator-associated pneumonia: a pilot study. Am. J. Med. Sci. 336 (5), 397. PubMed PMID: 19011396.

Zumla, A., 2013. Current trends and newer concepts on diagnosis, management and prevention of respiratory tract infections. Curr. Opin. Pulm. Med. [Epub ahead of print] PubMed PMID: 23425919.

Zumla, A., et al. 2013. Tuberculosis. N. Engl. J. Med. 368 (8), 745. doi: 10.1056/NEJMra1200894. Review. PubMed PMID: 23425167.

APPENDIX 15.1 OCCUPATIONAL LUNG DISEASES

Disorder	Source of causal agent	Group at risk	Clinical significance of pneumoconiosis
Anthracosis	Soot, carbon smoke	Urban dwellers	Benign
Asbestosis	Asbestos, insulation, fertilizers, explosives	Asbestos workers	Pulmonary fibrosis (crocidolite) predisposes to cor pulmonale) or amosite (bronchial carcinoma, mesothelioma)
Bagassosis	Mouldy sugar cane	Farmers	Acute pneumonia or fibre bronchiolitis
Barilosis	Barium	Barium miners	Benign
Berylliosis	Beryllium	Those using fluorescent lamps, various alloys	Chronic respiratory disease leading to cor pulmonale
Byssinosis	Cotton, flax or hemp	Cotton workers	Periodic bronchospasm leading to obstructive airways disease
Coal miner's lung	Coal dust	Coal miners	Largely asymptomatic but may cause fibrosis and emphysema
Kaolin	China clay	China-clay workers	Resembles silicosis (see below)
Siderosis	Iron dust	Welders, grinders	Benign
Silicosis	Silica (quartz) dust	Miners, sandblasters, potters	Pulmonary fibrosis leading to cor pulmonale, tuberculosis
Stannosis	Tin dust	Tin refiners	Benign

BONE

Bone morphogenetic proteins (BMPs) affect bone formation and are available as recombinant proteins, sometimes used in repair of periodontal defects, other bone defects and in implantology. Bone organic matrix consists largely of collagen produced by osteoblasts rich in alkaline phosphatase. Osteoblasts secrete osteoid, which mineralizes by deposition of calcium phosphate, largely as hydroxyapatite, together with smaller amounts of amorphous calcium phosphate, magnesium, sodium and other ions. Mineralization depends on the extracellular fluid calcium and phosphate levels.

Bone is a dynamic tissue, constantly remodelling, with deposition mediated by osteoblasts, and resorption mediated mainly by osteoclasts (also by prostaglandins and some cytokines). When osteoblastic activity rises, the serum level of alkaline phosphatase rises. When bone is resorbed, calcium and phosphate are removed and released into the extracellular fluid and serum. Osteoclasts are rich in acid phosphatase (particularly tartrate-resistant acid phosphatase), which may also be released into the serum when there is widespread osteolysis. Bone formation, metabolism and blood calcium levels are affected mainly by parathyroid hormone, vitamin D and calcitonin. Parathyroid hormone (PTH; parathormone) is regulated by blood calcium, vitamin D levels and phosphate levels. When PTH is secreted, intestinal transport of calcium and phosphate is promoted, and removal of calcium from bones accelerated.

Dietary vitamin D is fat-soluble and absorbed from the upper small intestine, promoting intestinal absorption of calcium and phosphate. Vitamin D is also synthesized in the skin from 7-dehydrocholesterol under the influence of sunlight, and converted by liver and then kidney to the most active metabolite, 1,25-dihydroxycholecalciferol (DHCC: calcitriol – the hormonal form of vitamin D), a process enhanced by PTH and low phosphate levels. The active metabolite (active vitamin D or DHCC) is a hormone that controls bone metabolism and enhances calcium absorption (Fig. 16.1). DHCC also, incidentally, affects the proliferation of various cells other than bone and enhances immunity. Vitamin D exerts its influence on many physiological processes, including the immune system; both the adaptive and innate immune systems are impacted by the active metabolite of vitamin D, 1,25(OH)(2)D, and individuals with vitamin D deficiency are prone to infectious diseases such as tuberculosis, as well as to autoimmune diseases such as type 1 diabetes mellitus, and to multiple sclerosis. Calcitonin opposes the action of PTH and lowers the blood calcium level, mainly by promoting deposition of calcium in the bones.

Bone growth varies throughout life; it is rapid in the fetus and infant, but slows somewhat during childhood until an adolescent growth

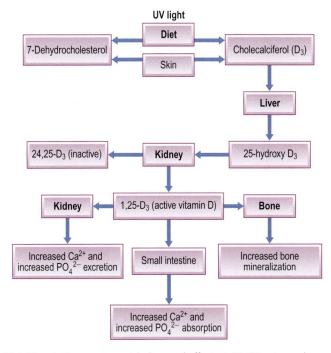

Fig. 16.1 Vitamin D: sources, metabolism and effects. 1,25-D3 acts as a hormone.

spurt. Several other hormones affect bone formation and metabolism to varying degrees, especially during the first two decades of life, including growth hormone, oestrogens in females and testosterone in males. Adult levels of bone mass are achieved by age 18 or so.

Lifestyle, especially physical activity and adequate nutrition, promotes the formation of bone, whereas smoking may impair it. Osteoblasts are also less efficient at laying down bone than are osteoclasts at removing it and, although the difference is slight, there is a gradual loss of bone mineral density (BMD) as a person ages (osteopenia). Anything that accelerates the rate of bone remodelling ultimately leads to a more rapid loss of bone mass and thus more fragile bones (osteoporosis).

BONE DISEASES

Acquired disorders of the skeleton are common. Genetic disorders are rare; the more important examples are discussed here and main features of others summarized in Appendix 16.1.

GENETIC DISORDERS

Osteogenesis imperfecta (fragilitas ossium; brittle bone syndrome)

General aspects

Osteogenesis imperfect (OI) is a rare, usually autosomal dominant, condition characterized by brittle bones that are susceptible to fracture. The underlying defect appears to be in type I collagen formation and, although osteoblasts are active, the amount of bone formed is small and mostly woven in type. This disorder, with a frequency of 1 in 12 000 births, has several variants (Table 16.1). The gene for dentinogenesis imperfecta, one of the more common heritable defects of the teeth, is closely related – and some patients (OI types I and IV) have both conditions.

Clinical features

The long bones are normal in length, with epiphyses of normal width but slender shafts, giving a trumpet-shaped appearance. The bones are fragile and multiple fractures can follow minimal trauma; healing is rapid but usually with distortion, so the ultimate effect in severe cases is gross deformity and dwarfism. The frequency of fractures usually tends to diminish after puberty.

The parietal regions of the skull may bulge outwards, causing eversion of the upper part of the ear. Other features are blue sclerae, deafness, easy bruising, and weakness of tendons and ligaments, causing loose-jointedness and often hernias. Cardiac complications, such as mitral valve prolapse or aortic incompetence, may be present.

Dental aspects

It is important not to confuse children with OI with those who have been subjected to physical abuse (Ch. 24). The management problems relate to bone fragility and careful handling of the patient. Despite the brittleness of most of the skeleton, however, the jaws rarely fracture and therefore dental extractions can usually be carried out safely; care should obviously be taken to use minimal force, to support the jaws and to ensure haemostasis if there is any bleeding tendency (Ch. 8). GA is a risk if there are chest deformities or cardiac complications.

When dentinogenesis imperfecta is associated, the teeth may have the characteristic abnormal translucency, brown or purplish colour and tendency to wear readily. The enamel may adhere poorly to the dentine and be progressively shed under the stress of mastication. By adolescence, the teeth may be worn down to the gingival margins but obliteration of the pulp chamber by dentine usually prevents pulp

exposure. The soft dentine makes the fitting of post crowns impractical so that steel crowns on primary molars and crowns in the permanent dentition, or even extraction and replacement by dentures, may be needed in severe cases. Bisphosphonate treatment may have implications (see Osteonecrosis of the jaw)

Dentinogenesis imperfecta can appear as an isolated abnormality without OI.

Achondroplasia

The achondrodysplasias are heritable disorders of skeletal growth, presenting typically with dwarfism, high forehead, cleft palate and various ocular anomalies.

General and clinical aspects

There are defects in cartilaginous bone formation, often inherited as an autosomal dominant trait. The phenotypic appearance is of dwarfism with a head of normal size but appearing large, and short limbs, which has traditionally led to many achondroplastics becoming circus clowns. Nasal septal and base of skull growth is impaired so that the bridge is depressed and skull bossed. Lumbar lordosis can be severe and occasionally causes spinal cord compression. Many patients with achondroplasia are otherwise completely healthy but diabetes is occasionally associated.

Dental aspects

The only significant dental aspects are orthodontic in nature as a result of malocclusion, but short stature, diabetes and kyphosis may affect management. Surgery is usually required for the cleft palate and other deformities.

Cleidocranial dysplasia (cleidocranial dysostosis)

General aspects

Cleidocranial dysplasia is a rare defect, mainly of membrane bone formation, involving especially the skull and clavicle. It is an autosomal dominant trait related to chromosome 6 and a defect in the signal transduction SH3-binding protein. There are also sporadic cases.

Clinical features

The clavicles are either absent or defective, thus conferring the unusual and pathognomonic ability to approximate the shoulders anteriorly (Fig. 16.2). The head is large but brachycephalic, with persistent fontanelles, a persistent metopic (frontal) suture, numerous Wormian bones and bulging frontal, parietal and occipital bones. The middle facial third is hypoplastic, leading to a depressed nasal bridge and relative mandibular protrusion. The mandibular symphysis may close late. Cranial base abnormalities and clefts of the hard and soft palate have been recorded. Other skeletal defects may be associated, such as kyphoscoliosis or pelvic anomalies.

Dental aspects

Apart from the facial anomalies, there may be excess teeth (hyperdontia, supernumeraries; Fig. 16.3) with persistence of the deciduous dentition, multiple unerupted permanent teeth, twisted roots, malformed crowns and dentigerous cysts.

Table 16.1 Osteogenesis imperfecta: subtypes

Type	Inheritance	Bone disease	Stature	Extraskeletal involvement
Iᵃ	AD	Mild: fractures in childhood	Almost normal	Common. Blue sclerae; otosclerosis; thin aortic valves; hypermobile joints; ± dentinogenesis imperfecta
II	AR	Severe: skull virtually unossified; multiple fractures; lethal	Low	No dentinogenesis imperfecta
III	AR, some sporadic	Progressive: few can walk unaided	Low	Blue sclerae; no dentinogenesis imperfecta
IV	AD	Severe	Low	Sclerae not blue; dentinogenesis imperfecta common
V	Variable	Mild	Almost normal	Loose-jointedness prominent

AD/AR = autosomal dominant/recessive.
ᵃConstitutes 80% of all cases.

Osteopetrosis (Albers–Schönberg disease; marble-bone disease)

General aspects

Osteopetrosis is a rare genetic disorder of variable severity characterized by excessive bone density, probably as a result of a defect in osteoclastic activity and hence of bone remodelling. The bones, though dense, are weak and can fracture easily, but usually heal normally.

Clinical features

In mild osteopetrosis, there may be no symptoms and the diagnosis is made by chance by radiography. In severe osteopetrosis (malignant infantile osteopetrosis), patients may suffer bone pain, fractures or osteomyelitis; added complications can be cranial neuropathies leading, for example, to optic atrophy. Anaemia is common, as the medullary cavities are filled with bone, despite extramedullary haemopoiesis in liver, spleen and lymph nodes, and there is a susceptibility to infections, since macrophages and neutrophils are defective. Hydrocephalus, epilepsy and learning disability are less frequent.

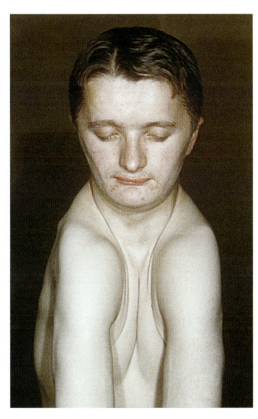

Fig. 16.2 Cleidocranial dysplasia.

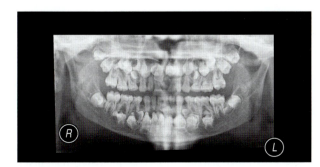

Fig. 16.3 Cleidocranial dysplasia (dysostosis).

General management

Serum levels of acid phosphatase are raised but calcium and phosphate levels are normal. Corticosteroid therapy may help but bone marrow transplantation (BMT) may be the best hope.

Dental aspects

The face may be broad, with hypertelorism, snub nose and frontal bossing. There may be retarded tooth eruption. Radiography shows excessive bone density and thickness, especially obvious in the skull. Trigeminal or facial neuropathies may complicate the disease.

Fracture of the jaw or osteomyelitis may complicate dental extractions. Eruption of posterior teeth may be complicated by osteomyelitis. Once established, infection is difficult to eradicate, so that surgery should be minimally traumatic; mucoperiosteal flaps should preferably not be raised and antibiotic cover should be given. Management problems may include anaemia (Ch. 8), corticosteroid therapy (Ch. 6) or complications of BMT (Ch. 35).

ACQUIRED DISORDERS

Rickets and osteomalacia

General aspects

Rickets is a disease of childhood characterized by inadequate skeletal mineralization. Osteomalacia has the same pathogenesis but affects adults, in whom there is failure of mineralization of replacement bone (osteoid) in the normal process of bone turnover. Both rickets and osteomalacia are largely related to a lack of vitamin D or calcium, due to the causes shown in Box 16.1. Rickets and osteomalacia are commonly results of a dietary deficiency in poorly nourished communities nowadays; South Asian immigrants living in northern Europe are particularly at risk. Contributory factors may be lack of sunshine exposure and eating chapattis made from wholemeal flour containing phytates, which impair calcium absorption.

Clinical features

In rickets, the bones are weak and readily deformed, fracturing easily but incompletely (greenstick or pseudofractures). Affected infants and young children are often also listless and irritable, with weak and hypotonic

---

Box 16.1 *Risk factors for rickets and osteomalacia*

- Dietary deficiency of vitamin D – abundant in fish liver oil and animal livers
- Failure of skin vitamin D synthesis from lack of sunlight exposure
- Vitamin D or calcium malabsorption – obstructive liver or biliary disease may lead to impaired absorption of vitamin D because of a lack of bile salts in the small intestine. The liver is also central to the conversion of vitamin D to its active forms. Phytates, in wholemeal flour, bind calcium and impair its absorption
- Excessive calcium demands in pregnancy and lactation
- Renal disease, with loss of calcium, loss of phosphate, acidosis and impaired synthesis of the active metabolite of vitamin D (1,25-dihydroxycholecalciferol)
- Vitamin D-dependent rickets – due to a defect of the enzyme required to form 1,25-dihydroxycholecalciferol
- Vitamin D-resistant rickets – an X-linked defect of renal reabsorption of phosphate (familial hypophosphataemia)
- Prolonged treatment with drugs that accelerate vitamin D metabolism – particularly phenytoin

muscles, and they suffer bone pains. Excess formation of osteoid matrix causes a 'rachitic rosary' (swellings at costochondral junctions).

General management

Plasma alkaline phosphatase levels are usually raised, calcium levels low (in 50%), and phosphate levels normal or low. The underlying cause should be rectified where possible. Vitamin D and calcium should be given.

Dental aspects

Dental defects are seen only in unusually severe cases but eruption may be retarded. The jaws may show abnormal radiolucency. Vitamin D deficiency is not a contributory cause of dental caries.

In malabsorption syndromes, there may be secondary hyperparathyroidism or vitamin K deficiency, with endocrine or bleeding disorders, respectively, and oral manifestations of malabsorption.

In vitamin D-resistant rickets (familial hypophosphataemia), the skull sutures are wide and there may be frontal bossing. Dental complaints frequently bring attention to the disease, since the teeth have large pulp chambers and abnormal dentine calcification, and are liable to pulpitis and multiple dental abscesses. Since even minimal caries or attrition can lead to pulpitis, preventive care and fissure sealing or prophylactic occlusal coverage are needed.

Osteoporosis

General aspects

Osteoporosis is a very common condition of diminished bone mass and low bone density, which leads to fragile bones, usually in the elderly. Factors that lead to limited formation of bone early in life or loss of bone structure later in life lead to osteoporosis. The same factors that encourage bone formation in youth affect the maintenance of bone mass during the adult years, particularly calcium intake, reproductive hormone status, normal parathyroid gland function and physical activity (Fig. 16.4). The difference between how much healthy bone is formed during the first 28 or so years of life and the rate at which it is remodelled and removed later determines how much osteoporosis or osteopenia (see later) results. From age 30 years, about 1% of bone is lost per year, rising to about 5% after the menopause. During the first 20 years of life, formation of bone is the most important factor preventing osteoporosis, but after that point it is prevention of bone loss that becomes most important. Risk factors for osteoporosis are shown in Box 16.2.

Clinical features

Mildly traumatic or non-traumatic injuries in osteoporosis can cause fractures. The chief complications are fractures of the femoral neck, distal radius or humerus, or of the vertebral bodies (causing gradual collapse of the spine – hence the shrinking size of some older women). Low back pain is common.

General management

Diagnosis of osteoporosis is mainly from bone densitometry – a radiographic technique that gives accurate and precise measurements of the amount of bone (not the *quality*), termed 'bone mineral density' (BMD). Dual X-ray energy absorptiometry (DXA or DEXA) or sometimes dual

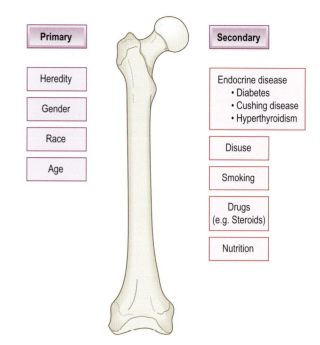

Fig. 16.4 Osteoporosis.

Box 16.2 *Risk factors for osteoporosis*

- Advanced age – over the age of 60 years, nearly one-third of the population has osteoporosis – at least 1 in three women and 1 in 12 men
- Female gender and early menopause – the most common form of osteoporosis is post-menopausal and affects 50% of women over 70 years of age. It is due to loss of oestrogen production by the ovaries, which accelerates bone loss. In terms of bone remodelling, the lack of oestrogen promotes the ability of osteoclasts to absorb bone
- Positive family history
- Lifestyle factors
  - Lack of exercise – when the normal stresses placed upon bones by normal physical activity are removed, bones lose density, best illustrated in a significant loss of bone density in patients with spinal injuries. Athletes have stronger bones than normal sedentary adults
  - Diet low in calcium or vitamin D
  - Excess alcohol intake
  - Smoking
- Drugs and disease
  - Drugs such as corticosteroids, heparin, ciclosporin and anticonvulsants
  - Malignant disease
  - Chronic inflammatory states, such as rheumatoid arthritis or ulcerative colitis
  - Endocrine disorders (Cushing syndrome, hyperthyroidism, hypogonadism)

---

photon absorptiometry (DPA) is used. BMD values that fall well below the average for the 25-year-old female (stated statistically as 2.5 standard deviations below the average) are diagnosed as 'osteoporotic'. BMD values less than those in the normal 25-year-old female, but not 2.5 standard deviations below the average, are diagnosed as 'osteopenic'. Initial screening for osteoporosis should be performed according to National Osteoporosis Foundation recommendations. The optimal interval for repeating DXA scans is uncertain, but because changes in bone density over short intervals are often smaller than the measurement error of most DXA scanners, frequent testing (e.g. at less than 2-year intervals) is unnecessary in most patients. Even in high-risk patients receiving drug therapy for osteoporosis, DXA changes do not always correlate

Table 16.2 Recommended calcium intake

Age	Amount of daily calcium
Infants	
Birth to 6 months	400 mg
6 months to 1 year	600 mg
Children/young adults	
1–10 years	800–1200 mg
11–24 years	1200–1500 mg
Adult women	
Pregnant or lactating	1200–1500 mg
25–49 years (pre-menopausal)	1000 mg
50–64 years (post-menopausal taking oestrogen or similar hormone)	1000 mg
50–64 years (post-menopausal not taking oestrogen or similar hormone)	1500 mg
Over 65 years	1500 mg
Adult men	
25–64 years	1000 mg
Over 65 years	1500 mg

with probability of fracture. Therefore, DXAs should only be repeated if the result will influence clinical management or if rapid changes in bone density are expected. Recent evidence also suggests that healthy women aged 67 and older with normal bone mass may not need additional DXA testing for up to 10 years, provided that osteoporosis risk factors do not change significantly. Poor BMD, raised serum alkaline phosphatase and urinary loss of calcium and hydroxyproline are risk markers but there are often no biochemical abnormalities. Bone biopsy is not practical or necessary.

The best management is to avoid falls and injuries and to consider use of hip protectors. Exercise has a positive effect on BMD, particularly in adults who have been sedentary and begin to exercise. Weight-bearing exercises, such as walking, running, jogging and dancing, are recommended. Additional calcium and 1-alpha-hydroxyvitamin D may also be helpful. The main sources of calcium are dairy products and green vegetables; the main sources of vitamin D are sun exposure (15 minutes exposure daily from April to October in the northern hemisphere is sufficient), margarine, breakfast cereals, oily fish, eggs and meat. Table 16.2 shows the recommended calcium intake according to age, gender and hormone status.

Hormone replacement therapy (HRT) may be effective in post-menopausal women and may also help relieve other symptoms, such as flushing (Ch. 25), but oestrogens can cause vaginal bleeding and increased risk of breast cancer. Raloxifene, given post-menopausally, may help to maintain BMD and assist the kidneys in producing vitamin D. Raloxifene also behaves like natural oestrogen in the liver, where it raises production of 'good' cholesterol (high-density lipoprotein; HDL) and lowers 'bad' cholesterol (low-density lipoprotein; LDL). Raloxifene appears to have no effect on the uterine endometrial lining growth, so there is no need for progestogen and there is no periodic bleeding. Raloxifene may also lower the breast cancer risk. The role of androgens (testosterone) in males is less clear, but the loss of testosterone promotes osteoporosis.

Anti-resorption drugs, which lower the rate at which osteoclasts reabsorb bone, include calcitonin, bisphosphonates and denosumab:

- Calcitonin is a thyroid hormone – a powerful inhibitor of osteoclastic activity that produces modest improvements in bone mass. A disadvantage has been that calcitonin had to be injected but a nasal spray has been developed.

- Bisphosphonates are adsorbed on to hydroxyapatite and can prevent or significantly slow normal osteoclastic activity; they can lead to a 50% reduction in fractures (including hip and spine), compared with women taking calcium only.
- Denosumab, a monoclonal antibody against receptor activator of nuclear factor kappa-B ligand (RANKL), is another potent inhibitor of osteoclastic bone resorption.

Strontium ranelate may inhibit osteoporosis but can cause serious drug rashes with eosinophilia and systemic symptoms (DRESS).

Dental aspects

There seems to be a correlation between osteoporosis and excessive alveolar bone loss in the elderly. Jaw osteoporosis is particularly a problem in women. Systemic treatment of osteoporosis may improve jaw bone density.

Patients with osteoporosis may have any of the problems of older people (Ch. 25). They may be at risk during general anaesthesia (GA) if there has been vertebral collapse and chest deformities.

Osteonecrosis of the jaw (ONJ; osteoclast modifier-related osteonecrosis of the jaws, OMRONJ)

Bisphosphonate-related or induced ONJ (BRONJ; BIONJ), defined as the presence of exposed bone in the mouth that fails to heal after appropriate intervention over a period of 6–8 weeks, has been reported in about 5% of patients with cancer who are receiving high-dose intravenous bisphosphonates. Use of oral bisphosphonates, such as alendronate and risedronate, results in an incidence of ONJ of about 1 case per 1500 patients to 2 cases per 100000 patient years.

Bisphosphonates, especially if used intravenously, may induce osteonecrosis of the jaws. These drugs are used to treat not only osteopenia/osteoporosis but also hypercalcaemia of malignancy, metabolic bone disease (hyperparathyroidism, Paget disease) and osteogenesis imperfecta, Gaucher disease and Langerhans histiocytosis. Bisphosphonates are pyrophosphate analogues that block the 3-hydroxy-3-methylglutaryl-coenzyme A (*HMG-CoA*) *reductase pathway* (mevalonate path) and inhibit osteoclasts, thereby decreasing bone resorption. However, bisphosphonates remain in bone for years and have an extremely long-lasting effect. Bisphosphonate potency varies enormously, from the lowest potency (etidronate, clodronate and tiludronate) to the highest nitrogenous bisphosphonates (risedronate, ibandronate and zoledronate). Intravenous bisphosphonates such as pamidronate and zoledronate, used in cancer patients, are a particularly high risk for producing BIONJ (ranging from 1 in 10 to 1 in 100 patients). However, in osteoporosis, in which the doses used are an order of magnitude lower, the prevalence appears to be very much lower. Oral bisphosphonates such as alendronate used for more than 3 years carry a risk between 1 in 10000 to 1 in 100000, the lowest risk being with the lower-potency agents etidronate and tiludronate.

ONJ has also been seen in patients treated with other drugs used in cancer patients, such as denosumab, bevacizumab and sunitinib.

Some 67% of ONJ cases are preceded by tooth extraction, whereas another factor, such as a denture pressure sore or a torus, is identified in 7%; no predisposing factor is found in 26% of patients. The mean time to development of ONJ in cancer patients treated with zoledronate is 1.8 years but ranges from 6 to 60 months.

Preventive dentistry prior to initiation of high-dose antiresorptive therapy is important in patients with cancer.

A working party from US National Institutes of Health and Canadian Institutes of Health Research recommendations (Khosla et al., 2007) defined a *confirmed case of BIONJ* as:

> *an area of exposed bone in the maxillofacial region that did not heal within 8 weeks after identification by a health care worker, in a patient who was receiving or had been exposed to a bisphosphonate and had not had radiation therapy to the craniofacial region*

and a *suspected case* as:

> *an area of exposed bone in the maxillofacial region that had been identified by a health care provider and had been present for < 8 weeks in a patient who was receiving or had been exposed to a bisphosphonate and had not had radiation therapy to the craniofacial region.*

Eighty per cent of cases present after surgery, as exposed necrotic bone, primarily mandibular alveolar bone (Fig. 16.5; Box 16.3). Lamina dura sclerosis or loss, and widening of the periodontal ligament space may well be early manifestations.

Prevention is by avoiding elective oral surgery; alternatively treatment should be carried out well before commencing bisphosphonates or after a drug holiday for 6 months. The patient must be counselled about risks and a risk assessment should be carried out. Risk factors include bisphosphonate type and dose (intravenous is worst), and dental co-morbidities (increase risk). Low bone turnover, as shown by low C-terminal cross-linking type 1 collagen telopeptides (CTX), increases risk. Recommendations for managing bisphosphonate patients are shown in Table 16.3.

If dental extractions become unavoidable in a patient taking bisphosphonates, the use of prophylactic antibiotics may be considered, but there are no controlled studies to support their use. The decision depends on the clinician's level of concern relative to the individual patient and their specific situation, including concomitant risk factors (e.g. prolonged use of oral bisphosphonates, intravenous bisphosphonates, older age and concomitant use of oestrogen or glucocorticoids).

Therefore, whenever possible, dentists should avoid performing extractions and elective oral surgery in patients taking bisphosphonates. If surgery is essential, the dentist must counsel the patient about the risks of use of intravenous or oral bisphosphonates taken for more than 3 years. Teriparatide has recently been introduced for treatment of ONJ.

Osteoradionecrosis (ORN)

See Chapter 22.

Osteomyelitis

General aspects

Osteomyelitis literally means 'inflammation of the bone marrow', although sometimes the subperiosteal bone is mainly affected.

Haematogenous osteomyelitis is an infection caused by bacterial seeding from the blood, involves a single species of microorganism (typically a bacterium), occurs primarily in children, and is most common in the rapidly growing and highly vascular metaphysis of growing bones.

Direct or contiguous inoculation osteomyelitis is usually caused by trauma or surgery, and tends to involve multiple microorganisms.

Acute osteomyelitis of the jaws primarily affects the mandible, usually in adults, and is essentially an osteolytic destructive process, but an osteoblastic response is typical of sclerosing osteomyelitis. In children, proliferative periostitis may occur. Predisposing factors for osteomyelitis are sources from which bacteria can spread to bone, from:

- local odontogenic infections (commonest cause)
- other adjacent structures (e.g. otitis media, tonsillitis, suppurative sialadenitis)
- haematogenous spread of organisms (rare in relation to the jaws).

When osteomyelitis of the mandible does occur, it may be a sign of an underlying debilitating disease, such as diabetes mellitus, an immune defect, an autoinflammatory condition or alcoholism. Alternatively, it may be related to reduced vascularity, such as after irradiation, or in rare bone conditions such as Paget disease or osteopetrosis.

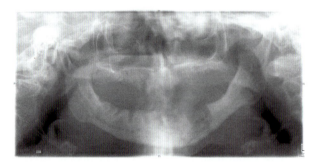

Fig. 16.5 Bisphosphonate-related osteonecrosis of the jaw (BRONJ).

Box 16.3 *Osteonecrosis of the jaws*

- Exposed bone
- Loose teeth
- Foul discharge
- Pain ±
- Fistula

Table 16.3 Recommendations for bisphosphonate patients[a]

	Patients with non-malignant disease on bisphosphonates > 3 y	Patients with malignancy, starting or already on bisphosphonates
Surgery	Conventional orthograde endodontics are recommended rather than extraction where possible	Conventional orthograde endodontics are recommended rather than extraction where possible
Periodontics	Periodontal surgery is appropriate if it reduces or eliminates disease	No periodontal surgery
Endodontics	No apical surgery	No apical surgery
Implants	Currently not contraindicated if taking bisphosphonates but prudent to gain informed consent, which should be documented (risk assessment)	Not recommended

[a]*From Khosla et al., 2007.*

Staphylococcus aureus is the commonest organism causing jaw osteomyelitis, but streptococci (both α- and β-haemolytic) and anaerobic organisms (e.g. *Bacteroides* and *Peptostreptococcus* species) are occasionally implicated. In acute osteomyelitis, the organisms excite acute inflammation in the medullary bone and the consequent oedema and exudation cause pus to be forced under pressure through the medullary bone, resulting in intrabone blood vessel (i.e. inferior dental artery) thrombosis, reducing the vascular supply to bone, which then necroses. Eventually, pus bursts through the cortical plate to drain via sinuses in the skin or mucosa. Where pus penetrates the cortex, it may spread subperiosteally, stripping the periosteum and thus further reducing the blood supply. Necrotic pieces of bone become sequestra, surrounded by pus, which either spontaneously discharge or remain and perpetuate infection. The periosteum lays down new bone to form an involucrum encasing the infected and sequestrated bone. The involucrum may prevent sequestra from being shed. Finally, if little new bone is formed, a pathological fracture may occur.

Clinical features

Jaw osteomyelitis presents with deep-seated, boring pain and swelling. Teeth in the affected area become mobile and tender to percussion, with pus oozing from the gingival crevices. The pain abates once pus penetrates the cortical plate, and discharges intraorally or extraorally, often through several sinuses. Labial anaesthesia is a characteristic feature because of pressure on the inferior alveolar nerve. The patient is often febrile and toxic with enlarged regional lymph nodes.

General management

Diagnosis is clinical, supported by imaging that, in established cases, shows marked bony destruction and sequestration. However, since radiographic changes are seen only after there has been significant decalcification of bone, early cases may not be detected; in these, isotope bone scanning using technetium diphosphonate may show increased uptake. Blood tests show a leukocytosis with neutrophilia and a raised erythrocyte sedimentation rate (ESR).

Treatment is with antibiotics and usually drainage. Penicillin was the drug of choice, but since many staphylococci are now penicillin-resistant, flucloxacillin or fusidic acid may be used. Lincomycin and clindamycin also give high bone levels but, because of a high incidence of pseudomembranous colitis, are now regarded as second-line drugs. Metronidazole gives good bone levels and is indicated for anaerobic infections. Drainage of pus follows the guidelines used for other infections. When dead bone is exposed in the mouth, it can often be left to sequestrate without surgical interference, but sequestrectomy should be undertaken if the separated dead bone fails to discharge; decortication of the mandible may be needed in order to allow this, along with drainage. Hyperbaric oxygen is an effective adjunct for recalcitrant osteomyelitis, especially where anaerobic organisms are involved.

Acute maxillary osteomyelitis is rare, and usually seen in infants, presumably because the lack of development of the antrum at this age means the maxilla is a dense bone.

Chronic osteomyelitis presents with intermittent pain and swelling, relieved by the discharge of pus through long-standing sinuses. Bone destruction is localized and often a single sequestrum may be the source of chronic infection. Removal of the sequestrum and curettage of the associated granulation tissue usually produces complete resolution.

Focal sclerosing osteomyelitis is usually asymptomatic and is revealed as an incidental radiographic finding. Most common in young adults, there is a dense, radio-opaque area of sclerotic bone caused by formation of endosteal bone – usually related to the apical area of a mandibular molar. This appears to be a response to low-grade infection in a highly immune host. Following tooth extraction, the infection usually resolves (but the sclerotic bone often remains).

Diffuse sclerosing osteomyelitis is a sclerotic endosteal reaction, which, like focal sclerosing osteomyelitis, appears to be a response to low-grade infection. However, the area of bone involved is widespread and sometimes involves most of the mandible or occasionally the maxilla. Sometimes the infection arises in an abnormally osteosclerotic mandible, such as in Paget disease, osteopetrosis or fibrous dysplasia. Intermittent swelling, pain and discharge of pus may go on for years. Management is difficult because of the extensive nature of the disease process. Long-term antibiotics, curettage and limited sequestrectomy all have their place.

Proliferative periostitis (*Garré osteomyelitis*) is more common in children than adults. The cellular osteogenic periosteum of the child responds to low-grade infection, such as apical infection of a lower first molar tooth, by proliferation and deposition of subperiosteal new bone. The subperiosteal bone may be deposited in layers, producing an onion-skin appearance radiologically, which can simulate Ewing sarcoma. The endosteal bone, however, may appear to be completely normal, but in severe cases also appears moth-eaten radiologically. Removal of the infective source is usually followed by complete resolution, although subsequent bone remodelling can take a considerable time.

Tumoral calcinosis

This rare disease is characterized by ectopic, soft tissue calcifications but normocalcaemia. Early-onset periodontitis may be a feature.

Fibrous dysplasia

General aspects

Fibrous dysplasia consists of replacement of an area of bone by fibrous tissue, causing a localized swelling that may affect a single bone (monostotic) or, less commonly, several bones (polyostotic).

The aetiology of fibrous dysplasia is unknown. The process typically starts in childhood and, as the skeleton matures, the lesions ossify progressively; ultimately, when skeletal growth ceases, they usually become stabilized.

Cherubism shares some features in common with fibrous dysplasia but may cause bilateral lesions of the maxilla causing the eyes to 'upturn towards heaven'.

Clinical features

Monostotic fibrous dysplasia is the most common type; it is more frequent in females and often involves the jaws, particularly the maxilla. *Polyostotic* fibrous dysplasia may affect either sex and may involve over 50% of the skeleton, but is uncommon. The lesions may be unilateral and 50% have abnormal skin hyperpigmentation of a café-au-lait colour, especially over the dorsum of the trunk and limbs, usually on the same side as the bone lesions (Jaffe syndrome). Albright syndrome is polyostotic fibrous dysplasia with skin hyperpigmentation and precocious puberty in females; there are episodic rises in serum oestrogen and falls in gonadotropin levels.

General management

Radiography typically shows a ground-glass appearance with no defined margins. Serum calcium and phosphate levels are normal, often with raised serum alkaline phosphatase level and raised urinary hydroxyproline.

Fibrous dysplasia is typically self-limiting and usually ceases to progress after adolescence. Patients are sometimes managed with calcitonin. Bisphosphonate treatment may have implications (see Osteonecrosis of the jaw). Testolactone is effective for the precocious puberty of Albright syndrome. Surgery can be used to correct any residual cosmetic defect but the bone tends to bleed a great deal. Radiotherapy should be avoided because of the risk of inducing osteosarcomas.

Dental aspects

The facial bones are frequently involved in monostotic fibrous dysplasia and in 25% of cases of polyostotic disease. Monostotic fibrous dysplasia is not a medical problem but it is possible for the polyostotic type of the disease to be unrecognized when the facial lesions are the most obvious feature. Hyperthyroidism or diabetes mellitus may occasionally be associated with polyostotic fibrous dysplasia and therefore may, rarely, complicate treatment. Mucosal pigmentation may be seen but is rare in Albright syndrome. In the differential diagnosis, it may be confused with that of Addison disease, while the skin pigmentation may simulate that of neurofibromatosis.

PAGET DISEASE OF BONE (OSTEITIS DEFORMANS)

General aspects

Paget disease is characterized by progressive deformity and enlargement of bones related to overactivity of osteoclasts and osteoblasts. There appears to be considerable geographical variation in the prevalence, disease being common in northern Europeans, and also in older age. Paget disease is rare in Africans, people from the Indian subcontinent, and other Asians.

The essential features are total disorganization of the normal orderly replacement of bone, and an anarchic alternation of bone resorption and apposition. In the earlier stages, resorption predominates (osteolytic phase) but later bone apposition takes over and, as disease activity declines, the affected bones become enlarged and dense (sclerotic stage).

There is a male predominance. The aetiology of Paget disease is unknown and a slow virus has been implicated. Inherited forms of Paget disease of bone, caused by mutations in genes such as *SQSTM1* that affect osteoclast differentiation and function, are recognized.

Clinical features

Symptoms are absent in the early stages, which can only be detected by imaging. Bone pain is the most common feature in older patients; it is usually felt around the hips or knees but is non-specific. One or many bones may be affected. In the polyostotic type, the axial skeleton is mainly involved but hands and feet are usually spared (Fig. 16.6). Other possible complications of Paget disease are deformities, pathological fractures, and constriction of skull foraminae – sometimes compressing cranial nerves and leading to effects such as deafness or impairment of vision. Rarely, there is brainstem or spinal compression.

If Paget disease is widespread, hypervascularity of the bones can produce, in effect, an arteriovenous fistula and high-output cardiac failure. Development of osteosarcoma is a recognized but rare complication.

General management

The differential diagnosis includes hyperostosis frontalis interna (a benign condition characterized by frontal bone sclerosis), fibrous

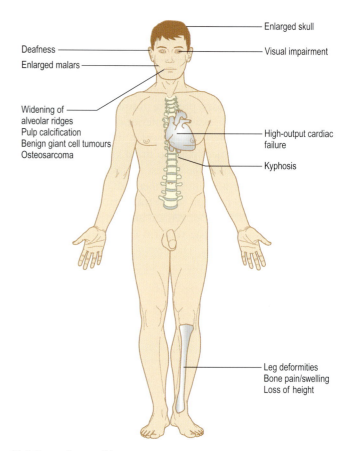

Fig. 16.6 Paget disease of bone.

dysplasia, pustulotic arthrosteitis (sclerotic lesions of clavicle and ribs) and osteosclerotic metastases. Diagnosis is from radiographs of affected bones, which show predominantly radiolucencies due to osteolysis early on but mixed areas of lysis with sclerosis later. Affected bones become thicker. Radionuclide bone scanning showing increased uptake of technetium diphosphonate helps define disease extent. The serum total alkaline phosphatase level is grossly raised when many bones are affected, but usually there is little or no change in calcium or phosphate levels. More specific is a rise in bone-specific alkaline phosphatase, procollagen type I N-terminal propeptide and osteocalcin. There is also raised urinary hydroxyproline and pyridinoline excretion. Biopsy is rarely indicated.

Currently, the most effective treatment of Paget disease is with bisphosphonates. Vitamin D deficiency is a common accompaniment.

Dental aspects

When the skull is affected, a typical early feature is a large irregular area of relative radiolucency (osteoporosis circumscripta; Fig. 16.7). Later, there is radio-opacity, with loss of the normal landmarks and an irregular cotton-wool appearance. Basilar invagination may be seen. The maxilla is involved occasionally and the mandible rarely. Typically, maxillary enlargement causes symmetrical malar bulging (leontiasis ossea; Fig. 16.8). The intraoral features are gross symmetrical widening of the alveolar ridges, loss of lamina dura and hypercementosis, often forming enormous craggy masses that may become fused to the surrounding bone. Pulpal calcification may be seen. Serious complications follow efforts to extract severely hypercementosed teeth. Attempts using forceps may fail to move the tooth or cause fracture of the alveolar bone. Alternatively, the tooth may be mobilized but retained, as if in a ball-and-socket joint. If hypercementosis is severe, a surgical approach with adequate exposure should be used for extractions.

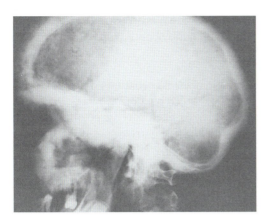

Fig. 16.7 Paget disease affecting the skull.

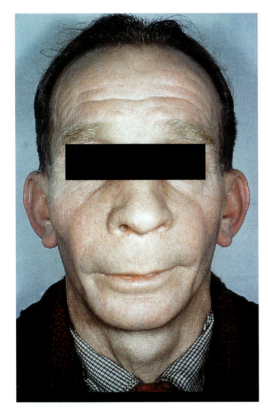

Fig. 16.8 Leontiasis ossea in Paget disease.

In the early stages of the disease, the highly vascular bone may bleed freely; later, the poor blood supply to the bone makes it susceptible to chronic suppurative osteomyelitis. Bisphosphonate treatment may have implications (see Osteonecrosis of the jaw). Prophylactic antibiotics, such as penicillin (immediately before and for 3 or 4 days after the operation), may help prevent postoperative infection. Dentures have to be replaced as the alveolar ridge enlarges. Benign giant cell tumours may be seen.

Patients with Paget disease involving facial or maxillo-mandibular parts of the skeleton have a higher prevalence of heart disease and of deteriorating hearing, sight and smell. Osteosarcoma is rare in the jaws. If the patient is in heart failure, the usual precautions have to be taken but, since GA may be needed for extractions, this aspect of the disease needs to be kept in mind. Chest deformity may also complicate GA.

Hyperparathyroidism

See Chapter 6.

THERAPEUTIC PROCEDURES

Guided bone regeneration (GBR)

Guided bone regeneration (GBR) is a surgical procedure that uses barrier membranes to direct new bone growth to sites having insufficient volumes or dimensions for function or prosthesis placement. Barrier membranes have been derived from a variety of sources, both natural and synthetic, and are marketed under various trade names. Membranes used in GBR may be of two principal varieties: non-resorbable (expanded polytetrafluoroethylene) and resorbable (collagen from various sources, ox caecum cargile membrane, poly-lactic acid, polyacetic acid, polyglycolic acid, polyglactin 910 (Vicryl), synthetic skin (Biobrane) and freeze-dried dura mater). A range of materials – from demineralized bone matrix formulations and bone morphogenic proteins to synthetic ceramic materials – are now being used. Animal studies have even enabled a hybrid tooth–bone construct to be developed.

Distraction osteogenesis

Distraction osteogenesis is a surgical process involving the gradual, controlled displacement of surgically created fractures, which permits simultaneous expansion of bone and soft tissue, in order to reconstruct combined deficiencies in bone and soft tissue. This is effective in orofacial skeletal reconstruction, including cleft palate reconstruction and alveolar ridge augmentation for placement of osseointegrated implants. Disadvantages are the expense, technical difficulty and the long training required. The most frequent complications are infection, and loosening and breaking of the introduced pins, with osteomyelitis and fracture of the newly generated bone.

JOINTS

A joint is the location at which two or more bones make contact. Joints can be:

- fibrous – joined by dense irregular connective tissue that is rich in collagen fibres
- cartilaginous – joined by cartilage
- synovial – not directly joined; the bones have a synovial cavity and are united by the dense irregular connective tissue that forms the articular capsule that is normally associated with accessory ligaments (e.g. temporomandibular joint; TMJ).

JOINT DISEASES

A joint disorder is termed an arthropathy; when it involves inflammation, it is called arthritis. Joints are considerably more frequently affected by disease than are bones or muscles. The jaws and TMJ are, however, rarely involved in systemic disease. Acquired disorders are the most common.

GENETIC DISORDERS

Marfan syndrome

The Marfan syndrome is most common genetic connective tissue disorder and has skeletal, cardiovascular, dermatological and ocular manifestations. It is an autosomal dominant condition involving the *FBN1* gene, which encodes connective tissue protein fibrillin-1 and is also a binding protein for transforming growth factor beta (TGF-β, which has a damaging effect on vascular smooth muscle development. Prevalence is 2–3 per 10 000 and disease affects both sexes equally. There is usually great variation in the phenotype within families whose members share the same genetic condition. The diagnosis of Marfan syndrome is usually clinical but may be difficult (Table 16.4). A Marfanoid body build may also be a feature of the benign joint hypermobility syndrome or multiple endocrine adenoma syndrome (MEA III; Ch. 6). The Marfan syndrome also shares the features of loose-jointedness, cardiac valvular defects and ocular lesions with various of the subtypes of Ehlers–Danlos syndrome; there can also be confusion with other rare disorders, particularly homocystinuria and congenital contractural arachnodactyly (long, spider-like fingers). However, the most obvious distinguishing feature of the Marfan syndrome is the long, thin body habitus and long slender fingers.

Clinical features

The condition can be asymptomatic, although patients are usually longer and thinner than average (Fig. 16.9). Fingers and toes are also usually long and thin. The following organs are affected:

- Skin – striae
- Cardiovascular system – abnormalities affect 90% of patients and aortic dissection can be life-threatening. There is often severe aortic and mild mitral incompetence. Death in the fifth decade is common. Mitral valve prolapse can lead to arrhythmias, embolism or sudden death; if it causes a systolic murmur, it can predispose to infective endocarditis, particularly in older persons. Thoracic aortic dilatation/rupture/dissection, aortic mitral valve/prolapse, mitral regurgitation, abdominal aortic aneurysm and cardiac arrhythmia may occur.
- Eyes – visual impairment is common due to lens subluxation or dislocation in 80%, glaucoma or myopia.
- Joints – arthralgia, lax ligaments are common, predisposing to joint hyperextensibility, subluxation or dislocation, and hernias.
- Skeleton – misshapen chest and excessive length of tubular bones so that patients are tall with a wide arm span (often exceeds the patient's height by a ratio of more than 1.03) and arachnodactyly.
- Lungs – function can be impaired by cysts, which lead to spontaneous pneumothorax and kyphoscoliosis.

Survival has been greatly improved with aortic graft surgery and the use of beta-blockers.

Dental aspects

Maxillary/mandibular retrognathia and long face are the main features. The palatal vault is high and TMJ dysfunction or recurrent subluxation may be troublesome. Bite problems may arise from malocclusion. Management may be complicated by chest deformities and cardiovascular abnormalities, which may be contraindications to GA, and by the risk of infective endocarditis (Ch. 5).

Ehlers–Danlos syndrome

General aspects

Ehlers–Danlos syndrome (EDS) is a group of rare disorders of collagen formation, characterized by hyperextensible skin, bleeding tendency and propensity to bruising and loose-jointedness. The most common forms are inherited as autosomal dominant traits, while the remainder are recessive.

Clinical features and general management

There is wide variation in the clinical features of the different EDS types (Table 16.5). Hypermobility of joints is the best-known manifestation of EDS and may be extreme (India-rubber man). Recurrent, semi-spontaneous dislocation may result. It may be possible to hyperextend the fingers until they are at right angles to the back of the hand, and the diagnosis is often made by the unusual ability of the patient to pull their thumb back to the forearm (Fig. 16.10).

The skin is typically soft, abnormally extensible, fine and thin, and may appear lax; even when it appears normal, it may be possible to pull the skin out for 2.5–5 cm (Fig. 16.11). Other, incidental oddities that may be seen in EDS include the ability to touch the nose with the tip of the tongue (Gorlin's sign). Wounds tend to gape or to split after slight trauma, while healing is slow and may leave fragile scars with a tissue-paper texture.

Easy ('spontaneous') bruising, though of vascular origin, may mimic purpura caused by haematological diseases but, unlike any of the latter, there is a combination of subcutaneous, submucosal and deep bleeding. Although platelet defects have occasionally been reported, haemostatic function is often normal, except in type IV. Weakness of the connective tissue component may cause lesions in the gastrointestinal tract, urinary tract and respiratory system. In the vascular type (type IV), spontaneous rupture of major arteries (dissecting aneurysm) can cause fatal haemorrhage and internal bleeding.

Table 16.4 Marfan syndrome		
Skeletal defects	**Cardiovascular defects**	**Neuro-ocular defects**
Disproportionately long limbs	Dilatation of ascending aorta	Ectopia lentis
		Blue sclerae in some
Arachnodactyly (spider fingers)	Dissecting aneurysm	Learning impairment (sometimes)
	Aortic regurgitation	
Loose joints	Mitral valve prolapse	
Pectus excavatum		
Temporomandibular joint subluxation		

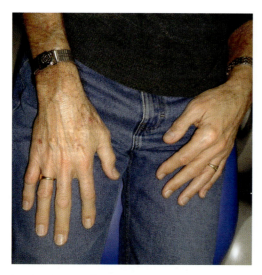

Fig. 16.9 Arachnodactyly in Marfan syndrome.

Table 16.5 Ehlers–Danlos syndrome: subtypes

Types	Inheritance	Hyper-extensibility	Skin fragility and bruising	Joint hypermobility	Special features
I (gravis) Classical type	AD	++	++	++	Parrot face. Frequent musculoskeletal disorders. Mitral valve prolapse
II (mitis) Classical type	AD	+	+	+ Hands and feet only	Mitral valve prolapse. Bruising common
III (benign hypermobility) Hypermobility type	AD	±	+	++	Dislocations, haemarthrosis, early-onset arthritis. Mitral valve prolapse
IV Vascular type	AR	±	+++	± Digits only	Bleeding from major arteries
V (sex-linked)	X-linked	++	+	±	Frequent musculoskeletal disorders. Males only
VI (ocular or hydroxylysine-deficient)	AR	++	±	++	Fragile cornea and sclera. Multiple ocular defects, deafness, often early loss of sight
VII (multiple congenital dislocation or arthrochalasis multiplex congenita)	AR	+	±	++	Early onset of multiple dislocations. Some laxity of ligaments, short stature
VIII (periodontal)	AD	±	±	±	Severe early-onset periodontitis and loss of teeth. Blue sclerae
IX (skeletal and urinary tract dysplasia)[a]	AR	–	±	±	Occipital exostoses, low copper levels
X (fibronectin deficiency)	AR	±	±	±	Bleeding tendency

AD/AR = autosomal dominant/recessive.
[a]No longer classified as Ehlers–Danlos syndrome.

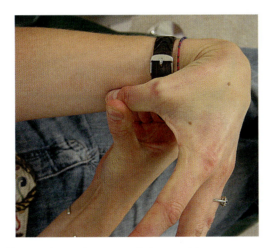

Fig. 16.10 Ehlers–Danlos syndrome. A typical party trick.

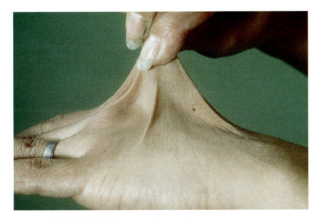

Fig. 16.11 Extensible skin in Ehlers–Danlos syndrome.

Mitral valve prolapse (floppy valve syndrome) is seen in many types of EDS, particularly type III, and may confer susceptibility to infective endocarditis or lead to rapid development of mitral insufficiency and heart failure. Cardiac conduction defects may be present.

Dental aspects

In EDS, the teeth may be small, with short or abnormally shaped roots and many pulp stones. The deciduous dentition shows abnormal morphology of the molars, obliteration of the tooth pulp and severe enamel attrition. The permanent dentition shows agenesis and microdontia of several teeth. Tooth discolouration, dysplastic roots and tooth pulp obliteration are present in a restricted number of permanent teeth:

- In types I, VI and VII EDS, joint hypermobility is severe and TMJ subluxation and dislocation is a possibility.
- In type III EDS, local anaesthetics may have less effect, though there is no satisfactory explanation.
- In type IV EDS (vascular type), post-extraction bleeding is likely to be most severe, with semi-spontaneous purpura, extensive ecchymoses and also weakness of arterial walls. Severe bleeding from the gingivae, especially after tooth-brushing or from extraction sockets, may sometimes be the main complaint.
- In type VII EDS, there may be micrognathia, an anterior open bite and gingival hyperplasia with varying degrees of hyperkeratosis.
- In type VIII EDS and possibly type IV, there is early onset of periodontal disease, with early loss of teeth.

Patients with mitral valve prolapse may develop heart failure with attendant risks during GA (Ch. 5).

Recurrent temporomandibular joint dislocation

Chronic recurrent TMJ dislocation is defined as the complete loss of articular relationships, during mouth wide-opening, between the temporal articular fossa and the condyle–disc complex. This may be seen in patients with EDS, those with internal derangements and those with other conditions. The classic treatment was the Dautrey operation (eminectomy), which modifies the bony obstacle, preventing condylar locking, but it does not have a therapeutic effect on TMJ ligament and capsular laxity or masticatory muscle incoordination, which seem to be the real causes of TMJ dislocation in most cases. Plication of the joint capsule may help.

ACQUIRED DISORDERS

ARTHRITIS

Osteoarthritis (osteoarthrosis)

General aspects

Osteoarthritis (OA) is the most common form of arthritis and is most frequently found in adults over the age of 45 years. It is especially painful in frequently used, weight-bearing or traumatized joints. OA is characterized by degeneration of articular cartilage with compensatory thickening of the exposed underlying bone and development of peri-articular cysts. Collapse of these peri-articular cysts, together with continued peripheral bone proliferation, causes progressive joint deformity. Risk factors for OA are shown in Box 16.4.

OA may affect any joint, but especially frequently used, weight-bearing or traumatized joints, such as those in the fingers, hips, knees, lower back and feet. Initially, it tends to strike only one joint but, if the fingers are affected, multiple hand joints may become arthritic, sometimes painlessly. The essential change in OA is degeneration of articular cartilage with compensatory thickening of the underlying bone, which becomes exposed and is at first smooth and shiny but later becomes roughened. Cystic spaces form beneath and bone proliferates at the joint margins. Exposure and collapse of the cystic cavities, together with continued peripheral proliferation, cause progressive deformity.

Clinical features

In OA there are no systemic symptoms, no obvious inflammation of affected joints or serological changes (Table 16.6) (in contrast to rheumatoid arthritis). Features of OA may include: pain with stiffness, progressively diminished function and deformity, particularly of larger joints, such as the hips or knees; pain, swelling and stiffness in a joint during or after use, or pain before or during a change in the weather; loss of joint flexibility; bony lumps on the fingers, on the middle (Bouchard nodes) or

> **Box 16.4** *Risk factors for osteoarthritis*
>
> - Age: most in people > 45 y
> - Gender: females more commonly affected
> - Genetic predisposition
> - Obesity
> - Malformed joints (hereditary or acquired)
> - Occupation (athletes)
> - Haemochromatosis
> - Paget disease
> - Gout

Table 16.6 Comparison of osteoarthritis and rheumatoid arthritis

Feature	Osteoarthritis	Rheumatoid arthritis
Age of onset	Late middle age or old age	Middle age
Pain and disability	+	++
Main joints affected	Weight-bearing or frequently used joints (hip, spine, knee, fingers)	Bilateral, interphalangeal
Clinical inflammation over joints	–	+
Joint deformities	Heberden or Bouchard nodes	Swelling and deviations
Morning stiffness	Some	Pronounced
Systemic problems, malaise, fatigue	–	+
Erythrocyte sedimentation rate	Normal	Raised
Rheumatoid factor	–	+ Usually

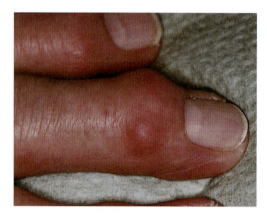

Fig. 16.12 Heberden nodes in osteoarthritis.

end joints (Heberden nodes; Fig. 16.12), or the first metacarpophalangeal joint at the thumb base (Fig. 16.13).

General management

The diagnosis is usually made on clinical grounds, supported by imaging. The characteristic radiographic features include narrowing of the joint space, marginal osteophyte formation (lipping), subchondral bone sclerosis, bone 'cysts' (rounded areas of radiolucency just beneath the joint surface) and deformity.

Physical methods of treatment are important and include a number of factors shown in Box 16.5. Medical methods of treatment are less important but include: topical pain relievers (counterirritant medications, such as trolamine salicylate, methyl salicylate, menthol and camphor, or capsaicin), which may relieve pain in joints close to the skin surface, such as fingers, knees and elbows; anti-inflammatory drugs (non-steroidal anti-inflammatory drugs; NSAIDs); licofelone or cyclo-oxygenase 2 (COX-2) inhibitors, such as celecoxib; glucosamine as a food supplement – said to provide moderate pain relief comparable to that from NSAIDs; antidepressants, which, independent of their antidepressant properties, can help lessen chronic pain; and intra-articular injections with a corticosteroid or hyaluronate, which can give pain relief for a time.

Surgical methods of treatment include joint replacement surgery – the most important surgical treatment for arthritis. The damaged joint is removed and replaced with a plastic or metal prosthesis. The hip

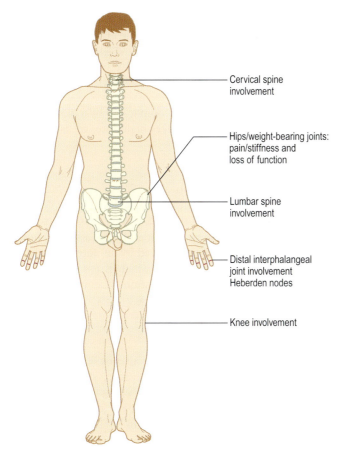

Fig. 16.13 Osteoarthritis.

- Cervical spine involvement
- Hips/weight-bearing joints: pain/stiffness and loss of function
- Lumbar spine involvement
- Distal interphalangeal joint involvement Heberden nodes
- Knee involvement

Box 16.5 *Physical aids to osteoarthritis*

- Regular exercise – to help maintain joint mobility
- Weight control – to minimize stress on joints
- Appropriate footwear – if there is arthritis in weight-bearing joints or back
- A walking stick – to ease the load on a damaged joint
- Heat application – to ease pain, relax tense, painful muscles, and increase the regional flow of blood
- Cold application – for occasional flare-ups

---

joint is most commonly replaced, but implants are available for knee, shoulder, elbow, finger or ankle joints. Completely normal function is usually restored. Arthroscopy can be used to remove loose fragments of bone or cartilage that may cause pain or mechanical symptoms, such as 'locking', but there is rarely significant improvement in pain relief or function 2 years afterwards. Surgery can also reposition bones to help correct deformities and can permanently fuse bones in a joint to improve stability and reduce pain.

Dental aspects

OA affects the TMJ in some older patients but is typically painless. Those with OA of other joints also do not appear to have significantly more TMJ involvement than controls. The radiographic severity of TMJ OA does not correlate with symptoms. Since TMJ OA is rarely clinically significant, patients should not be made unnecessarily anxious. A syndrome of dry mouth and OA has been described (sialoadenitis, osteoarthritis, xerostomia – SOX) but whether this is a true entity rather than simple coincidence needs confirmation.

Age and immobility may influence access to dental care. Patients with OA may also experience restricted manual dexterity, which may compromise their ability to maintain adequate oral hygiene. These patients may need toothbrushes with specially adapted handles (such as a handle with a ball added to help the patient grip) or may benefit from using electric toothbrushes. Since joint stiffness tends to improve during the day, short appointments in the late morning or in the early afternoon are recommended for patients with arthritis. Supine positioning may be uncomfortable for them and they may need neck and leg supports.

Dentists should consider a patient's tendency to bleed and any need for corticosteroid supplementation or antibiotic coverage before performing any invasive procedures. There is no reliable evidence of a need for antibiotic prophylaxis before dental treatment in most patients with prosthetic joints, and the risks from adverse reactions to antibiotics probably exceed any benefit. Infections of prosthetic joints are usually due to non-oral organisms such as staphylococci and are only caused by oral bacteria exceptionally rarely. Even where viridans streptococci have been found in infected joints, they could have come from non-oral sources, or simply from a bacteraemia associated with chewing. The same arguments as to the risk:benefit of antimicrobial prophylaxis in OA apply as for endocarditis (Ch. 5). Antibiotic prophylaxis is therefore not indicated for dental surgery on most patients with bone pins, plates and screws or with total joint replacements. The overall infection risk in hip replacement is less than 1% and in knee replacement less than 2%. Only rarely are these infections caused by oral streptococci and only a few have been attributed to recent dental procedures. Since the degree of the bacteraemia is reduced by good oral hygiene, best practice should incorporate dental screening to eliminate current dental disease before the replacement procedure, with advice on good oral hygiene maintenance following surgery.

Since the administration of antibiotic prophylaxis is likely to be ineffective, it should not be given routinely. The possible adverse effects and the risks of creating antibiotic resistance must also be considered. Gastrointestinal upsets and rashes are relatively common (1–10%). Anaphylaxis is rare but associated with a significant mortality rate of approximately 10%, and would result in more deaths than might occur as a consequence of infected replacements. There is a risk of developing *Clostridium difficile* infection, which is associated with significant morbidity and mortality, especially in people over 65 years, who are the ones most likely to need prostheses.

In 2012, the American Academy of Orthopedic Surgeons and American Dental Association (AAOS/ADA) released the first co-developed evidence-based guidelines on the prevention of orthopaedic implant infection in patients undergoing dental procedures (Appendix 16.2). Of note, that review found *no* direct evidence that dental procedures cause orthopaedic implant infections and concluded that antibiotic prophylaxis does not reduce the risk of subsequent implant infection. Three recommendations were drawn up:

1. The practitioner *might* consider discontinuing the practice of routinely prescribing prophylactic antibiotics for patients with hip and knee prosthetic joints undergoing dental procedures (strength of recommendation: limited).
2. The work group was unable to recommend for or against the use of topical oral antimicrobials in patients with prosthetic joint implants or other orthopaedic implants undergoing dental procedures (strength of recommendation: inconclusive).
3. In the absence of reliable evidence linking poor oral health to prosthetic joint infection, it was the opinion of the work group that patients with prosthetic joint implants or other orthopaedic implants maintain appropriate oral hygiene.

Another publication, a 'Shared decision-making tool' (http://ebd. ada.org/contentdocs/DentalSDMTool.pdf; accessed 30 September 2013), has been released as an aid to the AAOS/ADA *Prevention of orthopaedic implant infection in patients undergoing dental procedures* clinical practice guideline. It states:

- Patients who have compromised immune systems (diabetes mellitus, rheumatoid arthritis, cancer, chemotherapy, chronic steroid use) might be at greater risk for implant infections.
- Patients who are immune-compromised might wish to consider antibiotics before dental procedures because of their greater risk for infection.
- Thus, if there is any doubt on the management of such patients, the patient's orthopaedic surgeon should be consulted.
- Ideally, patients who are to undergo a total joint arthroplasty/ replacement should undergo dental evaluation and any oral disease present should be eliminated before the scheduled surgery.
- Patients with prosthetic joint implants should be encouraged to practise effective daily oral hygiene procedures and seek regular professional dental care.
- Patients who develop oral infections should be treated aggressively with antibiotics, incision and drainage, endodontics and extractions.

Thus, although the evidence may be controversial, medico-legal and other considerations suggest that dental professionals should err on the side of caution and fully inform and have discussions with the patient; take medical advice in any case of doubt; and give antibiotic prophylaxis only for at-risk procedures in patients at high risk for infection. Antibiotic prophylaxis 1–1.5 hours before dental treatment likely to initiate a bacteraemia (Box 16.6) may be considered where

dental at-risk procedures are to be carried out in patients who have recent new joints (within 2 years), or in haemophiliacs, or where the joint has previously been infected, or where patients are immuno-compromised, such as those with diabetes or rheumatoid disease. Antibiotic regimens are shown in Box 16.6; cephradine 1g orally or intravenously is a further choice.

Dental management may also be complicated by a bleeding tendency if the patient is anticoagulated or takes high doses of aspirin (Ch. 8).

Rheumatoid arthritis

Rheumatoid arthritis (RA) affects about 2% of the population in the West, and women approximately three times as frequently as men, typically between the ages of 30 and 40 years. RA is a multisystem, immuno-logically mediated disease seen in genetically predisposed individuals (HLA-DR4 genotype). It is characterized by an autoantibody directed against IgG (rheumatoid factor, RF), which is usually IgM; it forms immune complexes and leads to activation of complement, synovial inflammation and destructive joint disease.

Clinical features

RA often has an insidious onset, with increasing stiffness of the hands or feet; it is worse in the morning. In the acute stage, there is aching, swelling, redness, tenderness and limitation of movement of small joints of the wrists, hands and feet, which are typically affected first. The meta-carpophalangeal and interphalangeal joints typically become spindle-shaped as a result of joint swelling with muscle wasting on either side (Fig. 16.14). Ulnar deviation of the fingers may develop later. Eventually, the wrists, elbows, ankles and knees also may be involved and the patient becomes disabled (Fig. 16.15). The cervical spine is involved in 30% and there may be atlanto-axial subluxation (Fig. 16.16). Other common manifestations are tenosynovitis or subcutaneous nodules, but clinically apparent effects on other systems are less common (Table 16.7).

Box 16.6 *Prophylactic antibiotics in patients with prosthetic joints[a]*

Dental at-risk procedure

- Tooth removal
- Oral or periodontal surgery or raising of mucogingival flaps for any other purpose (including implants)
- Subgingival procedures, including probing, scaling, root planing, subgingival fibre placement or any form of periodontal surgery
- Intraligamentary injections
- Reimplantation of avulsed teeth
- Endodontic manipulation beyond the root apex
- Orthodontic banding

Joint at risk

- Joint placed within previous 2 years
- History of previous infection
- Patient with haemophilia
- Patient with type 1 diabetes
- Patient with rheumatoid arthritis
- Patient on immunosuppressive therapy

Antibiotic prophylaxis regimens

- Cefalexin 2g *or*
- Clindamycin 600mg *or*
- Azithromycin 500mg *or*
- Clarithromycin 500mg *or*
- Amoxicillin 2g

[a]Modified from American Association of Orthopedic Surgeons and American Dental Association guidelines (2012).

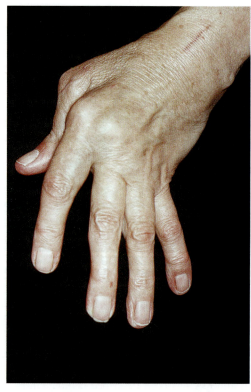

Fig. 16.14 Rheumatoid arthritis.

General management

RA is diagnosed if at least four of the features shown in Box 16.7 are present and is confirmed by finding a raised ESR and other inflammatory markers, and positive RF (present in about 70%; sensitive but not specific). The autoantibodies may occasionally be IgG and therefore not detected by the routine agglutination tests (latex and sheep-cell agglutination test; SCAT); in this case, the term 'seronegative' is used. However, radioimmunoassay (RIA) and enzyme-linked immunosorbent assay (ELISA) detect either class of RF.

Antiperinuclear factor (APF) and antikeratin antibodies (AKA), identified by immunofluorescence, have a specificity of close to 90% for RA and react with the same antigen, a citrullinated form of filaggrin (citrulline is an unusual amino acid formed by post-translational modification of arginine residues by the enzyme peptidyl arginine deaminase). Recombinant filaggrin fragments, after enzymatic deamination *in vitro*, react with autoantibodies in RA sera. Synthetic cyclic

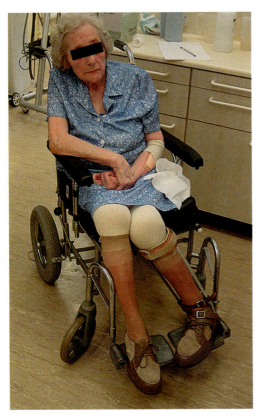

Fig. 16.15 Patient wheelchair-bound by severe rheumatoid disease.

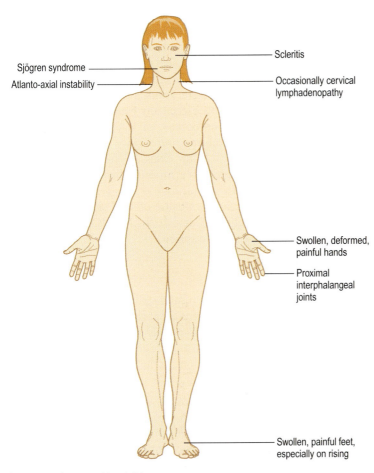

Fig. 16.16 Rheumatoid arthritis.

Sjögren syndrome
Atlanto-axial instability
Scleritis
Occasionally cervical lymphadenopathy
Swollen, deformed, painful hands
Proximal interphalangeal joints
Swollen, painful feet, especially on rising

Table 16.7 Rheumatoid arthritis: features and complications

System	Features/complications
Cardiovascular	Cardiac conduction defects
	Myocarditis
	Pericarditis
	Valvulitis
	Vasculitis
Dermal, oral and para-oral	Oral drug lesions
	Palmar erythema
	Sjögren syndrome
	Subcutaneous rheumatoid nodules
	Temporomandibular arthritis
	Vasculitis and various rashes
Haematological	Anaemia
	Leukopenia
	Thrombocytopenia
Hepatic	Abnormal liver function
Joints	Arthritis
	Laxity of ligaments
	Spinal nerve root compression
	Subluxation
	Tenosynovitis
Muscular	Wasting
	Weakness
Neurological	Benign trigeminal neuropathy
	Carpal tunnel syndrome
	Glove-and-stocking anaesthesia
	Various neuropathies
Non-specific features	Fatigue
	Fever
	Malaise
	Weight loss
Ocular	Episcleritis, scleritis or scleromalacia
	Sjögren syndrome
Osseous	Osteoporosis
Renal	Amyloidosis
	Various nephropathies
Respiratory	Bronchiolitis
	Fibrosis
	Lung nodules (rheumatoid lung disease)
	Pleurisy and pleural effusion

Box 16.7 *Diagnostic features of rheumatoid arthritis*

- Morning joint stiffness
- Arthritis affecting more than three joint areas
- Arthritis of hand joints
- Symmetrical arthritis
- Rheumatoid nodules
- Positive rheumatoid factor
- Radiographic changes consistent with rheumatoid arthritis

Table 16.8 *Laboratory findings in rheumatoid arthritis*

Test	Typical findings
Full blood count	Normocytic anaemia
	Mild leukocytosis (or leukopenia)
	Mild thrombocytopenia
Erythrocyte sedimentation rate*	Raised
Protein electrophoresis	Hypergammaglobulinaemia
Rheumatoid factor – latex agglutination	Positive usually
Antinuclear antibodies	Positive in 20–60%

*= or CRP

---

citrullinated peptide (CCP) variants also react with anti-filaggrin autoantibodies and serve as the substrate for detecting anti-CCP antibodies serologically. Most studies of anti-CCP antibodies demonstrated that these autoantibodies have much improved specificity for RA compared to RF. Anticyclic citrullinated peptide (anti-CCP) antibody can also help determine which patients may benefit from treatments such as anti-tumour necrosis factor alpha (TNFα) monoclonal antibodies; can be predictive of the progression of patients, indicating more erosive disease or increased joint involvement; and is more predictive of erosive arthritis measures, such as matrix metalloproteinases-3, ESR, and C-reactive protein (CRP). Antinuclear antibodies (ANA) are also often found but are usually in low titre (Table 16.8).

The Simplified Disease Activity Index DAS28) uses 28 tender and swollen joint counts, physician's and patient's global assessments, and CRP.

Radiographic features include widening of the joint space (in early disease); joint erosion, destruction and deformity; and peri-articular osteoporosis. Later, there is narrowing of the joint spaces, cyst-like spaces in the bone and subluxation. Ultimately, there may be severe bone destruction and deformity, but ankylosis is rare. Factors associated with a poor prognosis in RA include positive RF, extra-articular disease, HLA-DR4, early erosions and severe disability at presentation.

The main aspects of treatment include rest in the acute phases, but between these episodes maintenance of mobility of affected joints is important. Drugs used include symptom-modifying drugs, such as simple analgesics or NSAIDs, and disease-modifying antirheumatic drugs (DMARDs), which may relieve painful swollen joints and slow joint damage; the most commonly used are methotrexate, sulfasalazine and leflunomide (others include gold, penicillamine, minocycline, antimalarials, corticosteroids, azathioprine, ciclosporin and cyclophosphamide). A Prosorba column, a blood-filtering technique used weekly to remove autoantibodies, is sometimes available.

Biological response modifiers may include anakinra (a direct and selective blocker of interleukin-1 [IL-1] receptor – now rarely used) and TNF inhibitors – both first-generation (etanercept, infliximab and adalimumab) and second-generation agents (certolizumab and golimumab). Other drugs include tocilizumab (anti–IL-6); abatacept (a T-cell co-stimulator blocker) and rituximab (a monoclonal antibody against cluster of differentiation [CD]20 antigen on B lymphocytes). Biological therapies may be effective and given for severe active disease, as they are costly and can cause severe toxic effects.

Management of RA also includes general supportive measures, such as splints and appliances to facilitate mobility, reduce pain and preserve function. Surgery may be indicated for replacement of severely damaged joints.

Dental aspects

Sjögren syndrome is the most common oral complication. RA has a predilection for small joints, including the TMJ, but though there may be limitation of opening or stiffness, these are often painless. Radiographic changes are common in the TMJ and consist of erosions, flattening of the joint surfaces and marginal proliferation. Even when disease is severe, pain from the TMJ appears to trouble only a minority. Occasionally, an anterior open bite or even sleep apnoea may result.

Intubation for GA can be difficult. In some patients, dislocation of the atlanto-axial joint or fracture of the odontoid peg can readily follow sudden jerking extension of the neck, as a result of weakness of the ligaments. Disastrous accidents of this sort have been known to follow adjustment of the headrest on older types of dental chair, or sudden extension of the neck during the induction of GA.

Patients with RA may experience restricted manual dexterity, which may compromise their ability to maintain adequate oral hygiene. These individuals may need toothbrushes with specially adapted handles (such as a handle with a ball added to help the patient grip) or may benefit from using electric toothbrushes. Since joint stiffness tends to improve during the day, short appointments in the late morning or in the early afternoon are recommended for patients with arthritis. Supine positioning may be uncomfortable for them, and they may need neck and leg supports. Dentists should consider a patient's tendency to bleed and any need for corticosteroid supplementation or antibiotic coverage before performing any invasive procedures. There is no reliable evidence of a need for antibiotic prophylaxis before dental treatment in most patients with prosthetic joints, and the risks from adverse reactions to antibiotics probably exceed any benefit.

Patients with joint prostheses because of RA may possibly require antibiotic cover before surgical procedures since they are regarded as mildly immunocompromised. A few cases are treated with corticosteroids. Some treatments induce neutropenia, thrombocytopenia or a bleeding tendency.

The drugs used in RA can be a cause of oral side-effects, such as ulcers and lichenoid reactions (Table 16.9). NSAIDs, gold and low-dose methotrexate may cause ulceration.

Felty syndrome

Felty syndrome comprises RA, splenomegaly and lymphadenopathy, and is managed as RA. These patients are at risk from infections because of leukopenia. Management can also be complicated by anaemia and mild thrombocytopenia. Orofacial manifestations may include severe ulceration or oropharyngeal infections, including chronic sinusitis.

Juvenile rheumatoid arthritis

General aspects

There are many types of juvenile arthritis, one of which resembles adult RA; another has features in common with ankylosing spondylitis. Juvenile rheumatoid arthritis (JRA) is uncommon compared with adult RA, but can be considerably more severe.

Table 16.9 Drugs in rheumatoid arthritis: oral adverse effects

Drugs	Adverse effects
Antimalarials	Lichenoid reactions
	Hyperpigmentation
Anti-tumour necrosis factor (TNF) agents	Candidosis
	Other infections
	Erythema multiforme
	Ulceration
	Cancer?
Corticosteroids	Candidosis
Gold	Lichenoid reactions
	Ulceration
Leflunomide	Candidosis
	Salivary swelling
	Taste disturbance
Methotrexate	Ulceration
Non-steroidal anti-inflammatory drugs (NSAIDs)	Lichenoid reactions
	Ulceration
Pencillamine	Lichenoid reactions
	Loss of taste
	Severe ulceration

Clinical features

One important form of JRA predominantly affects girls in late childhood, involves virtually any joint and is associated with rheumatoid nodules, mild fever, anaemia and malaise. Over 50% develop severe arthritis and deformity.

General management

RF is positive in most cases and ANA are present in 75%. Management is as for RA.

Dental aspects

Damage to the TMJ of various types has occasionally been described. Complete bony ankylosis has been reported and micrognathia may develop in 4–25%. Chronic use of aspirin may occasionally cause tooth erosion.

Psoriatic arthritis

Psoriatic arthritis can affect the lower spine and sacroiliac joints in particular. Joint disease can closely resemble RA but is usually milder. There are no characteristic serological abnormalities. General management is with NSAIDs or methotrexate. Anti-TNF agents are available for use in psoriatic arthritis.

Psoriatic arthritis of the TMJ is rare. Oral mucosal lesions, histologically verified as oral psoriasis, are occasionally seen. Methotrexate or anti-TNF agents may cause oral ulcers.

Temporomandibular pain–dysfunction syndrome

See Chapter 13.

Gout

In gout, deposits of sodium urate monohydrate crystals in the joints result in the release of lysosomal enzymes from polymorphonuclear leukocytes, causing acute inflammation. Gout may be primary or secondary.

Primary gout is an inborn error of metabolism causing raised plasma urate levels (hyperuricaemia). It mainly affects adult men; food or drink rich in purines (e.g. fish roe) can precipitate an attack in those with the underlying metabolic disorder. Ethanol favours conversion of pyruvate to lactate, which impairs renal excretion of urate, so an alcoholic 'binge' (especially with beer) can precipitate an attack. Some forms of primary gout are inherited in an autosomal dominant manner, while in others there is evidence of polygenic inheritance.

Secondary gout is usually caused by cell breakdown from drug treatment or radiotherapy for myeloproliferative diseases, which releases large amounts of purines into the blood. Hyperuricaemia is common but usually symptomless.

Gout of either type is aggravated or can be caused by diuretics (thiazides and loop diuretics), which impair renal excretion of uric acid. Women are not significantly at risk from gout until after the menopause.

Lesch–Nyhan syndrome, deficiency of hypoxanthine–guanine phosphoribosyltransferase (HGPRT), is a rare cause of gout, associated with learning impairment, choreoathetosis and compulsive self-mutilation. The lips are chewed and self-inflicted injuries, especially to the face and head, despite the pain it obviously causes, are typical.

Clinical features

Many gouty patients are obese, and there is a high incidence of hyperlipidaemia, hypertension, diabetes and atherosclerosis. An acute attack of gout causes sudden and intensely severe joint pain, usually in the large toe, associated with fever, leukocytosis and raised serum uric acid. Gouty tophi are masses of urate crystals, which, in joints, interfere mechanically with function and also destroy bone and cartilage to cause a severe deforming arthritis. Extra-articular tophi typically form in the helix of the ear as conspicuous, almost white, hard, subcutaneous nodules. Chronic tophaceous gout is often associated with renal disease (gouty nephropathy), which, unless treated, leads to fatal renal failure in up to 25%.

General management

Blood chemistry shows raised uric acid levels. Secondary gout should be investigated to establish the underlying disorder.

Colchicine, etoricoxib, naproxen and indometacin relieve an acute attack but can cause severe adverse effects. Anti-inflammatory analgesics are therefore used but aspirin, which interferes with uricosuric agents, should not be given. Allopurinol reduces the frequency of acute gouty attacks by inhibiting xanthine oxidase, conversion of xanthine to uric acid, and purine synthesis. In severe cases, uricosuric agents, such as probenecid or sulfinpyrazone, can be used in addition to increase urate excretion. In very few patients (less than 1%) with diminished HGPRT activity, allopurinol does not work and the drug can, rarely, cause xanthine renal stones to form. Activation of 6-mercaptopurine and azathioprine, both purine antimetabolites, depends on HGPRT; consequently, these drugs are not effective in Lesch–Nyhan syndrome.

Dental aspects

Gout affects the TMJ only rarely. Drugs used for the treatment of gout, particularly allopurinol, can occasionally cause oral ulceration.

Hypertension, ischaemic heart disease, cerebrovascular disease, diabetes and renal disease may affect dental management. Aspirin is contraindicated, as it interferes with uricosuric drugs. The incidence

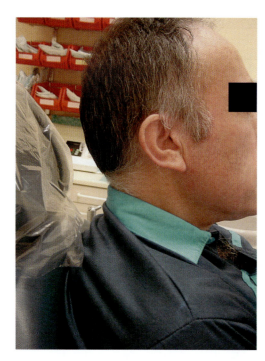

Fig. 16.17 Ankylosing spondylitis in this patient did not permit him to place his neck on the headrest.

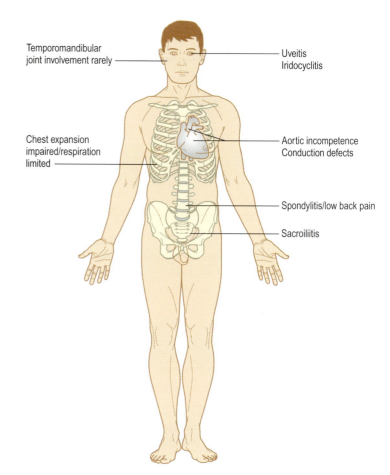

Fig. 16.18 Ankylosing spondylitis.

of rashes with ampicillin, but not other penicillin allergies, is greater in patients on allopurinol.

Calcium pyrophosphate deposition disease involves deposition of calcium pyrophosphate in and around joints in conditions of high plasma calcium, low phosphate or low magnesium. It manifests similarly to gout and is treated with NSAIDs and by correction of the metabolic disturbance.

Ankylosing spondylitis

General aspects

Ankylosing spondylitis is a seronegative spondyloarthropathy (predominantly affecting the spine), seen mainly in young males. The inflammation involves the insertions of ligaments and tendons, and is followed by ossification, forming bony bridges that fuse adjacent vertebral bodies or other joints. Ankylosing spondylitis is genetically determined in part; the family history may be positive and in Caucasians over 90% are positive for HLA-B27.

Clinical features

Ankylosing spondylitis onset is usually insidious, with low back pain (spondylitis) and stiffness, followed by worsening pain and tenderness in the sacroiliac region due to sacroiliitis. Hip joints may also be involved. Over the course of years, the back becomes fixed (Fig. 16.17), usually in extreme flexion, and chest expansion becomes limited and respiration impaired. About 25% develop eye lesions (acute uveitis or iridocyclitis) and about 10% develop cardiac disease (aortic incompetence or conduction defects; Fig. 16.18).

General management

ESR is raised, HLA-B27 is often positive and there is a mild anaemia, but no other significant laboratory findings – and no autoantibodies. Radiography shows progressive squaring-off of vertebrae (which become

rectangular), intervertebral ossification ('bamboo spine'), calcification of tendon/ligament insertions and obliteration of the sacroiliac joints.

Treatment consists of: physiotherapy and exercises; anti-inflammatory analgesics to control pain and allow the back to be kept as mobile as possible (indometacin may be used); and anti-TNF agents. Radiotherapy to the spine is occasionally given but carries the risk of leukaemia.

Dental aspects

Ankylosing spondylitis can affect the TMJ in about 10%, especially those aged over 40 with widespread disease, but symptoms are usually mild. GA can be hazardous because of severely restricted opening of the mouth, impaired respiratory exchange associated with severe spinal deformity or cardiac disease (aortic insufficiency).

Reactive arthritis or seronegative spondyloarthropathy (Reiter disease)

This comprises arthritis, urethritis and conjunctivitis, but there are numerous other effects and it is more appropriate to speak of reactive arthritis or seronegative spondyloarthropathy. It may follow a range on infections (Box 16.8).

Box 16.8 *Aetiology of reactive arthritis*

- Sexually transmitted infections with *Chlamydia trachomatis* (urogenital reactive arthritis)
- Gut infections, such as with *Shigella flexneri*, *Salmonella typhimurium*, *Yersinia* or *Campylobacter* (enteric or gastrointestinal reactive arthritis)
- Respiratory infections with *Chlamydia pneumoniae*

Reactive arthritis typically begins about 1–3 weeks after infection; it is itself not contagious but the causative bacteria can be passed from person to person or affect many individuals who acquire it from the same source. It most often targets males between 20 and 40 years of age, about 80% of whom are HLA-B27–positive.

Clinical features

Seronegative spondyloarthropathy often affects and causes symptoms in the urogenital tract, particularly the prostate or urethra in men, and the urethra or, rarely, the uterus or vagina in women. Joint symptoms typically include pain and swelling in the knees, ankles and feet. Approximately 50% have low back and buttock pain. Eye involvement usually takes the form of conjunctivitis and uveitis, with eye redness, pain and irritation, and blurred vision. Characteristic skin lesions are small, hard nodules of hyperkeratotic thickening, which can be gross, and affect the palms and soles (keratoderma blenorrhagica). The penis may show painless circinate lesions (circinate balanitis), and similar lesions may be seen in the mouth. The symptoms usually last 3–12 months, although they can return or develop into long-term disease in a few.

General management

There is no specific diagnostic test for seronegative spondyloarthropathy, which is usually diagnosed by the exclusion of other arthritides, the finding of a raised ESR and leukocytosis, and the demonstration of causal microorganisms or antibodies to them.

Treatment may include antibiotics for up to 3 months to eliminate the triggering of bacterial infection. Anti-inflammatory analgesics help control the acute phase. Corticosteroid injections are used if NSAIDs are unsuccessful. Other immunosuppressives, TNF inhibitors, sulfasalazine, methotrexate, etanercept or infliximab may be effective if other treatments fail.

Dental aspects

The most characteristic lesion is a pattern of painless scalloped white lines surrounding reddish areas and closely resembling one variant of migratory glossitis (geographic tongue), but affecting any part of the mouth. Oral ulcers or other lesions may be frequent but are transient and often unnoticed.

Infective arthritides

Infective (pyogenic) arthritides are rare but may follow penetrating wounds, extension from adjacent septic areas or extension by bloodstream spread. Possible causal agents include *Neisseria gonorrhoeae*, *Haemophilus influenzae*, *Staphylococcus aureus*, *Mycobacterium tuberculosis*, *Salmonella* or *Borrelia* (Lyme disease). Oral microorganisms are only rarely implicated.

Pain, limitation of movement, swelling and erythema may be evident (Fig. 16.19). Ankylosis can be a complication.

Infective arthritides are an emergency; joint fluid should be sent for microbiological examination and culture, and antibiotics given. Empirical treatment, given until the causal agent is known, is flucloxacillin intravenously plus fusidic acid or, in penicillin-allergic patients, clindamycin. Gentamicin is added if the patient is immunocompromised.

Lyme disease

General aspects

Lyme disease is caused by the spirochaete *Borrelia burgdorferi*, transmitted mainly by insects (*Ixodes* ticks from deer mainly). It is

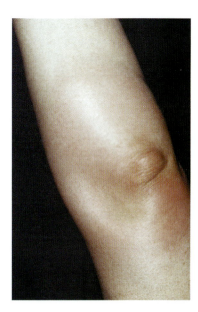

Fig. 16.19 Infective arthritis.

considerably more common in the USA (first described in Lyme, Connecticut) than in other countries, but cases are seen in most parts of the world and it is spreading in most areas, possibly as global warming increases the range of habitats of the vectors.

The risk of Lyme disease is mainly to those who live or work in or close to areas surrounded by tick-infested woods or overgrown brush. Lyme disease is not transmitted between humans.

Clinical features

The first sign is usually a red 'bull's-eye' rash (erythema migrans) that spreads outwards from the site of the insect bite. Tiredness, fever, headache, stiff neck and muscle aches are common. Arthritis may develop in the acute phase and be transient, or later persistent, most typically affecting the knees severely. Chronic arthritis can be a late complication. Neurological involvement may result in facial palsy. Cardiac disease, such as atrioventricular block, myopericarditis or cardiomegaly, is uncommon.

General management

Antibiotic treatment for 3–4 weeks with doxycycline or amoxicillin is generally effective in early disease but early treatment does not necessarily prevent development of chronic arthritis.

Cefuroxime axetil or erythromycin can be used for persons allergic to penicillin or who cannot take tetracyclines.

Dental aspects

Facial palsy and lymphadenitis may be seen. TMJ involvement is rare, even in endemic areas.

MUSCLE

Muscle fibres contain specialized structures for excitation–contraction coupling to ensure that a contractile stimulus (received at the synapse) is quickly and evenly communicated to the whole fibre. Force production occurs in the *myofibrils*, which are chains of sarcomeres running from one end of the fibre to the other. Contractile forces are closely linked to the myosin heavy chain isoform expressed by the fibre responsible for force generation. Myosin is a protein composed of a globular head with adenosine triphosphate (ATP) and actin binding sites, and a long tail involved in its polymerization into myosin filaments. Actin is the other major protein in force production. Troponin is the major regulator of force production. Titin maintains the neatly ordered striation pattern of skeletal (striped) muscles by anchoring myosin to actin. Nebulin acts as a molecular ruler, regulating the length of actin filaments.

ATP is the immediate source of energy for muscle contraction. Energy for contraction comes from the metabolism of fatty acids and sugars. Fatty acids are the major source of energy during normal activities and are derived from fats broken down to acetyl coenzyme A, which is then oxidized by the same citric acid cycle involved in the metabolism of glucose. Blood glucose diffuses into the muscle cytoplasm and is locked there by phosphorylation. A glucose molecule is then rearranged slightly to fructose and phosphorylated again to fructose diphosphate. Glucose is metabolized anaerobically in the cytoplasm but this is only moderately efficient. Aerobic metabolism is more efficient, but requires oxygen and takes place in the mitochondria. Creatine phosphate is one of the other important energy stores, a source for high-energy phosphate groups with which to replenish ATP, particularly in fast-twitch glycolytic fibres.

Anabolic steroids work by increasing synthesis of muscle proteins. Muscle cells are embedded in a basal lamina of collagen and large glycoproteins, between which are satellite cells important in the growth and repair of the fibres.

MUSCLE DISEASES

When weakness is limited to one side of the body, a stroke may be responsible (Ch. 13); weakness that affects the body below a certain level may be caused by a spinal cord disorder (Ch. 13).

Weakness that affects muscles of the upper arms and legs more than the hands and feet may indicate a disorder that affects all muscles (myopathy). Myopathies tend to affect the largest muscles first; the person may have difficulty combing hair or climbing stairs. When the hands and feet are weaker than the upper arms and legs, the problem is often a polyneuropathy, which tends to affect the longest nerves first (those in the hands and feet). The affected person may thus have the most trouble with fine finger movements. Strength that decreases with repetitive activity suggests myasthenia gravis.

Muscle diseases (myopathies) are uncommon and rarely cause oral manifestations or affect dental management. The genetic myopathies, which comprise the muscular dystrophies and the myotonic disorders, have the most significance but are uncommon. Acquired myopathies are rare but significant; metabolic myopathies are tabulated in Appendix 16.3.

GENETIC MYOPATHIES

Muscular dystrophies

General and clinical aspects

Muscular dystrophies, the main crippling diseases of childhood, are a group of uncommon genetically determined diseases characterized by degeneration of muscle leading to progressive weakness (Table 16.10).

Duchenne muscular dystrophy – a recessive sex-linked disorder that results from lack of a specific muscle protein, dystrophin – is the most common. Complications include loss of ability to walk, deterioration of lung and cardiac function, and, often, early death. The pelvic girdle is affected first and the disease becomes evident as the infant begins to walk with a waddling gait and severe lumbar lordosis. The child has difficulty in standing and, after lying down, typically has to climb up his legs in order to stand (Gower sign). The shoulder girdle is also weak and winging of the scapulae is characteristic. Weakness spreads to all other muscles but tends to spare those of the head, neck and hands.

The affected muscles enlarge (pseudohypertrophy) but the child is crippled and, before puberty, becomes confined to a wheelchair. Cardiac disease (cardiomyopathy), respiratory impairment and intellectual deterioration appear at an early stage, and patients usually die in their twenties.

Table 16.10 Muscular dystrophies

Type	Inheritance	Muscles affected	Pseudo-hypertrophy	Onset	Progress	Other features
Duchenne	X-linked	All	Usual	Early childhood	Rapid	Cardiomyopathy
						Death in early adulthood
Becker	X-linked	All	Usual	Late childhood	Variable	More benign than Duchenne type
Childhood	AR	All	Usual	Late childhood	Variable	More benign than Duchenne type
Limb girdle	AR	Pelvic and shoulder girdles	Occasional	Adolescence	Variable	Severely disabling
						May be cardiomyopathy
Facioscapulohumeral	AD	Starts in face and shoulder	Rare	Adolescence	Slow	Most benign type
						Normal life expectancy
						Pouting of lips with facial weakness
Scapuloperoneal	AD or X-linked	Scapular	Occasional	Adolescence	Slow	Cardiac conduction defects
		Peroneal				Relatively benign
		All				
Congenital muscular	AR	All	Rare	Birth	Variable	Possible joint deformities
Distal myopathy	AD	Distal	Rare	Any age	Slow	–
Oculopharyngeal	AD	Facial and sternomastoid	Rare	Adult	Slow	Dysphagia may be prominent
						Weakness of masticatory muscles and tongue

AD/AR = autosomal dominant/recessive.

Dental aspects

In those muscular dystrophies where there is facial myopathy (classically in the facioscapulohumeral type), there is lack of facial expression and, often, inability to whistle. Malocclusions, especially expansion of the arches, may be seen, but there is no abnormal susceptibility to dental disease. Cardiomyopathies and respiratory disease are contraindications to GA. Muscular dystrophy may also predispose to malignant hyperthermia (Ch. 23).

Myotonic disorders

Myotonic disorders are characterized by abnormally slow relaxation after muscle contraction. *Dystrophia myotonica* – the most disabling myotonic disorder – can lead to ptosis (Fig. 16.20), progressive facial weakness, cataracts, testicular atrophy and frontal baldness. The onset is typically in the third decade. Complications include cardiac conduction defects, respiratory impairment, mild endocrinopathies, intellectual deterioration and personality changes.

Myotonia congenita (Becker type) appears late in childhood and is characterized by muscle hypertrophy.

Myotonia congenita (Thomsen disease), a generalized myotonia without weakness, starting in infancy.

Paramyotonia congenita causes myotonia and weakness after exposure to cold.

Dental aspects

In dystrophia myotonica, there is atrophy of the temporalis, masseter and sternomastoid muscles (producing a swan-neck appearance), and sometimes distal limb weakness and wasting. Myotonia in the tongue causes difficulty in speaking (dysarthria) and there may also be problems with masticating food. Atrophy of the masticatory muscles leads

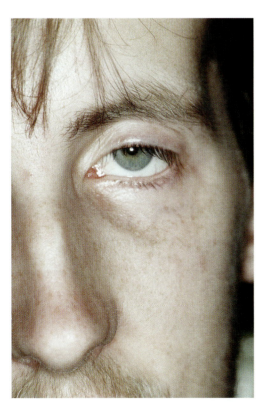

Fig. 16.20 Ptosis in dystrophia myotonica.

to an open mouth posture. There may also be dysphagia, dysarthria and dental caries.

GA may be a risk because of cardiac conduction defects, suxamethonium sensitivity, respiratory impairment, behavioural problems or malignant hyperthermia. Patients may have dental management problems resulting from treatment with corticosteroids or phenytoin.

ACQUIRED MYOPATHIES

Polymyalgia rheumatica

General aspects

Polymyalgia rheumatica is an uncommon disorder characterized by muscle pain and stiffness, which is sometimes accompanied by cranial arteritis (Ch. 13). Women are predominantly affected, usually after the age of 55.

Clinical features

There is pain, stiffness and weakness across the shoulders, in the upper arms and in the pelvic region, radiating into the thighs.

General management

The ESR is typically raised and electromyography (EMG) normal. Biopsy may be helpful. Small doses of corticosteroids usually give rapid relief but in most cases the disease is ultimately self-limiting after 1–2 years or longer.

Dental aspects

Orofacial manifestations are present if cranial arteritis is associated.

LA is safe. CS can be given if required. Corticosteroid treatment may be associated with its usual problems (Ch. 6).

Myasthenia gravis

General aspects

Myasthenia gravis (MG) is a chronic autoimmune disorder that causes weakness and rapid fatigue of voluntary muscles, and usually affects women between 20 and 30. Circulating autoantibodies to the nicotinic acetylcholine (ACh) receptor proteins on the post-synaptic membrane of the neuromuscular junction, detected in 85%, damage the receptor so that the response of the muscle to ACh is weak. These autoantibodies in 75% of cases suggest thymic hyperplasia and, in the remainder, a thymoma.

Occasional cases of MG are associated with carcinoma (Eaton–Lambert syndrome), drugs (penicillamine can also result in anti-ACh receptor antibodies) or other diseases.

Clinical features

Typically, the extraocular muscles and the muscles of face, tongue, neck and extremities are severely affected. Ptosis and diplopia are common early features. Disability is worsened by fatigue of the muscles, particularly towards the end of the day, but improves with rest. Other factors that can make MG worse include illnesses such as a cold, stress and overexertion.

MG can cause difficulties with speech, chewing and swallowing, as well as weakness of limbs. Speech may have a nasal quality. Problems

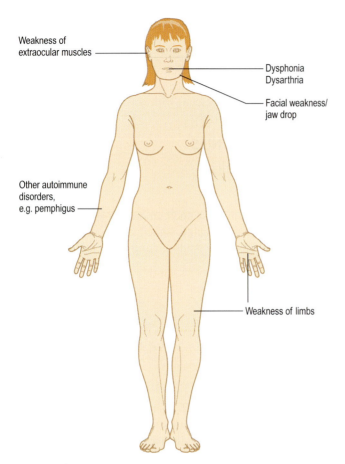

Weakness of
extraocular muscles

Dysphonia
Dysarthria

Facial weakness/
jaw drop

Other autoimmune
disorders,
e.g. pemphigus

Weakness of limbs

Fig. 16.21 Myasthenia gravis.

with swallowing, with nasal regurgitation of food and drink, may also develop (Fig. 16.21). The muscle weakness can lead to a variety of symptoms, including difficulties in:

- swallowing or mastication, causing frequent gagging, drooling or choking
- climbing stairs, lifting objects or rising from a seated position
- talking
- holding the head up
- maintaining a steady gaze
- breathing.

The Myasthenia Gravis Foundation of America Clinical Classification is as follows:

- Class I: Any eye muscle weakness, possible ptosis, no other evidence of muscle weakness elsewhere
- Class II: Eye muscle weakness of any severity, mild weakness of other muscles
- Class IIa: Predominantly limb or axial muscles
- Class IIb: Predominantly bulbar and/or respiratory muscles
- Class III: Eye muscle weakness of any severity, moderate weakness of other muscles
- Class IIIa: Predominantly limb or axial muscles
- Class IIIb: Predominantly bulbar and/or respiratory muscles
- Class IV: Eye muscle weakness of any severity, severe weakness of other muscles
- Class IVa: Predominantly limb or axial muscles
- Class IVb: Predominantly bulbar and/or respiratory muscles (can also include feeding tube without intubation)
- Class V: Intubation needed to maintain airway.

There is a potentially fatal complication of MG respiratory muscle involvement, particularly in the older patients: respiratory insufficiency may result from either the disease (myasthenic crisis) or treatment (cholinergic crisis).

Thymic disease is common and can also depress immunological responses; 10–25% have thymoma. There is also an uncommon syndrome of thymoma, myasthenia gravis, depressed cell-mediated immunity, chronic mucocutaneous candidosis and haematological disease (Good syndrome; Ch. 20).

General management

Examination may show muscle weakness – eye muscles are usually affected first – with normal reflexes and sensation. The diagnosis is made from the clinical features and confirmed by an edrophonium (anticholinesterase) test, sometimes supported by electrodiagnostic tests and detection of serum antibodies to ACh receptors. Other investigations that may be helpful include:

- antibodies against MUSK (muscle-specific kinase); these patients do not have evidence of thymus pathology
- HLA-B8 and DR3, with DR1 more specific for ocular myasthenia
- EMG and nerve conduction studies
- chest imaging: thymic disease should be excluded by mediastinal CT or MRI.

Myasthenia gravis very occasionally remits spontaneously but in those with thymoma the prognosis is poor. The following may be recommended:

- Scheduling of rest periods
- An eye patch (if diplopia is bothersome)
- Avoidance of stress and heat exposure (which can aggravate symptoms)
- Neostigmine or pyridostigmine
- Corticosteroids and other immunosuppressants
- Plasmapheresis
- Thymectomy.

Dental aspects

The most obvious features are facial muscle weakness, diplopia, ptosis and voice changes. Facial weakness may cause a snarling appearance as the patient attempts to smile. Weakness of the masticatory muscles may cause the mouth to hang open (hanging or lantern jaw sign) and patients typically tend to support the jaw with their hand. Occasionally, there is also furrowing, atrophy or paresis of the tongue or uvula palsy.

Occasionally, Sjögren syndrome or other autoimmune disorders, particularly pemphigus, may be associated. If there is a thymoma, there may be chronic candidosis. Salivation is increased if an anticholinesterase is being taken.

Dental treatment is best carried out during a remission, preferably early in the day, within 1–2 hours of routine medication with anticholinesterases, and with short appointments, since weakness increases during the day and fatigue or emotional stress may precipitate a myasthenic crisis.

LA is preferred but minimal doses should be given: lidocaine, prilocaine or mepivacaine can safely be used. A small oral dose of a benzodiazepine may be given if the patient is anxious, but intravenous sedation must not be given in the dental surgery since bulbar or respiratory involvement impairs respiration. GA is an issue. Many drugs used in GA, such as opioids, barbiturates, suxamethonium, curare or anaesthetic agents, are potentiated by or aggravate the myasthenic state. Postoperative respiratory infection can result and may also cause myasthenia to worsen.

Drugs that can also worsen myasthenia and should be avoided include beta-blockers, lithium, phenytoin and some antimicrobials (aminoglycosides, clindamycin, lincomycin, quinolones, sulphonamides, tetracyclines). Penicillin or erythromycin can be used safely unless there are other issues. Occasionally, aspirin has caused a cholinergic crisis in those on anticholinesterases; paracetamol (acetaminophen) and codeine do not have this potential disadvantage.

Corticosteroids, other immunosuppressants or emotional lability may also complicate dental treatment.

Myositis ossificans

Myositis ossificans is a rare condition in which there is ossification in muscles (muscles turn to bone). Two types are recognized.

Myositis ossificans is an autosomal dominant genetic disorder with overexpression of bone morphogenetic protein 4 (BMP4) mapped to chromosome 14. The most common sites affected are the sternomastoid, paraspinal, masticatory, shoulder and pelvic girdle muscles. The abdominal muscles, extraocular muscles and gastrointestinal tract and tongue muscles are spared. ECG findings may be abnormal, while spirometry may demonstrate a restrictive pattern.

Myositis ossificans circumscripta develops in response to soft tissue injury (blunt trauma, stab wound, fracture/dislocation or surgical incision) or without known injury. Non-documented trauma, repeated small mechanical injuries and non-mechanical injuries caused by ischaemia or inflammation may also be implicated. Most ossifications (80%) arise in the thigh or arm but intercostals, erector spinae, pectoralis and gluteal muscles may be affected.

In both types of myositis ossificans the diagnosis is made by serial radiography. There is no definitive treatment; immediate immobilization with a regime of gradually increased exercise should be arranged. Analgesics, corticosteroids and adrenocorticotropin may be indicated. Genetic counselling is indicated.

KEY WEBSITES

(Accessed 27 May 2013)
BMJ. <http://www.bmj.com/specialties/rheumatology>.
Centers for Disease Control and Prevention. <http://www.cdc.gov/arthritis/index.htm>.
National Institutes of Health: National Institute of Arthritis and Musculoskeletal and Skin Diseases. <http://niams.nih.gov/Health_Info/default.asp>.

USEFUL WEBSITES

(Accessed 27 May 2013)
Arthritis Foundation. <http://www.arthritis.org>.
MedlinePlus. <http://www.nlm.nih.gov/medlineplus/encyclopedia.html>.
National Institutes of Health: Osteoporosis and Related Bone Diseases National Resource Center. <http://www.niams.nih.gov/Health_Info/Bone/>.

FURTHER READING

Abel, M.D., Carrasco, L.R., 2006. Ehlers–Danlos syndrome: classifications, oral manifestations, and dental considerations. Oral Surg. Oral Med. Oral Pathol. Oral Radiol. Endod. 102, 582.

Bagan, J.V., et al. 2005. Avascular jaw osteonecrosis in association with cancer chemotherapy: series of 10 cases. J. Oral Med. Pathol. 34, 120.
Bagan, J.V., et al. 2006. Jaw osteonecrosis associated with bisphosphonates: multiple exposed areas and its relationship to teeth extractions. Study of 20 cases. Oral Oncol. 42, 327.
Bagan, J., et al. 2008. Collagen telopeptide (serum CTX) and its relationship with the size and number of lesions in osteonecrosis of the jaws in cancer patients on intravenous bisphosphonates. Oral Oncol. 44, 1088.
Baltali, E., et al. 2008. A method for quantifying condylar motion in patients with osteoarthritis using an electromagnetic tracking device and computed tomography imaging. J. Oral Maxillofac. Surg. 66, 848.
Baltali, E., et al. 2008. Kinematic assessment of the temporomandibular joint before and after partial metal fossa eminence replacement surgery: a prospective study. J. Oral Maxillofac. Surg. 66, 1383.
Cagla Ozbakis Akkurt, B., et al. 2008. Disease activity in rheumatoid arthritis as a predictor of difficult intubation? Eur. J. Anaesthesiol. 19, 1.
Cartsos, V.M., et al. 2008. Bisphosphonate use and the risk of adverse jaw outcomes. J. Am. Dent. Ass. 139, 23.
Cascone, P., et al. 2008. A new surgical approach for the treatment of chronic recurrent temporomandibular joint dislocation. J. Craniofac. Surg. 19, 510.
De Paepe, A., Malfait, F., 2004. Bleeding and bruising in patients with Ehlers–Danlos syndrome and other collagen vascular disorders. Br. J. Haematol. 127, 491.
Eppley, B.L., et al. 2005. Allograft and alloplastic bone substitutes: a review of science and technology for the craniomaxillofacial surgeon. J. Craniofac. Surg. 16, 981.
Epstein, M., et al. 2012. The effects of osteoclast modifiers on the oral cavity: a review for prescribers. Curr. Opin. Support Palliat. Care 6, 337.
Expert panel recommendations. Dental management of patients receiving oral bisphosphonate therapy. Am. Dent. Assoc. 2006; 137, 1144.
Kao, S.T., Scott, D.D., 2007. A review of bone substitutes. Oral Maxillofac. Surg. Clin. North Am. 19, 513. vi
Khosla, S., et al. 2007. Bisphosphonate-associated osteonecrosis of the jaw: report of a task force of the American Society for Bone and Mineral Research. J. Bone Miner. Res. 22, 1479.
Legout, L., et al. 2012. Antibiotic prophylaxis to reduce the risk of joint implant contamination during dental surgery seems unnecessary. Orthop.Traumatol. Surg. Res. 98, 910.
Little, J.W., et al. 2010. The dental treatment of patients with joint replacements: a position paper from the American Academy of Oral Medicine. J. Am. Dent. Assoc. 141 (6), 667.
Malfait, F., et al. 2004. The natural history, including orofacial features of three patients with Ehlers–Danlos syndrome, dermatosparaxis type (EDS type VIIC). Am. J. Med. Genet. A 131, 18.
Marx, R.E., 2006. Oral and intravenous bisphosphonate-induced osteonecrosis of the jaws: history, etiology, prevention and treatment. Quintessence, Illinois.
National Institute for Health and Clinical Excellence (NICE), 2005. Bisphosphonates (alendronate, etidronate, risedronate), selective oestrogen receptor modulators (raloxifene) and parathyroid hormone (teriparatide) for the secondary prevention of osteoporotic fractures in postmenopausal women. Technology appraisal guidance 87. NICE, London.
Oswald, T.F., Gould, F.K., 2008. Dental treatment and prosthetic joints antibiotics are not the answer!. J. Bone Joint Surg. [Br] 90-B, 825.
Ozcan, I., et al. 2008. Temporomandibular joint involvement in rheumatoid arthritis: correlation of clinical, laboratory and magnetic resonance imaging findings. B-ENT 4, 19.
Ralston, S.H., 2013. Clinical practice. Paget's disease of bone. N. Engl. J. Med. 368 (7), 644.10.1056/NEJMcp1204713 PubMed PMID: 23406029
Reid, I.R., Cornish, J., 2011. Epidemiology and pathogenesis of osteonecrosis of the jaw. Nat. Rev. Rheumatol. 8 (2), 90.
Scott, D.L., 2012. Biologics-based therapy for the treatment of rheumatoid arthritis. Clin. Pharmacol. Ther. 91 (1), 30.10.1038/clpt.2011.278 Epub 2011 Dec 14. Review. PubMed PMID: 22166850
Scully, C., Chaudhry, S., 2008. Aspects of human disease 28. Osteoarthritis. Dent. Update 35, 709.
Scully, C., Chaudhry, S., 2009. Aspects of human disease 29. Rheumatoid arthritis. Dent. Update 36, 61.
Scully, C., et al. 2006. Dental endosseous implants in patients on bisphosphonate therapy. Implant Dent. 15, 212.
Scully, C., et al. 2007. Special care in dentistry: handbook of oral healthcare. Churchill Livingstone/Elsevier, Edinburgh.
Shirota, Y., et al. 2008. Biologic treatments for systemic rheumatic diseases. Oral Dis. 14, 206.
Straub, A.M., et al. 2002. Severe periodontitis in Marfan's syndrome: a case report. J. Periodontol. 73 (7), 823.
Van Sickels, J.E., 2007. Distraction osteogenesis: advancements in the last 10 years. Oral Maxillofac. Surg. Clin. North Am. 19, 565. vii

APPENDIX 16.1 SOME GENETICALLY DETERMINED SKELETAL DISORDERS

Disorder	Features
Achondroplasia	See main text
Albers–Schönberg syndrome	Ch. 37
Albright syndrome	Ch. 37
Apert syndrome	Craniostenosis; syndactyly
Cheney syndrome	Osteoporosis; early loss of teeth
Cherubism	Familial symmetrical self-limiting soft-tissue jaw lesions
Cleidocranial dysplasia	See main text
Congenital hyperphosphatasia	Thickened calvarium; early loss of teeth; visual or hearing defects; blue sclerae
Crouzon syndrome	Hypoplastic mid-face; proptosis; craniostenosis; hearing defects
Ellis–van Creveld syndrome	Atrial septal defect; dwarfism; polydactyly
Gardner syndrome	Ch. 37
Gaucher disease	Ch. 37
Goldenhar syndrome	Same as Treacher Collins syndrome plus epibulbar dermoids
Gorlin syndrome	Ch. 37
Hallermann–Streiff syndrome	Cataracts; mandibular retrognathism; scanty hair
Holt–Oram syndrome	Abnormalities of thumb, wrist and clavicle; atrial septal defect
Hypophosphataemia	Vitamin D-resistant rickets; dentinal anomalies leading to early pulp involvement in caries
Klippel–Feil deformity	Ch. 37
Maffucci syndrome	Ch. 37
Mucopolysaccharidoses	Ch. 23
Noonan syndrome	Ch. 37
Odontomatosis	Multiple odontomas; cirrhosis; oesophageal stenosis
Ollier disease	Multiple enchondromas
Orofacial digital syndromes	Facial anomalies; fraenal hyperplasia; tongue hamartomas; digital anomalies
Osteogenesis imperfecta	See main text
Pierre Robin syndrome	Micrognathia; cleft palate; glossoptosis
Rubinstein–Taybi syndrome	Broad thumbs and toes; maxillary hypoplasia; patent ductus arteriosus
TAR syndrome	Thrombocytopenia, absent radius; atrial septal defect or tetralogy of Fallot
Treacher Collins syndrome	Hypoplastic malars and mandible; palpebral fissures slope down and out; colobomas; hearing defects
van Buchem syndrome	Generalized cortical hyperostosis; facial palsy; optic atrophy; hearing defects

APPENDIX 16.2 AMERICAN ACADEMY OF ORTHOPEDIC SURGEONS AND AMERICAN DENTAL ASSOCIATION (AAOS/ADA) CLINICAL PRACTICE GUIDELINE, 2012

The full guideline is available at: http://www.aaos.org/research/guidelines/PUDP/PUDP_guideline.pdf (accessed 30 September 2013)

SUMMARY OF RECOMMENDATIONS

The following is a summary of the recommendations of the AAOS-ADA clinical practice guideline, Prevention of orthopaedic implant infection in patients undergoing dental procedures. This summary does not contain rationales that explain how and why these recommendations were developed; nor does it contain the evidence supporting these recommendations. All readers of this summary are strongly urged to consult the full guideline and evidence report for this information. We are confident that those who read the full guideline and evidence report will see that the recommendations were developed using systematic evidence-based processes designed to combat bias, enhance transparency, and promote reproducibility.

This summary of recommendations is not intended to stand alone. Treatment decisions should be made in light of all circumstances presented by the patient. Treatments and procedures applicable to the individual patient rely on mutual communication between patient, physician, dentist and other healthcare practitioners.

1. The practitioner might consider discontinuing the practice of routinely prescribing prophylactic antibiotics for patients with hip and knee prosthetic joint implants undergoing dental procedures.
    Grade of recommendation: Limited
    Definition: A Limited recommendation means the quality of the supporting evidence that exists is unconvincing, or that well-conducted studies show little clear advantage to one approach versus another.
    Evidence from two or more "Low" strength studies with consistent findings, or evidence from a single Moderate quality study recommending for or against the intervention or diagnostic.
    Implications: Practitioners should be cautious in deciding whether to follow a recommendation classified as Limited, and should exercise judgment and be alert to emerging publications that report evidence. Patient preference should have a substantial influencing role.
2. We are unable to recommend for or against the use of topical oral antimicrobials in patients with prosthetic joint implants or other orthopaedic implants undergoing dental procedures.
    Grade of recommendation: Inconclusive
    Definition: An Inconclusive recommendation means that there is a lack of compelling evidence resulting in an unclear balance between benefits and potential harm. Evidence from a single low quality study or conflicting findings that do not allow a recommendation for or against the intervention.
    Implications: Practitioners should feel little constraint in deciding whether to follow a recommendation labelled as Inconclusive and should exercise judgment and be alert to future publications that clarify existing evidence for determining balance of benefits versus potential harm. Patient preference should have a substantial influencing role.
3. In the absence of reliable evidence linking poor oral health to prosthetic joint infection, it is the opinion of the work group that patients with prosthetic joint implants or other orthopaedic implants maintain appropriate oral hygiene.
    Grade of recommendation: Consensus
    Definition: A Consensus recommendation means that expert opinion supports the guideline recommendation even though there is no available empirical evidence that meets the inclusion criteria.

(Continued)

The supporting evidence is lacking and requires the work group to make a recommendation based on expert opinion by considering the known potential harm and benefits associated with the treatment.

Implications: *Practitioners should be flexible in deciding whether to follow a recommendation classified as Consensus, although they may set boundaries on alternatives. Patient preference should have a substantial influencing role.*

APPENDIX 16.3 METABOLIC MYOPATHIES

- Endocrine
  - Acromegaly
  - Diabetes mellitus
  - Hyperthyroidism
  - Hypothyroidism
  - Cushing syndrome and steroid therapy
  - Hyperaldosteronism
- Bone disease
  - Hyperparathyroidism
  - Osteomalacia
  - Chronic renal failure
- Drugs
  - Alcohol
  - Diuretics
  - Carbenoxolone
  - Vincristine
  - Cimetidine
  - Tryptophan
- Malignant hyperthermia
- Neuromuscular disorders
  - Peroneal muscular atrophy (Charcot–Marie–Tooth disease)
  - Hypertrophic polyneuritis (Dejerine–Sottas disease)
  - Glycogen storage diseases
  - Mitochondrial myopathies

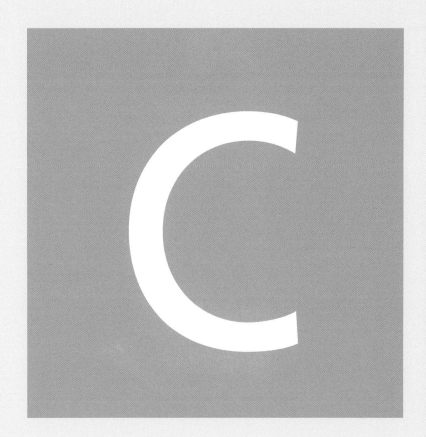

Other systems medicine

KEY POINTS

- Allergic reactions are common and increasing; some are potentially fatal
- Latex allergy is increasingly common
- Allergies may underlie asthma – and many other diseases
- Local anaesthetic allergies are rare

Allergy is an abnormal immune response (usually a type I or type IV hypersensitivity response) to an antigen – a protein or allergen. Many allergies have a hereditary component but the prevalence of allergies appears to be increasing. People who suffer allergies to one type of substance are more likely to suffer allergies to others.

Hypersensitivity responses are summarized in Table 17.1 and common allergens are shown in Table 17.2. Allergies to dental materials are discussed in Chapter 29.

Common allergens are pollen, dust mites, mould, pet dander, milk and egg proteins but, in many cases, the allergen cannot be reliably identified. The most common types of allergic type I hypersensitivity reactions include allergic rhinitis (hay fever), some asthma, eczema and urticaria – so-called 'atopic reactions', which affect about 10% of the population, have a strong genetic basis (and family history), and are related to antibody of immunoglobulin E (IgE) class. The first time an allergy-prone person is exposed to the allergen, T-helper (Th2) lymphocytes produce interleukin-4 (IL-4) and interact with B cells, stimulating them to produce large amounts of IgE antibody. This attaches to receptors on basophils (in the circulation) and mast cells (in the lungs, skin, tongue and linings of the nose and intestinal tract; Fig. 17.1). When the specific allergen is encountered again, the IgE antibody–antigen reaction on basophils and/or mast cells signals them to synthesize chemical mediators (prostaglandins and leukotrienes) and to release others (histamine and heparin, as well as substances that activate platelets and later on attract eosinophils and neutrophils). This produces a rapid type I hypersensitivity response within minutes, which may be anaphylactic and cause bronchospasm and hypotension (Fig. 17.2).

Type IV (delayed) hypersensitivity, seen mainly in contact allergies, arises more slowly and less dramatically, often more than 24 hours after exposure to the allergen; it is mediated by sensitized T lymphocytes, which release cytokines that attract macrophages to the site of exposure. Table 17.3 shows common contact allergens.

Type IV reactions also appear to be involved in the pathogenesis of some chronic diseases that result in granulomas (e.g. tuberculosis, leprosy, sarcoidosis, orofacial granulomatosis and Crohn disease) characterized by foci of chronic inflammatory cells, especially macrophages, that may fuse to produce giant cells, which arise in response to certain antigens (sometimes of an unidentified nature; Box 17.1).

Why allergies appear to be increasing is unclear, but alterations in exposure to microorganisms may be an explanation. Children who live in crowded households, or who attend day care, have fewer allergies, a fact that has been attributed to microbial exposure somehow protecting against allergies. Exposure to bacterial endotoxins reduces release of inflammatory cytokines such as tumour necrosis factor alpha (TNF-α), interferon gamma (IFN-γ), IL-10 and IL-12. Toll-like receptors (TLR), which respond to microorganisms, may also be involved.

CLINICAL FEATURES OF ALLERGIES

Clinical manifestations of an allergic reaction are dependent upon the nature of the response, the antigenic challenge and the individual's allergic predisposition. Early symptoms and signs of a type I (immediate) hypersensitivity reaction include wheezing, breathlessness, sneezing, runny eyes, itching and urticaria, which typically occur within a few minutes to an hour. As the reaction progresses, bronchospasm, acute hypotension and angioedema of the face and laryngopharynx may result in life-threatening anaphylactic shock (Table 17.4).

Contact allergy (type IV delayed hypersensitivity), being a T-cell-mediated process, is characterized by local inflammation at the allergen contact site (skin or mucous membrane), and is usually slower and less profound. Metals, disinfectants, rubber, detergents and bonding agents can cause allergic contact (and irritant contact) dermatitis. Rashes are seen in many allergies (Fig. 17.3).

GENERAL MANAGEMENT OF ALLERGIES

Physical factors (thermal stimuli, sunlight, water, pressure) and drugs may also release histamine in susceptible individuals and cause features

Table 17.1 *Hypersensitivity reactions*

Type	Alternative nomenclature	Mechanisms	Examples
I	Immediate (anaphylactic)	IgE-mediated via mast cell degranulation	Atopic disorders
			Anaphylaxis
II	Cytotoxic	Antibody against membrane-bound surface antigens	Pemphigus
			Idiopathic thrombocytopenic purpura
			Blood transfusion reactions
III	Immune complex	Immune complexes deposited in tissues	Systemic lupus erythematosus
			Rheumatoid arthritis
IV	Cell-mediated	T-lymphocyte–mediated	Contact allergies
			Graft rejection

Table 17.2 *Common allergens*

Source of allergen	Hypersensitivity	Examples
Food products	I	Milk, nuts, egg, shellfish
Drugs	I, III	Aspirin, penicillins, sulphonamides
Environmental	I, IV	Animal hair, dust mite, pollen
Latex	IV, I (rare)	Condoms, dressings, elastic bands, gloves
Dental materials	IV	Amalgam alloy, gold, mercury, resin-based materials

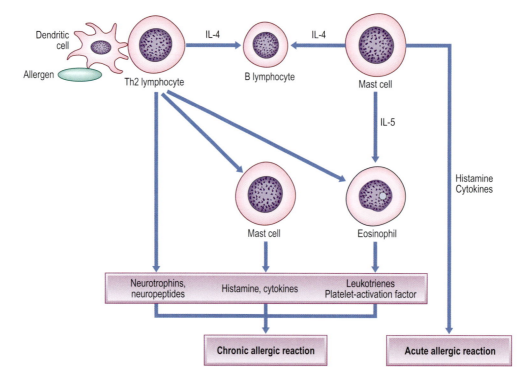

Fig. 17.1 Immunopathogenesis of allergic reactions. IL = interleukin.

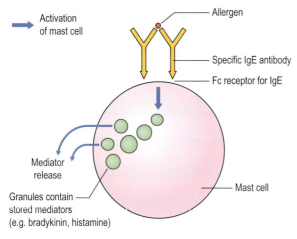

Fig. 17.2 Mast cell involvement in allergies. IgE = immunoglobulin E.

similar to allergies. For example, morphine can directly trigger mast cell histamine release and occasionally causes anaphylactoid reactions.

Diagnosis of an allergy is based on clinical history and presentation, including a family history of allergy; skinprick or patch testing to identify contact allergens using a battery of test allergens (*European Standard Contact Dermatitis Testing Series*; Table 17.5); or an elimination diet to identify food allergens. Patch testing is usually carried out with Finn chambers on Scanpor, a non-woven adhesive skin-friendly tape that contains no colophony. Assays of serum IgE levels (PRIST: *p*aper *r*adio-*i*mmuno*s*orbent *t*est) and serum specific IgE antibodies (RAST: *r*adio*a*llergo*s*orbent *t*est) can help. In the RAST, purified extracts of a range of allergens are coupled to cellulose or paper discs to which the patient's serum is applied. Its ability to react with one or more of these allergens is tested by adding rabbit anti-IgE labelled with radioactive iodine. The level of radioactivity then indicates the levels of specific IgE antibodies.

The *British Standard Series* of 12 allergens, used in addition to those already in the European Standard Series, includes carba mix,

Table 17.3 *Common contact allergens*

Allergens	Sources
Balsam of Peru	Cosmetics, perfumes
Chromate	Bleaches, cement, dental alloys, leather, matches, tattoos
Cobalt	Dental alloys, dental and other prostheses, jewellery, polish stripper
Colophony	Polish, solder flux, sticking plaster, varnishes
Epoxy resins	Glues, resins, PVC products, surface coatings
Ethylenediamine	Antifreeze, creams, paints, rubber
Formaldehyde	Clothing, cosmetics, deodorant, newsprint, shampoo
Mercaptobenzothiazole	Catheters, glues, rubber boots and gloves
Nickel	Clothing clasps, coins, dental alloys, earrings, jewellery, spectacles
Parabens	Cosmetics, skin creams
Paraphenylenediamine	Clothing colour, hair dyes, henna, rubber
Plant allergens	Blister bush (*Diplolophium buchananii*), dahlia, garlic, onion, poison ivy, primula, sesquiterpene lactones (artichoke, boneset, burdock, chamomile, chrysanthemum, cocklebur, gailladrin, lettuce, marsh elder, mugwort, parthenium, poverty weed, pyrethrum, ragweed, sagebrush, sneezeweed, spinach, sunflower, wormwood), tulip bulbs
Plant phototoxins	Celery, fennel, orange, parsley, parsnip
Thiurams	Clothing dyes, fungicides, hair dye, rubber, stockings
Topical medications	Antihistamines (antazoline), benzocaine, chloramphenicol, neomycin, quinoline
Wool alcohols	Cosmetics, skin creams, emollients, lanolin

ethylenediamine, cetearyl alcohol, 2-bromo-2-nitropane-1,3-diol, diazolidinyl urea, chlorocresol, fusidic acid, imidazolidinyl urea and chloroxylenol.

The *Dental Series* typically includes amalgam, amalgam alloying metals, ammoniated mercury, ammonium tetrachloroplatinate,

- Infections
  - Tuberculosis and non-tuberculous mycobacterial infections
  - Leprosy
  - Syphilis
  - Deep mycoses
  - Cat-scratch disease
  - Toxoplasmosis
- Foreign body reactions
  - To zirconium, beryllium, silicone or others
- Disorders of uncertain aetiology
  - Crohn disease
  - Orofacial granulomatosis, cheilitis granulomatosa and Melkersson–Rosenthal syndrome
  - Sarcoidosis
  - Granulomatosis with polyangiitis (formerly called Wegener granulomatosis)
- Some malignant diseases

Table 17.4 *Common clinical features of allergy*

Affected organ	Features
Nose	Sneezing, congested or runny nose and rhinorrhoea (allergic rhinitis)
Sinuses	Post-nasal drip and pain (allergic sinusitis)
Airways	Coughing, wheezing and dyspnoea (asthma or angioedema)
Eyes	Red, itchy, runny eyes (allergic conjunctivitis)
Ears	Discomfort and impaired hearing, due to blocked Eustachian tube (allergic rhinitis)
Skin	Eczema and hives (urticaria)
Gastrointestinal	Abdominal pain, bloating, vomiting, diarrhoea (food allergies)

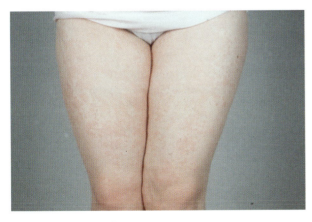

Fig. 17.3 Rash from penicillin allergy.

benzoyl peroxide, bisphenol A (Bis-GMA), diurethane dimethacrylate, ethylene glycol dimethacrylate, eugenol, 2-hydroxyethyl methacrylate (2-HEMA), hydroquinone, menthol, methyl methacrylate, palladium chloride peppermint oil, potassium dicyanoaurate, *N,N*-dimethyl-*p*-toluidine, sodium thiosulfatoaurate and triethylene glycol dimethacrylate.

Table 17.5 *The European Standard Contact Dermatitis Testing Series: some allergens and their sources*

Allergen	Source
Benzocaine	Benzocaine (local anaesthetic)
Cl + Me-isothiazolinone	Isothiazolinone (preservative)
Clioquinol	Clioquinol (antibacterial)
Cobalt chloride	Cobalt (metal)
Colophonium	Rosin and colophony (adhesive)
Epoxy resin	Epoxy resin (adhesive)
Formaldehyde	Formaldehyde and formalin (in clothing, cosmetics, household products)
Fragrance mix	Fragrance and perfume
Lanolin alcohol	Wool fat
Mercaptobenzothiazole	Rubber
Mercapto mix	Rubber
Methyldibromo-glutaronitrile	Preservative
Myroxylon pereirae resin	Balsam of Peru (fragrance)
Neomycin sulfate	Neomycin (topical antibiotic)
Nickel sulfate	Nickel (metal, coins, jewellery)
N-isopropyl-*N*-phenyl-4-phenylenediamine	Rubber
Parabens mix	Parabens (preservative)
4-Phenylenediamine base	Hair dye
Potassium dichromate	Chrome (cement, shoes, metal)
Primin	*Primula obconica* (plant)
Quaternium-15 (Dowicil 200)	Quaternium-15 (preservative)
Sesquiterpene lactone mix	Plant dermatitis (daisies)
4-tert-butylphenol formaldehyde resin	Para-tertiary butylphenol formaldehyde resin (adhesive)
Thiuram mix	Rubber
Budesonide	Topical corticosteroid
Tixocortol pivalate	Topical corticosteroid

No tests, however, can *reliably* predict the possibility of allergic or anaphylactic reactions. Many cases of 'local anaesthesia (LA) allergy' represent untoward events, such as the unintended intravenous injection of the drug, while many cases of 'food allergy' are of food intolerance or occasionally food poisoning only. Supposed phenomena such as systemic 'allergy' to amalgam restorations, 'candida syndrome' and 'total allergy syndrome' are myths.

Medications such as antihistamines or antidepressants that interfere with allergy tests must be stopped from 2 days to 6 weeks or more before testing. Resuscitation facilities must be available during allergy testing, since anaphylactic reactions can occasionally follow intradermal skin test doses, particularly of penicillin. The test procedure includes a positive control (usually histamine), a negative control – a solution without allergens, and then the test – the various suspect allergens. If the test substance provokes an allergic reaction, a raised, red, itchy wheal may develop within about 20 minutes; in general, the larger the reaction, the more sensitive is the patient. A negative skin test means that the patient is not allergic to that particular allergen. A complication of skin testing is that it can induce sensitivity to the test compound.

To avoid future allergic reactions, known allergens should be avoided, which is easier said than done, since sensitive individuals may react to minute traces and allergens can be present in the most unexpected places (more likely in commercially prepared foods and drinks than in natural products).

Table 17.6 *Management of allergies*

Allergen	Avoidance	Other measures
Any	Warning wristbands or bracelets detailing an individual's allergies. Avoid allergens	Patients at risk of anaphylaxis should carry adrenaline (epinephrine) in an EpiPen, Anapen or Twinject for immediate self-administration
Drugs	Accurate documentation of drug allergies in medical notes	Antileukotrienes (leukotriene receptor antagonists), such as montelukast or zafirlukast
Food products	Systematic elimination diets	Corticosteroids
House dust mite	Mite-proof bed linen and wooden floors	Cromoglicate to prevent mediator release
Pets	Avoid or exclude	Antihistamines to relieve itching and oedema
Pollens	Windows should be kept shut and grassy spaces avoided	Bronchodilators for the management of bronchospasm

Table 17.7 *Main precipitants of anaphylaxis*[a]

Latex	Drugs	Foods	Hymenoptera stings
–	Radiocontrast media	Eggs	Ants
	Chemotherapeutic agents	Fish	Bumble bees
	Asparaginase	Milk	Honey bees
	Ciclosporin	Peanuts	Hornets
	Fluorouracil	Shellfish	Wasps
	Methotrexate	Soy	
	Vinca	Tree nuts	
	Antimicrobials	Wheat	
	Cephalosporins		
	Ciprofloxacin		
	Penicillins		
	Sulphonamides		
	Tetracyclines		
	Vancomycin		
	Analgesics		
	Non-steroidal anti-inflammatory drugs (NSAIDs)		
	Opiates		
	Anaesthetics		
	Local anaesthetics		
	Intravenous anaesthetics		
	Heparin		
	Vaccines		
	Immune globulins		
	Insulin		

[a]See also Table 17.9.

Individuals with a complex history of allergy should be referred to a specialist allergy clinic for careful assessment and management. Treatments include drugs to block allergic mediators, or the activation of cells and degranulation (Table 17.6). These include antihistamines, corticosteroids and cromoglicate. Antileukotrienes (leukotriene receptor antagonists, e.g. montelukast or zafirlukast) are also effective. Intravenous injection of monoclonal anti-IgE antibodies (omalizumab), which bind to free and B-cell–associated IgE, causes their destruction. Immunotherapy by desensitization or hyposensitization is a treatment in which the patient is gradually vaccinated with progressively larger doses of the responsible allergen for at least a year – but this is potentially hazardous, as it can induce anaphylaxis.

Patients who have had serious allergic reactions are also usually advised *always* to carry adrenaline (epinephrine) with them, for subcutaneous self-administration in the event of a reaction (e.g. EpiPen; see below).

There is no reliable evidence that supports the use of alternative medicine in the control of allergies.

ANAPHYLAXIS

General aspects

Anaphylaxis is a severe life-threatening type I hypersensitivity reaction, which may affect up to 15% of the population. Hyper-IgE syndromes predispose to anaphylaxis and it is caused mainly by food, drugs, latex and insect stings (Table 17.7).

Clinical features

Bronchospasm, acute hypotension and angioedema of the face and laryngopharynx are the critical features, but there may also be flushing, dizziness and urticaria. The condition may progress to arrhythmias or cardiac arrest. The time to onset is usually indicative of the severity of the reaction (i.e. the more rapid the onset, the more severe the reaction). Most reactions occur within seconds to 30 minutes of exposure to the responsible precipitant.

General management

People at risk *must* avoid the allergens responsible and carry adrenaline (epinephrine) for immediate use to inject into the outer thigh

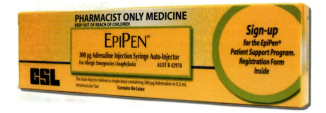

Fig. 17.4 EpiPen.

muscle. Patients should carry 2 EpiPens® with them because >35% of patients may require more than one adrenaline dose and up to 20% of patients will go on to develop a biphasic anaphylactic response sometimes hours later (Fig. 17.4).

ALLERGIC RHINITIS (HAY FEVER)

General aspects

There is often a positive family history. The common specific allergens are inhaled and include pollen, mould, dust mites and pet dander. Pollen from trees such as birch, alder, cedar, hazel, hornbeam, horse chestnut, willow, poplar, plane, linden/lime and olive can be responsible; in northern latitudes, birch is the most important. Grasses, especially ryegrass and timothy, may be responsible, as may various weeds.

Clinical features

Features typically include: itchy eyes, nose, roof of mouth or throat; frequent sneezing, nasal congestion and discharge; lacrimation; and cough. Nasal polyps often develop. In the northern hemisphere, symptoms are particularly prevalent from late May to the end of June.

General management

The best management is to avoid the allergens, if possible, but this can be difficult. Medications include: topical cromoglicate (which inhibits mast-cell release of chemicals) as prophylaxis to nose and eyes or lungs; corticosteroids, such as beclometasone (which suppress the response but take 3–10 days to provide maximum relief); leukotriene receptor antagonists; or antihistamines (which suppress the symptoms but many cause sedation). Non-sedating preparations include fexofenadine, loratadine and terfenadine.

Dental aspects

Patients with allergic rhinitis may be mouth-breathers and develop mild gingival hyperplasia. No oral diseases are known to have any significant direct association with atopic disease, although aphthae and geographic tongue may possibly be more frequent. Antihistamines can cause a dry mouth. Cromoglicate was once used in an attempt to control aphthae. Corticosteroids occasionally induce candidosis.

Azole antifungals, macrolide antibiotics such as erythromycin, human immunodeficiency virus (HIV) protease inhibitors and grapefruit juice can impair metabolism of the antihistamine terfenadine and can lead to arrhythmias (torsades de pointes).

ASTHMA

See Chapter 15.

ECZEMA

See Chapter 11.

ANGIOEDEMA

Causes of angioedema include:

- allergic angioedema:
  - food (fish, shellfish, tree nuts, groundnuts [peanuts])
  - hymenoptera (sawflies, wasps, bees and ants) stings
  - latex
  - medications
- non-allergic angioedema(chronic, recurrent forms):
  - hereditary angioedema (HAE; HANE)
  - idiopathic angioedema
  - medication-acquired angioedema (angiotensin-converting enzyme inhibitors [ACEIs], non-steroidal anti-inflammatory drugs [NSAIDS]).

General aspects

Acute urticaria ('nettle rash') and angioedema are potentially dangerous reactions, which can be triggered when mast cells release histamine and other chemicals into the bloodstream, causing increased blood vessel dilatation and permeability. About 1 in 5 people will experience one of these at one time or another. The risk of urticaria and angioedema is greater if there is a history of urticaria and angioedema, other allergies or a positive family history of allergies.

Angioedema can be life-threatening if swelling blocks the airway.

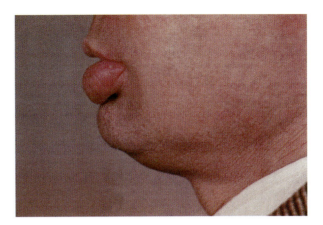

Fig. 17.5 Angioedema.

Table 17.8 *Laboratory findings differentiating the various forms of angioedema*

Type	C4 level	C1-esterase level	C1-esterase function	C1q level
Hereditary angioedema type 1	Raised	Raised	Raised	Normal
Hereditary angioedema type 2	Raised	Normal	Raised	Normal
Acquired angioedema	Raised	Raised	Raised	Raised
Other forms of angioedema	Normal	Normal	Normal	Normal

Allergens that precipitate acute angioedema and urticaria can be: latex; foods (shellfish, peanuts, eggs and milk); drugs (e.g. penicillin, aspirin, ibuprofen, ACEIs and opioids); and animal allergens (mainly pollen, animal dander and insect stings). Physical factors that can release histamine in susceptible individuals (heat, cold, sunlight, water, pressure on the skin, emotional stress and exercise) and immune factors (e.g. blood transfusions, immune disorders, such as lupus or cancer, thyroid disorders and infections, such as hepatitis A or B) are occasionally responsible.

Clinical features

Allergic angioedema typically occurs within several minutes of exposure to an identifiable allergic trigger, including food, medications and insect stings often with acute swelling of the lips, face and tongue. Depending on the severity of the reaction, urticaria, diarrhoea, cough, wheeze, conjunctivitis and rhinitis may also be present. Characteristically, neither ACEI-induced angioedema nor HAE is associated with urticaria, but patients with HAE may have a prodromal serpiginous rash, known as erythema marginatum. Features of urticaria include raised, red, often itchy skin wheals that appear and disappear most commonly where clothes rub the skin. Features of angioedema include non-pitting, asymmetric swelling of the face, lips, tongue, larynx, genitalia and extremities, especially near the eyes and lips, but also inside the throat (Fig. 17.5). Complications can include dyspnoea and anaphylaxis – bronchospasm and hypotension, sometimes causing loss of consciousness or death.

General management

Allergy tests should be made to determine the cause. Blood assays of C4 and C1inh may be indicated (Table 17.8). The standard treatment of allergic angioedema is with antihistamines such as loratadine or cetirazine. H$_2$-receptor antagonists such as cimetidine and ranitidine may help control symptoms. Occasionally, for severe urticaria, systemic corticosteroids of adrenaline given subcutaneously or intramuscularly may be indicated. Montelukast or omalizumab (anti-IgE) are increasingly used.

Dental aspects

Angioedema is characterized by rapid development of oedematous swelling, particularly of the head and neck region. It is the only type of allergy that can involve the oral tissues by causing swelling, particularly the lips or the floor of the mouth. When oedema affects the neck and extends to the larynx, it can cause rapidly fatal respiratory obstruction.

There is possibly a greater risk of sensitization or of acute allergic reactions to drugs used in dentistry. Dental materials (such as mercury), which accidentally come into contact with the patient's skin, can very occasionally provoke contact dermatitis but do *not* affect the oral mucosa.

There are anaesthetic hazards in asthma, and severe asthma or anaphylaxis can occur in the dental surgery (Ch. 15). Problems may be caused by drugs, particularly corticosteroids. Beclometasone dipropionate and betamethasone valerate inhalers can cause oropharyngeal thrush in a minority. Corticosteroids absorbed from ointments used for eczema can cause adrenal suppression. Dry mouth and drowsiness affect patients taking antihistamines.

Although there may be a slightly greater prevalence of allergic diseases associated with aphthous stomatitis, there is little evidence for an allergic mechanism (Ch. 11), though in a very few patients ulceration appears to be precipitated by foods – especially walnuts, chocolate or citrus fruits.

FOOD ALLERGY AND INTOLERANCE

True food allergy, primarily mediated by IgE antibodies to food proteins, is present in 3–4% of adults and the incidence appears to be increasing. There may be a positive family history but the cause is otherwise unclear. There is evidence that breast-feeding for at least 4 months prevents or delays the occurrence of cows' milk allergy, as well as childhood atopic dermatitis and wheezing. Symptoms range from mild mouth-itching ('oral allergy syndrome') to anaphylaxis. Peanut and shellfish allergies, in particular, can be dangerous or even fatal. However, many cases of suspected 'food allergy' are actually due to food intolerance or occasionally food poisoning.

General aspects

Food allergy is an abnormal immune response to a food but is comparatively rare. There may be a positive family history of atopic disease. The most common food allergens are eggs, milk and peanuts in children; and shellfish, fish, nuts and eggs in adults (Table 17.9). Gluten intolerance is discussed in Chapter 7.

Food allergens are proteins that usually are not broken down by the heat of cooking or by gastric acid or digestive enzymes; as a result, they enter the bloodstream, to reach target organs.

Other reactions include allergic eosinophilic reactions that present with oesophagitis, gastritis or gastroenteritis; reactions such as food protein-induced enteropathy (e.g. coeliac disease; Ch. 7), proctocolitis or enterocolitis syndrome (FPIES); milk soy protein intolerance (MSPI); and Heiner syndrome – a lung disease resulting from formation of milk protein/IgG antibody immune complexes.

Table 17.9 *Important allergens in foods*

Food	Main types implicated
Eggs	Hens'
Fish	Cod
Fruit	Apple, cherry, peach, nectarine
Gluten	Wheat, barley, rye
Milk	Cows'
Moulds	–
Mustard	–
Nuts	Peanuts and tree nuts (e.g. walnuts, brazil nuts, almonds, hazelnut)
Sesame	–
Shellfish	Crab, crayfish, lobster, mussels, prawns, shrimp, squid
Soya	
Sulphites	
Vegetables	Carrot, celery, potato

Clinical features

The symptoms may begin as itching in the mouth as the person starts to eat the food responsible, followed by abdominal symptoms (vomiting, diarrhoea or pain). Then, as the food allergens enter the bloodstream, hypotension, urticaria or eczema and bronchospasm can appear.

General management

A detailed patient history and diet diary or an elimination diet, together with skin tests, PRIST and RAST, are needed but confirmation is by double-blind food challenge. Food allergy is treated by dietary avoidance, which is possible if labels are read carefully and care is taken in choosing restaurant-prepared foods. However, many allergy-inducing foods, such as peanuts, eggs and milk, can appear and be unsuspected in prepared dishes.

Symptoms can be relieved by antihistamines and bronchodilators, but patients with severe food allergies can react to minute traces of the allergen. Such patients must always avoid the allergen and should wear medical alert bracelets or necklaces stating that they have a food allergy. If subject to severe reactions, they should always carry a syringe of adrenaline (epinephrine) to self-administer and be prepared to treat an inadvertent exposure instantly.

ORAL ALLERGY SYNDROME

General aspects

Oral allergy syndrome (pollen food allergy syndrome) is an uncommon variant of the reactions described above, usually preceded by hay fever typically associated with birch-pollen allergies, but it can also affect people with allergies to the pollens of grass, mugwort (more common in Europe) and ragweed (more common in North America; Table 17.10).

The precipitating antigens are commonly Proline Rich Polypeptides (PRPs). It can arise as a cross-reaction to proteins in a variety of fresh fruits or their juices (mainly apple, orange, grape and strawberry), vegetables (particularly tomato) and nuts. Cooking often destroys the allergens (except with celery and nuts, which may cause reactions even after being cooked).

Oral allergy syndrome occasionally causes urticaria or anaphylaxis; beans, celery, cumin, hazelnut, kiwi fruit, parsley and white potato are then typically responsible.

Table 17.10 *Causes of oral allergy syndrome*

Pollens	Foods that may trigger an allergic reaction
Birch	Fruits: apple, apricot, cherry, kiwi, nectarine, peach, pear, plum, prune
	Nuts: almond, hazelnut, walnut
	Seeds: sunflower
	Vegetables: anise, beans, caraway, carrot, celery, coriander, cumin, dill, fennel, green pepper, lentils, parsnips, parsley, peas, peanuts, potato, tomato
Grass	Fruits: kiwi, melon, orange, tomato, watermelon
Mugwort	Fruits: apple, melon, watermelon
	Vegetables: celery, carrot
Ragweed	Fruits: banana, cantaloupe, honeydew, watermelon
	Vegetables: cucumber, courgettes

Box 17.2 *Dental materials and health-care products that may cause allergic reactions*

- Denture fixatives
- Essential oils
- Iodides
- Latex
- Metals (amalgam, gold and other alloys, nickel, wires)
- Methylmethacrylate
- Oral health-care products – mouthwashes (including chlorhexidine), toothpastes
- Periodontal dressings
- Resins (colophony, composite and epoxy)
- Rubber base materials

Box 17.3 *People at high risk of latex allergy*

- People with regular occupational exposure: health-care workers, car mechanics, caterers and electronics tradespeople
- People with atopy or dermatitis/eczema (can facilitate the transfer of antigens across the skin)
- Patients frequently exposed to latex: pre-term infants; patients who have undergone multiple surgical procedures; those with spina bifida (up to 60% may be allergic), urogenital anomalies, imperforate anus, tracheo-oesophageal fistula, ventriculo-peritoneal shunts, paraplegia, learning impairment and cerebral palsy
- People allergic to foods with known latex cross-reactivity (see Box 17.4)

Clinical features

Symptoms usually develop within minutes but occasionally more than an hour later. Irritation, pruritus and swelling of the lips, tongue, palate and throat are sometimes associated with other allergic features, such as rhinoconjunctivitis, asthma, urticaria–angioedema and anaphylactic shock.

Some individuals, after peeling or touching the offending foods, may develop a rash, itching or swelling where the juice touches the skin.

General management

Individuals hypersensitive to the foods in Table 17.10 usually find that they can eat them provided that they are well cooked, tinned or microwaved. People who develop symptoms when touching or peeling these foods may prevent them by wearing gloves. Consultation with an allergologist is recommended.

FOOD INTOLERANCE

Food intolerance symptoms can resemble food allergy but enzyme defects, chemicals, additives, toxins or infections are implicated rather than the immune system.

Lactase (a gut enzyme that degrades milk lactose) deficiency is the most common; it is almost universal in people of Chinese origin and common in people of southern European or African descent, affecting at least 1 out of 10 other people. In lactase deficiency, lactose cannot be digested and remains in the gut to be used by bacteria, which produce gas, causing bloating, pain and sometimes diarrhoea.

Histamine (often along with tyramine) is a chemical present in foods such as some cheese, wines and fish (particularly tuna and mackerel); it can provoke a reaction mimicking food allergy.

Additives that may cause reactions that can be confused with food allergy include mainly caffeine, yellow dye number E5, benzoates, salicylates, tartrazine, monosodium glutamate (MSG) and sulphites.

Toxins found in some foods, such as mushrooms and potatoes, and from bacteria in putrefying meat and fish, can cause similar symptoms.

Infections are discussed in Chapter 21.

HYPERSENSITIVITY TO DRUGS AND MATERIALS

*L*atex allergy has become a significant clinical problem, along with *i*odine, *E*lastoplast and *d*rug allergies (hence the acronym LIED). The drugs causing the most severe and potentially fatal reactions are penicillins and intravenous anaesthetic agents. Allergies to other drugs and materials are uncommon.

Patients may be more likely to develop hypersensitivities if they are from an affected family, have atopic disease, have HIV disease or have Sjögren syndrome.

Of the dental materials that can induce reactions (Box 17.2), latex is particularly important. Thus many clinicians have switched to using non-latex (nitrile) gloves and latex-free equipment.

Adverse reactions to other materials and drugs are discussed in Chapter 29.

LATEX ALLERGY

See also Appendices 17.1 and 17.2.

Natural rubber latex (NRL) is manufactured from the sap (latex) of *Hevea brasiliensis*, which is found in Africa and South-East Asia; it is allergenic, as are some of the chemicals added during production. NRL products that are dipped or stretchy (e.g. athletic shoes, babies' bottles, rubber toys, balloons, condoms, gloves, teats and dummies, rubber bands, underwear, waistbands) more frequently cause allergic reactions than do dry rubber products (e.g. tubing, tyres) but by far the most common sensitizer is the rubber in the soles of shoes. Synthetic rubber is made from chemicals and does not trigger allergic reactions in people who are allergic to NRL products. Latex products are common in the home and workplace, including clinics, wards and operating theatres, where allergy is an important occupational problem, especially with abrasive hand-washing, which increases the risk of sensitization.

Allergic reactions have become increasingly common since the widespread use of protective medical/dental gloves following the advent of HIV/AIDS. Latex allergies are also now common in patients who have been frequently exposed to rubber gloves or long-term indwelling urinary catheters (Box 17.3). Latex allergy affects approximately 1%

- Apricots
- Avocados
- Bananas
- Celery
- Cherries
- Chestnuts
- Figs
- Grapes
- Kiwi fruit
- Melons
- Nectarines
- Papaya
- Passion fruit
- Peaches
- Pineapples
- Pistachios
- Plums
- Potatoes
- Strawberries
- Tomatoes

Box 17.5 *Latex in medical items*

- Equipment previously handled with latex gloves
- Anaesthetic masks, props, intubation tubes, airways and other equipment
- Catheters and cannulae
- Tourniquets
- Rubber gloves
- Rubber surgical drains
- Sphygmomanometer cuffs
- Stethoscopes

Box 17.6 *Latex in dental items*

- Equipment and laboratory work previously handled with latex gloves
- Adhesive dressings and their packaging
- Amalgam carrier tips
- Bandages and tapes
- Chip syringes
- Dappens pot
- Endodontic stops
- Gloves
- Gutta percha and gutta balata
- Headgear and head positioners
- Induction masks
- Latex ties on face masks
- Local anaesthetic cartridges[a]
- Mixing bowls
- Needle guards
- Orthodontic elastics
- Prophylaxis cups and polishing wheels and points
- Protective eyewear
- Rubber dam
- Rubber gloves
- Rubber sleeves on props and bite blocks
- Spatula
- Suction tips
- Surgical face masks and other protective items of clothing (e.g. gowns, overshoes)
- Tourniquets and blood pressure cuffs
- Wedges

[a]Latex is present in some rubber dental LA cartridges, stoppers or plungers – either where the harpoon penetrates or where the flat piston end of a self-aspirating syringe rests. At the other end of the cartridge is the diaphragm, which the needle penetrates. Any of these components may contain latex. Although there are no documented reports of allergy due to the latex component of cartridges of dental LA, the UK preparation of prilocaine (Citanest) contains no latex.

of the general population and up to 15% of health-care workers, and is usually due to a contact allergy (type IV delayed hypersensitivity) and only rarely to a type I immediate hypersensitivity reaction. Latex exposure may occur via the skin, mucous membranes or bronchial tree with inhalation of latex glove powder (NRL allergens may attach to lubricating powder and become aerosolized, causing sensitization or, in those allergic, respiratory, ocular or nasal symptoms).

Patients with food allergies to avocado, banana, chestnut, kiwi, papaya, tomato and others (Box 17.4) may show allergen cross-reactivity to latex.

Clinical features

Usually, latex allergy develops after several previous exposures. Symptoms begin within minutes of exposure to latex and may include itching, redness and swelling of skin that touched the item. Anaphylaxis and severe asthmatic reactions have been caused by inhaling latex proteins arising from powder in the latex glove. Latex causes immediate allergic reactions ranging from pruritus to urticaria and, rarely, anaphylaxis (type I) or, more commonly, slower contact dermatitis reactions (type IV), which appear after 24–48 hours and are eczematous. 'Allergic contact dermatitis', caused by chemicals such as thiurams and carbamates used in the manufacture of rubber gloves, manifests with eczema and blisters on the hands starting 1–3 days after wearing the gloves.

General management and dental aspects

Persons with symptoms of type I latex hypersensitivity should be regarded as truly allergic, since testing for latex allergy is problematic; intradermal injection carries the risk of inducing anaphylactic shock and false positives are not uncommon in patients with RAST. Individuals with type IV reactions can have patch testing, but this is difficult to standardize because of variations in latex preparations. Skinprick tests or RAST assays can also be used.

Anything containing, or contaminated by, latex should be avoided; a latex-free clinic and environment is ideal. Latex is found in many items used in hospital clinics, wards and operating theatres (Box 17.5), and even equipment and laboratory work previously handled with latex gloves may elicit an allergic response.

Many items used in dental practice can contain latex (Box 17.6).

Patients with latex type I hypersensitivity (category A)

Latex antigens must particularly be avoided for type I hypersensitivity patients. People with severe allergy reactions should:

- warn clinicians
- wear medical alert identification

Table 17.11 *Treatment of latex-sensitive patients*

History of latex allergy	Drug prophylaxis	Drug regimen
Previous anaphylaxis	Methylprednisolone	1 mg/kg 6-hourly i.v.
		Max. dose 50 mg
	Chlorphenamine	1 month–1 year 250 mcg/kg
		1–5 years 2.5–5 mg
		6–12 years 5–10 mg
Previous allergy with no anaphylaxis (e.g. urticaria, central dermatitis, facial swelling, bronchospasm)	Methylprednisolone	1-mg/kg 6-hourly i.v.
		Max. dose 50 mg
	Chlorphenamine	1 month–1 year 250 mcg/kg
		1–5 years 2.5–5 mg
		6–12 years 5–10 mg

■ carry an adrenaline (epinephrine) auto-injector for emergency treatment.

They should be treated by latex avoidance and in an environment where staff are confident in their ability to manage such problems, particularly anaphylaxis. NRL-free gloves and equipment *must* be used, which may mean specialist management in a hospital latex-free environment; affected persons should contact only latex-free vinyl (polyvinyl chloride), nitrile (acrylonitrile butadiene), vitrile (a blend of vinyl and nitrile), polychloroprene (Neolon), polystyrene–poly(ethylene–butylene)–polystyrene (Tactylon), styrene butadiene, polyurethane or other polymer gloves, medical or dental products. Treatment should be scheduled for the first case of the day, when airborne latex particles should be at the lowest level. Minimum staff should be present.

If there is any possibility of contact with traces of latex, pre-medication prophylaxis with corticosteroids and/or antihistamines may be indicated (Table 17.11).

Patients with unproven latex hypersensitivity (category B)
If the history of latex allergy is dubious, treatment is best carried out as above but without pre-medication. In the absence of a latex-free clinic, care is best offered at the beginning of the day, before environmental levels of latex allergens rise as activity in the surgery continues.

USEFUL WEBSITES

(Accessed 27 May 2013)
Allergy UK. <http://www.allergyuk.org/>.
Anaphylaxis Campaign. <http://www.anaphylaxis.org.uk/what-is-anaphylaxis/signs-and-symptoms>.
British Association of Dermatologists. <http://www.bad.org.uk//site/578/default.aspx>.
Centers for Disease Control and Prevention. http://www.cdc.gov/niosh/topics/asthma/
Health and Safety Executive. <http://www.hse.gov.uk/guidance/index.htm>.
National Institutes of Health: National Institute of Allergy and Infectious Diseases. <http://www.niaid.nih.gov/topics>.
NHS Choices. <http://www.nhs.uk/conditions/Allergies/Pages/Introduction.aspx>.

FURTHER READING

Bhole, M.V., et al. 2012. IgE-mediated allergy to local anaesthetics: separating fact from perception: a UK perspective. Br. J. Anaesth. 108 (6), 903. doi: 10.1093/bja/aes162. Review. Erratum in: Br J Anaesth 2012 Oct; 109(4):669. PubMed PMID: 22593127.

Bismil, Q., et al. 2007. Detecting patient allergy: beware the LIE. Ann. R. Coll. Surg. Engl. 89, 603.
Bush, R.K., 2008. Approach to patients with symptoms of food allergy. Am. J. Med. 121, 376.
Canter, L.M., 2005. Anaphylactoid reactions to radiocontrast media. Allergy Asthma Proc. 26, 199.
Chin, S.M., et al. 2004. Latex allergy in dentistry: review and report of case presenting as a serious reaction to latex dental dam. Aust. Dent. J. 49, 146.
Ciaccio, C.E., 2011. Angioedema: an overview and update. Mo. Med. 108, 354.
Clarke, A., 2004. The provision of dental care for patients with natural rubber latex allergy: are patients able to obtain safe care? Br. Dent. J. 197, 749.
DePestel, D.D., et al. 2003. Cephalosporin use in treatment of patients with penicillin allergies. J. Am. Pharm. Assoc. 2008 (48), 530.
Desai, S.V., 2007. Natural rubber latex allergy and dental practice. N. Z. Dent. J. 103, 101.
Fan, P.L., Meyer, D.M., 2007. FDI report on adverse reactions to resin-based materials. Int. Dent. J. 57, 9.
Field, E.A., et al. 1998. The dental management of patients with natural rubber latex allergy. Br. Dent. J. 185, 65.
García, J.A., 2007. Type I latex allergy: a follow-up study. J. Invest. Allergol. Clin. Immunol. 17, 164.
Garn, H., Renz, H., 2007. Epidemiological and immunological evidence for the hygiene hypothesis. Immunobiology 212, 441.
Greer, F.R., et al. 2008. Effects of early nutritional interventions on the development of atopic disease in infants and children: the role of maternal dietary restriction, breastfeeding, timing of introduction of complementary foods, and hydrolyzed formulas. Pediatrics 121, 183.
Hain, M.A., et al. 2007. Natural rubber latex allergy: implications for the orthodontist. J. Orthod. 34, 6.
Hamann, C.P., et al. 2005. Occupation-related allergies in dentistry. J. Am. Dent. Assoc. 136, 500.
Huber, M.A., Terezhalmy, G.T., 2006. Adverse reactions to latex products: preventive and therapeutic strategies. J. Contemp. Dent. Pract. 7, 97.
Issa, Y., et al. 2005. Oral lichenoid lesions related to dental restorative materials. Br. Dent. J. 198, 361.
Jee, R., et al. 2009. Four cases of anaphylaxis to chlorhexidine impregnated central venous catheters: a case cluster or the tip of the iceberg? Br. J. Anaesth. 103 (4), 614. PubMed PMID: 19749118.
Karabucak, B., Stoopler, E.T., 2007. Root canal treatment on a patient with zinc oxide allergy: a case report. Int. Endod. J. 40, 800.
Kelso, J.M., 2007. Allergic contact stomatitis from orthodontic rubber bands. Ann. Allergy Asthma Immunol. 98, 99.
Kerosuo, H.M., Dahl, J.E., 2007. Adverse patient reactions during orthodontic treatment with fixed appliances. Am. J. Orthod. Dentofacial Orthop. 132, 789.
Kitaura, H., et al. 2007. Treatment of a patient with metal hypersensitivity after orthognathic surgery. Angle Orthod. 77, 923.
Leggat, P.A., Kedjarune, U., 2003. Toxicity of methyl methacrylate in dentistry. Int. Dent. J. 53, 126.
Locke, M., Longman, L., 2012. Latex allergy and dentistry: a review. J. Disability Oral Health 13, 147.
McEntee, J., 2012. Dental local anaesthetics and latex: advice for the dental practitioner. Dent. Update 39, 508.
Morris, D.A., 2004. Contact dermatitis. Curr. Allergy Clin. Immunol. 17, 190.
Noble, J., et al. 2008. Nickel allergy and orthodontics: a review and report of two cases. Br. Dent. J. 204, 297.
Pandis, N., et al. 2007. Occupational hazards in orthodontics: a review of risks and associated pathology. Am. J. Orthod Dentofacial Orthop. 132, 280.
Schweikl, H., et al. 2006. Genetic and cellular toxicology of dental resin monomers. J. Dent. Res. 85, 870.
Scully, C., Chaudhry, S., 2006. Aspects of human disease 7. Allergy. Dent. Update 33, 637.
Sharma, P.R., 2006. Allergic contact stomatitis from colophony. Dent. Update 33, 440.
Torgerson, R.R., et al. 2007. Contact allergy in oral disease. J. Am. Acad. Dermatol. 57, 315.
Trattner, A., et al. 2008. Occupational contact dermatitis due to essential oils. Contact Dermatitis 58, 282.
Vamnes, J.S., et al. 2004. Four years of clinical experience with adverse reaction unit for dental biomaterials. Community Dent. Oral Epidemiol. 32, 150.
Vozza, I., et al. 2005. Allergy and desensitization to latex: clinical study on 50 dentistry subjects. Minerva Stomatol. 54, 237.

APPENDIX 17.1 LATEX ALLERGY

(Adapted from: http://www.hse.gov.uk/latex/dental.htm)

Natural rubber latex products may impact on dental health-care workers (i.e. dentists, nurses, hygienists) because:

1. they are at greater risk of developing NRL allergy through the frequent use of NRL gloves
2. they may need to manage NRL-sensitive patients, which may be either known in advance or previously undiagnosed
3. they have a statutory responsibility to reduce risk of sensitization in themselves, their colleagues and their patients.

Ensure you have and are familiar with:

- a written *policy* – on action to protect staff from developing NRL allergy; on safe accommodation of NRL-sensitive members of staff; for the safe dental management of patients with known or suspected NRL allergy
- an *education programme* to inform new and existing staff
- *posters* for patient and staff information, clearly displayed and on file
- an *occupational health* surveillance programme, which includes pre-employment screening
- a named *responsible person* for managing health and safety.

PREVENTION OF NRL ALLERGIES

It is important that you protect yourself against breaches of the skin barrier that can result from frequent use of skin cleansers and occlusive glove-wear, especially if you have an atopic background (asthma, hay fever or flexural eczema) where damage to the skin from irritants is more common. A compromised skin barrier will increase your chances of developing type IV rubber chemical or type I NRL allergy. Hand-disinfectant agents and protective gloves need to be selected with great care and it is also important to use a suitable aqueous-based emollient at the end of the session and also at other times if your skin has any tendency to dry out.

The British Dental Association (BDA) offers the following tips on hand care:

- Don't wear jewellery (e.g. rings).
- Wash and disinfect hands at the beginning and end of each session, as well as between each glove change.
- Use cool/tepid water when washing, to keep hand temperature down.
- Use hand-wash agents sparingly.
- Rinse thoroughly to remove all traces of hand wash.
- Pat skin dry rather than rubbing it.
- Use soft towels (disposable).
- Ensure hands are dry before putting on gloves.
- Use non-powdered gloves with low levels of NRL proteins and residual chemicals.
- Choose the right size of gloves.
- Minimize contact with other potential irritants/allergens in the surgery (e.g. acrylic powders/antimicrobial solutions).
- Outside work, don't forget to protect hands when gardening/doing household chores, etc.

The Faculty of General Dental Practice UK is presently developing NRL guidelines.

If you or your patients are not NRL-sensitive and you choose to wear NRL gloves to protect yourself from blood-borne pathogens, choose powder-free and low-protein (<50 mcg/g) gloves only.

Ensure that gloves comply with national and international standards of performance (British and European Standard BSEN 455, 1993). These should carry the 'CE' mark.

(See Hand dermatitis and latex allergy, BDA Fact File, May 2008; https://www.bda.org/Images/hand_dermatitis_factfile.pdf; accessed 30 September 2013.)

MANAGEMENT OF SENSITIZED WORKERS

If you suspect that you may be allergic to NRL, it is best to seek a referral to a dermatologist or immunologist via your general practitioner or occupational health physician so that this can be appropriately investigated as soon as signs and symptoms develop.

If you are found to be NRL-sensitive, then it is essential that your work environment is adapted as soon as possible to avoid unnecessary exposure to NRL, which would increase your sensitivity and put you at risk of more severe reactions.

Type I NRL allergy

If you are diagnosed with type I allergy, it may be possible for you to continue to work in the clinical environment, although this depends on the severity of reactions you experience (see earlier).

It is important that you learn to avoid NRL proteins in consumer and medical products both at home and at work. As gloves are the main cause of allergic reactions to NRL, it is essential that you replace NRL gloves with suitable *NRL-free gloves* for yourself and ensure that you are not working in powdered NRL environments (i.e. from the use of powdered NRL gloves worn by colleagues).

A minority of allergic workers can only work symptom free in a strict NRL-free glove environment so it may become necessary for colleagues to switch to using NRL-free gloves too or other modifications to the work environment may be required.

It is recommended that you wear a Medic-Alert® bracelet.

If you have been advised to carry adrenaline (epinephrine) for self-administration (e.g. EpiPen® or Anapen®), colleagues should be instructed on how to use it.

Type IV allergy

If you are diagnosed with type IV allergy to a rubber chemical, then you need to find a glove that does not contain the chemical to which you are allergic. The dermatologist who has diagnosed this should be able to help you with appropriate glove selection.

MANAGEMENT OF A PATIENT WITH TYPE I NRL ALLERGY

(See Field EA, et al. 1998.)

Establish a *patient history* to identify whether your patient needs to be treated in an NRL-safe environment. Questions include the following:

- Has the patient ever experienced an adverse reaction (itch or swelling) to balloons, condoms or household gloves, or associated with surgery, internal examination or dental treatment?

■ Does the patient have an allergy to foods cross-reacting with NRL (e.g. banana, kiwi, avocado, chestnut)?

■ Has the patient experienced hives, asthma or hay-fever symptoms as a result of their work, where latex gloves are used?

Contact with natural rubber latex in dental equipment and products (including medicines) must be avoided in patients with diagnosed or suspected type 1 NRL allergy, and NRL-free alternatives used instead.

Treatment at the beginning of the working day is preferred, before environmental levels of NRL allergens rise with increased activity in the surgery.

Patients with NRL allergy have often been treated in a general dental practice without significant problems when adjustments have been made by the dental team to manage the patient's allergy. However, if the dentist is in doubt or lacks confidence (e.g. managing a highly reactive patient), the patient may need to be referred for appropriate management, possibly in a Community and Primary Dental Services or hospital setting.

All forward planning and documentation should inform future carers of the patient's sensitization by effective recording in notes and the use of *labels for patient notes*.

Possible sources of NRL in dental practice include the following:

■ General:
   Gloves
   Rubber dam and some wedges
   Local anaesthetic cartridges
   Prophylaxis polishing cups
   Orthodontic elastics
   General anaesthesia/sedation equipment, including tubing, face masks, props
   Endodontic stops
   Amalgam carrier tips
   Adhesives and dressings and their packaging
   Equipment and laboratory work previously handled with latex gloves
■ Emergency equipment:
   Oral and nasal airways
   Oxygen masks and nasal cannulae
   Self-inflating bag
   Blood pressure monitor
   Emergency medication

For the more reactive patient or member of staff, other items should be checked for their latex content (e.g. mixing bowls, spatula, chip syringes, needle guards, dappens pot).

MANAGEMENT OF ALLERGIC REACTIONS DURING DENTAL TREATMENT

Ensure that NRL-free emergency equipment and medicines are readily available to treat any allergic reaction from mild (e.g. urticaria and asthma) to severe (i.e. laryngeal oedema/bronchospasm/cardiovascular collapse from anaphylaxis) and that staff are fully trained in resuscitation techniques.

APPENDIX 17.2 LATEX AND LOCAL ANAESTHESIA (LA)

Type	Composition	Dosage
Latex-free LA		
Articaine		
Artikent	Articaine 4% with adrenaline (epinephrine) 1:100 000	2.2 mL cartridge
Bartinest	Articaine 4% with adrenaline 1:100 000	2.2 mL cartridge
Espestesin	Articaine 4% with adrenaline 1:100 000	1.8 mL cartridge
	Articaine 4% with adrenaline 1:200 000	1.8 mL cartridge
Isonest	Articaine 4% with adrenaline 1:100 000	2.2 mL cartridge
Septanest	Articaine 4% with adrenaline 1:100 000	2.2 mL cartridge
	Articaine 4% with adrenaline 1:200 000	2.2 mL cartridge
Lidocaine		
Eurocaine	Lidocaine 2% with adrenaline 1:80 000	2.2 mL cartridge
Lignokent	Lidocaine 2% with adrenaline 1:80 000	2.2 mL cartridge
Lignospan Special	Lidocaine 2% with adrenaline 1:80 000	1.8 and 2.2 mL cartridge
Rexocaine	Lidocaine 2% with adrenaline 1:80 000	2.2 mL cartridge
Utilycaine	Lidocaine 2% with adrenaline 1:80 000	2.2 mL cartridge
Oraqix periodontal gel	Lidocaine 2.5% and prilocaine	2.5% 25 g tube
Xylonor gel	Lidocaine 5% 15 g tube	
Xylonor spray	Lidocaine 10% spray	36 g bottle
Mepivacaine		
Scandonest	Special mepivacaine 2% and adrenaline 1:100 000	2.2 mL cartridge
Scandonest	Plain mepivacaine 3%	2.2 mL cartridge
Prilocaine		
Citanest with Octapressin	Prilocaine 3% and felypressin 0.03 units/mL	2.2 mL standard and 2.2 mL self-aspirating cartridge
Latex-containing LA		
Lidocaine		
Xylocaine	Lidocaine 2% with adrenaline 1:80 000	2.2 mL standard and 2.2 mL self-aspirating cartridge
LA that possibly contains latex		
Emla cream	Lidocaine 2.5% (with or without prilocaine 2.5%	5 g tube
Xylocaine spray	Lidocaine 10% spray	50 mL bottle
Ametop gel	Tetracaine 4%	1.5 g tube

Sources: www.lasg.org.uk/information/aboutnrl-natural-rubber-latex, www.nhsplus.nhs.uk/providers/images/library/files/guidelines/Latex_allergy_guidelines.pdf and www.nelm.nhs.uk/en/NeLM-Area/Evidence/Medicines-Q--A/Which-dental-local-anaesthetics-are-latexfree/

18 Autoimmune disease

KEY POINTS

- Autoimmune conditions are seen mainly in women and with increasing age
- Autoimmune diseases are often associated one with another, and with Raynaud disease and Sjögren syndrome

The normal immune response and tests are summarized in Chapter 19.

Many diseases are immunologically mediated and this is especially notable in allergies and autoimmunity. A genetically determined susceptibility to immunologically mediated diseases is often suggested by a positive family history, and by significant associations with certain major histocompatibility complex (MHC) histocompatibility (human lymphocyte antigen, or HLA) antigens. The genes for histocompatibility antigens are identified by a letter (A–D) and a number (e.g. HLA-D2). This chapter discusses autoimmune disorders – mainly those that affect multiple tissues; organ-specific disorders are discussed in the appropriate chapters (Table 18.1). Autoimmunity is an immune response that destroys normal body tissues. There are more than 80 different autoimmune disorders and they may result in: destruction of body tissue; abnormal growth of or changes in organ function.

The causes of autoimmune disease are unclear but heredity appears to play a role; several polymorphic genes (i.e. *HLA-DRB1*, tumour necrosis factor [*TNF*] and *PTPN22* [protein tyrosine phosphatase non-receptor 22]) influence the susceptibility to different autoimmune diseases. Regulatory T cells (Treg) fail in their function. Many organ-specific autoimmune diseases are associated with HLA-B8 and DR3, but the association is not sufficiently strong to help in the diagnosis. Rheumatoid arthritis, by contrast, is associated with HLA-DR4.

General aspects

Autoimmune diseases are caused by antibodies and T cells directed against self, produced when immune system recognition fails or malfunctions. Autoimmune diseases may be initiated by viruses, drugs, chemicals or other factors, and affect the immune system at several levels. In patients with systemic lupus erythematosus, for instance, B cells are hyperactive while suppressor cells are underactive; it is not clear which defect comes first. Moreover, production of interleukin-2 (IL-2) is low, while levels of interferon-gamma (IFN-γ) are high. Patients with rheumatoid arthritis, who have defective suppressor T cells, continue to make antibodies to common viruses, a response that would normally cease after about 14 days. Some autoantibodies are directed against specific antigens and cause localized disease (e.g. autoantibodies to desmoglein in epithelial intercellular cement, which cause pemphigus; autoantibodies to red blood cells, which cause anaemia; autoantibodies to pancreatic islet cells, which contribute to juvenile diabetes; and autoantibodies to acetylcholine receptors, which are present in myasthenia gravis). Polyglandular autoimmune diseases are examples of autoimmune attack on many organs.

Where autoantibodies are directed against several types of cell and cellular components, including nuclear components such as deoxyribonucleic acid (DNA), ribonucleic acid (RNA) or proteins, then generalized disease, such as systemic lupus erythematosus, may result (see Table 18.1).

Clinical features

Autoimmune diseases share common features (Table 18.2).

General management

The blood picture may show results of autoantibodies against haematological factors (e.g. haemolytic anaemia, thrombocytopenia or leukopenia). Alternatively, there may be leukocytosis associated with inflammatory processes. The erythrocyte sedimentation rate (ESR) and C-reactive protein (CRP) are is often raised. Serum protein levels are also typically increased because of immunoglobulin overproduction. Specific tests for autoimmune disease include assays for serum autoantibodies (see Ch. 2 and Table 18.3). Specific autoantibodies

---

Table 18.1 *Types of autoimmune disease*

Non-organ-specific autoantibodies: the connective tissue diseases[a]	Organ or cell-specific autoantibodies[b]
Raynaud disease	Autoimmune haemolytic anaemia
Lupus erythematosus	Chronic atrophic gastritis (pernicious anaemia)[c]
Rheumatoid arthritis	Hashimoto thyroiditis
Sjögren syndrome	Idiopathic Addison disease
Scleroderma	Idiopathic hypoparathyroidism
Dermatomyositis	Idiopathic thrombocytopenic purpura
Mixed connective tissue disease	Myasthenia gravis
Antiphospholipid syndrome	Pemphigoid
	Pemphigus vulgaris

[a] Probably mediated by immune complex reactions: discussed in this chapter.
[b] Discussed elsewhere in this book (Section B).
[c] Not all chronic atrophic gastritis.

Table 18.2 *Typical features of autoimmune diseases*

Clinical features	Laboratory features[a]
Female predisposition	Hypergammaglobulinaemia
Family history often positive	Autoantibodies specific to tissue under attack sometimes present in the circulation. Circulating autoantibodies often detectable in apparently unaffected relatives. Multiple autoantibodies often detectable but frequently without clinical effect
Response to immunosuppressive treatment in many	Immunoglobulin and complement deposits sometimes detectable by immunofluorescence microscopy at sites of tissue damage (e.g. damaged blood vessels)
Patients especially liable to develop further autoimmune diseases	Associations with HLA-B8 and DR3 in some

Table 18.3 *Significance of the more common antinuclear antibodies related to connective tissue diseases*[a]

Autoantibodies	Main associations
Anti-Jo 1 (GAD65; histidine tRNA ligase)	Polymyositis, dermatomyositis, anti-synthetase syndrome
Anti-Ku	Polymyositis/scleroderma (PM/Scl) overlap syndrome
Anti- double-stranded (anti-ds) DNA	Antibody with the highest specificity for systemic lupus erythematosus (SLE) and found in most patients
Anti-extractable nuclear antigen (anti-ENA antibodies)	SLE
Anti-Sm antibody (snRNP)	
Anti-extractable nuclear antigen (anti-ENA antibodies) directed against RNP	Sjögren syndrome
Anti-Ro (Robair) = SS-A	
Anti-extractable nuclear antigen (anti-ENA antibodies) directed against RNP	Sjögren syndrome
Anti-La (Lattimer) = SS-B	
Anti-extractable nuclear antigen (anti-ENA antibodies)	Mixed connective tissue disease (MCTD), SLE
Anti-snRNP70	
Anti-PM/Scl (anti-exosome)	PM/Scl overlap syndrome
Anti-histone	Drug-induced lupus, SLE
Anti-Scl 70	
Anti-topoisomerase	Scleroderma
Anti-centromere	CREST syndrome (calcium deposits; *Raynaud* phenomenon; oesophageal dysfunction; *s*clerodactyly; and *t*elangiectasias)

[a]See Appendix 2.6.

can be identified by special tests but often an autoantibody profile is carried out (this includes the most common abnormalities – namely, rheumatoid and antinuclear factors and thyroid microsomal, gastric parietal cell, mitochondrial, smooth muscle and reticulin antibodies). Serum complement levels may show the complement consumed when the cascade is activated by antigen/antibody reactions or other triggering factors, with complement levels (CH50) often depressed. Biopsy and tissue immunostaining may show immunoglobulin or complement deposits. Vasculitis with deposits of immunoglobulins and complement in the damaged vessel walls strongly suggests immune complex injury.

Treatments for autoimmune diseases include mainly anti-inflammatory and immunosuppressive drugs (including biologics) or plasmapheresis (removal of the antibodies).

THE CONNECTIVE TISSUE DISEASES

The connective tissue diseases (collagen diseases) are autoimmune diseases that share, to a variable degree, common features, such as: multiple autoantibodies, often against nuclear components (antinuclear antibodies [ANAs]; see Table 18.3); immune complex reactions; associations with Raynaud phenomenon and Sjögren syndrome; responsiveness to immunosuppressives; and malignancy as a possible late complication.

Antinuclear antibodies

ANAs are found in a number of different autoimmune diseases (such as systemic lupus erythematosus, Sjögren syndrome, rheumatoid arthritis, polymyositis, scleroderma, juvenile diabetes mellitus, Addison disease, vitiligo, pernicious anaemia, glomerulonephritis); infections (viral or bacterial, mainly); lung diseases (primary pulmonary fibrosis, pulmonary hypertension); gastrointestinal diseases (ulcerative colitis, Crohn disease, primary biliary cirrhosis, alcoholic liver disease); hormonal diseases (Hashimoto autoimmune thyroiditis, Graves disease); blood diseases (idiopathic thrombocytopenic purpura, haemolytic anaemia), cancers (melanoma, breast, lung, kidney, ovarian and others); and skin diseases (psoriasis, pemphigus). They are also found in those people with a family history of rheumatic diseases and in older patients, and in association with some drugs, including procainamide, hydralazine and phenytoin. Since ANAs appear in several types of disease, they have a low specificity.

ANAs can present different 'patterns' on histology, depending on the staining of the cell nucleus in the laboratory – homogeneous or diffuse; speckled; nucleolar; and peripheral or rim – but these patterns are not specific for any particular illness, though (for example) the nucleolar pattern is more commonly seen in scleroderma. ANAs can be found in approximately 5% of the normal population, usually in low titres; these people rarely have disease. ANA titres of 1:40 or below are considered negative. Titres lower than 1:80 are unlikely to be significant. Higher titres may be indicative of disease, but even these levels are often insignificant in patients over 60 years of age. Nevertheless, the sensitivity and simplicity of an ANA test makes it popular as a screen for lupus in particular, since most affected people (more than 95%) test positive, and thus a negative ANA test can be helpful in excluding lupus. Only about 11–13% of people with a positive ANA test do have lupus and up to 15% of completely healthy people have a positive ANA test. Thus a positive ANA test does not necessarily mean a diagnosis of lupus or, indeed, any autoimmune disease. Tests for ANA sub-serologies (including antibodies to double-stranded DNA, Smith, RNP, SSA, SSB, Scl-70 and centromere) are usually negative if ANA is negative. Exceptions include anti-Jo1, which can be positive in some forms of myositis, or occasionally anti-SSA, in the setting of lupus or Sjögren syndrome. Broad testing of autoantibodies should be avoided; instead, the choice of autoantibodies should be guided by the specific disease under consideration.

RAYNAUD DISEASE AND RAYNAUD PHENOMENON

Raynaud phenomenon manifests as recurrent vasospasm of the fingers and toes – usually in response to stress or cold exposure. Raynaud phenomenon is characterized by skin arteries that over-respond to cold, contracting briefly and limiting blood flow (vasospasm), so that the skin first turns white, then blue and finally red, as the arteries relax and blood flows again. Women are mainly affected.

Primary Raynaud disease (idiopathic Raynaud disease) is characterized by vasospasm alone and has no obvious cause, but 10–30% eventually progress to secondary Raynaud disease. Older patients and males often have vasospastic symptoms that predate systemic disease by as many as 20 years. Young female patients who have had Raynaud phenomenon alone for more than 2 years and have not developed any additional manifestations are, however, at low risk for developing autoimmune disease.

Secondary Raynaud disease is a term used when vasospasm is associated with another condition – most commonly an autoimmune disease, and usually progressive systemic sclerosis and mixed connective-tissue disease. Raynaud phenomenon has also been described with disorders such as cryoglobulins, vibration injury, polyvinyl chloride (PVC) exposure and drugs (e.g. some cardiovascular drugs and ergotamine). In older patients with recent-onset Raynaud phenomenon and no obvious underlying cause, malignancy must also be excluded.

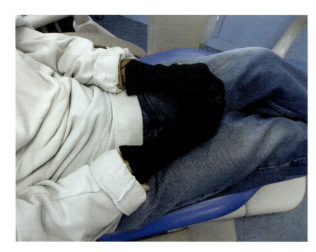

Fig. 18.1 Raynaud syndrome. Patients often wear gloves.

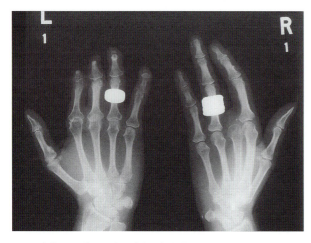

Fig 18.2 Loss of digit and atrophy of distal phalanges in severe Raynaud syndrome.

Clinical features

Symptoms include changes in skin colour (white to blue to red) and coldness (Fig. 18.1). Both hands and feet are usually affected. Raynaud phenomenon can sometimes attack other areas too, such as the nose and ears. It is common for the affected area to feel numb or prickly. Primary Raynaud disease usually affects both hands and both feet, while secondary Raynaud phenomenon may affect either both hands or both feet only.

The condition tends to be slowly progressive, with more frequent and prolonged episodes of spasm. Ischaemia can cause atrophy of the fat pads or ulceration at the tips of the fingers or toes, sometimes with the loss of more tissue (Fig. 18.2).

General management

Diagnosis is made from the fact that the attacks are triggered by exposure to cold and/or stress, symmetric bilateral involvement, an absence of necrosis, no detectable underlying cause, normal capillaroscopy findings, normal laboratory findings for inflammation, and an absence of antinuclear factors.

People suffering from Raynaud phenomenon should stop smoking (nicotine is vasoconstricting), protect themselves from cold, keep all their body warm – not just their extremities – and guard against cuts, bruises and other injuries to affected areas.

Primary Raynaud disease
Pharmacological therapy may include:

- angiotensin-receptor antagonists (losartan)
- calcium-channel blockers (e.g. nifedipine)
- fluoxetine
- iloprost (prostacyclin analogue)
- inositol nicotinate
- naftidrofuryl
- nitroglycerin (topically)
- prostaglandins (intravenously)
- reserpine.

Secondary Raynaud disease
Therapy should be tailored to the underlying disorder:

- Hyperviscosity syndromes and cryoglobulinaemia improve with treatments that decrease blood viscosity (e.g. plasmapheresis).
- Hepatitis B, hepatitis C and *Mycoplasma* infections need treating.

Pharmacological therapy is as for primary Raynaud disease.

Dental aspects

The dental environment should be kept at a comfortable temperature and humidity. Nifedipine may cause gingival swelling. Sjögren syndrome may be present.

LUPUS ERYTHEMATOSUS

Lupus can be categorized as systemic lupus erythematosus (SLE), drug-induced SLE or discoid lupus erythematosus (DLE).

Systemic lupus erythematosus
General aspects

SLE is a potentially fatal disease characterized by autoantibodies to DNA (anti-dsDNA [double strand DNA] antibody is peculiar to SLE). The immune complex reactions, in particular vasculitis, result in multisystem disease. Lupus susceptibility relates to several genes, including *HLA-DR3* and *B8*, *HLA-DR2*, complement C4 genes and a polymorphism of the T-cell receptor that has been associated with Ro (SS-A) antibodies.

Clinical features

SLE can cause a variety of clinical manifestations, which differ greatly in severity, ranging from mild to significant and potentially fatal lesions. The onset may be acute, resembling an infection, or there may be vague symptoms that may progress over many years (Table 18.4). The acronym SOAPBRAIN may serve as an *aide-mémoire* (*s*erositis; *o*ral ulcers; *a*rthritis; *p*ericarditis; *b*lood problems; *r*enal; *A*NA; *i*mmune; *n*eurological).

The classic picture of SLE is that of a young woman with fever, malaise, anaemia, joint pains, Raynaud phenomenon and a rash variable in character but erythematous, often with raised margins and scaling (Fig. 18.3). The well-known rash, with a butterfly pattern extending over both cheeks and bridge of the nose, is relatively uncommon and not specific to lupus erythematosus. Photosensitivity rashes are common. Renal involvement (proteinuria and haematuria) is frequently seen and often associated with hypertension. Relatively

Table 18.4 *Manifestations of systemic lupus erythematosus*

System	Main lesions
Skin	Rash
Joints	Arthritis
	Polyarthralgia
Serous membranes	Pericarditis
	Pleurisy
Cardiovascular	Endocarditis (Libman–Sacks)
	Myocarditis
	Raynaud phenomenon
Lungs	Pneumonitis
Kidney	Nephritis
Neurological	Cranial nerve palsies
	Neuroses
	Psychoses
	Strokes
Eye	Conjunctivitis
	Retinal damage
Gastrointestinal	Hepatomegaly
	Pancreatitis
	Sjögren syndrome
Blood	Anaemia
	Purpura

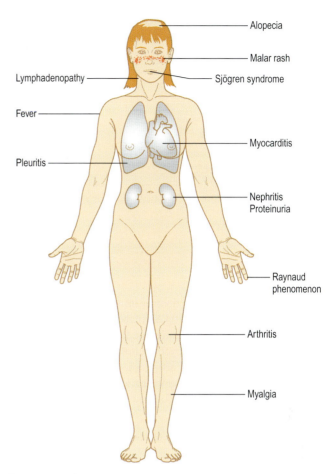

Fig. 18.4 Lupus erythematosus.

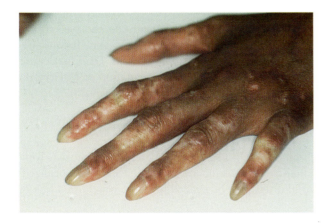

Fig. 18.3 Raynaud syndrome in lupus.

minor disturbances of mood, and depressive or hysterical behaviour, are common, while central nervous system (CNS) involvement is potentially fatal. Ocular lesions may affect 20–25%, and serositis can cause pleurisy or occasionally pericarditis and peritonitis (polyserositis) (Fig. 18.4).

Cardiac lesions typically cause myocarditis, which leads to cardiac failure; there is a higher risk of infarction, and a characteristic (Libman–Sacks) endocarditis can also develop. Murmurs are more often caused by anaemia.

Women who have SLE can pass antibodies across the placenta, which can cause fetal heart block (see Sjögren syndrome).

General management

The American College of Rheumatology diagnostic criteria for SLE are based on the presence of at least four of the following:

- Malar rash
- Discoid rash
- Photosensitivity
- Oral ulcers
- Arthritis
- Serositis (pleurisy or pericarditis)
- Renal disorder (persistent proteinuria or cellular casts)
- Neurological disorder (seizures or psychosis)
- Haematological disorder (anaemia, leukopenia or lymphopenia on two or more occasions, thrombocytopenia)
- An immunological disorder (positive lupus erythematosus cell preparation, anti-DNA or anti-Sm, false positive Venereal Disease Reference Laboratory [VDRL] test).

Initial screening includes ESR, autoantibodies (e.g. ANA; Box 18.1), a full blood count, liver and kidney function tests, syphilis screen (VDRL), lupus erythematosus cell test, urinalysis and blood chemistries. No single laboratory test can definitely prove or exclude SLE, but anti-Sm antibody or high-titre anti-native DNA antibody is an important indication (see Table 18.3); anti-dsDNA is peculiar to SLE and the titre of anti-DNA antibodies correlates well with disease activity. About 70% of patients have antibodies against double-stranded RNA (anti-dsRNA) or against hybrid RNA/DNA molecules. Other autoantibodies (e.g. anti-SS-A and anti-SS-B) may be helpful. About 40% of patients also have antibodies directed against phospholipid – and about 15% of patients have the antiphospholipid syndrome (APS; see later).

Biopsies of skin or kidney using immunofluorescent staining techniques can support the diagnosis of SLE.

Most patients appear to do well in the long term either with non-steroidal anti-inflammatory drugs (NSAIDs) or, if these are

- Antinuclear antibodies
  - Anti-DNA antibodies, especially anti-double-stranded DNA (crithidial)
  - Anti-RNA antibodies
- Circulating antibodies to platelets and other blood cells
- Raised erythrocyte sedimentation rate
- Hypergammaglobulinaemia
- Hypocomplementaemia
- Lupus erythematosus cell phenomenon
- Rheumatoid factor (30%)
- Venereal Disease Reference Laboratory (VDRL) false positive

Table 18.5 *Drugs associated with lupoid reactions*

Drugs having a proven association with LE	Drugs having a possible association with LE
Chlorpromazine	Beta-blockers
Hydralazine	Captopril
Isoniazid	Carbamazepine
Methyldopa	Cimetidine
Procainamide	Etanercept
	Ethosuximide
	Methimazole
	Phenazine
	Phenytoin (diphenylhydantoin)
	Quinidine

ineffective, on low doses of corticosteroids taken on alternate days. Other treatment options currently available include hydroxychloroquine and other immunosuppressive medications (e.g. azathioprine, ciclosporin, cyclophosphamide, mycophenolate or sirolimus), as well as a range of biological agents (abatacept, abetimus, anakinra, atacicept, belimumab, edratide, efalizumab, epratuzumab, infliximab, rituximab, rontalizumab, sifalimumab and tocilizumab). SLE has a 5-year survival rate of more than 90%.

Dental aspects

Oral lesions, which typically consist of erythematous areas, erosions or white patches, fairly symmetrically distributed and resembling lichen planus, may be seen in 10–20% of patients with SLE and are rarely an early feature. Slit-like ulcers may also be seen near the gingival margins. The best management of erosive lesions of SLE in the oral mucosa is uncertain but corticosteroids, often in high doses, may be the only effective treatment. Biopsies of oral lesions show irregular epithelial thinning and acanthosis, basement membrane thickening, liquefaction degeneration of the basal cell layer and an irregularly distributed chronic inflammatory infiltrate. Vasculitis is inconstant. Immunofluorescent staining shows lumpy deposits of immunoglobulins and complement perivascularly and along the basement membrane of lesions, and under normal skin or mucosa in up to 90% of patients with SLE. Sjögren syndrome is associated in up to 30%. Antimalarials, sometimes used to control SLE, can cause lichenoid oral lesions or occasionally oral hyperpigmentation.

Surgery may exacerbate SLE symptoms and, if elective, should therefore be postponed until lupus activity subsides. Hospitalization may be required for otherwise minor procedures and postoperative discharge may be delayed.

Tetracyclines may cause photosensitivity rashes while sulphonamides or penicillins may lead to deterioration in SLE. Bleeding tendencies are caused by thrombocytopenia; circulating anticoagulants rarely cause a bleeding tendency – rather they predispose to thrombosis. Other aspects to consider are corticosteroid or other immunosuppressive therapy (Ch. 35), renal disease (Ch. 12) and anaemia (Ch. 8).

Drug-induced lupus (Table 18.5) has some features similar to those of SLE, particularly pleuropericardial inflammation, fever, rash, arthritis and serological changes. The clinical and serological signs of the lupus erythematosus usually subside gradually after the offending drug is discontinued.

Discoid lupus erythematosus

General aspects

Discoid lupus erythematosus (DLE) is essentially a mucocutaneous disease in which the rashes may be indistinguishable from those of SLE, but serological abnormalities are typically absent or minor, there are no serious systemic effects and it only rarely progresses to SLE.

Clinical features

DLE is characterized by a rash, usually on the face or other sun-exposed areas, or by mucosal lesions. The skin lesions are patchy, crusty, sharply defined plaques that may scar. DLE may cause patchy, bald areas on the scalp, and hypopigmentation or hyperpigmentation in older lesions. Arthralgia is a frequent complaint.

General management

Lesional biopsy will usually confirm the diagnosis. Topical and intralesional corticosteroids are usually effective for localized lesions; antimalarial drugs may be needed for more generalized lesions.

Dental aspects

Oral mucosal lesions can be a feature of DLE and may also simulate lichen planus, but the lesions are less often symmetrically distributed and the pattern of striae is typically less well defined or conspicuous. Nevertheless, differentiation can be difficult and biopsy is essential. Even this may not be diagnostic and, occasionally, histological appearances that are intermediate between those of lichen planus and lupus erythematosus are seen. Management is as for the oral lesions of SLE but DLE may have some malignant potential.

RELAPSING POLYCHONDRITIS

Relapsing polychondritis (RP) is a severe, episodic and progressive inflammatory condition associated with antibodies to cartilage-specific collagen types II, IX and XI. RP affects cartilaginous structures, predominantly those of the ears, nose and laryngotracheobronchial tree. Other affected structures may include the eyes, cardiovascular system, peripheral joints, skin, middle and inner ear, and CNS. Aphthous-like oral ulceration has been described and the MAGIC variant of Behçet syndrome is a differential diagnosis. Management is with systemic corticosteroids.

RHEUMATOID ARTHRITIS

See Chapter 16.

SJÖGREN SYNDROME

General aspects

Sjögren syndrome (SS) is the association of dry mouth (hyposalivation) with dry eyes. It mainly affects middle-aged or older women. SS affects up to 5% of women and 0.5% of men.

Primary SS ('sicca syndrome') is the association of dry mouth with dry eyes in the absence of any connective tissue disease. Secondary SS refers to the association of dry mouth and dry eyes with another connective tissue disease – usually rheumatoid arthritis (RA) and, less frequently, thyroiditis, primary biliary cirrhosis, SLE, progressive systemic sclerosis or polymyositis. It is unclear how distinct the various forms are. The initial definition and diagnostic criteria for SS were the presence of 'keratoconjunctivitis sicca ("dry eyes"), xerostomia ("dry mouth") and RA or other connective tissue disease', and 'two of the three are generally considered sufficient for the diagnosis'. Patients who developed the dry eye/mouth components of SS without developing RA were initially labelled as having the 'sicca syndrome', and later 'primary SS', while those with RA who usually developed the dry eye/mouth components after onset of their joint disease were labelled as having 'secondary SS'.

SS is an autoimmune exocrinopathy. Lacrimal, salivary and other exocrine glands are infiltrated by lymphocytes and plasma cells, causing progressive acinar destruction and often multisystem disease. The aetiology may involve genetic factors; a range of loci have been implicated (Box 18.2). SS-A and SS-B autoantibodies activate caspase-3 and apoptosis, which could be responsible for impaired salivary secretory function. In SS, several neuroendocrine system functions are also impaired. Anti-muscarinic type 3 receptor (a-M3R) autoantibodies in SS inhibit intracellular trafficking of aquaporin-5 (AQP5), the water transport protein, leading to secretory dysfunction. Raised T-helper 1 (Th1) cytokines (IL-10 and IL-6) are seen in SS and correlate with the clinical manifestations of disease. High levels of cytokines from Th1 (IL-2, IL-2) and Th2 (IL-6, IL-10), and chemokines (CKs) CXCL13, CCL21 and CXCL12, which play roles in lymphoid tissue organization and the development of lymphoid malignancies, are expressed in salivary glands of patients with SS and mucosa-associated lymphoid tissue (MALT) lymphoma. Th1, Th2, Th17 and Reg (the regenerating gene) may also be involved in SS pathogenesis.

Clinical features

SS is characterized by dryness of all mucosae. Dry mouth can be a real complaint and salivary glands may swell (see below), but the most important effects are on the eyes, where drying causes keratoconjunctivitis

sicca. This can ultimately lead to impairment or loss of sight. Patients with dry eyes may have no symptoms or may complain of grittiness, burning, soreness, itching or inability to cry. They may wake in the morning with a pustular exudate in the eyes or crusting at the canthus, or have infections of the lids (Fig. 18.5). Lacrimal glands may swell.

Raynaud phenomenon or other autoimmune manifestations are common. Multisystem disease can manifest with extraglandular complications, as shown in Table 18.6 and Figure 18.6.

Extraglandular disease may precede exocrine problems by years and is found in 50% of SS-1. Fatigue, fever and Raynaud phenomenon are common early on; later complications include glomerulonephritis, lymphoma and skin problems (itching or cracking). Vaginal dryness causing painful intercourse is a frequent complaint. Lung disease can result from aspiration or bronchial dryness. Bronchitis, tracheobronchitis and laryngotracheobronchitis are common. Renal disease (interstitial nephritis) is an important complication. Peripheral nervous system involvement may present with carpal tunnel syndrome, peripheral neuropathy or cranial neuropathy such as trigeminal neuropathy. Gastrointestinal complaints may include dysphagia, heartburn, abdominal pain and swelling, anorexia, diarrhoea and weight loss.

Autoimmune thyroid disorders can appear as either an overactive thyroid (Graves disease) or an underactive thyroid (Hashimoto thyroiditis). Nearly half of the people with autoimmune thyroid disorder also have SS, and many people with SS show evidence of thyroid disease.

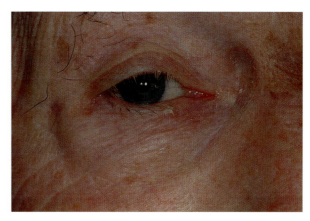

Fig. 18.5 Sjögren syndrome: dry eyes.

Box 18.2 *Some gene loci implicated in Sjögren syndrome*

- HLA-DQ: DQ1, DQ2 and DQB1*02/DQB1*0602
- Interleukin-10
- Immunoglobulin kappa-chain allotype KM1
- SS-A1
- STAT4
- Tumour necrosis factor

Table 18.6 *Sjögren syndrome*

Ocular	Oral	Vaginal	Autoimmune disorders	Extraglandular disease
Kerato-conjunctivitis sicca	Hyposalivation	Vaginal dryness	Mainly rheumatoid arthritis	Cutaneous
	Lobulated tongue			Gastrointestinal
				Haematological
	Infections (candidosis, caries, sialadenitis)			Joints
				Neurological
				Pancreatic
				Psychiatric
				Pulmonary
				Renal
				Respiratory
				Reticulo-endothelial
				Vascular

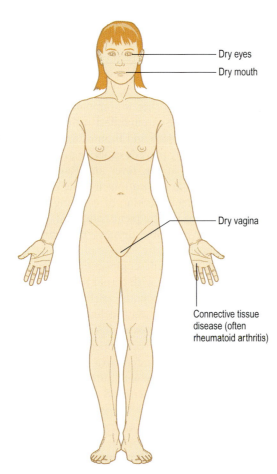

Fig. 18.6 Sjögren syndrome.

- Dry eyes
- Dry mouth
- Dry vagina
- Connective tissue disease (often rheumatoid arthritis)

Women who have SS can pass autoantibodies across the placenta into the fetal circulation, which can lead to heart block. Though it can be fatal, the long-term outlook for the child with heart block is generally good, but most require pacemakers, usually for life.

About 5% of people with SS develop lymphomas, mainly people with SS-1. Most (45–75%) are MALT lymphomas, usually affecting the parotid salivary glands. Risk factors for lymphoma are shown in Box 18.3.

Allergic drug reactions are frequent to penicillins and cephalosporins. Systemic reactions to trimethoprim present with CNS symptoms or aseptic meningitis. There are also rare associations of SS with a number of conditions (Box 18.4).

General management

Screening questions to assess ocular and oral symptoms (Box 18.5) may help identify patients. Dehydration, drugs, irradiation and infections can also cause dry mouth and dry eyes, and should be ruled out (Box 18.6).

There is no single gold standard test or agreement on criteria for diagnosing SS. Diagnosis is often based on American–European Consensus criteria (Table 18.7).

An ophthalmological examination is important; a Schirmer test shows impaired lacrimation (Fig. 18.7) and an ocular staining score and tear break-up time are useful. Serum autoantibodies, especially antinuclear antibodies SS-A (Ro: Robair) or SS-B (La: Lattimer), are a common diagnostically helpful and non-invasive approach. Hypergammaglobulinaemia is seen mainly as a result of rheumatoid factor.

Salivary flow rates can confirm the presence and degree of hyposalivation but are non-specific. Whole saliva collected without stimulation by allowing the patient to dribble into a sterile container over a measured period is now regarded as the best form of sialometry. A value below 1.5 mL/15 min is regarded as abnormal. Parotid output after stimulation with 10% citric acid can also be objectively determined by using a suction (Lashley or Carlsson–Crittenden) cup over the parotid duct orifice or by cannulation of the duct, but has no advantage. A value below 1.0 mL/min is regarded as abnormal.

Table 18.7 *Diagnostic criteria (American–European) for Sjögren syndrome*[a]

Type	Criteria	Detail
I Ocular symptoms	A positive response to at least one of the following questions:	1. Have you had daily ocular symptoms or persistent, troublesome dry eyes for >3 months? 2. Do you have a recurrent sensation of sand or gravel in the eyes? 3. Do you use tear substitutes >3 times a day?
II Oral symptoms	A positive response to at least one of the following questions:	1. Have you had a daily feeling of dry mouth for >3 months? 2. Have you had recurrently or persistently swollen salivary glands as an adult? 3. Do you frequently drink liquids to aid in swallowing dry food?
III Ocular signs	That is, objective evidence of ocular involvement defined as a positive result for at least one of:	1. Schirmer's 1 test, performed without anaesthesia (<5 mm in 5 min) 2. Rose Bengal score or other ocular dye score (>4 according to van Bijsterveld's scoring system)
IV Histo-pathology	In minor salivary glands (obtained through normal-appearing mucosa)	Focal lymphocytic sialadenitis evaluated by an expert histopathologist, with a focus score > 1, defined as a number of lymphocytic foci (which are adjacent to normal-appearing mucous acini and contain more than 50 lymphocytes) per 4 mm^2 of glandular tissue
V Salivary gland involvement	Objective evidence of salivary gland involvement, defined by a positive result for one of the following:	1. Unstimulated whole salivary flow, 1.5 mL in 15 min 2. Parotid sialography showing the presence of ductal sialectasis (punctate, cavitary or destructive pattern) without evidence of obstruction in the major ducts 3. Salivary scintigraphy showing delayed uptake, reduced concentration and/or delayed excretion of tracer
VI Auto-antibodies	Presence in the serum of the following autoantibodies:	Antibodies to Ro (SS-A) or La (SS-B) antigens, or both

[a]Not universally accepted. Many now undertake ultrasonography.

Table 18.8 *Sjögren syndrome – comparison of subtypes*

Feature	Primary	Secondary
Other connective tissue disease	–	+
Ocular involvement	More severe	Less severe
Extraglandular manifestations	More common	Less common
Oral involvement	More severe	Less severe
Recurrent sialadenitis	More common	Less common
Risk of lymphoma	More common	Less common
Human leukocyte antigen (HLA) associations	HLA-DR3	HLA-DR4, HLA-B8
Rheumatoid factor	50%	90%
Anti-SS-A (Ro)	5–10%	50–80%
Anti-SS-B (La)	50–75%	1–5%
Rheumatoid arthritis precipitin (RAP)[a]	5%	75%

[a]Also known as SS-C.

Labial gland biopsy is one of the more specific investigations. The parotid glands are chiefly affected but the changes usually are also present in the other glands, including the minor labial glands (such as in the lower lip). Labial gland biopsy is easier and safer, and usually reflects the parotid changes. Ultrasound in particular is non-invasive and inexpensive, and is considered positive for SS if the major glands show hypoechoic areas, echogenic streaks and/or irregular gland margins. It is also helpful in excluding lymphoma.

Other investigations may include sialography, scintigraphy and magnetic resonance imaging (MRI). Sialography, though non-specific and time-consuming, is helpful but is of course contraindicated if there is acute parotitis. Hydrostatic instillation of contrast medium typically shows a snowstorm appearance (punctate sialectasis) in well-established cases. Scintigraphy measures radioactive pertechnetate uptake and concentration in the major glands, but involves the use of radioisotopes, depends on the availability of specialized equipment and appears to have little place. MRI is helpful.

Sialochemistry is theoretically helpful; SS alters the protein profile and brings about a change in the composition of saliva with an increase in the levels of lactoferrin, beta$_2$-microglobulin, sodium, lysozyme C and cystatin C, and a decrease in salivary amylase and carbonic anhydrase.

Primary SS (SS-1) tends to be a more aggressive disorder than secondary SS (SS-2; Table 18.8). Management is largely symptomatic, though there have been attempts at immunosuppression to control the disease process. This may increase the risk of lymphomatous change. Cyclophosphamide may help control renal and vascular disease, and polyneuropathy. Mizoribine, a nucleoside produced by *Eupenicillium brefeldianum* with antibiotic, cytotoxic and immunosuppressive activity, may be effective. Mycophenolate, epratuzumab (anti-CD22 monoclonal antibody) and rituximab (anti-CD20 monoclonal antibody) may be helpful. Anti-TNF biological agents (infliximab, etanercept), ciclosporin, azathioprine, hydroxychloroquine, methotrexate and NSAIDs are of no reliable value.

Lymphoma predictors include swelling of salivary glands, lymph nodes, liver or spleen; vasculitis; lung infiltrates; fever; neuropathy or purpura; or blood changes (hypergammaglobulinaemia, anaemia, hypocomplementaemia, cryoglobulinaemia or hypocomplementaemia). Lymphomas may be best diagnosed with high-resolution computed tomography (CT), MRI, MRI contrast sialography (gadolinium MRI with fat subtraction) or ultrasonography and biopsy. They may respond to chemotherapy but rituximab may also be used.

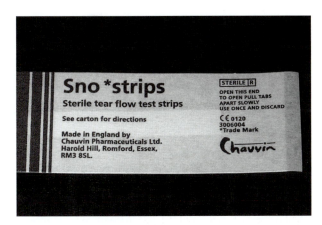

Fig. 18.7 Schirmer strip to test lacrimal flow.

Dental aspects

Oral involvement in SS results in discomfort caused by the poor salivary flow, obvious dryness of the mucosa in severe cases, and erythema and lobulation of the tongue. Apart from its dryness, the oral mucosa may appear normal but the supervention of candidal infection causes redness and soreness.

The other main effects of persistent hyposalivation can include difficulty in speaking, swallowing or managing dentures; disturbed taste sensation; accelerated caries; and susceptibility to oral candidosis and ascending (bacterial) sialadenitis.

Swelling of the parotid salivary glands is seen in a minority. Rarely, these glands can also be persistently painful. Late onset of salivary gland swelling, especially in sicca syndrome, may indicate development of a lymphoma (see Box 18.3).

Dry mouth may be helped symptomatically by simple methods. Frequently sipping water or sugar-free drinks, sucking ice or using frequent, liberal rinses of a salivary substitute (mouth-wetting agent) containing carboxymethyl cellulose or mucin may help.

Salivation may be stimulated by sialogogues. Simply chewing sugar-free gum or sucking citrus or malic acid lozenges may help salivation. Pilocarpine 5 mg three times daily with meals, or pyridostigmine, may improve salivation if any functional tissue remains, but systemic effects such as sweating, diarrhoea and blurred vision may be troublesome and there may be arrhythmias. Cevimeline is a newer alternative.

Preventive dental care is important. Patients have a tendency to consume a cariogenic diet because of the impaired sense of taste. This must be avoided and caries should also be controlled by fluoride applications and amorphous calcium phosphate. Use of a chlorhexidine mouthwash will help to control periodontal disease and other infections. Denture hygiene is important because of susceptibility to candidosis; antifungal treatment is often also needed.

Infections should be treated. Generalized soreness and redness of a dry oral mucosa is typically caused by *Candida albicans* and often associated with angular stomatitis. Antifungal treatment is given as rinses of nystatin, or topical miconazole or fluconazole. Acute complications, such as ascending parotitis, should be treated with antibiotics. Pus should be sent for culture and antibiotic sensitivities, but in the interim, a penicillinase-resistant penicillin, such as flucloxacillin in combination with metronidazole, should be started because of the possible presence of anaerobes.

No crowns should be constructed until caries is controlled and there are no new lesions for more than 1 year.

Patients with SS who need dental treatment may not be good candidates for general anaesthesia (GA) because of the tendency to respiratory infections. It is important to lubricate the eyes and throat, to humidify the gases, to avoid drying agents (e.g. nicotine, atropine, phenergan), to be conscious of the possibility of cervical spine involvement in RA, to maintain body heat (because of Raynaud disease) and to consider renal function.

There may also be problems in management related to the associated connective tissue disease and complicating factors such as anaemia (Ch. 8).

There is a higher incidence of drug allergies in SS. Trimethoprim may induce a systemic reaction of fever, headache, backache and meningeal irritation (trimethoprim-induced aseptic meningitis).

IGG₄ SYNDROME

Mikulicz disease (MD) was the term given to the condition of persistent salivary and lacrimal gland enlargement. MD has been included in the differential diagnosis of SS-1, but it represents a unique condition

---

Box 18.7 *Diagnostic features of IgG₄ disease*

- Visual confirmation of symmetrical and persistent swelling in more than two lacrimal and major salivary glands
- Prominent IgG₄-positive mononuclear cell infiltration of lacrimal and salivary glands
- Exclusion of other diseases that present with glandular swelling, such as Sjögren syndrome, sarcoidosis and lymphoproliferative disease
- IgG₄ raised serum levels

---

with persistent lacrimal and salivary gland enlargement, few autoimmune reactions and good responsiveness to glucocorticoids, leading to the recovery of gland function. The diagnostic features are shown in Box 18.7.

Many cases previously classified as Mikulicz disease, Küttner tumour and orbital pseudotumour (idiopathic orbital inflammation), however, show increased numbers of IgG₄-positive plasma cells, and some also show elevated levels of serum IgG₄, supporting the concept of IgG₄-associated sialadenitis/dacroadenitis. Complications include autoimmune pancreatitis, retroperitoneal fibrosis, tubulo-interstitial nephritis, autoimmune hypophysitis and Riedel thyroiditis, in all of which IgG₄ is involved. IgG₄ syndrome thus differs from SS, and is associated with raised serum IgG₄ concentrations and a prominent infiltration of IgG₄-expressing plasmacytes in the lacrimal and salivary glands. Mikulicz disease is therefore now termed systemic IgG₄-related plasmacytic disease.

In IgG₄ syndrome, the incidence of dry eyes, dry mouth and arthralgias is lower compared to SS, while allergic rhinitis, bronchial asthma, sclerosing pancreatitis, interstitial nephritis and interstitial pneumonitis are more common. Also, IgG₄ syndrome is *not* associated with anti-Ro/SS-A and anti-La/SS-B autoantibodies; and only a few patients have rheumatoid factor (RF) and ANA (low serum titres). There is good responsive to systemic corticosteroids or anti-CD20 (rituximab).

SCLERODERMA

General aspects

Scleroderma, from the Greek, means hard skin (*skleros* – hard; *derma* – skin), and is an uncommon disorder affecting about 2 in 10 000 people. It results from antinuclear antibodies against topoisomerase or centromeres causing fibroblasts to produce excess collagen. A gene that codes for fibrillin-1 may put some people at risk for scleroderma. Perivascular macrophage infiltration and endothelial cell damage with increased collagen and extracellular matrix are the main features.

Suspected triggers for scleroderma include viral infections (especially cytomegalovirus), drugs (e.g. taxanes or bleomycin), and adhesive and coating materials or organic solvents (e.g. vinyl chloride or trichloroethylene).

Women develop scleroderma at a rate up to ten times higher than men, possibly because of oestrogen; silicone breast implants have been blamed but no evidence found.

Clinical features

Scleroderma can be localized, which can be incapacitating, or systemic, which affects a number of organs and can be life-threatening. *Localized scleroderma* is limited to the skin and related tissues and, in some cases, the underlying muscle, but never progresses to a systemic form.

Localized types of scleroderma are recognized. *Morphoea* (from the Greek for 'form' or 'structure') is characterized by local patches

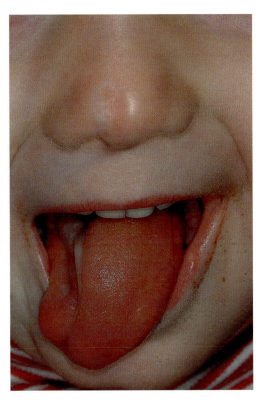

Fig. 18.8 *Coup de sabre*.

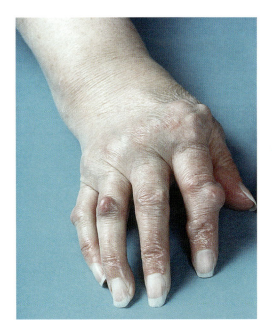

Fig. 18.9 CREST syndrome. Calcinosis and Raynaud phenomenon are shown here.

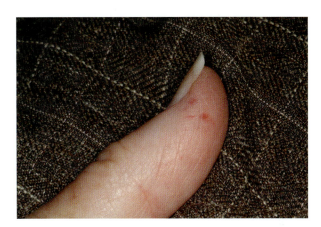

Fig. 18.10 Scleroderma. Finger telangiectasia.

of scleroderma. The first signs of the disease are reddish patches of skin, most often on the chest, stomach and back, that thicken into firm oval-shaped areas. The centre of each patch becomes whitish with violet borders. These patches sweat very little and have little hair growth. Morphoea generally fades out in 3–5 years, but patients are often left with darkened skin patches and, in rare cases, muscle weakness.

Linear scleroderma (*coup de sabre* or 'sword cut') has a single line or band of thickened and/or abnormally coloured skin that usually runs down an arm or leg, but in some cases runs down the side of the face (Fig. 18.8).

Scleroderma (systemic sclerosis; SSc) involves deeper tissues (blood vessels and major organs) and often the skin. It appears in one of three forms:

■ *Limited scleroderma* typically comes on gradually and affects the skin only in certain areas: the fingers, hands, face, lower arms and legs. Many people with limited disease have CREST: calcinosis – *c*alcium deposits typically on the fingers, hands, face and trunk, and on the skin above the elbows and knees; *R*aynaud phenomenon; *o*esophageal dysfunction; *s*clerodactyly – thick and tight skin on the fingers, making it difficult to bend or straighten the fingers; and *t*elangiectasias (Fig. 18.9).

■ *Diffuse scleroderma* typically develops suddenly, affecting the hands, face (Figs 18.10 and 18.11), upper arms, upper legs, chest and stomach in a symmetrical fashion (e.g. if one arm or one side of the trunk is affected, the other is also affected). About one-third develop severe renal, pulmonary, gastrointestinal or cardiac disease.

■ *Sine scleroderma* resembles either limited or diffuse systemic sclerosis, causing changes in the lungs, kidneys and blood vessels, but not the skin. However, it is heterogeneous with two main subsets. One is a diffuse cutaneous form with early onset of pulmonary, cardiac and renal complications and associated in 30% with anti-topoisomerase antibodies. The other is a limited

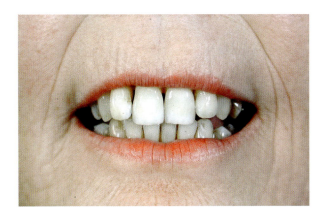

Fig. 18.11 Scleroderma. Fish-mouth.

cutaneous form of disease with somewhat similar features but with sclerosis limited to the skin, such as CREST, with late visceral complications, and often (70%) associated with anti-centromere antibodies.

Systemic scleroderma classically presents with Raynaud phenomenon, often associated with joint pains (polyarthralgia) and skin becoming thinned, stiff, tethered, pigmented and marked by prominent fine

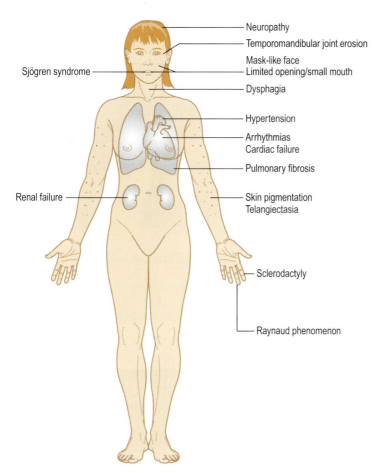

Fig. 18.12 Scleroderma.

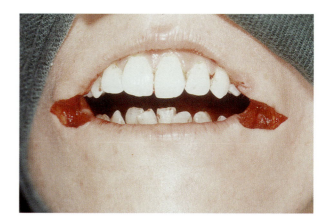

Fig. 18.13 Lip splitting during surgery in scleroderma (courtesy JP Shepherd).

blood vessels (telangiectases or spider naevi) and eventually limiting movement. There is also dysphagia and reflux oesophagitis; pulmonary involvement, which leads to impaired respiratory exchange and, eventually, dyspnoea and pulmonary hypertension; and renal damage secondary to vascular disease – typically a late feature, leading to hypertension, and an important cause of death (Fig. 18.12). There appears also to be an increased incidence of cancer of the oesophagus and of oral cancer.

General management

Scleroderma should be differentiated from undifferentiated connective tissue disease, overlap syndromes and eosinophilic fasciitis (EF); the latter involves the fascia, causing muscles to become encased in collagen, with contractures, and sometimes leading to disfigurement and problems with joint motion and function.

Diagnostically useful autoantibodies include anti-centromere antibodies (in up to 90% of people with limited systemic sclerosis) and anti-topoisomerase-1 antibodies (in 40% of people with diffuse SSc). PM-Sc1 antibodies suggest muscle involvement. Other laboratory findings are a raised ESR, normochromic anaemia and abnormal nailfold capillaroscopy.

There is no specific treatment, though hydroxychloroquine, methotrexate, ciclosporin, IFN-α and mycophenolate have been used; newer therapies include anti-transforming growth factor-beta (anti-TGF-β), stem cell transplantation and antagonists to endothelin. Medications for specific problems include iloprost to treat pulmonary hypertension, cyclophosphamide for lung fibrosis, angiotensin-converting enzyme inhibitors (ACEIs) for scleroderma-related kidney disease and nifedipine for Raynaud phenomenon.

The 5-year survival rate in severe forms is about 50%.

Dental aspects

Some 80% of patients have manifestations in the head and neck region; in 30% the symptoms start there. Involvement of the face causes characteristic changes in appearance, notably narrowing of the eyes and mask-like restriction of facial movement (Mona Lisa face). Constriction of the oral orifice can cause progressively limited opening of the mouth (fish-mouth; see Fig. 18.11). The submucosal connective tissue may also be affected and the tongue may become stiff and less mobile (chicken tongue).

The mandibular angle, condyle or coronoid process may be resorbed or rarely there is gross extensive resorption of the jaw. Occasionally, involvement of the peri-articular tissues of the temporomandibular joint together with the microstomia so limit access to the mouth as to make dental care and/or treatment more or less impracticable (Fig. 18.13).

Sjögren syndrome develops in a significant minority, but very frequently when systemic sclerosis is associated with primary biliary cirrhosis. Since self-care can be challenging and there may be xerostomia, it is not surprising that there are often more decayed, missing or filled teeth. Toothbrush-handle modifications or powered brushes and flosses, fluorides, dietary control and management of dry mouth may help. The dental facility should be kept at a temperature and humidity that the patient finds comfortable. Otherwise, the main problems of systemic sclerosis are caused by dysphagia and pulmonary, cardiac or renal disease as potential contraindications for GA.

A recognized but uncommon feature seen in fewer than 10% of cases is widening of the periodontal membrane space without tooth mobility. Trigeminal neuropathy may occur. There may be a predilection to carcinoma of the tongue.

Penicillamine therapy may cause loss of taste, oral ulceration, lichenoid reactions and other complications. Nifedipine for Raynaud phenomenon may cause gingival swelling.

A typical manifestation of morphoea is involvement of the side of the face, causing an area of scar-like contraction aptly described as *coup de sabre*. Morphoea in childhood is believed to be one cause of facial hemiatrophy.

POLYMYOSITIS AND DERMATOMYOSITIS

General aspects

Polymyositis and dermatomyositis are rare, immunologically mediated inflammatory myopathies. Polymyositis, if associated with skin lesions, is known as dermatomyositis. The conditions usually develop between the fifth and sixth decades, women being affected twice as often as men.

Clinical features

Polymyositis onset is characteristically insidious with pain and weakness, usually of the pelvic girdle and proximal limb muscles, especially the legs. Eventually, in severe cases, speaking and swallowing may become difficult and weakness may make patients bedridden. Ultimately, atrophy, contracture and calcinosis of muscles can develop. Other complications may include myocarditis and fibrosing alveolitis.

Dermatomyositis is characterized by a dusky and violaceous (Gottron, or heliotrope) rash with a butterfly distribution across the bridge of the nose and adjacent cheeks. This may spread to the upper part of the body or hands. Small, ulcerated skin lesions may develop over bony prominences. In a minority, Raynaud phenomenon is associated and there can be features of other connective tissue diseases, particularly scleroderma, myasthenia gravis or Hashimoto thyroiditis, especially in those with dermatomyositis.

Malignant disease may arise, particularly in dermatomyositis – typically, ovarian, lung, pancreatic, stomach and colorectal cancers, Waldenström macroglobulinaemia or non-Hodgkin lymphoma.

General management

Serum enzymes aldolase, creatinine phosphokinase [CPK] and aspartate transaminase [AST] may be raised, but the diagnosis is confirmed by electromyography (EMG) and muscle biopsy (shows muscle necrosis and regeneration and inflammation).

Treatment is with immunosuppressants (corticosteroids or others) but these are less effective when there is malignant disease.

Dental aspects

Oral lesions in polymyositis/dermatomyositis may be present in 10–20%; they are are variable in character and mainly comprise dark or purplish mucosal erythema and oedema. Small whitish patches, occasionally with shallow ulceration, may also develop and bear some resemblance to lichen planus or lupus erythematosus.

Dental management may be complicated by corticosteroid therapy or associated disorders, such as other connective tissue diseases, including Sjögren syndrome. A minority have pharyngeal weakness.

MIXED CONNECTIVE TISSUE DISEASE

Mixed connective tissue disease (MCTD) is an undifferentiated connective tissue disease presenting as a multisystem disorder with Raynaud phenomenon and features of two or more of the following connective tissue diseases: SLE, scleroderma and polymyositis. MCTD may evolve into one of several major connective tissue diseases or to an overlap syndrome. Patients have anti-ribonucleoprotein antibody (anti-U1-68kD antibody) but no anti-Smith autoantibody (anti-Sm Ab).

Sjögren syndrome is the main complication of dental interest, but mouth ulcers or sensory changes may be seen.

ANTIPHOSPHOLIPID SYNDROME (HUGHES SYNDROME)

Antiphospholipid syndrome (APS) is characterized by persistently raised antibodies against membrane anionic phospholipids (i.e. the antiphospholipid antibodies [aPL], anticardiolipin antibody [aCL] and antiphosphatidylserine) or their associated plasma proteins, predominantly beta$_2$ glycoprotein I (apolipoprotein H). The antibodies are deposited in small vessels, leading to intimal hyperplasia and hypercoagulability due to lupus 'anticoagulant', and causing venous or arterial thromboses in cerebral, renal, pulmonary, cutaneous and cardiac arteries. Transient ischaemic attacks, migrainous headaches, Raynaud syndrome and livedo reticularis are thus common. Primary APS is seen in isolation; secondary APS is associated with SLE or another connective tissue disease such as Sjögren syndrome.

Warfarin is the most effective treatment known. Thromboses or a bleeding tendency, and pulmonary and systemic hypertension are the main factors possibly complicating dental care.

ANTI-SYNTHETASE SYNDROME

Anti-synthetase syndrome is a rare, chronic inflammatory muscle disease characterized by myositis (polymyositis, dermatomyositis), arthritis, interstitial lung disease and Raynaud phenomenon. There are elevated muscle enzymes and anti-Jo-1 antibodies, directed against aminoacyl-tRNA synthetase. Corticosteroids and cyclophosphamide produce symptomatic improvement.

VASCULITIS SYNDROMES

Vasculitis (blood-vessel inflammation, which may affect the veins, arteries and capillaries) is characterized by an inflammatory infiltrate in and around blood vessels, and secondary narrowing or blockage of the vessels, which can cause manifestations in any organ system, including the CNS and peripheral nervous system. Under normal conditions, immune complexes of interlocking antigens and antibodies are rapidly removed from the bloodstream by splenic macrophages and liver Kupffer cells. If, however, they continue to circulate, they become trapped in blood vessels, kidneys, lungs, skin or joints, activating complement and thus initiating vasculitis and tissue damage. Immune complexes may form in autoimmune diseases; in persistent low-grade infections (e.g. malaria and viral hepatitis); or in response to environmental antigens, such as mouldy hay (e.g. farmer's lung) or drugs (e.g. serum sickness). Vasculitic disorders are rare but include:

- Behçet disease (Ch. 11)
- eosinophilic polyangiitis with granulomatosis (formerly called Churg–Strauss syndrome)
- CNS angiitis (granulomatous angiitis)
- giant cell arteritis (temporal or cranial arteritis; Ch. 13)
- Kawasaki disease (Chs 5 and 37)
- periarteritis nodosa
- rheumatoid arthritis (Ch. 16)
- scleroderma (see earlier)
- Sjögren syndrome (see earlier)
- SLE (see earlier)
- Takayasu disease (Ch. 37)
- polyangiitis with granulomatosis (formerly called Wegener granulomatosis).

Clinical features

Vasculitis disorders, or syndromes, give rise to a range of symptoms. Those affecting the CNS and PNS can cause: headaches; fever; weight loss; confusion leading to dementia; joint and muscle pains; paralyses or numbness; and visual disturbances. Vasculitis may be potentially fatal.

General management

Treatment for a vasculitis syndrome often includes corticosteroids, but some may also require other immunosuppressive drugs, such as cyclophosphamide.

ANTINEUTROPHIL CYTOPLASMIC ANTIBODY (ANCA)-ASSOCIATED VASCULITIDES

Antineutrophil cytoplasmic antibody (ANCA)-associated vasculitis affects small to medium-sized blood vessels and causes chronic inflammatory diseases. Possible causal factors include occupational exposure to silica (e.g. farming, construction work), antithyroid and antihypertensive drugs (propylthiouracil and hydralazine), and microbial agents, particularly *Staphylococcus aureus* (chronic nasal carriage has been associated with a higher incidence of relapse in granulomatosis with polyangiitis).

General aspects

Neutrophil priming causes the cytoplasmic ANCA (c-ANCA) antigens proteinase 3 (PR3) and myeloperoxidase (MPO) to be expressed on the neutrophil cell membrane, where they are accessible to ANCA. Neutrophils activated by ANCA degranulate, produce reactive oxygen species, and release proteolytic enzymes that damage blood vessel walls.
ANCA-associated systemic diseases include:

- granulomatosis with polyangiitis (formerly Wegener granulomatosis)
- microscopic polyangiitis
- eosinophilic granulomatosis with polyangiitis (formerly Churg–Strauss syndrome).

Prevalence is generally higher in men over 65 years.

Clinical features

Manifestations may include destructive upper airway disease, pulmonary nodules, renal and pulmonary inflammatory disease, rapidly progressive glomerulonephritis, skin vasculitis with systemic illness, mononeuritis multiplex, subglottic stenosis of the trachea, and retro-orbital mass leading to end-organ damage, particularly renal disease.
Presentation is often with prodromal ''flu-like'' generalized symptoms lasting weeks or months, such as fever, polymyalgia, polyarthralgia, headache, malaise, anorexia and weight loss. Some patients present with focal disease, such as rash, bloody–purulent rhinitis, scleritis, arthritis, ear, nose and throat problems (hearing loss, otalgia, bloody rhinorrhoea, otorrhoea, sinusitis, nasal crusting and recurrent otitis media), or mouth ulcers or characteristic gingival swelling. About 50% of patients have skin manifestations, such as rash or tender nodules. Other symptoms include:

- eyes and nervous system: unexplained conjunctivitis combined with general symptoms, uveitis, unilateral proptosis, and paresis of the ocular motor nerves (granulomatosis with polyangiitis)
- lungs: slowly developing cough and shortness of breath, possibly with bloody-purulent sputum, bilateral infiltrates on radiography that do not respond to antibiotics, non-tuberculous cavitating lesions (granulomatosis with polyangiitis), alveolar haemorrhage (microscopic polyangiitis)

- skin: bursts of small cutaneous vasculitis elements, pyoderma gangrenosum and oedema
- kidneys: haematuria, proteinuria, hypertension, decreasing renal function (granulomatosis with polyangiitis and microscopic polyangiitis). Renal involvement manifests with early detectable haematuria, red cell and other casts, and proteinuria.

General management

Blood tests may show leucocytosis, thrombocytosis, normochromic–normocytic anaemia and a raised serum creatinine. Urinalysis should be performed, for haematuria and proteinuria. Chest radiography may show infiltrates, nodules or cavitations in the lung parenchyma.

Although the ANCA test is positive in most cases, 5–10% of patients do not develop ANCA. Neither does a negative ANCA test exclude the presence of other non-ANCA-associated small- and medium-vessel vasculitic syndromes. ANCA assay is associated with a raised ESR or C-reactive protein (CRP). Indirect immunofluorescence (IIF) is more sensitive but enzyme-linked immunosorbent assay (ELISA) is more specific. Other conditions that can be associated with a positive ANCA test result include:

- inflammatory bowel disease
- chronic infections
- autoimmune conditions
- use of several drugs.

A diagnosis of ANCA-associated vasculitis is confirmed by biopsies obtained from sites of active disease, showing vasculitis, giant cells, 'geographical necrosis' and granulomas.

Remission is usually induced with high-dose corticosteroids and cyclophosphamide, followed by remission maintenance treatment.

GRANULOMATOSIS WITH POLYANGIITIS (FORMERLY WEGENER GRANULOMATOSIS: WG)

General aspects

Granulomatosis with polyangiitis is an uncommon, potentially fatal disease characterized by vasculitis associated with giant cells, necrotizing granulomatous lesions in the respiratory tract (Fig. 18.14) and glomerulonephritis. A limited form of the disease is confined primarily to the lung or oral cavity.

WG is an autoimmune inflammatory disease, involving c-ANCA directed at neutrophil proteinase 3 (PR-3). Neutrophils and endothelial cells are involved in early lesions as both targets and promoters of inflammation.

Many patients are nasal carriers of *Staph. aureus*.

Clinical features

Granulomatosis with polyangiitis comprises the triad of nasopharyngeal inflammation, pulmonary cavitation and renal disease. Upper respiratory involvement typically presents as chronic sinusitis that fails to respond to treatment. The lungs are involved in more than 90% and the kidneys in 75%. It typically terminates in a focal necrotizing glomerulonephritis.

General management

In granulomatosis with polyangiitis the cytoplasmic type of ANCA is found in more than 88% of patients and is virtually diagnostic.

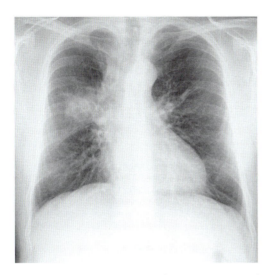

Fig. 18.14 Granuloma in polyangiitis with granulomatosis. Lung involvement.

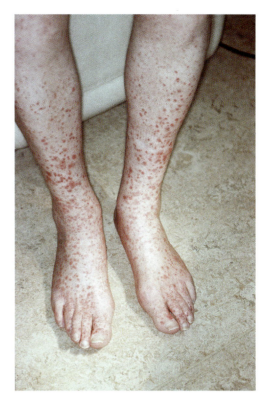

Fig. 18.15 Purpura due to vasculitis.

p-ANCA (directed at myeloperoxidase) is not found. Chest radiography and examination of urine for blood or sediment can indicate pulmonary or renal involvement. Biopsy shows inflammatory changes with giant cells. A necrotizing vasculitis is the main pathological feature but is not seen in gingival biopsies, where small arteries are lacking. This arteritis may, however, be seen in palatal lesions caused by downward spread of the disease from the nasopharynx. Granuloma formation is characteristic but the granulomas may be difficult to see.

Corticosteroids and cyclophosphamide are effective if given early enough. Trimethoprim–sulfamethoxazole may be effective used alone in disease restricted to the upper aerodigestive tract. In others, it may mitigate some of the adverse effects of cytotoxic agents and may prevent relapse. Etanercept and infliximab are under trial as therapies.

Dental aspects

Granulomatosis with polyangiitis can occasionally produce a characteristic and apparently pathognomonic form of gingivitis as its initial manifestation, where the gingivae are swollen and red, and have a strawberry-like texture. Mucosal ulceration and delayed healing of extraction sockets are complications of the later stages of disease, particularly if renal failure develops.

Dental management may be complicated by renal failure, respiratory disease or corticosteroid, other immunosuppressive or cytotoxic therapy.

POLYARTERITIS NODOSA (PERIARTERITIS NODOSA)

General aspects

Polyarteritis nodosa (PAN) is a multisystem immune-complex disease characterized by necrotizing vasculitis affecting mainly small and medium-sized arteries; it most frequently targets middle-aged men. ANCA appears to play a significant role in causing endothelial damage; perinuclear ANCA (p-ANCA; antimyeloperoxidase) is often found in microscopic polyarteritis (MPA). c-ANCA (antiproteinase 3) has also been described but is more often seen in polyangiitis with granulomatosis. Increased serum IFN-α and IL-2, and a moderate rise in TNF-α and IL-1β, may enhance endothelial damage by activating endothelial cells and polymorphonuclear neutrophil leukocytes (PMNLs).

The precipitating factor is often unidentified but may be microbial or a drug. Hepatitis B virus has been implicated in up to 40% of patients, and other infective agents occasionally involved include hepatitis C virus, human immunodeficiency virus (HIV), cytomegalovirus, parvovirus B19, human T-lymphotropic virus 1 (HTLV-1) or *Streptococcus* species. Drugs (e.g. thiouracil, iodides and sulphonamides) may occasionally be responsible.

Clinical features

PAN has protean manifestations as a result of the capricious distribution of the lesions anywhere in the body. Fever, anorexia, weight loss, myalgia, arthralgia, purpura (Fig. 18.15) and peripheral neuropathies are common but non-specific. Abdominal involvement, with pain, nausea, vomiting or diarrhoea, is seen in over 60%. Renal disease affects 50%. Tender skin nodules may be palpable over inflamed vessels. Hypertension and angina are common.

General management

Leukocytosis, eosinophilia, raised ESR, pANCA, hypergammaglobulinaemia and sometimes a false positive test for rheumatoid factor may be found. Albuminuria or haematuria is common. Angiography may demonstrate arterial aneurysms (early PAN) or vascular occlusions (late PAN). Histological examination of clinically involved tissue is needed to confirm the diagnosis.

The prognosis is poor in untreated disease; up to 60% die within 1 year. Systemic corticosteroids give a 5-year survival rate of over 40%. Cyclophosphamide may also be of value.

Allergic granulomatosis is a closely related disease characterized by fever, asthma and eosinophilia.

Dental aspects

Dental management may be complicated by corticosteroid therapy and immunosuppression; hepatitis B antigen carriage; hypertension and cardiac disease; or renal disease. Submucosal nodules, haemorrhage or oral ulcers are rare manifestations. Facial palsy or other cranial neuropathies may be occasional complications.

KEY WEBSITES

(Accessed 27 May 2013)
Leeds Teaching Hospitals NHS Trust Pathology Services. <http://www.pathology.leedsth.nhs.uk/pathology/ClinicalInfo/Immunology/Autoimmunedisease.aspx>.
MedlinePlus. <http://www.nlm.nih.gov/medlineplus/ency/article/000816.htm>.
National Institutes of Health. <http://health.nih.gov/topic/AutoimmuneDiseasesGeneral>.

USEFUL WEBSITES

(Accessed 27 May 2013)
British Sjögren's Syndrome Association. <http://www.bssa.uk.net>.
Dry.Org – Internet resources for Sjögren's syndrome. <http://dry.org>.
Lupus Foundation of America. <http://www.lupus.org/answers/topic/understanding-lupus>.
National Institute of Allergy and Infectious Diseases. <http://www.niaid.nih.gov/Pages/default.aspx>.
National Institute of Neurological Disorders and Stroke. <http://www.ninds.nih.gov/disorders/Sjogrens/sjogrens.htm>.
Sjögren's Syndrome Foundation. <http://www.sjogrens.org/index.php>.

FURTHER READING

Aframian, D., et al. 2013. Urban legends series: Sjögren's syndrome. Oral Dis. 19 (1), 46. doi: 10.1111/j.1601-0825.2012.01930.x. Epub 2012 Apr 11. PubMed PMID: 22490059.

Amital, H., et al. 2008. Role of infectious agents in systemic rheumatic diseases. Clin. Exp. Rheumatol. 26 (1 Suppl. 48), S27.

Barone, F., et al. 2008. CXCL13, CCL21, and CXCL12 expression in salivary glands of patients with Sjögren's syndrome and MALT lymphoma: association with reactive and malignant areas of lymphoid organization. J. Immunol. 180, 5130.

Barry, R.J., et al. 2008. The Sjögren's Syndrome Damage Index – a damage index for use in clinical trials and observational studies in primary Sjögren's syndrome. Rheumatology (Oxford) 47, 1193.

Berden, A., et al. 2012. Diagnosis and management of ANCA associated vasculitis. Br. Med. J. 344, e26. doi: 10.1136/bmj.e26. Review. PubMed PMID: 22250224.

Bischoff, L., Derk, C.T., 2008. Eosinophilic fasciitis: demographics, disease pattern and response to treatment: report of 12 cases and review of the literature. Int. J. Dermatol. 47, 29.

Boström, E.A., et al. 2008. Salivary resistin reflects local inflammation in Sjögren's syndrome. J. Rheumatol. 35, 2005.

Carr, A.J., et al. 2012. Sjögren's syndrome – an update for dental practitioners. Br. Dent. J. 213 (7), 353. doi: 10.1038/sj.bdj.2012.890 PubMed PMID: 23059671.

Ceribelli, A., et al. 2008. Hepatitis C virus infection and primary Sjögren's syndrome: a clinical and serologic description of 9 patients. Autoimmun. Rev. 8, 92.

Coaccioli, S., et al. 2007. The therapy of Sjögren's syndrome: a review. Clin. Ter. 158 (5), 453.

Derk, C.T., et al. 2005. Increased incidence of carcinoma of the tongue in patients with systemic sclerosis. J. Rheumatol. 32, 637.

Derk, C.T., et al. 2006. A cohort study of cancer incidence in systemic sclerosis. J. Rheumatol. 33, 1113.

Fedele, S., et al. 2008. Neuroelectrostimulation in treatment of hyposalivation and xerostomia in Sjögren's syndrome: a salivary pacemaker. J. Rheumatol. 35, 1489.

Furness, S., et al. 2011. Interventions for the management of dry mouth: topical therapies. Cochrane Database Syst. Rev. (12), CD008934. doi: 10.1002/14651858.CD008934.pub2. Review. PubMed PMID: 22161442.

Hansen, A., et al. 2003. New concepts in the pathogenesis of Sjögren syndrome: many questions, fewer answers. Curr. Opin. Rheumatol. 15, 563.

Ittah, M., et al. 2008. Viruses induce high expression of BAFF by salivary gland epithelial cells through TLR- and type-I IFN-dependent and -independent pathways. Eur. J. Immunol. 38, 1058.

Jorkjend, L., et al. 2008. Effect of pilocarpine on impaired salivary secretion in patients with Sjögren's syndrome. Swed. Dent. J. 32, 49.

Mathews, S.A., et al. 2008. Oral manifestations of Sjögren's syndrome. J. Dent. Res. 87 (4), 308.

Mignogna, M.D., et al. 2005. Sjögren's syndrome: the diagnostic potential of early oral manifestations preceding hyposalivation/xerostomia. J. Oral Pathol. Med. 34, 1.

Moutsopoulos, H.M., Fragoulis, G.E., 2008. Is mizoribine a new therapeutic agent for Sjögren's syndrome? Nat. Clin. Pract. Rheumatol. 4, 350.

Porter, S., Scully, C., 2008. Connective tissue disorders and the mouth. Dent. Update 35 294, 298, 302.

Postal, M., et al. 2012. Biological therapy in systemic lupus erythematosus. Int. J. Rheumatol. 2012, 57864.10.1155/2012/578641 Review article.

Ramos-Casals, M., et al. 2012. Primary Sjögren syndrome. Br. Med. J. 344, e3821. doi: 10.1136/bmj.e3821 Review. PubMed PMID: 22700787.

Ramos-Casals, M., et al. 2012. Topical and systemic medications for the treatment of primary Sjögren's syndrome. Nat. Rev. Rheumatol. 8 (7), 399. doi: 10.1038/nrrheum.2012.53 PubMed PMID: 22549247.

Sakai, A., et al. 2008. Identification of IL-18 and Th17 cells in salivary glands of patients with Sjögren's syndrome, and amplification of IL-17-mediated secretion of inflammatory cytokines from salivary gland cells by IL-18. J. Immunol. 181, 2898.

Salaffi, F., et al. 2008. Ultrasonography of salivary glands in primary Sjögren's syndrome: a comparison with contrast sialography and scintigraphy. Rheumatology (Oxford) 47, 1244.

Shiboski, S.C., et al. 2012. American College of Rheumatology classification criteria for Sjögren's syndrome: a data-driven, expert consensus approach in the Sjögren's International Collaborative Clinical Alliance cohort. Arthritis. Care Res. 64 (4), 475.10.1002/acr.21591.

Stewart, C.M., et al. 2008. Labial salivary gland biopsies in Sjögren's syndrome: still the gold standard? Oral Surg. Oral Med. Oral Pathol. Oral Radiol. Endod. 106, 392.

Thieblemont, C., et al. 2003. Nongastric mucosa-associated lymphoid tissue lymphomas. Clin. Lymphoma 3, 212.

Triantafyllopoulou, A., Moutsopoulos, H., 2007. Persistent viral infection in primary Sjögren's syndrome: review and perspectives. Clin. Rev. Allergy Immunol. 32, 210.

Triantafyllopoulou, A., Moutsopoulos, H.M., 2005. Autoimmunity and coxsackievirus infection in primary Sjögren's syndrome. Ann. N. Y. Acad. Sci. 1050, 389.

Tzioufas, A.G., Voulgarelis, M., 2007. Update on Sjögren's syndrome autoimmune epithelitis: from classification to increased neoplasias. Best Pract. Res. Clin. Rheumatol. 21, 989.

Tzioufas, A.G., et al. 2008. Neuroendocrine dysfunction in Sjögren's syndrome. Neuroimmunomodulation 15, 37.

Vitali, C., et al. 2013. Classification criteria for Sjögren's syndrome: we actually need to definitively resolve the long debate on the issue. Ann. Rheum. Dis. 72 (4), 476. doi: 10.1136/annrheumdis-2012-202565. Epub 2012 Dec 22.

Yamamoto, M., et al. 2006. A new conceptualization for Mikulicz's disease as an IgG4-related plasmacytic disease. Mod. Rheumatol. 16, 335.

This chapter discusses innate and acquired immunity and inflammation, autoinflammatory disorders and immunosuppressive therapy.

INNATE IMMUNITY AND INFLAMMATION

Innate immunity includes basic mechanisms of resistance to infection, such as epithelial anatomical barriers of skin and mucous membranes, cilia, secretions such as saliva and tears, and the innate inflammatory response. The latter is characterized by increased localized blood flow and capillary permeability (inflammation), releasing soluble factors that recruit phagocytes (neutrophils and macrophages), which restrict and engulf invasive microorganisms.

Inflammation is initiated and maintained by mediators, especially complement and cytokines – small proteins that specifically also affect the behaviour of immune cells (immunocytes). Cytokines, including interleukins, lymphokines and cell signal molecules such as tumour necrosis factors and interferons, regulate the intensity or duration of immune responses by stimulating or inhibiting proliferation of various immunocytes, or by modulating their secretion of other cytokines or antibodies.

COMPLEMENT

The complement system is a plasma protein sequence (cascade) involving at least nine plasma proteins. When activated, this sequence releases important mediators of inflammation and chemotaxis (C3a and C5a), compounds capable of opsonizing microorganisms for phagocytosis (C3b), and an attack complex (C5–9) capable of damaging cell membranes (Fig. 19.1). There are three complement pathways – classical, lectin and alternative – that differ in the manner in which they are activated (triggering agents include bacterial lipopolysaccharides [LPS] and immune [antigen/antibody] complexes), though all produce C3 convertase – the key enzyme. The system is controlled by inhibitors such as C1 esterase inhibitor, decay accelerating factor (DAF), membrane inhibitor of reactive lysis (MIRL) and homologous restriction factor (HRF).

CYTOKINES

Cytokines are a family of proteins – interferons, tumour necrosis factors, transforming growth factors, interleukins, chemokines and colony-stimulating factors – that act in concert with inhibitors and soluble receptors to regulate immune responses.

Interferons (IFNs) are one of the most important natural defences against viral infection. IFN-α and IFN-β are antiproliferative for virally infected and other cell types. IFN-γ is involved in cell-mediated immune responses, via Th1 lymphocytes; is antagonistic to interleukin 4 (IL-4); activates macrophages; and induces expression of class II major histocompatibility complex (MHC) antigens.

Tumour necrosis factors (TNFs) are important in inflammation and antitumour immunity. *TNF-α* is secreted by a variety of cells, including T and B lymphocytes, macrophages, natural killer (NK) cells, endothelial cells and keratinocytes. TNF-α primes both endothelial cells and neutrophils for adhesion, is chemotactic for inflammatory cells and can signal cells to begin apoptosis (programmed cell death). It is a death activator, triggering the proteolytic caspase cascade that culminates in apoptosis. It can also activate nuclear factor kappa B (NF-κB) and activator protein 1 (AP-1), leading to the induction of several genes and inflammation. It can also initiate and perpetuate an inflammatory response through upregulating adhesion molecules on microvascular endothelial cells, and enhance expression of MHC class I and II antigens, and co-stimulatory molecules on dendritic cells (DCs) and macrophages. Matrix metalloproteinase (MMP) production by stromal cells is induced, which may lead to tissue remodelling

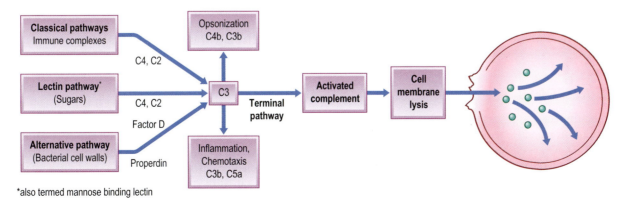

Fig. 19.1 Complement pathways.

Table 19.1 *Main cytokines*

Proinflammatory cytokines	Anti-inflammatory cytokines
Tumour necrosis factor (TNF-alpha)	IL-4, IL-10 and IL-11
Interferons (IFNs)	
Alpha	
Beta	
Interleukins (ILs)	
1	
6, 15, 17 and 18	

Box 19.2 *Colony-stimulating factors (CSFs)*

- CSF1: macrophage CSF (M-CSF)
- CSF2: granulocyte–macrophage CSF (GM-CSF; sargramostin)
- CSF3: granulocyte CSF (G-CSF; filgrastim)

Table 19.2 *Acute-phase reactants*

Protein	Main functions
Alpha$_1$-antichymotrypsin	A serpin, which downregulates inflammation
Alpha$_1$-antitrypsin	A serpin, which downregulates inflammation
Alpha$_2$-macroglobulin	Inhibits coagulation and fibrinolysis
Caeruloplasmin	Inhibits microbial iron uptake
Complement	See text
C-reactive protein (CRP)	Binds to phosphorylcholine in bacterial membranes and phosphatidyl ethanolamine in fungal membranes activating the classical complement pathway
D-dimer protein	Fibrin degradation product
Factor VIII	Coagulation factor
Ferritin	Inhibits microbial iron uptake
Fibrinogen	Coagulation factor
Haptoglobin	Inhibits microbial iron uptake
Mannan-binding protein (MBP) or lectin (MBL)	Binds to microbial mannose-rich glycans to act as an opsonin, and also activates the lectin pathway
Plasminogen	Coagulation factor
Prothrombin	Coagulation factor
Serum amyloid A	Recruits immunocytes to inflammatory sites
von Willebrand factor	Coagulation factor

Box 19.1 *Chemokines*

- C chemokines – attract T-cell precursors to the thymus
- CC chemokines – induce migration of monocytes, and dendritic and natural killer (NK) cells
- CXC chemokines – specifically induce the migration of neutrophils
- CX3C chemokines – chemoattractant and adhesion molecule

and the enhanced TNF-mediated secretion of keratinocyte growth factor (KGF). TNF can also induce fever, either directly via stimulation of prostaglandin E2 (PGE2) synthesis by the hypothalamic vascular endothelium, or indirectly by inducing release of the pyrogen interleukin 1 (IL-1), and can stimulate collagenase and PGE2 production. TNF also induces hepatic acute-phase reactant protein production.

TNF-β – from T and B cells, NK cells and astrocytes – mediates fibroblast and endothelial cell proliferation, important in wound healing.

Transforming growth factor beta (TGF-β) is part of a protein superfamily that includes inhibins, activins and bone morphogenetic protein (BMP), which can affect development, haemopoiesis, wound healing and tissue repair. TGF-β has a crucial role in cell-cycle regulation and apoptosis, via the SMAD (name derived from a fusion of gene names sma [in Caenorhabditis elegans] and Mad [in Drosophila]) or the DAXX (death domain-associated protein) pathways.

Interleukins and their functions are diverse. Over 33 interleukins have been identified, most originating from T cells, some macrophages and mast cells, or from B cells or other cells (Appendix 19.1).

Cytokines that promote inflammation are termed proinflammatory cytokines; others are anti-inflammatory (Table 19.1).

Chemokines (chemoattractant cytokines)

Historically known under names such as the SIS family of cytokines, SIG family of cytokines, SCY family of cytokines, platelet factor-4 superfamily or intercrines, chemokines are classified into four groups (Box 19.1).

Colony-stimulating factors (CSFs) are glycoproteins that bind to haemopoietic cell receptors to drive differentiation. Those most relevant to the immune response are shown in Box 19.2.

ACUTE-PHASE RESPONSE

In response to injury, infection, physical trauma or malignancy, neutrophils and macrophages secrete several cytokines (most notably IL-1, IL-6, IL-8 and TNF-α), which cause the liver to produce *acute-phase reactants* – proteins whose plasma concentrations increase in response to, and suppress, inflammation (Table 19.2).

C-reactive protein (CRP) and serum amyloid A protein (SAA) are critical in the innate immune response. CRP can bind to some bacteria

and fungi, activating complement and inflammation, as can SAA, which can also stimulate macrophages to phagocytose debris. Most organisms that tend to be invasive are ingested by phagocytes, including blood neutrophils (polymorphonuclear neutrophilic leukocytes) and tissue macrophages ('phage' = eating up), which kill most organisms. However, some (i.e. all viruses, and bacteria such as those causing tuberculosis or brucellosis) survive inside cells, including phagocytes, and then the immune system is the main defence. Clinically, this positive acute-phase response appears within 12 hours and can be measured by determining CRP levels or the erythrocyte sedimentation rate (ESR). The acute-phase response is also characterized by leukocytosis, fever, and alterations in the metabolism of many organs. In contrast, there is a negative acute-phase response with decreases in albumin, transferrin, transthyretin and insulin growth factor I.

ACQUIRED IMMUNE RESPONSE

The main activity of the immune system is protection against infections. Immunocytes (leukocytes) are mainly lymphocytes and they produce humoral (antibody; mainly B-cell) or cell-mediated (mainly T-cell) responses that are central to the immune defences. B lymphocytes evolve into plasma cells, which produce antibodies to protect against extracellular organisms (Fig. 19.2). Antigens are processed by antigen-presenting cells (APC) and presented to T lymphocytes, which fulfil most other immune functions (i.e. cell-mediated immunity [CMI]). Macrophages and polymorphs are the main professional phagocytes; macrophages and macrophage-like cells

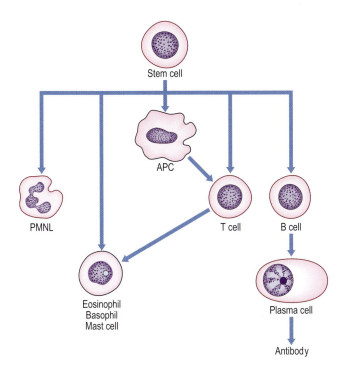

Fig. 19.2 Essentials of immunity. APC = antigen-presenting cell; PMNL = polymorphonuclear leukocyte.

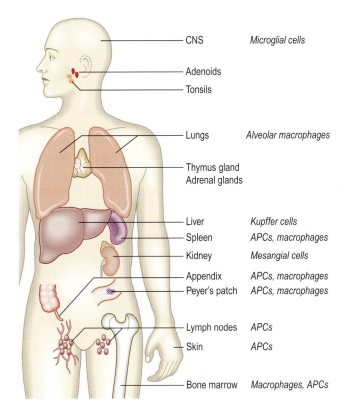

Fig. 19.3 Reticuloendothelial system. APC = antigen-presenting cell.

are widely distributed in the lymphoreticular (reticuloendothelial) system (Fig. 19.3).

More than 70 types of leukocyte are recognized and defined by their cluster of differentiation (CD) antigens, which in turn are recognized by monoclonal antibodies.

Immunocytes are, in large part, regulated by cytokines produced by a variety of cells. Cytokines produced by lymphocytes are termed lymphokines, and those that act between leukocytes are called interleukins

Table 19.3 *Immunoglobulins*

Classes	Comments
IgA	Secreted by exocrine glands and helps to protect mucosal surfaces
IgD	Of unclear function
IgE	Important in the mediation of atopic allergy but has a role in the defence against parasites
IgG	Essential for protection against bacterial infections, by such functions as neutralizing toxins, activating complement or promoting phagocytosis
IgM	(opsonization)

(see Appendix 19.1). Cytokines may also induce systemic effects, such as the acute-phase response (see above).

The movement of leukocytes between the blood and tissues depends on leukocyte–endothelial cell adhesion molecules known as selectins, integrins and the immunoglobulin gene superfamily (IgSF; intercellular adhesion molecules [ICAMs] and lymphocyte functional antigen 3), and over 20 other proteins.

HUMORAL IMMUNITY

Antibodies are immunoglobulins. B cells carry surface immunoglobulins and also receptors for immunoglobulin G (IgG; CD32) and complement-activated components C3d (CD21) and C3b (CD35). Antibody production is modulated by T lymphocytes, which either assist (T-helper cells) or moderate (T-suppressor cells). The many cytokines involved include IL-1 to IL-7 and B-cell growth factor (BCGF). Immunoglobulins (antibodies) are of different classes (Table 19.3).

Complement and polymorphonuclear leukocytes (PMNLs) are essential to phagocytosis and inflammation. Cell-mediated responses are usually protective, and macrophages are also phagocytic.

PHAGOCYTES AND OTHER CELLS

Macrophages and dendritic cells intimately involved in antigen processing and the transference of information to lymphocytes are called antigen-processing cells (APCs). Phagocytes (PMNLs and macrophages) are attracted towards antigens, via activated complement after an antigen–antibody reaction, and can ingest and often kill microbes that are opsonized (i.e. coated by specific antibody and activated complement components). During phagocytosis or attempted phagocytosis of, for example, immune complexes, these phagocytes may discharge degradative enzymes (lysosomal enzymes), which can cause local tissue damage.

Large granular lymphocytes (LGLs; or null cells) are non-phagocytic cells that mediate NK cell activity and antibody-dependent cellular cytotoxicity (ADCC) – the binding and lysis of antibody-coated target cells. NK cells recognize malignant or foreign cells by a non-immune mechanism.

Basophils and mast cells have surface receptors for IgE, and contain histamine, prostaglandins, leukotrienes and proteases. They are involved in immune responses to parasites and in the immediate type of hypersensitivity responses (Ch. 17).

Prostaglandins (Table 19.4) and leukotrienes (Table 19.5) are produced from eicosanoids – lipids produced by the oxygenation of arachidonic acid from omega-3 fatty acids in fish oils, or released from cells by phospholipase A2. The enzyme cyclo-oxygenase (COX) produces prostaglandins and thromboxane, while the enzyme 5-lipoxygenase produces leukotrienes.

Table 19.4 *Important prostaglandins (PGs)*

Prostaglandin	Sites of origin	Effects
PGD$_2$	Mast cells	Bronchoconstriction, vasodilatation and inhibition of platelet aggregation
PGI$_2$ (prostacyclin)	Endothelium	Vasodilatation and inhibition of platelet aggregation
PGE$_2$	Epithelium, dendritic cells	Inhibition of lymphocyte proliferation, cytokine production and neutrophil function

Table 19.5 *Leukotrienes (LTs)*

Leukotriene	Causes
LTB4	Neutrophil chemotaxis, mucus secretion, cell growth
LTC4 (formerly termed slow-reacting substance A)	Vascular permeability, smooth muscle contraction, mucus production
LTD4	
LTE4	

CELL-MEDIATED IMMUNITY

Antigens are processed by antigen-presenting cells, such as macrophages and Langerhans cells in epithelia, and presented to T cells in association with class I or II MHC molecules. T lymphocytes originate in bone marrow but differentiate within and are under the control of the thymus (hence T), acquiring immunological competence there, a process that requires the normal functioning of purine metabolism. T cells all have T-cell receptors, highlighted by the CD3 surface marker. When activated by antigens, T lymphocytes produce lymphokines, which, among other activities, can modulate nearby cells, particularly macrophages, resulting in CMI (type IV immune responses). These are particularly important in the defence against some intracellular bacteria, such as mycobacteria, and against viruses and fungi, graft rejection, graft-versus-host reaction, delayed hypersensitivity and defences against cancer cells.

Circulating T lymphocytes differentiate into CD4 cells – mainly helper T cells that are antigen-processing and can recognize MHC class II antigens, and can induce B-cell differentiation, induce CD8 cytotoxic T-cell proliferation, produce various soluble mediators (lymphokines) and regulate erythropoiesis. Healthy adults usually have CD4+ T-cell counts of 1000 or more per mm^3 of blood. CD4 helper T cells are either Th1 or Th2. Th1 cells secrete IL-2 and IFN-γ; they provide help for the generation of cytotoxic T cells involved in type IV immune responses (Ch. 17) and are suppressed by IL-10. Th2 secrete IL-4, 5, 6 and 10, which both help B cells to produce IgG, IgA and IgE, and regulate the production of other cytokines – and thereby the immune response. Th2 cells are involved in type II and type III immune reactions and are suppressed by interferon.

Circulating T lymphocytes can also differentiate into CD8 cells, which recognize MHC class I antigens and are one type of cytotoxic or suppressor T cell; they are important in eliminating virus-infected cells.

To summarize, T-cell proliferation and differentiation are regulated by many cytokines, including interleukins, interferons, tumour necrosis factors and transforming growth factors. Cytokines generally function as local signals for cell growth, differentiation, activation, inhibition, apoptosis or chemotaxis, but may also induce systemic effects such as acute-phase responses (fever, CRP, osteoclast activation, platelet release) induced by IL-1, IL-6 and TNF.

EVALUATION OF B-LYMPHOCYTE FUNCTION

The initial screening for B-lymphocyte function is an assay of serum IgG, IgA and IgM. There are four subclasses of IgG, and selective deficiencies of these can develop. Thus, when there is a strong suspicion of a humoral immunodeficiency based on clinical grounds but the total IgG is normal, quantitative measurement of individual subclasses is indicated.

Assessment of antibody function is necessary. Antibody titres after immunization with protein antigens (e.g. tetanus or diphtheria toxoids) and polysaccharide (e.g. pneumococcal capsular polysaccharides) are most convenient (immunization with live viral vaccines must be avoided, as the person may be immunocompromised). If immunoglobulin levels and/or antibody titres are low, more advanced tests of B-lymphocyte numbers and function are needed.

EVALUATION OF T-LYMPHOCYTE FUNCTION

Indirect information about T-lymphocyte function may be obtained by counting peripheral blood T lymphocytes. The total number of T lymphocytes (CD2 or CD3), T-helper lymphocytes (CD4) and T-suppressor/cytotoxic lymphocytes (CD8) in peripheral blood can be quantified with appropriate monoclonal antibodies.

Delayed-type hypersensitivity (DTH) skin tests use a panel of ubiquitous antigens to screen for T-cell function. A positive test generally indicates intact T-cell function and CMI, but requires prior exposure and sensitization to the antigen, which may not have happened. Also, a positive DTH skin test to some antigens does not guarantee that the patient will have normal CMI to all. Furthermore, some normal individuals may have transiently depressed DTH reactions during viral infections. Skin testing for DTH measures not only T-lymphocyte responses but also the afferent (receptor) arc of the cell-mediated immune response. Thus, most adults show DTH to tuberculin in the tuberculin (Mantoux) test, since they have had previous contact with *Mycobacterium tuberculosis* or bacilli Calmette–Guérin (BCG). A positive response in apparently well people is generally an index of 'waiting immunity' to the disease and usually does not mean that mycobacteria are actively causing cell-mediated tissue damage. A recent change from negative to positive in the absence of vaccination implies recent exposure, and prophylactic treatment may be indicated. By contrast, a negative tuberculin reaction indicates susceptibility to infection or occasionally that overwhelming infection is established – all CMI has been used up in an attempt to combat the infection. In such cases, successful treatment may allow CMI to return and a negative Mantoux test can then become positive.

It is possible also, in specialized laboratories, to measure several different cytokines involved in T- and B-lymphocyte regulation (e.g. IL-2, IFN-γ).

EVALUATION OF PHAGOCYTIC FUNCTION

A white blood cell count and differential are the first essentials. Assessment of phagocyte function requires *in vitro* assays of directed cell movement (chemotaxis), ingestion (phagocytosis) and intracellular killing (bactericidal activity).

EVALUATION OF THE COMPLEMENT SYSTEM

Most complement components can be detected using antibody-sensitized sheep erythrocytes in a total haemolytic complement assay (CH50 assay), since this assay requires the functional integrity of C1 to C9.

Table 19.6 *Main autoinflammatory syndromes*

Disease	Inheritance	Acronym	Gene and protein defect	Main features apart from fever and rashes	Management
Familial Mediterranean fever	AR	FMF	MEFV	Serositis, synovitis, amyloidosis	Colchicine
Tumour necrosis factor receptor-associated periodic syndrome	AD	TRAPS	TNFRS1A	Abdominal pain, migratory myalgia, rash, periorbital oedema, mouth ulcers, amyloidosis	Corticosteroids Etanercept (TNF inhibitor) Colchicine
Hyperimmunoglobulin D syndrome	AR	HIDS	MVK	Abdominal pain, diarrhoea, arthralgia, mouth ulcers	Simvastatin, anakinra (IL-1 receptor antagonist)
Mevalonate aciduria	AD	MA		Learning disability, failure to thrive, progressive visual impairment and cerebellar ataxia, dysmorphic features	Corticosteroids
Neonatal-onset multisystem inflammatory disease	AD	NOMID	CIAS1	Chronic meningitis, hearing and vision loss	Anakinra
Muckle–Wells syndrome	AD	MWS		Urticaria, arthralgia, deafness, amyloidosis	
Familial cold autoinflammatory syndrome	AD	FCAS		Urticaria, amyloidosis	
Pyogenic sterile arthritis, pyoderma gangrenosum, acne	AD	PAPA	PSTPIP1/CD2BP1	Arthritis, headache, abdominal pain, mouth ulcers	Anakinra Etanercept
Blau syndrome	AD	–	CARD15 or NOD2	Arthritis, uveitis	Anakinra
Periodic fever, aphthous stomatitis, pharyngitis, adenitis	Not known	PFAPA	Not known	Pharyngitis, adenitis, mouth ulcers	Corticosteroids Cimetidine
Chronic recurrent multifocal osteomyelitis	AD	CRMO	LPIN2 and Lipin2	Chronic recurrent multifocal osteomyelitis	Antimicrobials

AD/AR = autosomal dominant/recessive.

Deficiencies of alternative pathway components factors D, H and I and properdin can be detected by a haemolytic assay using activators of the alternative pathway, such as unsensitized rabbit erythrocytes. Individual components are detected by specialized functional and immunochemical tests.

AUTOINFLAMMATORY DISEASES (PERIODIC SYNDROMES)

General aspects

The autoinflammatory diseases (periodic syndromes) are rare disorders of innate immunity, often hereditary, which involve an ongoing imbalance between factors promoting and those inhibiting inflammation. The abnormalities seen include aberrant responses to pathogen-associated molecular patterns (PAMPs), including lipopolysaccharide (LPS) and peptidoglycan; neutrophilia; and dysregulation of the proinflammatory cytokines IL-1β and/or TNF-α, or the receptors for these cytokines.

Clinical features

Periodic syndromes usually begin from childhood and are characterized by fluctuating or recurrent episodes of fever and generalized inflammation, affecting the surfaces, joints, eyes and/or skin.

Patients with the autoinflammatory syndromes generally are well between abrupt episodes of fever and systemic inflammation, but some develop amyloidosis.

General management

Diagnosis is supported by evidence of elevated acute-phase response during attacks, and often a positive family history and ethnic background. Genetic testing is indicated. Many of the syndromes have a specific treatment (Table 19.6).

Dental aspects

Aphthous-like oral ulceration has been reported as one manifestation in periodic fever, aphthous stomatitis, pharyngitis, adenitis (PFAPA); familial Mediterranean fever (FMF); hyperimmunoglobulinaemia D and periodic fever syndrome; tumour necrosis factor receptor-associated periodic syndrome (TRAPS); and pyogenic sterile arthritis, pyoderma gangrenosum, acne (PAPA).

Chronic recurrent osteomyelitis has been recorded in the jaws in chronic recurrent multifocal osteomyelitis. There is a suggested association of FMF with Behçet disease.

PERIODIC FEVER, APHTHOUS STOMATITIS, PHARYNGITIS, ADENITIS (MARSHALL SYNDROME)

PFAPA is not a familial disease. Attacks usually appear in pre-school children as recurrent fever with aphthous-like stomatitis, pharyngitis and cervical lymphadenitis. Long-term sequelae have not been reported and most children eventually grow out of it. Diagnostically, raised ESR, leukocyte count, fibrinogen and serum IgD have been found. PFAPA often responds well to corticosteroids, cimetidine or tonsillectomy.

DEFICIENCY OF THE INTERLEUKIN-1 RECEPTOR ANTAGONIST (DIRA)

Deficiency of interleukin-1 receptor antagonist IL-1Ra (DIRA) is caused by inherited mutations in the gene *IL1RN* that encodes IL-1Ra. This antagonist binds to the same cell receptors as does IL-1 and blocks its inflammatory actions, so without IL-1Ra, the IL-1–induced systemic inflammation is uncontrolled. Mutations causing DIRA are rare, but more common in people of Puerto Rican or Dutch descent. Features include serious and potentially fatal bone swelling, pain and deformity; periosteitis; and skin pustulosis. Most children develop features from birth to 2 weeks of age and most respond to anakinra.

DEFICIENCY OF THE INTERLEUKIN-36–RECEPTOR ANTAGONIST

Aberrant interleukin-36Ra structure and function cause secretion of proinflammatory cytokines, hyperleukocytosis and raised C-reactive protein and generalized pustular psoriasis.

IMMUNOSUPPRESSIVE THERAPY

See also Chapter 35.

Where inflammation can become harmful, attempts can be made to suppress the immune response or block cytokine action. Most immunosuppressive drugs predominantly depress cell-mediated responses and autoantibody production more strongly than normal antibody production.

Immunosuppressive therapy is widely used, especially to suppress rejection in transplant recipients (bone marrow, kidney, liver, pancreas, heart and heart–lung; Ch. 35), to treat autoimmune and connective tissue diseases, and to control tumours – especially lymphoproliferative neoplasms (Ch. 8).

Immunosuppressive therapy inevitably predisposes patients significantly to infections, particularly viral, fungal, mycobacterial and protozoal ones, since T-cell immunity is largely depressed; patients are also predisposed to malignant disease (Kaposi sarcoma, lymphomas and squamous cell carcinomas of the skin, cervix and lip), most of which are virally related. Infections may be opportunistic (i.e. involve microorganisms that are normally commensal), may spread rapidly and often may be clinically silent or atypical.

Immunosuppressive strategies now attempt to be more selective in their effects on the immune response by using biological agents (also termed targeted immune modulators [TIMs]) and biological response modifiers [BRMs]) designed to inhibit the harmful effects of upregulated proinflammatory cytokines (e.g. TNF-α, IL-1 and receptor, IFN-β, IFN-α, IL-6, IL-15, IL-17 and IL-18). Potential therapeutic strategies may augment the activity of anti-inflammatory cytokines (e.g. IL-4, IL-10 and IL-11) (see below).

Systemic non-biological immunomodulators are used in oral health care in mucosal disease:

- Pemphigus
- Severe, resistant or systemic lesions in:
  aphthae or aphthous-like ulceration
  Behçet disease
  Crohn disease/orofacial granulomatosis (OFG)
  erythema multiforme
  lichen planus
  pemphigoid, etc.

They are also used in other conditions:

- Bell palsy
- Giant cell arteritis
- Vasculitis.

Most affect cytochrome P450-3A4 and P-glycoprotein drug pathways, and interact with foods/medications. All may have serious adverse effects, including:

- teratogenicity
- infections
- malignant disease:
  basal cell carcinomas
  Kaposi sarcomas (KS)
  lymphomas and lymphoproliferative disorders (e.g. post-transplant lymphoproliferative disease [PTLD])
  melanomas
  squamous cell carcinomas of skin, lip, cervix, external genitalia and perineum.

SYSTEMIC NON-BIOLOGICAL IMMUNOMODULATORS

Drugs such as azathioprine, cyclophosphamide and chlorambucil are cytotoxic to cells, including some immunocytes; they thus act as fairly crude immunosuppressive agents and adverse effects are common (Appendix 19.2). *Calcineurin inhibitors* bind to immunophilins (cyclophilin and macrophilin) and block receptor expression, T-cell activation and cytokine release. Calcineurin inhibitors (ciclosporin and tacrolimus) may enhance tumour development through mechanisms independent of host immunity. In contrast, inhibitors of the mammalian target of rapamycin (mTOR), including sirolimus and everolimus, are newer immunosuppressants that have antineoplastic properties.

BIOLOGICS (BIOLOGICAL RESPONSE MODIFIERS)

(Appendix 19.3; see also Chapter 35.)

Biologics are produced mainly by recombinant DNA technology and are usually:

- substances almost identical to key signalling proteins
- monoclonal antibodies (mAbs)
- receptor constructs, or fusion proteins.

Biological response modifiers (BRMs) block the inflammatory and immune responses, acting on immunocytes directly or via cytokines, inhibiting cellular activation and inflammatory gene transcription by various means.

Some are antibodies, soluble receptors or natural antagonists; others are small molecules that specifically inhibit intracellular, cell–cell and cell–matrix interactions intrinsic to inflammatory and immune processes. Examples are shown in Appendices 19.3 and 19.4.

Biologic therapies aim to modulate lymphocytes or cytokines. They include:

- TNFα inhibitors
- lymphocyte modulators
- interleukin inhibitors.

TNFα inhibitors (etanercept, adalimumab, infliximab, golimumab, certolizumab, natalizumab) bind and/or neutralize soluble (both circulating and within tissue) and membrane-bound TNFα, so blocking its effects upon target inflammatory cells.

T-cell modulators act on specific CD antigens. Alefacept targets CD2+ on memory T and NK cells. B-cell modulators, such as rituximab, act by targeting CD20, selectively depleting circulating B cells. An anti-CD28 is also available (abatacept).

Interleukin inhibitors include an IL-1 antagonist (anakinra) and an IL-6 antagonist (tocilizumab).

Labelled indications for use of BRMs include rheumatoid arthritis, ankylosing spondylitis, psoriasis, Crohn disease, ulcerative colitis and malignancies such as non-Hodgkin lymphoma. Off-label applications include pemphigus, recurrent aphthous stomatitis and Behçet disease, mucous membrane pemphigoid, lichen planus, orofacial granulomatosis and Sjögren syndrome.

One of the advantages of BRMs is that they act specifically to neutralize targeted immune components so there *should*, in theory, be relatively few adverse effects. They are administered by injection or infusion, and the most common adverse effect is a mild skin reaction at the injection site. All are injected preparations, with schedules varying with the condition being treated. Infliximab and rituximab must be given as periodic intravenous infusions; etanercept and adalimumab are given as regular subcutaneous injections; and alefacept is given as weekly intramuscular injections. Some patients develop headaches during infusion, and there may be an increased susceptibility to infection – a serious risk to patients already prone to infection (e.g. diabetics) or who have an active infection such as tuberculosis or hepatitis B virus (Tables 19.7 and 19.8). Immunomodulatory mAbs have an inherent risk for adverse immune-mediated drug reactions in humans, such as infusion reactions, cytokine storms, immunosuppression and autoimmunity. Other long-term effects are not yet clear (see also Chs 29 and 35). At least 30 therapeutic mAbs are marketed in a variety of indications, and have already had profound impacts on fields such as oncology, rheumatology, neurology, cardiology and gastroenterology. However, biologics can have a high cost and significant adverse effects, and the efficacy of murine human mAbs can be limited by development of human antichimeric antibodies.

Biologics suppress the immune system and carry an increased risk of infections, which, in rare cases, can be serious. These agents undoubtedly can have serious potential adverse effects but they are generally considered safe. People with tuberculosis, heart failure or multiple sclerosis should not take biologics because they can bring on these conditions or make them worse. In rare cases, some people taking TNF inhibitors have developed certain cancers such as lymphoma. Natalimumab increases the risk of a rare, potentially fatal brain infection – progressive multifocal leukoencephalopathy (PML). Common side-effects from biologic use include headache, 'flu-like symptoms, nausea, rash, injection site pain and infusion reactions.

Use of biologics does require precautionary considerations, including screening for coexisting medical conditions. Before prescribing biologics, it is crucial to check for potential problems, such as active liver infection or tuberculosis. Monitoring includes include laboratory tests and possibly regular checks for cancer (Box 19.3).

Screening for, and use in, comorbid conditions are described below.

Viral infections

In patients with hepatitis B virus (HBV), hepatitis C virus (HCV) and human immunodeficiency virus (HIV) infection receiving biologics, viral reactivation may occur, with specific cautions and caveats related to use. Recommendations are that screening for risk factors for HBV, HCV and HIV should be carried out before commencing therapy with either TNFα inhibitors or rituximab. If previous viral infection is diagnosed, a full risk/benefit assessment should be undertaken before any proposed use, and HBV

Table 19.7 *Main groups of biological response modifiers*

Actions	Examples	Names
Antibodies against immunocytes	Anti-B-lymphocyte CD20, proliferation and activation	Rituximab
	Anti-T-lymphocyte migration and cytotoxicity	Alefacept
		Efalizumab
	Anti-CD3	Visilizumab
	Anti-T-cell activation	Abatacept
	Anti-CD22	Epratuzumab
Cytokine inhibitors	Anti-tumour necrosis factor (TNF)	Adalimumab
		Certolizumab
		Etanercept
		Infliximab
		Onercept
	Anti-interferon-gamma (IFNλ)	Apilimod
		Fontolizumab
	Anti-interleukin 1 (IL-1)	Anakinra
Others	Anti-IL-2 receptors	Basiliximab
		Daclizumab
	Anti-alpha$_4$-integrin	Natalizumab
	Selectin inhibitors	Efomycine

immunization should be considered in prospective patients considered at risk. However, most authorities advocate significant caution in patients with HBV or HCV and HIV infection, and use of any agents in active disease is generally contraindicated. If used, where relevant, HBV serology titres, serum aminotransaminases and HCV-RNA should be monitored. While anti-TNF therapy has been given in HIV infection, only those with controlled disease and whose immune competence is not especially low (e.g. CD4 count over 200 and HIV viral load below 60 000 mm^3) should be considered eligible. Therapy must be given in combination with antiretroviral therapy (ART), and viral load and CD4 count should be monitored during biological therapy. Although rituximab can be used in HIV infection, limited data are available for its use in autoimmune conditions with coexistent HIV infection, and there are no clear recommendations for such use. As such, use of any agents is generally contraindicated. Alefacept is specifically contraindicated in HIV infection, as it reduces CD4 count.

Bacterial infections

Reactivation of mycobacterial infections with anti-TNF therapy is well recognized, and indeed, this can present with orofacial manifestations. It is crucial, therefore, that all patients in whom these agents may potentially be used should be screened for mycobacterial infections, especially tuberculosis, with consideration of prophylactic anti-tuberculosis therapy if there is evidence of latent disease and definitive anti-tuberculosis treatment in active disease. In contrast, there is no evidence of an increased frequency of tuberculosis with rituximab. It has been suggested that serious infections with rituximab may be more likely in patients being treated for mucocutaneous disease. Consequently, biological therapy should not be started in the presence of significant infection and clinical vigilance for such events is advocated; treatment should be stopped if serious infection develops. In clinical practice, any potential source of infection should be treated prior to initiation of anti-TNF therapies. An increased risk of surgical site perioperative infection has also been reported with anti-TNFα therapy; the general guidance is that, where possible, biological

Table 19.8 *Biological response modifiers in current clinical use*

Agent	Actions	Administration	Adverse effects	Monitoring
Adalimumab	Tumour necrosis factor alpha (TNFα) inhibitor; initiates complement-mediated cell lysis	Subcutaneous	Respiratory tract infections, dizziness, headache, neurological sensation disorders, cough, nasopharyngeal pain, diarrhoea, abdominal pain, mouth ulcers, increased hepatic enzymes, rash, pruritus, musculoskeletal pain, injection site reaction, pyrexia, fatigue	Pre-treatment purified protein derivative (PPD) screening, other recommended screening Liver function texts (LFTs), full blood count (FBC), antinuclear antibodies (ANA), anti-double-stranded (anti-ds) DNA, hepatitis B and C viruses (HBV/HCV), human immunodeficiency virus (HIV)
Alefacept	CD2 antagonist fusion protein; impairs memory T cells	Intramuscular	Lymphopenia, malignancies, infections, hypersensitivity reactions	CD4+ T lymphocyte counts every 2 weeks
Anakinra	Interleukin 1 (IL-1) inhibitor	Subcutaneous	Neutropenia, 'flu-like symptoms, infections	Pre-treatment PPD screening Blood platelets White cell count (WBC) Haemoglobin and haematocrit LFTs C-reactive protein (CRP) Other
Efalizumab	CD11a inhibitor; blocks interaction of lymphocyte function-associated antigen 1 (LFA-1) and intercellular adhesion molecule 1 (ICAM-1)	Subcutaneous	Leukocytosis and lymphocytosis, 'flu-like symptoms, infections, hypersensitivity, psoriasis, arthralgia, arthritis, back pain, raised alkaline phosphatase, thrombocytopenia, injection site reactions	Pre-treatment PPD screening Blood platelets WBC Haemoglobin and haematocrit LFTs CRP Other
Etanercept	TNFα inhibitor; blocks TNF receptor	Subcutaneous	Infections, reactions at injection site, allergic reactions, cardiac failure, lupus-like syndrome	Pre-treatment PPD screening/possible screening for tuberculosis FBC LFTs ANA and anti-ds DNA
Infliximab	TNFα inhibitor; initiates complement-mediated cell lysis	Intravenous	Infusion reaction and hypersensitivity, infections, respiratory infection, hepatitis B reactivation, serum sickness-like reaction, headache, vertigo, dizziness, nausea, abdominal pain, raised hepatic transaminases, urticaria, rash, hyperhidrosis, lymphoma and other malignancies	Pre-treatment PPD screening Possible monitoring and screening for: LFTs ANA and anti-DNA HBV, HCV, HIV FBC
Rituximab	Anti-CD 20; depletes B cells	Intravenous	Infections, human anti-chimeric antibodies, leukopenia, neutropenia, infusion-related reactions, angioedema, nausea Cardiac reactions, dyspnoea, bronchospasm, gastrointestinal effects, progressive multifocal leukoencephalopathy (PML) due to JC virus	FBC with differential and platelets, peripheral CD20+ cells HBV screening Signs or symptoms of PML (focal neurological deficits: hemiparesis, visual field deficits, cognitive impairment, aphasia, ataxia and/or cranial nerve deficits) Cardiac monitoring

treatment should be stopped prior to surgery and reintroduced following satisfactory postoperative healing. When rituximab is used in the organ transplant setting, numerous reports exist of postsurgical infection; some studies identifying at least a trend towards increased risk, although some report that the incidence may be no greater than that for other transplant regimens. However, with such insufficient data available, it remains true that a potential impact on wound healing and infectious complications exists with rituximab, and similar cautions as for TNFα blockers should be applied. Concerns have been raised regarding reports of infective endocarditis in patients receiving biological therapies. Although some of these have included infection with atypical organisms, others have been caused by oral commensals such as *Streptococcus intermedius*.

Other effects

TNFα inhibitors may also be associated with an increased risk of malignancy. They should not be given in patients with multiple sclerosis and must used with caution in patients with a history of other demyelinating diseases, such as optic neuritis and Guillain–Barré syndrome. Cardiac failure is aggravated during TNFα blockade.

TNFα inhibitors use in pregnancy may cause fetal adverse effects, in particular those of the VACTERL spectrum – a syndrome usually seen in embryos and fetuses, characterized by abnormalities of *v*ertebrae, *a*nus, *c*ardiovascular tree, *t*rachea, *oe*sophagus, *r*enal system and *l*imb-buds, and associated with the administration of sex hormones during early pregnancy. Rituximab treatment during pregnancy is

Box 19.3 *Uses of, concerns about and contraindications to biological therapies*

Eligibility

- Disease that is severe, or intolerant of or resistant to standard systemic therapy
- Patients fully informed of risks and benefits, and the fact that treatment is off label

Contraindications

- Hypersensitivity to agent
- Active infections
- Severe heart failure
- Pregnancy and lactation (rituximab)
- Demyelinating disease (tumour necrosis factor alpha [TNFα] inhibitors)
- Active or recent (10 y) malignancy (except non-melanoma skin cancer)

Pre-treatment screening

- History and physical examination
- Blood tests:
  - Full blood picture
  - Liver function tests
  - Screen for viruses (human immunodeficiency virus, hepatitis B or C virus)
  - Serum immunoglobulin levels
- Chest radiograph
- Purified protein derivative (PPD)
- Assess vaccination necessity; no live vaccines; give inactivated vaccines

Adverse events

- Hypersensitivity reactions (including anaphylaxis)
- Reactivation of latent tuberculosis, or progression of recently acquired infection
- Viral reactivation
- Exacerbation of cardiac failure
- Potential for malignancy, especially lymphoma (TNFα inhibitors)
- Cutaneous and mucocutaneous reactions
- Opportunistic infections (particularly fungal)
- Progressive multifocal leukoencephalopathy (PML)

Monitoring

- Infection throughout treatment
- New or exacerbation of cardiac dysfunction
- Central nervous system demyelinating disorders
- Malignancy (compliance with national screening programmes)

specifically contraindicated and should be avoided in lactating women. A variety of adverse effects has been reported with administration of TNFα blockers, involving approximately 20% of patients, and ranging from minor reactions at injection sites to hypersensitivity reactions and anaphylaxis. Mucocutaneous drug eruptions may be seen in patients receiving biological therapies.

Monitoring during biological therapy

Monitor the following every 3–6 months:

- Cardiac function
- Neurological status
- Full blood count
- Liver function tests
- In patients taking alefacept, CD4+ T-cell count every 2 weeks.

Screen for tuberculosis annually.

KEY WEBSITES

(Accessed 29 May 2013)
National Institute for Health and Care Excellence. <http://www.nice.org.uk/usingguidance/commissioningguides/biologicaltherapies/CommissioningBiologicDrugs.jsp>.
National Institutes of Health: National Institute of Arthritis and Musculoskeletal and Skin Diseases. <http://www.niams.nih.gov/Health_Info/Autoinflammatory/default.asp>.
Wikidoc. Immunosuppressive drug. <http://wikidoc.org/index.php/Immunosuppressive_drug>.

USEFUL WEBSITES

(Accessed 29 May 2013)
About.com. Aids/HIV. <http://aids.about.com/od/otherconditions/a/immunerecon.htm>.
Drug Effectiveness Review Project (DERP): Drug class review on targeted immune modulators. <http://www.ohsu.edu/drugeffectiveness>.
Kimball's Biology Pages. <http://users.rcn.com/jkimball.ma.ultranet/BiologyPages/I/Inflammation.html>.
Medscape Reference: Nonsteroidal anti-inflammatory agent toxicity. <http://emedicine.medscape.com/article/816117-overview>.
Todar's Online Textbook of Bacteriology. <http://www.textbookofbacteriology.net/innate.html>.
Wikipedia: Immunosuppressive drug. <http://en.wikipedia.org/wiki/Immunosuppressive_drug>.
Wikipedia: Inflammation. <http://en.wikipedia.org/wiki/Inflammation>.

FURTHER READING

Ahmed, A.R., et al. 2006. Treatment of pemphigus vulgaris with rituximab and intravenous immunoglobulin. N. Engl. J. Med. 26 (355), 1772.
Almoznino, G., Ben-Chetrit, E., 2007. Infliximab for the treatment of resistant oral ulcers in Behçet's disease: a case report and review of the literature. Clin. Exp. Rheumatol. 25 (4 Suppl 45), S99.
Antonucci, A., et al. 2007. Treatment of refractory pemphigus vulgaris with antiCD20 monoclonal antibody (rituximab): five cases. J. Dermatol. Treat. 18, 178.
Arin, M.J., et al. 2005. AntiCD20 monoclonal antibody (rituximab) in the treatment of pemphigus. Br. J. Dermatol. 153, 620.
Arin, M.J., Hunzelmann, N., 2005. Anti B-cell-directed immunotherapy (rituximab) in the treatment of refractory pemphigus – an update. Eur. J. Dermatol. 15, 224.
Atzeni, F., et al. 2005. Successful treatment of resistant Behçet's disease with etanercept. Clin. Exp. Rheumatol. 23, 729.
Azimzadeh, A.M., et al. 2011. Immunobiology of transplantation: impact on targets for large and small molecules. Clin. Pharmacol. Ther. 90, 229.
Barnadas, M., et al. 2006. Therapy of paraneoplastic pemphigus with rituximab: a case report and review of literature. J. Eur. Acad. Dermatol. Venereol. 20, 69.
Berookhim, B., et al. 2004. Treatment of recalcitrant pemphigus vulgaris with the tumor necrosis factor alpha antagonist etanercept. Cutis 74, 245.
Böhm, M., Luger, T.A., 2007. Lichen planus responding to efalizumab. J. Am. Acad. Dermatol. 56 (Suppl. 5), S92.
Bonilla, F.A., et al. 2005. Practice parameter for the diagnosis and management of primary immunodeficiency. Ann. Allergy Asthma Immunol. 94 (5 Suppl 1) S1, S63.
Canizares, M.J., et al. 2006. Successful treatment of mucous membrane pemphigoid with etanercept in 3 patients. Arch. Dermatol. 142, 1457.
Chang, A.L., et al. 2008. Alefacept for erosive lichen planus: a case series. J. Drugs. Dermatol. 7, 379.
Cheng, A., Mann, C., 2006. Oral erosive lichen planus treated with efalizumab. Arch. Dermatol. 142, 680.
Cianchini, G., et al. 2007. Treatment of severe pemphigus with rituximab: report of 12 cases and a review of the literature. Arch. Dermatol. 143, 1033.
Devauchelle-Pensec, V., et al. 2007. Improvement of Sjögren's syndrome after two infusions of rituximab (antiCD20). Arthritis Rheum. 57, 310.
Diaz, L.A., 2007. Rituximab and pemphigus – a therapeutic advance. N. Engl. J. Med. 357, 605.
Dupuy, A., et al. 2004. Treatment of refractory pemphigus vulgaris with rituximab (antiCD20 monoclonal antibody). Arch. Dermatol. 140, 91.
España, A., et al. 2004. Long-term complete remission of severe pemphigus vulgaris with monoclonal antiCD20 antibody therapy and immunophenotype correlations. J. Am. Acad. Dermatol. 50, 974.
Esposito, M., et al. 2006. Long-lasting remission of pemphigus vulgaris treated with rituximab. Acta Derm. Venereol. 86, 87.
Faurschou, A., Gniadecki, R., 2008. Two courses of rituximab (antiCD20 monoclonal antibody) for recalcitrant pemphigus vulgaris. Int. J. Dermatol. 47, 292.

Fivenson, D.P., Mathes, B., 2006. Treatment of generalized lichen planus with alefacept. Arch. Dermatol. 142, 151.

Foulon, G., et al. 2004. Sarcoidosis in HIV-infected patients in the era of highly active antiretroviral therapy. Clin. Infect. Dis. 38, 418.

Gaya, D.R., et al. 2006. Anti TNF-alpha therapy for orofacial granulomatosis: proceed with caution. Gut 55, 1524.

Goh, M.S., et al. 2007. Rituximab in the adjuvant treatment of pemphigus vulgaris: a prospective open-label pilot study in five patients. Br. J. Dermatol. 156, 990.

Gottenberg, J.E., et al. 2005. Tolerance and short term efficacy of rituximab in 43 patients with systemic autoimmune diseases. Ann. Rheum. Dis. 64, 913.

Graves, J.E., et al. 2007. Off-label uses of biologics in dermatology: rituximab, omalizumab, infliximab, etanercept, adalimumab, efalizumab, and alefacept (part 2 of 2). J. Am. Acad. Dermatol. 56, e55.

Guba, M., 2004. Pro- and anti-cancer effects of immunosuppressive agents used in organ transplantation. Transplantation 77, 1777.

Heffernan, M.P., Bentley, D.D., 2006. Successful treatment of mucous membrane pemphigoid with infliximab. Arch. Dermatol. 142, 1268.

Heffernan, M.P., et al. 2007. A single-center, open-label, prospective pilot study of subcutaneous efalizumab for oral erosive lichen planus. J. Drugs Dermatol. 6, 310.

Huang, W., et al. 2008. To test or not to test? An evidence-based assessment of the value of screening and monitoring tests when using systemic biologic agents to treat psoriasis. J. Am. Acad. Dermatol. 58, 970.

Jackson, J.M., 2007. TNF-alpha inhibitors. Dermatol. Ther. 20, 251.

Jacobi, A., et al. 2005. Rapid control of therapy-refractory pemphigus vulgaris by treatment with the tumour necrosis factor-alpha inhibitor infliximab. Br. J. Dermatol. 153, 448.

Joly, P., et al. 2007. A single cycle of rituximab for the treatment of severe pemphigus. N. Engl. J. Med. 9 (357), 545.

Mariette, X., et al. 2004. Inefficacy of infliximab in primary Sjögren's syndrome: results of the randomized, controlled trial of remicade in primary Sjögren's syndrome (TRIPSS). Arthritis Rheum. 50, 1270.

Meijer, J.M., et al. 2007. The future of biologic agents in the treatment of Sjögren's syndrome. Clin. Rev. Allergy Immunol. 32, 292.

Mestas, J., Hughes, C.W., 2004. Of mice and men: differences between mouse and human immunology. J. Immunol. 172, 2731.

Morrison, L.H., 2004. Therapy of refractory pemphigus vulgaris with monoclonal antiCD20 antibody (rituximab). J. Am. Acad. Dermatol. 51, 817.

Moutsopoulos, N.M., et al. 2008. Lack of efficacy of etanercept in Sjögren syndrome correlates with failed suppression of tumour necrosis factor alpha and systemic immune activation. Ann. Rheum. Dis. 67, 1437.

Niedermeier, A., et al. 2006. Delayed response of oral pemphigus vulgaris to rituximab treatment. Eur. J. Dermatol. 16, 266.

Ozkurede, V.U., Franchi, L., 2012. Immunology in clinic review series; focus on autoinflammatory diseases: role of inflammasomes in autoinflammatory syndromes. Clin. Exp. Immunol. 167 (3), 382. doi: 10.1111/j.1365-2249.2011.04535.x Review. PubMed PMID: 22288581; PubMed Central PMCID: PMC3374270.

Pardo, J., et al. 2005. Infliximab in the management of severe pemphigus vulgaris. Br. J. Dermatol. 153, 222.

Peitsch, W.K., et al. 2007. Infliximab: a novel treatment option for refractory orofacial granulomatosis. Acta Derm. Venereol. 87, 265.

Pijpe, J., et al. 2005. Rituximab treatment in patients with primary Sjögren's syndrome: an open-label phase II study. Arthritis Rheum. 52, 2740.

Robinson, N.D., Guitart, J., 2003. Recalcitrant, recurrent aphthous stomatitis treated with etanercept. Arch. Dermatol. 139, 1259.

Sacher, C., et al. 2002. Treatment of recalcitrant cicatricial pemphigoid with the tumor necrosis factor alpha antagonist etanercept. J. Am. Acad. Dermatol. 46, 113.

Sankar, V., et al. 2004. Etanercept in Sjögren's syndrome: a twelve-week randomized, double-blind, placebo-controlled pilot clinical trial. Arthritis Rheum. 50, 2240.

Scheinberg, M.A., 2002. Treatment of recurrent oral aphthous ulcers with etanercept. Clin. Exp. Rheumatol. 20, 733.

Schmidt, E., et al. 2005. Long-standing remission of recalcitrant juvenile pemphigus vulgaris after adjuvant therapy with rituximab. Br. J. Dermatol. 153, 449.

Schmidt, E., et al. 2007. Rituximab in autoimmune bullous diseases: mixed responses and adverse effects. Br. J. Dermatol. 156, 352.

Scully, C., et al. 2008. Auto-inflammatory syndromes and oral health. Oral Dis. 14, 690.

Scully, C., et al. 2007. Special care in dentistry: handbook of oral healthcare. Churchill Livingstone/Elsevier, Edinburgh.

Seror, R., et al. 2007. Tolerance and efficacy of rituximab and changes in serum B cell biomarkers in patients with systemic complications of primary Sjögren's syndrome. Ann. Rheum. Dis. 66, 351.

Sfikakis, P.P., et al. 2007. Anti TNF therapy in the management of Behçet's disease – review and basis for recommendations. Rheumatology (Oxford) 46, 736.

Shetty, K., Achong, R., 2005. Dental implants in the HIV-positive patient – case report and review of the literature. Gen. Dent. 53, 434. quiz 438, 446

Sommer, A., et al. 2005. A case of mucocutaneous Behçet's disease responding to etanercept. J. Am. Acad. Dermatol. 52, 717.

Steinfeld, S.D., et al. 2006. Epratuzumab (humanised antiCD22 antibody) in primary Sjögren's syndrome: an open-label phase I/II study. Arthritis Res. Ther. 8, R129.

Steinfeld, S.D., et al. 2002. Infliximab in primary Sjögren's syndrome: one-year follow up. Arthritis Rheum. 46, 3301.

Stevenson, G.C., et al. 2007. Short-term success of osseointegrated dental implants in HIV-positive individuals: a prospective study. J. Contemp. Dent. Pract. 8, 1.

Strietzel, F.P., et al. 2006. Implant-prosthetic treatment in HIV-infected patients receiving highly active antiretroviral therapy: report of cases. Int. J. Oral Maxillofac. Implants 21, 951.

Tayal, V., Kalra, B.S., 2008. Cytokines and anticytokines as therapeutics – an update. Eur. J. Pharmacol. 579, 1.

Vinuesa, C.G., Goodnow, C.C., 2004. Illuminating autoimmune regulators through controlled variation of the mouse genome sequence. Immunity 20, 669.

Vujevich, J., Zirwas, M., 2005. Treatment of severe, recalcitrant, major aphthous stomatitis with adalimumab. Cutis 76, 129.

APPENDIX 19.1 INTERLEUKINS (ILS)

(Modified from Wikipedia)

Name	Main sources	Functions
IL-1	Macrophages	Activates T cells. Induces IL-6. Generates prostaglandins. Induces acute-phase reaction and fever
IL-2	Th1 cells	T-cell growth and apoptosis
IL-3	T cells	Haemopoietic cell growth
IL-4	Th2 cells, just activated naive CD4+ cell, memory CD4+ cells, mast cells	Proliferation of B cells, and development of T cells and mast cells. Important role in allergic response (immunoglobulin E [IgE])
IL-5	Th2 cells	B-cell and eosinophil differentiation and IgA production
IL-6	Macrophages, Th2 cells	Activates many cells inducing acute-phase reaction and inflammation
IL-7	Stromal cells of the red marrow and thymus	B-, T- and natural killer (NK)-cell survival, development and homeostasis
IL-8	Macrophages, epithelial cells, endothelial cells	Neutrophil chemotaxis
IL-9	T cells, specifically by CD4+ helper cells	T-cell and mast-cell growth
IL-10	Monocytes, Th2 cells, mast cells	T-cell and mast-cell growth
IL-11	Bone marrow stroma	Plasma-cell growth
IL-12	Macrophages	Induces interferon-gamma (IFN-γ)
IL-13	Th2 cells	Induces IgE
IL-14	T cells and certain malignant B cells	B-cell growth
IL-15	Mononuclear phagocytes (and some other cells) following infection by virus(es)	Induces production of T and B cells, and NK-cell growth

Name	Main sources	Functions
IL-16	A variety of cells (including lymphocytes and some epithelial cells)	CD4-cell chemoattractant
IL-17	T cells	Induces IL-6, IL-8 and granulocyte colony-stimulating factor inflammatory cytokines
IL-18	Macrophages, liver	Induces production of IFN-γ
IL-19	T cells	–
IL-20	Monocytes	Regulates keratinocyte proliferation and differentiation
IL-21	T cells	Induces proliferation in NK cells and cytotoxic T cells
IL-22	T cells	Activates signal transducers and activators of transcription (STAT)1 and STAT3, and increases production of acute-phase proteins such as serum amyloid A, alpha$_1$-antichymotrypsin and haptoglobin in hepatoma cell lines
IL-23	Macrophages	Increases angiogenesis but reduces CD8 T-cell infiltration
IL-24	T cells, macrophages	Tumour suppression, wound-healing and psoriasis
IL-25	Mast cells	Induces IL-4, IL-5 and IL-13 production, which stimulates eosinophil expansion
IL-26	T cells	Enhances IL-10 and IL-8 secretion, and epithelial cell expression of CD54
IL-27	Dendritic cells	Regulates B- and T-lymphocyte activity
IL-28	Dendritic cells	Defence against viruses
IL-29	Dendritic cells	Defences against microbes
IL-30	–	Is one chain of IL-27
IL-31	T cells	Possible role in skin inflammation
IL-32	T cells	Induces monocytes and macrophages to secrete tumour necrosis factor alpha, IL-8 and CXCL2
IL-33	Stroma cells, fibroblasts	Induces helper T cells to produce cytokines

APPENDIX 19.2 IMMUNOMODULATORY NON-BIOLOGICAL AGENTS

Mode of action	Main adverse effects	Main interactions with	Main contraindications	Monitoring/cautions
Azathioprine				
Thiopurine methyltransferase (TPMT) metabolizes to active mercaptopurine (MP), which acts as a purine analogue and blocks nucleotides and DNA synthesis, and inhibits lymphocyte division	Arrhythmias	Allopurinol	Absolute:	Assay TPMT in whites/ blacks, inosine triphosphate pyrophosphatase (ITPA) in Japanese
	Fatigue	Angiotensin-converting enzyme inhibitors (ACEIs)	Bone marrow hypofunction	Bone marrow suppression in low TPMT or ITPA
	Gastrointestinal	Aspirin	Low enzyme TPMT	Blood (full blood count [FBC] every 2 weeks, then every 3 months) irrespective of TPMT status
	Haematological (leukopenia early, usually)	Ciclosporin	Hepatic disease	Blood pressure
	Hypersensitivity (in 3–42 days fever, myalgia, arthralgia, liver/kidney)	Clozapine	Hypersensitivity to azathioprine/6-MP	Hypersensitivity
	Hypotension	Co-trimoxazole	Infections	Infections (viruses: HBV, HCV, HIV, VZV)
	Liver damage (hepatitis)	Cyclophosphamide	Pancreatitis	Liver damage (liver function tests)
	Nausea	Febuxostat	Pregnancy and lactation	Malignancy (examination, Pap test, faecal occult blood [FOB])
	Pancreatitis	Immunosuppressants	Vaccines (live)	Renal damage (renal function tests)
	Renal damage (nephritis)	Mesalazine	Relative:	
	Carcinogenicity	Methotrexate	Pre-malignancy: skin, cervix, ?oral	
	Non-melanoma skin cancer (>10 y and ultraviolet radiation)	Osalazine	Renal disease	

(Continued)

Mode of action	Main adverse effects	Main interactions with	Main contraindications	Monitoring/cautions
	Non-Hodgkin lymphoma (often year 1 and Epstein–Barr virus or inflammatory bowel disease)	Ribavirin	Viruses: hepatitis B/C (HBV/HCV), human immunodeficiency virus (HIV), varicella zoster (VZV), herpes simplex (HSV), human papillomavirus (HPV)	
	Teratogenicity	Sulfasalazine		
		Trimethoprim		
		Warfarin		
		Grapefruit juice and cytochrome P450 inhibitors		
		Cytostatic drugs		
		Muscle relaxants		
Ciclosporin				
Calcineurin inhibitor Binds to immunophilin (cyclophilin) and resultant complex inhibits calcineurin and thus interleukin 2 (IL-2)	Allergy	Allopurinol	Hypertension	Blood (FBC and lipids)
Ciclosporin prevents dephosphorylation of nuclear translocation of nuclear factor of activated T cells (NFAT) and thus blocks cytokine IL-2	Blood dyscrasias (anaemia, thrombocytopenia)	Aminophylline	Porphyria	Blood pressure
	Gingival swelling (drug-induced gingival overgrowth; DIGO)	Analgesics	Pregnancy	Infections
	Hearing defects	Antibiotics (doxycycline, erythromycin)	Renal disease	Liver damage (liver function tests)
	Hepatotoxicity	Anticonvulsants		Neoplasia
	Hirsutism	Antifungals (azoles)		Renal damage (renal function tests)
	Hyperglycaemia	Carbamazepine, phenytoin, isoniazid, rifampicin, phenobarbital and other drugs that induce CYP3A4 – may lower ciclosporin concentrations. Drugs that inhibit cytochrome P450-3A4 may raise ciclosporin levels and risks of toxicity		
	Hypertension	Acute renal failure, rhabdomyolysis, myositis, and myalgias when taken concurrently with statins		
	Hypomagnesaemia			
	Muscle pain			
	Nephrotoxicity			
	Neurotoxicity/fits/tremors			
	Peptic ulceration			
	Teratogenicity			
Colchicine				
Interferes with tubulin and polymorphonuclear leukocyte (PMNL) motility, and blocks IL-1 via NALP3 inflammasome	Diarrhoea	Antibiotics (clarithromycin, erythromycin, telithromycin)	Cardiac disease	Blood (FBC)
	Hair loss	Antifungals (fluconazole, itraconazole, ketoconazole)	Hepatic disease	Infections
	Myelotoxicity (anaemia; neutropenia)	Ciclosporin	Older patient	Liver damage (liver function tests)
	Neuromyopathy	Fibrates	Pregnancy	Neoplasia
		Protease inhibitors	Renal disease	
		Statins		
		Grapefruit juice and cytochrome P450 inhibitors		

(Continued)

Mode of action	Main adverse effects	Main interactions with	Main contraindications	Monitoring/cautions
Corticosteroids				
Transactivate IL-10	Immunosuppression	Acetazolamide	Diabetes	Blood glucose
Annexin A1 (lipocortin-1)	Adrenal insufficiency	Aminoglutethimide	Hypertension	Blood pressure
IκB (inhibitor of nuclear factor kappa B)	Hyperglycaemia (increased gluconeogenesis, insulin resistance and impaired glucose tolerance – 'steroid diabetes')	Antacids	Osteoporosis	Bone mineral density
Tyrosine aminotransferase	Appetite stimulation and weight gain – visceral and truncal fat deposition (central obesity), expansion of malar fat pads, increased plasma amino acids, increased urea formation, negative nitrogen balance	Antihypertensives	Peptic ulcer	Eyes
Trans-repression of IL-1, 2, 6, 8	Raised blood pressure	Carbamazepine	Tuberculosis	Infections
Vascular endothelial growth factor (VEGF)	Increased skin fragility, dilatation of small blood vessels and easy bruising	Carbenoxolone		Urea and electrolytes
Cyclo-oxygenase-1 (COX-1)	Reduced bone density (osteoporosis, osteonecrosis, higher fracture risk)	Coumarin anticoagulants		Weight
Prostaglandins (PGs)	Muscle breakdown (proteolysis), weakness	Diuretics		Cautions required include:
Tumour necrosis factor (TNF)	Anovulation, menstrual period irregularity, pubertal delay	Hormonal contraceptives		Calcium supplements
Interferon-gamma (IFNγ)	Growth failure	Hypoglycaemics		Vitamin D
Inducible nitric oxide synthetase (INOS)	Central nervous system excitation (euphoria, psychosis)	Insulin		Antiresorptive medication (bisphosphonates)
Chemokines	Glaucoma, cataracts	Liver enzyme inducers/inhibitors		Warning card
Adhesion molecules	Bone: avascular necrosis/osteoporosis	Non-depolarizing muscle relaxants		
Glucocorticoid response elements	Eyes: cataract/central serous retinopathy/glaucoma	Oestrogens		
Anti-inflammatory genes/molecules, e.g. lipocortin-1, IL-10 and IL-1ra	Gastrointestinal	Phenobarbital		
Lipocortin (macrocortin) upregulated	Growth impairment	Phenytoin		
Leukotrienes, PGs and thromboxanes	Hepatic	Primidone		
COX-1 and COX-2 expression also suppressed	Hyperglycaemia, hyperlipidaemia, hypertension	Rifabutin, rifampicin		
Corticosteroids also induce IκB subtype a, reducing NF-κB translocation to the nucleus, thus decreasing proinflammatory cytokines	Infections (tuberculosis, etc.)	Salicylates		
Glucocorticoids also reduce microvascular permeability, mast cells and eosinophils	Malignancy?	Vaccines		
Corticosteroids may reduce inflammation by reversing increased capillary permeability, suppressing PMNLs and decreasing inflammatory cytokines	Mental			
	Renal			
	Skin: bruising, hirsutism, striae			
	Teratogenicity?			
	Weight gain			

(Continued)

Mode of action	Main adverse effects	Main interactions with	Main contraindications	Monitoring/cautions
Dapsone				
Blocks PMNL adherence, chemotaxis, prostaglandin E$_2$ release, lysosomal enzyme release, and myeloperoxidase–hydrogen peroxide–halide-mediated cytotoxicity	Haematological	Acetohydroxamic acid	Allergies to dapsone, naphthalene, niridazole, nitrofurantoin, phenylhydrazine, primaquine, sulfa drugs	FBC
	Headaches	Aminobenzoate potassium	Anaemia	G6PD level
	Hepatic dysfunction	Aminobenzoic acid	Cardiac disease	Haptoglobin
	Hypersensitivity	Clofazimine	Glucose-6-phosphate dehydrogenase (G6PD) deficiency	Liver function every 3 months
	Photosensitivity	Didanosine	HIV	Renal function every 3 month
	Renal dysfunction	Furazolidone	Liver disease	Reticulocyte count
	POTENTIALLY FATAL	Methotrexate	Methaemoglobin reductase deficiency	Hypersensitivity (mainly in first 6 weeks)
		Methyldopa	Porphyria	Blood: weekly for month 1, then alternate weeks during next 2 months, and every 3 months thereafter
		Nitrofurantoin	Pregnancy and breast-feeding	Methaemoglobin levels in patients symptomatic for methaemoglobinaemia
		Oral antidiabetics		Cimetidine and vitamin E minimize haemolysis (inhibit dapsone conversion to toxic hydroxylamine)
		Primaquine		Clothing, sunglasses and sunscreen are needed to avoid sun exposure
		Probenecid		
		Procainamide		
		Trimethoprim		
		Vitamin K		
		Grapefruit juice and cytochrome P450 inhibitors		
Mycophenolate mofetil				
Inhibits inosine monophosphate dehydrogenase	Compared with azathioprine:	Antiepileptics	Children	
Impairs cytotoxic T cells	Overall less toxic	Antivirals (aciclovir, ganciclovir)	Gastrointestinal disease	
	No kidney damage	Aspirin	Older patients	
	Less liver damage	Clozapine	Pregnancy and breast-feeding	
	Potentially less mutagenic	Colestyramine		
	More gastrointestinal, haematological effects and infections	Metronidazole		
	Expensive (15 times more)	Rifampicin		
	Nausea, vomiting	Grapefruit juice and cytochrome P450 inhibitors		
	No liver or kidney damage	Iron		
	Common adverse reactions include diarrhoea, nausea, vomiting, infections, leukopenia, anaemia, fatigue, headache and/or cough			
	Intravenous administration is commonly associated with thrombophlebitis and thrombosis			
	Infrequent adverse effects include oesophagitis, gastritis, gastrointestinal tract haemorrhage and/or invasive cytomegalovirus (CMV) infection			

(Continued)

Mode of action	Main adverse effects	Main interactions with	Main contraindications	Monitoring/cautions
	Blood dyscrasias (anaemia, neutropenia, marrow suppression)			
	Gastrointestinal (nausea, vomiting, diarrhoea, gastritis, oesophagitis and gastrointestinal bleeding)			
	Genitourinary (urgency, frequency, dysuria, haematuria)			
	Hypocalcaemia, hypomagnesaemia, hypophosphataemia			
	Hyperglycaemia, hyperkalaemia, hyperlipidaemia			
	Infections (including CMV, herpes simplex virus [HSV], VZV, BK nephropathy, John Cunningham polyomavirus [progressive multifocal leukoencephalopathy])			
	Neoplasms			
	Neurological			
	Rash			
Sirolimus				
A non-calcineurin inhibitor. Inhibits lymphocyte proliferation and impairs cytotoxic T cells	Hyperlipidaemia	Ch. 29		
Tacrolimus				
Calcineurin inhibitor similar to ciclosporin	Allergies	Aciclovir	Pregnancy	Blood (FBC)
Blocks T-cell activation and cytokines IL-2, 3, 4, 5, 8; TNF; IFN; granulocyte–macrophage colony stimulating factor (GM-CSF); intercellular adhesion molecule 1 (ICAM-1); E selectin; PMNL; mast cell/eosinophil recruitment; and release of histamine	Cardiomyopathy	Antacids	Metabolized by liver CYP1A and CYP111A; does not accumulate in blood or skin	Blood glucose
	Diabetes	Azathioprine		Blood pressure
	Hypertension	Colestyramine		Hypersensitivity
	Hyperglycaemia	Probenecid		Infections
	Neurotoxicity	Ch. 29		Liver damage (liver function tests)
	Renal			Neoplasia
				Renal damage (renal function tests)
Tetracyclines				
Downregulate proinflammatory cytokines	Anorexia	Zinc, iron and antacids inhibit absorption	Children	
Inhibit matrix metalloproteinases (including collagenases MMP-1, MMP-8 and MMP-13)	Gastrointestinal discomfort		Liver disease	
Inhibit PG synthesis	Hypersensitivity		Lupus erythematosus	
Inhibit nitric oxide release (and minocycline inhibits caspase activation)	Lupoid reactions		Myasthenia gravis	
	Nausea		Porphyria	
	Photosensitivity			
	Serum sickness-type reaction			
	Tooth-staining			

(Continued)

Mode of action	Main adverse effects	Main interactions with	Main contraindications	Monitoring/cautions
Thalidomide				
TNF inhibitor; modulates IFNγ–producing CD3+ cells	Adverse effects: major	Alcohol	Pregnancy	Pregnancy test
	Bradycardia and syncope	Bortezomib		Effective contraceptive measures
	Neuropathy	Carbamazepine		Sensory nerve action potentials (SNAP) before treatment, at start and every 6 months
	Neutropenia	Hydroxychloroquine		Anti-thrombotic prophylaxis for >5 months
	Stevens–Johnson syndrome	Paroxetine		Blood (FBC)
	Teratogenicity	Does not interact with grapefruit juice and cytochrome P450 inhibitors		Blood pressure
	Thrombocytopenia			Hypersensitivity
	Thromboses			Infections
	Adverse effects: minor			Liver damage (liver function tests)
	Constipation			Neoplasia
	Drowsiness			Renal damage (renal function tests)
	Hypersensitivity			
	Lymphopenia (reversible)			
	Oedema			

APPENDIX 19.3 BIOLOGIC AGENTS, TARGETS AND APPLICATIONS

Monoclonal antibody/fusion protein	Common names	Targets	Applications
Abatacept	Orencia	CD80, CD86	Transplant rejection, RA
Abciximab	ReoPro	gpII/IIIa	Coronary interventions
Adalimumab	Humira	Tumour necrosis factor alpha (TNFα)	Crohn disease, RA, psoriasis
Alefacept	Amevive	CD2	Psoriasis
Alemtuzumab	Campath	CD52	Chronic lymphoid leukaemia, RA
Anakinra	Kineret	Interleukin (IL)-1R	RA
Basiliximab	Simulect	IL-2R	Transplant rejection
Belatacept	Nulojix	CD80, CD86	Transplant rejection
Belimumab	Benlysta	Soluble B-lymphocyte stimulator (BLyS)	Transplant rejection
Bevacizumab	Avastin	Vascular endothelial growth factor (VEGF)	Cancers (various)
Bortezomib	Velcade	Proteasome	Multiple myeloma
Canakinumab	Ilaris	IL-1β	Juvenile arthritis
Catumaxomab	Removab	Epithelial cell adhesion molecule	Cancers
Certolizumab	Cimzia	TNFα	Crohn disease, RA, psoriasis
Cetuximab	Erbitux	Epidermal growth factor receptor (EGFR)	Head and neck cancer
Daclizumab	Zenapax	IL-2R	Transplant rejection
Denosumab	Prolia	Receptor activator of nuclear factor kappa-B ligand (RANKL)	Osteoporosis
Eculizumab	Soliris	C5	Paroxysmal nocturnal haemoglobinuria
Efalizumab	Raptiva	CD11a	Psoriasis
Etanercept	Enbrel	TNFα	Crohn disease, RA, psoriasis, sarcoid
Gemtuzumab	Mylotarg	CD33	Acute myeloid leukaemia
Golimumab	Simponi	TNFα	Crohn disease, RA, psoriasis,
Ibritumomab	Zevalin	CD20	Non-Hodgkin lymphoma (NHL)
Infliximab	Remicade	TNFα	Crohn disease, RA, psoriasis, sarcoid
Muromonab	Orthoclone OKT3	CD3	Transplant rejection
Natalizumab	Tysabri	Integrin receptor antagonist	Multiple sclerosis, Crohn disease
Omalizumab	Xolair	Immunoglobulin E (IgE)	Asthma

(Continued)

Monoclonal antibody/fusion protein	Common names	Targets	Applications
Palivizumab	Synagis	Respiratory syncytial virus	Respiratory syncytial virus
Panitumumab	Vectibix	EGFR	Cancers
Ranibizumab	Lucentis	VEGF	Age-related macular degeneration
Raxibacumab	ACthrax	*Bacillus anthracis*	Anthrax
Rilonacept	Arcalyst	IL-1	Autoinflammatory disease
Rituximab	Rituxan or Mabthera	CD20	NHL, RA
Sunitinib	Sutent	Tyrosine kinase	Cancers (renal)
Tocilizumab	Actemra	IL-6R	RA
Tofacitinib	Xeljanz	Janus kinases	RA
Tositumomab	Bexxar	CD20	NHL
Trastuzumab	Herceptin	ErbB2 (Her 2)	Breast cancer
Ustekinumab	Stelara	IL-12, IL-23	Psoriasis

APPENDIX 19.4 USES OF BIOLOGICS IN ORGAN DISEASE

Cytokines
- Interferons (IFNs)
- Interleukins (ILs)

Haematopoietic growth factors
- Erythropoietins
- Colony-stimulating factors (CSFs)

Enzymes
- Thrombolytics
- Aldurazyme
- Rasburicase

Monoclonals
- Anti-IL2R (basiliximab)
- Anti-immunoglobulin E (IgE; omalizumab)

Fusion proteins
- Tumour necrosis factor receptor (TNFR) linked to Fc of IgG (etanercept)
- Lymphocyte function-associated antigen 3 (LFA3TIP) fused IgG1 heavy chain (alefacept)

Oncology
- Alemtuzumab (Campath)
- Bavacizumab (Avastin)
- Cetuximab (Erbitux)
- Ibritumomab (Zevalin)
- Rituximab (Rituxan)
- Trastuzumab (Herceptin)

Cardiology
- Abciximab (ReoPro)
- Fibrinolytics

Pulmonary system
- Omalizumab (anti-IgE)
- Dornase alfa (Pulmozyme)

- Lebrikizumab (humanized monoclonal antibody that binds IL-13 – being developed for asthma treatment)
- Montelukast (leukotriene receptor antagonist)

Infections
- IFNα (hepatitis C virus)
- Palivizumab (Synagis; antibody to respiratory syncytial virus)

Dermatology
- Alefacept (anti-LFA3)
- Efalizumab (Raptiva; anti-CD11a)
- Becaplermin (Regranex; platelet-derived growth factor)
- Palifermin (keratinocyte growth factor)

Hereditary disorders
- IFNγ

Arthritis
- Infliximab (Remicade; anti-TNF)
- Etanercept (Enbrel; Fc TNFR)
- Anakinra (IL-1RA)
- Adalimumab (Humira; anti-TNF)

Neurology
- IFNβ
- Tissue plasminogen activator
- Botulinum toxin

Autoimmune disorders
- Etanercept
- Adalimumab
- Infliximab
- Rilonacept
- Canakinumab
- Epratuzumab

Immunodeficiencies are states that result from a defect in the immune response, and predispose to recurrent infections, especially of skin, mucosae and respiratory tract (Fig. 20.1). An immunodeficient patient is often somewhat ponderously referred to as an 'immunocompromised host'. Human immunodeficiency virus (HIV) disease and the resultant acquired immune deficiency syndrome (AIDS) constitute a major immunodeficiency and public health issue worldwide but other important and common causes of secondary immune defects are immunosuppressive therapy and malnutrition (Table 20.1). Vitamin D deficiency is also now recognized as causing failure of immune activation. Primary (genetically determined) immune defects are mostly rare, apart from selective immunoglobulin A (IgA) deficiency.

The most important consequence of all immunodeficiencies is an abnormal susceptibility to infections, frequently caused by organisms of such low pathogenicity as rarely to affect the normal individual (opportunistic infections). Candidosis, herpetic infections and *Pneumocystis jiroveci* (*P. carinii*) pneumonia (Table 20.2) are common. Immunocompromised people are also prone to various malignant neoplasms, some virally related.

Immunodeficiency diseases can affect any component of the immune system but often do not produce clinical pictures that are precisely

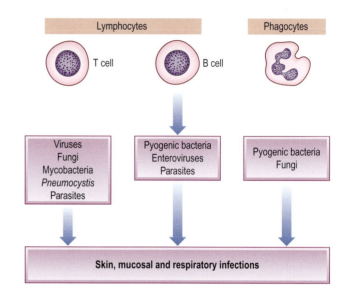

Fig. 20.1 Immune defects and infections.

Table 20.1 *Causes of immunodeficiency*

Primary	Secondary	
	Disease causes	Iatrogenic causes
Genetic	Diabetes mellitus	Chemotherapy
	HIV disease	Immunosuppressive drugs
	Leukaemias	Radiotherapy
	Lymphomas	Splenectomy
	Neutrophil defects	
	Vitamin D deficiency	

Table 20.2 *Complications in immunodeficient or immunosuppressed patients*

Infections				Neoplasms	Others
Mucocutaneous	Gastrointestinal	Respiratory	Meningitis; encephalitis		
Herpes simplex	Cryptosporidiosis	*Pneumocystis jiroveci* (*P. carinii*)	Creutzfeldt–Jakob agent	Kaposi sarcoma (Kaposi sarcoma herpesvirus, KSHV)	Thrombocytopenia
Herpes zoster	Microsporidiosis	Aspergillosis	Papova viruses	Lymphomas (EBV)	Lupus erythematosus
Cytomegalovirus (CMV)	Isosporiasis	Candidosis	*Cryptococcus neoformans*	Squamous cell carcinoma (cervix, anus) (HPV)	Encephalopathy
Epstein–Barr virus (EBV)	Giardiasis	Cryptococcosis	*Toxoplasma gondii*		Drug allergies
Human herpesvirus 8		Histoplasmosis			
Human papilloma viruses (HPV)		Zygomycosis (mucormycosis)			
		Strongyloidiasis			
Molluscum contagiosum		Tuberculosis			
Non-tuberculous mycobacteria		Non-tuberculous mycobacterioses			
Candida species		Legionellosis			
Staphylococcus aureus		*Pseudomonas aeruginosa*			
Histoplasmosis		*Staphylococcus aureus*			
		Streptococcus pneumoniae			
		Haemophilus influenzae			
		Toxoplasmosis			
		CMV			

predictable from the immune defect. Infections do vary in character as a consequence of the nature of the immune defect; the kinds of microorganisms to which the patient is exposed; and attempts at treatment (for example, broad-spectrum antibiotics used to control bacterial infections increase the risk of fungal infections such as candidosis). Thus, in T-cell disorders (such as HIV disease), cell-mediated immunity is principally affected but antibody production may also be impaired, so common infections are with fungi, viruses and certain bacteria - such as candida, herpesviruses and mycobacteria.

SECONDARY IMMUNE DEFECTS

HUMAN IMMUNODEFICIENCY VIRUS (HIV) INFECTION AND THE ACQUIRED IMMUNODEFIENCY SYNDROME (AIDS)

HIV is the virus that can lead to AIDS. HIV (a lentivirus or retrovirus) infects CD4+ helper T lymphocytes, causing AIDS after an average of 10 years in the untreated, and has spread worldwide to create a global pandemic. In 2012 there were over 2 million new infections and 34 million infections recorded worldwide; there was a three-fold rise in individuals over 50 years of age in the UK and one-third of those infected in the UK remained undiagnosed. HIV is found worldwide, and disease patterns are changing as a result of increasing travel and the emergence of new pathogens, such as multidrug-resistant tuberculosis, and the appearance of exotic infections in temperate zones. HIV weakens the immune system, putting persons with HIV or AIDS at risk for many different types of infections. In untreated AIDS, the mortality rate is virtually 100%, although antiviral drugs can significantly impede disease progress.

GENERAL ASPECTS

AIDS was first recognized in 1981 in young men who have sex with men (MSM) in the USA. Sporadic cases have since been identified as long ago as 1959 in Central Africa (where the virus appears to have crossed the species barrier from chimpanzee monkeys).

In June 1981, five cases of *Pneumocystis carinii* (now *jiroveci*) pneumonia were reported in five young males; all suffered from cytomegalovirus infections. Later the same year in the USA, a series of previously healthy MSM who developed *Pneumocystis carinii* pneumonia and mucosal candidiasis were reported, with the suggestion that infection could have been caused by a cellular immunodeficiency. These publications present the first proven cases of what later was termed AIDS. As the first AIDS patients were MSM, it was initially believed that the illness was provoked by peripheral vasodilator drugs ('poppers'), especially amyl nitrite, used by male homosexuals to increase sexual activity. Nevertheless, by the end of 1981, a few cases of AIDS appeared in intravenous drug users, suggesting an infectious aetiology. AIDS was also recognised in all populations, mainly in heterosexuals. After the discovery of the aetiological virus (then termed human T-lymphotropic virus: HTLV-3), retrospective analyses confirmed the presence of the causal virus, which became known as HIV, in the tissues of a Norwegian sailor who died in 1976 and an Afro-American adolescent who died in 1969, and in the plasma of a Congolese male obtained from 1959.

Ten years after HIV was defined, the use of a standardized method to quantify its plasma concentration (viral load) became adopted worldwide. The viral replication rate is stable at every stage of the disease, being estimated at about 10^{9-10} new virions a day. Its assessment is important in the follow-up of infected patients and in the choice of therapeutic approach.

HIV transmission

HIV is transmitted via body fluids, mostly by:

- sexual intercourse – semen, blood and possibly saliva may contain HIV
- contaminated blood, blood products and donated organs
- contaminated needles – intravenous drug users and needlestick injuries
- vertical transmission (mother to child) – *in utero*, during childbirth and via breast milk.

HIV is spread primarily by sexual intercourse, via:

- having unprotected sex with someone who is HIV-infected: Not using a condom when having sex with a person who has HIV is a risk.
  Unprotected anal sex is riskier than unprotected vaginal sex. Among MSM, unprotected receptive anal sex is riskier than unprotected insertive anal sex.
  Unprotected oral sex can be a risk, but is a much lower risk than anal or vaginal sex.
- having multiple sex partners or another sexually shared infection (SSI). This can increase the risk of HIV infection.
- sharing needles, syringes, rinse water or other equipment used to prepare drugs of abuse for injection.
- being born to an infected mother. HIV can be passed from mother to child during pregnancy, birth or breast-feeding.

Less common modes of HIV transmission include:

- being damaged or 'stuck' with an HIV-contaminated needle or other sharp object
- receiving HIV-contaminated blood transfusions, blood products or organ/tissue transplants
- receiving unsafe or unsanitary injections or other medical or dental practices
- eating food that has been pre-chewed by an HIV-infected person
- being bitten by an HIV-infected person
- being in contact with HIV-infected blood or blood-contaminated body fluids and broken skin, wounds or mucous membranes
- engaging in 'French' or deep open-mouth kissing with an HIV-infected person if there is bleeding in the latter's mouth (this presents an extremely remote chance that HIV could be transmitted)
- undergoing tattooing or body piercing using unsafe or unsanitary procedures.

HIV cannot reproduce outside the body and is *not* spread by:

- air
- water
- insects, including mosquitoes
- social contact, like shaking hands or sharing cups or dishes
- closed-mouth or 'social' kissing
- saliva, tears or sweat – provided blood is absent; there is no documented case of HIV being transmitted by spitting.

The virus is transmitted mainly by intimate sexual contact and can infect anyone who practises risky behaviours, such as having sexual contact with an infected person or someone whose HIV status is unknown without using a condom. Sexual transmission of HIV is more likely during HIV seroconversion or in advanced AIDS, by receptive anal intercourse, or where there is genital ulceration. Saliva and breast milk may contain HIV, but transmission via the orogenital route is uncommon. Reports that HIV virions are present in a cell-free state in saliva have not been confirmed and saliva contains inhibitory factors. However, saliva transmission may result from human bites.

Heterosexual intercourse is the main mode of transmission worldwide; it is an important route in developing countries in Africa and Asia, and is increasingly important in the developed world, where it is responsible for 25–50% of cases. MSM remain a major risk group in developed countries. In the UK, the number of young men diagnosed with HIV has more than doubled in the last decade and, in 2012, almost half of new cases were infected through sex between men. With antiretroviral therapy, more people with HIV now survive and this has resulted in a rise in the number of new cases of HIV infection – especially in MSM – along with increasing use of the Internet to make contact with new partners; greater substance abuse and use of medications to treat erectile dysfunction; and a rise in unsafe sexual practices. Unfortunately, multidrug-resistant HIV (MDR-HIV) has appeared, with a rapid progression to AIDS.

HIV spread by contaminated needles and syringes is an important route in injecting drug users. Persons infected with HIV, especially those who abuse drugs intravenously or/and are sexually promiscuous, may also be co-infected with other agents, including viruses, such as HTLV-1, HTLV-2 and hepatitis viruses, and other SSIs (Ch. 32). Transmission by needlestick injury is an occasional risk for health-care professionals (HCPs; see later and Ch. 31) and others.

Transmission of HIV can also occur via infected blood or blood products, including plasma, or tissues, such as in transplantation, but screening of blood and plasma for HIV antibody and heat treatment of clotting factor concentrates have substantially reduced the risk in developed countries. All HIV antibody-positive individuals are potentially infective and must not be allowed to donate blood, organs for transplantation or semen for artificial insemination. Rarely, some seronegative but infected blood (collected during the incubation period before antibodies are detectable) can still transmit HIV. Haemophiliacs, initially a risk group for HIV, now form only a small proportion of HIV patients.

Children can contract HIV intrapartum or via breast milk; approximately one-quarter of all untreated pregnant women infected with HIV pass the infection to their babies, and the figure rises to one-third if the infant is breast-fed. Antiretroviral drugs reduce this type of transmission (Box 20.1).

There is no reliable evidence for transmission of HIV by non-sexual social contact or by insect vectors such as mosquitoes or bedbugs. Studies of families of HIV-infected people have shown clearly that HIV is not spread through casual contact, such as the sharing of food utensils, towels and bedding, swimming pools, spas, telephones or lavatory seats.

Prevention of HIV/AIDS can thus be achieved by measures such as the use of condoms, the cessation of needle-sharing, screening blood and tissue before transfer to a recipient, and the use of antiretroviral drugs for children born to HIV-infected mothers.

HIV pre-exposure prophylaxis

Daily oral tenofovir disoproxil fumarate 300 mg (TDF)/emtricitabine 200 mg (FTC) is available as antiretroviral pre-exposure prophylaxis (PrEP) to reduce the risk for HIV acquisition. By 2013, four trials had compared HIV infection rates in participants randomized to receive PrEP compared with rates in participants on placebo. No serious toxicities were identified, efficacy was around two-thirds and there was no evidence of adverse effects among fetuses exposed to TDF or FTC. Daily oral TDF/FTC use has been shown to be safe in reducing the risk for sexual HIV acquisition when used consistently. The efficacy

of TDF/FTC for HIV prevention is dependent on adherence to daily doses of medication; PrEP long-term safety in HIV-uninfected adults or following fetal exposure is not yet determined.

Centers for Disease Control and Prevention (CDC) guidance for clinicians considering using PrEP for adults at very high risk for HIV acquisition through heterosexual sex is as follows:

- TDF/FTC is contraindicated for PrEP in persons with unknown or positive HIV status.
- TDF/FTC daily can be safe and effective in reducing HIV infection in women and men at very high risk for acquiring HIV from penile–vaginal sex.
- PrEP use may be one option to help protect HIV-negative partners in discordant couples during attempts to conceive.
- Before beginning PrEP and if not pregnant at initiation, women of reproductive age should have a regular documented pregnancy test while receiving PrEP.

Further information is available at: http://www.cdc.gov/hiv/prep/ (accessed 30 September 2013).

Box 20.1 *Main antiretroviral agents*

1. Reverse transcriptase inhibitors

Nucleoside/nucleotide reverse transcriptase inhibitors (NRTIs)

- Abacavir (ABC)
- Didanosine (ddI)
- Emtricitabine (FTC)
- Lamivudine (3TC)
- Stavudine (d4T)
- Tenofovir (TDF)
- Zidovudine (AZT, ZDV)

Non-nucleotide reverse transcriptase inhibitors (NNRTIs)

- Delavirdine (DLV)
- Efavirenz (EFV)
- Etravirine (ETR)
- Nevirapine (NVP)
- Rilpivirine (RPV)

2. Protease inhibitors (PIs)

- Atazanavir (ATV)
- Darunavir (DRV)
- Fosamprenavir (FPV)
- Indinavir (IDV)
- Lopinavir (LPV)
- Nelfinavir (NFV)
- Ritonavir (RTV)
- Lopinavir/ritonavir (LPV/r)
- Saquinavir (SQV)
- Tipranavir (TPV)
- Amprenavir (APV)

3. Integrase inhibitor
Raltegravir (RAL)

4. Entry inhibitor

Fusion inhibitors

- Enfuvirtide (ENF, T-20)

CCR5 antagonist

- Maraviroc (MVC)

HIV epidemiology

HIV-1, the most common virus causing AIDS, has spread to all continents to create a global pandemic with the most devastating consequences ever known to humankind. A further virus, HIV-2, which originated in sooty mangabee monkeys, predominates in West Africa, and has also now spread to many countries, including Central Africa, Europe, the USA and South America; at present, however, there are few HIV-2 infections in developed countries.

An estimated 20 million people have died from AIDS since the epidemic was recognized. Estimates are that over 40 million HIV cases had developed worldwide by 2008 – more than 1 in every 100 sexually active adults. The difference between numbers estimated and reported is due to underdiagnosis (especially in the developing world); underreporting and delayed reporting; and false extrapolation of basic information derived from Africa and MSM.

Probably 75% of cases worldwide are located in Africa, about 10% in Latin America, about 7% in the USA, about 5% in Asia and slightly less in Europe. However, epidemics are progressing in Asia, especially India and China, and in Eastern Europe. In the USA, the CDC estimated that, by 2008, gay and bisexual men of all races were the group most heavily affected by HIV, accounting for 53% of all new infections, and the impact of HIV was greater among blacks than any other racial or ethnic group, with an HIV incidence rate seven times higher than that of whites and almost three times higher than that of Latinos. Currently, HIV infection is the commonest cause of death in US men aged 25–44 years, and the third commonest cause of death in women of this age.

In the UK, HIV infection is the fourth most common cause of death in men aged 25–44 years. New HIV diagnoses in the UK in 2011 showed a slight decrease on 2010 and continued a year-on-year decline from the peak in 2005. The overall decline in new diagnoses is largely due to fewer reported cases among heterosexuals, who probably acquired their infection abroad. The number of new HIV diagnoses in MSM surpassed new diagnoses in heterosexuals. Half of those diagnosed in 2011 probably acquired their infection through sex between men. Continued low numbers of HIV diagnoses were made in people who inject drugs and through other exposures. All infections acquired through receipt of blood/tissue products diagnosed since 2002 were acquired outside of the UK.

Pathogenesis

The HIV viruses are ribonucleic acid (RNA) viruses. HIV-1 and HIV-2 differ in antigens and nucleic acids but are transmitted similarly, have similar biological properties and are both capable of causing disease. HIV-2 may progress more slowly and cause less profound immunosuppression. HIV-1/HIV-2 co-infection can occasionally be acquired. However, the remaining discussion relates to HIV-1.

HIV-1 can be classified into two major groups: M, which contains ten genetically distinct subtypes (A to J), and O, which contains several very heterogeneous viruses. The B virus is found in USA, Europe and Central Africa.

HIV contains several so-called 'core' proteins and is surrounded by an envelope made up of 'coat' proteins; one of these, the viral cover glycoprotein (gp 120), interacts with a cell surface protein receptor (CD4). The external layer or cover presents 72 external projections where glycoproteins (gp41, gp120) are placed, as well as a number of proteins derived from the host cells, such as beta$_2$-microglobulin and the alpha and beta chains of the human leukocyte antigen (HLA)-DR. Chemokine (co-)receptors are also involved, the most important being CCR5, the main monocytotropic cell receptor; chemokines (RANTES, MIP-1α MIP-2β); and the CXCR4 (fusine), which is inside the lymphotropic cells and whose natural linkage is stromal-derived factor 1 (SDF1) chemokine. There are several viral variants with different trophisms to CCR5 and CXCR4, which have the capacity for interaction with different co-receptors such as CCR2, CCR3, BONZO and BOB; they are sometimes capable of penetrating a cell using multiple co-receptors. The importance of RANTES and SDF lies in their capability to compete for the same HIV receptors, blocking the viral cycle by preventing virus penetration.

CD4 cells are mainly helper-inducer T lymphocytes, monocytes and macrophages, Langerhans cells, brain glial cells and some colonic cells. Brain tissue, in particular the cells of monocyte–macrophage lineage, can become infected with HIV. Neurological damage may also be mediated by the production of factors that affect neuronal cell function or neural transmitters by HIV-infected macrophages. Most HIV is tropic for various chemokines such as CC CKR-5 (CCR5-tropic virus or R5), involved in HIV–cell attachment; a few patients appear able to resist infection because of altered expression of this chemokine or the emergence of CXCR4-tropic virus strains (X4). Some HIV strains show dual tropism. HIV-1 variants that use the co-receptor CCR5 for entry (R5; macrophage tropic) predominate in early infection, while variants that use CXCR4 emerge during disease progression. Some late-stage variants use CXCR4 alone (X4; T-cell tropic), while others use both CXCR4 and CCR5 (R5X4; dual tropic). One coat protein, p24, is particularly antigenic and antibodies to p24 form the basis for most serological testing (the HIV test). The coat proteins are subject to considerable variability, making vaccine development difficult.

After interaction of the viral particle and receptors, the virus coat merges with the cell membrane, losing the external capsule, while the nucleocapsid penetrates the cytoplasm, releasing viral RNA. The genetic material is set inside the core, constituted by two identical RNA strands of positive polarity, nucleoproteins and several enzymes necessary to complete the viral cycle which eukaryote cells lack. HIV also contains enzymes involved in its pathogenicity – reverse transcriptase (which can transcribe DNA from RNA, i.e. in the reverse direction; hence 'retrovirus') and proteases. A retrotranscription is produced in the infected cell by a number of reactions in which DNA polymerase, RNAase and inverse transcriptase (from the virion) are involved. A DNA double strand develops from the RNA genome of the virus. This viral DNA is carried to the cell core, forming part of the host genome, due to the action of the viral integrase and other proteins such as Vpr, p17 and Nef, and becoming the integrated provirus. In the CD4 lymphocytes at rest, the viral genome is incompletely retrotranscribed and the integration process ends only when the cell becomes active. These proviruses lack pathogenic capability and, thus, preventing cellular activation would avoid the virus cytopathic effect.

The messenger RNA is carried to the cytosol and processed in different transcripts of different sizes, via the action of the Rev viral protein, leading to the synthesis of viral proteins by the polysomes. The absence of Rev protein would provoke the gathering of messenger RNA in the cell core.

Viral proteins synthesized and forming a single long chain have to be processed (cut) in order to become structural elements of the nucleocapsid and the viral coat, as well as to form proteins of enzymatic activity (transcriptase, ribonuclease, integrase and protease). In this process, although it is the protease action that is essential in the production of viral particles, turning the p55 pre-proteic precursors into p24, p17, p9, p6 nucleocapsid proteins and the gp160 ones into gp41 and gp120, different viral proteins such as Vif and Vpu are also involved. These are potential targets for therapy.

Finally, the viral genome, covered by the nucleocapsid, projects into the cellular membrane within a layer of proteins, such as viral beta$_2$-microglobulin and gp41 and gp120; the virus is then released.

After primary infection with HIV, acute viraemia results in widespread dissemination of HIV. The virus is trapped in follicular dendritic cells in lymphoid tissue germinal centres and there is expansion of a subset of CD8 cells that are precursors of HIV-specific cytotoxic T cells. Proinflammatory cytokines, including interleukin-6 (IL-6), tumour necrosis factor, gamma-interferon and IL-10, are also over-expressed and may represent an unsuccessful attempt at a protective response. Dendritic cells are involved in the initiation and propagation of HIV infection in CD4 cells.

Antibodies to HIV develop and appear in the serum within 6 weeks to 6 months from infection (seroconversion) but, within this window, the patient may be seronegative (though HIV may be detected by the polymerase chain reaction; PCR). The seroconversion clinical illness is a battle between the virus and the host. Usually, the virus has been proliferating unchecked prior to this point; therefore infectivity is maximal and thereafter wanes (although never dropping to zero). There is then a variable latent period that can last years, until HIV infection manifests with HIV disease and, ultimately, with AIDS.

CLINICAL FEATURES

Infection with HIV may be staged according to its clinical features (Table 20.3). After primary infection with HIV, an acute viraemia results in widespread dissemination of the virus. Antibodies to HIV develop and appear in the serum within 6 weeks to 6 months of infection (seroconversion). One-third of individuals develop a clinical seroconversion illness 3–6 weeks after infection, resembling glandular fever; this is often severe and is termed the acute retroviral syndrome (ARS). Sometimes there is neurological involvement or a rash or mouth ulcers (Fig. 20.2). HIV infection may then remain asymptomatic for a median time of about 10 years. However, despite having circulating (and thus diagnostic) antibodies, people are also able to transmit the disease in the interim. Persistent generalized lymphadenopathy may become evident (Fig. 20.3). As HIV damages CD4 cells in the immune and nervous systems, the risk of development of severe immunodeficiency, and symptoms of disease, rises. HIV damage to CD4+ lymphocytes leads to a lymphopenia over about 6 months to 10 years, a fall in the ratio of helper (CD4+) to suppressor (CD8+) lymphocytes, a profound defect in cell-mediated immune reactivity, and *HIV disease*, which manifests with infections (see Fig. 20.2) as the CD4 count falls to about 500/mm^3, and the CD4+ to CD8+ T-lymphocyte ratio falls. HIV disease manifests in a variety of clinical syndromes, commonly including infections (Fig. 20.4), neoplasms, and neurological and autoimmune disorders (Table 20.4). The CDC definition of *AIDS* comprises a CD4 count of less than 200/mm^3 of blood in a patient infected with HIV and a clinical condition associated

with advanced HIV disease – such as pulmonary tuberculosis (TB), *Pneumocystis* pneumonia, recurrent episodes of pneumonia or invasive cervical carcinoma.

Patients can, however, develop a range of infections (viral, mycobacterial, fungal and parasitic), malignancies (malignant neoplasms,

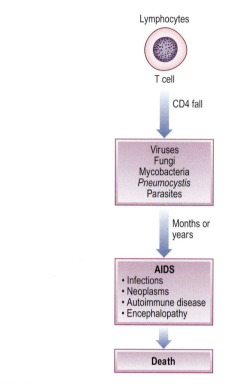

Fig. 20.2 HIV progression.

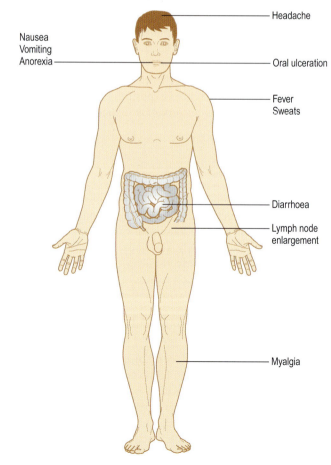

Fig. 20.3 Acute HIV infection – seroconversion illness.

CDC stage	Presentation
1	Primary seroconversion illness
2	Asymptomatic disease
3	Persistent generalized lymphadenopathy (PGL)
4a	AIDS-related complex (ARC) but no AIDS-defining conditions
4b–d	AIDS (AIDS-defining illness)

Table 20.3 *Centers for Disease Control and Prevention (CDC) classification of HIV infection*

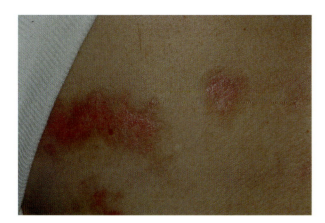

Fig. 20.4 Herpes zoster in HIV/AIDS.

Table 20.4 *Main manifestations of HIV/AIDS*

Main manifestations	Comments
Opportunistic infections	Mainly fungal and viral
Neoplasms	Mainly Kaposi sarcoma and lymphoma
Neurological disorders	Mainly dementia
Autoimmune disorders	Mainly purpura

including melanoma, basal cell carcinoma, Kaposi sarcoma, lymphomas and squamous cell carcinomas of the skin and lip, and carcinoma of the cervix, external genitalia and perineum) and encephalopathy. Loss of weight and wasting are common in AIDS and, in Africa, is called 'slim disease' (Figs 20.5 and 20.6). The onset of AIDS may be influenced by the HIV virus titre, patient age, gender, drug habits, immunogenetics and other factors. Clinical disease is most likely to appear when the CD4 counts fall to low levels, where the infected person has depressed defences for other reasons (e.g. diabetes or malnutrition), and where there is high exposure to potential pathogens (e.g. TB, cryptosporidiosis or histoplasmosis).

In the developed world, about 20% of HIV-infected people develop AIDS within 5 years, and 50% at 10 years; nearly all will have developed AIDS at 20 years unless treated. Some HIV-infected individuals have, or are vulnerable to, a host of co-morbid conditions, including other infections (e.g. fungal/viral infections, hepatitis, SSIs, TB), substance abuse, mental illness and homelessness.

A very small minority of people appear resistant to HIV infection, mostly because of a mutation in the *CCR5* gene called CCR5-delta32, which inhibits HIV binding to CD4 cells. A very few HIV-infected persons (about 2%) inherently appear not to develop AIDS over periods as long as 15 years, mostly because they retain active cytotoxic T cells.

The 2008 CDE Case Definition for HIV infection in adults is as follows (http://www.cdc.gov/osels/ph_surveillance/nndss/casedef/aids2008.htm; accessed 30 September 2013):

- Stage 1:
  No AIDS-defining condition (see below), and either CD4+ T-lymphocyte count of more than 500 cells/microlitre or CD4+ T-lymphocyte percentage of total lymphocytes of ≥29
- Stage 2:
  No AIDS-defining condition, and either CD4+ T-lymphocyte count of 200–499 cells/microlitre or CD4+ T-lymphocyte percentage of total lymphocytes of 14–28

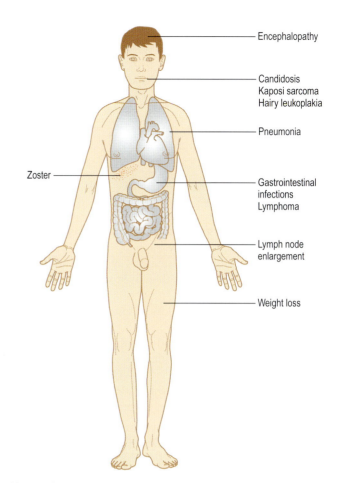

Fig. 20.5 AIDS.

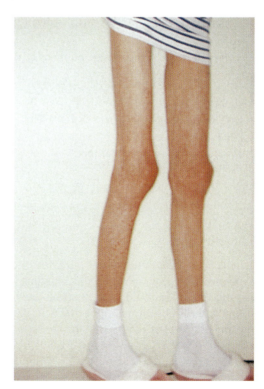

Fig. 20.6 Slim disease in HIV/AIDS.

- Stage 3 (AIDS):
  CD4+ T-lymphocyte count of <200 cells/microlitre or CD4+ T-lymphocyte percentage of total lymphocytes of <14 or documentation of an AIDS-defining condition. Documentation of an AIDS-defining condition supersedes a CD4+

T-lymphocyte count of ≥200 cells/microlitre and a CD4+ T-lymphocyte percentage of total lymphocytes of >14

Or criteria for HIV infection are met and at least one of the AIDS-defining conditions has been documented.

AIDS-defining conditions

These are listed as:

- candidiasis of bronchi, trachea or lungs
- candidiasis of oesophagus
- cervical cancer, invasive
- coccidioidomycosis, disseminated or extrapulmonary
- cryptococcosis, extrapulmonary
- cryptosporidiosis, chronic intestinal (>1 month's duration)
- cytomegalovirus disease (other than liver, spleen or nodes), onset at age >1 month
- cytomegalovirus retinitis (with loss of vision)
- encephalopathy, HIV-related
- herpes simplex: chronic ulcers (>1 month's duration) or bronchitis, pneumonitis or oesophagitis (onset at age >1 month)
- histoplasmosis, disseminated or extrapulmonary
- isosporiasis, chronic intestinal (>1 month's duration)
- Kaposi sarcoma
- lymphoid interstitial pneumonia or pulmonary lymphoid hyperplasia complex
- lymphoma, Burkitt (or equivalent term)
- lymphoma, immunoblastic (or equivalent term)
- lymphoma, primary, of brain
- *Mycobacterium avium* complex or *Mycobacterium kansasii*, disseminated or extrapulmonary
- *Mycobacterium tuberculosis* of any site, pulmonary, disseminated or extrapulmonary
- *Mycobacterium*, other species or unidentified species, disseminated or extrapulmonary
- *Pneumocystis jiroveci* pneumonia
- pneumonia, recurrent
- progressive multifocal leukoencephalopathy
- *Salmonella* septicemia, recurrent
- toxoplasmosis of brain, onset at age >1 month
- wasting syndrome attributed to HIV.

Opportunistic infections

Opportunistic infections are common and resistant to treatment. The pattern of infections varies geographically and with time. For example, histoplasmosis affects mainly AIDS patients from endemic areas of the USA and tuberculosis is seen mainly in AIDS in Africa. Fungal, bacterial, protozoal and viral infections that may be seen are described below.

Fungi

Pneumocystis jiroveci (*P. carinii*) *pneumonia* is a common fungal (previously thought to be a protozoon) lung infection in patients with HIV/AIDS; it is seen up to 80% and is the immediate cause of death in up to 20%. Features include cough, dyspnoea, fever and malaise. Treatment is often with co-trimoxazole or pentamidine. Clindamycin/primaquine, atovaquone and dapsone/trimethoprim are alternatives. *Pneumocystis*

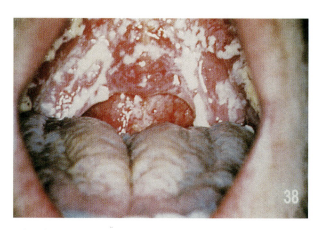

Fig. 20.7 Thrush in HIV/AIDS.

pneumonia is the most common opportunistic infection in people with HIV disease. People with CD4 cell counts under 200/mm^3 have the highest risk of developing it.

Candidosis (candidiasis) is extremely common in the mouth (Fig. 20.7) and vagina, and virtually all patients experience it. HIV infection should be suspected in a young or youngish person who develops thrush without any apparent precipitating factor.

Cryptococcus neoformans is a mycosis that is the main cause of meningitis in AIDS and is especially common in Africa. It is treated with amphotericin or/and an azole.

Histoplasmosis, usually as disseminated disease, mainly affects persons from endemic areas in the Americas. The same applies to coccidioidomycosis. Both infections are treated with amphotericin or/and an azole.

Penicillosis (infection with *Penicillium marneffei*) is seen in some areas of Thailand.

Bacteria

Tuberculosis is particularly common in Africa and is spreading in the West, where some 5% of patients now have lung infection with *Mycobacterium tuberculosis*, which is increasingly multidrug-resistant. TB can affect other sites, including the central nervous system (CNS). Since it can spread by droplets, it is becoming a major public health problem.

Atypical mycobacteria are found in about 40% of AIDS patients in the West, though double that number are actually infected. Over 95% of these are *Mycobacterium avium* complex (MAC) infections – *M. avium* and *M. intracellulare*.

Protozoa

Toxoplasmosis, due to the protozoon *Toxoplasma gondii*, affects about 15% of AIDS patients, and particularly involves the CNS. It is treated with pyrimethamine and sulfadiazine. Leishmaniasis may be seen.

Gastrointestinal protozoal infections (cryptosporidia, microsporidia, *Isospora belli*) often cause intractable diarrhoea.

Viruses

Herpes simplex virus can produce severe erosive lesions around the mouth, genitals, anus or other orifices, and may be seen intraorally and in the oesophagus. It can involve the skin and eyes. It is treated with aciclovir or foscarnet.

Herpes zoster can be severe, painful and incapacitating. It is treated with aciclovir or foscarnet.

Cytomegalovirus (CMV) is the most dangerous viral infection, capable of widespread lesions, especially ulceration throughout the gastrointestinal tract, and retinitis. It is treated with ganciclovir, foscarnet or cidofovir.

Epstein–Barr virus (EBV) is associated with oral hairy leukoplakia (Fig. 20.8) and with lymphomas.

Human papillomavirus (HPV) infections produce warty lesions.

Neoplasms

Various neoplasms are seen in HIV/AIDS – often virally related.

Kaposi sarcoma (an otherwise exceedingly rare tumour of endothelial cells among elderly persons) is seen almost exclusively in sexually transmitted HIV infection in MSM, associated with human herpesvirus 8 (HHV-8; Kaposi sarcoma herpesvirus, KSHV) and accounts for about 80% of neoplasms in AIDS. It often affects the gastrointestinal tract, skin, respiratory tract, mouth or lymph nodes. It is atypical in its early age of onset, distribution (particularly in the head and neck area) and greater malignancy (Fig. 20.9).

Lymphomas, mostly non-Hodgkin B cell lymphomas, are also seen in AIDS (Fig, 20.10); they frequently affect the brain and are often related to EBV. A diffuse infiltrative lymphocytosis syndrome (DILS) can cause asymptomatic bilateral parotid swelling; since patients with DILS can develop lymphomas, periodic observation is mandatory.

Carcinomas of the cervix and of the anus are increased in HIV disease and caused by HPVs.

Neurological disorders

HIV can cause a variety of neurological symptoms, culminating in encephalopathy (AIDS-related dementia) and death. In addition, intracranial infections (mainly parasitic, viral or fungal) are common. Up to two-thirds of AIDS patients develop a dementia complex, with personality changes, ataxia and convulsions; about 15% of AIDS patients develop CNS toxoplasmosis, while 10% develop cryptococcal meningitis. Spinal cord disease is seen in about 20% and may progress to bladder and bowel dysfunction.

Neurological manifestations can be acute, with fever, malaise, depression, fits, facial palsy and neuropathies affecting the extremities. Myelopathy or neuropathy can cause weakness of the legs, sometimes paraesthesiae and, in severe cases, ataxia and incontinence. Subacute encephalopathy affects about 30% of AIDS patients, who gradually develop a confusional state associated with fever and depression; the patient eventually may become bedridden and incontinent. Chronic meningitis may precede more typical features of AIDS and is characterized by fever, headache, meningeal signs and cranial nerve palsies (typically affecting nerves V, VII and VIII). Brain tumours, particularly lymphomas, are also common complications of HIV/AIDS. Peripheral and cranial neuropathies, and myopathy, are relatively common.

Autoimmune disorders

Autoimmune disorders, particularly thrombocytopenic purpura, are relatively common in HIV disease. Drug allergic reactions are common, mostly to co-trimoxazole, and may cause erythema multiforme.

HIV infection in children

Infection with HIV in children causes them to appear ill and stunted, and promotes staphylococcal and streptococcal infections, such as otitis media, rashes and diarrhoea, as well as fungal and viral infections.

Normal CD4/CD8 ratios may persist late in the disease and lymphopenia is uncommon. Humoral immunity is more severely affected than in adult HIV disease and may long precede changes in T-lymphocyte subsets. Bacterial infections are relatively more common because of depressed humoral immunity. Generalized lymphadenopathy and hepatosplenomegaly are often the first signs and chronic parotitis is a common presenting feature. Neurological disease develops in the great majority. Interstitial lymphoid pneumonitis is particularly

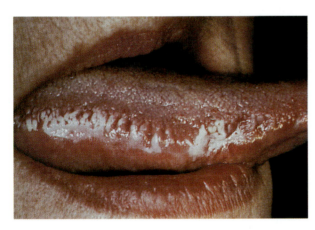

Fig. 20.8 Hairy leukoplakia in HIV/AIDS.

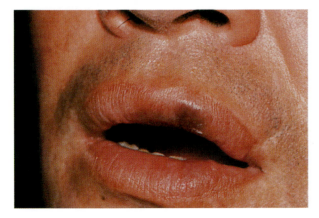

Fig. 20.9 Kaposi sarcoma in HIV/AIDS.

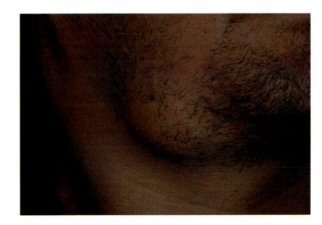

Fig. 20.10 Lymphoma in HIV/AIDS.

characteristic. Hypergammaglobulinaemia is also severe and 13% have thrombocytopenic purpura.

B-cell lymphomas are the most common tumours but Kaposi sarcoma is rare and affects the skin particularly infrequently. Other systemic effects of HIV infection in children include renal disease and cardiomyopathy.

GENERAL MANAGEMENT

Diagnosis of HIV infection

Diagnosis of HIV infection is made on suspicion, especially if there is a supportive history; clinical criteria, if present; and, after appropriate consent, laboratory investigations. Lymphopenia, low CD4 counts in the blood, and a low CD4:CD8 ratio (normal value is about 2, which falls to about 0.5 in AIDS) are typical but not specific findings. HIV infection must be confirmed by testing for HIV and all results must be kept confidential. Relatives *cannot* give consent for an HIV test. Most HIV tests detect HIV serum antibodies, but it takes some time – 2–8 weeks – to produce enough antibodies to be detected by the antibody test. This 'window period' can vary from person to person and the HIV viral load may be very high at this time, as is the likelihood of transmitting HIV to sex or needle-sharing partners. Most HIV-infected people (97%) will develop detectable serum antibodies in the first 3 months, but a few will take longer, so a follow-up test more than 3 months after the last potential exposure to HIV is prudent. All those infected will have detectable serum antibodies to HIV by 6 months.

Conventional HIV serological tests sent to a laboratory give results within a week or two; rapid HIV tests can produce results in as little as 20 minutes. A positive HIV serological test result means that a person may have been infected with HIV, but all positive HIV test results, whether from conventional or rapid tests, must be verified by a second 'confirmatory' HIV test. Thus HIV antibody screening tests (e.g. reactive enzyme immunoassay [EIA]) should be confirmed by a positive result from a supplemental HIV antibody test (e.g. Western blot or indirect immunofluorescence assay test) *or* a positive result or report of a detectable quantity from any of the following HIV virological (i.e. non-antibody) tests:

- HIV nucleic acid (DNA or RNA) detection test (e.g. PCR)
- HIV p24 antigen test, including neutralization assay
- HIV isolation (viral culture).

Note that a negative (i.e. undetectable or non-reactive) result from an HIV virological test (e.g. viral RNA nucleic acid test) does *not* rule out the diagnosis of HIV infection.

HIV testing should be offered not only as part of a sexual health screen but also to:

- anyone with one of a number of 'clinical indicator diseases'
- patients with specific lifestyle or demographic characteristics
- all adults in all health-care services if HIV prevalence is high.

No patient with signs of HIV infection should be discharged as uninfected solely on the basis of one negative HIV test result; neither should they be told that they have HIV infection without the knowledge that the laboratory has confirmed the test result using the above criteria. Treat the results of any HIV tests and a diagnosis of HIV infection or AIDS with confidentiality. Considerable care is needed regarding the social and psychological consequences of HIV infection. More information on HIV testing is available at: http://www.aidsmap.com/UK-guidelines/page/1321555/ (accessed 30 September 2013).

The mortality rate from AIDS was virtually 100% but, although there is still no effective treatment for the underlying immune defect, antiretroviral therapy (ART) employs drugs that can significantly impede the progress of HIV infection; these include nucleoside analogues, non-nucleoside reverse transcriptase inhibitors, protease inhibitors, entry/fusion inhibitors and integrase inhibitors. Treatment with a combination of these drugs is termed active ART. Early intervention with ART (Tables 20.5, 20.6, 20.7 and 20.8) is usually beneficial.

Table 20.5 *Antiretroviral drugs, cautions and adverse effects: nucleoside reverse transcriptase inhibitors (NRTIs)[a]*

Generic name (abbreviation)	Trade name	Possible orofacial adverse effects	Other main adverse effects	Cautions with drugs used in oral health care
Abacavir (ABC)	Ziagen	Erythema multiforme, ulcers	Lactic acidosis, nausea, diarrhoea, life-threatening rash; human leukocyte antigen (HLA)-B*5701 screening (for hypersensitivity reaction), lipodystrophy	No significant interactions
Didanosine (ddl)	Videx	Erythema multiforme, dry mouth, facial lipoatrophy	Nausea, diarrhoea, lactic acidosis, mitochondrial dysfunction leading to pancreatitis, abnormal liver function, peripheral neuropathy, retinal damage	Ciprofloxacin Ganciclovir Itraconazole Ketoconazole
Emtricitabine (FTC)	Emtriva	Hyperpigmentation, swelling	Lactic acidosis, pruritus, hyperpigmentation, lipodystrophy	No significant interactions
Lamivudine (3TC)	Epivir	Dry mouth	Nausea, diarrhoea, mitochondrial dysfunction leading to pancreatitis, abnormal liver function, neuropathy, lipodystrophy, clefts	No significant interactions
Stavudine (d4T)	Zerit	Facial lipoatrophy	Neuropsychiatric reactions, mitochondrial dysfunction leading to pancreatitis, abnormal liver function, lactic acidosis, neuropathy	No significant interactions
Tenofovir disoproxil (TDF)	Viread	Facial lipoatrophy	Renal tubular damage, hypophosphataemia	No significant interactions
Zidovudine (azidothymidine; AZT, ZDV)	Retrovir	Erythema multiforme, hyperpigmentation, lichenoid drug reaction, facial lipoatrophy	Nausea, diarrhoea, myelotoxicity, lactic acidosis, myopathy	Fluconazole Ganciclovir

[a]There are also combinations of these; zalcitabine (dideoxycytidine; DDC) is no longer marketed.

Table 20.6 *Antiretroviral drugs, cautions and adverse effects: non-nucleoside reverse transcriptase inhibitors (NNRTIs)*

Generic name (abbreviation)	Trade name	Possible orofacial adverse effects	Other main adverse effects	Cautions with drugs used in oral health care
Delavirdine (DLV)	Rescriptor (not licensed in UK)	Erythema multiforme, ulcers	Interference with liver drug-metabolizing enzymes	Carbamazepine Clarithromycin Dapsone Midazolam
Efavirenz (EFV)	Sustiva	Erythema multiforme, swelling, burning mouth, clefts	Interference with liver drug-metabolizing enzymes, lipodystrophy, neuropsychiatric reactions	Buprenorphine Carbamazepine Itraconazole Ketoconazole Midazolam Prednisolone (prednisone) Voriconazole
Etravirine (ETR)	Intelence	Erythema multiforme, ulcers	Hypersensitivity	Clarithromycin Fluconazole Itraconazole Posaconazole Voriconazole
Nevirapine (NVP)	Viramune	Erythema multiforme, ulcers, swelling, taste disturbance, lichenoid drug reaction, dry mouth, burning mouth	Induction of liver drug-metabolizing enzymes, abnormal liver function, lipodystrophy	Fluconazole Ketoconazole
Rilpivirine (RPV)	Edurant	Swelling	Liver problems, lipodystrophy, severe depression and suicidal thoughts	Ketoconazole

Table 20.7 *Antiretroviral drugs, cautions and adverse effects: protease inhibitors (PIs)[a]*

Generic name (abbreviation)	Trade name	Possible orofacial adverse effects	Other main adverse effects	Cautions with drugs used in oral health care
Atazanavir (ATV)	Reyataz	Erythema multiforme, swelling, ulcers	Nephrolithiasis, prolongation of QR interval, lipodystrophy, interference with liver drug-metabolizing enzymes, dyslipidaemia, neurological effects	Clarithromycin Colchicine Midazolam Paracetamol (acetaminophen) Posaconazole Voriconazole
Darunavir (DRV)	Prezista	Erythema multiforme, swelling, dry mouth	ECG changes, neuropathy, weight changes, lipodystrophy, interference with liver drug-metabolizing enzymes, dyslipidaemia	Carbamazepine Ciclosporin Clarithromycin Colchicine Fluticasone Itraconazole Ketoconazole Midazolam Voriconazole
Fosamprenavir (FPV)	Telzir/Lexiva	Erythema multiforme, swelling, perioral paraesthesia, parotid lipomatosis	Nephrolithiasis, lipodystrophy, interference with liver drug-metabolizing enzymes, dyslipidaemia	Colchicine Posaconazole
Indinavir (IDV)	Crixivan	Cheilitis (retinoid-like effect), parotid lipomatosis, dry mouth, taste disturbance	Nephrolithiasis in 40%, interference with liver drug-metabolizing enzymes, oesophagitis, haemolysis, lipodystrophy	Carbamazepine Clarithromycin Colchicine Ketoconazole Itraconazole Midazolam
Nelfinavir (NFV)	Viracept	Parotid lipomatosis, dry mouth, clefts	Nausea, diarrhoea, interference with liver drug-metabolizing enzymes, dyslipidaemia, lipodystrophy	Carbamazepine Colchicine Ciclosporin Desipramine Ketoconazole Midazolam Tacrolimus

(Continued)

Table 20.7 (Continued)

Generic name (abbreviation)	Trade name	Possible orofacial adverse effects	Other main adverse effects	Cautions with drugs used in oral health care
Ritonavir (RTV)	Norvir	Perioral paraesthesia, parotid lipomatosis, dry mouth, taste disturbance, swelling	Nausea, diarrhoea, interference with liver drug-metabolizing enzymes, flushing, dyslipidaemia, lipodystrophy, arrhythmias	Amitriptyline Carbamazepine Clarithromycin Colchicine Diazepam Fentanyl Fluoxetine Fluticasone Itraconazole Ketoconazole Metronidazole Midazolam Phenytoin Prednisolone Tacrolimus
Saquinavir mesylate (SQV)	Invirase	Erythema multiforme, ulcers, parotid lipomatosis, dry mouth, taste disturbance	Nausea, diarrhoea, interference with liver drug-metabolizing enzymes, dyslipidaemia, lipodystrophy, arrhythmias	Alprazolam Amitriptyline Carbamazepine Dexamethasone Diazepam Fluticasone Itraconazole Midazolam Tacrolimus
Tipranavir (TPV)	Aptivus	Erythema multiforme, swelling, ulcers	Hepatotoxicity and bleeding tendency, lipodystrophy, dyslipidaemia	Carbamazepine Clarithromycin Colchicine Fluconazole Midazolam

[a]There are also combinations; amprenavir (trade name Agenerase) is no longer marketed; saquinavir (trade name Fortovase) is no longer marketed.

Table 20.8 *Newer antiretroviral drugs, cautions and adverse effects*

Generic name (abbreviation)	Trade name	Possible orofacial adverse effects	Other main adverse effects	Cautions with drugs used in oral health care
Fusion inhibitor				
Enfuvirtide (ENF)	Fuzeon	Swelling, sinusitis	Hypersensitivity, neuropathy, hypotension, interference with liver drug-metabolizing enzymes, pneumonia	No significant interactions
Entry inhibitors: CCR5 co-receptor antagonist				
Maraviroc (MVC)	Selzentry/Celsentri	Taste disturbance	Liver problems, cardiovascular problems	Ketoconazole
Integrase strand transfer inhibitor				
Raltegravir (RAL)	Isentress	Erythema multiforme, dry mouth	Diarrhoea, abdominal pain	No significant interactions

Patients on ART are monitored by regular CD4 counts and plasma viral load levels, which correlate well with clinical response. Adverse effects are common and adherence to therapy is important to avoid the development of drug-resistant variants.

Patients with low CD4 counts are given antimicrobials as prophylaxis against opportunistic infections. Individuals should also be offered psychological support to help them come to terms with their illness and should be educated on measures necessary to prevent further spread of infection. At CD4 counts below 200/microlitre, patients are at high risk of *Pneumocystis jiroveci* infection; at counts below 100/microlitre, CMV and *Mycobacterium avium–intracellulare* are risks.

Antimicrobial prophylaxis

Antimicrobial prophylaxis and therapeutic and supportive treatment may help prolong and improve the quality of life in HIV disease. Drugs available to help treat opportunistic infections are shown in Table 20.9.

Table 20.9 *Antimicrobial agents for infections in HIV disease*

Antimicrobial	Used for
Aciclovir	Herpes simplex and zoster infections
Foscarnet and ganciclovir	Cytomegalovirus infections
Fluconazole	Yeast and other fungal infections
Trimethoprim/sulfamethoxazole (TMP/SMX), atovaquone or pentamidine	*Pneumocystis jiroveci* pneumonia
Rifabutin	Prophylaxis against *Mycobacterium avium* complex (MAC) infection
Isoniazid	Tuberculosis

Table 20.10 *Manifestations of immune reconstitution inflammatory syndrome (IRIS)*

Known infections	Other conditions
Cryptococcus	Aphthous-like ulcers
Cytomegalovirus	Castleman disease
Hepatitis viruses	Eosinophilic folliculitis
Herpes simplex	Graves disease
Herpes zoster	Myopathy
Histoplasmosis	Non-Hodgkin lymphoma
Human herpesvirus 8	Progressive multifocal leukoencephalopathy
Leprosy	Sarcoidosis
Mycobacterium avium	Systemic lupus erythematosus
Papillomavirus	
Pneumocystis	
Tuberculosis	

Vaccines

Attempts to produce a safe and effective vaccine against HIV encounter development problems, not least because the proteins of HIV can undergo changes. Some candidate vaccines are currently in the initial phases of testing in humans. Post-exposure vaccination (e.g. with killed virus, envelope subunits or recombinant vaccinia vectors in combination with viral subunits) may have provided some clinical benefit, but long-term detailed trials are still required before it is known whether such vaccines can provide reliable control of HIV.

Immune Reconstitution Syndrome (IRIS)

Profoundly immunodeficient people treated with ART may develop the immune reconstitution inflammatory syndrome (IRIS) – a paradoxical worsening or recurrence of opportunistic infections and symptoms. IRIS can be seen in HIV/AIDS, where it affects 8% to over 30% of patients, and also may affect immunosuppressed individuals.

General aspects of IRIS

IRIS development appears to be linked not only to increases in CD4 cells, but also to higher CD8 cell counts induced by ART. Raised CD8 cells may be a prime factor contributing to worsening of both herpes zoster and hepatitis B or C symptoms after the initiation of ART. Increased activity of IL-2 and IL-12 may contribute. Though most individuals starting ART are not likely to experience IRIS, AIDS patients are more at risk if they are put on ART for the first time, or if they have recently been treated for an opportunistic infection.

Clinical features of IRIS

While IRIS, by definition, heralds a return to a healthier immune system, a range of common conditions can occur or be exacerbated (Table 20.10); these can be serious, even fatal.

The two common IRIS scenarios are the 'unmasking' of occult opportunistic infectious pathogens, which needs appropriate antimicrobial therapy, and the 'paradoxical' symptomatic relapse of a prior infection despite microbiological treatment success, which usually resolves spontaneously. IRIS can have a range of effects, including TB, MAC infections, cytomegalovirus retinitis, disseminated cryptococcosis and Kaposi sarcoma. IRIS is characterized by a greater disease burden, a low CD4-cell nadir and, for *M. tuberculosis*, a shorter time period between diagnosis and initiation of ART. Many cases of IRIS have atypical presentations. For example, the hallmarks of IRIS in a person previously responding to treatment for TB might be a new or worsening fever, new effusions, new or worsening lymphadenopathy, and other uncharacteristic reactions, rather than progression of lung disease itself. Mild shingles or a local *M. avium* infection without bacteraemia, both seen in IRIS, would be unusual in an HIV-positive person not taking ART.

GENERAL MANAGEMENT OF IRIS

Treatment of IRIS is continuation of the current HIV medication regimen; antimicrobial medications to treat infection; and corticosteroids to suppress the inflammatory process temporarily.

DENTAL ASPECTS OF HIV/AIDS

Immunologically stable (undetectable viral load and T-cell (CD4) count over 200/mL) HIV-positive patients on ART may be considered the best dental treatment risk. However, patients with profound immunodeficiency (those with neutropenia and/or CD4 T-lymphocyte count below 200/mL) may require antibiotic cover with metronidazole, amoxicillin plus clavulanic acid, or clindamycin before surgery or after maxillofacial injuries.

There is a theoretical interaction of local anaesthesia (LA) with PIs, and PIs such as indinavir and nelfinavir can enhance benzodiazepines. Bleeding can be aggravated by non-steroidal anti-inflammatory drugs (NSAIDs) such as aspirin or indometacin; codeine and paracetamol (acetaminophen) are safer analgesics (the interaction with zidovudine, inducing granulocytopenia, appears rarely to be clinically significant). Of note, however, HIV disease is a major risk factor for adverse drug reactions; the incidence of reactions to ampicillin is inversely proportional to CD4+ cell counts. Dental treatment should be carried out with the standard precautions and additional attention given to the possibility, though small, of postoperative infection and prolonged haemorrhage.

It is unethical to withhold treatment from any patient on the basis of a moral judgment that the patient's activities or lifestyle might have contributed to the condition for which treatment was being sought. There is a move towards normalization and mainstreaming of oral health-care provision but many HIV-infected individuals have concerns about privacy; the additional stigma and social implications of their infection may prevent them from accessing general dental services – at least in their locality. It is therefore critical to ensure that there is a strict adherence to data protection and patient confidentiality; the patient should be reassured that none of their details will be discussed, even with their physicians, unless permission is sought from the patient.

Medical consultation is mandatory for symptomatic HIV-infected patients before any dental surgical procedure, although no serious postoperative complications have been found in most instances. There have been no systematic studies involving dental implants, orthognathic surgery, periodontal therapy, prophylaxis, or scaling and root planing, and only one study on endodontics, which reported few immediate complications. Prospective studies on dental implants showed a 100% success rate at 6 months for both HIV and controls, with no difference in clinical outcomes. The prevalence of complications following tooth extractions in HIV-infected persons overall is estimated at about 5%, similar to that achieved in HIV-negative patients, and most complications are mild (alveolitis and delayed healing) and easily treated. Postoperative bleeding is unusual, even in thrombocytopenic patients. Factors increasing the potential for postoperative complications are shown in Box 20.2.

Box 20.2 *Factors increasing the potential for postoperative complications in HIV/AIDS*

- Low CD4 count
- High viral load
- Low lymphocyte count
- Neutropenia
- Bleeding tendency (i.e. thrombocytopenia, liver damage, etc.)
- Another concomitant infection

Most patients with HIV disease have head and neck and oral manifestations at some time (Table 20.11). Oral lesions are most likely to appear when the CD4 cell count is low and are often controlled, at least temporarily, by ART. Cervical lymphadenopathy is an almost invariable feature at some stage of HIV disease and AIDS. Persistent generalized lymphadenopathy (PGL) is common. Oral features are classified as strongly, less commonly or possibly associated with HIV infection (Table 20.12). Oral candidosis (usually thrush or erythematous candidosis) is common; it is often the initial manifestation and seen in 50% of patients. Oral candidosis is frequently associated with oesophageal candidosis and is also a predictor of liability to systemic opportunistic infections; the latter, but not the former, is an AIDS-defining illness. Conventional antifungal treatment is indicated initially, although fluconazole may be required, especially if there is oesophageal infection. Azole resistance is a growing problem.

Infections with herpes simplex virus, varicella zoster virus, CMV, EBV, human herpesvirus 6 (HHV-6) and KSHV are common. Herpes simplex infections are usually intraoral, sometimes severe and persistent, but rarely disseminate; they usually respond well to aciclovir. Severe herpes zoster may be seen. CMV may cause mouth ulcers. EBV has been implicated in hairy leukoplakia and some lymphomas (see later). Hairy leukoplakia, though characteristic of HIV, can be seen very rarely in other patients, mainly those who are immunocompromised. It derives its name from the raised white areas of thickening, usually on the lateral borders of the tongue. The EBV capsid antigen can be identified in the prickle cell layer. It appears not to be pre-malignant. Less common oral and perioral infections include venereal warts. Mycobacterial oral ulcers and oral histoplasmosis or

---

Table 20.11 *Features, diagnosis and management of orofacial lesions of HIV infection*

Frequency	Condition	Clinical features	Diagnosis	Management
Common	Candidosis[a]	White removable lesions or red lesions, typically in the palate	Clinical plus investigations; smear, culture, rinse or biopsy	Antifungals (fluconazole most effective)
	Hairy leukoplakia[a]	White non-removable lesions, almost invariably bilaterally on the tongue	Clinical plus cytology; deoxyribonucleic acid (DNA) studies or biopsy	None usually but podophyllin or aciclovir effective
	Kaposi sarcoma[a]	Purple macules leading to nodules, seen mainly in the palate	Clinical plus investigations; biopsy	Liposomal anthracyclines or paclitaxel chemotherapy. Vinblastine intralesionally. Alitretinoin gel, interferon-alpha intralesionally; cryotherapy and photodynamic therapy reportedly effective
Uncommon	Periodontal disease	Linear gingival erythema, necrotizing gingivitis or periodontitis	Clinical	Oral hygiene, plaque removal, chlorhexidine, metronidazole
	Aphthous-like ulcers	Recurrent ulcers anywhere but especially on mobile mucosae	Clinical plus investigations; possibly biopsy	Corticosteroids or thalidomide or granulocyte colony-stimulating factor
	Herpesvirus infections (herpes simplex, cytomegalovirus, varicella zoster)	Chronic ulcers often on tongue, hard palate or gingivae Zoster increased by ART	Clinical plus investigations; cytology, electron microscopy, DNA studies or biopsy	Antivirals
	Papillomavirus infections	Warty lesions, increased by ART	Clinical plus investigations; DNA studies, possibly biopsy	Excise or remove with heat, laser or cryoprobe, imiquimod, interferon-alpha or podophyllin
	Salivary gland disease	Hyposalivation and sometimes salivary gland enlargement	Clinical plus investigations; sialometry, possibly biopsy	Salivary substitutes and/or pilocarpine or cevimeline
	Lymphomas	Lump or ulcer in fauces or gingivae	Clinical plus investigations; biopsy	Chemotherapy or radiation or both. Ifosfamide, mesna and rituximab on trial
Rare	Mycobacterial infections, deep fungal infections			
	Osteomyelitis, neuropathies			

[a]Antiretroviral therapy (ART) reduces manifestations.

Table 20.12 *World Health Organization classification of oral lesions in HIV/AIDS*

Group I lesions strongly associated with HIV infection	Group II lesions less commonly associated with HIV infection	Group III lesions possibly associated with HIV infection
Candidosis	Atypical ulceration (oropharyngeal)	A miscellany of rare diseases
Erythematous	Idiopathic thrombocytopenic purpura	
Hyperplastic	Dry mouth	
Thrush (pseudomembranous)	Salivary gland diseases	
Hairy leukoplakia (Epstein–Barr virus; EBV)	Unilateral or bilateral swelling of major salivary glands	
HIV gingivitis	Viral infections (other than EBV)	
Necrotizing ulcerative gingivitis	Cytomegalovirus	
HIV periodontitis	Herpes simplex virus	
Kaposi sarcoma (human herpesvirus 8)	Human papillomavirus (warty-like lesions): condyloma acuminatum, focal epithelial hyperplasia and verruca vulgaris	
Non-Hodgkin lymphoma (EBV)	Varicella zoster virus: herpes zoster and varicella	

Table 20.13 *Possible oral health-care drug interactions in HIV-infected patients[a]*

Drug used in oral health care	May interact with	Possible consequences
Azole antifungals: Miconazole Fluconazole Itraconazole Ketoconazole	Terfenadine (astemizole and cisapride withdrawn because of interaction)	Arrhythmias and cardiotoxicity
	Anticoagulants	Anticoagulants potentiated
	Antacids	Azole absorption impaired
	Didanosine	
	H$_2$ antagonists	
	Omeprazole	
Benzodiazepines	Azole	Benzodiazepines enhanced
	Indinavir	
	Ritonavir	
Carbamazepine	Indinavir	Antiretroviral reduced
	Lopinavir	
	Nevirapine	
	Saquinavir	
Corticosteroids	Ritonavir	Corticosteroids enhanced
Erythromycin	Ritonavir	Erythromycin enhanced
	Saquinavir	Arrhythmias
Fluconazole	Rifabutin	Uveitis from rifabutin toxicity
	Zidovudine	Zidovudine enhanced
Ganciclovir	Zidovudine	Zidovudine enhanced; haematological toxicity
Metronidazole	Ritonavir	Disulfiram-like reaction
Midazolam	Efavirenz	Midazolam enhanced
	Indinavir	
	Nelfinavir	
	Ritonavir	
	Saquinavir	
Non-steroidal anti-inflammatory drugs (NSAIDs)	Ritonavir	NSAIDs enhanced
	Saquinavir	
	Zidovudine	NSAIDs enhanced; haematological toxicity

[a]See also http://www.medadvocates.org/drugs/haart/druginteractions.html and HIV and AIDS Activities at http://www.fda.gov/ForConsumers/byAudience/ForPatientAdvocates/default.htm (both accessed 30 September 2013).

cryptococcosis, as well as sinusitis, gingivitis or periodontitis, may be seen. Major aphthae increase in frequency and severity with the severity of the immunodeficiency. Giant persistent aphthous-like ulcers respond to thalidomide (which needs to be given with caution and never to potentially pregnant women). Post-extraction infections, osteomyelitis after jaw fractures and cancrum oris (noma) have very occasionally been seen.

Kaposi sarcoma in 50% of patients is oral or perioral, and often an early oral manifestation, presenting as a red or purple macule or a nodule, usually on the palate. Oral and salivary gland lymphomas also develop more frequently in patients with AIDS than in a normal population; EBV is implicated.

In childhood HIV disease, chronic parotitis is common and virtually pathognomonic (see Table 20.12). Chronic oral candidosis is present in 75% and is the single most common mucocutaneous manifestation. Most types of oral candidosis may be seen, most frequently in the form of persistent thrush. Difficulties in swallowing usually indicate candidosis of the oesophagus. Unlike normal children, those with AIDS are frequently subject to recurrent intraoral as well as labial herpetic infection. Initially, the infection responds to intravenous aciclovir but becomes more resistant as AIDS progresses. Shingles is rare in normal children but can be an early sign of AIDS in a child, and tends to be more severe and painful.

Drug interactions

Possible drug interactions with drugs used in oral health care are shown in Table 20.13.

Anaesthetic agents may induce pharmacodynamic changes to affect the efficacy and toxicity of antiretrovirals (ARVs), and pharmacokinetic effects of ARVs can affect the absorption, distribution, metabolism and elimination of anaesthetic drugs. Pharmacodynamic interactions can be managed by avoiding anaesthetic agents such as halothane or methoxyflurane that cause hepatic or renal dysfunction. Propofol and NRTIs may both potentially promote mitochondrial toxicity and lactic acidosis, and it may be wise to avoid propofol infusions in patients receiving ARVs. Pharmacokinetic interactions are more complicated and are primarily due to liver enzyme induction or inhibition, particularly the CYP450 3A4 enzyme. PIs and NNRTIs are the most commonly implicated group of ARVs in drug interactions. Enzyme induction or inhibition can affect the action of several classes of anaesthetic drugs, including:

■ *opioids*. Fentanyl may be enhanced by ritonavir due to both liver enzyme inhibition and induction. Enzyme inhibition reduces fentanyl clearance and enzyme induction increases metabolism to active metabolites such as normeperidine.
■ *benzodiazepines*. Saquinavir may inhibit midazolam metabolism.
■ *calcium-channel blockers*. These may have enhanced hypotensive effects due to enzyme inhibition.

- *local anaesthetics*. Agents such as lidocaine may have increased plasma levels due to enzyme inhibition.
- *neuromuscular blockers*. Effects may be prolonged, even by a single dose of vecuronium, for instance.

More information is available at www.hiv-druginteractions.org (accessed 30 September 2013).

Regional anaesthesia

The presence of HIV infection is not an absolute contraindication to regional anaesthesia and there is no evidence that HIV progression is increased by central neuraxial blockade. However, the presence of HIV complications may pose relative contraindications to regional anaesthesia:

- myelopathy
- vertebral or spinal neoplasms
- CNS infections
- coagulopathy.

It is essential to conduct a full preoperative neurological assessment and to document any neurological deficit.

Anaesthetic management plan

Thorough preoperative assessment for status of HIV infection includes:

- history, including risk factors
- physical examination
- laboratory tests
- organ involvement
- drug history and side-effects.

Investigations should include:

- full blood count
- clotting function – to exclude coagulation abnormalities (consideration of use of thromboelastography (TEG)/platelet mapping if available)
- biochemical tests, including glucose, electrolytes, renal and liver function – to exclude possible metabolic, liver or renal disturbances
- viral load and CD4+ count
- chest radiography – screen for opportunistic infections and TB
- cardiac evaluation with electrocardiography and echocardiography (if possible) – to screen for cardiomyopathy.

Perioperative management of ART

Due to increasing problems of drug resistance in the treatment of HIV, it is recommended that ART therapy be continued throughout the perioperative period if at all possible. Naturally, this needs to be compatible with surgery and the patient's gastrointestinal function. Some ARVs are available in liquid form, enabling administration via feeding tube or gastrostomy. Parenteral preparations are limited to zidovudine and enfuvirtide only.

Consider drug interactions between ART and drugs affected by hepatic enzyme inhibition and/or induction.

Employ a strict aseptic technique; HIV-infected patients are immunocompromised and are susceptible to infections.

Periodontal disease in HIV

Bacterial species other than the classical periodontal pathogens may be involved in periodontal diseases since the classical putative periodontal pathogens, *Treponema denticola*, *Porphyromonas gingivalis* and *Tannerella forsythia* may be below the limit of detection. Putative periodontal pathogens are more prevalent in the subgingival microbiota of HIV-seronegative patients with chronic periodontitis, whereas species not usually associated with periodontitis are detected in higher frequency in HIV-seropositive subjects under ART. Species of *Gemella*, *Dialister*, *Streptococcus* and *Veillonella* are predominant. Species or phylotypes most commonly detected are *Bulleidia extructa*, *Dialister*, *Fusobacterium*, *Selenomonas*, *Peptostreptococcus*, *Veillonella* and the phylum TM7.

There is significant prevalence of *Porphyromonas gingivalis* and *Treponema denticola* among HIV-negative patients compared to HIV-positive patients. Odds ratio analysis revealed a statistically significant positive association between 3 of the 28 possible combinations in the HIV-positive group. They included *Prevotella nigrescens/Campylobacter rectus*, *P. nigrescens/P. gingivalis* and *P. nigrescens/T. denticola*. Although the prevalence of periodontal pathogens is similar in both groups, the combination of certain periodontal pathogens may be responsible for chronic periodontitis seen in HIV-infected adults.

Periodontal attachment loss in HIV-infected patients is associated with the major histocompatibility (MHC) complex 8.1 haplotype (HLA-A1,B8,DR3). Periodontal attachment loss is mediated by overproduction of tumour necrosis factor (TNF) and IL-1, and appears to have a genetic component. The 8.1 MHC ancestral haplotype (HLA-A1,B8,TNFA-308(2),DR3) is associated with raised TNF production and predisposes carriers to several autoimmune/immunopathological disorders, including rapid progression of HIV disease, but not early-onset periodontal disease in healthy individuals. Rather a high proportion of subjects with severe periodontal disease carry allele 2 at IL-1A-889 and IL-1B + 3953.

ART may affect the prevalence of some orofacial manifestations (Table 20.14) but may also cause adverse reactions (Table 20.15).

Transmission of HIV to or from health-care professionals

Accidental exposure to blood following a needlestick (sharps) injury is one of the most common occupational accidents in health care. The highest reported risks are after a needlestick incident, especially with:

- devices that are visibly contaminated with blood
- hollow-bore needles that have been in an artery or vein
- deep injuries
- exposure to blood from patients with terminal infection.

Exposure-prone procedures (EPPs) are those where there is a risk that injury to the HCP may result in exposure of the patient's open tissues to the blood of the HCP. These procedures include those where

Table 20.14 *Effect of antiretroviral therapy on orofacial manifestations of HIV/AIDS*

Declined	Increased
Candidosis	Salivary gland disease
Hairy leukoplakia	Warts and zoster
Kaposi sarcoma	Drug adverse effects

[a] See also HIV Drug Chart/Overview at http://www.thewellproject.org/en_US/Treatment_and_Trials/index.jsp (accessed 30 September 2013).

Table 20.15 *Management problems related to HIV infection or the adverse effects of antiretroviral therapy, chemotherapy or anti-infective agents*

System	Possible lesions	Possible treatment influences
Cardiac	Endocardial, myocardial, pericardial or vascular lesions, or neoplasms	Acute coronary syndrome
		Dilated cardiomyopathy
		Endocarditis and valvular lesions
		Pericardial effusions
		Pulmonary hypertension
		Vasculitis
Gastrointestinal	Diarrhoea	Bleeding: electrolyte loss and dehydration
	Hepatobiliary impairment	
	Pancreatitis	Difficulty or pain on swallowing
		Delayed gastric emptying
Haematological	Anaemia	Bleeding tendency
	Coagulation abnormalities	Infections
	Haematological malignancies	
	Neutropenia	
	Persistent generalized lymphadenopathy	
	Thrombocytopenia	
Metabolic	Hypo- or hyperthyroidism	Corticosteroid cover
	Hyponatraemia from syndrome of inappropriate antidiuretic hormone	
	Hypothalamo–pituitary–adrenal axis disorders	
	Lactic acidosis	
	Lipodystrophy (truncal obesity, buffalo hump)	
	Metabolic syndrome (raised plasma triglycerides, cholesterol)	
	Cushing syndrome and Addison disease	
Neurological	Direct infection, inflammation, demyelination or opportunistic infections, neoplasms or immune deficiency	Autonomic neuropathy
		Encephalopathy
		Neurocognitive impairment (with implications for consent)
		Seizures
Renal	Hypertension	Drug-induced nephrotoxicity
	Diabetes	Renal impairment
	HIV-associated nephropathy	
Respiratory	Both upper and lower airway can be involved with infection, malignancies, opportunistic infections or adverse effects of medication	Obstruction (by Kaposi sarcoma, lymphoma or infections)
		Atypical infections (commonly tuberculosis, other mycobacteria and fungal infections)
		Bronchitis
		Sinusitis
		Pneumonia
		Pneumonitis

the worker's gloved hands may be in contact with sharp instruments, needle tips or sharp tissues (spicules of bone or teeth) inside a patient's open body cavity, wound or confined anatomical space, where the hands or fingertips may not be completely visible at all times.

All employers should have an acceptable policy for managing occupational injuries, and could be answerable to the Health and Safety Executive, the General Dental Council or the civil courts.

The risk of HIV transmission from an occupational exposure to HIV-infected blood is dependent upon the titre of HIV in the blood (viral load), the volume of the blood that is transmitted and whether the virus is still infective. The risk of transmission of HIV from an occupational exposure among dental health workers is low; no occupational exposure has as yet resulted in HIV transmission to a member of the dental team. HIV infection of a clinician therefore no longer precludes clinical work in many countries.

Needlestick injuries are most likely in the following situations:

- During needle recapping
- During surgery, especially wound closure
- When an uncapped needle has ended up in linen, etc.
- When taking an unsheathed used needle to the sharps container
- During the cleaning and transporting of waste material
- When using more complex collection and injection techniques
- In accident and emergency departments
- In high-stress interventions.

See also Chapter 31. More information is also available at: https://www.gov.uk/government/organisations/department-of-health (search on 'HIV post-exposure prophylaxis'; accessed 30 September 2013).

The risk of transmission of HIV from an infected patient through a needlestick (inoculation) injury is less than 1%: around 1 in 300 – far lower than the nearly 26% of persons who develop HBV infection or the 10% who contract HCV infection after needlestick injuries involving those agents (see Fig. 20.11 and Ch. 31).

The chief occupational risk of acquiring infection is as a result of injury by a sharp instrument, particularly an LA needle, which can contain a significant amount of contaminated fluid. Though needlestick

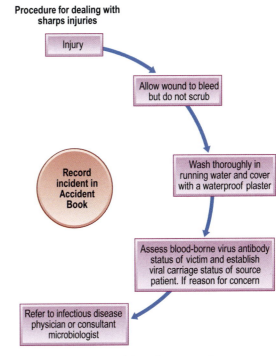

Procedure for dealing with sharps injuries

Injury → Allow wound to bleed but do not scrub → Wash thoroughly in running water and cover with a waterproof plaster → Assess blood-borne virus antibody status of victim and establish viral carriage status of source patient. If reason for concern → Refer to infectious disease physician or consultant microbiologist → Record incident in Accident Book

Fig. 20.11 Needlestick injury protocol (see also Fig. 31.2).

injuries can transmit the virus, infection among dental health personnel caring for HIV-infected patients is rare, despite reports of many such injuries. In most HCPs who have acquired HIV, the infection has been sexually transmitted. By 2008, there had only been two reports of dental staff contracting HIV as a consequence of occupation, even in endemic areas.

The virus does appear to have been transmitted within healthcare facilities on rare occasions. One dentist with HIV infection in Florida, USA, appears to have transmitted it to at least six patients as a consequence of invasive dental procedures. That the dentist was the source of the infection was suggested by the fact that the strain of the virus was the same; the circumstances surrounding transmission remain uncertain, as the dentist has since died. An outbreak of 14 cases of HIV infection was discovered in May 1993 among haemodialysis patients at a university hospital in Bucaramanga, Colombia, and seems most likely to have been transmitted by contaminated dental instruments. Many other studies, however, have shown no evidence of any transmission of HIV from HIV-infected dentists to patients.

TRANSFUSION-RELATED IMMUNOMODULATION (TRIM)

Red blood cell transfusion in any patient may be associated with immunosuppressive or proinflammatory effects that may increase morbidity; older transfused red blood cells are a risk factor for poorer outcomes in certain groups, such as cardiac surgery and trauma patients. Allogeneic blood transfusion (ABT) in an HIV-infected patient can lead to transfusion-related immunomodulation (TRIM), with effects attributable to ABT by immunomodulatory mechanisms (e.g. cancer recurrence, postoperative infection, or virus activation and increased HIV viral loads), plus effects attributable to ABT by pro-inflammatory mechanisms (e.g. multiple-organ failure or mortality). TRIM may be mediated by allogeneic mononuclear cells; white-blood-cell-derived soluble mediators; and/or soluble HLA peptides circulating in allogeneic plasma. Blood should therefore only be transfused where unavoidable to maintain patient safety.

IDIOPATHIC CD4 T-LYMPHOCYTOPENIA (ICL)

Idiopathic CD4 T-lymphocytopenia (ICL) is a rare syndrome that appears to represent a variety of disorders not related to HIV or any known transmissible agent. It causes a generalized immunodeficiency state similar to that seen with HIV infection, with CD4 counts around 300/microlitre, but differs from HIV infection in that all lymphocyte cell lines tend to fall (low CD8 and B cells) and the lymphopenia is usually transient. In addition, immunoglobulin levels are normal or low.

There is no evidence for transmissibility but ICL has been associated with many infectious entities not related to AIDS and with non-infectious diseases, such as autoimmune disorders, malnutrition, drugs and skin disorders. About 40% of patients with ICL have developed AIDS-defining illnesses, including cryptococcal meningitis, histoplasmosis and MAC. Some persons are healthy but have had idiopathic CD4+ lymphocytopenia diagnosed by the more frequent screening for lymphocyte subsets. Finally, ICL does not progress and may even improve spontaneously.

ANTI-INTERFERON IMMUNODEFIENCY

Neutralizing anti-IFNγ autoantibodies have been found in 88% of Asian adults with multiple opportunistic infections and associated with a recently reported adult-onset immunodeficiency syndrome akin to that of advanced HIV infection.

OTHER SECONDARY IMMUNODEFICIENCIES

Worldwide, most immune defects are secondary and one of the most common causes is malnutrition. Immunosuppressive and other drugs, other iatrogenic causes and various chronic diseases are increasingly important (Table 20.16). Immunodeficiency can also be caused by hypercatabolism of immunoglobulin or excessive loss of immunoglobulins (nephrosis, severe burns, lymphangiectasia or severe diarrhoea).

AGRANULOCYTOSIS, LEUKOPENIA AND NEUTROPENIA

General aspects

Agranulocytosis is the name given to the clinical syndrome resulting from leukopenia or neutropenia. It is characterized by abnormal susceptibility to infection and oropharyngeal ulceration.

Leukopenia refers to low levels of circulating functional leukocytes, either in absolute numbers or as functionally effective cells. It is a feature of cytotoxic drug therapy and many diseases.

Neutropenia refers to low levels of circulating functional polymorphonuclear leukocytes, either in absolute numbers or as functionally effective cells. It is also a feature of cytotoxic drug therapy and many diseases. Some cases are genetically determined.

These states can develop in isolation or they can be associated with other effects of depressed bone marrow function, notably anaemia and bleeding tendencies, as in acute leukaemia and aplastic anaemia.

Table 20.16 *Some causes of white cell defects*

| Congenital defects | Bone marrow disease | Acquired defects | | | |
		Drugs	Autoimmune disorders	Viral infections	Others
See Appendix 20.1	Leukaemia, other marrow infiltrations and myelofibrosis	Antithyroid drugs	Systemic lupus erythematosus	HIV infection	Diabetes
		Cefalothin	Felty syndrome	Others	Crohn disease
		Chloramphenicol	Others		
	Aplastic anaemia (Ch. 8)	Cytotoxic agents			
		Phenothiazines			
		Phenylbutazone			
		Phenytoin			
		Sulphonamides			

Clinical features

There is often a sudden onset and fever, weakness or prostration, and sore throat are characteristic. Gingival, oral and pharyngeal ulceration with pseudomembrane formation are typical features but ulceration can affect any mucous membrane. Lymphadenopathy and sometimes rashes are also features. Later, haemorrhagic necrosis of mucous membranes and respiratory infection may go on to septicaemia as the terminal event. Purpura and bleeding as a result of thrombocytopenia are also a common early manifestation.

In neutropenia, even a minor infection can quickly become serious. Reasons for special concerns include:

- fever that is 100.4°F (38°C) or higher for more than 1 hour, or a one-time temperature of 101°F or higher
- chills and sweats
- change in cough or new cough
- sore throat or new mouth sore
- shortness of breath
- nasal congestion
- stiff neck
- burning or pain with urination
- unusual vaginal discharge or irritation
- increased urination
- redness, soreness or swelling in any area, including surgical wounds and ports
- diarrhoea
- vomiting
- pain in the abdomen or rectum
- new onset of pain
- changes in skin, urination or mental status.

General management

The diagnosis is confirmed by blood examination and bone marrow biopsy.

Treatment depends on the underlying cause. In the case of drugs, the triggering agent must be stopped and this may sometimes allow bone marrow function to recover. The main measure is to control infections. Septicaemia is a hazard, particularly in neonates and patients treated with cytotoxic chemotherapy.

Gram-negative infections should be treated with antibiotics such as ticarcillin, mecillinam or one of the third-generation cephalosporins, such as ceftazidime or cefotaxime. Complications of septicaemia include acute respiratory distress syndrome, pneumonia or shock, but endocarditis is rare. Mortality rates may be as high as 30%. Patients should therefore be nursed in laminar-airflow rooms and surgical procedures should be carried out under antibiotic cover.

Gram-positive oral microorganisms, such as viridans streptococci – mainly *Streptococcus mitis* and *S. sanguis*, are increasingly frequently implicated and may lead to serious morbidity and mortality. Predisposing factors appear to be mucositis, the use of high doses of cytosine arabinoside, and the failure to use intravenous antibiotics at the time of bacteraemia. Viridans streptococci are sensitive to many antibiotics but there is increasing resistance to penicillin after prolonged exposure. Penicillin, vancomycin and roxithromycin are usually effective in lowering the incidence of viridans streptococcus bacteraemia but co-trimoxazole is not.

If patients develop a fever, samples of blood, urine, sputum and faeces should be taken for culture lest there be septicaemia, and the patient started on systemic antibiotics; initially, piperacillin/tazobactam plus gentamicin is usually given, or ceftazidime if the patient is penicillin-allergic.

> **Box 20.3** *Management modifications for dental care in neutropenias*
>
> - Consider delaying treatment until recovery
> - Consider colony stimulating factors
> - Consider antimicrobial cover
> - Strict asepsis

Granulocyte colony-stimulating factors (filgrastim, lenograstim, molgramostim) are now available and may be of benefit.

Dental aspects

Infections and ulcers are the main oral manifestations; periodontal disease may be accelerated and minor oral infections may result in gangrenous stomatitis in severe cases. Oral infections can be painful and a potential source of metastatic infections or septicaemia, sometimes fatal. Oral infections can usually be controlled with topical or systemic antibiotic therapy or sometimes with antiseptics such as chlorhexidine. Mixed infections can often be controlled by a broad-spectrum antibiotic, such as topical tetracycline, but this should be given together with an antifungal drug because of the risk of candidal superinfection. Failure to respond to such treatment indicates that the causative bacteria are not sensitive and bacteriological investigation is required. Clindamycin may be a more suitable choice for anaerobic infections.

Dental surgical procedures should be covered with an antibiotic and particular attention should be paid to the possibility of thrombocytopenia with haemorrhagic tendencies and to the risks associated with corticosteroid treatment (Box 20.3).

CHRONIC DISEASES WITH IMMUNE DEFECTS

Diabetes mellitus is the most common chronic disease associated with immune defects, mainly defective phagocytosis. Cancers of lymphoid or haemopoietic tissues are also linked with immune defects, especially as a consequence of their treatment. Many infections, particularly viral, produce some degree of immune defect.

For dental surgical procedures, particular attention should be paid to the possibility of thrombocytopenia with haemorrhagic tendencies and to the risks associated with corticosteroid treatment.

ASPLENIC PATIENTS

General aspects

The spleen is essential for controlling the quality of erythrocytes in the circulation by sequestrating effete erythrocytes. It is also essential for the production of opsonins, thereby having an important function in antibody production and phagocytosis of microorganisms. The opsonins properdin and tuftsin protect against bacteria such as pneumococci.

Asplenia may be caused by splenectomy (e.g. after serious splenic injuries in abdominal trauma, for some haemolytic anaemias, in idiopathic thrombocytopenic purpura and in some lymphomas). The spleen becomes hypofunctional in sickle cell disease and other disorders.

Clinical features

Asplenia predisposes to infections, which usually appear within the first 2 years after splenectomy, though up to one-third may manifest at least 5 years later, and some have developed more than 20 years later. Children are ten times more likely than adults to develop sepsis. Patients may become predisposed to infection with encapsulated bacteria and other microbes. *Streptococcus pneumoniae* (pneumococcus) is

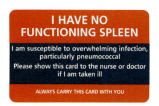

Fig. 20.12 Asplenia.

the most common pathogen and, together with *Haemophilus influenzae* and *Neisseria meningitidis* (meningococcus), accounts for 70–90% of cases. Other infections can include *Capnocytophaga canimorsus* (from dog bites), babesiosis (from tick bites), hepatitis C, tuberculosis and malaria. Infection after splenectomy only rarely emanates from the oral flora.

After splenectomy, patients may also be predisposed to develop malignant neoplasms.

General management

Patients having splenectomy should therefore be immunized 2 weeks beforehand, against pneumococci, *H. influenzae* type b and meningococcus. Post-splenectomy, for at least the first 2 years, and especially for other immunocompromised patients and for children under 16, daily penicillin or erythromycin prophylaxis is advised. Patients are usually advised to carry a warning card (Fig. 20.12).

If patients who have had splenectomy in the past become acutely unwell, they should be given benzyl penicillin promptly.

Dental aspects

There is no indication for antimicrobial prophylaxis before dental procedures unless there are other reasons and, in any event, such prophylaxis might fail.

It is important, however, to consider thrombocytopenia and corticosteroid therapy.

PRIMARY (CONGENITAL) IMMUNODEFICIENCY DISEASES

Primary immunodeficiency diseases are due to abnormalities of one or more genes that are important in immunity. There are over 100 different immune defects, mostly rare, and most can be categorized according to the main type of immune cell that is defective (Appendix 20.1, Table 20.17 and Fig. 20.13). These are also comprehensively outlined by the International Union of Immunological Societies Expert Committee on Primary Immunodeficiencies (2009).

General aspects

Some primary immune defects are inherited as autosomal recessive traits, some as X-linked recessive traits, and at least one as an autosomal dominant trait. Others are not inherited as single-gene defects. Two of the most common primary immunodeficiency diseases, selective IgA deficiency and common variable immunodeficiency, considered later, are frequently sporadic.

Immune defects are also common in some chromosomal anomalies, including Down syndrome (Ch. 28), Fanconi anaemia and Bloom syndrome, and in various rare hereditary metabolic defects.

Clinical features

Primary immune defects should be suspected if there are recurrent or persistent infections or other features.

The main features suggestive of an immune defect are summarized in Box 20.4 and features of the main primary immune defects in Appendix 20.1.

General management

Antibody deficiency is most frequently encountered and commonly presents with sinopulmonary bacterial infections. If these are the only types of infection under consideration, screening for antibody deficiency is appropriate. Other forms of primary immunodeficiency may present with distinct infectious complications with or without sinopulmonary bacterial disease. Some of these forms of infection are more or less characteristic of specific categories of immunodeficiency.

Some primary immune defects are treated by replacement of defective immunocytes or their products with immunoglobulin or bone marrow transplantation (haematopoietic cell transplantation [HCT] – which has the potential to cure primary immune deficiency syndromes that primarily affect a single lineage, e.g., lymphoid or myeloid lineage), and gene transfer is being developed to correct several defects. Immune system molecules, such as IFNγ, can be injected to improve immune function and control infection.

Infections must be treated by accepted means.

Dental aspects

The more severe congenital immune defects often cause early death, so that they are not relevant to dental care, except in so far as some are treated by bone marrow transplantation.

T-LYMPHOCYTE DEFECTS

CHRONIC MUCOCUTANEOUS CANDIDOSIS

General aspects and clinical features

Chronic mucocutaneous candidosis (CMC or CMCC) is a group of disorders in which candidosis is the main or a prominent feature. Defects of cell-mediated immunity can sometimes be detected, particularly in the more severe cases (Table 20.18).

Early-onset CMC (types 1–3) typically begins in infancy, often as persistent thrush; the candidosis is mainly or entirely oral, and immunological defects are sometimes associated.

Familial candidosis in an adult with chronic oral candidosis can escape diagnosis until middle age. Enquiry should be made as to whether siblings are affected and if there was any parental consanguinity, as the disease appears to be autosomal recessive. In familial candidosis, investigation for iron deficiency should be carried out, and treatment with iron may improve the response to antifungal drugs.

The diffuse type of CMC presents with particularly severe candidosis that can give rise to gross proliferative and disfiguring lesions of the skin (so-called granulomas), as well as widespread oral lesions. Immunological defects are frequently found and there is also susceptibility to bacterial infections of the respiratory tract or elsewhere. Even in this unusually severe form of the disease, candidosis remains superficial and does not progress to candidal septicaemia or other types of disseminated infection.

Candidosis–endocrinopathy syndrome (autoimmune polyendocrinopathy candidosis–ectodermal dystrophy [APECED]) has usually

Table 20.17 *Main primary immune defects*[a]

Main defect	Includes	Manifestations
Severe combined immune deficiencies	Includes mutations in relation to DNA ligase IV and CD3δ deficiencies	Recurrent serious infections
Predominantly T-cell deficiencies	Chronic mucocutaneous candidiasis DiGeorge anomaly	Usually present as recurrent or persistent fungal infections
Predominantly B-cell deficiencies	Autosomal recessive agammaglobulinaemia X-linked agammaglobulinaemia Common variable immunodeficiency Inducible co-stimulator (ICOS) deficiency Selective antibody deficiency (such as IgA deficiency) Hyper-IgM syndrome – includes activation-induced cytidine deaminase (AID) and uracil-DNA glycosylase (UNG) deficiencies	Usually present as recurrent bacterial infections
Other well-defined immunodeficiency syndromes in which there are non-immunological features	Includes syndromes with defects in DNA repair mechanisms. This group has included Bloom syndrome	The immune defects associated with non-immunological features, such as Wiskott–Aldrich syndrome, DNA repair defects and thymic defects, have traditionally been classified together
Diseases of immune dysregulation	Includes defects of apoptosis resulting in lymphoproliferative or autoimmune syndromes. Autoimmune lymphoproliferative syndrome (ALPS) Immune dysregulation, polyendocrinopathy, enteropathy, X-linked syndrome (IPEX) – a recessive disorder	ALPS presents with lymphadenopathy, autoimmunity and expansion of a normally infrequent population of CD4⁻ CD8⁻ T cells IPEX presents with protracted diarrhoea, ichthyosiform dermatitis, type 1 diabetes mellitus, thyroiditis and haemolytic anaemia
Defects of phagocytic cell number, function or both	Chédiak–Higashi syndrome Chronic granulomatous disease Hyperimmunoglobulinaemia E (Job) syndrome Leukocyte glucose-6-phosphate dehydrogenase deficiency Myeloperoxidase deficiency Leukocyte adhesion defects – include LAD types 1–3, Rac2 deficiency, β-actin deficiency and localized juvenile periodontitis Papillon–Lefèvre syndrome	Range from defects of wound healing or localized infections or periodontitis, to severe clinical phenotypes requiring bone marrow transplantation
Defects of innate immunity relating to monocyte and dendritic cell functions	Defects in nuclear factor kappa B or other signals	Various
Autoinflammatory disorders	Periodic fever, aphthous stomatitis, pharyngitis, adenitis (PFAPA) syndrome) – not inherited Hereditary conditions, including: 1. Familial Mediterranean fever (FMF) 2. Mevalonate kinase deficiencies (including hyperimmunoglobulinaemia D and periodic fever syndrome [HIDS] and mevalonate aciduria) 3. Tumour necrosis factor receptor-associated periodic syndrome (TRAPS) 4. Pyogenic sterile arthritis, pyoderma gangrenosum, acne (PAPA) 5. Chronic recurrent multifocal osteomyelitis (CRMO) 6. Blau syndrome 7. Cryopyrin-associated periodic syndromes (CAPS)	The periodic fevers
Complement deficiencies	Complement component 1 (C1) inhibitor deficiency (hereditary angioedema) C3 deficiency C6 deficiency C7 deficiency C8 deficiency New complement-related deficiencies – mannose-binding protein (MBP) deficiency and MBP-associated serine protease 2 (MASP2) deficiency	Various

[a]For fine detail, see Notarangelo L, et al. 2004.

mild but persistent candidosis as the initial feature; endocrine disorders appear but often not until 10 or 15 years later. Occasionally, this sequence is reversed. There is no evidence that candidosis causes the endocrine disorders or vice versa. Hypoparathyroidism or Addison disease, or both, is the most commonly associated endocrinopathy. The endocrine disorders in candidosis–endocrinopathy syndrome are associated with multiple organ-specific autoantibodies both in patients and in unaffected relatives. Patients may long appear to be quite well, apart from chronic oral candidosis. If, therefore, a patient, particularly a child or adolescent with chronic oral candidosis, has a family history of any of the associated disorders, and autoantibodies (particularly to glandular tissues) are found, endocrine disease will probably develop in the future.

Candidosis–thymoma syndrome presents with late-onset CMC, when evidence of impaired cell-mediated immunity, particularly to

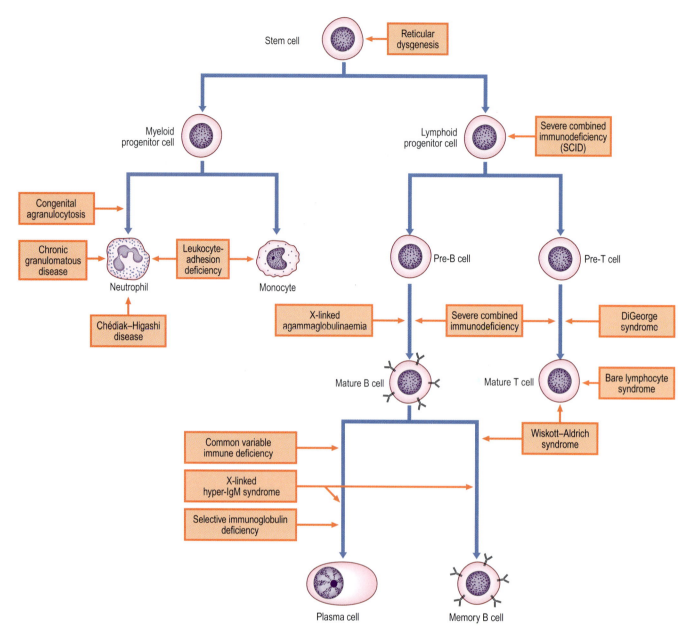

Fig. 20.13 Primary immune defects.

Table 20.18 *Chronic mucocutaneous candidosis syndromes*

Type	Clinical features
1. Familial	Persistent oral candidosis
	Often iron deficiency
2. Diffuse (candida granuloma)	Severe chronic candidosis
	Susceptibility to bacterial infections
3. Candidosis–endocrinopathy syndrome (polyendocrinopathy syndrome)	Mild chronic oral candidosis
	Hypoparathyroidism
	Hypoadrenocorticism
4. Candidosis–thymoma syndrome	Chronic oral candidosis
	Myasthenia gravis
	Haematological disorders
5. Chronic mucocutaneous candidosis in HIV disease or hyperimmunoglobulin E syndrome	Recurrent candidosis

Candida albicans, may be found. In such a case, investigation for a thymoma should be carried out, as early excision may improve the prognosis.

General management

Candidosis is persistent and responds poorly to topical treatment with nystatin or amphotericin, but topical antifungal agents, such as miconazole, or systemic ketoconazole, fluconazole, itraconazole or voriconazole, may be helpful.

DIGEORGE ANOMALY

The coincidental association between chronic candidosis and hypoparathyroidism (type I polyendocrinopathy syndrome), also seen in the DiGeorge syndrome (CATCH 22), has given rise to the myth that hypoparathyroidism predisposes to candidosis. However, treatment of hypoparathyroidism has no effect on candidosis, and hypoparathyroidism from any other cause is not associated with candidosis. Branchial arch defects in DiGeorge syndrome affect both thymus (and thymocytes) and parathyroids.

ANTIBODY DEFICIENCY SYNDROMES

Hypoimmunoglobulinaemia can have several causes and can also be caused by hypercatabolism, or excessive loss, of immunoglobulins (Table 20.19).

COMMON VARIABLE IMMUNODEFICIENCY

General aspects

Also known as adult-onset agammaglobulinaemia, late-onset hypogammaglobulinaemia or acquired agammaglobulinaemia, common variable immunodeficiency (CVID) is relatively common. Serum IgG is low with a marked decrease in IgM or IgA. The serum IgM concentration is normal in about half of the patients. Most patients have normal B-cell numbers, though some do have low or absent B cells. Abnormalities in T-cell numbers or function are common.

Clinical features

Symptoms are mainly frequent bacterial infections of ears, sinuses, bronchi and lungs. Viral, fungal and parasitic infections, as well as bacterial ones, may be problematic. Pneumonias are common and approximately 50% of patients have autoimmune disease. Gastrointestinal disease, including chronic diarrhoea, affects as many as 30% and there is a high incidence of inflammatory bowel disease, gluten-sensitive enteropathy and nodular lymphoid hyperplasia. *Giardia lamblia* and bacterial overgrowth of the small bowel are the most frequently identified pathogens. Haematological abnormalities may include autoimmune haemolytic anaemia, immune thrombocytopenia, leukopenia and pernicious anaemia. Arthralgia in the knee, ankle, elbow or wrist is common, and rheumatoid arthritis and other collagen vascular diseases are also more common than expected. Splenomegaly and lymphadenopathy may be seen. Patients are usually recognized to be immunodeficient by the second, third or fourth decade of life.

General management

Diagnosis is confirmed by finding low serum IgG, IgA and possibly IgM. B cells still produce antibodies after a common vaccination such as tetanus. Antibody levels can be normalized by intravenous immunoglobulin every 3–4 weeks. Bacterial infections are treated with antibiotics. Physical therapy and daily postural drainage may help clear respiratory infections.

SELECTIVE IgA DEFICIENCY

General aspects

Selective IgA deficiency is the most common congenital immunodeficiency, affecting 1 in 600 in the normal population. IgA is deficient in both serum and secretions.

Table 20.19 *Differential diagnosis of hypogammoglobulinaemia*

Genetic disorders	Drug-induced	Infections	Malignancy	Immunoglobulin loss or degradation
Ataxia telangiectasia	Antimalarials	Congenital rubella or cytomegalovirus or *Toxoplasma gondii*	Chronic lymphocytic leukaemia	Lymphangiectasia
				Nephrosis
Autosomal severe combined immunodeficiency (SCID)	Captopril	HIV	Immunodeficiency with thymoma	Severe burns
	Carbamazepine	Epstein–Barr virus	Non-Hodgkin lymphoma	Severe diarrhoea
	Glucocorticoids		B-cell malignancy	
	Fenclofenac			
Hyper immunoglobulin M (IgM) immunodeficiency	Gold salts			
	Penicillamine			
	Phenytoin			
Transcobalamin II deficiency and hypogammaglobulinaemia	Sulfasalazine			
X-linked agammaglobulinaemia				
X-linked lymphoproliferative disorder				
X-linked SCID				
Chromosome 18q– syndrome				
Monosomy 22				
Trisomy 8				
Trisomy 21				

Clinical features

Many individuals with IgA deficiency are asymptomatic if the levels of other classes of immunoglobulin are normal or raised. Others have persistent or recurrent infections and some develop CVID over time. Some have an increased incidence of upper respiratory tract infections, allergies and autoimmune disease but a normal IgG antibody response to vaccination.

Where IgA deficiency is associated with deficiency of IgG2, there is a definite predisposition to recurrent bacterial or viral respiratory infections, and small intestine infections – usually with *Giardia lamblia* (a protozoon causing diarrhoea and malabsorption, although the disease is often unrecognized because the symptoms are chronic and indolent). Atopic disease, coeliac disease, lupus erythematosus, rheumatoid arthritis and Sjögren syndrome are abnormally frequent.

General management

IgA replacement is difficult since autoantibodies frequently form against IgA when blood transfusions or immunoglobulins are given, and can sometimes cause anaphylactic reactions.

Bacterial infections should be treated with antibiotics. Giardiasis needs treatment with metronidazole or quinacrine hydrochloride.

Dental aspects

Despite the fact that IgA is the main salivary antibody, reported effects of IgA deficiency on dental caries and other oral disease are conflicting. Part of the reason for this apparently anomalous situation is that other immunoglobulins may be secreted in saliva. IgA deficiency may be associated occasionally with oral ulcers and herpes labialis.

X-LINKED AGAMMAGLOBULINAEMIA (BRUTON SYNDROME)

Patients with X-linked agammaglobulinaemia (XLA) are male with low CD19+ B cells and low serum IgG, IgM and IgA, no isohaemagglutinins and/or a poor response to vaccines. They develop recurrent bacterial infections in the first 5 years of life, particularly otitis, sinusitis and pneumonia. The most common organisms are *Streptococcus pneumoniae* and *Haemophilus influenzae*. Approximately 20% of patients present with a dramatic, overwhelming infection, often also with neutropenia. Another 10–15% have higher concentrations of serum immunoglobulin than expected or are not recognized to have immunodeficiency until after 5 years of age.

B- AND T-LYMPHOCYTE DEFECTS

ATAXIA TELANGIECTASIA

Ataxia telangiectasia (AT) is progressive cerebellar ataxia with walking difficulty presenting at the end of the first year of life; by the teenage years, most patients are wheelchair-bound. Ocular or facial telangiectasia is usually seen at 4–8 years of life. Serum IgA is low and alpha-fetoprotein high. Many patients have recurrent respiratory infections. Radiation-induced chromosomal breakages may culminate in leukaemia or lymphomas.

SEVERE COMBINED IMMUNODEFICIENCY (SCID)

Patients with SCID have low CD3+ T cells. They usually fail to thrive, and develop persistent diarrhoea, respiratory infections and/or thrush in the first 7 months of life. *Pneumocystis* pneumonia, significant bacterial infections and disseminated bacille Calmette-Guérin (BCG) infection are common. SCID is fatal in the first 2 years of life, unless the patient is treated with extremely restrictive isolation, haemopoietic stem cell transplant, or therapy that replaces the abnormal gene or gene product. Transplantation in early life offers a survival now approaching 90%.

WISKOTT–ALDRICH SYNDROME

Wiskott–Aldrich syndrome (WAS) presents in males with congenital thrombocytopenia, small platelets and abnormal antibody response to polysaccharide antigens. Many patients have increased IgE and IgA, with low IgM, and T-cell numbers and function decline with age. The main features include eczema, recurrent bacterial or viral infections, autoimmune diseases (vasculitis, haemolytic anaemia and glomerulonephritis) and lymphoma, leukaemia or brain tumour. Otitis and sinusitis, and infections due to herpes simplex virus and EBV are particularly troublesome.

X-LINKED LYMPHOPROLIFERATIVE SYNDROME

Males with X-linked lymphoproliferative syndrome (XLP) are usually asymptomatic until they develop EBV infection, which may cause fulminant hepatitis (60% of patients), particularly in young children. Lymphoma/Hodgkin disease, immunodeficiency, aplastic anaemia or lymphohistiocytic disorders may be fatal in childhood. Less common manifestations include EBV-associated haemophagocytic syndrome and vasculitis.

PHAGOCYTE DEFECTS

CHÉDIAK–HIGASHI SYNDROME

Chédiak–Higashi syndrome (CHS) is caused by impaired polymorphonuclear leukocyte function related to abnormal microtubular assembly. It is a rare autosomal recessive disorder that manifests with: hypopigmentation of skin, eyes and hair; bleeding tendency and easy bruisability; recurrent infections; abnormal natural killer (NK) cell function; and peripheral neuropathy. Most patients who do not undergo bone marrow transplantation die from a lymphoproliferative syndrome.

CHRONIC GRANULOMATOUS DISEASE

Patients with the X-linked form of chronic granulomatous disease (CGD; 60–70%) usually present earlier and with more severe disease than patients with autosomal recessive forms. Abnormal respiratory burst in activated neutrophils characterizes CGD. Clinically, there are deep-seated infections (liver, perirectal or lung abscess; lymphadenitis; or osteomyelitis) due to catalase-positive organisms such as staphylococci, *Serratia marcescens*, *Candida* or *Aspergillus*; diffuse granulomas in the respiratory, gastrointestinal or urogenital tract; failure to thrive; and hepatosplenomegaly or lymphadenopathy.

HYPERIMMUNOGLOBULINAEMIA E SYNDROME (JOB SYNDROME; BUCKLEY SYNDROME)

Patients with hyperimmunoglobulinaemia E syndrome (HIES) appear to have T-cell abnormalities, including a decrease in IFNγ and an increase in IL-4, and an inadequate inflammatory response that may delay recognition of infections. HIES is characterized by eczema, recurrent skin abscesses, cystic lung infections (primarily *Staphylococcus aureus* and *Candida* species [chronic mucocutaneous candidosis]), eosinophilia and raised IgE. Non-immunological features include multiple bone fractures, joint hyperextensibility and other skeletal abnormalities, coarse facial features, retained primary teeth, palatal keratosis or ridging, and tongue-fissuring.

LEUKOCYTE ADHESION DEFICIENCY (LAD)

Decreased expression of CD18 on neutrophils with mutation in the beta2-integrin gene leads to recurrent or persistent bacterial or fungal infections, leukocytosis, and delayed separation of the umbilical cord and/or defective wound-healing. Infections with *Staphylococcus*, Gram-negative enteric bacteria and fungi are particularly troublesome. Periodontitis is a common finding. In the severe form of LAD, with no CD18 expression on neutrophils, the patient usually succumbs without bone marrow transplantation. In the moderate form, patients can survive to adulthood.

LEUKOCYTE GLUCOSE-6-PHOSPHATE DEHYDROGENASE DEFICIENCY

Glucose-6-phosphate dehydrogenase (G6PD) is one of the pentose phosphate pathway enzymes, involved in maintaining adequate coenzyme nicotinamide–adenine dinucleotide phosphate (NADPH) in cells. G6PD deficiency can lead to meningitis, septicaemia or osteomyelitis.

MYELOPEROXIDASE DEFICIENCY

Myeloperoxidase (MPO) is an enzyme in the neutrophil azurophilic granules and in lysosomes of monocytes, which has a major role in killing some bacteria (*Staphylococcus aureus*, *Serratia* species and *Escherichia coli*), fungi, parasites, protozoa, viruses and tumour cells. Most individuals with partial or total MPO deficiency have no increased frequency of infections but recurrent infections may be seen, especially where there is coexistent diabetes.

COMPLEMENT DEFECTS

Defects in complement components tend to be associated with autoimmune disease, especially lupus erythematosus, and increased susceptibility to meningococcal and gonococcal infections.

HEREDITARY ANGIOEDEMA (C1 ESTERASE INHIBITOR DEFICIENCY)

General aspects

Hereditary angioedema (HANE) is caused by continued complement activation resulting from a mainly genetically determined deficiency of an inhibitor of the enzyme C1 esterase (Fig. 20.14); thus C4 is consumed and its plasma level falls. The level of C3 is usually normal. Complement activation is associated with release of kinin-like substances, such as bradykinin, which are the probable cause of the sudden increase in capillary permeability.

Despite its hereditary nature, usually as an autosomal dominant trait, the disease may not present until later childhood or adolescence, and nearly 20% of cases are caused by spontaneous mutation. Rare cases are acquired.

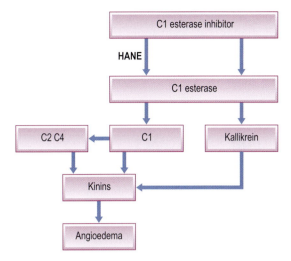

Fig. 20.14 Hereditary angioedema (HANE).

Clinical features

Blunt injury is the most consistent precipitating event and the trauma of dental treatment is a potent trigger of attacks. Some attacks follow emotional stress.

Hereditary angioedema mimics allergic angioedema, though it causes a more severe reaction. Abdominal pain, nausea or vomiting, diarrhoea, rashes and peripheral oedema sometimes herald an attack. Oedema typically affects the mouth, face and neck region, can persist for up to 4 days and may involve the airway. The extremities and gastrointestinal tract may be involved.

The mortality may be as high as 30% in some families but the disease is compatible with prolonged survival if emergencies are effectively treated.

General management

Initial screening should include a C4 level, which will be depressed during and between attacks. If a C4 level is found to be low or clinical suspicion of hereditary or acquired angioedema is high, testing of C1-inhibitor (INH) level and function is warranted. C4 levels are often low due to improper handling; therefore, repeating a C4 level when further testing is performed is also advisable. In types 1 and 2 HANE, as well as acquired angioedema, the C1 INH level will be low, typically less than 30% of normal (see Table 20.17). A C1q level will differentiate these acquired and hereditary angioedema, as it will only be low in acquired angioedema but not type 1 HANE. In 85% of cases, the C1 esterase levels are low (type 1 HANE); in 15% this inhibitor is present but dysfunctional (type 2 HANE). In both types the C4 level falls. C1 esterase inhibitor concentrates are available for replacement of the missing factor. Type 3 HANE is related to pregnancy and C1 inhibitor levels are usually normal but bradykinin levels high.

Management of HANE may include both short-term and long-term prophylaxis, as well as treatment of acute episodes. Plasma or plasminogen inhibitors, such as tranexamic acid, can mitigate attacks and may be life-saving. The androgenic steroids, danazol and stanozolol, raise plasma C1 esterase inhibitor levels to normal. Stanozolol needs to be given for 5 days to be effective and should not be used during pregnancy. Oligomenorrhoea may be induced in women and there may be acne, hirsutism, hypercalcaemia or headache. Androgens may cause virilization, weight gain and hypertension; antifibrinolytic agents have been reported to cause muscle necrosis, hypotension and menorrhagia. Plasma-derived C1 INH concentrates have good efficacy and tolerability, adverse effects (headache and fever) are rare, and the primary limitation is cost. Icatibant (a bradykinin antagonist) can be helpful. Ecallantide, a plasma kallikrein inhibitor given subcutaneously, is an efficacious alternative to C1 INH therapy. Adverse effects are mild and similar to C1 INH concentrate but there is a risk of anaphylaxis.

MUCOCILIARY SYNDROMES

Cilia in the respiratory tract normally clear mucus and act as a defence mechanism. If they are impaired, as in some genetic and acquired disorders, this may lead to chronic sinusitis or other respiratory infections. Examples are Kartagener syndrome (mucociliary disease and dextrocardia) and intolerance of NSAIDs in the Fernand–Widal syndrome.

EMERGING IMMUNE DEFECTS

Emerging primary immune defects are increasingly recognised, and these include:

- Herpes simplex encephalitis may arise as a result of impaired intrinsic signalling in neurons and oligodendrocytes from a variety of gene mutations affecting innate immunity (which include; unc-93 homolog B1 (*UNC93B1*), TIR-domain-containing adaptor protein inducing IFNβ (*TRIF*), TNF receptor-associated factor 3 (*TRAF3*), TANK-binding kinase 1 (*TBK1*) and Toll-like receptor 3 [*TLR3*]).
- Defects in the innate generation of dendritic cells (DCs), monocytes, neutrophils, B lymphocytes and natural killer (NK) cells, lead to viral, fungal and mycobacterial infections as well as myelodysplasia and are seen in mutations of the GATA-binding protein 2 (*GATA2*) gene.
- The development and immune activation of DCs and other myeloid cells, are impaired by interferon-regulatory factor 8 (*IRF8*) mutations.
- Mutations affecting interleukin-10 (IL-10)-mediated signalling in myeloid cells and other haematopoietic cells seems to be essential to prevent the early onset of colitis.
- Mast cells are susceptible to spontaneous activation and degranulation in cold temperatures where mutations affect phospholipase Cγ2 (PLCG2).
- Mutations in PIK3CD gene lead to PASLI (p110 delta activating mutation causing senescent T cells, lymphadenopathy, and immunodeficiency) with impaired T and B cell immune responses, predisposing patients to chronic respiratory bacterial infections, Epstein-Barr virus infection and lymphoma. mTOR, is excessively activated by p110 delta in PASLI patients.

KEY WEBSITES

(Accessed 29 May 2013)
Centers for Disease Control and Prevention. <http://www.cdc.gov/osels/ph_surveillance/nndss/casedef/aids2008.htm>.
Great Ormond Street Hospital for Children NHS Foundation Trust. <http://www.gosh.nhs.uk/medical-conditions/>.
Immune Deficiency Foundation: About primary immunodeficiency diseases, with a link to Specific disease types. <http://primaryimmune.org/about-primary-immunodeficiency-diseases>.
NHS Choices. <http://www.nhs.uk/conditions/HIV/Pages/Introduction.aspx>.

USEFUL WEBSITES

(Accessed 29 May 2013)
AIDSPortal. <http://www.aidsportal.org/>.
Centers for Disease Control and Prevention. <http://www.cdc.gov/hiv/default.htm>.
Crown Prosecution Service. <http://www.cps.gov.uk/legal/h_to_k/intentional_or_reckless_sexual_transmission_of_infection_guidance/>.
European Society for Immunodeficiencies. <http://www.esid.org>.
Hivatis.org. <http://www.hivatis.org>.
HIVdent. <http://www.hivdent.org>.

FURTHER READING

Achenbach, C.J., et al. 2012. Paradoxical immune reconstitution inflammatory syndrome in HIV-infected patients treated with combination antiretroviral therapy after AIDS-defining opportunistic infection. Clin. Infect. Dis. 54 (3), 424.
Achong, R.M., et al. 2006. Implants in HIV-positive patients: 3 case reports. J. Oral Maxillofac. Surg. 64 (8), 1199.
Bohjanen, P.R., Boulware, D.R., 2007. Immune reconstitution inflammatory syndrome Chapter 18. In: Volberding, P. (Ed.), Global HIV/AIDS medicine. Elsevier, Philadelphia, pp. 193.
Bonilla, F.A., et al. 2005. Practice parameter for the diagnosis and management of primary immunodeficiency. Ann. Allergy Asthma Immunol. 94 (5 Suppl 1), S1.
Browne, S.K., et al. 2012. Adult-onset immunodeficiency in Thailand and Taiwan. N. Engl. J. Med. 367, 725.
Centers for Disease Control and Prevention, 2007. Notice to readers: updated information regarding antiretroviral agents used as HIV postexposure prophylaxis for occupational HIV exposures. MMWR 56 (49), 1291.
Chapel, H.M., 2003. IUIS report on immunodeficiency disease: an update. Clin. Exp. Immunol. 132, 9.
Chapel, H.M., 2005. Primary immune deficiencies – improving our understanding of their role in immunological disease. Clin. Exp. Immunol. 139, 11.
Collaborative Group for HIV and STI Surveillance, 2006. A complex picture: HIV and other sexually transmitted infections in the United Kingdom. Health Protection Agency, Centre for Infections, London.
Dios, D., et al. 2000. Changing prevalence of human immunodeficiency virus-associated oral lesions. Oral Surg. Oral Med. Oral Pathol. Oral Radiol. Endod. 90, 403.
Dios, P.D., Scully, C., 2002. Adverse effects of antiretroviral therapies: focus on orofacial effects. Expert Opin. Drug Safety 1, 304.
Freeman, A.F., et al. 2009. Hyper IgE (Job's) syndrome: a primary immune deficiency with oral manifestations. Oral Dis. 15, 2.
Fukui, N., et al. 2000. Oral findings in DiGeorge syndrome: clinical features and histologic study of primary teeth. Oral Surg. Oral Med. Oral Pathol. Oral Radiol. Endod. 89, 208.
HPA Centre for Infection. Testing times – HIV and other sexually transmitted infection in the United Kingdom 2007. London, 2007, UK Collaborative Group for HIV and STI Surveillance.
International Union of Immunological Societies Expert Committee on Primary Immunodeficiencies, 2009. Primary immunodeficiencies: 2009 update. J. Allergy Clin. Immunol. 124, 1161.
Isgrò, A., et al. 2005. Idiopathic CD4+ lymphocytopenia may be due to decreased bone marrow clonogenic capability. Int. Arch. Allergy Immunol. 136, 379.
Lucas, C.L., et al., 2014. Dominant-activating germline mutations in the gene encoding the PI(3)K catalytic subunit p110δ result in T cell senescence and human immunodeficiency. Nat. Immunol. 15 (1), 88–97. doi: 10.1038/ni.2771. Epub 2013 Oct 28. PubMed PMID: 24165795.
Malaspina, A., et al. 2007. Idiopathic CD4+ T lymphocytopenia is associated with increases in immature/transitional B cells and serum levels of IL-7. Blood 109, 2086.
Markowitz, M., et al. 2005. Infection with multi-drug resistant dual-tropic HIV-1 and rapid progression to AIDS: a case report. Lancet 365, 1031.
Mazer, B., et al. 2005. Practice parameter for the diagnosis and management of primary immunodeficiency. Ann. Allergy Asthma Immunol. 94 (5 Suppl 1), S1.
Milner, JD., Holland, SM., 2013. The cup runneth over: lessons from the ever-expanding pool of primary immunodeficiency diseases. Nat. Rev. Immunol. 13, 635–648.
Notarangelo, L., et al. 2004. Primary immunodeficiency diseases: an update. J. Allergy Clin. Immunol. 114, 677.
Parisi, E., Glick, M., 2003. Immune suppression and considerations for dental care. Dent. Clin. N. Am. 47, 709.
Patel, A.S., Glick, M., 2003. Oral manifestations associated with HIV infection: evaluation, assessment, and significance. Gen. Dent. 51, 153.
Patton, L.L., et al. 2002. A systematic review of complication risks for HIV-positive patients undergoing invasive dental procedures. J. Am. Dent. Assoc. 133, 195.
Price, P., et al. 2002. Polymorphisms in cytokine genes define subpopulations of HIV-1 patients who experienced immune restoration diseases. AIDS 16, 2043.
Satterthwaite, A.B., White, O.N., 2000. The role of Bruton's tyrosine kinase in B-cell development and function: a genetic perspective. Immunol. Rev. 175, 120.

Saurborn, D., Boiselle, P.M., 2003. Recognizing the radiologic signs of mycobacterial infections: pleural effusion may be the only sign in some patients. J. Res. Dis. 24, 454.

Scully, C., Chaudhry, S., 2009. Aspects of human disease 30. HIV infection and AIDS. Dent. Update. 36, 125.

Scully, C., Dios, P.D., 2001. HIV topic update: orofacial effects of antiretroviral therapies. Oral Dis. 7, 205.

Scully, C., et al. 2008. Autoinflammatory syndromes and oral health. Oral Dis. 14, 690.

Scully, C., et al. 2002. Complications in HIV-infected and non-HIV-infected hemophiliacs and other patients after oral surgery. Int. J. Oral Maxillofac. Surg. 31, 634.

Scully, C., et al. 2007. Special care in dentistry: handbook of oral healthcare. Churchill Livingstone/Elsevier, Edinburgh.

Shelburne, S.A., et al. 2005. Incidence and risk factors for immune reconstitution inflammatory syndrome during highly active antiretroviral therapy. AIDS 19, 399.

Shetty, K., Achong, R., 2005. Dental implants in the HIV-positive patient – case report and review of the literature. Gen. Dent. 53, 434. quiz 438, 446.

Stevenson, G.C., et al. 2007. Short-term success of osseointegrated dental implants in HIV-positive individuals: a prospective study. J. Contemp. Dent. Pract. 8, 1.

Strietzel, F.P., et al. 2006. Implant-prosthetic treatment in HIV-infected patients receiving highly active antiretroviral therapy: report of cases. Int. J. Oral Maxillofac. Implants. 21, 951.

Vinuesa, C.G., Goodnow, C.C., 2004. Illuminating autoimmune regulators through controlled variation of the mouse genome sequence. Immunity 20, 669.

Walker B.D. Immune reconstitution and immunotherapy in HIV infection. Medscape Clin. Update. <www.medscape.com/viewprogram/2435_pnt>. 2003.

Wilson S. HIV and anaesthesia. Update in anaesthesia. <www.anaesthesiologists.org>

Yin, M.T., et al. 2007. Epidemiology, pathogenesis, and management of human immunodeficiency virus infection in patients with periodontal disease. Periodontol 2000 44, 55.

APPENDIX 20.1 MAIN FEATURES OF MAJOR PRIMARY (GENETICALLY DETERMINED) IMMUNODEFICIENCY DISORDERS

Type or name of syndrome	Immunological phenomena	Clinical effects	Possible orofacial features
Predominantly B-cell defects			
Transient hypogammaglobulinaemia of infancy	Hypogammaglobulinaemia in early childhood only	Eczema, food allergies	NR
X-linked infantile hypogammaglobulinaemia (XLA; Bruton syndrome)	Immunoglobulins of all classes deficient or absent	Recurrent pyogenic infections	Sinusitis, absent tonsils, cervical lymph node enlargement, ulcers
		Infants develop pus-producing infections of the inner ear and lungs	
		Hepatitis, central nervous system (CNS) viral infections	
X-linked hyper-immunoglobulin M (IgM) syndrome	IgA, IgG and IgE low	Recurring upper and lower respiratory infections in first year of life. Enlarged liver and spleen, chronic diarrhoea, and increased risk of unusual or opportunistic infections and non-Hodgkin lymphoma	Enlarged tonsils
		Recurrent bacterial infections in the first 5 years of life	Over 50% of patients have chronic or intermittent neutropenia, often associated with oral ulcers
		Pneumocystis carinii infection in the first year of life	
		Neutropenia	
		Cryptosporidium-related diarrhoea. *Cryptosporidium* infection may lead to severe bile duct disease and hepatic cancer	
		Sclerosing cholangitis	
		Parvovirus-induced aplastic anaemia	
Non–X-linked hyper-IgM syndrome	IgA and IgE low	Neutropenia, thrombocytopenia, liver disease	Mouth ulcers
Nijmegen breakage syndrome	Serum IgG and IgA more than 2 SD below normal for age	Increased radiation-induced chromosomal breakage on chromosome 8q21	Microcephaly
		Additional features are café-au-lait spots, vitiligo, and clinodactyly and syndactyly	Typical facial appearance (receding forehead, prominent midface with long nose and long philtrum and a receding mandible)
		More than 50% develop B- or T-origin lymphomas before 18 y of age	
		Many have recurrent bacterial and viral respiratory infections (56%) associated with antibody deficiencies	
WHIM (warts, hypogammaglobulinaemia, infections, myelokathexis) syndrome	Chronic neutropenia (absolute neutrophil count <500/L)	Male or female patient	Facial warts
	Myelokathexis (retention of senescent neutrophils in the bone marrow)		
	Chronic lymphopenia (absolute lymphocyte count <1500/L)	Autosomal dominant disorder	
	Serum IgG at or below the normal range for age	Most patients present with recurrent infections at less than 3 y of age	
		Warts generally begin to appear after 5 y of age and some patients have hundreds of warts	
	Hypogammaglobulinaemia may be present, but the serum immunoglobulin concentrations do not correlate with the number of B cells	Increased susceptibility to infection from members of the herpesvirus family can be seen	
		Most patients develop a normal neutrophil count during infection	

(Continued)

Type or name of syndrome	Immunological phenomena	Clinical effects	Possible orofacial features
Common variable immunodeficiency	Variable deficiency of different immunoglobulins	Respiratory infections starting in childhood	Sinusitis, hyperplastic tonsils, cervical lymph node enlargement, oral ulceration
Wiskott–Aldrich syndrome	Deficiency mainly of IgM and IgA	Recurrent infections, especially by pneumococci, meningococci and *Haemophilus influenzae*, thrombocytopenia, eczema	Purpura, candidosis, herpetic infections
		Severe infections with herpesviruses and *Pneumocystis jiroveci (carinii)*	
	IgE may be increased	High incidence of malignancies, particularly lymphomas and autoimmune diseases	
Hypogammaglobulinaemia after intrauterine viral infections (e.g. rubella)	Deficiency usually of only one Ig class (e.g. IgA)	Occasionally increased susceptibility to infection	Enamel hypoplasia
IgA deficiency	Variable. Deficient IgA and sometimes IgE or IgG_2	Recurrent respiratory infections or atopic allergy or autoimmune disease or normal health	Tonsillar hyperplasia, possibly oral ulceration, herpetic infections
IgG_2 subclass deficiency	Defective humoral immunity	Recurrent respiratory infections	Sinusitis
T- and B-cell defects			
Congenital thymic aplasia (DiGeorge syndrome)	Deletion of chromosome 22q11.2	Viral and fungal infections starting in infancy	Dysmorphic facies or palatal abnormalities, bifid uvula
	Defective cell-mediated immunity; reduced numbers of CD3+ T cells ($<500/mm^3$). Ig production also impaired	Cardiovascular defects: conotruncal cardiac defect (truncus arteriosus, tetralogy of Fallot, interrupted aortic arch or aberrant right subclavian)	Candidosis, herpetic infection
		Hypoparathyroidism with hypocalcaemia of >3 weeks' duration	
		The severity of the T-cell defect varies greatly;	
		in many patients the immunodeficiency resolves in the first few years of life	
		Autoimmune disorders may be seen in older patients	
Major histocompatibility complex (MHC) class II deficiency (base lymphocyte syndrome)	Subtype of severe combined immunodeficiency (SCID)	Seen most often in patients from around the Mediterranean Sea; results in a clinical phenotype similar to SCID with severe infections and protracted diarrhoea in the first 6 months of life	Candidosis
		Pseudomonas, cytomegalovirus and *Cryptosporidium* infections are common	
		Hepatic abnormalities, particularly sclerosing cholangitis, are frequent	
Severe combined immunodeficiency (SCID)	Defective cell-mediated immunity and hypogammaglobulinaemia	Lack of resistance to all types of infection	Candidosis, herpetic infections
	Two types:	In the first 3 months of life, babies get serious or life-threatening infections, especially pneumonia, meningitis and sepsis	Oral ulceration
	Patients lack adenosine deaminase (ADA)	Common infections like chickenpox, measles or herpes can overwhelm them	
	Patients lack the ability to produce the IL-2 receptor gamma chain, a molecule that T cells need to communicate with B cells	Chronic skin infections, candidosis, chronic hepatitis, diarrhoea and blood disorders	
X-linked SCID	Defective cell-mediated immunity and hypogammaglobulinaemia	Onset of failure to thrive before 1 y of age, serum IgG and IgA more than 2 SD below normal for age	Thrush
		Persistent or recurrent diarrhoea, urinary tract infection or thrush	
		Many patients have normal serum IgM	
		Some show signs of graft-versus-host disease	
Deficiencies of MHC class II CD3, ZAP-70 or TAP-2	Decreased CD4 cells, CD8 cells	Recurrent infections	NR
Immunodeficiency with ataxia telangiectasia	Defective cell-mediated immunity	Respiratory infections starting in infancy	Sinusitis, oral ulceration
	Ig production impaired	Ataxia telangiectasia, learning impairment	
Late-onset immunodeficiency	Defective cell-mediated or hypogammaglobulinaemia	Susceptibility to various infections starting late in life	Chronic candidosis

(Continued)

Type or name of syndrome	Immunological phenomena	Clinical effects	Possible orofacial features
Complement deficiencies			
C1, C2 or C4 deficiencies	Defects in complement pathways	Autoimmune disease, especially lupus erythematosus	Possibly oral lesions of lupus erythematosus
C1, C3 or C5 deficiencies	Defects in complement pathways	Increased susceptibility to meningococcal and gonococcal infections	NR
C1 esterase inhibitor deficiency	Abnormal complement activation	Swelling of face and neck Airway obstruction	Swellings
Granulocyte defects			
Interferon-gamma receptor (IFNGR) deficiency	Granulocytes have protein that rejects interferon	Infections with mycobacteria and *Salmonella*	NR
Cyclical neutropenia	Depression of neutrophil count at 21-day intervals	Periodic infections – especially bacterial	Recurrent oral ulceration Periodontitis
Chronic granulomatous disease	Leukocyte killing defect	Catalase-positive bacterial infections, *Escherichia coli*, *Staphylococcus aureus*, *Pseudomonas*, *Serratia* and *Aspergillus* Lymph node abscesses	Cervical lymphadenopathy and suppuration Enamel hypoplasia
Myeloperoxidase deficiency	Leukocyte killing defect	Candidosis	Candidosis
Chédiak–Higashi syndrome	Leukocyte defect of chemotaxis and phagocytosis	Albinism, recurrent infections, hepatosplenomegaly, thrombocytopenia	Cervical lymph node enlargement, oral ulceration, periodontitis
Leukocyte adhesion defect (LAD) 1	Adhesion defect (deficiency of beta2-integrin; also called CD18, Mac1 or p150, 95)	Umbilical cord does not detach Severe infections of soft tissue Eroding skin sores without pus Infections of the gastrointestinal tract Wounds that heal slowly and may leave scars Poor prognosis	Periodontitis
LAD 2	Adhesion defect (failure to convert mannose to fucose)	Recurrent infection	Periodontitis
Papillon–Lefèvre syndrome	Chemotactic defect	Recurrent infection	Periodontitis
Job syndrome	HIE with neutrophil defects	Recurrent infection by *Staphylococcus aureus*	Asymmetry or uneven facial features
Hyperimmunoglobulinaemia E (HIE)	In about half of the cases, linked to chromosome 4. In most, it is autosomal dominant	HIE patients may also have scoliosis (curvature of the spine), weak bones and recurrent bone fractures, strokes or other brain problems, severe itching and inflamed skin	Prominent forehead Deep-set eyes Broad nasal bridge Wide, fleshy nasal tip Protruding lower jaw Periodontitis Ulcers
Glycogen storage disease b	Leukopenia and defect of chemotaxis	Recurrent infection	Periodontitis Ulcers
Schwachman syndrome (lazy leukocyte syndrome)	Leukocyte defect of chemotaxis	Recurrent infection	Periodontitis Ulcers

NR = not recorded; SD = standard deviation.

KEY POINTS

- Increasing population mobility means that a wide range of infections is seen globally
- Infections are especially common in immunodeficient people

An enormous range of infections is recognized; many are prevalent in the tropics and developing countries, and some are fatal. Global travel and global warming increasingly bring contact with these infections to the rest of the world. Concern has been expressed about more than a dozen potentially fatal infections that appear to be increasing in their geographical range (Box 21.1).

Bacteria, viruses and fungi are common in the external and internal environment, however, and most cause problems only if they secrete noxious substances, become invasive or elicit inappropriate host defence responses. Protection against most bacteria involves largely B cells and plasma cell production of antibodies, together with phagocytes (neutrophils and macrophages). Protection against mycobacteria, viruses and fungi is largely via T lymphocytes.

EMERGING INFECTIONS

Emerging infections (see also Appendix 21.1 and Ch. 33) may be:

- a recognized infection spreading to new areas or populations
- a hitherto known disease that is discovered to be caused by infection
- a previously unrecognized infection appearing where the habitat is changing (e.g. deforestation)
- a new infection resulting from change(s) in pre-existing microorganisms
- a known infection re-emerging because it has become resistant to treatment, or because of a breakdown in public health measures.

Box 21.1 *Possible fatal diseases increasing with global warming*

- Avian flu
- Babesiosis
- Cholera
- Dengue fever
- Ebola fever
- Lyme disease
- Malaria
- Parasitic infections
- Plague
- Red tides
- Rift valley fever
- Sleeping sickness
- Tuberculosis
- West Nile fever
- Yellow fever

INFECTION CONTROL

Guidelines to prevent transmission of infections are found at http://www.bda.org/dentists/advice/ba/ic.aspx (accessed 30 September 2013).

DISEASE NOTIFICATION

Notification of a number of specified infectious diseases is required in UK under the Public Health (Infectious Diseases) 1988 Act and the Public Health (Control of Diseases) 1984 Act. New (amended) regulations for clinical notifications came into force on 6 April 2010 (Box 21.2). Registered general *medical* practitioners (GMPs) in England and Wales

---

Box 21.2 *Notifiable diseases*

UK

- Acute bacterial meningitis (urgent)
- Acute viral meningitis (not Scotland)
- Acute encephalitis (not Scotland)
- Acute infectious hepatitis (not Scotland, urgent)[a]
- Acute poliomyelitis (urgent)
- Anthrax (urgent)
- Botulism (urgent)
- Brucellosis (urgent if UK-acquired)
- Cholera (urgent)
- Diphtheria (urgent)
- Enteric fever (typhoid or paratyphoid, urgent)
- Food poisoning (not Scotland, urgent if clusters or outbreaks)
- Haemolytic uraemic syndrome (urgent)
- Infectious bloody diarrhoea (not Scotland unless caused by *Escherichia coli* O157, urgent)
- Invasive group A streptococcal disease (Scotland any necrotizing fasciitis, urgent)
- Scarlet fever (not Scotland)
- Legionnaires' disease (not Scotland, urgent)
- Leprosy (not Scotland or Northern Ireland)
- Malaria (not Scotland, urgent if UK-acquired)
- Measles (urgent)
- Meningococcal septicaemia (urgent)
- Mumps
- Plague (urgent)
- Rabies (only urgent if seen at time of bite rather than with symptoms)
- Rubella
- Severe acute respiratory syndrome (SARS) (urgent)
- Smallpox (urgent)
- Tetanus (urgent if intravenous drug user)
- Tuberculosis (urgent if health worker, case cluster or multiple drug resistance)
- Typhus
- Viral haemorrhagic fever (urgent)
- Whooping cough (urgent in acute phase)
- Yellow fever (urgent if UK-acquired)

USA

- Anthrax
- Arboviral neuroinvasive and non-neuroinvasive diseases:
    - California serogroup virus disease
    - Eastern equine encephalitis virus disease
    - Powassan virus disease
    - St Louis encephalitis virus disease
    - West Nile virus disease
    - Western equine encephalitis virus disease
- Babesiosis
- Botulism:
    - Botulism, food-borne
    - Botulism, infant
    - Botulism, other (wound and unspecified)
- Brucellosis
- Chancroid
- Chlamydia trachomatis infection
- Cholera
- Coccidioidomycosis
- Cryptosporidiosis
- Cyclosporiasis
- Dengue:
    - Dengue fever
    - Dengue haemorrhagic fever
    - Dengue shock syndrome
- Diphtheria
- Ehrlichiosis/Anaplasmosis:
    - *Ehrlichia chaffeensis*
    - *Ehrlichia ewingii*
    - *Anaplasma phagocytophilum*
    - Undetermined
- Giardiasis
- Gonorrhea
- Haemophilus influenzae, invasive disease
- Hansen disease (leprosy)
- Hantavirus pulmonary syndrome
- Haemolytic uremic syndrome, post-diarrhoeal
- Hepatitis:
    - Hepatitis A, acute
    - Hepatitis B, acute
    - Hepatitis B, chronic
    - Hepatitis B virus, perinatal infection
    - Hepatitis C, acute
    - Hepatitis C, past or present
- HIV infection:
    - HIV infection, adult/adolescent (age ≥13 y)
    - HIV infection, child (age ≥18 months and <13 y)
    - HIV infection, paediatric (age <18 months)
- Influenza-associated paediatric mortality
- Legionellosis
- Listeriosis
- Lyme disease
- Malaria
- Measles
- Meningococcal disease
- Mumps
- Novel influenza A virus infections
- Pertussis
- Plague
- Poliomyelitis, paralytic
- Poliovirus infection, non-paralytic
- Psittacosis
- Q fever:
    - Acute
    - Chronic
- Rabies:
    - Rabies, animal
    - Rabies, human
- Rubella
- Rubella, congenital syndrome
- Salmonellosis
- Severe acute respiratory syndrome-associated coronavirus (SARS-CoV) disease
- Shiga toxin-producing *E. coli* (STEC)
- Shigellosis
- Smallpox
- Spotted fever rickettsiosis
- Streptococcal toxic shock syndrome
- *Streptococcus pneumoniae*, invasive disease
- Syphilis:
    - Primary
    - Secondary
    - Latent
    - Early latent
    - Late latent
    - Latent, unknown duration
    - Neurosyphilis
    - Late, non-neurological
    - Stillbirth
    - Congenital
- Tetanus
- Toxic shock syndrome (other than streptococcal)
- Trichinellosis (trichinosis)
- Tuberculosis
- Tularaemia
- Typhoid fever
- Vancomycin-intermediate *Staphylococcus aureus* (VISA)
- Vancomycin-resistant *Staph. aureus* (VRSA)
- Varicella (morbidity)
- Varicella (deaths only)
- Vibriosis
- Viral haemorrhagic fevers, due to:
    - Ebola virus
    - Marburg virus
    - Crimean–Congo haemorrhagic fever virus
    - Lassa virus
    - Lujo virus
    - New World arenaviruses (Guanarito, Machupo, Junin and Sabia viruses)
- Yellow fever

[a] Acute infective hepatitis but not HIV is notifiable in the UK.

have 'a statutory duty to notify a "proper officer" of the Local Authority of suspected cases of certain infectious diseases' – usually the consultant in communicable disease control (CCDC). The GMP should fill out a notification certificate immediately on diagnosis without waiting for laboratory confirmation and ensure that it reaches the officer within 3 days (telephone if urgent). The proper officers are required weekly to inform the Health Protection Agency (HPA) Centre for Infections (CfI) of the details of each case of each disease that has been notified.

As well as notifications of the infectious diseases specified below, the 2010 regulations also require GMPs to notify cases of 'other infections or of contamination which they believe present, or could present, a significant risk to human health', e.g. emerging or new infections, or cases of contamination (such as with chemicals or radiation) – particularly if there is a risk of transmission to others. Diagnostic laboratories also have a requirement to notify the HPA of specified causative agents they identify in tests on human samples.

Notification requires completion of the appropriate form, but urgent cases should be notified by telephone as well (certainly within 24 hours of any suspicions arising).

The following details are required:

- Patient's name, date of birth, sex and home address with postcode
- Patient's National Health Service number
- Ethnicity (used to monitor health equalities)
- Occupation, and/or place of work or educational establishment if relevant
- Current residence (if it is not the home address)
- Contact telephone number
- Contact details of a parent (for children)
- The disease or infection, or nature of poisoning/contamination being reported
- Date of onset of symptoms and date of diagnosis
- Any relevant overseas travel history
- If in hospital, also:
  hospital address
  day admitted
  whether the disease was contracted in hospital.

There is no fee payable for notification.

In Scotland, written notification should be undertaken electronically via the Scottish Care Information (SCI) Gateway (http://www.hps.scot.nhs.uk/publichealthact/NotifiableInfectiousDiseaseData.aspx; accessed 30 September 2013).

Diseases that are notifiable to the local authorities in the UK and USA are shown in Box 21.2. Incubation times are shown in Appendix 21.2.

Further information may be found at: http://www.hpa.org.uk/infections/topics_az/noids/archive.htm (accessed 30 September 2013).

BACTERIAL INFECTIONS

Bacterial infections and therapy are discussed here and in other chapters (Table 21.1) and in Appendices 21.3, 21.4 and 21.5.

Bacterial infections are common. Most are transient with few untoward sequelae but some can cause serious, recurrent, disseminated or persistent lesions – especially in immunocompromised persons (particularly in neutropenic patients, those with organ transplants, and those with human immunodeficiency virus/acquired immunodeficiency syndrome [HIV/AIDS]) – or can be life-threatening immediately (e.g. meningococcal meningitis), less immediately (e.g. diphtheria) or in the longer term (e.g. tuberculosis, syphilis).

Bacterial infections are often diagnosed on clinical grounds, supported by smears, culture, testing for immune responses (serology) and, increasingly, examining for nucleic acids.

Antibacterial drugs can often be effective therapy (see Appendix 21.3) but drainage of pus is often more important. Antibiotic resistance is increasingly a serious problem (e.g. *Staphylococcus aureus*, *Clostridium difficile*, *Mycobacterium tuberculosis*) and is encouraged by unwarranted use of antibiotics. Uncommon bacterial infections

Table 21.1 Bacterial infections

Bacterial infection	Chapter location
Bartonella infections (*Rochalimaea*)	This chapter
Brucellosis	This chapter
Chlamydia	Ch. 32
Cholera	This chapter
Diphtheria	This chapter
Gonorrhoea	Ch. 32
Granuloma inguinale	Ch. 32
Haemophilus	This chapter
Legionella	Ch. 15
Leprosy	This chapter
Leptospirosis	This chapter
Listeria	This chapter
Lyme disease	This chapter
Meningococci	Ch. 13
Paratyphoid	This chapter
Pertussis	This chapter
Plague	This chapter
Pneumococci	This chapter
Q fever	This chapter
Rickettsia	This chapter
Salmonella	This chapter
Staphylococci	This chapter
Streptococci	This chapter
Syphilis	Ch. 32
Tetanus	This chapter
Trichomoniasis	Ch. 32
Tuberculosis	Ch. 15
Tularaemia	This chapter
Typhoid	This chapter
Yersinia	This chapter

are shown in Appendix 21.6. Immunization against various bacteria is available and should be taken up (Appendix 21.7).

A wide range of bacterial infections are recognized (see Table 21.1). This chapter discusses odontogenic and orofacial bacterial infections; most cause lesions of limited duration but some are life-threatening. Nosocomial infections (health-care associated infections; HCAIs), tetanus, puncture wounds and bites, and other infections not discussed elsewhere are then summarized.

OROFACIAL AND ODONTOGENIC BACTERIAL INFECTIONS

PERIODONTAL INFECTIONS

Abscesses

A gingival abscess may arise from infection or a foreign body. A lateral periodontal abscess (parodontal abscess) is seen almost exclusively in patients with chronic periodontitis but may follow impaction of a foreign body or, rarely, can be related to a lateral root canal on a non-vital tooth.

Clinical features

Erythema and swelling are the main features. Lateral periodontal abscesses may be painful and eventually may discharge – either through the pocket or buccally, but more coronally than a periapical abscess.

General management

Drainage is needed, and sometimes antibiotics (Table 21.2).

Acute necrotizing ulcerative gingivitis

Acute necrotizing ulcerative gingivitis (ANUG) is a non-contagious anaerobic infection associated with proliferation of *Borrelia vincentii* and fusiform bacteria. It is typically an infection of young adults, found especially in institutions, the armed forces, etc., and predisposing factors include poor oral hygiene, smoking, viral respiratory infections and immune defects such as in HIV/AIDS.

Clinical features

Characteristic features of ANUG include profuse gingival bleeding, severe soreness from gingival ulceration, halitosis and a bad taste. Malaise, fever and cervical lymph node enlargement are rare.

General management

Diagnosis is usually clinical. Smears show fusospirochaetal bacteria and leukocytes. Occasionally, ANUG may be confused with acute leukaemia or herpetic stomatitis, and a full blood picture may be needed. HIV infection may need to be considered.

Management is by oral debridement, metronidazole (penicillin, if pregnant) and improved oral hygiene.

Noma (cancrum oris; gangrenous stomatitis)

Noma can result from ANUG in malnourished, debilitated or immunocompromised patients, especially in children in developing areas. Anaerobes have been implicated, particularly *Bacteroides* (*Porphyromonas*) species, *Fusobacterium necrophorum* (an animal pathogen), *Prevotella intermedia*, *Actinomyces* and alpha-haemolytic streptococci. In cases following ANUG, *Streptococcus anginosus* and *Abiotrophia* species are the predominant organisms. In early noma, predominant species include *Ochrobactrum anthropi*, *Stenotrophomonas maltophilia*, an uncharacterized species of *Dialister* and an uncultivated phylotype of *Leptotrichia*. A range of species or phylotypes

is found in advanced noma, including *Propionibacterium acnes*, *Staphylococcus* species, *Stenotrophomonas maltophilia*, *Ochrobactrum anthropi*, *Achromobacter* species, *Afipia* species, *Brevundimonas diminuta*, *Capnocytophaga* species, *Cardiobacterium* species, *Eikenella corrodens*, *Fusobacterium* species, *Gemella haemolysans* and *Neisseria* species. Phylotypes unique to noma infections include those in the genera *Eubacterium*, *Flavobacterium*, *Kocuria*, *Microbacterium* and *Porphyromonas*, and the related *Streptococcus salivarius* and genera *Sphingomonas* and *Treponema*. Spreading necrosis penetrates the buccal mucosa, leading to gangrene, an orocutaneous fistula and scarring.

Diagnosis is clinical; an immune defect should always be excluded. Management includes improving nutrition, systemic antibiotics (clindamycin, penicillin, tetracyclines or metronidazole) and plastic surgery.

Pericoronitis

Acute pericoronitis is inflammation of the operculum over an erupting or impacted tooth, usually a mandibular third molar. It appears in relation to the accumulation of plaque and trauma from the opposing tooth. A mixed flora with *Fusobacterium* and *Bacteroides* is recognized to be important. Immune defects may predispose.

Clinical features

Acute pericoronitis manifests with pain, trismus, swelling and halitosis. The operculum is swollen, red and often ulcerated, and there may be fever and regional lymphadenitis. Pus usually drains from beneath the operculum but, in a migratory abscess of the buccal sulcus, may track anteriorly.

General management

Diagnosis is from clinical features. Radiology is usually indicated to confirm the position and root formation of the underlying partially erupted tooth.

Initial management comprises local debridement and application of antiseptics such as chlorhexidine. Reduction of the occlusal surface (or extraction) of an opposing tooth may be helpful if there is local trauma. Pyrexia, trismus or cervical lymphadenopathy may be indications for use of systemic antibiotics, typically metronidazole. Long-term treatment may include extraction of the associated impacted tooth, particularly when this is a lower third molar.

Dental abscess (periapical abscess, odontogenic abscess)

General aspects

A dental abscess is often a sequel of pulpitis caused by dental caries, but may arise in relation to any non-vital tooth. A mixed bacterial flora, especially anaerobes such as *Fusobacterium* and *Bacteroides* (*Porphyromonas*), is implicated.

Clinical features

The causal tooth is non-vital but tender to palpation. Most dental abscesses produce an intraoral swelling, typically on the labial or buccal gingival; those on maxillary lateral incisors and those from palatal roots of the first molar tend to present palatally. Occasionally, abscesses track or discharge elsewhere; for example, lower incisors or molars may discharge extraorally, and maxillary premolars and molars may discharge into the maxillary sinus (Fig. 21.1). Pain and

Table 21.2 Antimicrobials for odontogenic and antral infections[a]

Condition	In non-allergic individuals, antimicrobial for >3 days or until symptoms resolve	Comments
Acute necrotizing gingivitis	Metronidazole or amoxicillin	Only if systemic involvement
Bites	Co-amoxiclav	Ch. 24
Cellulitis	Benzyl penicillin plus flucloxacillin	–
Periapical abscess	Amoxicillin or metronidazole for 5 days	Only if systemic involvement or cellulitis
Pericoronitis	Metronidazole or amoxicillin	Only if systemic involvement or trismus
Periodontal abscess	Amoxicillin or metronidazole for 5 days	Only if systemic involvement or cellulitis
Periodontitis	Metronidazole or doxycycline	Only for severe disease
Sinusitis	Amoxicillin or doxycycline or erythromycin for 7 days	Only for symptoms >7 days

[a]After British National Formulary 2009.

facial swelling are characteristic but, once the abscess discharges, the acute inflammation, pain and swelling resolve and a chronic abscess develops discharging from a sinus – usually buccally and intraorally. Acute periapical suppuration may track through the cortical plate and may be limited by fascial planes within anatomical spaces or spread beyond them, as in the case of Ludwig's angina. Spread may also be lymphatics to regional lymph nodes, or haematogenously leading to thrombophlebitis, bacteraemia or even septicaemia.

General management

Diagnosis is from clinical features plus imaging. Extraction or endodontic therapy of the affected tooth removes the source of infection. Analgesics may be indicated. Antimicrobials are required only in the circumstances outlined below.

ODONTOGENIC INFECTIONS

Odontogenic infections are mainly a consequence of pulpitis that leads initially to periapical infection and a dental abscess. Most odontogenic (and many orofacial) infections arise from the commensal oral mixed flora, with a substantial proportion of anaerobes. Most odontogenic and orofacial infections respond to drainage, by either endodontic treatment, incision or tooth extraction. A drain usually needs to stay in place for 24–48 hours until most/all of the pus has discharged. Analgesics also may be required. Antimicrobials may be indicated in a number of circumstances (Table 21.3).

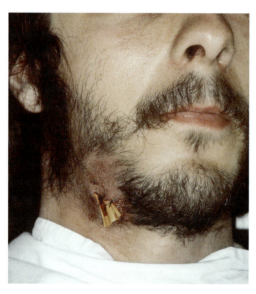

Fig. 21.1 Odontogenic infection.

Table 21.3 Indications for antimicrobial therapy

Patient status	Infections
Any patient with:	Fascial space infections in the neck
	Necrotizing fasciitis
	Osteomyelitis; removal of affected tissue is mandatory
	Serious or life-threatening infections
Ill or immunocompromised persons with:	Acute sinusitis
	Acute ulcerative gingivitis
	Dental abscess
	Dry socket
	Oral surgery
	Pericoronitis

Most odontogenic infections respond well to penicillin or metronidazole, but increasing rates of resistance due to production of beta-lactamase (an enzyme that degrades penicillins) have lowered the usefulness of many penicillins. Amoxycillin (± metronidazole) is a common first choice: second choices include cefuroxime, erythromycin, or clindamycin. Co-amoxiclav plus clindamycin are increasingly used first-line because of their broad spectrum of activity and resistance to beta-lactamase.

Anaerobic infections

Most head and neck infections are endogenous and mixed, with anaerobes, two-thirds containing more than one anaerobic species. Predominant anaerobes include *Prevotella*, *Fusobacterium* species, *Actinomyces* species (about 50% are *Actinomyces odontolyticus*), anaerobic cocci and *Eubacterium* species. *Prevotella intermedia*, *Fusobacterium nucleatum*, *Prevotella melaninogenica* and the *Bacteroides fragilis* group are the most common Gram-negative anaerobic species. Microaerophilic streptococci are often associated with anaerobes. Gram-positive anaerobic cocci (GPAC) are detected in about 15% of specimens – *Finegoldia magna* accounting for about one-third. Among aerobic/facultative isolates are Gram-positive cocci, Gram-negative bacteria and *Candida* species.

Treatment involves surgical procedures and antibacterial agents, which should cover both aerobes and anaerobes. Resistance rates to some agents (such as ampicillin/sulbactam and clindamycin) have increased.

Group A streptococcus (GAS) infections

People may carry group A streptococci in the throat or on the skin without symptoms of illness. Streptococcal oral or head and neck infections are shown in Table 21.4 (see also Fig. 21.2). Most streptococci are highly susceptible to penicillin. Some pneumococci (mostly imported) are increasingly resistant. Few people who come in contact with GAS will develop invasive GAS disease, but people with chronic illnesses like cancer, diabetes and chronic heart or lung disease, and those on

Table 21.4 Streptococcal infections in the head and neck

Bacteria	Found in/on	May cause
Streptococcus viridans	Normal oral flora	Caries and, rarely, infective endocarditis
Strep. pyogenes	Skin and pharynx	Cellulitis, impetigo (Fig. 21.2), necrotizing fasciitis, pharyngitis, scarlet fever or erysipelas, rheumatic fever and carditis
Strep. pneumoniae (pneumococci)	Upper respiratory tract	Acute glomerulonephritis, meningitis, sinusitis, otitis media, bronchitis and pneumonia

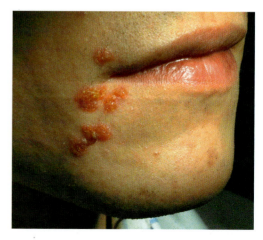

Fig. 21.2 Impetigo can mimic herpes simplex infections.

immunosuppressive medications such as steroids, have a higher risk. Persons with skin lesions (such as cuts, chickenpox or surgical wounds), the elderly, and adults with a history of alcohol abuse or injection drug use also have a higher risk for disease. Infection with GAS can result in a range of symptoms ranging from mild illness (streptococcal throat or a skin infection such as impetigo) to severe disease (necrotizing fasciitis, streptococcal toxic shock syndrome [STSS]). About 25% of those with necrotizing fasciitis and more than 35% with STSS die (see below).

Staphylococcal infections

Staphylococcal oral or head and neck infections may be caused by *Staphylococcus aureus*; most are minor (such as furuncles and boils) and most can be treated without antibiotics, but *S. aureus* can also cause serious infections such as surgical wound infections, sinusitis, tonsillitis, otitis externa or media, tracheitis, cellulitis, necrotizing fasciitis and toxic shock syndrome (caused by a staphylococcal-produced toxin that has resulted from nasal packing, and by tampon use). Infection is characterized by fever, hypotension, flushing of the skin followed by desquamation, shock and sometimes death.

Up to 80% of the *S. aureus* isolates in the West are resistant to penicillin, primarily due to production of beta-lactamase, but these will usually respond to lactamase-stable antibiotics such as flucloxacillin and meticillin. Meticillin-resistant *S. aureus* (MRSA) is resistant to these, however, and often to other antibiotics. Culture is essential to guide treatment of MRSA infections.

SERIOUS SEQUELAE OF ODONTOGENIC OR OROFACIAL INFECTIONS

Fatal dental or orofacial infections are rare unless there is an immune defect, but may include progression to mediastinitis, infective endocarditis, necrotizing fasciitis, brain abscess and disseminated intravascular coagulation. Patients with advanced infections need urgent admission for intravenous antibiotics and urgent surgery to remove the cause as well as for incision and drainage of tissue spaces involved. ICU may be needed until the airway is assured. Fibreoptic endotracheal intubation or occasionally emergency surgery (cricothyrotomy or tracheostomy) may be indicated.

Cellulitis

Cellulitis is usually an acute streptococcal or staphylococcal skin infection. It normally resolves on treatment with benzyl penicillin plus flucloxacillin or, if the patient is penicillin-allergic, clarithromycin, erythromycin, clindamycin or vancomycin/teicoplanin. Cellulitis can spread locally or systemically.

Buccal cellulitis is usually caused by *Haemophilus influenzae* type B, spread by bacteraemia, by lymphatics from, for example, otitis media, or more probably from direct invasion through the oral mucosa. It is an uncommon but distinctive infection, characterized by swelling, tenderness, induration and warmth of the cheek soft tissues in the absence of an adjacent oral or skin lesion; it almost invariably affects children under the age of 5 years. A minority develop meningitis. Blood and cerebrospinal fluid cultures should be taken and treatment with intravenous cefuroxime started.

Lymphangitis

Lymphangitis (inflammation of the lymphatics with pain and systemic symptoms) is commonly secondary to an acute streptococcal or staphylococcal cellulitis, or to an abscess in the skin or soft tissues. Lymphangitis may be confused with thrombophlebitis and suggests

that an infection is progressing, and may lead to bacteraemia, septicaemia and life-threatening infection.

Fascial space infections

Fascial space infections of the neck are dangerous, since they can embarrass the airway, erode the carotid vessels, cause toxicity, or spread to the mediastinum or intracranially. They usually arise from the oral flora and are polymicrobial, involving predominantly anaerobes, including Gram-positive cocci and bacilli, as well as Gram-negative bacilli.

Patients with fascial space infections must be admitted for hospital care, which may involve drainage and usually high-dose antibiotics.

Necrotizing fasciitis (Fournier gangrene, Meleney ulcer, postoperative progressive bacterial synergistic gangrene, flesh-eating bacteria, Cullen ulcer)

More information about necrotizing fasciitis is available at: http://www.nnff.org/ (accessed 30 September 2013).

General aspects

Necrotizing fasciitis is a dangerous, rapidly progressive, and spreading infection in the deep fascia, with secondary necrosis of subcutaneous tissues, which destroys muscles, fat and skin. The speed of spread along the deep fascial plane is directly proportional to the thickness of the subcutaneous layer. Most patients are middle-aged or older but, though the condition has become more frequent because of an increase in immunocompromised patients with diabetes, cancer, alcoholism, vascular insufficiencies, transplants, neutropenia or HIV, few have such detectable underlying predisposing factors.

Group A haemolytic streptococci and *S. aureus*, alone or in synergism, are often the initiating causal bacteria, but other aerobic and anaerobic pathogens, such as *Bacteroides* (*Porphyromonas*), *Clostridium*, *Peptostreptococcus*, Enterobacteriaceae, coliforms, *Proteus*, *Prevotella*, *Pseudomonas*, *Klebsiella*, *Bacteroides fragilis*, *Fusobacterium necrophorum* and *Escherichia coli* may be present.

Some men who have sex with men (MSM) have suffered outbreaks of necrotizing fasciitis caused by community-associated MRSA – distinct from health-care-associated strains. Anaerobic streptococci, occasionally seen in drug users, cause many forms of non-clostridial myonecrosis. Necrotizing fasciitis can also be caused by *Vibrio vulnificus*, often following the consumption of raw seafood – especially in patients with chronic liver disease. There may also be a relationship between the use of non-steroidal anti-inflammatory drugs (NSAIDs) and the development of necrotizing fasciitis during varicella infections.

Clinical features

There is often a history of trauma or recent surgery to the area. Features of necrotizing fasciitis include the following:

- *Early* (usually within 24 hours):
  Usually a minor trauma or other skin opening (the wound does not necessarily appear infected)
  Pain in the general area of the injury, not necessarily at the site of the injury but in the same region or limb of the body; it is usually disproportionate to the injury and may start as something akin to a muscle pull, but becomes more and more painful
  'Flu-like symptoms, such as diarrhoea, nausea, fever, confusion, dizziness, weakness and malaise

Intense thirst

■ *Advanced* (usually within 3–4 days):
Swelling of the limb or area of body experiencing pain, possibly accompanied by a purplish rash
Large, dark marks on the limb, which will become blisters filled with blackish fluid
Necrotic appearance of the wound, with a bluish, white or dark, mottled, flaky surface

■ *Critical* (usually within 4–5 days):
Severe drop in blood pressure
Signs that the body is entering toxic shock
Unconsciousness.

The lesion begins with an area of thrombosis and skin necrosis, which is initially red, painful and oedematous. Erythema quickly spreads over hours to days, and rapidly turns purplish, dusky and then black, with gas and exudate, and pain disproportionate to the clinical appearance. The margins of the infection move into surrounding skin without being raised or sharply demarcated. Over the next several hours to days, despite severe pain, there may be cutaneous anaesthesia – an unusual combination, as the cutaneous nerves are damaged by the infection (hence anaesthesia) but the proximal stump is irritated (hence the pain). Multiple patches develop to produce a large area of gangrenous skin.

Early on, the patient may look deceptively well but, within 24–48 hours, fever appears with rapidly spreading tissue necrosis, so that the patient usually appears moderately to severely toxic.

General management

Necrotizing fasciitis is uncommon but potentially fatal; if from a dental source, it can also spread and may threaten the airway. The mortality can sometimes reach 30%.

The gas-forming organisms may release subcutaneous gas that may be seen on radiography. Absence of gadolinium contrast enhancement in magnetic resonance imaging (MRI) T1 images reliably detects fascial necrosis. Thoracic computed tomography (CT) may be required to detect mediastinal spread.

Necrotizing fasciitis requires early aggressive treatment. The patient should be admitted to hospital and intubated; the affected area is opened to drain, and necrotic tissue excised. High doses of penicillin or clindamycin are given, plus metronidazole or a cephalosporin, or gentamicin, combined with clindamycin or chloramphenicol. Hyperbaric oxygen, if available, should be given.

Streptococcal toxic shock syndrome (STSS) results in acute hypotension and organ (e.g. kidney, liver, lungs) failure. STSS is not the 'toxic shock syndrome', which is due to *S. aureus* associated with tampon usage.

Recommended therapy for necrotizing fasciitis and STSS is early aggressive surgery plus high-dose antimicrobials (penicillin plus clindamycin). Supportive care in an intensive care unit may also be needed.

Lemierre syndrome (post-anginal septicaemia)

Lemierre syndrome is a rare, potentially fatal, acute anaerobic oropharyngeal infection, the classical presentation of human necrobacillosis. The main pathogen is *Fusobacterium necrophorum*, an obligate anaerobic, pleomorphic, Gram-negative rod.

The primary infection is in the head in a young, previously healthy person, who subsequently develops persistent high fever and disseminated metastatic abscesses, frequently including septic thrombophlebitis of the internal jugular vein. Lemierre syndrome is often complicated by septic pulmonary emboli and distant metastatic infections.

Surgical drainage and intravenous antibiotics are indicated. *F. necrophorum* is typically susceptible to penicillin, cephalosporins, metronidazole,

clindamycin, tetracyclines and chloramphenicol. Some beta-lactamase–producing strains of *F. necrophorum* have been reported.

Septicaemia

Septicaemia can arise from odontogenic or orofacial infections, but more commonly from infections of the urinary tract, gallbladder or chest. Immunosuppressed patients are particularly susceptible and oral bacteria are sometimes responsible.

Blood, urine and sputum should be cultured and the patient started on ceftriaxone (a once-daily dose), or cefuroxime plus metronidazole if anaerobic sepsis is suspected.

Actinomycosis (lumpy jaw)

Actinomycosis is a rare chronic infection, usually of the face and neck. It is caused by *Actinomyces israelii*, a Gram-positive, non-contagious anaerobic bacillus with filamentous growth and mycelia-like colonies bearing a striking resemblance to fungi; it is primarily a commensal found in normal oral cavities, tonsillar crypts, dental plaque and carious teeth. There are three main presentations.

Cervicofacial actinomycosis is the most common and typically causes a red or purplish, somewhat indurated, subcutaneous mass of abscesses and open draining sinuses, usually in the submandibular area near the angle of the mandible, arising a few weeks after an antecedent local lesion (dental or periodontal infection or tooth extraction). Tenderness is slight or absent. Microscopic examination of drained fluid shows 'sulphur granules' and *Actinomyces*, and culture of the fluid or tissue shows *Actinomyces* species.

Pulmonary actinomycosis causes fever and general malaise, cough and purulent sputum. Cutaneous sinuses may form.

Abdominal actinomycosis may cause pain and a palpable mass in the abdomen.

Treatment of actinomycosis is at least 1–2 months of penicillin or tetracycline. Surgical drainage may be indicated.

Osteomyelitis

See Chapter 16.

ANTIMICROBIAL PROPHYLAXIS

Antimicrobial cover may be required for bites; for contact with certain infections (e.g. open tuberculosis, meningitis, *Haemophilus influenzae* B infections or group A streptococci); and for oral-health-care invasive procedures in people with sickle cell anaemia or asplenia (usually phenoxymethyl penicillin or erythromycin – plus relevant vaccinations). It is sometimes suggested for various procedures or in various other conditions, but otherwise is infrequently indicated (Box 21.3).

Box 21.3 *Conditions in which antibiotic prophylaxis for oral health care is not usually considered essential*

- Augmentation procedures (e.g. lips, breasts)
- Cardiac surgery
- Immunocompromising states unless severe
- Indwelling intraperitoneal catheters
- Intraocular lenses
- Pacemakers and other cardiac devices
- Penile prostheses
- Prosthetic joint implants
- Ventriculo-peritoneal shunts

HEALTH-CARE-ASSOCIATED (NOSOCOMIAL) INFECTIONS (HCAIs)

HCAIs are an increasing problem across the world (Box 21.4). Box 21.5 shows precautions against them. A number of microorganisms can be involved in HCAIs, usually bacteria, and many are antimicrobial-resistant ('super-bugs'). HCAIs may affect wounds (surgical site infections), the skin, the respiratory tract, the gastrointestinal tract, the urinary tract, catheters, ventilators or any implanted device. Central line-associated bloodstream infections, catheter-associated urinary tract infections and ventilator-associated pneumonia account for about two-thirds of all HCAIs that are not in surgical sites.

WOUND INFECTIONS (SURGICAL SITE INFECTIONS)

General aspects

Infections (surgical wound infections; surgical site infections, SSIs) can be a problem in terms of morbidity and mortality. Postoperative bacterial infection rates vary from 3% to 21%, with SSIs accounting for up to 34% of the total (probably underestimated since most wound infections start after the patient is discharged). SSIs have significant morbidity and mortality, accounting for approximately 77% of deaths of general surgical patients.

Surgical wounds have been classified as clean, clean-contaminated, contaminated and dirty-infected (Table 21.5). Most head and neck surgery involves class I or II wounds.

Most SSIs arise from the patient's own flora, from health-care workers and articles brought into the operative field, and from the operating room air. The usual pathogens on skin surfaces are Gram-positive aerobic cocci (mainly staphylococci), but anaerobes and Gram-negative aerobes may be involved. The normal oral flora is 90% anaerobes and 10% Gram-positive aerobic cocci. Gram-negative aerobes may be a problem in patients who have been hospitalized or treated with radiotherapy. Factors promoting wound infection include preoperative removal of hair, especially when there is skin abrasion, inadequate skin preparation with bactericidal solution, poor surgical technique, lengthy operation (over 2 hours), intraoperative contamination, prolonged stay in hospital,

Box 21.4 *Main health-care-acquired infections (HCAIs)*

- *Acinetobacter*
- *Burkholderia cepacia*
- *Clostridium difficile*
- *Clostridium sordellii*
- Enterobacteriaceae (carbapenem-resistant)
- *Escherichia coli*
- Glycopeptide-resistant enterococci (GRE)
- Hepatitis
- Human immunodeficiency virus (HIV)
- Influenza
- *Klebsiella*
- Meticillin-resistant *Staphylococcus aureus* (MRSA)
- *Mycobacterium abscessus*
- Norovirus
- Pencillin-resistant *Streptococcus pneumoniae* (PRSP)
- *Staphylococcus aureus*
- Tuberculosis
- Vancomycin-intermediate *Staphylococcus aureus* and vancomycin-resistant *Staphylococcus aureus*
- Vancomycin-resistant enterococci (VRE)

Box 21.5 *Prevention of health-care-associated infection transmission*

- Follow good hygiene and standard infection control procedures
- Avoid contact with wounds or material contaminated from wounds
- Use alcohol-based waterless antiseptic agents for routinely decontaminating hands, when hands are not visibly soiled
- Wash hands thoroughly with a non-antimicrobial soap and water, or an antimicrobial soap and water, when hands are visibly dirty or contaminated with proteinaceous material such as blood
- Keep cuts and abrasions clean and covered with a proper dressing until healed, when hands are cut or abraded
- Use a moisturizer to prevent skin cracking

Table 21.5 Surgical wound classification and subsequent risk of infection (no antibiotics used)

Classification	Oral or perioral example	Description	Infective risk (%)
Clean (Class I)	Excision of a facial skin lesion	Uninfected operative wound	<2
		No acute inflammation	
		Closed primarily	
		Respiratory, gastrointestinal, biliary and urinary tracts not entered	
		No break in aseptic technique	
		Closed drainage used if necessary	
Clean-contaminated (Class II)	Parotid surgery	Elective entry into respiratory, biliary, gastrointestinal or urinary tracts and with minimal spillage	<10
		No evidence of infection or major break in aseptic technique	
Contaminated (Class III)	Third molar surgical removal	Non-purulent inflammation present	About 20
		Spillage from gastrointestinal tract	
		Penetrating traumatic wounds <4h	
		Major break in aseptic technique	
Dirty-infected (Class IV)	Incision and drainage of a submandibular abscess	Purulent inflammation present	About 40
		Preoperative perforation of viscera	
		Penetrating traumatic wounds >4h	

From Cruse 1980.

hypothermia, trauma, non-viable tissue in the wound, haematoma, foreign material (including drains and sutures), dead space, pre-existing sepsis (local or distant), immunocompromised or malnourished host, hypovolaemia, poor tissue perfusion or obesity, and delayed prophylaxis with, or incorrect choice of, antibiotics.

Prophylaxis

Prophylactic antibiotics are indicated for clean-contaminated and contaminated trauma, for clean procedures in which prosthetic devices are inserted and, more controversially, for clean procedures such as orthognathic surgery.

The concentration of prophylactic antibiotic should be at therapeutic levels by the time of incision, during the surgical procedure and for a few hours postoperatively, and this is achieved by intravenous administration of the antibiotic 30 minutes before incision (but not more than 2 hours before surgery). For head and neck surgery, *S. aureus*, streptococci, anaerobes and streptococci can be present in an oropharyngeal approach; examples of antibiotics shown to be effective in class II head and neck wound prophylaxis include cefazolin 1–2 g alone or in combination with metronidazole, or clindamycin alone or with gentamicin or amikacin, amoxicillin/clavulanate, ampicillin/sulbactam and ticarcillin/clavulanate.

Clinical features

SSI is suggested by features such as pus draining from the wound, the wound becoming excessively tender, progressive swelling starting about 48 hours after surgery, increasing redness around the wound (cellulitis), a red streak from the wound toward the heart (lymphangitis), lymphadenitis or fever. The wound may fail to heal within 10 days after the injury, the scab increases in size, and a pimple or yellow crust may form on the wound (impetigo).

General management

Treatment of SSI often involves antibiotics after opening the wound, evacuating pus and cleansing the wound – inspecting deeper tissues for integrity and for deep space infection or source. Dressing changes allow the tissues to granulate, and the wound heals by secondary intention over several weeks.

The antibiotic choice depends on the known or probable infecting microorganism, and factors such as severity of SSI, patient's age, hepatic and renal function, allergies and other medication(s). First choices are flucloxacillin in the absence of allergy if staphylococci or streptococci are implicated; metronidazole or clindamycin for anaerobic infections; cefuroxime for Gram-negative organisms; and amoxicillin or co-amoxiclav for enterococcal infection. For pain relief, paracetamol (acetaminophen), ibuprofen or an opioid is indicated.

CENTRAL LINE-ASSOCIATED BLOODSTREAM INFECTION (CLABSIs)

CLABSI is a serious infection that may present with fever, skin erythema and soreness around the central line entry point. CLABSIs must be prevented in the following manner:

- Follow recommended central line insertion practices:
  Hand hygiene
  Skin antiseptic
  Barrier precautions: sterile gloves, sterile gown, cap, mask, sterile drape.

- Once the central line is in place, wash hands with soap and water or an alcohol-based handrub before and after touching the line.
- Remove a central line as soon as it is no longer needed.

More than 50% of all *S. aureus* CLABSI isolates are MRSA but the incidence is decreasing. In contrast, *Klebsiella pneumoniae* and *E. coli* resistance to third-generation cephalosporins has increased significantly, as has imipenem and ceftazidine resistance in *Pseudomonas aeruginosa*, and *Candida* spp. are increasingly fluconazole-resistant.

Guidelines for the prevention of intravascular catheter-related infections are available at: http://www.cdc.gov/hicpac/BSI/BSI-guidelines-2011.html (accessed 30 September 2013).

ANTIBIOTIC-RESISTANT INFECTIONS

The main antibiotic-resistant infections are meticillin-resistant *S. aureus* (MRSA) and clindamycin-resistant *Clostridium difficile*, but there are several others; many of these arise as HCAIs and the most important are discussed here, alphabetically. Six of these bacteria have been dubbed ESKAPE (*Enterococcus faecium*, *S. aureus*; *Klebsiella* species, *Acinetobacter baumannii*, *Pseudomonas aeruginosa* and *Enterobacter* species). Some of these infections are with multidrug-resistant organisms (MDROs); see http://www.cdc.gov/hicpac/mdro/mdro_toc.html (accessed 30 September 2013).

ACINETOBACTER

Acinetobacter are commonly found in soil and water. *Acinetobacter* infections in the community are rare and most strains are sensitive to antibiotics. Infections are usually HCAIs and are typically found in intensive care units, in very ill patients and with resistant organisms. *A. baumannii* accounts for about 80% of reported infections and these include pneumonia, bacteraemia (bloodstream infection), wound infections and urinary tract infections. They are often resistant to antibiotics and are increasingly difficult to treat. *A. baumanii* wound infections have been found in US military personnel deployed to Iraq and Afghanistan. Of the beta-lactamase inhibitors, sulbactam possesses the greatest intrinsic bactericidal activity against *A. baumannii*. Carbapenems (imipenem, meropenem or doripenem) are the most important other options for serious infections caused by multidrug-resistant *A. baumannii*. Amikacin and tobramycin are aminoglycosides that appear to retain activity against *A. baumannii*. Other possibilities include polymyxin E, polymyxin B, colistin, minocycline and doxycycline. Tigecycline may be used, as may extended-infusion β-lactams, cefepime and piperacillin–tazobactam.

BURKHOLDERIA CEPACIA

Burkholderia cepacia is a group of bacteria found in soil and water; they are often resistant to common antibiotics but pose little risk to healthy people. However, *B. cepacia* can cause infections in people with immune defects or chronic lung disease (particularly cystic fibrosis/bronchiectasis). Treatment typically involves multiple antibiotics and may include ceftazidime, doxycycline, piperacillin, meropenem, chloramphenicol or co-trimoxazole.

CLOSTRIDIUM DIFFICILE

Clostridium difficile (also called *C. diff*) is the major organism linked with antibiotic-associated diarrhoea and colitis, usually caused by expanded-spectrum and broad-spectrum cephalosporins and clindamycin, though the role of fluoroquinolones is less clear. An HCAI that mostly affects older patients with other underlying disorders in hospital environments, the disease usually develops after cross-infection from another patient, either through direct contact, or via health-care staff or via a contaminated environment. Community-acquired *C. difficile* infection (CDI) has also emerged.

Diagnosis is from the presence of *C. difficile* toxins in a faecal sample. The emergence and epidemic spread of a novel strain, known as PCR ribotype 027 (BI/NAP1/027), resistant to clindamycin, is an issue. Type 027 produces many more of the toxins than most other types.

Prevention and control of *C. difficile* is by reduction of the use of broad-spectrum antibiotics, isolation of patients with *C. difficile* diarrhoea, good infection control nursing (alcohol gel does not destroy the spores), and enhanced environmental cleaning using a chlorine-containing disinfectant. Metronidazole and vancomycin are the treatments of choice but some strains are now resistant. More information on epidemiology can be found by searching on *C. difficile* at http://cmr.asm.org (accessed September 2013).

CLOSTRIDIUM SORDELLII

Clostridium sordellii is a rare bacterial cause of pneumonia, endocarditis, arthritis, peritonitis and myonecrosis. *Cl. sordellii* bacteraemia and sepsis are usually seen in people with other health conditions – mostly after trauma, childbirth and gynaecological procedures – but they have recently been associated with medically induced abortions and injection drug use. Mortality is very high; *Cl. sordellii* is typically susceptible to beta-lactams, clindamycin, tetracycline and chloramphenicol but resistant to aminoglycosides and sulphonamides. Further details may be found at: http://www.cdc.gov/hai/organisms/csordellii.html (accessed September 2013).

EXTENDED-SPECTRUM BETA-LACTAMASE (ESBL) PRODUCERS

Gram-negative enteric bacilli (Enterobacteriaceae) are producers of enzymes that destroy beta-lactam antibiotics and mediate resistance to extended-spectrum (third-generation) cephalosporins (e.g. ceftazidime, cefotaxime and ceftriaxone) and oxyimino-monobactams (e.g. aztreonam) but do not affect cephamycins (e.g. cefoxitin and cefotetan) or carbapenems (e.g. meropenem or imipenem). ESBL enzymes are most commonly produced by *E. coli* and *K. pneumoniae*, but other bacteria that may do so include *Enterobacter cloacae*, *Citrobacter freundii*, *Serratia marcescens*, *Pseudomonas aeruginosa*, *Salmonella* species and *Proteus mirabilis*. *K. pneumoniae* most commonly produce *K. pneumoniae* carbapenemase (KPC). Resistance of *Enterobacter* species to third-generation cephalosporins is most typically caused by overproduction of AmpC beta-lactamases. Some *E. cloacae* strains are now ESBL- and AmpC-producers, conferring resistance to both third- and fourth-generation cephalosporins.

Quinolone resistance in Enterobacteriaceae is usually the result of chromosomal mutations leading to alterations in target enzymes or drug accumulation. More recently, however, plasmid-mediated quinolone resistance has been reported in *K. pneumoniae* and *E. coli*, associated with acquisition of the *qnr* gene. The vast majority of Enterobacteriaceae, including ESBL-producers, remain susceptible to carbapenems, which are considered the preferred empirical therapy for serious infections.

ESBL infection may stem from infected chicken meat and outbreaks have originated in hospitals and nursing homes, and increasingly in the community, typically with urinary tract infections and bacteraemia. Persistent oral carriage may be seen in immunocompromised persons, in advanced age and in dry mouth. Until recently, the numbers of patients affected remained small and the problem showed little sign of growing. However, a new class of ESBL (CTX-M enzymes) has emerged and has been widely detected among hospital *E. coli* but also found in the community. These ESBL-*E. coli* are found most often in urinary tract infections and are resistant to penicillins and cephalosporins. Carbapenems, such as meropenem, are usually the effective treatment for ESBL. However, *carbapenem-resistant Enterobacteriaceae (CRE; glycopeptide-resistant enterococci [GRE])* may arise in *Klebsiella* species and *E. coli*. CRE infections are most common in patients receiving treatment involving devices such as catheters or ventilators, and those who are on long antibiotic courses. New Delhi metallo-beta-lactamase (NDM-1), an enzyme that inactivates carbapenems, is most widespread in *Klebsiella* in the Indian subcontinent but has spread to the UK and elsewhere, often via patients previously treated in the subcontinent. Verona integron-encoded metallo-beta-lactamase (VIM) and imipenemase (IMP) metallo-beta-lactamases may also be seen.

CRE have been associated with high mortality rates (up to 40–50% in some studies). In addition to beta-lactam/carbapenem resistance, CRE often have high levels of resistance to many other antimicrobials. More information is available at: http://www.cdc.gov/hai/organisms/cre/index.html (accessed September 2013).

Most bacteria with NDM-1 remain susceptible to colistin and tigecycline. 'Pan-resistant' KPC-producing strains have been reported.

METICILLIN-RESISTANT *STAPHYLOCOCCUS AUREUS* (MRSA)

Meticillin-resistant *Staphylococcus aureus* (MRSA) is resistant to beta-lactam antibiotics (meticillin and other more common antibiotics, such as oxacillin, flucloxacillin, penicillin and amoxicillin). Most severe or potentially life-threatening MRSA infections occur among patients in health-care settings. The most common clones are E(pidemic)-MRSA 15 and E-MRSA16. Strains of *S. aureus* producing Panton–Valentine leukocidin (PVL) are especially virulent. About 1 in 3 people carry *S. aureus* on the skin surface or in the nose; if this enters the body through a break in the skin, it can cause infections such as abscesses or impetigo. MRSA is no more infectious than other types of *S. aureus* but infections are more difficult to treat, owing to their antibiotic resistance, and mortality is increased. The infection may simply require a much higher dose over a much longer period, or the use of an agent to which MRSA is not resistant.

MRSA is usually spread through person-to-person contact with someone who has an MRSA infection or who is colonized. It can also spread through contact with towels, sheets, clothes, dressings or other objects that have been used by someone with MRSA. *S. aureus* can also survive on objects or surfaces such as door handles, sinks, floors and cleaning equipment. MRSA infections are far more common in people who are in hospital; risk factors are shown in Box 21.6.

Box 21.6 *Risk factors for MRSA infection*

- Immune incompetence (e.g. elderly, newborn babies, patients with diabetes, cancer or HIV/AIDS)
- Open wound, catheter or intravenous tube
- Severe skin condition (e.g. burn or cut, ulcer or psoriasis)
- Recent surgery
- Frequent courses of antibiotics
- Prolonged hospital stay
- Asymptomatic MRSA nasal carriage

Community-associated MRSA infections typically involve the skin, and are usually transmitted from people with active MRSA skin infections. The strains causing these infections, designated community-associated MRSA (CA-MRSA), are distinct from health-care-associated strains (HA-MRSA). Infection with multidrug-resistant USA300 MRSA has emerged among MSM. Infection most often involves the buttocks, genitals or perineum. The risk is independent of HIV infection but the infection might be sexually transmitted in this population.

Community-associated MRSA spreads especially to:

- intravenous drug users
- children in day care
- athletes
- military personnel
- prison inmates.

Clinical features

Symptoms depend on the type of infection. Most *S. aureus* infections involve the skin, and include boils, abscesses, styes, carbuncles, cellulitis and impetigo, but infections are also able to enter the bloodstream (bacteraemia); these can cause septicaemia, septic shock, septic arthritis, osteomyelitis, abscesses, meningitis, pneumonia and endocarditis, and can be fatal. *S. aureus* can also cause scalded skin syndrome and, very occasionally, toxic shock syndrome.

General management

Many hospitals now test all people being admitted to see if they are colonized; swabs from the skin and nose, and urine and blood samples may be tested. It can take 3–5 days for the results to become available. People colonized with MRSA may still be admitted to hospital but treated to reduce or remove it by using antibiotic cream applied to the skin or the inside of the nose, and washing skin and hair with antiseptic shampoo and lotion. Health-care workers should use fast-acting, special alcohol rubs or gels, and wear disposable gloves when there will be physical contact with open wounds: for example, when changing dressings, handling needles or inserting intravenous lines.

MRSA infections are diagnosed by testing blood, urine or a tissue sample for the presence of the organism. Patients who are only *colonized* with MRSA usually do not need treatment. Infections often require hospital treatment in isolation for several weeks. Frank MRSA infections can sometimes be treated without antibiotics by draining and, in reality, most are resistant to multiple antibiotics as well as to meticillin.

Agents used to treat MRSA infections include vancomycin, or quinupristin combined with dalfopristin or linezolid, but resistance has been reported. Linezolid can also cause cytopenias, including pancytopenia, and optic neuropathy, and acts as a monoamine oxidase inhibitor. Teicoplanin, rifampicin and streptogramin may be effective.

People more at risk of MRSA are best advised not to visit an infected person and all visitors must wash their hands thoroughly before and after visiting. Mandatory MRSA bacteraemia surveillance and better infection control practices, such as universal hand hygiene, contact precautions and admission screening, have seen a dramatic reduction in MRSA infection. The intensive care unit (ICU), an important reservoir for seeding MRSA, has been at the forefront of MRSA control programmes. Decolonization with agents such as chlorhexidine and mupirocin has an important role in reducing transmission. Chlorhexidine particularly is being recommended in the ICU

for an increasing number of indications, including decolonization, universal patient bathing, oropharyngeal antisepsis in ventilated patients and antisepsis at vascular catheter insertion sites.

MRSA has rarely been transmitted to dental patients but oral infections have now been reported.

PENICILLIN-RESISTANT *STREPTOCOCCUS PNEUMONIAE* (PRSP)

Streptococcus pneumoniae (pneumococcus) is the major pathogen causing community-acquired infections such as acute otitis media, pneumonia, bacteraemia and meningitis. Penicillin resistance in seen in over 80%. The penicillin-resistant *S. pneumoniae* are usually also resistant to macrolides, tetracyclines, co-trimoxazole, chloramphenicol and clindamycin, and increasingly to fluoroquinolone. Treatment is generally with a third-generation cephalosporin, or vancomycin together with rifampicin for a serious infection such as meningitis.

STAPHYLOCOCCUS AUREUS

S. aureus is found on the skin and in the nose of about 30% of healthy individuals. Coagulase-positive (*S. aureus*) and coagulase-negative staphylococci are Gram-positive cocci – important causes of infection, primarily of the skin, bloodstream, native and prosthetic cardiac valves, and other implanted devices. Their progressively reduced susceptibility to penicillin, meticillin and glycopeptides makes treatment of staphylococcal infections difficult. Although the use of chlorhexidine-impregnated catheters has reduced catheter-related infections, chlorhexidine-resistant *S. aureus* has emerged. MRSA strains carrying the antiseptic resistance genes *qacA/B* can be clinically resistant to chlorhexidine.

The two most commonly used decolonization agents are mupirocin for nasal carriage and chlorhexidine for skin carriage, the latter applied either as a daily bath after dilution in water, where there is potential for variability in the applied concentration, or as disposable cloths saturated in 2% chlorhexidine. Triclosan, octenidine dihydrochloride and tea tree oil are alternatives to chlorhexidine.

Chlorhexidine is used for skin antisepsis prior to blood culture collection and the insertion of vascular catheters; applied to the catheter exit site in the form of impregnated sponges; impregnated into vascular catheters to prevent bloodstream infections; and for oropharyngeal antisepsis to prevent ventilator-associated pneumonias. Mupirocin resistance is well known, but chlorhexidine resistance is an emerging threat and of additional concern.

STENOTROPHOMONAS MALTOPHILIA ('STENO')

Stenotrophomonas (*Pseudomonas*) *maltophilia* is an aerobic, nonfermentative, Gram-negative bacterium of low virulence found in aquatic environments. It frequently colonizes fluids used in hospitals (e.g. irrigation solutions, intravenous fluids) and is found in patient secretions (e.g. secretions, urine, exudates).

S. maltophilia rarely causes disease in healthy hosts, unless invasive medical devices are present. Antimicrobial treatment is usually unnecessary and may be potentially harmful. Infections are, in any event, difficult to treat, but *S. maltophilia* is susceptible to trimethoprim–sulfamethoxazole (TMP-SMX), meropenem, minocycline, quinolones and colistin/polymyxin B.

TUBERCULOSIS

See Chapter 15.

VANCOMYCIN-RESISTANT BACTERIA

Vancomycin-resistant enterococci (VRE)

Vancomycin-resistant enterococci (VRE) are often present in the normal intestinal flora and in the female genital tract, as well as in the environment. Some of the other antibiotics that fail include some types of penicillin, cephalosporins, clindamycin, aminoglycosides, macrolides (such as erythromycin), tetracycline, quinolones and others.

Most VRE infections occur in hospitals and are often acquired from other people or from contaminated food or water. Up to 66% carry enterococci in the mouth, especially patients undergoing endodontic treatment. VRE may be associated with endodontic failures. It can cause diarrhoea, wound infection, bacteraemia or urinary tract infections, mainly in immunocompromised and medically ill patients. It may also give rise to endocarditis. Most VRE infections can be treated with antibiotics other than vancomycin.

Vancomycin-intermediate *Staphylococcus aureus* and vancomycin-resistant *Staphylococcus aureus*

Vancomycin-resistant (VRSA) and reduced susceptibility (vancomycin-intermediate) *S. aureus* (VISA) infections are usually seen in people with underlying health conditions (e.g. diabetes, chronic kidney disease), devices (e.g. catheters), previous infections with MRSA, and recent exposure to vancomycin and other antimicrobials.

Quinupristin–dalfopristin, linezolid, tetracycline, trimethoprim–sulfamethoxazole (TMP-SMX), tigecycline and daptomycin have been used for treatment of VISA infections.

TETANUS, PUNCTURE WOUNDS AND BITES

TETANUS

General aspects

Tetanus is a non-communicable infection caused by wound contamination with *Clostridium tetani* spores; it has a mortality of up to 60%. The spores are ubiquitous in soil or dust, particularly where there is faecal contamination, as on agricultural land. Tetanus is most likely to follow contaminated deep wounds, such as puncture wounds, especially if there is tissue necrosis, but it may also follow trivial wounds, or even bites or burns. The elderly, particularly women, are at greatest risk. Neonates may develop tetanus from contamination of the umbilical stump, a condition only found in the developing world.

Clinical features

The incubation period is between 4 and 21 days, commonly about 10 days.

C. tetani produces a neurotoxin (tetanospasmin) that is responsible for violent muscular spasms; trismus (lockjaw) due to masseteric spasm is the single most common early sign. Facial spasm produces a so-called sardonic smile (risus sardonicus), in which the eyebrows are raised with eyes closed and the lips are drawn back over clenched teeth. Spinal muscle spasm produces arching of the back (opisthotonos), while laryngeal spasm can lead to asphyxiation. Autonomic dysfunction can cause cardiac arrhythmias and fluctuations in blood pressure. Death may follow within 10 days of the onset of tetanus, usually from asphyxia, autonomic dysfunction or bronchopneumonia.

General management

Patients who have contaminated wounds, such as those associated with maxillofacial injuries caused by road traffic or riding accidents, are at greatest risk from tetanus. Situations that are considered tetanus-prone include any wound or burn sustained more than 6 hours before surgical treatment of the injury, or that shows a significant degree of devitalized tissue; a puncture wound; contact with manure or soil; or clinical sepsis.

Management of wounds where tetanus is likely includes active immunization with tetanus toxoid but it is *not* good practice to give toxoid after every *minor* injury, as severe allergic reactions can occasionally follow (Table 21.6).

The diagnosis of tetanus is clinical. There are no immediate tests that will help the diagnosis. Patients with tetanus should be admitted to an ICU for protection of the airway (tracheostomy should be carried out if the airway is endangered) and to facilitate artificial respiration, should it become necessary. They should be given anti-tetanus immunoglobulin (early, as it is ineffective after the toxin has become bound to nervous tissue) – human anti-tetanus immunoglobulin (ATG; Humotet, 500 units or more); if this is not available, animal anti-tetanus serum (ATS) should be used, after testing for hypersensitivity and with adrenaline (epinephrine) and corticosteroids available in case a severe reaction develops. Control of muscle spasms should be achieved by heavy sedation or, in severe cases, using general anaesthesia, muscle relaxants and mechanical ventilation; wound debridement should also be carried out, the purpose being to remove the source of toxin, as antibiotics alone are ineffective. Metronidazole is usually given.

Survivors suffer no after-effects but should have active immunization with toxoid.

Prophylaxis

Prophylaxis is active immunization in childhood, given as a triple vaccine (diphtheria, pertussis and tetanus antigens) starting at the age of 12 weeks, followed by further injections 6–8 weeks later and then after a further 4–6 months. Booster immunization (diphtheria, tetanus, pertussis and polio) is given at 3 years 4 months, and tetanus, diphtheria and polio at around 14 years old. The duration of immunity after such an immunization schedule is not known but current practice is to boost it every 10 years. Groups at highest risk (e.g. farm workers) should be given boosters every 5 years. Most cases of tetanus in developed countries are now seen in those who were never immunized, or in those whose immunity has declined – hence the risk in the elderly.

Table 21.6 Management of wounded patients at risk from tetanus

Wound type	Immune status	Course of action[a]
Superficial wound or abrasion	Immune[b]	–
	Not known to be immune	Active immunization with toxoid. Full three-dose course or, if partially immune, a reinforcing dose
Deep wounds, puncture wounds, or bites or burns	Immune	Give toxoid booster[c]
	Not known to be immune	Give antibiotics (metronidazole or penicillin) and start immunization with toxoid and: (1) if seen after 4h, give 250–500 units HTIG i.m.; (2) if seen after 24h, give 500 units HTIG i.m.

[a]Wound debridement in all.
[b]Last of three-dose course or reinforcing dose within past 10 y.
[c]Human tetanus immunoglobulin (HTIG; 250–500 units i.m.) should also be given if the wound is highly contaminated or there is any doubt about immune status.

Dental aspects

Trismus is usually caused by local irritation, such as pericoronitis or temporomandibular pain–dysfunction syndrome, but in the absence of a local cause, tetanus must always be considered. Such patients should therefore be asked whether they have had any recent wounds, particularly if they are farm workers or gardeners.

Dyskinesias due to phenothiazines include facial grimacing but rarely trismus – the mouth is usually opened forcefully.

PUNCTURE WOUNDS

A puncture wound is caused by an object *piercing* the skin and creating a small hole. Some punctures can be very deep, do not often result in obvious excessive bleeding and tend to close fairly quickly spontaneously. A puncture wound from a cause such as stepping on a nail can become infected. Treatment may be necessary to prevent tetanus or other infections. Most healthy people without signs of infection do not require antibiotics, but these may be given to people with diabetes, peripheral vascular disease, contaminated wounds or deep wounds to the foot.

BITES

Dogs and cats cause most animal bites. Dog bites may cause severe tissue injury, as well as infections. Cat bites are more frequently (approximately 50%) infected. Animal bite infections are usually bacterial – typically polymicrobial (staphylococci and anaerobes). Tetanus is rarely transmitted.

Bites from non-immunized domestic animals and wild animals may carry the risk of rabies, which is more common in raccoons, skunks, bats and foxes than in cats and dogs. Rabbits, squirrels and other rodents rarely carry rabies.

Human bites are discussed in Chapter 24. Bites from humans may carry the risk of blood-borne virus infections (e.g. hepatitis B or C, or HIV). Consideration of post-exposure prophylaxis is important.

Treatment of bites may include debridement; antimicrobial coverage for staphylococci (co-amoxiclav) and anaerobes; and consideration of the possibilities of tetanus, rabies and blood-borne viruses.

Cat scratch disease (CSD) is caused by a bacterium, *Bartonella henselae,* usually transmitted when a person is bitten or scratched by a cat. About 40% of cats carry *B. henselae* at some time in their lives but show no signs. Patients develop lymphadenopathy, especially around the head, neck and axilla, and may develop fever, headache, fatigue and anorexia. Immunocompromised people are more likely to have complications – bacillary angiomatosis and Parinaud oculoglandular syndrome.

FOOD POISONING

Food poisoning is common, especially where hygiene is lacking and in warmer climes. Prevention is by:

- washing hands thoroughly before preparing or eating food, particularly after using the bathroom, changing nappies or having contact with animals or their environments
- cooking meat, poultry and fish thoroughly, preferably using a thermometer
- preventing cross-contamination in food preparation areas by washing hands, working tops, cutting boards and utensils thoroughly – particularly after preparing raw meat
- avoiding unpasteurized dairy products and juices
- avoiding swallowing water when swimming or playing in lakes, ponds, streams, rivers or swimming pools.

CAMPYLOBACTER

Campylobacter is the commonest reported bacterial intestinal disease in the UK. Most infections are with *C. jejuni* or *C. coli*, which are found in the gastrointestinal tract of birds (particularly poultry), cattle and domestic pets. Raw or undercooked meat (especially poultry), unpasteurized milk, bird-pecked milk on doorsteps, untreated water, and domestic pets with diarrhoea are the usual sources. Occupational exposure when processing poultry in abattoirs has been implicated in some cases. However, most infections remain unexplained by recognized risk factors.

Clinical features and general management

After an incubation period of 1–11 days (usually 2–5 days), there is abdominal pain, profuse diarrhoea and malaise, but vomiting is uncommon.

Disease may be passed from person to person if personal hygiene is poor. The illness is contagious, and children must be kept at home until they have been clear of symptoms for at least 2 days. Treatment is with azithromycin.

ESCHERICHIA COLI

E. coli are bacteria that normally live in the intestines of humans and animals without causing problems. Some strains can cause food poisoning, however, and one (*E. coli* O157:H7) can cause severe food poisoning, releasing a verotoxin (verocytotoxic *E. coli* [VTEC]; enterohaemorrhagic *E. coli* [EHEC]; or 'Shiga toxin-producing' *E. coli* [STEC]) that binds to receptors on human kidney, brain and gut cells, damaging them.

STEC live in the guts of ruminant animals, including cattle, goats, sheep, deer and elk. The major source of human illnesses is cattle. STEC that cause human illness generally do not make animals sick. Other kinds of animals, including pigs and birds, sometimes pick up STEC from the environment and may spread it. Foods implicated can include unpasteurized (raw) milk, unpasteurized apple cider, and soft cheeses made from raw milk. Sometimes the contact is obvious (e.g. working with cows or changing nappies) but sometimes it is not (e.g. eating undercooked hamburger or contaminated lettuce). People have been infected by swallowing water while swimming, touching the environment in zoos, and eating food prepared by people who did not wash their hands well.

The strain of STEC O104:H4 that caused a large outbreak in Europe in 2011 was referred to as EHEC. The most common STEC in North America is *E. coli* O157:H7 (*E. coli* O157 or simply 'O157').

Other *E. coli* serogroups in the STEC group, including *E. coli* O145, are sometimes called 'non-O157 STECs'. Some types of STEC frequently cause severe disease, including bloody diarrhoea and haemolytic uraemic syndrome (HUS).

Clinical features

After an incubation period of 3–4 days (1–10 days), abdominal pain or non-bloody diarrhoea appears and worsens over several days. While people can become infected at any age, very young children and older people are more likely to develop severe illness and HUS. The symptoms of STEC infections vary but often include severe stomach cramps, diarrhoea (often bloody) and vomiting. If there is fever, it usually is not very high (less than 38.5°C). Most people recover within 5–7 days.

Around 5–10% of those who are diagnosed with STEC infection develop HUS and manifest decreased frequency of urination, malaise and anorexia. HUS, if it occurs, develops an average 7 days after the first symptoms, when the diarrhoea is improving. Persons with HUS should be hospitalized because renal failure is possible.

General management

STEC infections are usually diagnosed through laboratory testing of faecal specimens. Non-specific supportive therapy, including hydration, is important. There is no evidence that treatment with antibiotics is helpful, and taking antibiotics may increase the risk of HUS. Antidiarrheal agents may also increase that risk.

STEC typically disappear from the faeces by the time the illness is clinically resolved but may be shed for several weeks, even after symptoms go away. Young children tend to carry STEC longer than adults. A few people keep shedding these bacteria for several months.

INVASIVE MENINGOCOCCAL DISEASE

Meningococcal infection is typically caused by *Neisseria menigitidis*. Of the 13 *N. meningitides* serotypes, only A, B, C, W135 and Y are clinically important. *N. meningitides* serogroups A, B and C account for up to 90% of disease worldwide. W135 has emerged in recent years in Africa and the Middle East. Serogroups B and C are responsible for most cases in Europe and the Americas, serogroups A and C in Asia and Africa. Worldwide, the highest rates of infection occur in the meningitis belt of sub-Saharan Africa – from Senegal in the west, to Ethiopia in the east.

High-risk groups for invasive meningococcal disease include:

■ people living in dormitories
■ microbiologists who are routinely exposed to isolates of *N. meningitidis*
■ people visiting countries where *N. meningitidis* is hyperendemic or epidemic (e.g. for Haj), particularly if contact with the local population is prolonged
■ people who have terminal complement component deficiencies
■ people who have asplenia.

The reservoir for *N. menigitidis* is exclusively human, the bacteria being carried in the nasopharynx. Transmission is via the respiratory route, from coughing and sneezing, during close contact with a carrier. Epidemics are seen during the winter–spring period in temperate areas and during the dry season in tropical areas.

Clinical features

Infection risk is highest in the first 7 days after exposure to an infected person and falls rapidly during the following week. The incubation period is 2–10 days. Meningococcal infection can cause mainly:

■ meningitis (49% of cases)
■ septicaemia (33%)
■ pneumonia (9%).

Infection can have an abrupt onset, with a rapid disease course and a case fatality rate of up to 15%; up to 20% of survivors suffer serious sequelae, including deafness, neurological deficit or limb loss. Meningococcal meningitis usually presents with sudden onset of fever, intense headache, nausea and vomiting. Neck stiffness from meningeal irritation is characteristic. A non-blanching petechial or purpuric rash usually occurs with septicaemia. Delirium, coma and shock can ensue.

General management

Suspected meningococcal infection is a medical emergency. On admission to hospital, parenteral antibiotics should be commenced immediately. Intensive care, monitoring and supportive treatment are necessary.

For practical purposes, a 7-day period is considered sufficient to identify close contacts for prophylaxis. The ideal protection is provided by simultaneous administration of an antimicrobial drug and quadrivalent meningococcal vaccine. This approach is particularly suitable for outbreaks because of prolonged risk of transmission.

Antibiotic prophylaxis should be given as soon as possible after diagnosis of the index case. The drug of choice is rifampicin 600 mg b.i.d. for 2 days, but a single dose of ciprofloxacin 500 mg or an intramuscular injection of ceftriaxone 250 mg may also be used. The protection lasts for several days to a few weeks. The risk for contacts is still significant after 2 weeks and may persist for 6 months or even longer. Therefore immunization should be considered.

There is no vaccine to protect against all forms of meningitis and associated diseases, including the most common in the UK – meningococcal group B and streptococcal group B. Routine UK immunization programme protects against *Haemophilus influenzae* b, meningitis C and, most recently, pneumococcal meningitis.

Quadrivalent A/C/W135/Y and bivalent A/C meningococcal vaccines are available in the UK. ACWY is needed for Haj/Umrah pilgrims (http://www.nathnac.org/pro/factsheets/Hajj_Umrah.htm; accessed 30 September 2013). There are two quadrivalent vaccines available in the UK: ACWY Vax® and Menveo®. See also Chapter 33.

Information for health professionals is available at: http://www.nathnac.org/pro/factsheets/index.htm (accessed 30 September 2013).

OTHER BACTERIAL INFECTIONS

Many other infections are seen, especially in the developing world (see Appendix 21.5).

VIRAL INFECTIONS

Viral infections are often transmitted readily in saliva and other body fluids; where general hygiene is low and there is close contact with other persons or their secretions, infections are common. They thus mainly affect young children, who often thereby acquire immunity. In developed countries, children may not contract these infections and thus are non-immune, and may have a primary infection as adolescents and adults.

Rashes (exanthemata) are common in some viral infections (Table 21.7).

Most viral infections are transient with few untoward sequelae, though many cause malaise, fever and depression of the immune system. Some viral infections can be immediately life-threatening (e.g. severe acute respiratory syndrome; SARS), others can result in tumours (e.g. hepatitis C and B and liver cancer), and others can seriously damage the immune system (e.g. HIV/AIDS; Ch. 20). Many viral infections can cause severe, recurrent, disseminated or persistent lesions in immunocompromised persons, such as those with organ transplants or HIV/AIDS.

Viral infections are often diagnosed on clinical grounds, supported by testing for immune responses (serology) and, increasingly, by examining for viral nucleic acids.

Antiherpetic and antiretroviral drugs can be effective (see the Appendices in Ch. 21) but relatively few other effective antiviral agents are available. Immunization against various viruses is available and should be taken up.

A wide range of infections is recognized (Table 21.8). This chapter discusses the important common viral infections, alphabetically; see

Table 21.7 Common childhood infections with rashes (exanthemata)

	Name	Alternative term
First disease	Measles	Rubeola
Second disease	Scarlet fever	Streptococci
Third disease	German measles	Rubella
Fourth disease	Filatov–Dukes disease	Doubt exists over the existence of this
Fifth disease	Erythema infectiosum ('slapped cheek syndrome')	Parvovirus
Sixth disease	Herpesvirus 6 infection ('exanthem subitum')	Roseola infantum

Table 21.8 Viral infections

Viral infection	Chapter location
Arboviruses	This chapter
Arenaviruses	This chapter
Enteroviruses	This chapter
Hantaviruses	This chapter
Hepatitis viruses	Ch. 9
Herpesviruses	This chapter
Human immunodeficiency viruses	Ch. 20
Influenza	Ch. 15
Measles	This chapter
Molluscum contagiosum	This chapter
Mumps	This chapter
Papillomaviruses	This chapter
Parvovirus	This chapter
Poliomyelitis	Ch. 13
Rabies	This chapter
Rhabdoviruses	This chapter
Rubella	This chapter
Severe acute respiratory syndrome (SARS)	Ch. 15

Appendices 21.8 and 21.9 for serious life-threatening but fortunately uncommon viral infections.

CHIKUNGUNYA

This is a togavirus (RNA) transmitted by the Asian Tiger mosquito (*Aedes albopictus*), found mainly in areas in, and bordering, the Indian Ocean. Similar to dengue and O'nyong'nyong, the incubation is 2–4 days, and clinical features may include;

- Oral ulceration
- Rash; central maculopapular
- Headache, malaise
- Arthralgia
- Fever to 39 degrees.

There are neither cures nor antiviral drug treatments.

ENTEROVIRUSES

Enteroviruses multiply in the gut mucosa and are transmitted from person to person by the faecal–oral route. Most infections are in childhood, often as small epidemics. Enterovirus infections are usually

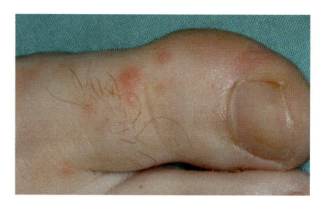

Fig. 21.3 Hand, foot and mouth disease.

transient but produce lifelong immunity to the strain. Clinical syndromes are generally mild but occasional infections may cause serious disease, such as paralytic poliomyelitis, meningitis or myocarditis.

Enterovirus diseases relevant to dentistry include hepatitis A (Ch. 9), poliomyelitis (Ch. 13), herpangina, and hand, foot and mouth disease.

HERPANGINA

Coxsackie viruses, usually A7 or B1, or echoviruses 9 or 17 cause infections, often subclinically. After an incubation of 2–9 days, clinical features may include mouth ulcers affecting the posterior mouth alone (soft palate and uvula) and causing sore throat, cervical lymphadenitis, fever, malaise, irritability, anorexia and sometimes vomiting. Diagnosis is from the clinical features. Management is symptomatic (see Herpes simplex).

HAND, FOOT AND MOUTH DISEASE

Picornaviruses (Coxsackie A and enterovirus [EV] 71) are responsible for most hand, foot and mouth disease (HFMD). Coxsackie (usually A16; rarely, A5 or 10) virus infections are often subclinical. However, the World Health Organization reported one outbreak in 2008 in China involving a total of 1884 cases, including 20 deaths, due to enterovirus EV-71.

Clinical features, after an incubation of 2–6 days, include mouth ulcers, resembling herpetic stomatitis, mild fever, malaise, anorexia and a rash. Red papules that evolve to superficial vesicles in a few days form mainly on the palms and soles (Fig. 21.3). Diagnosis is from the clinical features. Management is symptomatic (see Herpes simplex).

HERPESVIRUSES

The herpesviruses are DNA viruses, transmitted mainly in saliva and other body fluids (Table 21.9). They typically cause a short-lived primary clinical, or more often subclinical, infection, and remain latent thereafter. Reactivation is often because of immunosuppression and recrudescence can lead to protracted illness. Some herpesviruses can be oncogenic.

HERPES SIMPLEX VIRUS (HSV; HUMAN HERPESVIRUS TYPES 1 AND 2) INFECTIONS

General aspects

Type 1 herpes simples virus (HSV) typically causes primary oral infection with acute gingivostomatitis but may cause primary pharyngeal or anogenital infection. Type 2 HSV typically causes anogenital

Table 21.9 The herpesviruses

Herpesvirus type	Standard nomenclature	Abbreviation
1	Herpes simplex type 1	HSV-1
2	Herpes simplex type 2	HSV-2
3	Herpes varicella zoster	VZV
4	Epstein–Barr virus	EBV
5	Cytomegalovirus	CMV
6	Human herpesvirus type 6	HHV-6
7	Human herpesvirus type 7	HHV-7
8	Human herpesvirus type 8 (Kaposi sarcoma herpesvirus)	HHV-8 (KSHV)

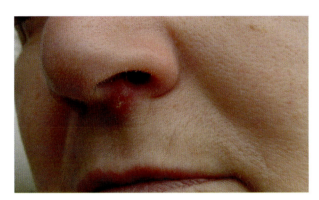

Fig. 21.4 Herpes simplex recurrent infection.

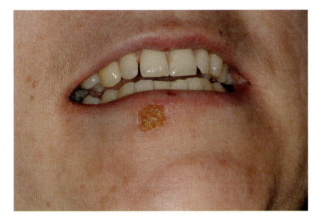

Fig. 21.5 Recurrent herpes labialis.

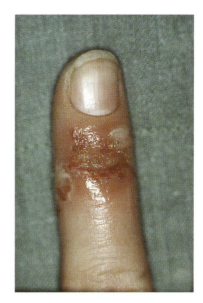

Fig. 21.6 Herpetic whitlow.

Table 21.10 Antiviral therapy considerations in common herpesvirus infections

Virus	Disease	Otherwise healthy patient	Immunocompromised patient
Herpes simplex	Primary	Consider oral aciclovir[a] 100–200 mg, five times daily as suspension (200 mg/5 mL) or tablets	Aciclovir 250 mg/m^2 i.v. every 8h
	Recurrent herpetic ulcers	Consider oral aciclovir[a] 100–200 mg, five times daily as suspension (200 mg/5 mL) or tablets	Consider aciclovir 250 mg/m^2 i.v. every 8h
	Recurrent herpes labialis	Penciclovir 1% cream or aciclovir 5% cream every 2h	Consider aciclovir 250 mg/m^2 i.v. every 8h
Herpes varicella	Chickenpox	–	Aciclovir 500 mg/m^2 (5 mg/kg) i.v. every 8h
	Zoster (shingles)	3% aciclovir ophthalmic ointment for shingles of ophthalmic division of trigeminal	Aciclovir 500 mg/m^2 (5 mg/kg) i.v. every 8h or famciclovir 250 mg three times daily, or 750 mg daily

Aciclovir: systemic preparations, caution in renal disease and pregnancy, occasional rise in liver enzymes and urea, rashes, CNS effects. Famciclovir: caution in renal disease and pregnancy. Occasional nausea and headache.
[a]In neonate, treat as if immunocompromised.

infections but may cause oral or oropharyngeal infections. HSV thereafter remains latent in the sensory ganglia but if reactivated may cause lesions. Recurrent infections typically affect the mucocutaneous junctions and are often precipitated by factors such as exposure to systemic infections, sunlight, trauma, stress, menstruation or immune incompetence (Figs 21.4 and 21.5).

Clinical features

Primary oral infection with HSV, usually type 1, typically causes acute gingivostomatitis, ulcers, fever, cervical lymph node enlargement and irritability. It is common in young children and sometimes misdiagnosed as 'teething', or may be subclinical. Primary herpetic gingivostomatitis is limited to the mouth and resolves within about 10 days but, in immunosuppressed patients or in those with eczema, disseminated infection may result.

Thereafter HSV remains latent, often in the trigeminal ganglia, but reactivates from time to time; it appears in the saliva and may cause

lesions. The virus can be spread by saliva and occasionally causes painful whitlows in dental staff not previously exposed to it (Fig. 21.6). A growing number of oral or oropharyngeal infections appear to be caused by HSV-2, which otherwise causes genital infections. Diagnosis is typically clinical.

Aciclovir is effective against HSV but many patients present with disease that is too far advanced for there to be any real benefit. Aciclovir, famciclovir and other antivirals are essential to control infection in immunocompromised patients (Table 21.10). Treatment is supplemented with supportive care, such as adequate fluid intake, antipyretics and analgesics (usually paracetamol [acetaminophen]), and good oral hygiene by mouth cleansing and use of aqueous chlorhexidine mouthwashes.

Recurrent infections appear in up to 30% of patients, typically at the mucocutaneous junction of the lip (herpes labialis; cold sores) or nose, and are often precipitated by exposure to systemic infections, sunlight, trauma, stress or menstruation. These factors stimulate HSV to reactivate by more than one mechanism. One way is by direct induction of viral genes such as *ICP4* and *VP16*. Heat can induce these viral genes either directly or via the by-products of heat. The activated viral gene products then overcome the effects of latent (LAT) RNAs. Another mechanism is an indirect one involving immunosuppression. Ultraviolet light is immunosuppressive and also induces cytokines that can trigger inflammation. These cytokines may affect dendrites that communicate the signal back to the neuron where the viral DNA is residing; *ICP4* and *VP16* are viral genes critical for reactivation.

Diagnosis is clinical. Recurrent labial infections respond well to penciclovir or aciclovir cream applied early. A patch with hydrocolloid particles and zinc sulphate is an alternative.

Intraoral recurrences appear as ulcers and seem to be more likely after trauma, such as in the palate, or in immunocompromised patients (e.g. leukaemia or HIV/AIDS). Aciclovir may be indicated but HSV is now showing starting to show resistance. Famciclovir, valaciclovir or even foscarnet may then be required.

Genital herpes

A person almost always contracts HSV-2 infection by sexual contact. HSV-1 infection of the genitals is almost always caused by oral–genital contact with a person who has oral HSV-1 infection. One out of five of the total adolescent and adult population in the USA are infected with HSV-2; the prevalence is rising but few have signs or symptoms. When signs of genital herpes do appear, they are typically as blisters on or around the genitals or rectum. The blisters break, leaving tender ulcers that may take 2–4 weeks to heal. It is important that women avoid contracting HSV-2 during pregnancy because a first episode during pregnancy causes a greater risk of transmission to the newborn. HSV-2 can cause potentially fatal infections in infants if the mother is shedding virus at the time of delivery. If a woman has active genital herpes at delivery, a Caesarean delivery is therefore usually performed.

Antiviral medications, such as aciclovir or famciclovir, can shorten and prevent outbreaks during the period the medication is being taken.

VARICELLA ZOSTER VIRUS (VZV; HUMAN HERPESVIRUS 3)

Chickenpox

General aspects

Varicella (chickenpox) is a highly contagious disease caused by the varicella zoster virus (VZV), spread readily by droplets. VZV is an exclusively human pathogen. The primary infection typically occurs during childhood and causes varicella. Patients are infectious from 1–2 days before the rash, until the rash scabs and dries.

During viraemia, VZV enters epidermal cells, causing the typical varicella rash; it then enters sensory nerves in mucocutaneous sites and travels through retrograde axonal transport to the sensory dorsal root ganglia adjacent to the spinal cord, where the virus establishes permanent latency in neuronal cell bodies. VZV then remains latent within dorsal root ganglia and, if reactivated, as can happen in older or immunocompromised people, can lead to shingles (zoster) – a painful unilateral rash.

More information on varicella and other infectious diseases may be found at: http://www.hpa.org.uk/Topics/InfectiousDiseases/InfectionsAZ/ (accessed September 2013).

Clinical features

Varicella is most common in children below the age of 10 years. There is fever, malaise and a centripetal rash (mainly on trunk and face), which passes through macular, papular, vesicular and pustular stages before scabbing. There are about 3–5 crops of lesions. There may be mouth ulcers.

Infants, adolescents, adults and immunocompromised persons are at higher risk for complications, such as disseminated or haemorrhagic varicella. Adults, especially those who are pregnant or who smoke, are at risk from fulminating varicella pneumonia. There is also a risk to the fetus and neonate if the mother contracts chickenpox. In the first 20 weeks of pregnancy, a congenital varicella syndrome with microcephaly, cataracts, growth retardation and limb hypoplasia may result, and the mortality rate is high. Later in pregnancy, chickenpox may result in zoster in an otherwise healthy infant. Chickenpox around the time of delivery may cause severe and even fatal infection of the neonate.

General management

Diagnosis is clinical. Varicella zoster immunoglobulin, or aciclovir, valaciclovir or famciclovir, may be indicated for non-immune persons who are pregnant or immunocompromised. Varicella vaccine is effective in preventing illness or modifying varicella severity if used within 3 days, and possibly up to 5 days of exposure.

Zoster

General aspects

VZV remains latent within dorsal root ganglia and may be reactivated, especially in the elderly or immunocompromised, leading to shingles (zoster). In about 8–10%, zoster may reflect an underlying immunodeficiency state, sometimes as a result of HIV/AIDS or a neoplasm, particularly a lymphoma.

Latent VZV infects approximately 98% of the adult population and is non-infectious but it can reactivate to migrate to the skin through axons, spread from cell to cell, and penetrate the epidermis, causing pain; this is followed by a vesicular rash distributed across closely overlapping dermatomes of the involved sensory nerve roots. VZV reactivation triggers are unclear but cell-mediated immunity (CMI) is important in controlling the development of zoster. The CMI components are partially or substantially maintained by periodic 'endogenous boosting' in response to subclinical reactivation or to 'exogenous boosting' in response to VZV circulating in the population as chickenpox.

Age is the most important risk factor for development of zoster. Approximately 50% of persons who live to the age of 85 years will have experienced zoster.

The incidence of zoster is increased substantially in persons with haematological malignancies and solid tumours. Patients with Hodgkin's disease are at particularly high risk for zoster. Zoster is common following haemopoietic stem cell transplantation (HSCT) and following solid organ transplants (renal, cardiac, liver and lung; 5–17%). Incidence is highest during the months immediately following the procedure, and the majority of zoster cases occur within a year of transplantation. The risk for zoster and its recurrence is elevated in persons infected with HIV.

The risk for zoster also appears to be higher in persons with inflammatory diseases. Zoster has been associated with systemic lupus erythematous (SLE), rheumatoid arthritis, granulomatosis with polyangiitis (formerly called Wegener granulomatosis), Crohn disease and ulcerative colitis, and possibly diabetes mellitus and multiple sclerosis.

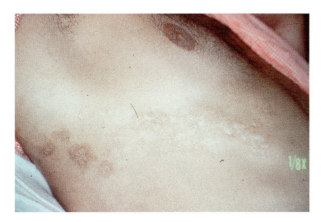

Fig. 21.7 Thoracic zoster.

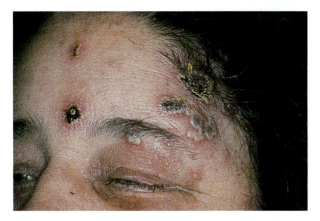

Fig. 21.8 Ophthalmic zoster.

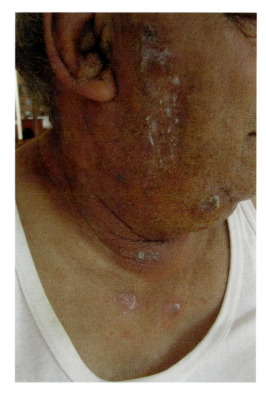

Fig. 21.9 Zoster in cervical nerves.

Zoster lesions contain high concentrations of VZV that can be spread, presumably by the airborne route, and cause primary varicella in exposed susceptible persons. Zoster is contagious after the rash erupts and until the lesions crust. It is less contagious than varicella, though transmission has been documented between patients or from patients to health-care personnel, but transmission from health-care personnel to patients has not been documented.

Clinical features

Zoster involves one or more contiguous sensory dermatomes, usually of the face or the chest, and causes severe pain and a rash similar to chickenpox but localized to the dermatome (Fig. 21.7). Trigeminal ophthalmic zoster may cause facial rash and pain, and ulcerate the cornea (Fig. 21.8). Zoster of the maxillary or mandibular divisions of the trigeminal nerve may cause facial rash and pain (sometimes simulating toothache) and oral ulceration – unilateral and in the nerve distribution.

Zoster is usually more severe in older adults, typically with a prodrome of headache, photophobia and malaise (Fig. 21.9). Abnormal skin sensations and aching, burning, stabbing or shock-like pain of varying severity are common and can precede the rash by days to weeks; rarely, they might constitute the only clinical manifestation (termed zoster sine herpete).

Zoster rash is typically unilateral and does not cross the midline, erupting in one or two adjacent dermatomes. Thoracic, cervical and ophthalmic involvement are most common. The rash is initially erythematous and maculopapular but progresses to coalescing clusters of clear vesicles over several days and then evolves through pustular, ulcer and crust stages over 7–10 days, with complete healing within 2–4 weeks.

A common consequence of zoster is post-herpetic neuralgia (PHN), a persistent pain after resolution of the rash. The duration of pain after rash resolution, used to define PHN, ranges from at least 30 days to 6 months or more after rash onset. PHN can last for weeks or months and occasionally for many years, and varies from mild to excruciating in severity; it may be constant, intermittent, or triggered by trivial stimuli.

Zoster may be associated with other complications too: 10–25% have eye involvement, called herpes zoster ophthalmicus (HZO). Keratitis occurs in approximately two-thirds of patients with HZO, often causing corneal ulceration. Other sequelae include conjunctivitis, uveitis, episcleritis and scleritis, retinitis, choroiditis, optic neuritis, lid retraction, ptosis and glaucoma. Extraocular muscle palsies also occur. Ramsay Hunt syndrome is an uncommon complication, in which there is a peripheral facial nerve palsy accompanied by reactivation of VZV in the geniculate ganglion of the facial nerve with zoster vesicles on the ear, hard palate or tongue. Occasionally, zoster can cause motor weakness in noncranial nerve distributions, called zoster paresis; this develops abruptly within 2–3 weeks of the rash and can involve upper or lower extremities. Diaphragmatic paralysis has also been described. Zoster can also result in autonomic dysfunction, causing urinary retention and colon pseudo-obstruction. Rarely, patients will experience acute focal neurological deficits weeks to months after resolution of the rash, with myelitis, aseptic meningitis, meningoencephalitis or Guillain–Barré syndrome.

In immunocompromised persons, the rash tends to be more severe and its duration prolonged; there may be dissemination and it is a marker for VZV viraemia that can seed the lungs, liver, gut and brain, and cause pneumonia, hepatitis, encephalitis and disseminated intravascular coagulopathy. Neurological zoster complications are increased in immunocompromised persons and can be aggressive and even fatal; they include myelitis, chronic encephalitis, ventriculitis, meningoencephalitis and cranial palsies.

General management

Diagnosis is clinical and might not be possible in the absence of a rash. VZV obtained from lesions can be identified using tissue culture, but this can take several days and false negative results occur because viable virus is difficult to recover from cutaneous lesions. Direct fluo-rescent antibody (DFA) staining of VZV-infected cells in a scraping of cells from the base of the lesion is rapid and sensitive. DFA and other antigen-detection methods can also be used on biopsy material, and eosinophilic nuclear inclusions (Cowdry type A) are observed on histopathology. Polymerase chain reaction (PCR) techniques can be used to detect VZV DNA rapidly and sensitively.

Treatment of zoster is with aciclovir, valaciclovir or famciclovir by mouth, given within 3 days of the appearance of the rash. Intravenous administration is needed in immunodeficient patients, particularly in those with HIV/AIDS, for whom it can be a life-threatening disease.

An urgent ophthalmological opinion should be sought for patients with ophthalmic zoster. Aciclovir, famciclovir and valaciclovir are approved by the US Food and Drug Administration (FDA) for treat-ment of zoster; they reduce the duration of viral shedding and lesion formation, and decrease the time to rash healing, the severity and duration of acute pain from zoster, and the risk for progression to PHN. Even with antiviral treatment, fatality from dissemination is 5–15%, with most deaths attributable to pneumonia.

The pain of herpetic neuralgia may not respond well to analgesics but tricyclic antidepressants, carbamazepine or capsaicin may be of value. Other treatments for postherpetic pain include skin stimula-tion of the painful area by prolonged rubbing with a soft cloth; firm pressure with the flat of the hand or the ball of the thumb; massage; acupuncture; local heat; a cold spray; or transcutaneous electric nerve stimulation (TENS).

Immunization of children against VZV reduces the risk of zoster at a later age. However, if immunity wanes with age, there may be epidem-ics of chickenpox in the middle-aged, and if the middle-aged who have had chickenpox do not receive occasional boosts of their immunity by exposure to chickenpox (which has been prevented in children by vac-cination), the incidence of shingles may rise. In immunocompromised patients who are exposed to VZV, it may be desirable to give zoster immunoglobulin or vaccine.

If a person susceptible to varicella infection has close exposure to a person with zoster, postexposure prophylaxis with varicella vaccine or VARIZIG™ should be considered. Zoster vaccine may be offered to older patients and is now offered in UK to those over 70.

EPSTEIN–BARR VIRUS (EBV; HUMAN HERPESVIRUS 4)

General aspects

Epstein–Barr virus (EBV) causes infectious mononucleosis (IM; clas-sic glandular fever). EBV also has epidemiological associations with Burkitt and some other lymphomas, and with nasopharyngeal car-cinoma. EBV may also cause sialadenitis (see later) and, in immuno-compromised patients, may be associated with hairy leukoplakia (Ch. 20) or lymphomas.

Clinical features

EBV is found in saliva during IM and for several months thereafter. It is also often in the saliva of immunocompromised persons. Though infectivity is low, EBV appears to be spread by close oral contact, such as kissing.

Infection is common among young adults but is often subclinical or unrecognized, especially in children. IM mainly causes lymphadeno-pathy, sore throat and fever but is protean in its manifestations (glan-dular fever). Glandular fever is a syndrome in which fever, malaise and lymph node enlargement are the main features; though typically

- Cytomegalovirus infection
- Epstein–Barr virus infection (infectious mononucleosis)
- HIV infection
- Human herpesvirus 6 infection
- Infectious lymphocytosis (babesiosis; *Bordetella pertussis*; brucellosis; cat scratch disease; Coxsackie, hepatitis, influenza, mumps, rubella, syphilis, TB; varicella)
- Toxoplasmosis
- Rarely: acute leukaemia; drug-induced hypersensitivity syndrome (DIHS; drug reaction with eosinophilia and systemic symptoms [DRESS] syndrome)

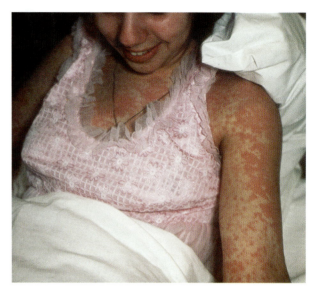

Fig. 21.10 Infectious mononucleosis.

caused by EBV, other infectious agents are occasionally responsible (Box 21.7).

IM can appear in many forms:

- *Febrile type IM* – high fever with rubelliform rashes and occasionally jaundice
- *Anginose type IM* – sore throat with soft palate petechiae and a whitish exudate confined to the tonsils, and pharyngeal oedema that may threaten the airway (to be distinguished from diphtheria) and petechiae on the palate. The latter are occasionally seen in other viral infections, such as rubella and HIV. Occasionally, there is mouth ulceration
- *Glandular type IM* – generalized, especially cervical lymph node enlargement and splenomegaly. IM is an important cause of enlarged cervical lymph nodes. Unfortunately, the lymph node histopathological changes closely resemble those in lymphomas and an expert opinion is needed.

Complications of IM include persistent fatigue, mild liver dysfunc-tion, ECG changes, depression, neurological syndromes and, rarely, nephritis, pancreatitis or lung infiltration. Ampicillin and amoxicillin frequently cause a maculopapular rash (which is not an allergy), affect-ing the extensor surfaces of limbs (Fig. 21.10).

General management

Characteristic blood changes of IM are an excess of atypical lympho-cytes (mononucleosis); these may cause confusion with leukaemia – but for the absence of anaemia. Occasionally, there is also mild neutropenia or thrombocytopenia.

Serological tests for IM include heterophile antibodies and EBV antibodies. Heterophile antibodies are immunoglobulin M (IgM) antibodies that agglutinate sheep and horse red blood cells. The Paul–Bunnell heterophile antibody test uses sheep erythrocytes, but a more rapid method identifies heterophile antibodies (to horse red blood cells) by detecting agglutination on a glass slide (Monospot test). Heterophile antibodies usually develop during the first or second week of the illness (60% of patients), and by 4 weeks up to 90% of patients have a titre before absorption of 224, which then declines and disappears over 3–6 months.

EBV-specific laboratory tests on a single acute-phase serum sample can help determine whether a person is susceptible to EBV, has had recent infection, has had past infection, or has reactivated EBV infection (Table 21.11).

When the Monospot (Paul–Bunnell) test is negative, the best testing combination is of:

- IgM and IgG to viral capsid antigen (VCA): IgM appears early in infection and disappears within 4–6 weeks. IgG to VCA appears in the acute phase, peaking at 2–4 weeks after onset, declining slightly and then persisting for life
- IgM to early antigen (EA), and IgG to EA: these appear in the acute phase and generally fall to undetectable levels after 3–6 months
- antibody to EBV nuclear antigen (EBNA): this slowly appears 2–4 months after onset and persists for life. Some EBNA enzyme immunoassays can detect antibody sooner.

However, even when EBV antibody tests suggest that reactivated infection is present, this does not necessarily indicate that the current illness is caused by EBV infection, since a number of healthy people continue to have antibodies to EBV EA for years. There may be a false positive Wassermann reaction.

Infection with EBV is usually acute and self-limiting, and no reliably effective specific treatment is available. As malaise and fatigue are frequent accompaniments, however, the patient may benefit from bed rest. Systemic corticosteroids are required if there is severe pharyngeal oedema that poses a hazard to the airway. Nearly 20% of patients have concurrent beta-haemolytic streptococcal pharyngeal infection, for which penicillin may be given. Tinidazole may improve the sore throat.

Burkitt lymphoma

Burkitt lymphoma, found predominantly in Africa in children below 12 years of age, presents with massive swellings that affect the mandible in particular; there is pain, paraesthesia and bone destruction, causing tooth mobility, jaw radiolucencies and destruction of the lamina dura. It appears to be related to EBV in association with malaria.

Table 21.11 Diagnosis in Epstein–Barr virus (EBV) infection

EBV nuclear antigen (EBNA) antibody	Other EBV antibodies	Interpretation
Absent	Viral capsid antigen (VCA) antibodies absent	Susceptible
Absent	VCA immunoglobulin M (IgM) antibody present	Primary infection
	VCA IgG antibody rising or high	
Present	VCA antibodies present	Past infection
Present	Early antigen (EA) antibodies present	Reactivation

Burkitt lymphoma may also be seen outside of Africa and can be a complication of HIV/AIDS. Chemotherapy is remarkably effective but relapse is common.

Hairy leukoplakia in HIV/AIDS
See Chapter 20.

Lymphomas
See Chapter 8.

Nasopharyngeal carcinoma
See Chapters 14 and 22.

CYTOMEGALOVIRUS (CMV; HUMAN HERPESVIRUS 5)

Cytomegalovirus (CMV) is a ubiquitous herpesvirus found in large quantities in the saliva and urine of infected persons.

Primary infections are mostly asymptomatic but some cause a glandular fever-like illness. Thereafter CMV remains latent in oropharyngeal and other epithelial cells, and may be reactivated by immunosuppression and other factors. Under these circumstances, disseminated infection can cause CMV retinitis in particular, often leading to blindness. CMV infection is a particular problem in HIV/AIDS (Ch. 20).

The other main problem identified in relation to CMV is its potential to cause fetal damage. A range of infections of the pregnant mother, especially in the first trimester, can cause fetal damage, that can sometimes be fatal. These include *to*xoplasmosis, *r*ubella, *c*ytomegalovirus and *h*erpes simplex virus (TORCH syndrome). When less severe, they may cause mild hearing loss; alternatively, they may result in learning disability, pneumonitis, cardiac malformations, microophthalmia, microcephaly, jaundice and low birth weight. CMV is thereafter excreted by the neonate in urine and saliva for many months.

Antiviral therapy for CMV includes ganciclovir or foscarnet.

HUMAN HERPESVIRUS 6

Human herpesvirus 6 (HHV-6) is a T-cell lymphotropic herpesvirus that is almost invariably contracted via oropharyngeal secretions within the first 2 years of life.

HHV-6 causes a febrile illness, sometimes with a macular or papular rash on the face and/or trunk (exanthema subitum; roseola infantum; sixth disease), mild diarrhoea, cough, oedematous eyelids and occasionally sialadenitis, hepatitis, meningitis or meningo-encephalitis or blood dyscrasias (particularly granulocytopenia). Erythematous papules (Nagayama spots) may appear on the soft palate and uvula and pharynx. Cervical lymphadenopathy is detectable in about one-third of patients. HHV-6 infection in later life may produce a glandular fever syndrome, persistent lymphadenopathy, chronic fatigue syndrome or hepatitis.

Thereafter, HHV-6 remains latent. Immunocompromised patients may suffer reactivation of HHV-6 with pneumonitis, retinitis, encephalitis or bone marrow failure, and it may have a cofactorial role in HIV infection. There are suggested but certainly unproven associations with multiple sclerosis and various neoplasms.

HHV-6 is inhibited by ganciclovir, foscarnet (phosphonoformate, PFA) and phosphonoacetic acid (PAA) but is relatively resistant to aciclovir.

HUMAN HERPESVIRUS 7

Human herpesvirus 7 (HHV-7) is T-lymphotropic; it is not known to be related to any human disease but might be a cofactor in HHV-6–related syndromes and may cause rashes.

HUMAN HERPESVIRUS 8

Human herpesvirus 8 (HHV-8; Kaposi sarcoma herpesvirus, KSHV) is a B-lymphotropic DNA virus, transmitted mainly by sexual contact. It is strongly associated with Kaposi sarcoma and body cavity-based lymphomas. It is present in saliva but there are as yet no documented cases of nosocomial transmission to health-care workers. There is no specific effective treatment but ART (Ch. 20) may play an indirect role in clearing HHV-8 from HIV-infected patients.

HUMAN IMMUNODEFICIENCY VIRUSES

See Chapter 20.

MEASLES

Measles is an acute infection with the measles virus, transmitted by droplet infection, with an incubation period of about 10–14 days. Whitish spots in the buccal mucosa (Koplik spots) herald the onset. The illness consists of fever, coryza, conjunctivitis and a maculopapular rash. Complications include bronchitis, pneumonia, otitis media, convulsions and encephalitis (which has a mortality of 15% – highest in infants – and leaves a neurological deficit in up to 40%). Subacute sclerosing panencephalitis (SSPE) is a late complication.

Immunization is indicated in early childhood (Appendix 21.7) and had almost abolished measles, until the recent decline over concerns about immunization.

MOLLUSCUM CONTAGIOSUM

Molluscum contagiosum is a viral infection that spreads easily among children; in adults, it may be sexually transmitted and is common in HIV/AIDS. Characteristic umbilicated papules may be seen on the face and elsewhere. Local application of trichloracetic acid effectively burns the lesions off.

MUMPS

Mumps was a common infection, usually caused by the mumps virus and spread by droplet infection; it is now mostly eliminated by vaccination. Of 101 specimens in a recent study on mumps, 38 were positive for a single virus: Epstein-Barr virus (in 23), human herpesvirus (HHV)-6B (10), human parainfluenza virus (HPIV)-2 (3), HPIV-3 (1), and human bocavirus (1). Mumps virus itself, enteroviruses (including human parechovirus), HHV-6A, HPIV-1, and adenoviruses were not detected. Mumps-like illnesses are occasionally caused by adenoviruses or echoviruses.

The incubation period is 14–21 days and mumps is transmissible from 2 or 3 days before parotitis appears until several days afterwards. Mumps causes swellings involving particularly the major salivary glands, usually the parotids (Fig. 21.11). One or both parotids become enlarged and tender (parotitis) with trismus, and oedema and erythema of the orifice of the parotid duct (papillitis). The other major salivary glands may also be affected but rarely in the absence of parotitis. Mumps should always be considered in the differential diagnosis of acute swellings of salivary glands, particularly in the young. Complications of mumps are uncommon but include deafness, pancreatitis, meningo-encephalitis, orchitis and oophoritis in particular. The latter conditions rarely cause sterility, even if bilateral.

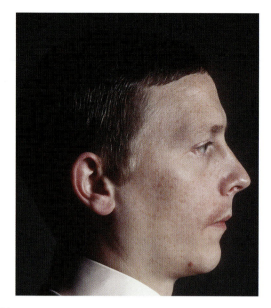

Fig. 21.11 Mumps.

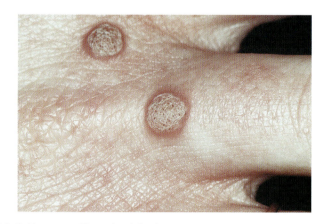

Fig. 21.12 Human papillomavirus infection: common warts.

There is no antiviral agent available for use against mumps. Mumps immunization is carried out in childhood.

PAPILLOMAVIRUSES (HUMAN PAPILLOMAVIRUSES; HPVS)

Human papillomaviruses (HPVs) are ubiquitous DNA viruses. Over 100 HPV types are recognized; they are transmissible and mostly cause benign warts and other epithelial lesions affecting skin and mucosae, including mouth and genitals. Skin warts (verruca vulgaris) are common (Figs 21.12 and 21.13), especially in children, and spread mainly from close contact or in wet environments such as changing rooms. Genital warts (condylomata acuminata) are caused by HPV and may be found on the penis, vulva or vagina or perianally, or may be unseen in the urethral meatus or cervix. Around one-third of young American women have genital HPV infection. About 65% of sexual contacts of patients with genital warts develop warts after an incubation period that may exceed 2 years.

Some HPVs cause oral warts (verruca vulgaris) and papillomas. Heck disease (focal epithelial hyperplasia) is an unusual oral condition caused by specific HPV (types 13 and 32), mainly in ethnic groups such as Inuits and American Indians.

Some HPVs are closely associated with malignant disease; for example, HPV-16, 18 and 33 appear to be associated with cervical carcinoma. HPVs may also be associated with some oropharyngeal carcinomas.

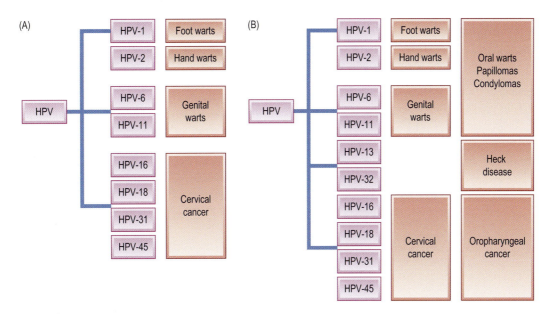

Fig. 21.13 Human papillomavirus infections.

Local surgery or podophyllum resin has been the usual treatments for non-malignant HPV-related lesions. Immune stimulators such as interferon-alpha and imiquimod are now available.

HPV vaccines protect against the types of HPV that cause most cervical cancers. There are two vaccines, both of which are safe and are usually given as a three-shot series:

■ Cervarix: recommended for females from 10 to 25 years of age, and protects against HPV 16 and 18.
■ Gardasil: recommended for 11–26-year-old females and also for 9- to 26-year-old males to protect against some genital warts. This vaccine protects against HPV 6, 11, 16 and 18.

There is no statistically significant increased risk for stroke, thromboembolism, appendicitis, seizures, syncope, allergic reactions, Guillain–Barré syndrome and anaphylaxis but the most common adverse events reported from vaccination have been:

■ syncope – common, especially in pre-teens and teens
■ local pain and redness at the site of immunization
■ dizziness
■ nausea
■ headache
■ venous thromboembolism – 90% had a known other risk factor, such as smoking, obesity or hormonal contraceptives.

PARVOVIRUSES

Parvoviruses are among the smallest, simplest DNA viruses and cause infections in a variety of birds and mammals. The only known human parvovirus is B19, which is transmitted by droplets, touch and occasionally in blood, and usually has an incubation period of 4–14 days. Parvoviruses tend to infect rapidly dividing tissues, most commonly the fetus, the intestinal epithelium or the haemopoietic system. A total of 70–90% of most adult populations is seropositive for B19.

Parvovirus commonly causes fifth disease (erythema infectiosum; slapped cheek syndrome), a mild illness with a lace-like rash on the face, trunk and extremities, usually in children. In approximately 80% of patients, there is also arthropathy – temporary arthritis-like joint involvement (particularly in adults). Since the vaccination-induced disappearance of rubella, parvovirus is the commonest cause of infection-related transitory arthritis, particularly if it affects the hands.

B19 also causes acute depression of red blood cell production, a transient event of little clinical significance, except in patients with other haematological diseases, particularly sickle cell disease, when haemolytic crises may be precipitated. B19 infection in pregnancy is associated with early fetal loss, although the probability of this appears to be low (less than 10%). There is no specific therapy for parvoviruses.

RUBELLA (GERMAN MEASLES)

ACQUIRED RUBELLA

Rubella, caused by rubella virus, is a highly infectious but usually mild disease, spread by droplet infection, with an incubation period of about 14–21 days.

In children, rubella causes a minor macular rash, starting on the face and behind the ears, mild fever, sore throat and enlarged lymph nodes (including the posterior auricular and suboccipital posterior cervical nodes). In adults, rubella may cause arthritis or arthralgia.

No antiviral treatment is available for rubella. Immunization is available and indicated for health-care workers. After rubella immunization, immunity is long-lasting.

CONGENITAL RUBELLA

Rubella infection during the first trimester of pregnancy can damage the fetus, causing problems ranging from deafness to death. If the fetus survives, learning disability, retinopathy and cataracts, cardiac malformations and deafness may result (major rubella syndrome). The infant may also have liver damage, bone defects and thrombocytopenic purpura. The virus is excreted, particularly in the urine, for months after birth (see TORCH syndrome). Pregnant females should thus consider whether or not they are immune to rubella. Rashes resembling rubella (rubelliform rashes) are also common in enterovirus and other infections, and thus a *clinical* diagnosis of rubella may not always be accurate unless confirmed serologically. Females who believe they have had rubella (and thus think they are immune) may in fact be non-immune and they and any fetus may be at risk. Antibody titres should be assayed to determine their actual immune status.

Rubella immunization of non-immune pre-pubertal females is the most effective prophylaxis and should be given to female health-care staff who are not known to be immune, who are seronegative, and who

Table 21.12 *Confirmation of diagnosis of rubella*

Suspected rubella infection of patient	Suspected rubella contact
1. Test acute serum for haemagglutination inhibition (HAI) antibody to rubella	1. Test acute serum for HAI antibody to rubella
2. If HAI-positive in acute serum, reassure. If HAI continues negative, reassure	2. Test serum of the contact for rubella. If HAI-negative, reassure
3. If HAI-negative but then rises, offer termination or rubella immunoglobulin	3. If pregnant woman has rubella antibodies already, reassure
	4. If pregnant woman has no immunity and contact is, or is suspected of being, rubella-positive, retest patient's sera for HAI. If HAI continues negative, reassure. If HAI becomes positive, offer termination or rubella immunoglobulin

Table 21.13 *Fungal infections*

Fungal infection	Chapter location
Aspergillosis	This chapter
Blastomycosis (North American blastomycosis)	This chapter
Candidosis	This chapter
Coccidioidomycosis	This chapter
Cryptococcosis	This chapter
Histoplasmosis	This chapter
Mucormycosis (zygomycosis)	This chapter
Paracoccidioidomycosis (South American blastomycosis)	This chapter
Pneumocystosis	This chapter
Rhinosporidiosis	This chapter
Sporotrichosis	This chapter
Tinea	This chapter

are not pregnant and are unlikely to become pregnant within the following 2 months. Rubella immunization should also be given to males who, as health-care workers, may come into contact with pregnant women.

Because of the danger to the fetus, pregnant patients exposed to, or developing, rubella or a similar rash should have serological investigation. The haemagglutination inhibition (HAI) test for rubella antibodies is rapid and reliable; antibody titre rises within 48 hours of illness or immunization, persists for years, and is useful for differentiating past infection from acute illness. Serum should be obtained within 2 days of the onset of the illness or within 2 weeks of exposure to the virus. If this acute serum is not available, complement fixation tests or assay of rubella-specific IgM antibody is required (Table 21.12).

OTHER VIRAL INFECTIONS

See Appendix 21.9.

MYCOSES (FUNGAL INFECTIONS)

Fungi are widespread and sometimes commensals, but infections may occur where general hygiene is low, where suitable local conditions (humid sites) are present and where people are immunocompromised, such as those with organ transplants or HIV/AIDS.

Fungal infections (Table 21.13) are often diagnosed on clinical grounds, supported by culture. Antifungal drugs can be effective therapy but resistance may arise, especially in long-term use or HIV/AIDS (Appendix 21.10). Most fungal infections have few untoward sequelae in otherwise healthy people but some can cause severe, recurrent, disseminated or persistent lesions in immunocompromised persons (Appendix 21.11).

SUPERFICIAL MYCOSES

The common superficial mycoses are candidosis and tinea.

CANDIDOSIS

Candidosis (candidiasis) is infection with *Candida* species, usually *Candida albicans*. Candidosis can produce a variety of clinical pictures but thrush is the best-known type. Thrush was aptly described in the nineteenth century as a 'disease of the diseased', and candidosis can

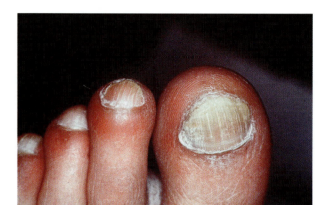

Fig. 21.14 Candidosis.

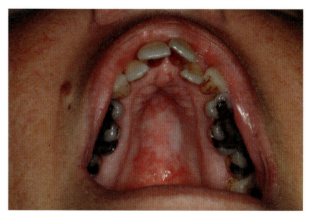

Fig. 21.15 Candidosis.

undoubtedly be a reflection of impaired immune responses. This has become particularly evident since HIV/AIDS was first recognized. *Candida* is one of many other fungi that can cause severe, recurrent, disseminated or persistent lesions in immunocompromised persons, such as those with AIDS (Figs 21.14 and 21.15).

Candida species other than *C. albicans* can cause candidosis (Table 21.14), particularly in immunocompromised individuals, and some, especially *C. krusei*, are resistant to conventional antifungal agents. Correction of any underlying local cause, and use of antifungals, is the usual treatment for candidosis. Topical gentian violet is now rarely used as an antifungal. Topical nystatin or an azole such as miconazole or fluconazole are the usual treatments. Nystatin is available as a suspension, miconazole as a gel or gingival muco-adhesive tablet.

Table 21.14 Candida *species*

Most common	Less common
Candida albicans	Candida zeylanoides
Candida tropicalis	Candida viswanathii
Candida glabrata	Candida rugosa
Candida parapsilosis	Candida lambica
Candida krusei	Candida norvegensis
Candida lusitaniae	Candida lipolytica
Candida kefyr	Candida famata
Candida guilliermondii	Candida ciferrii
Candida dubliniensis	

Table 21.15 *Factors predisposing to mycoses*

Predisposing factor	Aetiological agent(s)
Cell-mediated immune defects	Candida spp., Cryptococcus neoformans, Histoplasma capsulatum, Coccidioides immitis
	Paracoccidioides brasiliensis, Blastomyces dermatitidis
Chronic granulomatous disease	Aspergillus spp., Candida albicans, Torulopsis glabrata
Desferrioxamine therapy	Agents of zygomycosis
Intravenous drug abuse	Candida spp., agents of zygomycosis
Ketoacidosis	Agents of zygomycosis
Malnutrition	Candida spp., agents of zygomycosis
Moisture	Trichophyton spp.
Neutropenia	Candida spp., Aspergillus spp., agents of zygomycosis, Pseudallescheria boydii, Trichosporon spp., Fusarium spp.
Traumatized skin	Candida spp., Torulopsis glabrata, Malassezia furfur

Thrush

General aspects and clinical features

Thrush produces a highly characteristic picture of soft, creamy-coloured, slightly raised patches that *can be wiped off the mucosa*, leaving red areas. These lesions may form isolated flecks or large confluent areas. Typical sites are the vagina or mouth.

Thrush is common in the newborn, in whom it does not usually indicate any immunodeficiency and may resolve spontaneously or in response to topical antifungal treatment. In adults, unless they are known to be having immunosuppressive treatment, thrush is rare and should prompt investigation for an underlying cause. Thrush in a young or middle-aged adult must be regarded as a possible sign of HIV infection until proved otherwise. The other main predisposing factors are antibiotic treatment, anaemia, diabetes mellitus or an immunological defect, as shown in Table 21.15.

General management

The diagnosis is usually clinical but can be readily confirmed by taking a Gram-stained smear, which shows long tangled masses of candidal hyphae.

Superficial fungal infections often respond readily to topical treatment but deep-seated infections often require protracted systemic therapy. In addition to treatment of any underlying disorder, localized thrush should be manageable with topical antifungal drugs such as nystatin or amphotericin. Alternatively, a nystatin suspension or systemic fluconazole or suspension may be indicated.

Erythematous candidosis

General aspects and clinical features

Erythematous candidosis appears as mucosal erythema, in the mouth due to coverage of the mucosa with a denture (denture-related stomatitis; denture sore mouth), antibiotic treatment, xerostomia or immunodeficiency. Denture-related stomatitis (denture-associated stomatitis) is a common infection secondary to long-standing occlusion of part of the oral mucosa by a denture. Denture-related stomatitis typically develops beneath a well-fitting upper denture, which effectively cuts off the mucous membrane from the normal oral defence mechanisms. It is not seen under a lower denture, in spite of the fact that the latter is a common cause of trauma. The characteristic feature is uniform bright erythema of the whole of the upper denture-bearing area, limited by the denture margin. Occasionally, the erythema is patchy or there may be flecks of thrush. Symptoms are typically absent but occasionally there is soreness. Angular stomatitis is frequently associated. The vast majority of patients are healthy, as local factors alone determine the pathogenesis. Occasionally, patients may be anaemic but less frequently than might be expected from the fact that angular stomatitis is often regarded as a typical sign of iron deficiency. Other occasional contributory factors are dry mouth, diabetes mellitus or immune defects. It is, however, unjustifiable to screen all patients with denture-related stomatitis but investigation should be considered if the patient has any other complaints suggestive of such disorders or if the infection is particularly severe or intractable. Treatment includes leaving dentures out of the mouth at night and storing them in hypochlorite to clear the fungus from the denture surface. Topical antifungals should also be used, as suggested above, or the fitting surface of the denture can be coated with miconazole.

Antibiotic stomatitis occasionally follows the use of broad-spectrum antibiotics, particularly tetracycline used topically in the mouth. The whole of the oral mucosa is then typically red, oedematous and sore. One or two flecks of thrush may be found in protected situations, such as the posterior upper buccal sulcus. A similar picture of generalized redness and soreness of the oral mucosa is the typical manifestation of candidosis related to xerostomia. As with any other type of candidosis, angular stomatitis may be associated.

Xerostomia may also underlie erythematous candidosis. In HIV infection a patch of erythematous candidosis is sometimes seen on the palate or tongue.

General management

The treatment of erythematous candidosis is to deal with the underlying problem, if feasible, and to give antifungal drugs as described earlier.

Angular stomatitis

General and clinical aspects

Angular stomatitis (angular cheilitis; cheilosis) is most frequently seen as a complication of denture-related stomatitis but can be associated with any type of intraoral candidosis; in addition, it is a 'classic' sign of a deficiency anaemia.

General management

It is important to consider the possibility of underlying systemic disease, and treat it where possible.

Clearance of intraoral candidosis with adequate antifungal treatment typically leads to healing of the lesions at the angles of the mouth without any local treatment, but miconazole cream applied to the lesion may be useful. Occasionally, bacteriological examination may be necessary, as the cause may be staphylococcal, but imidazoles such as miconazole or clotrimazole also have antibacterial activity and may be effective.

Candidal leukoplakia

General aspects and clinical features

Candidal leukoplakia (chronic hyperplastic candidosis) appears as white plaques clinically indistinguishable from other types of keratotic lesion, though they may be speckled, tough and firmly adherent; they are seen mainly in men of middle age or over, many of whom are heavy smokers. Typical sites are the buccal mucosa just within the commissures, or the dorsum or edges of the tongue. Long-standing angular stomatitis and occasionally also denture-related stomatitis may be associated. Patients are usually otherwise well.

Candidal leukoplakia may account for up to 10% of leukoplakias and several reports of malignant transformation have appeared. However, the prevalence of candidal leukoplakia and its potentialities remain uncertain.

General management

Diagnosis depends on biopsy, showing *C. albicans* hyphae and a characteristic inflammatory reaction in the superficial epithelial plaque. Investigations should include a family history and haematological examination. Investigations for cell-mediated responses to *C. albicans* may be needed to exclude one of the rare mucocutaneous candidosis syndromes that show similar oral lesions, as described below, but in most cases no abnormality is detectable.

Treatment is difficult, since the response to topical antifungal drugs such as nystatin or amphotericin is poor, and excision is also followed by recurrence. Antifungals like miconazole topically or ketoconazole or fluconazole systemically appear to be more effective.

Persistent candidosis

General aspects and clinical features

Persistent candidosis is a well-recognized complication of defective cell-mediated immunity (Box 21.8).

Both thrush and herpetic infection may be present together and produce confluent lesions.

General management

Candidal infection usually responds eventually to antifungal drugs but sometimes immunosuppressive treatment has to be moderated for a time. Patients on long-term corticosteroid treatment for any of the immunologically mediated diseases are also susceptible to oral candidosis but not often as a serious complication.

Box 21.8 *Causes of persistent candidosis*

- HIV infection
- Primary immunodeficiencies, especially severe combined (Swiss) type or DiGeorge syndrome
- Chronic mucocutaneous candidosis (CMCC)
- Intense immunosuppression, particularly for organ grafts
- Resistant *Candida* species

Chronic mucocutaneous candidosis (CMC or CMCC)

See Chapter 20.

'Chronic candidiasis syndrome'

Many normal persons, around half the population, harbour *C. albicans* as part of their normal microflora. This finding has been exploited as a supposed explanation of such symptoms as headaches, fatigue and lassitude, rashes and gastrointestinal symptoms, but this so-called syndrome has absolutely no scientific basis, and there is no evidence that antifungal treatment is warranted. A controlled trial has shown that it has no effect on the symptoms.

TINEA

General aspects and clinical features

Tinea is a term for a range of common skin infections seen worldwide; they are caused by dermatophytes, usually *Trichophyton* (Table 21.16; Figs 21.16 and 21.17). Dermatophytes, specifically *Trichophyton*, *Epidermophyton* and *Microsporum* species, are responsible for most superficial fungal infections. Fungal transmission occurs through direct contact with infected persons, animals, soil or fomites.

General management

Treatment of tinea is with topical clotrimazole, miconazole or terbinafine, or oral fluconazole, itraconazole or terbinafine.

Dental aspects

Terbinafine may disturb taste. Azoles may enhance the effects of warfarin (Ch. 8).

Table 21.16 Forms of tinea

Tinea	Features	Organisms
Barbae	Beard area	*Trichophyton verrucosum*
Capitis ('ringworm')	Head; itchy, red areas, leaving bald patches	*Trichophyton tonsurans* *Microsporum andouinii* *Microsporum canis*
Corporis	Red spots growing into large rings on arms, legs or chest	*Trichophyton rubrum* *M. canis* *T. tonsurans* *T. verrucosum*
Cruris	Itchy erythema in moist, warm areas, e.g. the groin ('jock itch') or beneath the breasts (Fig. 21.16). Second most common tinea	*T. rubrum* *Epidermophyton floccosum*
Pedis (athlete's foot)	Most common tinea. Itchy and red moist skin between toes (Fig. 21.17), with a white, wet surface. Infection may spread to the toenails (tinea unguium – from Latin for nail). Toenails become thick and crumbly	*T. rubrum* *Trichophyton mentagrophytes var. interdigitale* *E. floccosum*
Versicolor	Patchy skin discolouration. Areas of infected face, for example, may appear lighter in colour (hypopigmented). Seen primarily in young adults	*Malassezia furfur*

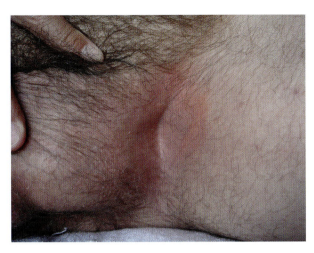

Fig. 21.16 Tinea cruris.

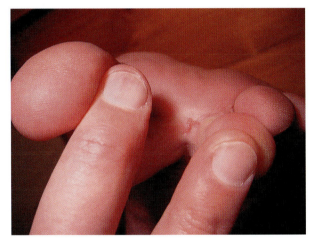

Fig. 21.17 Tinea pedis.

SYSTEMIC MYCOSES (DEEP MYCOSES)

Healthy individuals in endemic areas (often in the developing world) are often infected with fungi, typically involving the lungs but often asymptomatic. In otherwise healthy persons, even acute pulmonary and primary mucocutaneous symptomatic mycotic lesions may resolve spontaneously. Chronic pulmonary infections tend to progress and disseminated infections can be fatal. Immunocompromised persons are at particular risk from clinical disease. Equally, clinical infection with mycoses may be an indication of an underlying immune defect. Severe, recurrent, disseminated or persistent lesions appear in immunocompromised persons, particularly those with HIV/AIDS, organ transplants, leukaemia, leukopenia, solid tumours or burns, and in premature infants.

The proliferation of mycoses in immunocompromised persons includes 'new' opportunists such as new *Candida* species, *Torulopsis glabrata*, *Fusarium* and *Trichosporon beigelii*.

Orofacial lesions caused by the main systemic mycoses may occasionally be seen in isolation but they are typically associated with lesions elsewhere, often in the respiratory tract. The diagnosis may be suggested by a tumour-like nodule or mass, chronic oral ulceration, chronic sinus infection or bizarre mouth lesions, especially in immunocompromised patients or in those who have been in endemic areas, or where there is granuloma formation found on biopsy. Investigations include smear, biopsy, culture, sometimes serology, physical examination and chest radiography. Tissue forms of the fungus may be visible but special stains are often required.

Patients should be managed in consultation with a physician with appropriate expertise, usually with systemic antimycotics. Most systemic mycoses can be treated with systemic amphotericin given orally, liposomally or slowly intravenously, or with azoles. Adverse effects from intravenous amphotericin include thrombophlebitis, nephrotoxicity, chills, nausea, anaemia and hypokalaemia. The azoles are less toxic but the cost is prohibitive where they are most needed – in the developing world. Given orally, the adverse effects of ketoconazole include nausea, gynaecomastia and liver damage. The main adverse effects of miconazole include thrombophlebitis and ventricular tachycardia. Fluconazole and itraconazole are therefore now being used but fluconazole resistance can be a significant problem.

SYSTEMIC CANDIDOSIS

Candidosis is typically a superficial mycosis but, nevertheless, increasingly often causes invasion of deep organs, particularly in immunocompromised persons. Many *Candida* species are now responsible; some are resistant to fluconazole but voriconazole or caspofungin may be effective.

PNEUMOCYSTIS JIROVECI (CARINII)

General aspects and clinical features

Pneumocystis jiroveci (carinii) is now recognized to be a fungus rather than a protozoan. Some of the first patients recognized in the HIV epidemic were revealed because of *Pneumocystis* pneumonia (PCP); it is a common infection in AIDS and other severely immunocompromised patients.

General management

Treatment is with co-trimoxazole, inhaled pentamidine isetionate or atovaquone.

ASPERGILLOSIS

General aspects and clinical features

Aspergillus species are the most common environmental fungi and are prolific saprophytes in soil and decaying vegetation.

Aspergillosis is found worldwide; it is increasing in frequency and is the most prevalent mycosis after candidosis. Inhalation of *Aspergillus* spores and colonization of the respiratory tract are common but disease is rare. Types of aspergillosis include the following:

- *Allergic bronchopulmonary aspergillosis* – the most common disease
- *Invasive aspergillosis* – a rare lung infection that may spread to brain, bone or endocardium. Invasive sinus aspergillosis affects mainly immunocompromised hosts, though it is also seen in some apparently healthy individuals in subtropical countries, such as Sudan, Saudi Arabia or India
- *Aspergillus fumigatus* – the usual cause of invasive sinus aspergillosis, although *A. flavus* appears to predominate in immunocompromised patients. There is destruction of the antral wall and often antral pain, swelling or sequelae from orbital invasion (impaired ocular motility, exophthalmos or impaired vision) or intracranial extension (headaches, meningism)

- *Aspergillomas* – fungus balls that grow in pre-existing cavities, such as tuberculous lung cavities. Aspergilloma of the maxillary antrum is uncommon, typically appearing in a healthy host as a hyphal ball in a chronically obstructed sinus
- *Chronic sinus aspergillosis* – an uncommon cause of a diffusely radio-opaque antrum, sometimes with dense punctate radio-opacities. It is unresponsive to treatment used for bacterial sinusitis. Occasional cases of sinus aspergillosis are a result of metastasis from pulmonary aspergillosis or are iatrogenic, following dental procedures such as extractions
- *Allergic fungal sinusitis* – an uncommon problem, usually due to fungi other than *Aspergillus*.

General management

Diagnosis of antral aspergillosis is supported by MRI and CT (which are more sensitive than conventional radiography in detecting bone erosion) and confirmed by smear and lesional microscopy, staining with periodic acid–Schiff (PAS) or Gomori methenamine silver. Immunostains may help definitive diagnosis.

Prolonged conservative therapy may worsen the prognosis. Topical ketoconazole or clotrimazole may clear superficial infections. If there is no resolution in 72 hours, a course of systemic amphotericin should be tried. Miconazole is not active and ketoconazole is not particularly active against *Aspergillus*, but itraconazole may have a place in treatment. Fluconazole is under trial.

Non-invasive antral forms usually need treatment by antral debridement and drainage. Corticosteroids may also be indicated in allergic sinusitis.

Invasive aspergillosis should be treated by surgical debridement supplemented with amphotericin and, possibly, hyperbaric oxygen.

BLASTOMYCOSES

General aspects and clinical features

Blastomyces dermatitidis causes North American blastomycosis, seen predominantly in the USA and Canada. *Paracoccidioides brasiliensis* causes the South American form, seen especially in Brazil. Inhalation of spores, found in soil, leads to subclinical infection in up to 90% of the population in endemic areas. Outdoor workers are particularly affected.

Clinical illness is typically pulmonary. HIV infection and other immunocompromising states predispose to pulmonary and disseminated disease.

General management

Diagnosis is based on biopsy, smear or culture. Amphotericin, ketoconazole, miconazole, itraconazole and voriconazole can be effective.

COCCIDIOIDOMYCOSIS

General aspects and clinical features

Coccidioidomycosis is seen mainly in hot dry areas of the south-west USA, Mexico, Central America and parts of South America. Inhalation of spores of *Coccidioides immitis*, found in soil, produces subclinical infection in up to 90% of the population. Clinical illness is typically acute pulmonary disease and fever (San Joaquin valley fever). Chronic pulmonary disease is less common but pregnant women, blacks, Filipinos, Mexicans and immunocompromised persons are susceptible.

General management

Diagnosis is mainly by history and examination, supported by histology and the spherulin or coccidioidin skin tests. Management is with systemic amphotericin, sometimes supplemented with ketoconazole, itraconazole, fluconazole or voriconazole.

CRYPTOCOCCOSIS

General aspects and clinical features

Cryptococcosis is seen worldwide. Aspiration of spores of *Cryptococcus neoformans*, a yeast found especially in pigeon faeces and soil, may lead to infection. In healthy persons, infection is typically pulmonary and subclinical. Immunocompromised persons are liable to dissemination of infection to meninges, heart, spleen, pancreas, adrenals, ovaries, muscles, bones, liver and gastrointestinal tract. Most patients with disseminated cryptococcosis have meningoencephalitis and, untreated, this is fatal in over 70%.

Cryptococcosis is the most common systemic mycosis in AIDS.

General management

Diagnosis is confirmed by microscopy, culture and assay of serum or cerebrospinal fluid for capsular antigen and antibody. Systemic amphotericin is effective, best supplemented with flucytosine. Ketoconazole and itraconazole may be effective.

HISTOPLASMOSIS

General aspects and clinical features

Histoplasmosis is found worldwide and is the most frequent systemic mycosis in the USA. *Histoplasma capsulatum* is present especially in bird and bat faeces and is a soil saprophyte found particularly in the Ohio and Mississippi valleys, Latin America, India, the Far East and Australia. In endemic areas, over 70% of adults are infected, typically subclinically, by inhaling spores. Clinical histoplasmosis includes acute and chronic pulmonary and cutaneous forms. Disseminated and potentially fatal histoplasmosis, which can affect the reticuloendothelial system, lungs, kidneys and gastrointestinal tract, is rare and seen typically in immunocompromised patients, especially in HIV/AIDS.

General management

Diagnosis is confirmed by microscopy, culture and serotests. Amphotericin is the first line for treatment, followed by ketoconazole, fluconazole, itraconazole or voriconazole.

MUCORMYCOSIS (ZYGOMYCOSIS; PHYCOMYCOSIS)

General aspects and clinical features

Mucorales are responsible for most mucormycosis. *Mucor*, *Rhizopus* and many other species of the class Zygomycetes can be responsible and therefore the condition is probably better termed zygomycosis. These fungi are ubiquitous worldwide in soil, manure and decaying organic matter, and can commonly be cultured from the nose, throat, mouth and faeces of healthy individuals.

Immunocompromising conditions underlie most zygomycosis; diabetes mellitus and leukaemia are the most important underlying causes but cases are now appearing in HIV/AIDS and malnutrition. Rhinocerebral and pulmonary zygomycoses are the most common forms.

Rhinocerebral zygomycosis is usually caused by *Rhizopus oryzae*; it typically starts in the nasal cavity or paranasal sinuses with pain and nasal discharge, accompanied by fever, and may then invade the palate, orbit or skull. Orbital invasion may cause orbital cellulitis, impaired ocular movements, proptosis and ptosis. Intracranial invasion follows penetration of ophthalmic vessels or the cribriform plate.

General management

Zygomycosis used to be almost uniformly fatal and still has a mortality approaching 20%. Radiography or MRI typically shows thickening of the antral mucosa with patchy destruction of the walls, and may define the extent of the lesion.

Diagnosis is confirmed by smears and histological demonstration of tissue invasion by hyphae. Control of underlying disease is essential, if at all possible, together with systemic amphotericin and surgical debridement.

RHINOSPORIDIOSIS

Rhinosporidium seeberi can infect the nasal and other mucosae. It is particularly common in India and Sri Lanka, but also found in Latin America, Africa and South-East Asia. Mouth lesions are usually proliferative lumps on the palate. Diagnosis is by biopsy. Surgery is required for treatment.

SPOROTRICHOSIS

Sporothrix schenckii is found throughout the world, mainly as a saprophyte on plants and shrubs. Disease is seen almost exclusively in visitors to tropical and subtropical countries. Infection follows an injury to the epithelium resulting in a primary lesion – a sporotrichotic chancre. Lesions may then spread by the lymphatics. Pulmonary and disseminated sporotrichoses are rare and of uncertain origin.

Diagnosis is confirmed by histology and culture. Potassium iodide is effective treatment for superficial sporotrichosis, itraconazole or amphotericin for other forms.

CRYPTOSPORIDIOSIS ('CRYPTO')

Cryptosporidiosis is a diarrhoeal disease spread in animal and human faeces; it is one of the most frequent causes of water-borne disease among humans and can be spread by drinking and recreational water. *Cryptosporidium* is a parasite found throughout the world in soil, food, water or surfaces that have been contaminated with faeces from infected humans or animals. *Cryptosporidium* survives outside the body for long periods of time, and is resistant to chlorine disinfection. It is not spread by contact with blood but exposure to human faeces through sexual contact may transmit infection. People who are most likely to become infected with *Cryptosporidium* include:

- children who attend day-care centres
- child-care workers
- people who take care of others with cryptosporidiosis
- international travellers
- backpackers, hikers and campers who drink unfiltered, untreated water

- people who drink from untreated shallow, unprotected wells
- people, including swimmers, who swallow water from contaminated sources
- people who handle infected cattle
- people exposed to human faeces through sexual contact.

Although cryptosporidiosis can infect anyone, young children, pregnant women and the immunocompromised are likely to develop more serious illness.

Clinical features

The incubation period is 2–10 days (average 7 days). Some people with cryptosporidiosis have no symptoms but the most common symptom is watery diarrhoea. Other features include:

- abdominal pain
- nausea
- vomiting
- dehydration
- fever
- weight loss.

General management

Treatment for cryptosporidiosis is nitazoxanide.

INFESTATIONS

Parasitic infestations are endemic in the tropics and developing world, and are seen increasingly frequently in developed countries, in travellers or immigrants; infection is usually acquired from animals (zoonotic parasites), water or improperly prepared food. Common parasitic infestations include fleas, lice, mites and ticks, all transmitted between humans, particularly in conditions of poor hygiene and close-living and in war areas; sometimes disease can be fatal. Serious parasitic infections are shown in Box 21.9 and Appendix 21.12.

Since the appearance of the HIV/AIDS pandemic, parasitic infestations, especially toxoplasmosis and leishmaniasis, are now being recognized in HIV-infected patients.

Many parasitic infestations can be prevented by avoidance of insect bites (avoiding areas of high prevalence, maintaining good hand and food hygiene, and using protective clothing and insect repellents), especially at high-risk times (dusk is the worst time for many mosquitoes, though dengue is transmitted by mosquitoes that bite during the day). Many parasitic infestations are difficult to diagnose unless there is a high index of suspicion. Clinicians and pathologists should therefore

---

Box 21.9 *Main parasitic infestations*

- Amoebiasis – common in the developing world; causes gastrointestinal disease
- Giardiasis – common worldwide; causes gastrointestinal disease
- Leishmaniasis – common in the tropics and around the Mediterranean; may cause skin lesions
- Malaria – one of the more serious infestations worldwide; common in the tropics, where anopheline mosquitoes survive; causes haemolysis
- Toxoplasmosis – one of the more serious infestations worldwide; endemic in the developing world, relatively common in the developed world; causes eye and CNS disease
- Worms, fleas, lice, ticks, mites and maggots (Ch. 33)

be vigilant, especially when examining lesions in travellers or immigrants. Treatments include a range of medications, and patients should be managed in consultation with a specialist physician.

AMOEBIASIS

General aspects and clinical features

Entamoeba histolytica can cause amoebic dysentery or amoebic liver abscesses.

General management

Metronidazole is used. Diloxanide furoate clears cysts from symptomless patients.

GIARDIASIS

General aspects and clinical features

Giardia lamblia is a protozoon, cysts of which may be found in unfiltered drinking and recreational waters contaminated by faeces of humans or animals in many parts of the world. Features include anorexia, chronic diarrhoea, abdominal cramps, bloating, frequent loose greasy stools, fatigue and weight loss.

General management

Treatment is with metronidazole, tinidazole or mepacrine.

LEISHMANIASIS

General aspects and clinical features

A blood-sucking sandfly is the intermediate host; humans or other vertebrates, including dogs and cats, are the definitive hosts. The developmental stage is the amastigote in the vertebrate host and promastigote in the arthropod host. After inoculation into the skin, leishmanias multiply within histiocytes. Leishmaniasis is one of the most common HIV/AIDS-associated opportunistic infections in Spain. Human *Leishmania* species, although similar in morphology and life cycle to one another, produce different types of infection.

Mucocutaneous leishmaniasis usually has an incubation period of 2–8 weeks but it can be as long as 3 years. An itching papule at the site of the sandfly bite (usually on the face) becomes surrounded by gradually spreading erythema and induration. In a few days, the surface crusts, then breaks down to form a slowly extending ulcer that discharges fluid. Healing usually begins in 3–12 months, leaving a scar. Secondary lesions develop at the mucocutaneous junctions many years after the primary infection and are destructive. The nose is the site of predilection.

Visceral leishmaniasis causes fever, splenomegaly, anaemia, wasting, cough and diarrhea, and is potentially fatal.

General management

Clinical and serological tests are useful diagnostically but the demonstration of the parasite in biopsies or smears is definitive. A leishmanin skin test is also available. Mucocutaneous leishmaniasis may heal spontaneously but, since there can be extensive destruction of tissue, chemotherapy is indicated.

Pentavalent antimony as sodium stibogluconate or meglumine antimonate is usually effective. Alternatives are amphotericin or pentamidine isetionate. Miltefosine is the only available oral treatment for visceral, cutaneous, and mucosal leishmaniasis.

MALARIA

General aspects and clinical features

Malaria is the most serious and common parasitic infection worldwide; it still infects over 100 million persons, mainly in tropical areas of Africa, Latin America and Asia. It is transmitted by mosquito bites and is potentially fatal.

There are four main species of the protozoon, usually *Plasmodium falciparum* or *P. vivax*, sometimes *P. ovale* or *P. malariae*. In highly endemic areas, the patient may become infected with one, two or even more species of the malarial parasite. In India, 4–8% of cases are due to mixed infection. The plasmodium infects erythrocytes and damages them, causing haemolysis, as well as fever, myalgia, headaches and, in some cases, cerebral involvement. Infection with *P. falciparum* is the most dangerous (Table 21.17) and often fatal (malignant malaria) due to haemolysis and sludging in intracerebral vessels. Infection with *P. vivax*, *P. ovale* or *P. malariae* is usually benign.

Typical features of malaria are incapacitating episodes of hyperexia, rigors and chills, sometimes recurring for years.

Table 21.17 Malaria

Plasmodium	Comments	Chloroquine resistance
falciparum	Widespread. Results in the most severe infections and responsible for nearly all malaria-related deaths. 'Severe' and 'complicated' are the terms used more frequently than 'malignant' to describe this type of malaria	Chloroquine-resistant strains found in South America, Central America east of the Panama Canal, the Western Pacific, East Asia and sub-Saharan Africa. Resistance to combination of pyrimethamine and sulfadoxine in South-East Asia, Amazon Basin and sub-Saharan Africa. Variable degrees of resistance to quinine and quinidine in South-East Asia and Oceania, and in sub-Saharan Africa
malariae	Restricted distribution in India and responsible for less than 1% of infections	No chloroquine resistance
ovale	A rare parasite of humans; mostly confined to tropical Africa	No chloroquine resistance
vivax	The widest geographical distribution throughout the world. Causes much debilitating but relatively mild disease, which is seldom fatal. Also called benign or uncomplicated malaria	High levels of chloroquine resistance in Indonesia and Papua New Guinea, also Solomon Islands, Myanmar, Brazil, Colombia. Resistance to pyrimethamine and sulfadoxine, particularly in South-East Asia

General management

Diagnosis is made from the history of travel to a malarial area and from clinical features, confirmed by demonstrating the parasite in a blood smear. Repeated smears may be required.

Treatment of *P. malariae* disease is usually chloroquine; that of *P. ovale* and *P. vivax* malaria is usually chloroquine followed by primaquine; and that of *P. falciparum* infections (which are often drug-resistant, particularly in Asia and Latin America) is currently with quinine, mefloquine or artesunate or artemether or artemether with lumefantrine.

Prophylaxis

Specialist advice should always be sought before travel to the tropics. Disease is transmitted by the bite of an infected mosquito, and clothing, insect repellents and nets reduce the risk. Prophylactic chemotherapy does not guarantee total protection but may be life-saving. It may be with chloroquine and/or proguanil, but mefloquine or doxycycline or proguanil plus atovaquone is recommended where the malaria risk is high and chloroquine resistance likely; it should commence well before entering the malarial area and continue for 6 weeks after leaving.

TOXOPLASMOSIS

General aspects and clinical features

Toxoplasma gondii is a common intestinal parasite of many animals, particularly cats. Infection is contracted mainly from the ingestion of cysts, either from animal faeces or in inadequately cooked food (up to 10% of lamb and pork contains cysts). *Toxoplasma* may also be transmitted occasionally in infected blood or blood products.

T. gondii may cause a glandular fever-type of illness with fever and cervical lymphadenopathy, sometimes with rash, hepatosplenomegaly, myalgia and other minor features. Some patients may develop chorioretinitis, which threatens sight, severe pneumonia, necrotizing encephalitis or myocarditis, but such untoward sequelae are seen mainly if the patient is immunocompromised. Central nervous system (CNS) involvement is common, and can cause changes in mental status, headache, neurological defects and epilepsy. CT or MRI scans may demonstrate the lesions.

Toxoplasmosis in pregnancy may lead to chorioretinitis, or transplacental spread and fetal infection, with resultant congenital defects and blindness (TORCH syndrome; Fig. 21.18).

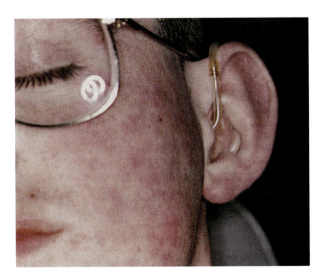

Fig. 21.18 Congenital toxoplasmosis causing learning impairment with visual and hearing defects.

General management

Toxoplasmosis is confirmed serologically by the Sabin–Feldman dye test, enzyme-linked immunosorbent assay (ELISA), indirect fluorescent antibody test or indirect haemagglutination test. The organism may be demonstrable in tissue sections or smears. Treatment is *not* usually required for asymptomatic healthy infected persons who are not pregnant. For immunocompromised patients with toxoplasmosis, treatment is a combination of pyrimethamine and sulfadiazine, together with folic acid (pyrimethamine is a folate antagonist), continued for at least 1 month after clinical resolution. Weekly full blood counts are essential.

For pregnant patients with toxoplasmosis, sulfadiazine alone is used since pyrimethamine may be teratogenic. Clindamycin, clarithromycin and azithromycin are alternatives.

WORMS

A range of helminths can occasionally infect humans (Table 21.18).

CYSTICERCOSIS

Cysticercus cellulosae (encysted larva of *Taenia solium*) can cause cysticercosis, which prevails in regions of poverty and where hygiene is insufficient, particularly Africa, the Far East, India, Latin America, Eastern Europe and the Iberian peninsula. It is rare in Jews and Muslims since they avoid pork.

General aspects and clinical features

The adult *T. solium* lives in the intestine of humans, the only definitive host. The stools release eggs, which, if they contaminate the ground,

Table 21.18 Worms (helminths)

Usual helminth	Geographical distribution	Therapy
Cestodes		
Cysticercus cellulosae (Taenia solium larvae)	Worldwide	Niclosamide Praziquantel
Echinococcus granulosus	Middle East, North and East Africa, Asia, Latin America, Australasia	Albendazole
Nematodes		
Ancylostoma duodenale	Mediterranean littoral, Middle East, China, India, South America	Mebendazole
Ascaris lumbricoides	Worldwide	Mebendazole Levamisole
Filariae	South-East Asia, India, East Africa, South America	Diethylcarbamazine Ivermectin
Gnathostoma spinigerum	South-East Asia	Albendazole Ivermectin
Gongylonema pulchrum	Former USSR, China, Sri Lanka	Albendazole
Onchocerca volvulus	Africa, Central America	Ivermectin Diethylcarbamazine
Schistosoma mansonii, S. haematobium or S. japonicum	Middle and Far East, Latin America, sub-Saharan Africa	Praziquantel
Trichinella spiralis	Worldwide	Mebendazole
Trichuris trichiura	South-East Asia	Mebendazole

can be swallowed by pigs. The eggs hatch in the pig's intestine, releasing oncospheres that enter the bloodstream and become encysted as cysticerci in muscle. Pork is then the intermediate host. The life cycle is completed when humans ingest inadequately cooked pork containing cysticerci (measly pork), which, upon reaching the human intestine, release the oncospheres. Oncospheres also penetrate the gut mucosa and are distributed to various tissues and organs, particularly muscles; here they develop into cysticerci, most commonly in the brain and eye, striated muscles in the tongue, neck and trunk, and skin and subcutaneous tissues.

General management

Prevention relies on thorough cooking of pork meat and good hygiene.

Diagnosis usually relies upon identification of the parasite. The appearance of the translucent membrane, with its central milky spot, is characteristic.

Praziquantel plus prednisolone (prednisone), or albendazole, or niclosamide can be curative. Single or even multiple parasites may be excised from tissues and organs.

ECHINOCOCCOSIS (ECHINOCOCCIASIS)

Echinococcosis (hydatid disease) is caused most often by larvae (cestodes) of the tapeworm *Echinococcus granulosus*. Echinococcosis has been a serious problem in many sheep-raising regions, most prevalently in Australia, New Zealand, South, East and North Africa, Mediterranean countries and parts of the Russian Federation, Middle East and Americas.

General aspects and clinical features

The adult tapeworm *E. granulosus* lives in the small intestine of sheep mainly, though many mammals can serve as intermediate hosts. The eggs hatch in the sheep's intestine, releasing oncospheres that penetrate the intestinal mucosa, enter the bloodstream and develop into hydatid cysts in various organs, particularly the liver and the lungs. Daughter cysts pass in the faeces. Dogs and wolves are infected by eating the discarded offal of sheep and deposit eggs in their faeces. Humans are an accidental intermediate host, usually infected by ingestion of eggs from the faeces of dogs, typically from improper hand-washing and, less often, by ingestion of contaminated water or food such as lamb or mutton containing cysts or eggs. The incubation is from 10 to 30 years. Only the larval stage, the hydatid cyst, develops in humans and there are no specific clinical signs until a cyst becomes large enough to act as a space-occupying lesion, causing compression of adjacent structures. Typically, the liver and sometimes the lungs, bone or brain are affected.

General management

A skin test (Casoni test) is available but not specific. Serology may be helpful. Eosinophilia is merely suggestive of a parasitic disease and not specific. The hydatid cyst can sometimes be demonstrated radiographically or by MRI or ultrasound, but a definitive diagnosis is often made only by identifying it at operation.

Prevention relies on protecting definitive hosts (dogs), as well as intermediate hosts (sheep), from contamination. Thorough hand-washing, washing of vegetables and wild berries located close to the ground, and elimination of contact with potentially contaminated dogs are the best measures. High doses of albendazole, mebendazole or flubendazole interfere with larval growth but are not curative. Only surgery is curative.

FILARIASIS

General aspects and clinical features

Filariae are helminths transmitted by the bite of blood-sucking insects, usually mosquitoes or black flies, whose adult and larval forms are found in humans. The main filariasis is onchocerciasis, seen mainly in tropical Africa but also in Saudi Arabia, Yemen and Latin America. It may involve the face, and eye lesions remain a major problem in Africa (river blindness). The diagnosis is made by identifying the worm in biopsies. Treatment is with ivermectin.

Lymphatic filariasis is infestation, particularly by *Wuchereria bancrofti* or *Brugia malayi*, transmitted by blood-sucking mosquitoes and most common in India, South-East Asia, the South Pacific, Latin America, East Africa and Egypt. The lymphatics are affected, causing obstructive oedema or elephantiasis. Diagnosis is from blood examination for filariae. Diethylcarbamazine is the treatment of choice.

GNATHOSTOMIASIS

Gnathostomiasis is a rare benign infestation, seen mainly in South and South-East Asia; it is caused by larvae of the nematode *Gnathostoma spinigerum*, harboured in chicken, snails or fish. The worm may cause swellings in the skin or mouth, or occasionally bleeding. Skin tests and serology help the diagnosis. Metronidazole, albendazole or ivermectin may be of some benefit or the worm can be excised.

LARVA MIGRANS

General aspects and clinical features

Adult hookworms live mainly in animal intestines and release ova into the faeces, which are then found in sand or soil contaminated by the animals. The ova hatch into infective larvae, which can infect human skin; here they fail to develop fully but may wander in the tissues, causing 'larva migrans'. Larva migrans is common in tropical climates, along the US coast from southern New Jersey to Florida, around the Caribbean and around the Mediterranean. It is seen especially in those working or playing in warm, moist, shaded sandy places.

There are two types of larva migrans:

- *Visceral larva migrans* is synonymous with toxocariasis – infection by larvae from roundworms of dogs, cats or wild carnivores
- *Cutaneous larva migrans* (creeping eruption) is caused by hookworms of dogs, cats and other mammals and characterized by itching serpiginous tracks, mainly on the feet, hands or buttocks.

Larva migrans is self-limiting but nearly 50% of patients can develop transient migratory pulmonary infiltrates with eosinophilia (Loeffler syndrome).

General management

Larva migrans can be prevented by stopping dogs, cats and other animals contaminating play areas. Treatments include thiabendazole, albendazole, ivermectin or mebendazole. Local application of 10% thiabendazole, ethyl chloride, chloroform, electrocoagulation and cryotherapy have been tried for cutaneous lesions.

THREADWORMS

General aspects and clinical features

Threadworms (*Enterobius vermicularis*; pinworms) are common infestations worldwide. The ova are swallowed and worms develop when

exposed to digestive juices of the upper gastrointestinal tract. Female worms lay ova on the anal skin, which cause intense peri-anal itching.

General management

Treatment must involve the whole family and includes mebendazole (or piperazine) and improved hygiene.

TRICHINOSIS

General aspects

Trichinosis is the most frequent roundworm infestation to affect muscles.

Trichinella spiralis is a nematode acquired through the ingestion of contaminated meat, usually pork products. Trichinosis is more prevalent in Central Europe and North America, where pork is widely consumed, than in Islamic or Jewish cultures or tropical countries. Both larval and adult forms of *T. spiralis* can parasitize humans as the definitive host but later they become the intermediate host when the larvae are established in the muscles. The same host sustains the adult worm temporarily, but the larvae for a long period of time. After ingestion of infected meat, the larvae mature to adult forms in the intestine in approximately 1 week. Adult female nematodes then deposit larvae in the gastrointestinal mucosa. The larvae penetrate and subsequently enter the bloodstream and pass to muscles such as the tongue, masseter, gastrocnemius, deltoid and diaphragm, where they grow and develop, and become encapsulated. Many infestations are subclinical but they can calcify and appear as radio-opaque nodules.

Clinical features

In mild infections, symptoms are often vague and transient. Acute trichinosis is characterized by myalgia, facial and palpebral oedema, and fever with eosinophilia. Myocarditis is present in up to 20% and there may be involvement of lungs, kidneys, pancreas and CNS.

General management

The diagnosis is clinical, supported by a history of ingestion of poorly cooked meat and by investigations. There is eosinophilic leukocytosis, serodiagnosis is feasible after the third week, and serum levels of muscle enzymes (such as creatine phosphokinase) are also raised. However, definitive diagnosis relies on biopsies from affected muscle or blind biopsies from the deltoid or gastrocnemius muscles.

Treatment is mebendazole or thiabendazole. Prevention requires meat to be cooked throughout at a temperature above 65°C.

TRICHURIASIS

General aspects and clinical features

Trichuriasis, infestation of the large intestine by the whipworm *Trichuris trichiura*, is common in the Caribbean and South-East Asia, especially in children, who contract the condition by ingesting eggs from contaminated soil.

General management

Trichuriasis is diagnosed by faecal examination for the worms. Treatment is mebendazole or albendazole.

MITES

General aspects and clinical features

Scabies is a common infestation with the mite *Sarcoptes scabiei*, which is transmitted by close contact, particularly in bed. The mite burrows into the superficial skin and lays eggs, which excite an inflammatory response and an itchy rash, typically interdigitally and on the wrists.

General management

Patient and family/partners need improved hygiene and treatment with malathion or permethrin.

MAGGOTS

General aspects and clinical features

Myiasis is the condition when fly maggots invade living tissue, most commonly the nose, or when they are harboured in the intestine or any part of the body and feed on the host's organs. Human myiasis is most common in the tropics.

Various flies can cause human myiasis; most troublesome in the New World is *Cochliomyia hominovorax* (screwworm). *Chrysomya bezziana* is seen in Africa, Asia, the Pacific Islands and the Old World.

Larvae burrow through tissue and may produce a type of larva migrans creeping eruption (see earlier); when they mature, they migrate out of the host in an effort to reach soil to pupate, and may then be visible.

General management

A few drops of turpentine or 15% chloroform in light vegetable oil should be instilled in the lesion and larvae should be removed with blunt tweezers.

PRION INFECTIONS

See Chapter 13.

KEY WEBSITES

(Accessed 29 May 2013)
Centers for Disease Control and Prevention. <http://www.cdc.gov/parasites/bedbugs/>.
National Center for Infectious Diseases. <http://www.cdc.gov/ncidod/diseases/eid/index.htm>.
National Institutes of Health: National Center for Biotechnology Information. <http://www.ncbi.nlm.nih.gov/books/NBK20370/>.
NHS Choices. <http://www.nhs.uk/conditions/Head-lice/Pages/Introduction.aspx>.
NHS Direct. <http://www.nhsdirect.nhs.uk/FemaleSexualHealthSelfCare/Worms>.

USEFUL WEBSITES

(Accessed 29 May 2013)
Centers for Disease Control and Prevention. <http://www.cdc.gov/Diseasesconditions>.
Department of Health's consultation draft of HTM 01-05 on Decontamination in primary care dental facilities. <https://www.gov.uk/government/publications/decontamination-in-primary-care-dental-practices>.
fitfortravel. <http://www.fitfortravel.nhs.uk/home.aspx>.
Medline Plus. <http://www.nlm.nih.gov/medlineplus/>.
Merck Manual Home Health Handbook for Patients & Caregivers. <http://www.merckmanuals.com/home/index.html>.

FURTHER READING

Almeida, O.D.P., et al. 2003. Paracoccidioidomycosis of the mouth: an emerging deep mycosis. Crit. Rev. Oral Biol. Med. 14, 377.

Barskey A.E., Juieng P., Whitaker B.L., Erdman D.D., Oberste M.S., Chern S.W., et al. Viruses detected among sporadic cases of parotitis, United States, 2009–2011. J. Infect. Dis. 2013;208(12):1979–1986. 10.1093/infdis/jit408. Epub 2013 Aug 9. PubMed PMID: 23935203.

Bedi, R., Scully, C., 2009. Tropical oral health. In: Cook, G.C., Zumla, A. (Eds.), Manson's tropical diseases (22nd ed.). WB Saunders/Elsevier, Edinburgh, pp. 499.

Berman, J., 2003. Current treatment approaches to leishmaniasis. Curr. Opin. Infect. Dis. 16, 397.

Beyari, M.M., et al. 2003. Multiple human herpesvirus-8 infection. J. Infect. Dis. 188, 678.

Bez, C., et al. 2000. Genoprevalence of TT virus among clinical and auxiliary UK dental health care workers: a pilot study. Br. Dent. J. 189, 554.

Boyanova, L., et al. 2006. Anaerobic bacteria in 118 patients with deep-space head and neck infections from the University Hospital of Maxillofacial Surgery, Sotia, Bulgaria. J. Med. Microbiol. 55, 1759.

Centers for Disease Control and Prevention, 2003. Guidelines for infection control in dental health care settings. MMWR 52, 10.

Cleveland, J.L., Cardo, D.M., 2003. Occupational exposures to human immunodeficiency virus, hepatitis B virus, and hepatitis C virus: risk, prevention and management. Dent. Clin. N. Am. 47, 681.

Cousin, G.C., 2002. Potentially fatal oro-facial infections: five cautionary tales. J. R. Coll. Surg. Edinb. 47, 585.

Cruse, P.J., 1970. Surgical wound sepsis. Can. Med. Assoc. J. 102, 251.

Cruse, P.J., Foord, R., 1980. The epidemiology of wound infection: a 10-year prospective study of 62,939 wounds. Surg. Clin. North Am. 60, 27.

Dawson, M.P., Smith, A.J., 2006. Superbugs and the dentist: an update. Dent. Update 33, 198.

Epstein, J.B., et al. 2003. Oral candidiasis in hematopoietic cell transplantation patients: an outcome-based analysis. Oral Surg. Oral Med. Oral Pathol. Oral Radiol. Endod. 96, 154.

Fishbain, J., Peleg, A.Y., 2010. Treatment of Acinetobacter infections. Clin. Infect. Dis. 51 (1), 79.

Garcia-Pola, M.J., et al. 2002. Submaxillary adenopathy as sole manifestation of toxoplasmosis: case report and literature review. J. Otolaryngol. 31, 122.

Groll, A.H., 2002. Itraconazole – perspectives for the management of invasive aspergillosis. Mycoses 45 (Suppl. 3), 48.

Gupta, A.K., Tomas, E., 2003. New antifungal agents. Dermatol. Clin. 21, 565.

Hay, R.J., 2003. Antifungal drugs used for systemic mycoses. Dermatol. Clin. 21, 577.

Hegarty, A.M., et al. 2008. Oral health care for HIV-infected patients: an international perspective. Expert Opin. Pharmacother. 9, 387.

Hodgson, T.A., Rachanis, C.C., 2002. Oral fungal and bacterial infections in HIV-infected individuals: an overview in Africa. Oral Dis. 8 (Suppl. 2), 80.

Holmstrup, P., et al. 2003. Oral infections and systemic diseases. Dent. Clin. North Am. 47, 575.

Karlsmark T., Goodman J.J., Drouault Y., Lufrano L., Pledger G.W. Cold Sore Study Group; Randomized clinical study comparing Compeed cold sore patch to acyclovir cream 5% in the treatment of herpes simplex labialis. J. Eur. Acad. Dermatol. Venereol. 2008;22(10):1184–1192.

Knouse, M.C., et al. 2002. Pseudomonas aeruginosa causing a right carotid artery mycotic aneurysm after a dental extraction procedure. Mayo Clin. Proc. 77, 1125.

Martin, S., 2001. Congenital toxoplasmosis. Neonatal. Netw. 20, 23.

Martins, M.D., et al. 2007. Orofacial lesions in treated southeast Brazilian leprosy patients: a cross-sectional study. Oral Dis. 13, 270.

Milian, M.A., et al. 2002. Oral leishmaniasis in an HIV-positive patient: report of a case involving the palate. Oral Dis. 8, 59.

Moraru, R.A., Grossman, M.E., 2000. Palatal necrosis in an AIDS patient: a case of mucormycosis. Cutis 66, 15.

Motta, A.C.F., et al. 2007. Oral leishmaniasis: a clinicopathological study of 11 cases. Oral Dis. 13, 335.

Nakamura, S., et al. 2002. Clostridial deep neck infection developed after extraction of a tooth: a case report and review of the literature in Japan. Oral Dis. 8, 224.

Nunez-Marti, J.M., et al. 2004. Leprosy: dental and periodontal status of the anterior maxilla in 76 patients. Oral Dis. 10, 19.

Ochandiano, S., 2000. Leprosy. Med. Oral 5, 316.

Phelan, J.A., 2003. Viruses and neoplastic growth. Dent. Clin. North Am. 47, 533.

Reichart, P.A., et al. 2002. High oral prevalence of Candida krusei in leprosy patients in northern Thailand. J. Clin. Microbiol. 40, 4479.

Reichart, P.A., et al. 2007. Prevalence of oral Candida species in leprosy patients from Cambodia and Thailand. J. Oral Pathol. Med. 36, 342.

Scott, L.A., Stone, M.S., 2003. Viral exanthems. Dermatol. Online J. 9, 4.

Silverman, S., Scully, C., 2000. Infectious diseases. In: Millard, D., Mason, D.K. (Eds.), 3rd World workshop on oral medicine. University of Michigan Press, Ann Arbor.

Sitheeque, M.A., Samaranayake, L.P., 2003. Chronic hyperplastic candidosis/candidiasis (candidal leukoplakia). Crit. Rev. Oral. Biol. Med. 14, 253.

Vargas, P.A., et al. 2003. Parotid gland involvement in advanced AIDS. Oral Dis. 9, 55.

Witherow, H., Swinson, B.D., Amin, M., Kalavrezos, N., Newman, L., 2004. Management of oral and maxillofacial infection. Hosp. Med. 65, 28–33.

APPENDIX 21.1 EMERGING INFECTIONS

Infection	Comments	Distributions
Acquired immunodeficiency syndrome (AIDS); human immunodeficiency virus (HIV)	Recognized in 1980s	Worldwide
Bovine spongiform encephalopathy (BSE; 'mad cow disease').	Prion disease first recognized in mid-1980s	UK mainly
Cholera new strain: 0139	Appeared in 1992 in south-eastern India	India, into western China, Thailand and other parts of South-East Asia
Cryptosporidiosis	Came to prominence in AIDs epidemic	Worldwide
Diphtheria	Epidemics since 1980s following lax vaccinations	Russian Federation and other former republics of the USSR
Ebola	Recorded in Zaire and Sudan in 1976; struck in Côte d'Ivoire in 1994 and 1995, Liberia in 1995, and again in Zaire in 1995	Africa, Asia, USA and Latin America
Enterococci strains	Outbreaks resistant to the main groups of antibiotics, such as the beta-lactams and the aminoglycosides	USA and other countries
Escherichia coli O157:H7 strain	Appeared in 1982	
Hantavirus pulmonary syndrome	First recognized in USA in 1993	Hantavirus infection has been detected in more than 20 US states, and has also surfaced in Argentina and Brazil. Other hantaviruses have been recognized for many years in Asia
Influenza pandemics	–	Worldwide
Resistant tuberculosis, malaria, cholera, dysentery, pneumonia, staphylococci, streptococci	–	Worldwide
		Resistance to multiple drugs is common in South-East Asia
Salmonella typhi, resistance to antibiotics	–	India and Pakistan in recent years
Salmonella typhimurium isolated from cattle is paralleled by increasing resistance among strains of human origin	–	Thailand
Shigella dysenteriae	–	Central and southern Africa

APPENDIX 21.2 SOME INFECTIOUS DISEASES: INCUBATION TIMES AND PERIOD OF INFECTIVITY

Incubation period	Disease	Incubation period	Period of infectivity
<1 week	Diphtheria	2–5 days	Until treated[a]
	Gonorrhoea	2–5 days	Until treated[a]
	Influenza	1–2 days	Until fever gone
	Scarlet fever	1–3 days	3 weeks after onset of rash
	Hand, foot and mouth	3–6 days	Until rash gone
1–2 weeks	Herpes	2–12 days	Until lesions gone[a]
	Measles	7–14 days	4 days after onset of rash
	Pertussis	7–10 days	21 days after onset of symptoms
2–3 weeks	Chickenpox	14–21 days	Until all lesions scab[a]
	Mumps	12–21 days	7 days after onset of sialadenitis
	Rubella	14–21 days	7 days after onset of rash
>3 weeks	Hepatitis A	2–6 weeks	Usually non-infective at diagnosis
	Hepatitis B	2–6 months	3 months after jaundice resolves[a]
	Hepatitis C	2–26 weeks	3 months after jaundice resolves[a]
	Human immunodeficiency virus (HIV)	Up to 5 y	Persists.[a] Average time from infection to acquired immunodeficiency syndrome (AIDS) is 10 y in the untreated
	Human papillomavirus (HPV)	30–180 days	While lesions present
	Infectious mononucleosis (Epstein–Barr virus)	30–50 days	Until fever resolved.[a] Once infected, patients intermittently excrete the virus asymptomatically for the rest of their lives. Thus most people who develop infectious mononucleosis have not had contact with someone who has had a recent illness
	Syphilis	10–90 days	Until treated[a]
	Tuberculosis	14–70 days	Until treated[a]

[a]Carrier states exist.

APPENDIX 21.3 SOME ANTIBACTERIALS

Antibacterial	Group	Examples
Aminoglycosides	–	Amikacin
		Gentamicin
		Neomycin
		Streptomycin
		Tobramycin
Beta-lactams	Penicillin	Benzyl penicillin
		Phenoxymethyl penicillin
	Penicillinase-resistant penicillins	Flucloxacillin
		Temocillin
	Broad-spectrum penicillins	Amoxicillin
		Ampicillin
		Co-amoxiclav
		Co-fluampicil
	Anti-pseudomonal penicillins	Piperacillin
		Ticarcillin
	Mecillinams	Pivmecillinam
	Cephalosporins	First-generation (cephalosporin)
		Second-generation (cefuroxime, cefamandole)
		Third-generation (cefotaxime, ceftazidime, ceftriaxone)
	Carbapenems	Imipenem–cilastatin
		Doripenem
		Ertapenem
		Meropenem
	Monobactams	Aztreonam
Glycopeptides	–	Teicoplanin
		Vancomycin
Lincosamides	–	Clindamycin

(Continued)

Antibacterial	Group	Examples
Macrolides	–	Azithromycin
		Clarithromycin
		Erythromycin
		Spiramycin
		Telithromycin
Nitroimidazoles	–	Metronidazole
Oxazolidinones	–	Linezolid
Quinolones (fluoroquinolones; 4-quinolones)	–	Ciprofloxacin
		Norfloxacin
		Ofloxacin
Sulphonamides and trimethoprim	–	Co-trimoxazole
Tetracyclines	–	Doxycycline
		Minocycline
		Tetracycline
		Tigecycline is related

APPENDIX 21.4 SUMMARY OF THE MAIN ANTIBACTERIAL AGENTS USED IN DENTISTRY

Antibacterial	Comments	Cautions and contraindications
Penicillins		
Amoxicillin	Given by mouth (absorption better than ampicillin)	Contraindicated in penicillin allergy
	Broad-spectrum (effective against many Gram-negative bacilli)	Rashes, particularly in infectious mononucleosis, lymphoid leukaemia, or during allopurinol treatment
	Staphylococcus aureus often resistant	May cause diarrhoea
	Not resistant to penicillinase	
Ampicillin	Less well absorbed than amoxicillin, otherwise similar (many analogues, such as bacampicillin and pivampicillin – but few advantages)	Contraindicated in penicillin allergy. Causes transient rashes if given to patients with glandular fever, leukaemia or cytomegalovirus infection
	Available with cloxacillin (Ampiclox) or flucloxacillin (co-fluampicil)	
Benzyl penicillin	Given i.m. or i.v.	Contraindicated in penicillin allergy
	Most effective penicillin when organism is sensitive	Large doses may cause K^+ to fall, Na^+ to rise
	Not resistant to penicillinase	
Co-amoxiclav	Mixture of amoxicillin and potassium clavulanate	Contraindicated in penicillin allergy
	Inhibits some penicillinases (beta-lactamases) and therefore active against most *Staph. aureus*; also active against some Gram-negative bacilli	May cause cholestatic jaundice
Flucloxacillin	Given by mouth	Contraindicated in penicillin allergy
	Effective against most penicillin-resistant staphylococci	Treatment in elderly, or for more than 2 weeks, may result in cholestatic jaundice
Phenoxymethyl penicillin (penicillin V)	Given by mouth	Contraindicated in penicillin allergy
	Not resistant to penicillinase	
	Used for prophylaxis of rheumatic fever, in sickle cell disease, and after splenectomy	
Procaine penicillin	Depot penicillin	Contraindicated in penicillin allergy
	Not resistant to penicillinase	Rarely, psychotic reaction due to procaine
Temocillin	Given by i.m. or i.v. injection	Contraindicated in penicillin allergy
	Active against penicillinase-producing Gram-negative bacteria	
Triplopen	Depot penicillin (benzyl penicillin 300 mg, procaine penicillin 250 mg, and benethamine penicillin 475 mg)	Contraindicated in penicillin allergy
	Not resistant to penicillinase	
Tetracyclines		
Tetracyclines	Very broad antibacterial spectrum. Little to choose between the many preparations, but doxycycline and minocycline (see later) are safer for patients with renal failure	Absorption impaired by iron, antacids, milk, etc.
	Given by mouth	May predispose to candidosis

(Continued)

Antibacterial	Comments	Cautions and contraindications
	Many bacteria now resistant but still useful for infections with *Chlamydia*, *Rickettsia*, *Brucella*, Lyme disease, acne, leptospirosis, *Haemophilus influenzae*, methicillin-resistant *Staph. aureus* (MRSA)	Contraindicated in pregnancy and children up to at least 7 y (tooth discolouration)
		Dose reduced in renal failure, liver disease and elderly
		Frequent mild gastrointestinal upsets
		May rarely cause intracranial hypertension
Doxycycline	Given by mouth in a single daily dose	Contraindicated in pregnancy and children up to at least 7 y (tooth discolouration)
		Safer than other tetracyclines in renal failure; may rarely cause intracranial hypertension
		Reduce dose in liver disease and elderly
		Mild gastrointestinal effects
Minocycline	Given by mouth	Safer than tetracycline in renal disease
	Active against some meningococci	May cause dizziness and vertigo
	Absorption not reduced by milk	Contraindicated in pregnancy and children up to at least 7 y (tooth discolouration)
		May also cause bone pigmentation
Macrolides		
Azithromycin	Slightly less active than erythromycin against Gram-positive bacteria	Reduced dose indicated in liver disease and long QT syndrome
	Long half-life (single daily dose)	With terfenadine and pimozide may cause arrhythmias
	Fewer gastrointestinal effects than erythromycin	
		Interacts with theophylline and lithium
		Caution in pregnancy
Erythromycin	Given by mouth but absorption erratic and unpredictable	Reduced dose indicated in liver disease and long QT syndrome
	Similar antibacterial spectrum to penicillin	With terfenadine and pimozide may cause arrhythmias
	Avoid erythromycin estolate, which may cause liver disturbance	Interacts with theophylline and lithium
	Useful in those hypersensitive to penicillin	Caution in pregnancy
	Effective against some staphylococci and most streptococci	
	May cause nausea or hearing loss in large doses	
	Rapid development of resistance	
Clarithromycin	Fewer gastrointestinal effects than with erythromycin	Reduced dose indicated in liver disease and long QT syndrome
		With terfenadine and pimozide may cause arrhythmias
		Interacts with theophylline and lithium
		Caution in pregnancy
Others		
Cephalosporins cephamycins and other beta-lactams	Rarely needed in dentistry; expensive	May cross-react with penicillins, causing hypersensitivity reactions in those allergic to penicillins
		Caution in pregnancy
Clindamycin	Given by mouth	Cross-resistance with erythromycin
	Very reliably absorbed	Mild diarrhoea common
		Repeated doses may cause pseudomembranous colitis (antibiotic-associated colitis), especially in the elderly and in combination with other drugs
		Caution in pregnancy
Gentamicin	Reserved for serious infections	Can cause vestibular and renal damage
		Contraindicated in pregnancy and myasthenia gravis
Metronidazole	Given by mouth	Use only for 7 days (or peripheral neuropathy may develop, particularly in patients with liver disease)
	Effective only against anaerobes	Avoid alcohol (disulfiram-type reaction)
	Available as i.v. preparation but expensive	May increase warfarin effect
		Avoid in pregnancy
Rifampicin	Reserved mainly for treatment of tuberculosis	May interfere with oral contraception
	May be used in prophylaxis of meningitis after head injury since *Neisseria meningitidis* and *Staph. aureus* are frequently resistant to sulphonamides	Occasional rashes, jaundice or blood dyscrasias
		Safe and effective but resistance rapidly develops
		Body secretions turn red
Sulphonamides	Main indication is for prophylaxis of post-traumatic meningitis but meningococci are increasingly resistant	Contraindicated in pregnancy and in renal disease

(Continued)

Antibacterial	Comments	Cautions and contraindications
	Adequate hydration essential to prevent (rare) crystalluria	
	Other adverse reactions include rashes, erythema multiforme and blood dyscrasias	
Teicoplanin	Reserved mainly for endocarditis and serious *Staph. aureus* infections, including some MRSA	Reduce dose in renal failure and elderly
	Occasional rashes, nausea, fever, anaphylaxis	
	May cause hearing loss or tinnitus	
Vancomycin	Reserved for serious infections (including MRSA)	Contraindicated in renal disease or deafness
	Given by slow (100-min) i.v. infusion	May cause nausea, rashes, 'red man syndrome', tinnitus, deafness when given intravenously
	Extravenous extravasation causes necrosis and phlebitis	
	Effective by mouth for pseudomembranous colitis	
Quinolones	Can induce fits	Contraindicated in patients with tendonitis, the elderly or those on steroids; epilepsy; diabetes; pregnancy; myasthenia gravis
	Can cause tendon damage	

Warn patients taking an oral contraceptive to use additional precautions if on antimicrobials for more than a single dose.

APPENDIX 21.5 BACTERIAL INFECTIONS SEEN MAINLY IN PEOPLE FROM THE DEVELOPING WORLD

Disease	Microorganism or parasite (areas of greatest risk)	Infection via	Possible outcomes	Prevention	Diagnostic aids	Management
Anthrax	*Bacillus anthracis* (Central Asia and worldwide)	Contact with contaminated products or soil infected by animals (mainly cattle, goats, sheep). Spores survive for decades	Untreated infections may spread to regional lymph nodes and bloodstream, and may be fatal	Avoidance of direct contact with soil and products of animal origin (e.g. souvenirs made from animal skins). Vaccine available for people at high risk	Isolation from blood, skin or respiratory secretions	Ciprofloxacin, doxycycline or erythromycin
Bartonella	*Bartonella* (*Rochalimaea*) *henselae*, Gram-negative bacilli that appear to be transmitted by ectoparasites (worldwide)	Contact with cats	Cat scratch disease lymphadenitis	Avoidance of cats	Warthin–Starry silver stain may show causal organisms, or they may be identified by in vitro DNA amplification or serological testing	Treatment, if required, involves use of tetracyclines, doxycycline or chloramphenicol, or erythromycin or other macrolides
			Most common in children, in the cervical region; the typical case presents with a tender papule about 3–10 days after contact with the animal, and this is followed by cervical lymphadenopathy after up to 6 weeks			
			Systemic features vary from none to a mild 'flu-like illness and only very rarely are there more serious sequelae such as encephalitis			
			B. henselae or sometimes *B. quintana* in immunodeficient patients may cause epithelioid (bacillary) angiomatosis; clinical resemblance of the lesions to Kaposi sarcoma, but they are benign			

(Continued)

Disease	Microorganism or parasite (areas of greatest risk)	Infection via	Possible outcomes	Prevention	Diagnostic aids	Management
	B. bacilliformis (in some valleys of Colombia, Ecuador and Peru)	Transmitted by sandflies	Carrion disease is either acute with severe infectious haemolytic anaemia (or Oroya fever), or appears as benign cutaneous tumours (verruga peruana). Healthy blood carriers of the bacterium exist	Avoidance of sandflies		
		Bacterial reservoir is in humans only				
	B. quintana (worldwide)	Transmitted by body louse	Trench fever, first described during the First World War, is a non-fatal disease of recurrent attacks of fever and bone pains. Can also cause endocarditis, bacillary angiomatosis and chronic or recurrent bacteraemia	Avoidance of lice		
		Humans seem to be the reservoir of *B. quintana*				
Brucellosis	*Brucella* species (worldwide, mainly in developing countries and around the Mediterranean)	From cattle (*B. abortus*), dogs (*B. canis*), pigs (*B. suis*), or sheep and goats (*B. melitensis*), by direct contact with animals, skin or unpasteurized milk or cheese	Continuous or intermittent fever and malaise	Avoidance of unpasteurized milk and milk products, and direct contact with animals, particularly cattle, goats and sheep	Blood or bone marrow culture and serology are required for diagnosis	Doxycycline and rifampicin are used in combination for 6 weeks to prevent recurring infection
			Acute form, symptoms are non-specific and 'flu-like, particularly fever, sweats, malaise, anorexia, headache, myalgia and back pain			
			Undulant form (<1 y from illness onset), symptoms include undulant fevers, arthritis and epididymo-orchitis in males. Neurological symptoms may develop rapidly in up to 5%			
			Chronic form (>1 y from onset), symptoms may include chronic fatigue syndrome-like depressive episodes and arthritis			
			Brucellosis may be associated with chronic or intermittent lymphadenopathy			
Cholera	*Vibrio cholerae*, serogroups O1 and O139 from contaminated water, occasionally from food (developing countries, particularly in Africa and Asia, and to a lesser extent in Central and South America; endemic in Bangladesh and common throughout the tropics, currently in South America, the Middle East, Africa and Asia)	Ingestion of food or water contaminated directly or indirectly by faeces or vomitus of infected persons	Acute enteric disease varying in severity	Oral cholera vaccines gave little protection and have been abandoned	Stool culture	Treatment is with electrolyte-containing solutions and, if necessary, ciprofloxacin

(Continued)

Disease	Microorganism or parasite (areas of greatest risk)	Infection via	Possible outcomes	Prevention	Diagnostic aids	Management
			Can cause massive diarrhoea with depletion of water and electrolytes, and can be fatal	All care should be taken to avoid consumption of potentially contaminated food, drink and drinking water		
Diphtheria	*Corynebacterium diphtheriae* (where immunization has been neglected, diphtheria continues to re-emerge, as in Eastern Europe, e.g. Ukraine 2008)	Human-to-human transmission by droplet infection and fomites	*C. diphtheriae* multiplies mainly on the nasal, pharyngeal or laryngeal mucous membranes to cause inflammation, surface necrosis and exudate (pseudomembrane)	Diphtheria immunization carried out in early childhood	Swabs should be taken for bacterial culture and for Gram and Kenyon staining	Antibiotics (usually penicillin or erythromycin) immediately
		Patients infectious for up to 4 weeks but carriers may shed for longer	Mild sore throat but disproportionate cervical lymph node enlargement, which in severe cases produces a bull neck. Nasal, laryngeal or tracheal diphtheria are variants			Diphtheria antitoxin if the patient has not been actively immunized
		Three biotypes – *gravis*, *intermedius* and *mitis*, the most severe disease being caused by the *gravis* biotype, but any strain may produce neurotoxin	Exotoxin causes potentially fatal myocardial, adrenal and neurological damage			Household contacts may need immunization
			Palatal paralysis is a possible manifestation			
Haemophilus meningitis	*Haemophilus influenzae* type b (Hib) (worldwide where vaccination against Hib is not practised)	Direct contact with infected person	Meningitis in infants and young children; may also cause epiglottitis, osteomyelitis, pneumonia, sepsis and septic arthritis	Vaccination against Hib	White cell count	
					Hib culture from blood	
Leprosy	*Mycobacterium leprae* (India alone accounts for 78% of new cases detected worldwide; endemic in tropical and subtropical areas of Asia, Africa and Latin America; also seen occasionally around the Mediterranean and Black Sea and in southern Europe)	*M. leprae* transmitted by direct contact and via the respiratory tract	Outcome of infection highly dependent upon cell-mediated immune reactions; if these are intact, infection results in localized form (tuberculoid leprosy); if deficient, generalized (lepromatous) leprosy	Hygiene	Based on one or more of three cardinal signs: hypopigmented or reddish hypo- or anaesthetic skin lesion(s); peripheral nerve involvement; and a positive smear from an open lesion, or biopsy, for acid-fast bacilli	Multidrug therapy (MDT) with clofazimine, rifampicin and prothionamide over 2 or more years; second-line drugs include ofloxacin, minocycline and clarithromycin
			Tuberculoid leprosy: a benign form and causes thickening of cutaneous nerves, flat and hypopigmented or raised and erythematous skin lesions, and enlarged lymph nodes		The lepromin test is of dubious value	

(Continued)

Disease	Microorganism or parasite (areas of greatest risk)	Infection via	Possible outcomes	Prevention	Diagnostic aids	Management
			Lepromatous leprosy: affects nerves (with hypoaesthesia); skin with macules progressing to papules and nodules or infiltration; lymph nodes; and other tissues, including bones, eyes, testes, kidneys and bone marrow		Serological diagnostic tests capable of identifying and allowing treatment of early-stage leprosy are appearing	
Leptospirosis	Spirochaetes of the genus *Leptospira* worldwide (most common in tropics)	Contact between the skin or mucosae and water, wet soil or vegetation contaminated by animal urine, notably rats and foxes	Sudden fever, headache, myalgia, chills, conjunctival suffusion and rash. May progress to meningitis, haemolytic anaemia, jaundice, haemorrhages and hepatorenal failure	Avoidance of contact with rodents and contaminated waters, including canals, ponds, rivers, streams and swamps	Enzyme-linked immunosorbent assay (ELISA) serology	Doxycycline, penicillin
Listeriosis	*Listeria monocytogenes* (worldwide)	*Listeria* multiplies readily in refrigerated foods that have been contaminated (e.g. unpasteurized milk, soft cheeses, vegetables and prepared meat products)	Newborn infants, pregnant women, older and immunocompromised individuals are particularly susceptible. In pregnancy, causes fever and abortion. Meningoencephalitis and/or septicaemia in adults and newborn infants. In others, disease may be limited to a mild acute febrile episode	Avoidance of unpasteurized milk and milk products	Culture blood, urine, cerebrospinal fluid or amniotic fluid	Ampicillin plus gentamicin
Lyme disease	*Borrelia burgdorferi* (first recognized in 1977 when arthritis was noted in children in and around Lyme, Connecticut, USA)	Bite of infected deer ticks, which have become infected by feeding on small rodents, such as white-footed mice	Some individuals have subclinical infection but presentation is most often with a 'bull's-eye' rash (erythema migrans) and non-specific features, e.g. fever, malaise, fatigue, headache, muscle aches (myalgia) and joint aches (arthralgia)	Avoidance of areas where there could be deer	Serological testing initially with a sensitive ELISA or indirect fluorescent antibody (IFA) test, followed by testing with the more specific Western immunoblot (WB), which is confirmatory	Doxycycline or amoxicillin for 3–4 weeks
	British Lyme disease differs from the USA version, in having fewer complications	Spirochaetes disseminate from the tick bite via lymphatics and blood to nervous or musculoskeletal systems, or heart	Rash usually appears 7–14 days after tick exposure			Cefuroxime or erythromycin for persons allergic to penicillin
			Early neurological manifestations may include lymphocytic meningitis, cranial neuropathy (especially facial nerve palsy) and radiculoneuritis			
			Musculoskeletal manifestations may include migratory joint and muscle pains			
			Cardiac manifestations rare but may include myocarditis and transient atrioventricular blocks			
Meningococcal disease	*Neisseria meningitides* (epidemics in Saudi Arabia during Haj)	Humans	Meningitis	Hygiene		

(Continued)

Disease	Microorganism or parasite (areas of greatest risk)	Infection via	Possible outcomes	Prevention	Diagnostic aids	Management
				Vaccination is indicated		
Paratyphoid	*Salmonella paratyphi*, *S. cholerae-suis* or *S. enteritidis*	Poultry, eggs, dairy products, other foods	Similar to typhoid but usually less severe	Hygiene	Culture stool	Supportive therapy
Pertussis	*Bartonella pertussis*	Nasopharyngeal secretions	Catarrh, recurrent cough	Hygiene	Culture nasopharyngeal swab	Erythromycin, azithromycin
Plague	*Yersinia pestis* (Asia, Africa, South America; epidemics)	*Xenopsylla cheopis* (oriental rat flea) is primary vector	*Bubonic plague*: lymphadenitis with swelling and suppuration – buboes. Untreated bubonic plague is often fatal	Avoidance of contact with rodents	Immunostain smear from affected tissues serology	Aminoglycosides, e.g. streptomycin and gentamicin
		Other routes of spread include direct contact with infected tissues or fluids from handling sick or dead animals or by droplets from cats	*Septicaemic plague*: may develop from bubonic plague or occur in the absence of lymphadenitis. Dissemination of infection in bloodstream causes meningitis, endotoxic shock and disseminated intravascular coagulation	Antibiotics for prophylaxis with tetracyclines or sulphonamides		
		Direct person-to-person transmission only in pneumonic plague	*Pneumonic plague*: results from secondary infection of lungs following dissemination from other sites. Direct infection of others may result. Untreated septicaemic and pneumonic plague are invariably fatal			
Q fever	*Coxiella burnetii* (worldwide)	Excreta or milk of cattle, sheep and goats	Fever, headache, malaise, myalgia, sore throat, chills, sweats, cough, nausea, vomiting, diarrhoea, abdominal and chest pain	Avoidance of contact with excreta or unpasteurized milk	Serology	Tetracycline, doxycycline
		Ticks				
Salmonellosis	*Salmonella* serotype *typhimurium* and *Salmonella* serotype *enteritidis* (outbreaks in developing world mainly, e.g. Kenya 2008, but also in developed world, e.g. USA 2008)	Contaminated foods are often of animal origin, such as beef, poultry, milk or eggs, but any food, including vegetables, may become contaminated	Diarrhoea, fever or abdominal cramps	Avoidance of contact with uncooked food and not eating raw or undercooked eggs, poultry or meat	Laboratory tests that identify *Salmonella* in the stool of an infected person	Usually resolves in 5–7 days and often does not require treatment other than oral fluids
				Thorough cooking kills *Salmonella*		Persons with severe diarrhoea may require rehydration with intravenous fluids
				Reptiles (turtles, iguanas, lizards, snakes) may harbour *Salmonella*. Chicks and birds may carry *Salmonella* in their faeces		Antibiotics, e.g. ampicillin, trimethoprim–sulfamethoxazole or ciprofloxacin, are not usually necessary
				Hands should be washed immediately after handling reptiles or birds		

(Continued)

Disease	Microorganism or parasite (areas of greatest risk)	Infection via	Possible outcomes	Prevention	Diagnostic aids	Management
Sodoku	*Spirillum minus* (Asia mainly)	From rat bites or scratches	High fever, headache and regionally swollen lymph nodes	Avoidance of rats, mice or squirrels	Darkfield microscopy	Penicillin
Tularaemia	*Francisella tularensis* (USA and other countries)	From ticks, water contaminated by rats, undercooked meat from an infected animal such as rabbit, and also from contaminated soil	High fever, generalized aching and swollen lymph nodes	Avoidance of rats	Serology	Aminoglycosides (e.g. gentamicin and streptomycin), chloramphenicol, fluoroquinolones and tetracyclines
Typhoid fever	*Salmonella typhi* (worldwide, especially North and West Africa, South Asia and Peru)	Contaminated water or food	Fever, rash, splenomegaly and leukopenia, and intestinal bleeding or perforation	Vaccination	Culture blood, vomit and stool	Chloramphenicol effective but toxic. *S. typhi* may be resistant in India, Middle East and South-East Asia, where ciprofloxacin is indicated
		A strict human pathogen, typhoid is always acquired from a human. Contact tracing is important		Hygiene		
				Avoidance of contaminated water or food		
Typhus fever (epidemic louse-borne typhus)	*Rickettsia prowazekii* (colder, i.e. mountainous, regions of Central and East Africa, Central and South America, and Asia. In recent years, most outbreaks have taken place in Burundi, Ethiopia and Rwanda)	Human body louse, rat or cat flea	Sudden fever, headache, chills, prostration, coughing and muscular pains	Avoidance of infestation by body lice	Serology after the first week	Doxycycline, azithromycin, rifampicin
			After 5–6 days, a macular skin eruption (dark spots) on the upper trunk and then rest of the body, except face, palms or soles		Polymerase chain reaction (PCR)	
			Case fatality rate up to 40%			
Yersiniosis	*Y. enterocolitica* (worldwide)	Eating contaminated food, especially raw or undercooked pork products	Features typically develop 4–7 days after exposure and may last 1–3 weeks or longer	Hygiene	Culture stool or body fluids	Uncomplicated cases usually resolve spontaneously
			Fever, abdominal pain, bloody diarrhoea and sometimes cervical lymphadenopathy			In severe or complicated infections, use aminoglycosides, doxycycline, trimethoprim–sulfamethoxazole or fluoroquinolones

APPENDIX 21.6 UNCOMMON BACTERIAL INFECTIONS THAT MAY HAVE IMPLICATIONS IN DENTISTRY

Organism	Main features	Orofacial lesions	Treatments
Bacillus anthracis	Anthrax	Painful or ulcerated swellings, mainly on palate	Penicillin
Brucella melitensis, suis and *abortus*	Brucellosis	Rare infections or cranial nerve palsies	Tetracycline with streptomycin
Clostridium botulinum	Botulism	Xerostomia, parotitis	Antitoxin
		Muscle weakness	
Clostridium perfringens (C. welchii), C. sporogenes, C. oedematiens and *C. septicum*	Gas gangrene	Gas gangrene	Antitoxin
			Penicillin
			Surgery
Escherichia coli	Enteric infections, mainly	Found in some oral infections, especially in denture wearers and immunocompromised	Ampicillin
	Also urinary tract, wound and other infection		Cefalexin
			Cefalotin
			Co-trimoxazole
Francisella tularensis	Tularaemia	Pharyngitis	Streptomycin
		Stomatitis (often ulcerative)	
		Faucial membrane	
		Cervical lymphadenopathy	
Mycoplasma hominis and *pneumoniae*	Pneumonia	Rare infections or cranial nerve palsies?	Tetracyclines
		Reiter syndrome	Erythromycins
Neisseria meningitidis	Meningitis	Petechiae	Penicillin
	Septicaemia	Occasionally, herpes labialis	
		Facial palsy	
Nocardia asteroides, brasiliensis and *caviae*	Nocardiosis	Ulceration	Co-trimoxazole
		Cheek or gingivae	
Proteus vulgaris	Urinary tract and wounds	Occasional infections	Ciprofloxacin
Pseudomonas aeruginosa	Skin and lungs	Opportunistic infections	Sulfadiazine
			Aminoglycosides
Pseudomonas mallei	Glanders (acute pneumonia)	Ulceration from nasal glanders	Penicillin
		Ulcers	Cephalosporins
Pseudomonas pseudomallei	Melioidosis (lung or other localized infections or septicaemia)	Oral abscesses, or other infections	Tetracyclines
		Parotitis	
Rickettsia rickettsiae	Rocky mountain spotted fever	Faucial gangrene	Tetracyclines
Rickettsia akari	Rickettsial pox	Vesicles	Tetracyclines
Salmonellae typhi, paratyphi, cholerae, suis and *enteritidis*	Typhoid and paratyphoid fever	Occasional infections	Co-trimoxazole
			Ampicillin

APPENDIX 21.7 IMMUNIZATION SCHEDULES (UK)[a]

When to immunize	Diseases protected against	Vaccine
2 months old	Diphtheria, tetanus, pertussis, polio and *Haemophilus influenzae* type b (Hib)	DTaP/IPV/Hib (Pediacel)
	Pneumococcal disease	PCV (Prevenar 13)
	Rotavirus	Rotavirus (Rotarix)
3 months old	Diphtheria, tetanus, pertussis, polio and Hib	DTaP/IPV/Hib (Pediacel)
	Meningococcal group C disease (MenC)	MenC (Neisvac-C or Menjugate)
	Rotavirus	Rotavirus (Rotarix)
4 months old	Diphtheria, tetanus, pertussis, polio and Hib	DTaP/IPV/Hib (Pediacel)
	Pneumococcal disease	PCV (Prevenar 13)
Between 12 and 13 months old – within a month of the first birthday	Hib/MenC	Hib/MenC (Menitorix)

(Continued)

When to immunize	Diseases protected against	Vaccine
	Pneumococcal disease	PCV (Prevenar 13)
	Measles, mumps and rubella	MMR (Priorix or MMR VaxPRO)
2 and 3 years old	Influenza	Flu nasal spray (Fluenz; annual)
		If Fluenz unsuitable, use inactivated flu vaccine
3 years 4 months old or soon after	Diphtheria, tetanus, pertussis and polio	dTaP/IPV (Repevax) or DTaP/IPV (Infanrix-IPV)
	Measles, mumps and rubella	MMR (Priorix or MMR VaxPRO; check first dose has been given)
Girls aged 12–13 years	Cervical cancer caused by human papillomavirus types 16 and 18 (and genital warts caused by types 6 and 11)	HPV (Gardasil)
Around 14 years old	Tetanus, diphtheria and polio	Td/IPV (Revaxis), and check MMR status
	MenC	MenC (Meningitec, Menjugate or NeisVac-C)
65 years old	Pneumococcal disease	PPV Pneumococcal polysaccharide vaccine (Pneumovax II)
65 years of age and older	Influenza	Flu injection (annual)
70 years old	Shingles	Shingles (Zostavax)
Immunizations for those at risk		
At birth, 1 month old, 2 months old and 12 months old	Hepatitis B	Hep B
At birth	Tuberculosis	BCG
6 months up to 2 years	Influenza	Inactivated flu vaccine (annual)
2 years up to under 65 years	Pneumococcal disease	PPV Pneumococcal polysaccharide vaccine (Pneumovax II)
Over 2 up to less than 18 years	Influenza	Flu nasal spray (Fluenz; annual)
		If Fluenz unsuitable, use inactivated flu vaccine
18 up to under 65 years	Influenza	Inactivated flu vaccine (annual)
From 28 weeks of pregnancy	Pertussis	dTaP/IPV (Repevax)

[a]Source: https://www.gov.uk/government/publications/the-complete-routine-immunisation-schedule-201314 (accessed 30 September 2013).

APPENDIX 21.8 COMMON VIRAL INFECTIONS THAT MAY HAVE IMPLICATIONS IN DENTISTRY[a]

Virus	Infection mainly in	Orofacial consequences	Antivirals that may have a role
Cytomegalovirus	Immunocompromised persons	Ulcers	Ganciclovir / Foscarnet / Valganciclovir
Epstein–Barr virus	Any	Ulcers	–
	Immunocompromised persons	Ulcers / Hairy leukoplakia / Lymphomas	Ganciclovir / Aciclovir
Hepatitis B	Any	–	Usually none. Interferon-alpha 2b, adefovir, entecavir, lamivudine, telbivudine or tenofovir
	Chronic infection or immunocompromised persons	–	Interferon-alpha 2b, adefovir, entecavir, lamivudine, telbivudine or tenofovir
Hepatitis C	Any	Lichenoid lesions/lichen planus	Usually none. Interferon-alpha 2b and ribivirin. A protease inhibitor (e.g. boceprevir or telaprevir) may also be given
	Chronic infection or immunocompromised persons	Sicca syndrome	
Herpes simplex	Primary infections	Gingivostomatitis	Aciclovir
	Secondary infections (labial or orogenital)	Blistering	Aciclovir / Penciclovir
	Secondary infections (oral)	Ulceration / Erythema multiforme / Bell palsy	Aciclovir
	Encephalitis	–	Aciclovir
HIV	See Ch. 20		
Influenza	Older or immunocompromised persons	–	Amantadine / Oseltamivir

(Continued)

Virus	Infection mainly in	Orofacial consequences	Antivirals that may have a role
			Rimantadine
			Zanamivir
Papillomaviruses	Any	Warty lesions	Interferon-alpha 2b
		Oropharyngeal carcinoma	Imiquimod
Respiratory syncytial virus	Young or immunocompromised persons	–	Ribavirin
Severe acute respiratory syndrome corona virus	Older or immunocompromised persons	–	Ribavirin
Varicella zoster virus	Chickenpox; any patient	Ulcers	Aciclovir
	Zoster; any patient	Pain	Famciclovir
		Ulcers	Valaciclovir
	Zoster in immunocompromised	Pain	Aciclovir
		Ulcers	

[a]See Table 21.10.

APPENDIX 21.9 VIRAL INFECTIONS PREVALENT MAINLY IN THE DEVELOPING WORLD

Disease	Virus	Infection via	Consequences	Epicentres of greatest risk	Prevention
Arboviruses	Many different arboviruses	Transmitted to humans by arthropods, mostly mosquitoes, sandflies or ticks	Fever with rashes, arthralgias, lymphadenopathy, CNS involvement or haemorrhagic features	Worldwide, especially Latin America, the southern USA, South-East Asia and Africa	Avoid insect bites (wear protective clothing and use insect repellants) and use prophylactic measures such as vaccination
Chikungunya	Togavirus	Mosquito	Similar to dengue; fever and joint pain, muscle pain, headache, nausea, fatigue and rash	Around Indian Ocean	Avoid mosquito bites
Dengue	Dengue virus – a flavivirus	*Aedes aegypti* mosquito, which bites during the day. There is no direct person-to-person transmission. Monkeys act as a reservoir host in South-East Asia and West Africa	Dengue fever – an acute febrile illness, macular skin rash and muscle pains ('breakbone fever')	Tropical and subtropical regions of Central and South America, South and South-East Asia, and Africa below 600 m	Avoid mosquito bites
			Dengue haemorrhagic fever		
			Dengue shock syndrome		
Ebola fever	See Haemorrhagic fevers				
Encephalitis viruses	Togaviridae or flaviviruses	Mosquito bites	Aseptic meningitis or encephalitis. Infections range from mild 'flu-like illness to frank encephalitis, coma and death, leaving mild to severe neurological deficits in survivors	Worldwide	Avoid bites of mosquitoes. A vaccine against tick-borne encephalitis is available for those walking or camping in forests in areas at risk
				Tick-borne encephalitis is seen in forested areas of Austria, northern Europe and Scandinavia	
				Japanese encephalitis virus is a flavivirus	
				St Louis encephalitis virus is a flavivirus seen in the southern USA and Caribbean	

(Continued)

Disease	Virus	Infection via	Consequences	Epicentres of greatest risk	Prevention
Haemorrhagic fevers: Crimean–Congo haemorrhagic fever (CCHF), dengue, Ebola and Marburg haemorrhagic fevers, Lassa fever, Rift Valley fever (RVF) and yellow fever	Most haemorrhagic fevers, including dengue and yellow fever, caused by flaviviruses	Most viruses transmitted by mosquitoes	Sudden onset of fever, malaise, headache and myalgia followed by pharyngitis, vomiting, diarrhoea, rash and haemorrhages, including from the mouth. Fatal in over 50%	Tropics and subtropical regions	Avoid mosquitoes, ticks and rodents
	Ebola and Marburg caused by filoviruses, CCHF by bunyavirus, Lassa fever by arenavirus, RVF by phlebovirus	Ebola or Marburg viruses acquired from bats or monkeys or direct contact with body fluids of infected patients		Ebola and Marburg haemorrhagic fevers in sub-Saharan Africa. Marburg virus has been of concern since first reports in 1967 in persons working with monkeys in Germany and Yugoslavia	Filoviruses have very high transmissibility, morbidity and mortality
		CCHF transmitted by a tick bite		Lassa fever, the most infamous arenavirus, is named after the Nigerian town where infection was first recorded in 1969. Cases since reported from Liberia, Sierra Leone and Uganda	
		Lassa fever virus carried by rodents and transmitted by excreta, either as aerosol or direct contact		CCHF in steppe regions of Central Asia and Central Europe (including Greece and Turkey in 2008), as well as in tropical and southern Africa	
		RVF acquired either by mosquito bite or by direct contact with blood or tissues of infected animals		RVF in Africa and Saudi Arabia	
				Other viral haemorrhagic fevers in Central and South America	
				Other arenavirus infections include Korean, Argentinian and Bolivian fevers	
Hantavirus diseases – haemorrhagic fever with renal syndrome (HFRS) and hantavirus pulmonary syndrome (HPS)	Hantaviruses – family bunyaviruses. HPS caused by sin nombre virus (SNV)	Direct contact with the faeces, saliva or urine of infected rodents such as deer, mice or by inhalation of the virus	Vascular endothelium is damaged, leading to vascular permeability, hypotension, haemorrhages and shock	Worldwide. New World hantaviruses with distinct rodent hosts. A pan-American zoonosis, with an expanding clinical spectrum. Seen also in Europe	Avoid exposure to rodents and their excreta
			Impaired renal function with oliguria characterizes HFRS; fatal in up to 15%		
			Respiratory distress due to pulmonary oedema in HPS; fatal in up to 50%		
Hepatitis viruses	Ch. 9				
Human immunodeficiency virus (HIV)	Ch. 20				
Influenza	Ch. 15				

(Continued)

Disease	Virus	Infection via	Consequences	Epicentres of greatest risk	Prevention
Japanese encephalitis	Japanese encephalitis (JE) virus – a flavivirus	Various mosquitoes of the genus *Culex*. Infects pigs and wild birds as well as humans	Fever, headache or aseptic meningitis. Severe cases rapid onset with headache, high fever and meningeal signs. May be neurological sequelae. Approximately 50% of severe cases are fatal	Asia, especially monsoon areas of South-East Asia	Vaccination. Avoid mosquito bites
Lassa fever	See Haemorrhagic fevers				
Marburg virus	See Haemorrhagic fevers				
Nipah and Hendra viruses	Paramyxoviruses	Animals (Nipah from fruit bats and pigs; Hendra from horses)		Nipah- Malaysia, Bangladesh; Hendra- Australia	Avoid excreta
Poliomyelitis	Ch. 13				
Rabies	Rhabdovirus of genus Lyssavirus	Bite of an infected animal such as a dog, fox or bat	Acute encephalomyelitis, which is almost invariably fatal. Initial signs include sense of apprehension, headache, fever, malaise and sensory changes around bite site. Excitability, hallucinations and aerophobia are common, followed in some cases by fear of water (hydrophobia) due to spasms of swallowing muscles, progressing to delirium, convulsions and death	Worldwide, especially in developing countries	Avoid contact with both wild and domestic animals, including dogs and cats. Vaccination
Severe acute respiratory syndrome (SARS)	Ch. 15				
Tick-borne encephalitis (spring–summer encephalitis)	Tick-borne encephalitis (TBE) virus – a flavivirus	Bite of infected ticks	Influenza-like illness, with a second phase of fever in 10% of cases. Encephalitis develops during the second phase and may result in paralysis or death	Below 1000 m in Eastern Europe, particularly Austria, Baltic States, Czech Republic, Hungary and Russian Federation	Avoid bites by ticks by wearing long trousers and closed footwear when hiking or camping in endemic areas
West Nile fever	West Nile virus (WNV)	Bite of an infected mosquito, and can infect people, horses, many types of birds and some other animals	Rarely, severe or sometimes fatal encephalitis	Africa, USA, southern Europe	Avoid mosquito bites
		The virus can be transmitted through contact with the blood or other tissues of infected animals			Avoid handling WNV-infected tissues or fluids from animals
Yellow fever	Yellow fever virus – an arbovirus of the Flavivirus genus	Bite of *Aedes aegypti* mosquitoes	Acute illness characterized initially by fever, chills, headache, muscular pain, anorexia, nausea and/or vomiting, with bradycardia. About 15% progress to second phase, with fever resurgence, jaundice, abdominal pain, vomiting and haemorrhages. 50% die after 10–14 days	Tropical areas of Africa and Central and South America below 2500 m	Vaccination. Avoid mosquito bites during the day, as well as at night
		Yellow fever virus infects humans and monkeys			

[a]See also Appendix 21.8 for the more common viral infections.

APPENDIX 21.10 MAIN ANTIFUNGAL DRUGS

Group	Examples	Comments	Oral dose
Polyenes	Amphotericin[a]	Active topically. Negligible absorption from gastrointestinal tract. Given i.v. for deep mycoses	10–100 mg 6-hourly
	Nystatin[a]	Active topically. Negligible absorption from gastrointestinal tract. Pastilles taste better than lozenges	500 000 unit lozenge, 100 000 unit pastille or 100 000 unit per mL of suspension 6-hourly
Imidazoles	Ketoconazole	Absorbed from gastrointestinal tract. Useful in intractable candidosis. Contraindicated in pregnancy and liver disease. May cause nausea, rashes, pruritus and liver damage. Interacts with anticoagulants, terfenadine, cisapride and astemizole	200–400 mg once daily with meal, for 14 days
	Miconazole[a]	Active topically. Also has antibacterial activity. Absorption from gastrointestinal tract. Theoretically the best antifungal to treat angular stomatitis. Interacts with anticoagulants, terfenadine, cisapride and astemizole. Avoid in pregnancy and porphyria	250 mg tablet 6-hourly or 25 mg/mL gel used as 5 mL 6-hourly, for 14 days
Triazoles	Fluconazole	Absorbed from gastrointestinal tract. Useful in intractable candidosis. Contraindicated in pregnancy and lactation, and liver and renal disease. Interacts with anticoagulants, terfenadine, cisapride and astemizole	50–100 mg daily for 14 days
	Itraconazole	Absorbed from gastrointestinal tract. Useful in intractable candidosis. May cause nausea, neuropathy, diarrhea and rash. In high dose, or in older people or those with cardiac disease or on calcium channel blockers, it may cause cardiac failure. Contraindicated in heart disease, pregnancy, liver disease. Interacts with terfenadine, cisapride and astemizole	100 mg daily for 14 days
	Posaconazole	Caution with cardiac patients. Contraindicated in porphyria	400 mg b.d.
	Voriconazole	Caution with cardiac patients, and liver or renal disease. Contraindicated in porphyria and breast-feeding	200 mg b.d.

[a]Dissolve in mouth slowly.

APPENDIX 21.11 IMPORTANT SYSTEMIC (DEEP) MYCOSES

Disease	Organism	Source	Main endemic areas	Clinical forms	Prognosis
Aspergillosis	*Aspergillus fumigatus*, *A. flavus*, *A. niger* and other *Aspergillus* spp.	Ubiquitous	Worldwide	Allergic bronchopulmonary, pulmonary, disseminated, aspergilloma	Variable
Blastomycosis	*Blastomyces dermatitidis*	Soil	Mississippi and Ohio valleys in USA, Canada, North Africa and Venezuela	Cavitary, pulmonary, disseminated, others	Often good, except in disseminated form
Coccidioidomycosis	*Coccidioides immitis*	Soil	South-western USA, Mexico, Latin America	Acute pulmonary, disseminated, chronic pulmonary, meningitis	Often good, except in disseminated or meningeal form
Cryptococcosis	*Cryptococcus neoformans*	Soil, pigeon droppings	Worldwide	Pneumonia, meningitis, disseminated, cryptococcoma	Poor in disseminated form
Histoplasmosis	*Histoplasma capsulatum*	Soil, bird and bat droppings	Mississippi and Ohio valleys in USA, Latin America, Africa, India, Far East, Australia	Benign pulmonary, disseminated, chronic pulmonary, cutaneous	Often good, except in disseminated form
Mucormycosis	*Mucor*, *Rhizopus* and *Absidia*	Ubiquitous	Worldwide	Rhinocerebral, pulmonary, gastrointestinal	Variable
Paracoccidioidomycosis (South American blastomycosis)	*Paracoccidioides brasiliensis*	Soil	South America, especially Brazil	Pulmonary, disseminated	Good in young patients
Pneumocystosis	*Pneumocystis jiroveci* (*carinii*)	Ubiquitous	Worldwide	Pulmonary, disseminated	Variable
Sporotrichosis	*Sporothrix schenkii*	Associated with thorny plants, wood, sphagnum moss	Worldwide	Lymphocutaneous, localized cutaneous, pulmonary, disseminated	Good

APPENDIX 21.12 MAIN PARASITIC INFESTATIONS[a]

Disease	Microorganism or parasite	Infection via	Consequence	Areas of greatest risk	Prevention	Treatment
Angiostrongyliasis	*Angiostrongylus cantonensis*	Rat lungworm	Eosinophilic meningitis	Asia, Africa, Caribbean, Hawaii and other Pacific islands	Avoid eating undercooked or raw snails and slugs. Fish do not spread this parasite	None
Filariasis	Nematodes (roundworms) of family Filarioidea	Lymphatic filariasis transmitted through bite of mosquitoes. Onchocerciasis transmitted through bite of blackflies	Lymphatic filariasis and onchocerciasis (river blindness)	Lymphatic filariasis throughout sub-Saharan Africa and South-East Asia. Onchocerciasis in western and Central Africa, Central and South America	Avoid bites of mosquitoes and/or blackflies	Diethylcarbamazine, ivermectin
Giardiasis	Protozoan parasite *Giardia lamblia*	Ingestion of *Giardia* cysts in water (unfiltered drinking and recreational waters) contaminated by faeces of humans or animals	Anorexia, chronic diarrhoea, abdominal cramps, bloating, frequent loose greasy stools, fatigue and weight loss	Worldwide	Avoid ingesting any potentially contaminated (i.e. unfiltered) drinking water or recreational water	Metronidazole
Leishmaniasis	See text					
Malaria	See text					
Schistosomiasis (bilharziasis)	Parasitic blood flukes (trematodes), of which the most important are *Schistosoma mansoni*, *S. japonicum* and *S. haematobium*	Infection occurs in fresh water containing larval forms (cercariae) of schistosomes, which develop in snails infected as a result of excretion of eggs in human urine or faeces. The free-swimming larvae enter the skin of individuals swimming or wading in water	*S. mansoni* and *S. japonicum* cause hepatic and intestinal signs. *S. haematobium* causes urinary dysfunction	*S. mansoni* in sub-Saharan Africa, Arabian peninsula, Brazil, Surinam and Venezuela. *S. japonicum* in China, Indonesia and Philippines (not Japan). *S. haematobium* in sub-Saharan Africa and eastern Mediterranean areas	Avoid swimming or wading in fresh water in endemic areas	Praziquantel
Strongyloidiasis	*Strongyloides stercoralis*, *Strongyloides fuelleborni*	Infection acquired by walking barefoot in contaminated soil. Larvae enter the body by burrowing into the skin	At entry site, larvae petechial haemorrhages and intense pruritus. Larvae migrate into pulmonary circulation via lymphatic system and venules, produce haemorrhages and alveolar inflammatory response with eosinophilic infiltration (pneumonitis). Larvae migrate up pulmonary tree, are swallowed and reach gastrointestinal system, where they embed and can produce inflammatory reaction and malabsorption syndrome	*Strongyloides* spp. distributed worldwide but endemic in tropical and subtropical regions. Most prevalent in South-East Asia, Sahara Desert, Colombia and tropical Brazil. Infection rates in these areas can be 60%	Avoid walking barefoot	Albendazole

(Continued)

Disease	Microorganism or parasite	Infection via	Consequence	Areas of greatest risk	Prevention	Treatment
		Humans are principal host. Dogs, cats and other mammals too			Persons in household contact not at risk for infection	Tiabendazole
					Proper disposal of human excreta reduces prevalence	
Trypanosomiasis:	Protozoan parasites *Trypanosoma brucei (T. b.) gambiense* and *T. b. rhodesiense*	Bite of infected tsetse flies	*T. b. gambiense* causes chronic illness after prolonged incubation period of weeks or months	*T. b. gambiense* present in foci in tropical countries of western and central Africa	Avoid contact with tsetse flies – bites are difficult to avoid because tsetse flies bite during day, can penetrate clothing and are not deterred by insect repellents	Consult experts
African trypanosomiasis (sleeping sickness)			*T. b. rhodesiense* causes more acute illness, with onset a few days or weeks after infected bite; often, a striking inoculation chancre. Initial signs include headache, insomnia, enlarged lymph nodes, anaemia and rash. In late stages, there is loss of weight and involvement of CNS. Without treatment, invariably fatal	*T. b. rhodesiense* in East Africa, extending south as far as Botswana		
Trypanosomiasis: American trypanosomiasis (Chagas disease)	Protozoan parasite *Trypanosoma cruzi*	Blood-sucking triatomine bugs ('kissing bugs'). Also by transfusion if blood is from infected donor	Chronic illness, progressive myocardial damage leading to cardiac arrhythmias and dilatation, and mega-oesophagus and megacolon	Mexico, Central and South America (to central Argentina and Chile)	Avoid exposure to blood-sucking bugs. Use bednets in houses and camps	Consult experts

aA more comprehensive list is available at: http://www.cdc.gov/parasites/az/index.html (accessed 30 September 2013).

KEY POINTS

- Lifestyle habits underlie several malignant diseases
- Tobacco is responsible for a very wide range of malignant diseases
- Alcohol is also responsible for some malignant disease
- Infections such as with viruses (herpesviruses and papillomaviruses) are responsible for some malignant disease.

GENERAL ASPECTS

Malignant neoplasms or 'cancers' develop because of deoxyribonucleic acid (DNA) mutations – some spontaneously (possibly due to oxygen radicals), others from chemical carcinogens (e.g. tobacco, alcohol or betel), ionizing and ultraviolet radiation, or oncogenic microorganisms (e.g. hepatitis, herpesviruses and human papillomaviruses (HPVs); Fig. 22.1). Important chemical carcinogens are aromatic amines (including arylamines and heterocyclic amines) found in tobacco smoke and cooked foods. The list of known carcinogens is long; the most important – relevant in tobacco and alcoholic beverages – are shown in Box 22.1.

Various liver enzymes termed xenobiotic-metabolizing enzymes (XMEs) are involved in the metabolism of carcinogens or pro-carcinogens (Table 22.1); several are polymorphic and they may be involved in carcinogen activation or degradation. Other enzymes can reverse or repair some of the damage from mutations (DNA repair enzymes) but, when mutations involve genes such as tumour suppressor genes, the cell may become autonomous, despite attempts at DNA and cell repair, and the cell then proliferates and invades – the hallmark of cancer. Eventually, the tumour spreads elsewhere (metastasizes) to lymph nodes and through the blood.

Carcinomas are malignant neoplasms that arise from epithelia; they are a leading cause of morbidity and mortality, mainly in persons who are middle-aged or older, and are most common in the lung, breast, colon, cervix, stomach, pancreas, ovary, prostate and skin. They metastasize mainly to the brain, liver and bones.

Oral cancer is discussed below. Lung tumours are discussed in Chapter 15, breast, ovary and prostate cancer in Chapter 25, gastrointestinal and pancreatic cancer in Chapter 7, haematological malignancies in Chapter 8, brain tumours in Chapter 13, liver cancer in Chapter 9 and skin cancer in Chapter 11.

CANCER PREVENTION

The prognosis of malignant disease is generally poor and unfortunately treatment can also have significant adverse effects, so prevention and early detection are important. The European Code against Cancer summarizes the preventive aspects (Box 22.2). The World Cancer Research Fund advocates measures in addition to not using tobacco and alcohol, and avoiding sun exposure, as in Table 22.2.

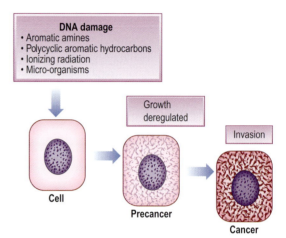

Fig. 22.1 Diagrammatic simplification of the process of carcinogenesis.

Box 22.1 *Some known common carcinogens*

- Acetaldehyde
- Alkyl halides
- Arylamines
- Nitrosamines
- Polycyclic aromatic hydrocarbon
- Urethane

Table 22.1 *Main xenometabolizing enzymes*

Enzyme	Abbreviation	Main activities of some genotypes
Alcohol dehydrogenases	ADH	Activate ethanol
Aldehyde dehydrogenases	ALDH	Inactivate ethanol
Cytochrome P450	CYP	Activate ethanol, benzpyrene and nitrosamines
Glutathione S-transferases	GST	Metabolize benzpyrene, alkyl halides, epoxides and lipid peroxides
N-acetyl transferases	NAT	Acetylate arylamines

AVOIDANCE OF TOBACCO

Tobacco is best avoided; up to 30% of cancers in developed countries are tobacco-related. Tobacco smoke is a mixture of at least 50 compounds, including polycyclic aromatic hydrocarbons (PAHs), nitrosamines, aldehydes and aromatic amines. Tobacco, acting either singly or jointly with the consumption of alcohol, is responsible for 87% of lung cancer, and between 43% and 60% of cancers in oesophagus, larynx and oral cavity. Tobacco consumption is also linked to cancers of the bladder and pancreas, a minority of cancers of the kidney, stomach, cervix and nose, and myeloid leukaemia. On smoking cessation, the risk of cancer rapidly declines; benefit is evident within 5 years and is progressively greater over time.

Many aspects of general health can be improved and many cancer deaths prevented if we adopt healthier lifestyles:

1. Do not smoke; if you smoke, stop doing so. If you fail to stop, do not smoke in the presence of non-smokers
2. Avoid obesity
3. Undertake some brisk physical activity every day
4. Eat a variety of vegetables and fruits every day; eat at least five portions daily. Limit your intake of foods containing fats from animal sources
5. If you drink alcohol, whether beer, wine or spirits, moderate your consumption to two drinks per day if you are a man, or one drink per day if you are a woman
6. Care must be taken to avoid excessive sun exposure. It is specifically important to protect children and adolescents. For individuals who have a tendency to burn in the sun, active protective measures must be taken throughout life
7. Comply strictly with regulations aimed at preventing occupational or environmental exposure to known cancer-causing substances. Follow the advice of National Radiation Protection Offices

There are public health programmes that could prevent cancers developing or increase the probability that a cancer may be cured:

8. Women from 25 years of age should participate in cervical screening. This should be within programmes with quality control procedures in compliance with *EU Guidelines for Quality Assurance in Cervical Screening*
9. Women from 50 years of age should participate in breast screening. This should be within programmes with quality control procedures in compliance with *EU Guidelines for Quality Assurance in Mammography Screening*
10. Men and women from 50 years of age should participate in colorectal screening. This should be within programmes with built-in quality control procedures
11. Participate in vaccination programmes against hepatitis B virus infection

^a Third version: Boyle et al., 2003.

Table 22.2 *Ten rules for reducing cancer risk*

Rule	Rationale
1. Be as lean as possible without being underweight	Convincing evidence shows that weight gain and obesity increase the risk of cancers, including bowel and breast. Maintain healthy weight through a balanced diet and regular physical activity to keep your risk lower
2. Be physically active for at least 30 min every day	Strong evidence shows that physical activity protects against cancers, including bowel and breast. Being physically active is also key to maintaining a healthy weight
3. Avoid sugary drinks. Limit consumption of energy-dense foods (particularly processed foods high in added sugar, or low in fibre or high in fat)	Energy-dense foods are high in fats and sugars, and often low in nutrients; especially when consumed frequently or in large portions, they increase the risk of obesity, which increases the risk of cancer. Fast foods like burgers, chips, fried chicken and pizzas, and snack foods like chocolate, crisps and biscuits tend to be energy-dense. Some energy-dense foods, such as nuts, seeds and vegetable oils, are important sources of nutrients, and have not been linked with weight gain as part of a typical diet
4. Eat more of a variety of vegetables, fruits, wholegrains and pulses such as beans	Evidence shows that vegetables, fruits and other foods containing dietary fibre (such as wholegrains and pulses) may protect against a range of cancers, including mouth, stomach and bowel. They also help protect against weight gain and obesity. As well as eating five portions a day, try to include wholegrains (e.g. brown rice, wholemeal bread and pasta) and/or pulses with every meal. Sugary drinks, such as colas and fruit squashes, can also contribute to weight gain. Fruit juices, even without added sugar, are likely to have a similar effect. Try to eat less energy-dense foods, such as vegetables, fruits and wholegrains instead. Opt for water or unsweetened tea or coffee in place of sugary drinks
5. Limit consumption of red meats (such as beef, pork and lamb) and avoid processed meats	There is strong evidence that red and processed meats are causes of bowel cancer. Aim to limit intake of red meat to less than 500 g cooked weight (about 700–750 g raw weight) a week. Try to avoid processed meats (bacon, ham, salami, corned beef, sausages)
6. If consumed at all, limit alcoholic drinks to 2 a day for men and 1 a day for women	There is evidence that alcoholic drinks can increase the risk of a number of cancers, including breast and colon. Any alcohol consumption can increase cancer risk. There is some evidence to suggest that small amounts of alcohol can help protect against heart disease. If you choose to drink, do so in moderation
7. Limit consumption of salty foods and food processed with salt (sodium)	Evidence shows that salt and salt-preserved foods probably cause stomach cancer and hypertension. Processed foods, including bread and breakfast cereals, can contain large amounts of salt
8. Do not use supplements to protect against cancer	High-dose nutrient supplements can affect cancer risk, so it is best to opt for a balanced diet without supplements. However, supplements are advisable for some groups of people
9. It is best for mothers to breast-feed exclusively for up to 6 months and then add other liquids and foods	Strong evidence shows that breast-feeding protects mothers against breast cancer and babies from excess weight gain
10. After treatment, cancer survivors should follow the recommendations for cancer prevention	Maintaining a healthy weight through diet and physical activity may help to reduce the risk of cancer recurrence

Although the greatest cancer hazard is caused by cigarette smoking, cigars can cause similar hazards, and both cigar smoking and pipe smoking are implicated in cancers of the oral cavity, pharynx, larynx and oesophagus. Bidi, a type of cigarette made of tobacco rolled in a dried temburni leaf, is smoked in India and is associated with a high incidence of oral leukoplakia and oral cancer. Tobacco smoke released to the environment by smokers, commonly referred to as environmental tobacco smoke (ETS) and which is responsible for 'passive smoking', has several deleterious effects on people who inhale it. It causes a small rise in the risk of lung cancer, and also some increase in the risk of heart disease and respiratory disease. It is particularly harmful to small children.

Tobacco-chewing in peoples from parts of Asia, along with a variety of ingredients in a 'betel quid' (betel vine leaf, areca nut, catechu and slaked lime, together with tobacco) appears to predispose to oral squamous cell carcinoma (OSCC). Smokeless tobacco, for example snuff-dipping in women in the south-eastern USA who place snuff in the buccal sulcus, predisposes to gingival and alveolar carcinoma close to where the snuff is placed, but the risk is low.

AVOIDANCE OF ALCOHOL

Alcoholic beverages may contain carcinogens or pro-carcinogens, including ethanol, nitrosamines and urethane contaminants. The total amount of ethanol ingested appears to be the key factor. Alcoholic beverages increase the risk of squamous cell cancers of the oral cavity, pharynx, larynx and oesophagus. Alcohol-drinking raises the risk of neoplasms, even in the absence of smoking, but alcohol-drinking and tobacco-smoking together greatly increase the risk. A probable carcinogenic mechanism of alcohol is the facilitation of the effect of tobacco and possibly of other carcinogens to which the upper digestive and respiratory tracts are exposed, particularly those of dietary origin. However, a direct carcinogenic effect of acetaldehyde, the main metabolite of ethanol, and of other agents present in alcoholic beverages, is likely. A diet poor in fruits and vegetables, typical of heavy drinkers, may also play a role.

Alcohol-drinking is also strongly associated with the risk of primary liver cancer, particularly among smokers and among people chronically infected with hepatitis C virus. A higher risk of colorectal cancer seems to be linearly correlated with the amount of alcohol consumed and independent of the type of alcohol. A greater risk of breast cancer has been consistently reported. More cases of breast cancer than of any other cancer are attributable to alcohol-drinking among European women. It has been suggested that alcohol acts on hormonal factors involved in breast carcinogenesis.

Few studies have analysed the relation between stopping alcohol-drinking and the risk of cancers of the upper respiratory and digestive tracts, but there is clear evidence that the risk of oesophageal cancer falls by 60%, 10 years or more after drinking cessation.

OTHER FACTORS

Weight reduction

Obesity is associated with a greater risk of cancer of the colon, breast (post-menopausal), endometrium, kidney and oesophagus (adenocarcinoma). In Western Europe, it has been estimated that being overweight or obese accounts for approximately 11% of all colon and breast cancers, 39% of endometrial cancers, 27% of oesophageal adenocarcinomas and 25% of renal cell cancers. A body mass index of below 25 kg/m2 should, if possible, be maintained.

Greater physical activity

There is consistent evidence that regular physical activity is associated with a 40% reduction in the risk of colorectal, breast and oesophageal cancer and may possibly also lower the risk of prostate cancer. The protective effect of physical activity improves with increasing levels of activity. One hour per day of moderate physical activity, such as walking, may also be needed to maintain a healthy body weight, particularly for people with sedentary lifestyles.

Greater intake of fruit and vegetables

A low-fat diet with at least 11 servings of fruits, vegetables, wholegrains and beans daily may reduce the chances of colon cancer by 75%, breast cancer by 50% and lung cancer by 30%. There may also be a protective effect on the risk of a wide variety of other cancers, in particular oral, oesophagus, stomach, rectum and pancreas.

'Five-a-day' (minimum 400 g/day, i.e. two pieces of fruit and 200 g of vegetables) is advocated to lead to a lower cancer risk. Vegetables and fruits contain many potentially anticarcinogenic agents. Antioxidant activity seems important in cancer protection but the exact molecule(s) in vegetables and fruits that confer(s) protection is/are unknown and the mechanism of action unclear.

Avoidance of sun exposure

Ninety per cent of skin cancers are seen in white-skinned peoples and are caused by the sun's ultraviolet rays (Ch. 11). Squamous cell carcinoma of the skin or lip shows the clearest relationship with sun exposure and the risk is greatest in outdoor workers. The recipients of transplanted organs are particularly at risk as a result of the combined effects of the unchecked growth of human papillomavirus (HPV) due to immunosuppression, and exposure to the sun (Ch. 35).

Malignant melanoma is more common in people of high socioeconomic status who work inside but who have the opportunity to spend leisure time in the sun, and this includes dentists. The incidence of melanoma has doubled in Europe in 30 years, and this is attributed to longer intense sun exposure. The fair-skinned are more susceptible, particularly those with red hair, freckles and a tendency to burn in the sun. These characteristics are genetically determined at least partially by the *MCIR* gene, which codes for the melanocyte-stimulating hormone receptor. Variants in the *MCIR* gene control the ratio of black melanin (eumelanin) to red (phaeomelanin) in the skin. The strongest phenotypic risk factor for melanoma, however, is the presence of large numbers of moles or melanocytic naevi, which may be normal in appearance but are also usually accompanied by so-called atypical moles. The latter are larger than 5 mm in diameter with variable colour and an irregular shape. The phenotype, described as the atypical mole syndrome (AMS) phenotype, is present in around 2% of the Caucasian population and is associated with an approximately tenfold higher risk of melanoma. Advice on sun protection is of particular importance to this population.

The best protection from the summer sun is to stay out of it. If outdoors, keep out of the sun between 11.00 a.m. and 3.00 p.m., wear close-weave heavy cotton and use sunscreens with high sun protection factor (SPF). Do not rely upon sunscreens for protection.

Avoidance of occupational exposures

The cancers that have most frequently been associated with occupational exposures are those of the lung, urinary bladder, mesothelioma, larynx, liver, nose and nasal cavity, and skin, as well as leukaemia (non-melanoma). The more common occupational exposures are solar radiation, passive smoking, crystalline silica, diesel exhaust, radon, wood dust, benzene, asbestos, formaldehyde, PAHs, chromium, cadmium and nickel compounds. There is no reliable evidence of a risk from power plants, power lines or mobile telephones.

Many chemicals are known or suspected carcinogens. Many are still widely used: for example, 1,3-butadiene and formaldehyde. Prevention of workplace exposures can be effective; the incidence of occupational bladder cancer fell after the ban on the use of beta-naphthylamine in the rubber and chemical industries.

Avoidance of environmental exposures

The term 'environmental exposures' usually refers to exposures of the general population that cannot be directly controlled by the individual; these include air pollution, drinking water contaminants, passive smoking, radon gas in buildings, exposure to solar radiation, food contaminants such as pesticide residues, dioxins or environmental oestrogens, chemicals from industrial emissions, ionizing radiation, waste from nuclear processes, and others. These exposures have been associated with cancers of the lung, urinary bladder, leukaemia and skin. The impact of several exposures that are widespread, such as disinfection by-products in drinking water, is still inconclusive. Agents in the general environment to which many are exposed for long periods (such as passive smoking or air pollution) may increase the relative risk for certain cancers only modestly, but may be responsible for a significant number of cases overall.

Table 22.3 *Cancer screening*[a]

Cancer site	Methods
Breast	Self-examination/mammography/*BRCA1* and *BRAC2* mutation in Jewish women
Cervix	Cervical cytology/human papillomavirus testing
Colon/rectum	Faecal occult blood/flexible sigmoidoscopy
Lung	Spiral computed tomography (CT) or chest radiography
Neuroblastoma	Urinary homovanillic acid (HVA) and vanillylmandelic acid (VMA)
Oral	Examination of the mouth
Ovary	Cancer antigen 125 (CA125) and/or ultrasonography
Prostate	Prostate-specific antigen (PSA)
Skin (melanoma)	Examination for moles
Stomach	*Helicobacter pylori* testing; breath test/endoscopy
Testis	Self-examination

[a]From Boyle, et al. 2003.

Box 22.3 *Common cancer types*

- Bladder cancer
- Breast cancer
- Colon and rectal cancer
- Endometrial (cervical) cancer
- Kidney (renal cell) cancer
- Leukaemia
- Lung cancer
- Melanoma
- Non-Hodgkin lymphoma
- Oral cancer
- Pancreatic cancer
- Prostate cancer
- Skin cancer (non-melanoma)
- Thyroid cancer

Box 22.4 *Features that may suggest cancer*

- Abdominal pain
- Abnormal vaginal bleeding
- Anorexia
- Blood in faeces
- Blood in sputum
- Blood in urine
- Change in bowel habits
- Change in size or colour of a skin lump
- Change in urination
- Chronic backache
- Chronic headaches
- Dysphagia
- Fever
- Finger clubbing
- Hoarseness
- Lump in breast
- Lump in testicle
- Lymph node enlargement
- Night sweats
- Persistent cough
- Unexplained anaemia
- Weight loss

stage. Because of this, 'tumour markers' are used mainly in patients who have already been diagnosed with cancer in order to monitor treatment response or detect recurrences. The most widely accepted tumour marker assessment is the prostate-specific antigen (PSA) blood test, which is used (along with the digital rectal examination) to screen for prostate cancer; it also suffers from the drawbacks outlined in Chapter 25. Others tumour markers are shown in Table 22.4.

Surgery, radiotherapy and chemotherapy are the main treatments for cancer.

Avoidance of hormones that may play a role

Hormone replacement therapy (HRT) for menopausal symptoms appears to raise the risk of breast cancer.

CANCER SCREENING

Table 22.3 shows cancer screening methods.

CLINICAL FEATURES

There is a range of different cancers (Box 22.3), each with specific manifestations (see relevant chapters). Features that may raise suspicion of cancer are shown in Box 22.4.

MANAGEMENT

Clinical examination, supplemented with imaging and biopsy, is invariably indicated to diagnose malignant disease. There is also considerable interest in tumour markers in blood or other body fluids, or in tissues; unfortunately, none of these tumour markers, including carcinoembryonic antigen (CEA), meets the goal of *reliably* finding cancer at an early

ORAL CANCER

GENERAL ASPECTS

Oral cancer is usually squamous cell carcinoma (OSCC) and is the predominant cancer in the head and neck. It is mainly a disease of older males. High rates of OSCC are seen particularly in India, Sri Lanka, Brazil, Hungary and France, and there is a wide geographical variation in incidence. Risk factors are shown in Box 22.5. The results of many studies of lifestyle risk factors have been summarized by the International Agency for Research on Cancer (IARC) and show the importance of specific factors (i.e. tobacco, betel and alcohol use).

Tobacco contains a number of addictive components, especially nicotine, and releases many carcinogens (see above). Tobacco use in all forms appears to carry a risk of OSCC. Oral cancer risks show a clear decline after stopping tobacco use. Snuff – finely powdered plant material, principally tobacco, used orally or nasally – is a risk factor for OSCC.

Betel quid (BQ) is probably used by 20% of the world's population and may lead to:

- cancer: oral, oesophageal, pancreatic, hepatocellular
- other conditions:
  oral submucous fibrosis
  hypertension

Table 22.4 *Tumour markers*

Marker	Abbreviation	Comments
Alpha-fetoprotein	AFP	Useful to follow treatment response and follow-up in liver cancer (hepatocellular carcinoma) and testicular cancers (embryonal cell and endodermal sinus types). Raised AFP levels also seen in rare ovarian and testicular cancers (yolk sac tumour or mixed germ-cell cancer)
Beta$_2$-microglobulin	B2M	Raised in multiple myeloma, chronic lymphocytic leukaemia (CLL) and some lymphomas
Bladder tumour antigen	BTA	Found in urine in bladder cancer
Calcitonin	–	Raised blood levels in cancer of parafollicular C cells (medullary thyroid carcinoma; MTC)
Cancer antigens	CA15-3	Breast cancer
	CA19-9	Developed to detect colorectal cancer, but more sensitive for pancreatic cancer
	CA27.29	Breast cancer
	CA72-4	Ovarian and pancreatic cancer and digestive tract cancers, especially stomach
	CA125	Ovarian cancer
Carcinoembryonic antigen	CEA	Used to monitor treatment and recurrence of colorectal carcinoma and breast, lung, pancreatic and gastric malignancies
Chromogranin A	CgA	Neuroendocrine tumours (carcinoid tumours, neuroblastoma and small-cell lung cancer)
Immunoglobulins	Igs	Bone marrow cancers (e.g. multiple myeloma and Waldenström macroglobulinaemia)
Neuron-specific enolase	NSE	Neuroendocrine tumours (small-cell lung cancer, neuroblastoma and carcinoid tumours)
Soluble 100% in ammonium sulphate	S-100	Found in most melanoma cells
Tissue polypeptide antigen	TPA	Follow-up of patients treated for cancers in lung or bladder
Thyroglobulin	–	Thyroid diseases, including some cancers

Box 22.5 *Risk factors for oral cancer*

- Age (advancing)
- Diet low in fruit and vegetables
- Gender: male
- Graft-versus-host disease
- Immunosuppression
- Infections with human papillomavirus, *Candida* or syphilis
- Ionizing radiation
- Lifestyle habits:
  - Alcohol
  - Betel (areca)
  - Tobacco
- Low socioeconomic status
- Sun exposure

Table 22.5 *Occupations associated with risk of oral cancer*

Occupations	Main countries
Exposure to wood-stove fumes	Brazil
Building industry	Italy
Electricity production	
Machinery operations	
Plumbing	
Textile industry	
Carpet installation	USA
Exposure to fossil fuels	
Furniture industry	
Machining	
Metalworking	
Painting	
Petroleum industry	
Woodworking	
Blacksmithing	Uruguay
Butchering	
Driving	
Electricity working	
Masonry	
Railway working	
Metalworking	Brazil
Exposure to horses on farms, employment on construction work, pesticide use, grain production	Norway
Exposure to benzene	UK

metabolic syndrome
adverse birth outcomes
liver cirrhosis
chronic kidney disease
contact dermatitis
periodontitis
urinary calculi.

Increased consumption of alcohol-containing beverages is associated with a risk of OSCC. The risk decreases after stopping alcohol use but the effects appear to persist for several years. The type of alcoholic beverage appears to influence the risk – hard liquors conferring higher risks. There have been reports of oral cancer in marijuana smokers and in users of alcohol-containing mouthwashes but any relationships have yet to be confirmed by full epidemiological studies.

Charcoal-grilled red meat and fried foods have been implicated as risk factors, but an increased consumption of fruits and vegetables is associated with lower risk of OSCC. Higher risks of oral cancer have also been found in a number of occupations (Table 22.5).

Microorganisms implicated in the aetiology of OSCC include syphilis, *Candida albicans* and viruses such as herpesviruses and HPV. Syphilis is discussed in Chapter 32. Candidal leukoplakias are potentially malignant and autoimmune polyendocrinopathy–candidiasis–ectodermal dystrophy (APECED), an autosomal recessive disease associated with a limited T-lymphocyte defect, seems to favour the growth of *C. albicans* and predisposes to OSCC. Viral infections, particularly with oncogenic HPV subtypes and possibly Epstein–Barr virus (EBV), can have a tumorigenic effect. Oropharyngeal cancer is significantly associated with oral HPV and also with a high lifetime number of vaginal-sex partners and oral-sex partners; HPV-16 DNA is detected in most.

Lip cancer is seen mainly in males with chronic sun exposure and in smokers. Antihypertensive agents increase the risk. Ionizing radiation exposure is a possible risk factor for second primary cancers.

Persons with poor oral hygiene appear to have an increased risk of OSCC, independent of any effect of tobacco, alcohol, or other well-proven risk factors; not all workers agree, however, so further studies are required. Polymicrobial supragingival plaque is a possible independent factor, as it possesses a relevant mutagenic interaction with saliva, and individual oral health is a cofactor in the development of OSCC. Viridans group streptococci of the normal oral flora can produce acetaldehyde *in vitro* during ethanol incubation via alcohol dehydrogenase. In particular, the clinical strain of *Streptococcus salivarius*, both clinical and culture collection strains of *Streptococcus intermedius* and the culture collection strain of *Streptococcus mitis* produced high amounts of acetaldehyde.

SYSTEMIC HEALTH AND ORAL SQUAMOUS CELL CARCINOMA

There is a highly significant increase in the incidence of OSCC in dyskeratosis congenita and systemic sclerosis, and an increase of potentially malignant lesions and OSCC in transplant recipients and in people with cancers elsewhere in the upper aerodigestive tract. There is a putative association of diabetes mellitus with oral cancer.

POTENTIALLY MALIGNANT DISORDERS

Some potentially malignant (pre-cancerous) oral clinical lesions that can progress to OSCC include the following, in particular:

- erythroplasia (erythroplakia) – the most likely lesion to progress to severe dysplasia or carcinoma
- leukoplakia, particularly where admixed with red lesions, as in speckled leukoplakia, and proliferative verrucous leukoplakia, sublingual leukoplakia, candidal leukoplakia and syphilitic leukoplakia (exceptionally rare now)
- lichen planus
- oral submucous fibrosis.

Apart from these lesions, most other potentially malignant lesions or conditions have only a very low incidence of dysplasia or malignant change (Table 22.6).

CLINICAL FEATURES

Common sites for OSCC are the lips, the lateral border of the tongue, and the floor of the mouth. There may be widespread dysplastic mucosa ('field change') or even a *second primary neoplasm* anywhere in the oral cavity, oropharynx or upper aerodigestive tract.

Cancer must be suspected, especially when there is a single oral lesion persisting for more than 3 weeks, and particularly when having the features shown in Box 22.6. Many OSCCs can be detected visually but early OSCC can be asymptomatic, may appear innocuous and can be overlooked, especially if the examination is not thorough. The whole oral mucosa should be examined, often along with the rest of the upper aerodigestive tract – and the cervical lymph nodes must always be carefully examined by palpation (Fig. 22.2). Various stains or lights purported to help diagnosis tend to lack sensitivity or specificity. Biopsy is invariably indicated.

CLASSIFICATION/GRADING

Oral cancer is a term that usually includes cancer of the lip, tongue, salivary glands and other sites in the mouth (gum, floor of the mouth and other unspecified parts of the mouth). Pharyngeal cancer is

Table 22.6 *Potentially malignant oral disorders*

Malignant potential	Lesion	Known aetiological factors
Very high (≥85%)	Erythroplasia	Tobacco/alcohol
High in some instances (≥30%)	Actinic cheilitis	Sunlight
	Chronic candidosis (candidal leukoplakia)	*Candida albicans*
	Dyskeratosis congenita	Genetic
	Leukoplakia (non-homogeneous)	Tobacco/alcohol
	Proliferative verrucous leukoplakia	Tobacco/alcohol/human papillomavirus (HPV)
	Sublingual keratosis	Tobacco/alcohol
	Submucous fibrosis	Areca nut
	Syphilitic leukoplakia	Syphilis
Low (<5%)	Atypia in immunocompromised patients	?HPV
	Leukoplakia (homogeneous)	Friction/tobacco/alcohol
	Discoid lupus erythematosus	Autoimmune
	Lichen planus	Idiopathic
	Paterson–Brown-Kelly syndrome (Plummer–Vinson syndrome)	Iron deficiency

Box 22.6 *Warning features of oral cancer*

- Red lesion (erythroplasia)
- Mixed red/white lesion, irregular white lesion
- Lump
- Ulcer with fissuring or raised exophytic margins
- Pain or numbness
- Abnormal blood vessels supplying a lump
- Loose tooth
- Extraction socket not healing
- Induration beneath a lesion (i.e. a firm infiltration beneath the mucosa)
- Fixation of lesion to deeper tissues or to overlying skin or mucosa
- Lymph node enlargement
- Dysphagia
- Weight loss

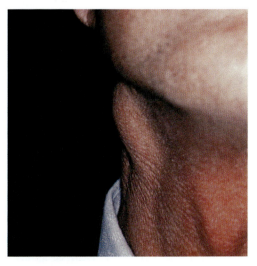

Fig. 22.2 Cervical lymph node enlargement in oral carcinoma.

Table 22.7 *TNM classification of malignant neoplasms*[a]

Stage	Criteria
Primary tumour size (T)	
Tx	No available information
T0	No evidence of primary tumour
Tis	Only carcinoma *in situ*
T1, T2, T3, T4[b]	Increasing size of tumour
Regional lymph node involvement (N)	
Nx	Nodes could not or were not assessed
N0	No clinically positive nodes
N1	Single ipsilateral node <3 cm in diameter
N2a	Single ipsilateral node 3–6 cm
N2b	Multiple ipsilateral nodes <6 cm
N2c	Bilateral or contralateral nodes <6 cm
N3	Any node >6 cm
Involvement by distant metastases (M)	
Mx	Distant metastasis was not assessed
M0	No evidence of distant metastasis
M1	Distant metastasis is present

[a]Several other classifications are available, e.g. STNM (S = site).
[b]T1 = maximum diameter 2 cm; T2 = maximum diameter 4 cm; T3 = maximum diameter >4 cm; T4, massive tumour >4 cm in diameter, with involvement of adjacent anatomical structures.

Table 22.8 *Prognosis for intraoral carcinoma*

Stage	TNM	Approximate 5-year survival (%)
I	T1 N0 M0	85
II	T2 N0 M0	65
III	T3 N0 M0, or T1, T2 or T3 N1 M0	40
IV	Any T4, N2, N3 or M1	10

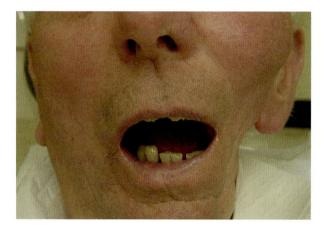

Fig. 22.3 Deformity after tumour resection.

a term that includes cancers of the nasopharynx, oropharynx and hypopharynx.

Staging of OSCC should be made according to the TNM classification of the International Union against Cancer (UICC) – tumour size (T), nodal metastases (N) and distant metastases (M; Table 22.7) – since this classification relates well to overall survival rate (i.e. the earlier the tumour is detected, the better the prognosis and the less complicated the treatment).

It is generally accepted that prognosis is best in early carcinomas, especially those that are well differentiated and not metastasized (Table 22.8).

GENERAL MANAGEMENT

Any lesion of a potentially malignant or dubious nature persisting for more than 3 weeks should be biopsied and second primary tumours should be excluded by chest radiography and endoscopy. Tumours are staged using the TNM system (tumour, nodes, metastases).

OSCCs are routinely discovered late and have one of the lowest 5-year survival rates of any major cancer site, at approximately 50%; this has not changed in the past 30 years. Localized cancers have the highest 5-year relative survival rates (80%), those with regional disease intermediate (40%) and cancers with distant metastasis the lowest (20%). OSCC is also particularly dangerous because it may be associated with second primary tumours.

Patients with oral cancer are best managed by a team of specialists that includes dental and maxillofacial surgeons, as well as oncologists, nurses, speech therapists and hygienists.

Cancer treatment can be with surgery, radiotherapy, chemotherapy (cytotoxic drugs singly or in combination), targeted therapy stem-cell transplantation, immunotherapy (monoclonal antibodies and, on the horizon, vaccines) and now gene therapy.

The choice of surgery in the treatment of oral cancer depends on tumour location, size, proximity to bone, and depth of infiltration. In most cases in which bone is involved, a segmental resection of the tumour is necessary with microvascular reconstruction using free flaps to restore mastication and facial contour, and allow for the placement of osseo-integrated implants for orofacial and dental rehabilitation. Transoral robotic surgery and transoral laser microsurgery and minimally invasive surgery with curative intent have increased. Surgery can lead to complications, which are discussed in standard textbooks of surgery – not least some defects of aesthetics and function (Fig. 22.3).

Radiotherapy and chemotherapy are used mainly to damage or destroy proliferating malignant cells (particularly in malignant disease affecting blood cells and lymphomas [Ch. 8]), but also for some more solid tumours such as OSCC. They can affect many tissues and can have severe adverse effects on health, health care and quality of life. These treatments can also damage the developing fetus.

Radiotherapy and cytotoxic chemotherapy can also have profound adverse effects on oral health and quality of life, and can give rise to the major complaints of the patient undergoing cancer treatment – especially when the radiotherapy field affects the head and neck, and involves the oral cavity and salivary glands. Chemoradiation therapy (CRT) is commonly used for locally advanced head and neck cancers or as adjuvant therapy. Altered fractionation plus concurrent CRT improves tumour control and reduces late toxicity but is associated with more severe acute oral toxicities, especially mucositis. Intensity-modulated radiotherapy (IMRT) offers advantages; arc therapy reduces IMRT delivery time from 20 minutes to less than 5 minutes, while optimizing dose homogeneity and sparing normal tissue, including parotid gland sparing. Opinion varies as to the relative value of radiotherapy or surgery.

The role of targeted agents, such as cetuximab, as part of a combined modality treatment approach for locally advanced cancer has yet to be clearly defined.

Treatment of patients with oral and oropharyngeal tongue cancers has not shown a significant improvement in 5-year disease-specific survival over decades. Poorer survival is significantly associated with ages of more than 45 years, oropharyngeal tongue cancers and advanced-stage disease. A multimodal approach of surgery for the primary tumour and the neck, followed by postoperative radio(chemo) therapy, seems superior to non-surgical treatment protocols, since it results in better disease-free and overall survival.

Many early carcinomas can be treated by either surgery or radiotherapy, but in the later stages surgery is the first option. Cancer of the floor of the mouth presents considerable problems in surgery and may necessitate partial mandibulectomy. Lingual and labial cancers are often managed with radiotherapy, which may also provide the best palliation in patients with advanced disease. Cytotoxic chemotherapy has not offered any better prognosis and, indeed, may cause greater morbidity and mortality, but newer drugs may help, as discussed below.

SURGERY

Surgery is the oldest form of treatment for oral cancer (see http://www. oralcancerfoundation.org/facts/surgery.htm; accessed 30 September 2013) and is often performed to achieve more than one of the following goals:

- *Curative surgery* – the removal of a tumour when it appears to be confined to one area. It may be used along with radiation therapy or chemotherapy, which can be given before or after the operation. In some cases, radiation therapy is actually used during an operation (intraoperative radiation therapy).
- *Debulking (or cytoreductive) surgery* – sometimes done when removing a tumour entirely would cause too much damage to an organ or surrounding areas. In these cases, radiation therapy or chemotherapy is also typically used.
- *Palliative surgery* – used to treat complications of advanced disease. It is not intended to cure the cancer.
- *Supportive surgery* – used to help with other types of treatment. For example, a vascular access device, such as a catheter port, can be placed into a vein to facilitate chemotherapy.
- *Restorative (or reconstructive) surgery* – used to restore aesthetics and function.

Transoral laser microsurgery is a new trend for complete resection of tumours with preservation of function. Advanced reconstructive techniques that allow free transfer of soft tissue and bone from all over the body improve the functional and aesthetic outcomes following major ablative surgery. With successful surgical reconstruction, dental and prosthetic rehabilitation choices are enhanced. Neck dissection has also greatly advanced – from radical to function-preserving surgery, with sensory and spinal accessory nerve-preserving neck surgery resulting in a lower incidence and severity of neck and shoulder pain and loss of function compared to patients who have the nerve removed, and less depression and better quality-of-life scores with lower pain intensity.

Wound infection is a common complication after OSCC surgery and may lead to significant functional morbidity, poor cosmetic results and prolonged hospitalization. The most important factors contributing to operative wound infections are male sex, tumour stage, reconstruction, tracheostomy, nasogastric tube or gastrostomy feeding, and the extent of surgery.

RADIOTHERAPY

Radiation therapy is commonly used to treat OSCC (see http://www.oral-cancerfoundation.org/facts/radiation.htm; accessed 30 September 2013). Prior to therapy, a planning session is required, including a computed tomography (CT) scan and measurements of the area to be treated, as well as skin markings to help with positioning during treatments. A porous mask is used in radiation treatment, to immobilize the patient's head so that radiation will only be delivered to the designated areas. The radiation therapy is given in small amounts (fractions) on a daily basis, usually 5 days in a row with a 2-day break each week. Normally, each daily treatment lasts about 10–15 minutes, with the majority of this time spent making sure that the radiation-blocking devices, which limit the radiation to the appropriate area, are properly in place, and the patient and machine are properly positioned. The daily dose must be great enough to destroy the cancer cells while sparing the normal tissues from excessive levels of radiation. Typically, 2 Gy is delivered five times a week to a total dose of 64–70 Gy.

Internal radiotherapy

Internal radiotherapy involves placing radioactive implants directly into a tumour or body cavity, resulting in less radiation exposure to other parts of the body. Brachytherapy, interstitial irradiation and intracavitary irradiation are types of internal radiotherapy.

External beam radiotherapy

This involves the use of machines to focus radiation on a cancer site. With modern radiation equipment, there is minimal scatter of X-ray energy outside the treatment beam.

X-rays were the first form of photon radiation to be used to treat cancer. Depending on the amount of energy they possess, the X-rays can be employed to destroy cancer cells on the surface of an area, or to penetrate to tissues deeper in the body. The higher the energy of the X-ray beam, the deeper the X-rays penetrate into the target tissue.

Linear accelerators produce X-rays of increasingly greater energy. Gamma rays are another available form of photon radiation and are produced spontaneously as certain elements (such as radium, uranium and cobalt 60) release radiation when they decompose or decay.

Intraoperative irradiation

In intraoperative irradiation, a large dose of external radiation is directed at the tumour and surrounding tissue during surgery.

Intensity-modulated radiotherapy

Intensity-modulated radiotherapy (IMRT) uses a different software programme to administer the radiation from multiple angles in smaller doses, with a new shuttering device to limit the size of the radiation beams, thus sparing the salivary glands.

Particle beam radiation therapy

This involves the use of fast-moving subatomic particles to treat localized cancers. A sophisticated machine is needed to produce and accelerate the particles required for this procedure. Some particles (neutrons, pions and heavy ions) deposit more energy along the path they take through tissue than do X-rays or gamma rays, thus causing more damage to the cells they hit. This type of radiation is often referred to as high linear energy transfer (high LET) radiation.

The consensus is that patients with OSCC with involved margins or extracapsular spread (ECS) should have adjuvant radiotherapy. IMRT, three-dimensional (3-D) conformal radiotherapy, and conventional radiotherapy provide similar disease control but IMRT produces less hyposalivation.

Chemoradiotherapy

Chemotherapeutic agents are increasingly used to enhance the effects of radiotherapy (chemoradiation) (see below).

DENTAL ASPECTS

Careful treatment planning, close monitoring and strict application of preventive measures can reduce the incidence of complications. Improved techniques, such as the application of lower radiation doses or IMRT, use of shielding, reduction in toxic drugs and improved oral hygiene, can also reduce complications. Pain control is of paramount importance; patients may need potent analgesics, such as opioids, sedatives or antidepressants, particularly if they have terminal cancer. Completion of dental treatment before cancer care benefits the patient greatly.

Patients with advanced disease have a high prevalence of oral treatment complications, particularly hyposalivation, which is seen in nearly three-quarters; often soreness, taste disturbances and difficulties with wearing dentures are also present. Candidosis is common.

The most obvious oral importance of tumours in other parts of the body is as a source of metastases that can form in the jaws or occasionally in soft tissues. Histological examination of all such swellings in a person with malignant disease elsewhere is therefore essential. Other oral manifestations of internal malignancy are summarized in Appendix 22.1.

RADIOTHERAPY INVOLVING THE ORAL CAVITY OR SALIVARY GLANDS

External beam radiotherapy is mostly used to treat oral cancer (Table 22.9). In the treatment of head and neck cancers, radiotherapy, despite being targeted at the cancer, inevitably damages surrounding normal tissues, causing mucositis, and often salivary damage and hyposalivation (Table 22.10). Hair loss and skin erythema are common in the path of the radiation beam (Fig. 22.4). Carotid stenosis may arise.

Careful treatment planning with precise dosimetry and careful shielding of the healthy tissues, as well as close monitoring of the oral cavity with application of preventive measures, can significantly reduce many complications.

Mucositis

Mucositis is virtually inevitable but can be mitigated by modifying the radiation schedule; protecting the mucosa with midline mucosa-sparing blocks; or, theoretically, by using amifostine, which, with its active metabolite, is a free-radical scavenger and is cytoprotective. However, amifostine is rarely used in clinical practice because of fears that the free-radical scavenging action may also reduce the effectiveness of radiotherapy on the cancer cells. Amifostine may cause severe nausea and vomiting, although it also reduces the risk of infection associated with neutropenia. Interventions apart from oral care protocols, that may help ameliorate symptoms in mucositis may include cryotherapy, laser therapy, recombinant human keratinocyte growth factor-1 (palifermin), benzydamine hydrochloride, systemic zinc supplements, and patient controlled analgesia with morphine/transdermal fentanyl/2% morphine mouthwash/0.5% doxepin mouthwash to treat pain.

Hyposalivation

Radiotherapy to tumours of the mouth, nasopharynx and oropharynx is especially liable to damage the salivary glands, depress salivary secretion and result in saliva of a higher viscosity but lower pH. The severity

Table 22.9 *Types of external beam radiotherapy used to treat head and neck cancer*

Type	Source	Used for
Electron beam	Electrical	Superficial lesions
Low-voltage	X-ray	Superficial lesions
Orthovoltage	X-ray	Skin lesions
Supervoltage	Cobalt-60	Deeper lesions
Megavoltage	Linear accelerator	Larger lesions

Table 22.10 *Oral complications of radiotherapy involving the mouth and salivary glands*

Week 1	Week 2+	Week 3+	Later
Nausea	Mucositis	Dry mouth	Infections
Vomiting	Taste changes		Caries
			Pulp pain and necrosis
			Tooth hypersensitivity
			Trismus
			Osteoradionecrosis
			Craniofacial defects

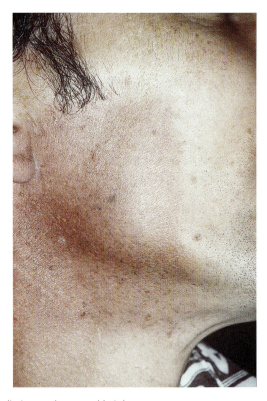

Fig. 22.4 Radiation erythema and hair loss.

experienced depends on a number of factors but especially the volume of salivary tissue irradiated (Table 22.11) and the dose. Salivary secretion diminishes within a week of radiotherapy in virtually all patients and the saliva becomes thick and tenacious. Some salivary function may return after many months. Doses greater than 30 Gy generally lead to a persistently, if not permanently, dry mouth.

Both acute and long-term hyposalivation can be reduced by using IMRT; sparing at least one parotid gland during irradiation of patients with head and neck cancer; stimulating salivation pre-radiotherapy with pilocarpine; or by giving amifostine. Occasionally, submandibular gland transfer is used.

Regimen	Approximate % fall in salivation
Mantle	30
Unilateral	50
Bilateral	75
Head and neck cancer	95
Nasopharynx	100

Table 22.11 *Fall in salivary flow with different radiotherapy fields*

Infections

Hyposalivation predisposes the patient to infections (caries, oral candidosis and acute ascending sialadenitis).

Loss of taste (hypogeusia)

Loss of taste follows radiation damage to the taste buds. Taste may start to recover within 2–4 months and is typically restored by 6 months, but if more than 6000 cGy have been given, loss of taste may be permanent.

Radiation caries

Caries and dental hypersensitivity may follow radiotherapy. Patients frequently take a softer, more cariogenic diet because of mouth dryness and soreness, and loss of taste. Salivary protection is diminished. There is a change to a more cariogenic oral flora and the hypersensitive teeth make oral hygiene difficult. These factors combine to cause rampant dental caries, including in areas such as incisal edges and cervical margins, which are normally free from caries. Caries begins at any time between 2 and 10 months after radiotherapy, and may eventually result in the crown breaking off from the root. A complete dentition may be destroyed within a year of irradiation.

Caries may be minimized by controlling sugar intake, protecting salivary function as above, and using fluorides, sialogogues and mouth-wetting agents.

Trismus

Trismus may result from replacement fibrosis of the masticatory muscles following progressive endarteritis of affected tissues, with reduction in their blood supply. Fibrosis becomes apparent 3–6 months after radiotherapy and can cause permanent limitation of opening. Fibrosis must be differentiated from recurrence of the tumour and from osteoradionecrosis.

Osteoradionecrosis

Radiation therapy induces endarteritis obliterans, which leads to progressive fibrosis and capillary loss, leaving bone susceptible to avascular necrosis. The latter predisposes to the late and more severe complication of osteoradionecrosis (ORN), which may occur months to years later. ORN is a potentially serious complication of radiotherapy involving the jaws and often results from dental extractions carried out after radiotherapy. Oral sepsis, particularly from periodontal disease, may contribute.

The mandible, a compact bone with high density and poor vascularity, is more prone than the maxilla to ORN, and risk is greatest when radiation dose exceeds 60 Gy, when the floor of mouth is irradiated, from 10 days before to several years after radiotherapy (especially at

3–12 months after radiotherapy), and in patients who are malnourished or immuno-incompetent. ORN may follow months or years after radiotherapy but about 30% of cases develop within 6 months and are heralded by pain and swelling. Presentation is with exposed bone in an irradiated mouth, with or without external sinuses, pain and pathological fracture. In severe cases, the whole of the body of the mandible may be destroyed, and the bone may become exposed internally and externally. The area involved is often small (less than 2 cm in diameter) and, with antibiotics, the signs and symptoms of inflammation may clear within a few weeks.

ORN may be prevented by avoiding operations such as dental extractions after the jaws have been irradiated – which is best achieved by removing unsalvageable teeth at least 2 weeks before starting radiotherapy.

New developments in radiotherapy, such as 3-D conformal radiotherapy and IMRT, have allowed radiation oncologists to escalate the dose of radiation delivered to tumours while minimizing the dose delivered to surrounding normal tissue/bone, contributing to a remarkable decline in the prevalence of ORN to less than 4%.

Local measures used to treat ORN include meticulous oral hygiene, chlorhexidine mouthwashes after meals, wound irrigation, removal of loose sequestrate and antibiotic therapy (tetracycline, clindamycin, metronidazole). It is possible that ultrasound and hyperbaric oxygen (HBO) may help. The 'Marx protocol' consists of 20 HBO sessions prior to surgery and 10 sessions afterwards. However, a high-quality trial has demonstrated that HBO alone is not effective in treating ORN of the mandible compared to placebo. There is a lack of evidence regarding the effect of HBO on dental implants/ORN risk. Complete resolution of ORN can, however, take 2 or more years, despite intensive treatment.

Craniofacial defects

Craniofacial defects, tooth hypoplasia and retarded eruption can follow irradiation of developing teeth and growth centres in children. Children treated for neuroblastoma, therefore, are at particularly high risk.

Dental management of patients receiving radiotherapy to the head and neck

Before radiotherapy

Meticulous oral hygiene should be implemented, preventive dental care instituted and restorative procedures carried out. Unsalvageable teeth in the radiation path should be extracted at least 2 weeks before starting radiotherapy and no bone should be left exposed in the mouth.

During radiotherapy

During radiotherapy, mucosal and salivary gland protection with amifostine can minimize mucositis and hyposalivation. Smoking and alcohol should be discouraged.

Mucositis may be relieved by using warm normal saline mouthwashes and benzydamine (which has anti-tumour necrosis factor activity) oral rinses, or lidocaine 2% gel. A 0.2% chlorhexidine mouthwash improves oral hygiene. Antifungal drugs, such as nystatin suspension as a mouthwash used four times daily, may be required. Palifermin, transforming growth factor beta (TGFβ), interleukin-1 (IL-1) and IL-11 show promise.

A saliva substitute, such as carboxymethylcellulose, may provide some symptomatic relief, as may salivary stimulants.

Table 22.12 *Chemotherapeutic drug groups*

Drug group	Actions	Administration route	Examples
Alkylating agents	Directly attack DNA	Oral or intravenous	Cyclophosphamide and mechlorethamine, cisplatin, chlorambucil or melphalan
Nitrosoureas	Inhibit DNA repair	Oral or intravenous	Carmustine and lomustine
Antimetabolites	Interfere with DNA synthesis	Oral or intravenous	6-Mercaptopurine, 5-fluorouracil, methotrexate, fludarabine and cytarabine
Antitumour antibiotics	Prevent RNA synthesis and DNA replication	Intravenous	Doxorubicin and mitomycin-C, daunorubicin, idarubicin and mitoxantrone
Plant (vinca) alkaloids	Prevent cell division	Intravenous	Vincristine and vinblastine
Taxanes	Stop microtubules from breaking down and thus prevent cancer cells from growing and dividing	Intravenous	Paclitaxel and docetaxel
DNA-repair enzyme inhibitors	Attack DNA repair mechanisms	Oral or intravenous	Etoposide or topotecan
Steroid hormones	Modify growth of hormone-dependent cancers	Oral	Tamoxifen and flutamide

Trismus may be improved by jaw-opening exercises with tongue spatulas, wedges or TheraBite®, used three times a day.

After radiotherapy

Oral hygiene and preventive dental care should be continued; dryness of the mouth is managed as for Sjögren syndrome (Ch. 18).

Radiation caries and dental hypersensitivity can be controlled with a non-cariogenic diet, high-fluoride dentifrice and daily topical fluoride applications, such as fluoride mouthwash. The standard of care for natural teeth is by daily application of fluoride by means of custom-fabricated carriers. Amorphous calcium phosphate may be indicated.

If extractions become unavoidable, trauma should be kept to a minimum, raising the periosteum as little as possible, ensuring that sharp bone edges are removed, suturing carefully and giving prophylactic antibiotics in adequate doses from 48 hours preoperatively, continued for at least 4 weeks to prevent ORN. Clindamycin 600 mg three times daily is an appropriate antibiotic since it penetrates bone well.

If dentures are required, they should be fitted at about 4–6 weeks after radiotherapy, when initial mucositis subsides and there is only early fibrosis.

CHEMOTHERAPY

Chemotherapy alone is rarely appropriate in OSCC but taxanes, cisplatin and 5-fluorouracil (TPF), or carboplatin, methotrexate and bleomycin may be used. Chemotherapy is used mainly for treating lymphoproliferative neoplasms. Mucositis may result.

Cytotoxic chemotherapy drugs act mainly by interacting with cancer cell DNA or RNA and affecting some phase of the cell's life cycle (http://www.oralcancerfoundation.org/facts/chemotherapy.htm; accessed 30 September 2013). The first phase of the cell cycle (G1) is when the cell prepares to replicate its chromosomes. The second stage (S) is when DNA synthesis occurs and the DNA is duplicated. The next phase (G2) is when the RNA and protein duplicate. The final (M) stage is the stage of actual cell division; the duplicated DNA and RNA split and move to separate ends of the cell, and the cell divides into two identical functional cells (mitosis). Chemotherapeutic drugs are divided into several broad categories, depending on their function (Tables 22.12 and 22.13).

Chemotherapy is given orally or, more usually, intravenously, then typically by catheter – a thin plastic tube – inserted into a central vein or artery and left in place throughout treatment; this eliminates the need for multiple needle insertions every time treatment is needed. Chemotherapy results in OSCC appear to be improving, and the technique of continuous intra-arterial infusion therapy may sometimes be

Table 22.13 *Other drugs used in the treatment of malignant disease*

Drug class	Examples
Aromatase inhibitors	Aminoglutethimide
	Anastrozole
	Formestane
	Letrozole
Hormones	For prostate carcinoma:
	Bicalutamide
	Cyproterone
	Flutamide
	Gonadotrophin-releasing hormone analogues (buserelin, goserelin, leuprorelin, triptorelin)
	Oestrogen
	For breast carcinoma:
	Progestogens
	Tamoxifen
	Toremifene
Recombinant interleukin-2	Aldesleukin
Somatostatin analogues	Lanreotide
	Octreotide

as effective as surgery or radiation therapy, with an excellent cosmetic result, preservation of function and minimal side-effects.

Complications from cytotoxic chemotherapy

Most cytotoxic agents cause complications, particularly if treatment is prolonged or in high dosage (see Tables 22.12 and 22.13); they include alopecia, nausea and vomiting, anorexia, bone marrow suppression, hyperuricaemia, reproductive function damage, especially in males, and mucositis (Fig. 22.5) in particular. Some 90% of children and approximately 50% of adults develop oral lesions, more frequently so when chemoradiotherapy is given.

Mucositis

Chemotherapy-induced mucositis typically appears from 7 to 14 days after the initiation of drug therapy. At least 90% of patients treated with fluorouracil and cisplatin develop mucositis (Table 22.14). Etoposide, melphalan, doxorubicin, vinblastine, taxanes and methotrexate are also particularly stomatotoxic. By contrast, mucositis is uncommon with asparaginase and carmustine.

Table 22.14 *Main chemotherapeutic agents responsible for oral mucositis*

Alkylating agents	Anthracyclines	Antibiotics	Antimetabolites	Taxanes	Microtubule disassemblers
Busulfan	Daunorubicin	Actinomycin D	Cytosine arabinoside	Docetaxel	Etoposide
Cyclophosphamide	Doxorubicin	Amsacrine	5-Fluorouracil	Paclitaxel	Vinblastine
Mechlorethamine	Epirubicin	Bleomycin	Hydroxycarbamide		Vincristine
Melphalan		Dactinomycin	Methotrexate		Vinorelbine
Procarbazine		Daunorubicin	6-Mercaptopurine		
Thiotepa		Doxorubicin	Tioguanine		
		Mithromycin			
		Mitomycin			
		Mitoxantrone			

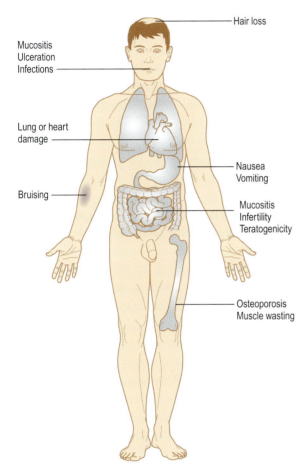

Fig. 22.5 Adverse effects from chemotherapy.

Table 22.15 *Oral assessment guide*

	1	2	3
Voice	Normal	Deeper or raspy	Difficulty talking
Swallow	Normal	Some pain	Inability to swallow
Lips	Smooth, pink and moist	Dry or cracked	Ulcerated or bleeding
Tongue	Pink and moist	Coated and shiny ± red	Blistered or cracked
Saliva	Watery	Thick	Absent
Mucous membranes	Pink and moist	Red and coated without ulcers	Ulcers
Gingivae	Pink and firm	Oedematous ± redness	Spontaneous or pressure-induced bleeding
Teeth/denture areas	Clean, no debris	Plaque and localized debris	Generalized plaque or debris

Table 22.16 *Diet in oral mucositis*

Diet that is typically acceptable	Foods to avoid	Lifestyle habits to avoid
Liquids	Rough food (chips, crisps, toast)	Smoking
Purées	Spices	Alcohol
Ice	Salt	
Custards	Acidic fruit (grapefruit, lemon, orange)	
Non-acidic fruits (banana, mango, melon, peach)		
Soft cheeses		
Eggs		

If associated with neutropenia, mucositis predisposes to septicaemia. Potential pathogens include alpha-haemolytic streptococci, especially *Streptococcus oralis* and *Strep. mitis*, *C. albicans*, other *Candida* species, *Aspergillus* and *Mucor*. Mucositis may be a predictor of gastrointestinal toxicity and, after haemopoietic stem-cell transplantation (HSCT), may predict the onset of hepatic veno-occlusive disease.

General management

It is helpful to attempt to score the degree of mucositis for monitoring progress and therapy. Several systems have been devised but most lack standardization or validation, and none thus far has found universal acceptance; an example is shown in Table 22.15.

Despite the numerous approaches tried for the prevention and treatment of mucositis, virtually nothing works consistently or predictably. However, there is benefit from a soft diet (Table 22.16). Ice chips sucked for 30 minutes before 5-fluorouracil, methotrexate or melphalan administration may be beneficial by reducing exposure of mucosae to the chemotherapy agent. Folinic acid (as calcium folinate), levofolinic acid or disodium folinate can reduce mucositis from methotrexate or fluorouracil. Palifermin, TGFβ, IL-1 and IL-11 show promise.

Mucositis often necessitates the use of opioid analgesics for pain control; tube feeding; and prophylaxis for infectious complications. Interventions that may ameliorate symptoms include oral care protocols, oral cryotherapy, laser therapy, recombinant human keratinocyte growth factor-1 (palifermin), benzydamine hydrochloride, systemic zinc supplements, and patient controlled analgesia with morphine/transdermal fentanyl/2% morphine mouthwash/0.5% doxepin mouthwash to treat pain.

Infections

Cytotoxic agents predispose to infections with fungi, viruses, toxoplasma or bacteria. Oral candidosis is common, usually caused by *C. albicans* or, less often, other *Candida* species. It is promoted especially by severe leukopenia and the use of antibiotics. Oral mucormycosis (phycomycosis) or aspergillosis is rare. Herpetic infections (herpes simplex or herpes zoster) are common and may cause chronic oral ulcers. Gram-negative oral infections may be caused by *Pseudomonas, Klebsiella, Escherichia, Enterobacter, Serratia* or *Proteus*, and dental infections may spread rapidly. Gram-positive bacterial infections (staphylococci) are less common as patients usually receive antibiotics prophylactically.

Bleeding

Drug-induced thrombocytopenia may cause gingival bleeding, mucosal petechiae or ecchymoses.

Hyposalivation

Cytotoxic agents (especially doxorubicin) can lead to hyposalivation, caries and other oral infections.

Craniofacial maldevelopment

Delayed and abnormal craniofacial, jaw and dentition development and abnormalities can follow prolonged chemotherapy.

Dental management of patients on cytotoxic chemotherapy

Before chemotherapy

A careful oral assessment should be carried out to enable extractions and any other surgery to be completed before cytotoxic treatment (Table 22.17). Oral hygiene should be improved as far as possible.

During chemotherapy

During chemotherapy, it may be possible to lessen the stomatitis by using ice-cold water or asking the patient to suck ice during infusion of the agent. Established mucositis or oral ulceration is managed by maintaining good oral hygiene with twice-daily 0.2% aqueous chlorhexidine mouth rinses; 2% lidocaine gel or benzydamine rinse or spray can lessen discomfort. Nystatin suspension as a mouthwash, 4–6 times daily, may be given prophylactically. Fluconazole may be more appropriate for patients with candidosis who develop fever. Dentures should be carefully cleaned and stored overnight in 1% hypochlorite to reduce candidal carriage. Prophylactic aciclovir has lowered the incidence of herpes simplex and zoster, and mortality from zoster. Oral herpetic infections should be treated with aciclovir suspension or

Table 22.17 *Dental treatment for patients on cytotoxic chemotherapy*

Blood cell type	Peripheral blood count	Precautions
Platelets	>50 × 10⁹/L	Routine management, though desmopressin or platelets needed to cover surgery
	<50 × 10⁹/L	Platelets needed for any invasive procedure[a]
Granulocytes	>2 × 10⁹/L	Routine management
	<2 × 10⁹/L	Prophylactic antimicrobials for surgery
Erythrocytes	>5 × 10¹²/L	Routine management
	<5 × 10¹²/L	Special care with general anaesthesia

[a]Any procedure where bleeding is possible.

systemic aciclovir or valaciclovir (tablets or infusion). Zoster immune globulin may ameliorate varicella or zoster.

Although patients are frequently on several antibiotics already, Gram-negative infections may need treatment with gentamicin or carbenicillin, as the oral lesions can act as portals for systemic spread.

Possible drug interactions should be considered. Aspirin should not be given to patients on methotrexate, as it may enhance its toxicity. Some cytotoxic drugs enhance the effects of suxamethonium (Ch. 23); others cause more serious complications that can influence dental management (Appendices 22.2, 22.3, 22.4 and 22.5).

After chemotherapy

After chemotherapy, there should still be close attention to oral hygiene and preventive dentistry, as many patients continue to have anaemia and bleeding tendencies and to be susceptible to infection.

TARGETED THERAPY

Therapies that specifically target cell-signalling pathways that are dysregulated in tumours have focused mainly on epidermal growth factor receptor (EGFR or HER1) inhibitors, particularly cetuximab. These appear not to exacerbate the common effects associated with radiotherapy, such as mucositis, hyposalivation, dysphagia or pain. An acneiform rash is common, xerosis cutis and paronychia may be seen, and oral ulceration has been reported.

HAEMOPOIETIC STEM CELL TRANSPLANTATION (BONE MARROW TRANSPLANTATION)

See Chapter 35.

SALIVARY NEOPLASMS

See Chapter 14.

CHILDHOOD NEOPLASMS

These include the following:

- Leukaemias – common in childhood (Ch. 8).
- Solid tumours – rare but most are treated with surgery plus radiotherapy and/or chemotherapy, which can damage craniofacial and dental development. They include:
  - brain tumours, especially gliomas, which are the most frequent solid tumours in childhood, and are usually low-grade astrocytomas or medulloblastomas found in the posterior cranial fossa.
  - Wilms tumour, which arises from the kidney, is often associated with aniridia, and may metastasize to the lungs, liver or bone.
  - retinoblastomas, which have a strong hereditary basis, appear in pre-school children and cause blindness.
  - neuroblastomas, which arise from neural crest cells, especially abdominally, and metastasize to lymph nodes, lungs, bone and liver.

END-OF-LIFE CARE

The quality of life is as important as, or more important than, its duration. Good communication with patient, partners, family and friends

Table 22.18 *Analgesics: routes of administration*

	Buccal	Intravenous	Per rectum	Subcutaneous	Sublingual	Transdermal
Fentanyl	+					+
Hydromorphone		+	+	+		
Morphine		+	+	+	+	
Oxycodone		+				

is essential. Many different people are involved, so that (providing the patient consents) all should be aware of:

- the prognosis
- how much patients understand about their disease
- their psychological reactions to cancer
- the side-effects of treatment.

PSYCHOLOGICAL CARE

Hope is all-important and management must include particular attention to psychological problems. Patients may or may not know, or may not want to know, that they have malignant disease; even if they are aware of it, they may not appreciate, or be willing to accept, the prognosis.

PAIN CONTROL

Pain control is of paramount importance. Potent analgesics, such as opioids, sedatives or antidepressants, may be needed and are warranted in terminal cancer. The World Health Organization's three-step analgesic ladder (Ch. 3) is a guideline for cancer pain management, and is effective in relieving pain for approximately 90% of patients with cancer and over 75% of cancer patients who are terminally ill.

The five essential concepts in drug therapy for cancer pain are:

- by the mouth
- by the clock
- by the ladder
- for the individual
- with attention to detail.

Adjuvant drugs to enhance analgesic efficacy, treat concurrent symptoms that exacerbate pain, and provide independent analgesic activity for specific types of pain may be used at any step.

Step 1 in this approach is to give paracetamol (acetaminophen), aspirin or another non-steroidal anti-inflammatory drug (NSAID) orally for mild to moderate pain.

Step 2, when pain persists or worsens, is an opioid such as codeine or hydrocodone, which should be added (not substituted) to the NSAID. Opioids at this step are often administered in fixed-dose combinations with paracetamol or aspirin because this combination provides additive analgesia. Fixed-combination products may be limited by the content of paracetamol or NSAID, which may cause dose-related toxicity. When higher doses of opioid are necessary, the third step is taken.

Step 3, for pain that is still persistent, or moderate to severe, involves giving separate dosage forms of the opioid and non-opioid analgesic in order to avoid exceeding maximally recommended doses of paracetamol or NSAID.

Patients who have moderate to severe pain when first seen should be started at the second or third step of the ladder. Pain that is severe at the outset should be treated by giving more potent opioids or using higher dosages. Drugs such as codeine or hydrocodone are replaced by more potent opioids (usually morphine, hydromorphone, methadone, fentanyl or levorphanol). Fentanyl transdermal patches can be helpful (Table 22.18).

Medications for persistent cancer-related pain should be administered on an around-the-clock basis, with additional 'as-needed' doses, because regularly scheduled dosing maintains a constant level of drug in the body and helps to prevent a recurrence of pain. Patient-controlled analgesia (PCA), usually delivered via continuous systemic intravenous infusion, allows patients to control the amount of analgesia they receive. PCA can also be accomplished by mouth, subcutaneously or epidurally. Patient-administered boluses are required to treat breakthrough pain, and to provide a basis for more accurate and rapid upward titration of the continuous infusion rate. Intravenous or subcutaneous PCA allows patients to accommodate transient changes in analgesic requirements (such as during dressing changes or positioning) and to tailor analgesic doses according to their own requirements. Intravenous and subcutaneous PCA is contraindicated for sedated and confused patients. Morphine and diamorphine, often by intravenous infusion, are the drugs of choice for severe pain in hospitalized patients. Phenazocine may be valuable in patients intolerant of, or allergic to, morphine. Pethidine has too short an action and the metabolite norpethidine can accumulate in renal failure and then cause convulsions. Buprenorphine is a partial agonist and should be avoided. Dextromoramide is only very short-acting but can be useful to 'cover' painful procedures. NSAIDs may help ease bone pain, while dexamethasone is valuable for headaches associated with raised intracranial pressure. Carbamazepine or tricyclic antidepressants may relieve pain due to tumour infiltrating nerves. Transdermal fentanyl (skin patches) is increasingly used since it has an effect comparable with morphine and a duration of action of around 3 days. In the past, doctors have been anxious about giving sufficient opioids to terminally ill patients. However, if patients know that they can have opioids or other analgesics whenever they feel the need, the demand for these drugs falls.

QUALITY OF LIFE

Patients with any cancer may have severe psychological disturbances in view of the nature of the illness; these problems are compounded in oral cancer since there are additional disabilities, particularly interference with speech and swallowing, and disfigurement (e.g. 'Andy Gump' facies). Percutaneous endoscopic gastrostomy (PEG; Fig. 22.6) is a feasible and effective option when adequate oral nutrition is not possible. Patients are thus subject to considerable distress and up to a third have anxiety or depression, which occasionally leads to suicide. Counselling is especially important preoperatively but should be continued postoperatively, and include family members and partners.

Most general quality-of-life issues (emotional functioning, pain, insomnia, constipation) do not change after treatment or improve compared to baseline scores; most head- and neck-specific quality-of-life issues deteriorate after treatment but return to pre-treatment levels at 12 months, except for senses, opening mouth, sticky saliva and coughing, which remain deteriorated in the long term. Tumour site and stage, co-morbidity and extensive resections are significantly associated with adverse quality-of-life outcomes, as are marital status and age.

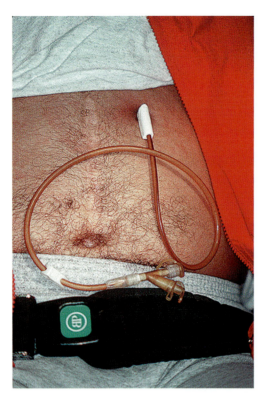

Fig. 22.6 Percutaneous endoscopic gastrostomy for feeding directly into the stomach.

PRESERVATION OF DIGNITY

Dignity is extremely important, and there are few other conditions that are as disfiguring as oral cancer. Feeding can be difficult, especially if there is dysphagia, when nasogastric (NG) intubation may be needed, but PEG is a better long-term solution, as it avoids the fear of choking and aspiration pneumonia. In some cases, hospice care is preferable.

The type of oral health care must be planned in relation to the interest that the patient has in their oral state. Just because patients are dying does not mean that they should be allowed to suffer from pain or that their appearance may be neglected. Indeed, the provision of oral hygiene, attention to halitosis and dental care (e.g. the construction of a new denture) may all help the patient's morale.

HEREDITARY CANCER SYNDROMES

These include:

- Cowden syndrome (gene; PTEN)
- Gardner syndrome or Familial Adenomatous Polyposis (FAP) (gene; APC)
- Gorlin syndrome (gene; PTCH1)
- Hereditary Breast And Ovarian Cancer (HBOC) (genes; BRCA1 and BRCA2)
- Li Fraumeni syndrome (gene; TP53)
- Lynch syndrome or Hereditary Nonpolyposis Colorectal Cancer (HNPCC) (genes; MLH1, MSH2, MSH6, PMS2, and EPCAM)
- Multiple Endocrine Neoplasia type 2 (MEN 2) (gene; RET)
- Peutz-Jegher syndrome (gene; STK11 or LKB1)

See http://www.cancer.gov/cancertopics/pdq/genetics/colorectal/HealthProfessional/page3

KEY WEBSITES

(Accessed 29 May 2013)
Cancer Research UK. <http://www.cancerresearchuk.org/cancer-help/>.
Macmillan. <http://www.macmillan.org.uk/Cancerinformation/Cancertypes/Headneck/Headneckcancers.aspx>.
MedlinePlus: Medical Encyclopaedia. <http://www.nlm.nih.gov/medlineplus/encyclopedia.html>.
National Institutes of Health: National Cancer Institute. <http://www.cancer.gov>.
Scottish Intercollegiate Guidelines Network: Diagnosis and management of head and neck cancer. <http://www.sign.ac.uk/guidelines/fulltext/90/index.html>.
Wikipedia. <http://en.wikipedia.org/wiki/Cancer>.

FURTHER READING

Accortt, N.A., et al. 2005. Cancer incidence among a cohort of smokeless tobacco users (United States). Cancer Causes Control 16, 1107.
Annane, D., et al. 2004. Hyperbaric oxygen therapy for radionecrosis of the jaw: a randomized, placebo-controlled, double-blind trial from the ORN96 study group. J. Clin. Oncol. 22, 4893.
Annertz, K., et al. 2002. Incidence and survival of squamous cell carcinoma of the tongue in Scandinavia, with special reference to young adults. Int. J. Cancer 101, 5.
Astsaturov, I., et al. 2007. EGFR-targeting monoclonal antibodies in head and neck cancer. Curr. Cancer Drug. Targets 7, 650.
Bagan, J.V., et al. 2009. Osteonecrosis of the jaws in intravenous bisphosphonate use: proposal for a modification of the clinical classification. Oral Oncol. 45, 645. Epub 2008 Aug 19.
Bagan, J.V., Scully, C., 2008. Recent advances in oral oncology 2007: epidemiology, aetiopathogenesis, diagnosis and prognostication. Oral Oncol. 44, 103.
Bagan, J.V., Scully, C., 2009. Recent advances in oral oncology 2008: squamous cell carcinoma aetiopathogenesis and experimental studies. Oral Oncol. 45, e45. Epub 2009 Feb 3.
Bedi, R., Scully, C., 2008. Tobacco-debate on harm reduction enters new phase as India implements public smoking ban. Lancet Oncol. 9, 1122.
Belusic-Gobic, M., et al. 2007. Risk factors for wound infection after oral cancer surgery. Oral Oncol. 43, 77.
Bennett, M.H., et al. 2005. Hyperbaric oxygen therapy for late radiation tissue injury. Cochrane Database Syst. Rev. 3, CD005005.
Bernier, J., 2006. Cetuximab in the treatment of head and neck cancer. Expert Rev. Anticancer Ther. 6, 1539.
Bernier, J., Schneider, D., 2007. Cetuximab combined with radiotherapy: an alternative to chemoradiotherapy for patients with locally advanced squamous cell carcinomas of the head and neck? Eur. J. Cancer 43, 35.
Blackburn, T.K., et al. 2007. A questionnaire survey of current UK practice for adjuvant radiotherapy following surgery for oral and oropharyngeal squamous cell carcinoma. Oral Oncol. 43, 143.
Blick, S.K., Scott, L.J., 2007. Cetuximab: a review of its use in squamous cell carcinoma of the head and neck and metastatic colorectal cancer. Drugs 67, 2585.
Borggreven, P.A., et al. 2007. Quality of life after surgical treatment for oral and oropharyngeal cancer: a prospective longitudinal assessment of patients reconstructed by a microvascular flap. Oral Oncol. 43, 1034.
Boyle, P., et al. 2003. European Code against Cancer and Scientific Justification: third version (2003). Ann. Oncol. 14, 973.
Braakhuis, B.J., et al. 2005. Head and neck cancer: molecular carcinogenesis. Ann. Oncol. 16 (Suppl 2), ii249.
Brown, J.S., et al. 2007. A comparison of outcomes for patients with oral squamous cell carcinoma at intermediate risk of recurrence treated by surgery alone or with post-operative radiotherapy. Oral Oncol. 43, 764.
Burtness, B., 2005. The role of cetuximab in the treatment of squamous cell cancer of the head and neck. Expert Opin. Biol. Ther. 5, 1085.
Chih-Fung Wu, 2007. Continuous intraarterial infusion chemotherapy for early lip cancer. Oral Oncol. 43, 825.
D'Souza, G., et al. 2007. Case-control study of human papillomavirus and oropharyngeal cancer. N. Engl. J. Med. 356, 1944.
Dahlstrom, K.R., et al. 2008. Squamous cell carcinoma of the head and neck in never smoker-never drinkers: a descriptive epidemiologic study. Head Neck 30, 75.
Derk, C.T., et al. 2005. Increased incidence of carcinoma of the tongue in patients with systemic sclerosis. J. Rheumatol. 32, 637.
Downer, M.C., et al. 2006. A systematic review of measures of effectiveness in screening for oral cancer and precancer. Oral Oncol. 42, 551.
Feng, F.Y., et al. 2007. Effect of epidermal growth factor receptor inhibitor class in the treatment of head and neck cancer with concurrent radiochemotherapy in vivo. Clin. Cancer Res. 13, 2512.
Fuwa, N., et al. 2007. Chemoradiation therapy using radiotherapy, systemic chemotherapy with 5-fluorouracil and nedaplatin, and intra-arterial infusion using carboplatin for locally advanced head and neck cancer – phase II study. Oral Oncol. 43, 1014.
Galeone, C., et al. 2005. Role of fried foods and oral/pharyngeal and oesophageal cancers. Br. J. Cancer 92, 2065.

Galimont-Collen, A.F., et al. 2007. Classification and management of skin, hair, nail and mucosal side-effects of epidermal growth factor receptor (EGFR) inhibitors. Eur. J. Cancer 43, 845.

Gandolfo, S., et al. 2006. Toluidine blue uptake in potentially malignant oral lesions in vivo: clinical and histological assessment. Oral Oncol. 42, 89.

Garavello, W., et al. 2007. Oral tongue cancer in young patients: a matched analysis. Oral Oncol. 43, 894.

Gebbia, V., et al. 2007. Cetuximab in squamous cell head and neck carcinomas. Ann. Oncol. 18 (Suppl 6), vi5.

Goldwaser, B.R., et al. 2007. Risk factor assessment for the development of osteoradionecrosis. J. Oral Maxillofac. Surg. 65, 2311.

Goutzanis, L., et al. 2007. Diabetes may increase risk for oral cancer through the insulin receptor substrate-1 and focal adhesion kinase pathway. Oral Oncol. 43, 165.

Grant, WBA, 2007. Meta-analysis of second cancers after a diagnosis of nonmelanoma skin cancer: additional evidence that solar ultraviolet-B irradiance reduces the risk of internal cancers. J. Steroid. Biochem. Mol. Biol. 103, 668.

Hashibe, M., et al. 2005. Radiotherapy for oral cancer as a risk factor for second primary cancers. Cancer Lett. 220, 185.

Ho, T., et al. 2007. X-ray repair cross-complementing group 1 (XRCC1) single-nucleotide polymorphisms and the risk of salivary gland carcinomas. Cancer 110, 318.

Karamouzis, M.V., et al. 2007. Therapies directed against epidermal growth factor receptor in aerodigestive carcinomas. JAMA 4 (298), 70.

Klug, C., et al. 2008. Preoperative chemoradiotherapy in the management of oral cancer: a review. J. Craniomaxillofac. Surg. 36, 75.

Koga, D.H., et al. 2008. Dental extractions and radiotherapy in head and neck oncology: review of the literature. Oral Dis. 14, 40.

Kujan, O., et al. 2005. Screening for oral cancer. Lancet 366, 1265. author reply 1266

Kujan, O., et al. 2006. Screening programmes for the early detection and prevention of oral cancer. Cochrane Database Syst. Rev. 3, CD004150.

Le Tourneau, C., et al. 2007. Molecular targeted therapy of head and neck cancer: review and clinical development challenges. Eur. J. Cancer 43, 2457.

McGurk, M.G., et al. 2007. Complications encountered in a prospective series of 182 patients treated surgically for mouth cancer. Oral Oncol. 43, 471.

Mehanna, H., et al. 2011. Head and neck cancer – part 1: epidemiology, presentation, and preservation. Clin. Otolaryngol. 36 (1), 65.http://dx.doi.org/10.1111/j.1749-4486.2010.02231.x Review. PubMed PMID: 21414154

Mehanna H., et al. Head and neck cancer – part 1: epidemiology, presentation, and prevention. BMJ 2010; 341: c4684. http://dx.doi.org/10.1136/bmj.c4684. Review. PubMed PMID: 20855405.

Mehanna H., et al. Head and neck cancer – part 2: treatment and prognostic factors. BMJ 2010; 341: c4690. http://dx.doi.org/10.1136/bmj.c4690. Review. PubMed PMID: 20876637.

Oliver, R.J., et al. 2007. Interventions for the treatment of oral and oropharyngeal cancers: surgical treatment. Cochrane Database Syst. Rev. 4, CD006205.

Panikkar R.P., et al. The emerging role of cetuximab in head and neck cancer: a 2007 perspective. Cancer Invest. 2008; 26: 96.

Penel, N., et al. 2007. A simple predictive model for postoperative mortality after head and neck cancer surgery with opening of mucosa. Oral Oncol. 43, 174.

Perez-Ordoñez, B., et al. 2006. Molecular biology of squamous cell carcinoma of the head and neck. J. Clin. Pathol. 59, 445.

Petti, S., Scully, C., 2005. Oral cancer: the association between nation-based alcohol-drinking profiles and oral cancer mortality. Oral Oncol. 41, 828.

Rades, D., et al. 2007. Prognostic factors in head-and-neck cancer patients treated with surgery followed by intensity-modulated radiotherapy (IMRT), 3D-conformal radiotherapy, or conventional radiotherapy. Oral Oncol. 43, 535.

Rapidis, A., et al. 2009. Major advances in the knowledge and understanding of the epidemiology aetiopathogenesis, diagnosis, management and prognosis of oral cancer. Oral Oncol. 45, 299.

Rapidis, A., et al. 2009. Oral cancer management. Oral Oncol. 45, 299.

Roh, J.L., et al. 2007. Cervical sensory preservation during neck dissection. Oral Oncol. 43, 491.

Ron, E., 2003. Cancer risks from medical radiation. Health Phys. 85, 47.

Sciubba, J.J., 2001. Oral cancer: the importance of early diagnosis and treatment. Am. J. Clin. Dermatol. 2, 239.

Sciubba, J.J., Goldenberg, D., 2006. Oral complications of radiotherapy. Lancet Oncol. 7, 175.

Scottish Intercollegiate Guidelines Network (SIGN), 2006. Diagnosis and management of head and neck cancer: a national clinical guideline. SIGN, Edinburgh.

Scully, C., 2010. Oral healthcare in people living with cancer. Oral Oncol. 46, 401. http://dx.doi.org/10.1016/j.oraloncology.2010.02.020. Epub 2010 Mar 29.

Scully, C., Bagan, J.V., 2009. Oral squamous cell carcinoma overview. Oral Oncol. 45, 301. http://dx.doi.org/10.1016/j.oraloncology.2009.01.004. Epub 2009 Feb 26.

Scully, C., Bagan, J.V., 2009. Oral squamous cell carcinoma: overview of current understanding of aetiopathogenesis, and clinical implications. Oral Dis. 15, 388. Epub April 2.

Scully, C., Bagan, J.V., 2008. Recent advances in oral oncology 2007: imaging, treatment and treatment outcomes. Oral Oncol. 44, 211.

Scully, C., Bagan, J.V., 2009. Recent advances in oral oncology 2008: squamous cell carcinoma imaging, treatment, prognostication and treatment outcomes. Oral Oncol. 45, e25.

Scully, C., Boyle, P., 2005. The role of the dental team in preventing and diagnosing cancer. 1. Cancer in general. Dent. Update 32, 204.

Scully, C., et al. 2008. Oral cancer: current and future diagnostic techniques. Am. J. Dent. 21, 199.

Scully, C., et al. 2004. Oral health care in patients with the most important medically compromising conditions. 6. Patients undergoing radiotherapy. CPD Dent. 6, 80.

Scully, C., et al. 2005. Oral health care in patients with the most important medically compromising conditions. 7. Patients undergoing chemotherapy. CPD Dent. 6, 3.

Scully, C., et al. 2006. Oral mucositis. Oral Dis. 12, 229.

Scully, C., et al. 2003. Oral mucositis: a challenging complication of radiotherapy, chemotherapy, and radiochemotherapy. Part 1. Pathogenesis and prophylaxis of mucositis. Head Neck 25, 1057.

Scully, C., et al. 2004. Oral mucositis: a challenging complication of radiotherapy, chemotherapy, and radiochemotherapy. Part 2. Diagnosis and management of mucositis. Head and Neck 26, 77.

Scully, C., et al. 2005. The role of the dental team in preventing and diagnosing cancer. 2. Oral cancer risk factors. Dent. Update 32, 261.

Scully, C., et al. 2005. The role of the dental team in preventing and diagnosing cancer. 3. Oral cancer diagnosis and screening. Dent. Update 32, 326.

Scully, C., Warnakulasuriya, S., 2010. Cancer of the mouth for the dental team: comprehending the condition, causes, controversies, control and consequences. 1. General principles. Dent. Update 37, 638.

Subramanian, S., et al. 2007. Second primary malignancy risk in thyroid cancer survivors: a systematic review and meta-analysis. Thyroid 17, 1277.

Tsantoulis, P.K., et al. 2007. Advances in the biology of oral cancer. Oral Oncol. 43, 523.

Warnakulasuriya, K.A.A.S., 2004. Smokeless tobacco and oral cancer. Oral Dis. 10, 1.

Warnakulasuriya, S., et al. 2005. Tobacco, oral cancer, and treatment of dependence. Oral Oncol. 41, 244.

Whatley, W.S., et al. 2006. Salivary gland tumors in survivors of childhood cancer. Otolaryngol. Head Neck Surg. 134, 385.

Worthington, H.V., et al. 2007. Interventions for treating oral candidiasis for patients with cancer receiving treatment. Cochrane Database Syst. Rev. 2

Yao, M., et al. 2007. Current surgical treatment of squamous cell carcinoma of the head and neck. Oral Oncol. 43, 213.

APPENDIX 22.1 ORAL MANIFESTATIONS OF INTERNAL CANCER

Metastases in jaws or (rarely) oral soft tissues, especially from cancer of:

- Breast
- Lung
- Prostate
- Thyroid
- Kidney
- Stomach
- Colon

Effects of tumour products

- Facial flushing (carcinoid syndrome)
- Pigmentations (ectopic adrenocorticotropic hormone-secreting tumours)
- Amyloidosis (multiple myeloma)
- Oral erosions (glucagonoma)
- Swellings (acanthosis nigricans)

Changes caused by other functional disturbances

- Purpura, anaemia, infections (leukaemia)
- Infections (lymphoma)
- Bleeding (liver cancer)
- Anaemia (bleeding from gastrointestinal tumours)

Mucocutaneous diseases

- Dermatomyositis (carcinoma)
- Acanthosis nigricans (abdominal carcinoma)
- Erythema multiforme (lymphoma, leukaemia or carcinoma, especially after radiotherapy)
- Paraneoplastic pemphigus (lymphomas or Castleman disease)
- Pemphigoid
- Dermatitis herpetiformis

(Continued)

Inherited disorders with predisposition to internal malignancy and oral lesions

- Cowden syndrome
- Dyskeratosis congenita
- Gardner syndrome
- Gorlin–Goltz syndrome
- Maffucci syndrome
- Multiple endocrine neoplasia
- Neurofibromatosis (von Recklinghausen disease)
- Peutz–Jeghers syndrome
- Tuberous sclerosis
- Tylosis

APPENDIX 22.2 CHEMOTHERAPEUTIC AGENTS: MAIN USES AND TOXICITIES[a]

Agent	Main uses	Main toxicities
Alkylating agents[b,c]		
Busulfan	Chronic myeloid leukaemia (CML)	Myelosuppression
		Hyperpigmentation
		Pulmonary fibrosis
Carmustine	Multiple myeloma	Nephrotoxicity
	Lymphomas	Pulmonary fibrosis
Chlorambucil	Chronic lymphocytic leukaemia (CLL)	Myelosuppression
	Lymphomas	Erythema multiforme
	Ovarian cancer	–
Cyclophosphamide	CLL	Cystitis (avoid with mesna)
	Lymphomas	Severe nausea and vomiting
Estramustine	Prostatic carcinoma	Angina
		Gynaecomastia
		Liver dysfunction
Ifosfamide	CLL	Cystitis (avoid with mesna)
	Lymphomas	–
Lomustine	Hodgkin disease	Nausea and vomiting
		Delayed myelosuppression
Melphalan	Multiple myeloma	Delayed myelosuppression
Mustine	Hodgkin disease	Severe vomiting
Thiotepa	Malignant effusions	Enhances suxamethonium
	Bladder carcinoma	–
Treosulfan	Ovarian carcinoma	Hyperpigmentation
		Pulmonary fibrosis
		Haemorrhagic cystitis
Cytotoxic antibiotics[b,d]		
Aclarubicin	Acute myeloid leukaemia (AML)	Nausea and vomiting
Bleomycin	Squamous carcinomas	Pulmonary fibrosis
Dactinomycin	Paediatric tumours	Similar to doxorubicin but no cardiotoxicity
Daunorubicin	Kaposi sarcoma	Cardiotoxicity
Doxorubicin (Adriamycin)	Acute leukaemias	Mucositis
	Lymphomas	Nausea and vomiting
	Ovarian cancer	Supraventricular tachycardia
		Cardiomyopathy
		Myelosuppression
Epirubicin	Breast carcinoma	Cardiotoxicity

Agent	Main uses	Main toxicities
Idarubicin	Breast cancer	Cardiotoxicity
	Acute leukaemias	–
Mitomycin	Upper gastrointestinal and breast carcinomas	Myelosuppression
		Nephrotoxicity
		Lung fibrosis
Mitoxantrone	Breast carcinoma	Myelosuppression
	Lymphomas	Cardiotoxicity
Plicamycin (mithramycin)	Hypercalcaemia in malignancy	Thrombocytopenia
Antimetabolites[b]		
Capecitabine	Colorectal cancer	Hand–foot syndrome (desquamation)
Cladribine	Hairy cell leukaemia	Myelosuppression
Cytarabine	Acute leukaemias	Myelosuppression
Fludarabine	CLL	Myelosuppression
		Immunosuppression
		CNS toxicity
		Pulmonary toxicity
Fluorouracil	Colon carcinoma	Mucositis
	Breast carcinoma	Myelosuppression
		Cerebellar syndrome
Gemcitabine	Non-small-cell lung carcinoma	Myelosuppression
Mercaptopurine	Acute leukaemias	Myelosuppression
		Hepatotoxicity
Methotrexate	Acute lymphocytic leukaemia (ALL)	Mucositis
	Rheumatoid arthritis	Myelosuppression (ameliorate with leucovorin)
	Psoriasis	
Raltitrexed	Colorectal cancer	Fever and cytokine release
Tegafur	Colorectal cancer	Nausea and vomiting
Tioguanine	Acute leukaemias	Myelosuppression
Mitotic inhibitors[b]		
Etoposide	Small-cell carcinoma or lung lymphomas	Nausea and vomiting
		Myelosuppression
Vinblastine	Acute leukaemias	Myelosuppression
	Lymphomas	Neurotoxicity
Vincristine	Acute leukaemias	Neurotoxicity
	Lymphomas	Inappropriate antidiuretic hormone (ADH) secretion
Vindesine	Acute leukaemias	Neurotoxicity
	Lymphomas	Myelosuppression
Vinorelbine	Breast cancer	Neurotoxicity
	Lung cancer	Myelosuppression
Other antineoplastic drugs[b]		
Aldesleukin (interleukin-2)	Renal cancer	Capillary leak
		Marrow, liver, CNS, thyroid and kidney toxicity
Alemtuzumab	CLL	Severe cytokine release syndrome (dyspnoea)
Amsacrine	AML	Mucositis
		Myelosuppression
		Arrhythmias
Bexarotene	T-cell lymphoma	Hyperlipidaemia
		Hypothyroidism
Carboplatin	Small oat cell carcinoma of lung	Myelosuppression
		Severe nausea and vomiting

(Continued)

Agent	Main uses	Main toxicities
Cisplatin	Ovarian carcinoma	Severe nausea and vomiting
	Testicular carcinoma	Ototoxicity
		Nephrotoxicity
Crisantaspase	ALL	Anaphylaxis
		Glucose intolerance
		CNS changes
		Liver dysfunction
Dacarbazine	Hodgkin lymphoma	Severe nausea and vomiting
		Myelosuppression
Docetaxel	Breast cancer	Fluid retention
Hydroxycarbamide (hydroxyurea)	CML	Nausea
		Rashes
		Myelosuppression
Irinotecan	Colorectal cancer	Acute cholinergic syndrome
Interferon-alpha	Kaposi sarcoma	'Flu-like symptoms
	Hairy cell leukaemia	Cardiotoxicity
	Non-Hodgkin lymphoma	Hepatotoxicity
		Depression
Oxaliplatin	Colorectal cancer	Neurotoxicity
		Myelosuppression
Paclitaxel	Ovarian cancer	Hypersensitivity
	Breast cancer metastases	Myelosuppression
		Arrhythmias
Pentostatin	Hairy cell leukaemia	Myelosuppression
		Immunosuppression
Porfimer	Lung cancer	Photosensitivity
Procarbazine	Hodgkin lymphoma	Myelosuppression
		Hypersensitivity
		Disulfiram reaction with alcohol
Razoxane	Leukaemia	Myelosuppression
Rituximab	Lymphoma	Cytokine release syndrome (dyspnoea)
Temozolomide	Glioma	Myelosuppression
Topotecan	Ovarian cancer	Diarrhoea
Trastuzumab	Breast cancer	Cardiotoxicity if used with anthracyclines
Tretinoin	Acute promyelocytic leukaemia	Dyspnoea
		Multiorgan failure

[a]See also Biologics, Chapter 19.
[b]All can produce mucositis, nausea, vomiting and alopecia.
[c]All can interfere with gametogenesis and predispose to acute leukaemias.
[d]Should not be used with radiotherapy, as they enhance radiation toxicity.

APPENDIX 22.3 MAIN CHEMOTHERAPY COMPLICATIONS AND RESPONSIBLE AGENTS

Complication	Agent responsible
Early	
Alopecia	Alkylating agents
	Anthracyclines
	Cisplatin
Diarrhoea	5-fluorouracil (5-FU)
	Ironotecan
Myelosuppression	Alkylating agents
	Anthracyclines
	Taxanes
Mucositis	Etoposide
	5-FU
	Methotrexate
Nausea	All
Nephrotoxicity	Cisplatin
Neurotoxicity	Cisplatin
	Taxanes
Ototoxicity	Cisplatin
Dark urine	Anthracyclines
Late	
Cardiotoxicity	Anthracyclines
Infertility	Alkylating agents
Menopause	Alkylating agents
Myelodysplasia	Etoposide
Pulmonary fibrosis	Bleomycin
	Mitomycin

APPENDIX 22.4 MANAGEMENT OF EARLY ADVERSE EFFECTS FROM CHEMOTHERAPY

Adverse effect	Management
Anorexia	Megestrol acetate
Bladder damage (cystitis)	Mesna
Constipation	Docusate sodium, milk of magnesia
Diarrhoea	Loperamide, co-phenotrope (Lomotil)
Dry skin, hair loss	Emollients, vitamin E, zinc supplements
Extravasation injury to soft tissue	Dimethyl sulfoxide (DMSO) topically
Heart injury	Dexrazoxane
Kidney injury	Sodium thiosulfate injection
Nausea and/or vomiting	Ondansetron, granisetron, dolasetron, metoclopramide, dexamethasone
Nerve injury	Amifostine

APPENDIX 22.5 COLONY-STIMULATING FACTORS

Factor	Marrow cell stimulated
Erythropoietin alpha	Erythrocytes
Filgrastim	Granulocytes
Sargramostim	Granulocytes and macrophages
Oprelvekin	Platelets

METABOLIC SYNDROME

Metabolic syndrome (metabolic syndrome X, insulin resistance syndrome, dysmetabolic syndrome, hypertriglyceridaemic waist, obesity syndrome, Reaven syndrome) is the name for a group of risk factors that increase the risk for ischaemic heart disease (IHD), diabetes and stroke (Fig. 23.1). The metabolic syndrome is diagnosed when at least three of the IHD risk factors listed in Table 23.1 are present. Whether the syndrome, which affects possibly 25% of the US population, is a specific syndrome, and nothing more than the sum of its parts, is controversial.

In general, a person with metabolic syndrome is twice as likely to develop IHD and five times as likely to develop diabetes as someone without it. The probability of developing metabolic syndrome is also closely linked to a lack of physical activity and the fact of being overweight/obese. Other causes include insulin resistance, ethnicity (often Asian), family history, older age and other factors (Box 23.1). Associated diseases and signs may be raised uric acid levels, hepatic steatosis, haemochromatosis and acanthosis nigricans. Metabolic syndrome may be associated with inflammatory periodontal disease.

Treatment of metabolic syndrome is to increase physical activity but to reduce weight, unhealthy diet, low-density lipoprotein cholesterol and high blood pressure; diabetes should also be controlled (Chs 5 and 6).

INBORN ERRORS OF METABOLISM

There are a vast number of rare metabolic disorders that result from inherited enzyme defects; some have a high prevalence in certain ethnic groups (Table 23.2). Most arise from recessive traits and thus manifest only when both parents are heterozygous carriers. They affect 1 in 4 of the offspring of heterozygous parents, often as a result of first-cousin marriage.

Some inborn errors of metabolism, especially suxamethonium sensitivity, malignant hyperpyrexia, hyperlipoproteinaemias and porphyria, can seriously complicate management if general anaesthesia (GA) is required (see Table 23.2 and Appendix 23.1). Many others are associated with learning impairment or neurological disease. Some others can also be relevant occasionally, such as haemochromatosis, homocystinuria and glycogen storage diseases. A few (e.g. hereditary pentosuria) are innocuous (see Appendix 23.1). Few inborn errors of metabolism will be encountered in primary care, but they are more common in paediatric or special care clinics.

DEFECTS IN CARBOHYDRATE METABOLISM

Gaucher disease

Gaucher disease is a rare lysosomal storage disease, common in Ashkenazi Jews; it is caused by glucocerebrosidase deficiency.

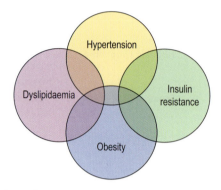

Fig. 23.1 Metabolic syndrome.

Table 23.1 *The metabolic syndrome*

Features	Detail[a]
Hypertension	Blood pressure ≥ 130/85 mmHg
Hyperglycaemia	Fasting blood glucose ≥ 5.6 mmol/L
Dyslipidaemia	Triglycerides ≥ 150 mg/dL
	High-density lipoprotein (HDL) < 50 mg/dL for women and < 40 mg/dL for men
Abdominal obesity	Large waistline: ≥ 35 inches for women and ≥ 40 inches for men

[a]Figures given by various expert bodies differ.

Box 23.1 *Groups at risk for metabolic syndrome*

- People with a sibling or parent with diabetes
- People with a personal history of diabetes
- Certain ethnic groups (e.g. South Asians)
- Women with a personal history of polycystic ovarian syndrome
- People with sleep apnoea
- People with a prothrombotic state (e.g. high blood fibrinogen or plasminogen activator inhibitor-1)
- People with a pro-inflammatory state (raised blood C-reactive protein)

Manifesting with hepatosplenomegaly, skeletal involvement (including honeycomb-like mandibular radiolucencies), anaemia and thrombocytopenia, it may present challenges with bleeding and – should the patient be splenectomized – a liability to infection.

Glycogen storage diseases

General aspects

Glycogen storage diseases (GSD) are rare disorders due to inherited defects in degradative enzymes that mobilize glycogen to glucose, so that it accumulates and hypoglycaemia results.

Table 23.2 *Inborn errors of metabolism*

Defect in	Diseases
Structural proteins	Clotting factor defects
	Connective tissue proteins
	Oxygen-carrying proteins – sickle-cell anaemia and thalassaemias
Carbohydrate metabolism	Fructose, galactose and glycerol disorders, glycogen storage diseases
Cholesterol and lipoprotein metabolism	Hyperlipoproteinaemias
	Hypolipoproteinaemias
Mucopolysaccharide and glycolipid	Mucolipidoses
	Mucopolysaccharidoses (MPS)
	Oligosaccharidoses
	Sphingolipidoses
Lysosomal storage	Lipid storage disorders (including Gaucher and Niemann–Pick diseases)
	Gangliosidosis (including Tay–Sachs disease)
	Leukodystrophies
	Mucopolysaccharidoses (including Hunter syndrome and Hurler disease)
	Glycoprotein storage disorders
	Mucolipidoses
Amino and organic acid metabolism	Amino-acid transport defects
	Specific amino acids
	Urea-cycle defects
Haem and bilirubin	Bilirubin metabolism disorders
	Porphyrias
Fatty acid metabolism	Disorders of beta-oxidation
	Disorders of carnitine-mediated transport and carnitine uptake
Metal metabolism and transport	Copper transport disorders (Wilson disease)
	Haemochromatosis
Peroxisomes	Disorders of peroxisome biogenesis
	Adrenoleukodystrophies
Nucleotide metabolism	Defects in purine nucleotide metabolism
	Lesch–Nyhan syndrome (hypoxanthine–guanine phosphoribosyltransferase [HGPRT] deficiency), severe combined immunodeficiency disease (SCID) – due to adenosine deaminase (ADA) deficiency; gout, renal lithiasis – due to adenine phosphoribosyltransferase (APRT) deficiency; xanthinuria – due to xanthine oxidase deficiency
	Defects in pyrimidine nucleotide metabolism
	Types I and II orotic aciduria, ornithine transcarbamylase deficiency
DNA or repair	Ataxia telangiectasia (AT)
	Bloom syndrome
	Cockayne syndrome
	Fanconi anaemia
	Xeroderma pigmentosum (XP)
Drug-metabolizing enzymes	Glucose-6-phosphate dehydrogenase (G6PD) deficiency
	Malignant hyperthermia
	Neuroleptic malignant syndrome (NMS)
	Suxamethonium sensitivity

Clinical features

Glycogen accumulates in liver and muscle, resulting in hepatomegaly, muscle pain, weakness, respiratory muscle weakness and cardiac failure. Hypoglycaemia is common, as are infections.

Dental aspects

Enlarged tongue, periodontal breakdown and masticatory muscle pain may be complaints. Patients with GSD type 1b have a bleeding tendency that can be corrected preoperatively by 24–48 hours of glucose infusion. Local anaesthesia (LA) appears to have no contraindications. Conscious sedation (CS) may be given if required. GA requires expert attention in hospital.

Defects in fructose metabolism

Hereditary fructose intolerance (aldolase B deficiency) and fructosuria – hepatic fructokinase deficiency – discourage the patient from ingesting sugar (sucrose) and are therefore associated with low dental caries rates.

DEFECTS IN CHOLESTEROL AND LIPOPROTEIN METABOLISM

Hyperlipoproteinaemia (hyperlipidaemia; hypercholesterolaemia)

General aspects

Cholesterol is found in some hormones, as well as in every cell, and thus is an essential element. However, high cholesterol (hypercholesterolaemia), which is directly related to hyperlipoproteinaemia (Table 23.3), predisposes to atherosclerosis (Ch. 5).

The lipoproteins consist of lipids (insoluble in plasma), phospholipids and apolipoproteins (apoproteins). Based on density and electrophoretic mobility, the lipoproteins are divided into four groups:

- *Chylomicrons* are large particles carrying mainly triglyceride to the liver, where lipoprotein lipase releases free fatty acids (Fig. 23.2).
- *Very low-density lipoproteins* (VLDLs) carry triglycerides and cholesterol from liver to the tissues, and are hydrolysed by lipoprotein lipase to free fatty acids and intermediate-density and low-density lipoproteins.
- *Low-density lipoproteins* (LDLs) are associated with a high risk of IHD; they contain a cholesterol core and are formed by hepatic lipase. LDLs bind to cell LDL receptors and are taken up by cells, especially when there is inhibition of 3-hydroxy-3-methylglutaryl coenzyme A reductase (HMG-CoA reductase), which raises cellular cholesterol. The LDL lipoprotein-alpha inhibits fibrinolysis but promotes atherosclerosis.
- *High-density lipoproteins* (HDLs), formed in liver and gut, carry cholesterol from intracellular tissue pools back to the liver and are associated with a lowered risk of IHD. The main plasma lipids transported are triglycerides, cholesterol ester and phospholipids (lecithin, sphingomyelin, etc.). Non-esterified fatty acids and cholesterol are also present.

Hypercholesterolaemia can be due to abnormalities in lipoprotein levels related to diet, or secondary to obesity, diabetes, hypothyroidism, nephrotic syndrome, chronic renal failure, liver disease, alcoholism, smoking (lowers HDL) and use of oral contraceptives. In primary (familial) hyperlipidaemia (FH), genetic factors play a role, with defects, for example, in the LDL receptor (*LDLR*), apolipoprotein B-100 (*APOB*) and proprotein convertase subtilisin/kexin type 9 (*PCSK9*) genes.

Table 23.3 *Primary hyperlipoproteinaemias*

Type	Name	Pathogenesis	Alternative name and lipid changes	Features in addition to atherosclerosis
I	Hypertriglyceridaemia	Autosomal dominant (AD). May occur as a secondary defect in diabetes mellitus, pancreatitis and alcoholism	Hyperchylomicronaemia Lipoprotein lipase deficiency Abnormality in chylomicron removal	Xanthomas Acute pancreatitis, hepatosplenomegaly
Ib	Hyperlipoproteinaemia	Apolipoprotein c-II deficiency	Reduced low-density lipoprotein (LDL) and high-density lipoprotein (HDL); high triglycerides	No xanthomas Acute pancreatitis
Ic	Hyperlipoproteinaemia	Circulating inhibitor of lipoprotein lipase	Chylomicronaemia	Xanthomas Acute pancreatitis
II	Hyperbetalipoproteinaemia	AD. Also may be secondary to hypothyroidism, plasma cell myeloma, macroglobulinaemia and obstructive liver disease	Hypercholesterolaemia: increase in plasma beta-lipoproteins	Xanthomas and xanthelasmas (common) Premature coronary, cerebral and peripheral vascular disease
IIa	Hyperlipoproteinaemia	AD. Also may be secondary to hypothyroidism, plasma cell myeloma, macroglobulinaemia and obstructive liver disease	LDL receptor disorder; increase in plasma LDLs	Xanthomas, corneal arcus Premature coronary, cerebral, and peripheral vascular disease
III	Dysbetalipoproteinaemia	Autosomal recessive (AR). Rarely, secondary to severe diabetes and hypothyroidism	Broad-beta disease Apolipoprotein E deficiency	Peripheral vascular disease, hyperglycaemia, xanthomas (rare)
IV	Endogenous hyperlipoproteinaemia	AR. Rarely, secondary to diabetes mellitus, pancreatitis, alcoholism, hypothyroidism, glycogen storage disease, Gaucher disease, gout and hypercalcaemia	Carbohydrate-inducible hyperlipaemia	Mild glucose intolerance, hyperuricaemia, atherosclerosis and ischaemic heart disease, xanthomas (common)
V	Mixed hyperlipidaemia	AD	–	Acute pancreatitis Xanthomas, hyperuricaemia, abdominal pain, hepatosplenomegaly, paraesthesias and lipaemia retinalis

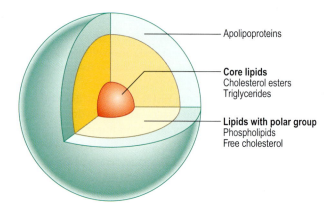

Fig. 23.2 Chylomicron structure.

Apolipoproteins

Core lipids
Cholesterol esters
Triglycerides

Lipids with polar group
Phospholipids
Free cholesterol

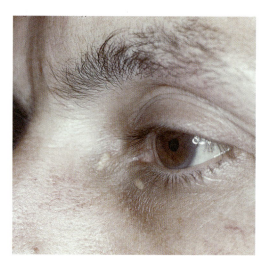

Fig. 23.3 Xanthelasma in familial hyperlipidaemia. Such lesions may suggest a high risk of ischaemic heart disease.

Clinical features

Gout, arthralgias, arthritis and premature IHD may result. Yellowish cutaneous plaques called xanthomas, in soft tissue, tendons and subperiosteal and intraosseous locations (xanthelasmas on the eyelids; Fig. 23.3), are associated with accelerated IHD. Prominent xanthomas on elbows and knees, especially with yellow to orange discolouration of palmar creases, are unique to type II hyperlipoproteinaemia.

General management

Around 75% of FH is undiagnosed, so screening for *LDLR*, *APOB* and *PCSK9* genes may help. Dietary intervention and lipid-lowering drugs (particularly statins – HMG-CoA reductase inhibitors) are essential to treatment (Ch 5). Ezetimibe is an option for primary hypercholesterolaemia.

Dental aspects

LA is the safest method of pain control. CS can be given if required. GA may be a risk because of IHD.

Facial xanthomas may help recognition of these potentially dangerous diseases. Types IV and V hyperlipoproteinaemias may be complicated by sicca syndrome.

Hypolipoproteinaemias

Pulpal calcifications, unusual odontomes and orange deposits in the tonsils may be found in HDL deficiency (Tangier disease).

ERRORS IN AMINO ACID AND ORGANIC ACID METABOLISM

Homocysteine (Hcy), a sulphur amino acid, is an intermediate product in conversion of methionine to cysteine; it participates in the re-methylation pathway, enabling maintenance of adequate cellular levels of methionine, or is catabolized by trans-sulphuration. Several hereditary defects in the enzymes involved and acquired deficiencies in the vitamin cofactors of these enzymes can cause hyperhomocysteinaemia.

Hyperhomocysteinaemia

An increased homocysteine level is associated with a higher risk of strokes. Carotid stenosis appears to have a graded response to increased levels of homocysteine; increased carotid plaque thickness has been associated with high homocysteine and low B_{12} levels. Homocysteine may also be a risk factor for Alzheimer disease. Dietary folate and B_{12} supplementation may normalize homocysteine levels and modify the risk of vascular disease.

Homocystinuria

Homocystinuria is a disorder of methionine metabolism, leading to an abnormal accumulation of homocysteine and its metabolites (homocystine, homocysteine–cysteine complex, and others) in blood and urine. Homocystinuria is an autosomal recessively inherited defect in the trans-sulphuration pathway (homocystinuria I) or methylation pathway (homocystinuria II and III).

Affected patients are tall with a Marfanoid appearance, joint hypermobility, ectopia lentis, and visual and mental deterioration. Blood vessel abnormalities, together with excessive platelet adhesiveness, predispose to thromboembolism, both spontaneously and postoperatively. Pyridoxine is the treatment. During and after surgery, aggressive hydration and prophylaxis for deep vein thrombosis (DVT) are recommended.

DEFECTS IN NON–AMINO-ACID NITROGEN METABOLISM

The porphyrias

General aspects

Porphyrias are rare inborn errors in enzymes involved in haem metabolism, which result in the accumulation of porphyrins, the intermediate

compounds in haem(oglobin) synthesis (Fig. 23.4). Classification is according to the principal site of enzyme defect: namely, liver (hepatic porphyrias) or erythrocytes (erythropoietic porphyrias; Table 23.4).

Most people with porphyrias enjoy entirely normal health. However, three porphyrias are significant clinically, since drugs precipitate acute illness. Patients may develop potentially fatal acute attacks of cardiovascular (hypertension and tachycardia) and gastrointestinal disturbances, accompanied by neuropsychiatric disturbance (porphyria in King George III of England probably explains his 'madness'). These

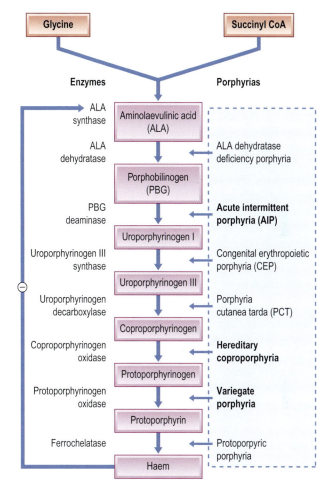

Fig. 23.4 Haem synthesis. (Bold disorders are most significant). Adapted from James MF, Hift RJ. Porphyrias. *Br J Anaesth* 2000; 85:143

Table 23.4 *Porphyrias*

Porphyrias	Type	Alternative name	Particular features
Acute	Acute intermittent porphyria[a]	Swedish porphyria	Acute, severe abdominal pain, cardiovascular disturbances, neuropsychiatric disturbance, autonomic dysfunction
	Hereditary coproporphyria[a]	Coproporphyria	Acute, severe abdominal pain, cardiovascular disturbances, neuropsychiatric disturbance, autonomic dysfunction
	Plumboporphyria	5-aminolaevulinic acid (ALA) dehydratase deficiency	Acute abdominal pain
	Variegate porphyria[a]	South African (Afrikaans) genetic porphyria	Acute, severe abdominal pain, cardiovascular disturbances, neuropsychiatric disturbance, autonomic dysfunction, rashes
Chronic	Congenital porphyria[b]	Erythropoietic porphyria	Red teeth, hypertrichosis, severe mutilating photosensitivity rashes and haemolytic anaemia
	Porphyria cutanea tarda	Cutaneous hepatic porphyria	Photosensitivity and iron overload. Drugs do not precipitate acute attacks but the condition is aggravated by alcohol, oestrogens, iron and polychlorinated aromatic compounds

[a]Clinically significant.
[b]Erythropoietic.

porphyrias are *variegate porphyria*, the commonest, found mainly in South Africans of Afrikaans descent; *acute intermittent porphyria*, seen less frequently but affecting all population groups; and *hereditary coproporphyria*, which is rare and may cause patients to appear normal, apart from severe photosensitivity rashes.

Most of the drugs that have been incriminated in attacks are enzyme inducers that also increase hepatic 5-aminolaevulinic acid (ALA) synthetase levels. Assessing drug safety in porphyria is an inexact science; for many drugs no such information is available, and for some others the data are of doubtful validity and often conflicting (Table 23.5). A wide array of other factors can cause exacerbations, including fasting, alcohol, infections and pregnancy.

Clinical features of attacks

Often a single dose of a drug of this type can precipitate an acute episode, but in some patients, repeated doses are necessary to provoke a reaction. Attacks are accompanied by cardiovascular disturbance (tachycardia and hypertension, sometimes followed by postural hypotension). Respiratory embarrassment or major convulsions and neuropsychiatric disturbance (typically a peripheral sensory and motor neuropathy, but sometimes agitation, mania, depression, hallucinations and schizophrenic-like behaviour) may occur. Autonomic dysfunction may cause profuse sweating, pallor and pyrexia. Severe hyponatraemia, due to inappropriate secretion of antidiuretic hormone, may cause convulsions or deteriorating consciousness.

General management

The essentials of treatment for attacks of porphyria are, if possible, to stop the administration of the triggering drug and to give an intravenous infusion of haem arginate, fluids, electrolytes and glucose. Alcohol is sometimes an important trigger and, in some, the disease may be controlled simply by its withdrawal. The diagnosis is confirmed by demonstrating ALA and porphobilinogen in urine, and attacks are accompanied by raised levels; the urine may turn red.

Dental aspects

Anaesthetics, analgesics, antimicrobials and anxiolytics (benzodiazepines) that are liable to precipitate attacks are absolutely contraindicated (see Table 23.5).

Congenital erythropoietic porphyria is characterized by red teeth (which fluoresce in ultraviolet light). Fewer than 100 cases have ever been reported, but it has been suggested that this disease might have been the source of the werewolf legend because of the red teeth (thought to be dripping with blood), the hairy facial features and avoidance of daylight.

DISORDERS OF METAL METABOLISM AND TRANSPORT

Haemochromatosis

Haemochromatosis is a disease that occurs as a result of significant iron overload.

General aspects

Iron overload causes high serum ferritin levels and deposition of iron as haemosiderin, and damages liver, abdominal lymph nodes,

Table 23.5 *Drug use in porphyria*[a]

Drug group	Contraindicated	Safer
Local anaesthetics	Articaine	Bupivacaine
	Mepivacaine	Lidocaine (used with caution)
		Prilocaine (used with caution)
Conscious sedation agents	Diazepam	Flumazenil
		Midazolam
General anaesthetics	Barbiturates	Nitrous oxide
	Enflurane	
	Halothane	
Analgesics	Dextropropoxyphene	Aspirin
	Diclofenac	Paracetamol (acetaminophen)
	Indometacin	
	Mefenamic acid	
	Opioids	
	Pentazocine	
Antibiotics	Cephalosporins	Metronidazole
	Clindamycin	Penicillin
	Co-trimoxazole	
	Doxycycline	
	Erythromycin	
	Flucloxacillin	
	Rifampicin	
	Sulphonamides	
	Tetracyclines	
Antifungals	Fluconazole	Nystatin
	Griseofulvin	
	Itraconazole	
	Ketoconazole	
	Miconazole	
	Voriconazole	
Psychoactive drugs	Amphetamines	
	Antidepressants	
	Antihistamines	
	Barbiturates	
	Calcium-channel blockers	
	Carbamazepine	
	Chlordiazepoxide	
	Contraceptive pill	
	Diazepam	
	Dichloralphenazone	
	Ergot	
	Meprobamate	
	Monoamine oxidase inhibitors	
	Phenytoin	
	Tricyclics	
Endocrine active drugs	Androgens	
	Chlorpropamide	
	Contraceptive pill	
	Oestrogens	
	Progestogens	
Others	Ethanol (alcohol)	
	Clonidine	
	Danazol	
	Pentoxifylline	
	Statins	

[a]List is not exhaustive.

joints, skin, adrenals, pancreas, salivary glands, pituitary and heart (Fig. 23.5). Haemochromatosis can have genetic and non-genetic causes. Acquired haemochromatosis may appear after repeated transfusions, as may be needed in haemoglobinopathies.

Hereditary haemochromatosis, the genetic disease caused by the *HFE* gene on chromosome 6, is one of the most common genetic disorders in the West, and most often affects Caucasians of northern European descent. The condition affects more than 1 in 200 of the population and often remains undetected. The *HFE* gene codes for a transmembrane glycoprotein highly expressed in intestinal cells, and modulates iron uptake. *HFE* gene mutations can lead to increased dietary iron absorption and overloading. Once iron is absorbed, there is no physiological mechanism for excretion of the excess from the body other than blood loss (i.e. pregnancy, menstruation or other bleeding). After several decades of increased absorption, symptoms appear once 15–20 g of iron have accumulated in the body. Men tend to become symptomatic in middle age (40s) and women who stop menstruating develop symptoms about 15 years later.

Clinical features

The fibrotic reaction to haemosiderin deposits can produce pigmentation, adrenocortical insufficiency, cardiomyopathy, cirrhosis or diabetes (bronze diabetes). The most common complaint is joint pain but non-specific symptoms, such as weakness, fatigue, abdominal pain, and loss of libido due to hypopituitarism and hypogonadism, are common. About 30% of patients with cirrhosis develop hepatocellular carcinoma.

General management

A sensitive and relatively inexpensive method of screening involves the transferrin saturation test (serum iron divided by the total iron-binding capacity). High serum ferritin levels may also suggest the diagnosis. Treatment is iron removal by venesection and chelation using desferrioxamine. Liver transplantation is needed for end-stage haemochromatosis.

Dental aspects

A sicca syndrome from salivary haemosiderin deposition may be seen.
LA is generally safe. CS can be given. Cirrhosis, adrenocortical insufficiency, diabetes or cardiomyopathy may complicate care.

Wilson disease

See Chapters 9 and 37.

DISEASES ASSOCIATED WITH DEFECTIVE DNA REPAIR

Several inborn errors predispose to malignancy because of impaired DNA repair mechanisms (Table 23.6; Chs 22 and 37). Xeroderma pigmentosum produces a liability to skin and lip cancers. Bloom syndrome, dyskeratosis congenita and Fanconi anaemia have a higher than normal risk of oral carcinomas.

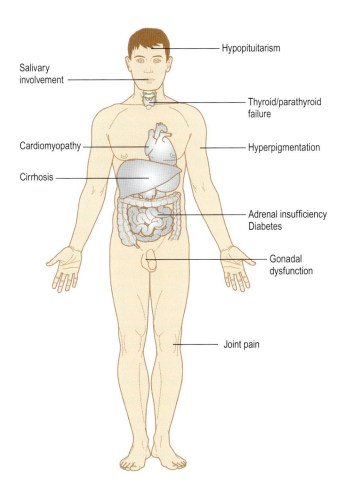

Fig. 23.5 Iron overload in haemochromatosis.

Table 23.6 *Diseases associated with defective DNA repair*

Disorder	Main genetics	Features
Ataxia telangiectasia (AT)	Autosomal recessive (AR)	Cerebellar ataxia, telangiectases, immune defects, neoplasms
Bloom syndrome	AR	Proportionate pre- and postnatal growth deficiency; sun-sensitive, telangiectatic, and hypo- and hyperpigmented skin
Cockayne syndrome	AR	Dwarfism, precociously senility, pigmentary retinal degeneration, optic atrophy, deafness, marble epiphyses in digits, photosensitivity and learning disability. Disproportionately long limbs with large hands and feet and flexion contractures of joints. Knee contractures result in a 'horseriding' stance
Dyskeratosis congenital	AR or autosomal dominant (AD)	Abnormal skin pigmentation and nail growth, premature ageing and a highly increased risk of malignancy (skin, gut and oral). Bone marrow failure (aplastic anaemia) affects 80%
Fanconi anaemia	AR	All bone marrow elements depressed with cardiac, renal and limb malformations, dermal pigmentary changes and oral cancer
Xeroderma pigmentosum (XP)	AR	Sensitivity to sunlight carcinomas at an early age. Starts with freckle-like lesions in exposed areas, usually in early years

ENZYME DEFECTS AFFECTING DRUG METABOLISM

Drug responses vary greatly between individuals, owing to genetic as well as environmental effects on drug absorption, distribution, metabolism or excretion (pharmacokinetics), and on receptor or post-receptor sensitivity (pharmacodynamics). Genetic differences in drug metabolism can have profound effects on treatment in terms of genetically determined variation in the activity of enzymes involved in detoxification, or of other abnormal proteins that render an individual especially susceptible to some adverse reaction.

Pharmacogenetic variation is sometimes due to the actions of a single mutant gene (as in genetic polymorphism, or Mendelian disorders that exhibit discontinuous variation), or polygenic influences. For example, some Asians metabolize carbamazepine poorly and can thus suffer from overdose or other adverse events, so they should be screened for human leukocyte antigen (HLA). The HLA-B*1502 allele has been shown to be strongly correlated with carbamazepine-induced Stevens–Johnson syndrome and toxic epidermal necrolysis (SJS-TEN) in the Han Chinese and other Asian populations but not in European populations. The presence of the HLA-A*3101 allele was associated with carbamazepine-induced hypersensitivity reactions among subjects of northern European ancestry.

Drug-metabolizing enzymes include glucose-6-phosphate dehydrogenase, *N*-acetyltransferase, and the superfamily of cytochrome P450 (CYP) isoenzymes (CYP2D6, CYP2C9, CYP2C19 and CYP3A). Table 23.7 shows examples of major disorders that influence drug responses.

Glucose-6-phosphate dehydrogenase deficiency

Glucose-6-phosphate dehydrogenase (G6PD) is the enzyme responsible for maintaining the nicotinamide–adenine dinucleotide phosphate (NADPH) needed to keep glutathione in its reduced form to act as a scavenger for dangerous oxidative metabolites. Low G6PD activity is the most common enzyme deficiency, affecting 400 million people worldwide, and is seen mainly in people of Mediterranean, Middle Eastern, African or Asian descent. G6PD deficiency results in haemolysis and methaemoglobinaemia when red blood cells are exposed to oxidation during intercurrent infection, exposure to various drugs, broad beans (*Vicia fava*) or naphthalene; it occasionally occurs spontaneously.

General aspects

Haemolysis follows when oxidizing drugs are taken.

General management

The diagnosis is confirmed by G6PD enzyme assays. Haemolysis is self-limiting and splenectomy is rarely needed. If there is acute severe haemolysis, the drug may have to be withdrawn and blood transfusion may be needed. Hydrocortisone is given intravenously and the urine alkalinized to reduce acid haematin deposition in renal tubules.

Prevention is crucial. Drugs that can be dangerous in G6PD deficiency and should be avoided are shown in Table 23.8 and Appendix

Table 23.7 *Variations in drug response due to genetic polymorphism*

Pharmacogenetic variation	Inheritance	Frequency	Drugs involved
Glucose-6-phosphate dehydrogenase (G6PD) deficiency	X-linked incomplete co-dominant	10 000 000 in the world	Many, including quinolines and most sulphonamides
Malignant hyperthermia	Autosomal dominant (AD)	1:20 000 of population	Anaesthetics, especially halothane and suxamethonium
Methaemoglobinaemia	Autosomal recessive (AR)	1:100 are heterozygotes	Same drugs as for G6PD deficiency
Neuroleptic malignant syndrome	AD	Seen in 0.02–3.23% of psychiatric patients receiving neuroleptics	Neuroleptics
Porphyria	AD	Acute intermittent type 15:1000 000 in Sweden; porphyria cutanea tarda 1:100 in Afrikaaners	Barbiturates, chloral, chloroquine, ethanol, sulphonamides, phenytoin and griseofulvin (many others)
Suxamethonium sensitivity	AR	Most common in Europeans and rare in Asians	Suxamethonium and mivacurium

Table 23.8 *Drugs that may precipitate haemolysis in glucose-6-phosphate dehydrogenase deficiency*

Analgesic/antipyretic	Antimalarial	Cardiovascular	Cytotoxic/antibacterial	Miscellaneous	Sulfonamides/sulfones
Aspirin	Chloroquine	Procainamide	Chloramphenicol	Alpha-methyldopa	Dapsone
Phenacetin	Hydroxychloroquine	Quinidine	Ciprofloxacin	Ascorbic acid	Most sulphonamides, including co-trimoxazole
Prilocaine	Mepacrine (quinacrine)		Furazolidone	Dimercaprol (BAL)	
	Pamaquine		Furmethonol	Hydralazine	
	Pentaquine		Moxifloxacin	Mestranol	
	Primaquine		Nalidixic acid	Methylene blue	
	Quinine		Neoarsphenamine	Naphthalene	
	Quinocide		Nitrofurantoin	Phenylhydrazine	
			Nitrofurazone	Pyridium	
			Norfloxacin	Toluidine blue	
			Ofloxacin	Trinitrotoluene	
			Para-aminosalicylic acid (PAS)	Urate oxidase	
				Vitamin K (water-soluble) and menadione	

Table 23.9 *Drugs contraindicated, and safer alternatives, in malignant hyperpyrexia in susceptible subjects*

Drug group	Contraindicated	Safer
General anaesthetics	Halothane	Local anaesthetics
	Ether	Thiopental
	Cyclopropane	Nitrous oxide
	Ketamine	
	Enflurane	
Conscious sedation agents	Benzodiazepines	Nitrous oxide
Muscle relaxants	Suxamethonium	Pancuronium
	Curare	
Antidepressants	Tricyclic antidepressants	
	Monoamine oxidase inhibitors (MAOIs)	Selective serotonin reuptake inhibitors (SSRIs)

23.2. Substances labelled 'low-risk' may often be given safely at normal therapeutic doses unless the patient is severely G6PD-deficient or has chronic non-spherocytic hemolytic anaemia, but there is no guarantee that they will not cause haemolysis. Avoid mothballs, artificial blue food colouring, legumes (broad beans, beans, peas, peanuts, soy, lentils, etc.), sulphites and tonic water. Read all labels on processed foods before feeding them to the patient. A diet rich in antioxidant foods is recommended to help minimize the effects of oxidative stress and the resultant hemolysis. Vitamins B_6, B_{12}, folic acid and *N*-acetyl cysteine (NAC) are also important.

Dental aspects

Aspirin up to at least 1 g a day is safe for most patients. Paracetamol (acetaminophen) also appears to be safe but doses should be limited. Codeine may also be used. LA with prilocaine may, in large doses, induce methaemoglobinaemia and should be avoided (see Table 23.8). CS is usually safely given as relative analgesia. GA is given in hospital. Metabolic acidosis causes haemolysis and must be avoided.

Malignant hyperthermia (malignant hyperpyrexia)

General aspects

Malignant hyperthermia (MH) is a rare, potentially fatal, inherited condition, related to the ryanodine receptor (*RYR1*) gene (the muscle sarcoplasmic reticulum calcium release channel) on chromosome 19. MH affects about 1 in 20 000, males predominantly. It is characterized by a rapid rise in temperature when the patient has a GA or other drugs that trigger an attack. The most common trigger is the combination of a halogenated volatile GA, such as halothane or enflurane, together with muscle relaxants such as suxamethonium and curare-like (non-depolarizing) agents (Table 23.9).

Clinical features

Suxamethonium, unlike pancuronium or vecuronium, causes jaw stiffness in many normal people, but poor muscular relaxation after induction of GA or complete failure of the jaw to relax after suxamethonium has been given can herald the onset of MH. However, it is controversial whether masseter spasm is a reliable early sign. The most reliable earliest signs of an MH reaction are rapid breathing and heart rate, and rising blood pressure. There is also a temperature rise, with arrhythmias. Hyperkalaemia, cardiac arrhythmias and disseminated intravascular coagulation (DIC) may occur and the mortality rate of MH may approach 80% in the absence of treatment.

Two forms of MH are recognized: an autosomal dominant type, in which patients are clinically normal between attacks; and a recessive type, which affects young boys with various congenital abnormalities such as myotonia congenita, myotonic dystrophy, central core disease and Evan syndrome (proximal wasting, short stature, kyphoscoliosis).

General management

The family history is important, as emphasized by the fact that a patient reported to the writer had had 14 relatives die under GA. Raised serum creatine kinase and pyrophosphate levels indicate susceptibility, though nearly one-third of patients have normal levels of creatine kinase. Muscle biopsy shows excessive *in vitro* response of muscle to halothane, suxamethonium or caffeine, and raised myophosphorylase A levels.

Malignant hyperthermia is a medical emergency; management includes stopping the trigger, correcting respiratory acidosis and using dantrolene. All trigger agents (i.e. all anaesthetic vapours) must be withdrawn, dantrolene given and temperature, arterial blood gases, K+ and creatine phosphokinase (CPK) measured. Surface cooling, avoiding vasoconstriction, is needed. Serious arrhythmias are treated with beta-blockers, and hyperkalaemia and metabolic acidosis corrected. A clotting screen is done to detect DIC, a urine sample taken for myoglobin estimation and output measured for developing renal failure. Diuresis is promoted with fluids/mannitol. The patient should be referred to an MH unit.

Dental aspects

Infections should be treated quickly and effectively since they also may precipitate attacks of MH.

Dantrolene given preoperatively and postoperatively for about 3 days may prevent hyperthermia. Plain LA is safe (amides, including lidocaine and prilocaine, were once thought to be weak triggering agents but this has been dismissed). Adrenaline (epinephrine) may cause signs similar to an attack of MH, confusing the diagnosis, and may enhance calcium release inside muscle cells and aggravate an MH episode. Endogenous adrenaline release should be minimized (avoid stress, anxiety and pain) and effective LA must be used (which may mean choosing an adrenaline-containing LA). Benzodiazepines are contraindicated; CS can usually be safely carried out using relative analgesia. MH has been reported after administration of nitrous oxide but this is rare. Inquiry into the family history is essential before giving GA, as there are no absolutely reliable predictive tests. Unfortunately, absence of reaction to a previous GA does not exclude the possibility of a reaction on the next occasion.

In the event of hyperthermia, surgery must be stopped and the patient cooled. Oxygen, and a bicarbonate intravenous infusion to counteract the metabolic acidosis, should be given. Dantrolene sodium or procainamide is effective in controlling the reaction.

Methaemoglobinaemia

Methaemoglobin is a haemoglobin that is not functional in oxygen carriage. A small amount of methaemoglobin is always present in erythrocytes but is usually converted back to haemoglobin through successive electron transfers, by nicotinamide adenine dinucleotide (NADH)–dependent methaemoglobin reduction (in the diaphorase pathway). Cytochrome b5 reductase is important in this process because it transfers electrons from NADH to methaemoglobin, and usually removes 95–99% of the methaemoglobin produced. Nicotinamide adenine dinucleotide phosphate (NADPH)–dependent methaemoglobin reduction, which utilizes glutathione production and G6PD to reduce methaemoglobin to haemoglobin, usually plays only a minor role – unless there are inherited cytochrome b5 reductase deficiencies.

There are two types of inherited methaemoglobinaemia:

- Type 1 (erythrocyte reductase deficiency) – red blood cells are affected.
- Type 2 (generalized reductase deficiency) – there are defects in the haemoglobin molecule itself; this is called haemoglobin M disease.

Methylene blue and ascorbic acid are used to treat severe methaemoglobinaemia. Alternative treatments include hyperbaric oxygen therapy and exchange transfusions.

Methaemoglobinaemia may also be caused by exposure to certain drugs, chemicals or foods (acquired), including paracetamol (acetaminophen) and local anaesthetics – benzocaine, lidocaine and prilocaine (Box 23.2). Acquired methaemoglobinaemia requires no treatment other than to avoid the agents implicated.

Neuroleptic malignant syndrome

Neuroleptic malignant syndrome (NMS) is a rare, potentially fatal complication due to a dopamine receptor blockade from the use of neuroleptics (Box 23.3). Although potent neuroleptics (e.g. haloperidol, fluphenazine) are causally associated with NMS more frequently, all antipsychotics may precipitate it. NMS has also been associated with non-neuroleptics that block central dopamine pathways, such as amoxapine, lithium and metoclopramide.

NMS is characterized by fever, muscular rigidity, altered mental status and autonomic dysfunction. The relationship of NMS to malignant hyperthermia is unknown. Features may develop dramatically within hours of drug exposure, or insidiously over several days; they may persist for several days, or death can result from renal failure. There are disturbances in mental state, temperature regulation, and autonomic and extrapyramidal functions. Hyperthermia, muscle rigidity, fluctuating consciousness, obtundation, catatonia, pallor, sweating, tachycardia, labile blood pressure, incontinence, tremors, dysarthria, dysphagia and drooling result.

NMS is an emergency; withdrawal of the neuroleptic agent and assessment of the airway, breathing and circulation (ABC) are crucial, as are exclusion of other medical conditions and aggressive supportive care. Any patient with altered mental status should receive thiamine, dextrose (or rapid glucose determination) and naloxone.

Dental aspects

In NMS, LA can usually be safely given. CS dentistry can usually be safely given using relative analgesia. Phenothiazines should be avoided for patients who have stopped their levodopa before a GA. Levodopa can be given before GA, apart from the fact that it may cause vomiting.

Serotonin syndrome

Serotonin syndrome is a constellation of muscle rigidity, headache and rises in blood pressure and temperature, induced by drugs such as antidepressants or 5-HT1 agonists (triptans) (Box 23.4).

Box 23.2 *Agents that may precipitate methaemoglobinaemia*

Inorganic agents

- Nitrates – fertilizers, contaminated well water, preservatives, industrial products
- Chlorates
- Copper sulphate – fungicides

Organic nitrites/nitrates

- Amyl nitrite
- Isobutyl nitrite
- Sodium nitrite
- Nitric oxide
- Nitrogen dioxide
- Nitroglycerin
- Nitroprusside
- Trinitrotoluene (TNT), combustion products

Others

- Local anesthetics – benzocaine, lidocaine, prilocaine, phenazopyridine
- Antimalarials – primaquine, chloroquine
- Rasburicase
- Antineoplastic agents – cyclophosphamide, ifosfamide, flutamide
- Analgesics/antipyretics – paracetamol (acetaminophen), acetanilide, phenacetin, celecoxib
- Zopiclone
- Herbicides – paraquat (dipyridylium)
- Methylene blue
- Indigo carmine (indigotindisulfonate)
- Resorcinol
- Antibiotics – sulphonamides, nitrofurans, P-amino-salicylic acid, dapsone
- Industrial/household agents – aniline dyes, nitrobenzene, naphthalene (mothballs), aminophenol, nitroethane (nail polish remover)

Box 23.3 *Precipitants of neuroleptic malignant syndrome*

- Alcohol
- Amphetamines
- Antidepressants (tricyclic or monoamine oxidase inhibitors)
- Benzodiazepines
- Metoclopramide
- Neuroleptics (e.g. phenothiazines, haloperidol or flupentixol)
- Tetrabenazine
- Abrupt withdrawal of L-dopa

Box 23.4 *Possible precipitants of serotonin syndrome*

- 5-HT1 agonists
- Antidepressants
- Buspirone
- Chlorphenamine
- Herbs (e.g. St John's wort)
- L-dopa
- Lithium
- Olanzapine
- Opioids
- Psychedelics
- Ritonavir
- Tramadol
- Valproate

- Inherited suxamethonium sensitivity (scoline sensitivity)
- Myopathies:
  - Malignant hyperpyrexia
  - Dystrophia myotonica
  - Myotonia congenita
  - Myasthenia gravis
- Liver disease
- Renal disease
- Burns
- Drugs:
  - Aprotinin (trasylol)
  - Cyclophosphamide
  - Cytotoxic drugs
  - Pancuronium
  - Phenothiazines
  - Procaine

Table 23.10 *Amyloid types*

Amyloid type	Deposit	Comments
Idiopathic (primary) amyloidosis	AL	Derived from immunoglobulin light chains plus serum amyloid P
Myeloma-associated amyloidosis	AL	Derived from immunoglobulin light chains
Hereditary amyloidosis	AA	Derived from other proteins (lyosozyme, fibrinogen, apolipoproteins)
Secondary amyloidosis	AA	The most common form of amyloid disease. Derived from serum amyloid A protein, an acute-phase protein released by the liver in chronic infections or inflammatory states such as rheumatoid arthritis and ulcerative colitis, via interleukin-1 from activated mononuclear phagocytes
Other forms of amyloidosis	Range of proteins	Mainly pre-albumin. A heterogeneous group, some related to senility, dialysis or drug abuse, and some localized to medullary carcinoma of thyroid or calcifying epithelial odontogenic tumour

Suxamethonium sensitivity (pseudocholinesterase deficiency; scoline apnoea)

Suxamethonium (scoline) is a depolarizing neuromuscular blocker widely used for muscle relaxation during GA induction. The usual response to a single intravenous dose of suxamethonium is muscular paralysis for about 6 minutes, after which it is rapidly destroyed by a plasma enzyme. About 1 in 2500 of the population has a defect in this enzyme (cholinesterase; butyrylcholinesterase; pseudocholinesterase) and are thus abnormally sensitive to the action of suxamethonium, so that muscle paralysis and apnoea persist. Suxamethonium sensitivity is an autosomal recessive trait due to mutant alleles of *CHE1* on chromosome 3; it is most common in Europeans and rare in Asians. Abnormal sensitivity to suxamethonium may also result from other diseases (Box 23.5) or may be a type of hypersensitivity reaction.

When given suxamethonium, patients with suxamethonium sensitivity remain unable to breathe and will die unless artificially ventilated until the drug action abates after 2 hours or more. Patients may also react similarly to other choline ester compounds, such as mivacurium, and can have severe reactions to cocaine.

LA action is occasionally prolonged. Nitrous oxide/oxygen sedation is preferable to GA.

ACQUIRED METABOLIC DISORDERS

AMYLOID DISEASE

General aspects

Amyloidosis is not a disease in itself, rather a manifestation of several diseases. Amyloid consists of deposits in tissues of an eosinophilic hyaline protein with a characteristic fibrillar structure on electron microscopy. Up to 60 types of amyloid protein are known, categorized as primary (AL), secondary (AA) and hereditary (ATTR). In addition, there are other forms of amyloidosis, including beta$_2$-microglobulin amyloidosis and localized amyloidoses.

In *primary amyloidosis*, AL protein deposition is seen in conditions with immunoglobulin overproduction, as in benign monoclonal gammopathy, and has a prominent immunoglobulin light-chain component (Table 23.10). Primary amyloidosis can also occur with multiple myeloma but is not associated with any other diseases. It is treated with chemotherapy.

Secondary amyloidosis may occur secondary to conditions of chronic excessive stimulation of the reticuloendothelial system (see Table 23.10), such as infections (e.g. tuberculosis or osteomyelitis) or inflammatory diseases (e.g. rheumatoid arthritis, ankylosing spondylitis or autoinflammatory syndromes); the deposits are AA proteins related to acute phase proteins such as serum amyloid P (SAP; Fig. 23.6). Amyloid is then deposited mainly in the heart, skeletal muscle and gastrointestinal tract, and affects their functions. Other secondary amyloid is of uncertain origin but involves the spleen, liver, kidney and adrenals predominantly. Treatment is directed to the underlying illness.

Localized amyloid may be seen in a range of disorders (see Fig. 23.6) including Alzheimer disease. In various tissues, often with ageing, amyloid can be locally deposited to cause tissue injury.

Deposits of a protein transthyretin (TTR) are found in the rare autosomal dominant condition called *familial amyloidosis* (TTR amyloid or ATTR). Sephardic Jews and Turks inherit familial Mediterranean fever (FMF), which is associated with this amyloidosis and characterized by episodes of fever, joint and abdominal pains; these can be prevented by colchicine. Armenians and Ashkenazi Jews also have a higher incidence of FMF attacks but do not suffer amyloid.

Beta$_2$-microglobulin amyloidosis occurs when amyloid deposits develop in dialysis patients and are often found around joints.

Clinical features

Amyloid is a great mimic in medicine. The widespread lesions and the possible involvement of virtually any system make amyloid disease protean in its manifestations. There may also be a bleeding tendency related to a coagulation factor X defect.

General management

The diagnosis is established by biopsy of lesional tissue or by rectal, gingival or salivary biopsy examined with Congo Red and polarized light or thioflavin T.

An underlying cause must be sought and treated where possible. Combination therapy is used, with corticosteroids, melphalan and fluoxymesterone.

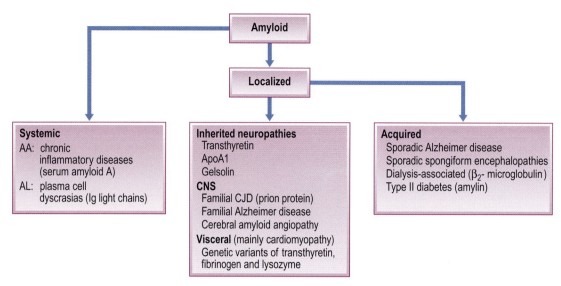

Fig. 23.6 Types of amyloid. ApoA1 = apolipoprotein A1; CJD = Creutzfeld–Jakob disease.

Dental aspects

Dental management may be influenced by the underlying disorder, or by cardiac, renal, adrenal or corticosteroid complications, or a bleeding tendency.

LA can safely be given. CS can be given if required.

Macroglossia, gingival swellings, oral petechiae, bullae or, rarely, a sicca syndrome may result from amyloidosis, but virtually only in the primary type.

TRIMETHYLAMINURIA (TMA-URIA; FISH-ODOUR SYNDROME)

Trimethylaminuria is a rare autosomal recessive syndrome in which there is abnormal trimethylamine (TMA) excretion. TMA is found in some foods and is produced by gut bacteria from foods rich in TMA-oxide, choline, lecithin or carnitine. TMA is found in milk from wheat-fed cows, TMA precursors in choline (eggs, liver, kidney, peas, beans, peanuts, soya and brassicas [Brussels sprouts, broccoli, cabbage, cauliflower]), lecithin and lecithin-containing fish oil supplements. TMA N-oxide is found in seafood (fish, cephalopods and crustaceans).

TMA is normally oxidized by liver flavin mono-oxygenase 3 (FMO3) to odourless trimethylamine N-oxide (TMAO). Trimethylaminuria is an inherited *FMO3* gene mutation leading to impaired TMA oxidation. Unoxidized TMA then appears in and causes odour from urine, sweat, genital secretions, saliva and breath. Other causes of excess TMA include:

- deficient nicotine N-oxidation
- disorders of carnitine and choline intake
- haematological abnormalities
- Noonan syndrome
- Prader–Willi syndrome
- renal and hepatic disease
- Turner syndrome.

Similar symptoms may appear in some normal people under conditions such as fever, stress, exercise or menstruation. Trimethylaminuria is managed by diet (avoid eggs, fish, brassicas); antimicrobials (e.g. metronidazole); lactulose; activated charcoal and copper chlorophyllin; and riboflavin.

USEFUL WEBSITES

(Accessed 29 May 2013)
National Institutes of Health: Offices of Rare Diseases Research. <http://rarediseases.info.nih.gov/>.
The Medical Biochemistry Page. <http://themedicalbiochemistrypage.org>.
Wikipedia: Inborn error of metabolism. <http://en.wikipedia.org/wiki/Metabolic_disorder>.
Wikipedia: Metabolic syndrome. <http://en.wikipedia.org/wiki/Metabolic_syndrome>.

FURTHER READING

Ayonrinde, O.T., et al. 2008. Clinical perspectives on hereditary hemochromatosis. Crit. Rev. Clin. Lab. Sci. 45, 451.
Cappellini, M.D., Fiorelli, G., 2008. Glucose-6-phosphate dehydrogenase deficiency. Lancet 371, 64.
Cassiman, D., et al. 2008. Porphyria cutanea tarda and liver disease. A retrospective analysis of 17 cases from a single centre and review of the literature. Acta Gastroenterol. Belg. 71, 237.
Chen, M., Wang, J., 2008. Gaucher disease: review of the literature. Arch. Pathol. Lab. Med. 132, 851.
Cope, T.M., Hunter, J.M., 2003. Selecting neuromuscular-blocking drugs for elderly patients. Drugs Aging 20, 125.
Di Mauro, S., 2007. Muscle glycogenoses: an overview. Acta Myol. 26, 35.
Dinauer, M.C., 2007. Disorders of neutrophil function: an overview. Methods Mol. Biol. 412, 489.
Friedlander, A.H., et al. 2007. Metabolic syndrome: pathogenesis, medical care and dental implications. J. Am. Dent. Assoc. 138, 179. quiz 248
Friedlander, A.H., Golub, M.S., 2006. The significance of carotid artery atheromas on panoramic radiographs in the diagnosis of occult metabolic syndrome. Oral Surg. Oral Med. Oral Pathol. Oral Radiol. Endod. 101, 95.
Galley, H.F., et al. 2005. Pharmacogenetics and anesthesiologists. Pharmacogenomics 6, 849.
Katzin, L.W., Amato, A.A., 2008. Pompe disease: a review of the current diagnosis and treatment recommendations in the era of enzyme replacement therapy. J. Clin. Neuromuscul. Dis. 9, 421.
Kopelman, P., 2004. The metabolic syndrome as a clinical problem. Nestle Nutr. Workshop Ser. Clin. Perform Programme 9, 77. discussion 88
Lajtman, Z., et al. 2002. 'Warning card' as a prevention of prolonged apnea in children. Coll. Antropol. 26 (Suppl), 129.
Lee, J.H., et al. 2002. Oral self-mutilation in the Lesch–Nyhan syndrome. ASDC J. Dent. Child. 69 (66), 12.
McCormack, M., et al. 2011. HLA-A*3101 and carbamazepine-induced hypersensitivity reactions in Europeans. N. Engl. J. Med. 364 (12), 1134. doi: 10.1056/NEJMoa1013297. PubMed PMID: 21428769; PubMed Central PMCID: PMC3113609.
Nishimura, F., et al. 2005. Periodontal disease as part of the insulin resistance syndrome in diabetic patients. J. Int. Acad. Periodontol. 7, 16.
Olynyk, J.K., et al. 2008. Hereditary hemochromatosis in the post-HFE era. Hepatology 48, 991.

Rosenberg, H., et al. 2007. Malignant hyperthermia. Orphanet J. Rare Dis. 2, 21.

Saranjam, H.R., et al. 2012. Mandibular and dental manifestations of Gaucher disease. Oral Dis. 18, 421.

Sarkany, R., 2008. Making sense of the porphyrias. Photodermatol. Photoimmunol. Photomed. 24 (2), 102.

Shimazaki, Y., et al. 2007. Relationship of metabolic syndrome to periodontal disease in Japanese women: the Hisayama Study. J. Dent. Res. 86, 271.

Taddei, T., et al. 2008. Inherited metabolic disease of the liver. Curr. Opin. Gastroenterol. 24, 278.

Thomas, C.L., et al. 2008. Sclerodermatous changes of face, neck and scalp associated with familial porphyria cutanea tarda. Clin. Exp. Dermatol. 33, 422.

Williams, D.S., 2007. Porphyria cutanea tarda. J. Insur. Med. 39, 293.

APPENDIX 23.1 INBORN ERRORS OF METABOLISM

Disease	Management problems
Abetalipoproteinaemia	Ataxia: haemorrhage
Acatalasaemia	Gingival ulceration
Acid lipase deficiency	Learning impairment; anaemia
Acrodermatitis enteropathica	Oral ulceration; neuropathies
Adenosine deaminase deficiency	Immunodeficiency
Alkaptonuria	Arthritis; aortic valve disease
Alpha1-antitrypsin deficiency	Hepatic disease; emphysema
Argininaemia	Spasticity; learning disability; epilepsy
Aspartylglucosaminuria	Learning impairment
Cerebrotendinous xanthomatosis	Dementia; ataxia; paresis; cataracts
Cholinesterase deficiency	Suxamethonium sensitivity
Chronic granulomatous disease	Lymph node abscesses (cervical, etc.); liability to severe bacterial infections
Combined hyperlipidaemia	Atherosclerosis
Congenital adrenal hyperplasia	Hypoadrenocorticism
Crigler–Najjar syndrome	Jaundice
Cystinosis	Renal disease
Cystinuria	Renal disease
Diphosphoglycerate mutase deficiency	Anaemia
Dubin–Johnson syndrome	Jaundice
Dysbetalipoproteinaemia	Atherosclerosis
Fabry disease	Neuropathy; thromboses; renal failure; pulmonary failure
Familial dysautonomia (Riley–Day syndrome)	Sensitivity to barbiturates; dysphagia; sialorrhoea; insensitivity to pain; learning impairment; epilepsy; labile blood pressure
Familial goitre	Hypothyroidism
Fanconi syndrome	Aminoaciduria; osteomalacia; oral cancer
Fucosidosis	Learning impairment
Galactosaemia	Learning impairment; hepatic disease; cataracts; hypoglycaemia
Gilbert disease	Jaundice
GM1 gangliosidosis	Learning impairment; epilepsy; blindness
GM2 gangliosidosis	Learning impairment; epilepsy; blindness
Tay–Sachs disease	Learning impairment; epilepsy; blindness
Sandhoff disease	Learning impairment; epilepsy; blindness
Gaucher disease	Learning impairment; spasticity; thrombocytopenia; leukopenia
Glucose-6-phosphate dehydrogenase deficiency	Haemolytic anaemia, care with drugs
Glutaric aciduria	Hypoglycaemia
Glycogen storage disease:	
Type I	Hypoglycaemia; caries; bleeding tendency
Type II	Cardiomyopathy; respiratory infection; neurological abnormalities
Type III	Hypoglycaemia
Type IV	Hepatic disease; cardiac failure
Type VI	Mild hypoglycaemia
Type VIa	Mild hypoglycaemia
Type O	Mild hypoglycaemia

Disease	Management problems
Gout	Renal disease; hypertension; atherosclerosis
Haemochromatosis	Diabetes; hepatic disease; cardiomyopathy
Hereditary angioedema	Airways obstruction
Hereditary fructose intolerance	Hepatic disease; hypoglycaemia
Hereditary oroticaciduria	Severe anaemia; leukopenia
Hereditary spherocytosis	Haemolytic anaemia
Hexokinase deficiency	Anaemia
Histidinaemia	Hearing deficit; speech deficit; infections; learning disability
Homocystinuria	Learning impairment; epilepsy; blindness; hepatic disease; chest deformities; thrombotic disease
Hypercalcaemia	Renal disease; cardiac subaortic stenosis; learning disability (William syndrome)
Hypercholesterolaemia	Atherosclerosis
Hypercystinuria	Renal disease
Hyperornithinaemia	Learning impairment
Hyperoxaluria	Renal disease
Hypertriglyceridaemia	Atherosclerosis; pancreatitis
Hypophosphatasia	Skeletal abnormalities; dental hypoplasia
Krabbe disease	Learning impairment; blindness
Lecithin/cholesterol/acetyltransferase deficiency	Haemolytic anaemia; atherosclerosis; renal disease
Lesch–Nyhan syndrome	Mutilation of tongue or lips; learning impairment; epilepsy; athetosis; renal failure
Lipoprotein lipase deficiency	Pancreatitis
Lysinuria	Epilepsy
Mannosidosis	Learning impairment
Metachromatic leukodystrophy	Learning impairment; blindness; psychoses
Methionine malabsorption	Epilepsy
Mucolipidosis (I-cell disease)	Learning impairment; blindness; valvular heart disease
Mucopolysaccharidosis (MPS) I Hurler syndrome	Learning impairment; blindness; cardiac impairment; trismus
MPS II Hunter syndrome	As in MPS I
MPS III Sanfilippo syndrome	Learning impairment
MPS IV Morquio syndrome	Blindness; chest deformity; aortic valve disease; enamel hypoplasia
MPS V Ullrich–Scheie syndrome	Blindness; valvular heart disease
MPS VI Maroteaux–Lamy syndrome	Learning impairment; blindness
MPS VII	Learning impairment
Myeloperoxidase deficiency	Candidosis
Neuronal ceroid lipofuscinoses	Learning impairment; epilepsy; blindness
Niemann–Pick disease	Learning impairment; epilepsy; pancytopenia
Oxalosis	Renal disease; cardiac disease
Phenylketonuria	Learning impairment; epilepsy

(Continued)

Disease	Management problems
Porphyrias	Drug sensitivities; neuropathies; hypertension
Primary hypophosphataemia (vitamin D-resistant rickets)	Dwarfism; rickets; dental abscesses
Prolinaemia	Epilepsy; deafness
Purine nucleoside phosphorylase deficiency	Immunodeficiency
Pyruvate kinase deficiency	Anaemia
Refsum disease	Blindness; deafness
Renal glycosuria	Glycosuria (confusion with diabetes)
Rotor syndrome	Jaundice
Sandhoff disease	Learning impairment; epilepsy; blindness
Tay–Sachs disease	Learning impairment; epilepsy; blindness
Transcobalamin II deficiency	Macrocytic anaemia; pancytopenia
Triosephosphate isomerase deficiency	Anaemia
Tyrosinaemia	Hepatic disease
Tyrosinosis	Myasthenia; epilepsy
Wilson disease (hepatolenticular degeneration)	Hepatic disease; renal disease; spasticity; tremor; mental problems
Wolman disease	Learning impairment
Xeroderma pigmentosum	Skin cancers

APPENDIX 23.2 DRUGS CONTRAINDICATED IN GLUCOSE-6-PHOSPHATE DEHYDROGENASE (G6PD) DEFICIENCY

Drug	Risk
Acetanilide	High
Acetylphenylhydrazine	High
Aminophenazone	Low
Antazoline	Low
Ascorbic acid	Low
Aspirin	High
Beta-naphthol	High
Chloramphenicol	High
Chloroquine	High
Ciprofloxacin	High
Colchicine	Low
Dapsone	High
Dimercaprol	High
Diphenhydramine	Low
Dopamine	Low
Doxorubicin	High
Ethanol	High
Furazolidone	High
Furosemide	High
Gadopentetate dimeglumine	High
Glibenclamide (glyburide)	High
Glucosulfone	High
Henna	High
Ibuprofen	Low
Isobutyl nitrite	High
Isoniazid	Low
Lamotrigine	High
Levofloxacin	High
Lisinopril	High
Mefloquine	High
Menadiol sodium sulfate (vitamin K_4 sodium sulfate)	High
Menadione	High

Drug	Risk
Menadione sodium bisulfite (Vitamin K_3 sodium bisulfite)	High
Menthol	High
Mesalazine	High
Metformin	High
Methylene blue	High
Mirtazapine	Low
Moxifloxacin	High
Nalidixic acid	High
Naphthalene	High
Nimesulide	High
Niridazole	High
Nitrofurantoin	High
Nitrofurazone	High
Norfloxacin	Low
Pamaquine	High
Para-aminobenzoic acid	Low
Paracetamol (acetaminophen)	Low
Pefloxacin	High
Pentaquine	High
Phenacetin	High
Phenazone (antipyrine)	Low
Phenazopyridine	High
Phenylbutazone	Low
Phenylhydrazine	High
Phenytoin	Low
Primaquine	High
Probenecid	High
Procainamide	Low
Proguanil	Low
Pyrimethamine	Low
Quinacrine	High
Quinidine	Low
Quinine	Low
Stibophen	High
Streptomycin	Low
Sulfacetamide	High
Sulfacytine	Low
Sulfadiazine	Low
Sulfadimidine	High
Sulfafurazole	High
Sulfaguanidine	Low
Sulfamerazine	Low
Sulfamethoxazole	High
Sulfamethoxypyridazine	Low
Sulfanilamide	High
Sulfapyridine	High
Sulfasalazine	High
Sulfathiazole	High
Sulfonylurea	Low
Sulfoxone	High
Tamsulosin	High
Tiaprofenic acid	Low
Toluidine blue	High
Trihexyphenidyl	Low
Trimethoprim	Low
Trinitrotoluene	High
Tripelennamine	Low
Vitamin K_1	Low

This chapter deals with: trauma to the head, maxillofacial area and spine; burns; gunshot and stab wounds; and human bites. Animal bites, sports injuries and child abuse are discussed elsewhere (Chs 25 and 33).

GENERAL ASPECTS

Injuries outrank cancer and heart disease as a leading cause of death in children, and in men up to the age of 35. It is males predominantly who are affected by trauma. Up to a third of these deaths are, theoretically, preventable. Violence (assaults or fights; Figs 24.1–24.3) and road traffic accidents are the major causes of trauma, with alcohol or other drugs being frequent cofactors. In the Western world, assaults are increasingly common but, in contrast, trauma from road traffic accidents (RTAs) has become less common since the institution of seatbelt-wearing. Nevertheless, 3500 people are killed and 40000 seriously injured each year from RTAs in Britain. Maxillofacial trauma is the single most common injury to occupants of vehicles involved in RTAs, even in seatbelted drivers. Airbags may be a supplemental restraint system but they themselves can cause injury – particularly in people of short stature, unrestrained or out of position within the vehicle. Industrial accidents, sport, falls, epilepsy and non-accidental injuries (child abuse) are other causes of trauma. Equine-related maxillofacial fractures mainly involve the young and predominantly females, and alcohol is rarely implicated.

The main causes of oral and craniofacial injuries are sports, violence, falls and RTAs. Cranial injuries are a leading cause of mortality and oral–facial injuries can result in disfigurement and dysfunction, greatly diminish quality of life and cause social and economic burdens.

Sports

Craniofacial sports injuries arise mainly in contact sports, but also in activities such as cycling, skating and gymnastics, especially on trampolines (Ch. 33).

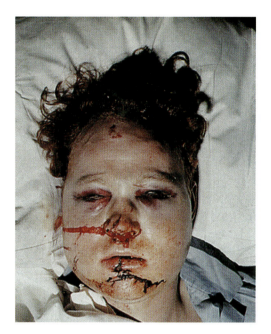

Fig. 24.2 Maxillofacial trauma.

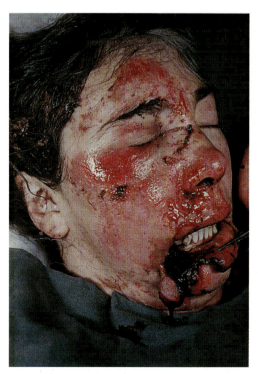

Fig. 24.3 Maxillofacial trauma.

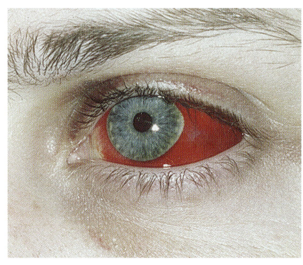

Fig. 24.1 Subconjunctival haemorrhage.

Violence

Domestic violence, including child abuse, spousal and elder abuse, and abuse of the disabled, is the single most common type of violence. Child abuse is of particular concern (Ch. 25) because more than 65% of cases involve head and oral–facial trauma, and in the young child, head injury is the most common cause of death. Dentists are required to report suspected cases. The incidence of specific injury patterns and outcomes of violence in adults are similar between the genders. Males, however, make up the majority of facial fracture cases (over 70%); the aetiology of their injuries includes altercations with strangers, often after consuming alcohol or using drugs, or violent gang activities. Males are more likely to be admitted with fracture but not soft-tissue injury only; more likely to be assaulted with a weapon; and more likely to be involved in an altercation, gang violence, arrest or robbery. Females are more prone to domestic violence and rape, and less likely to be involved in violent criminal activity or to have gang associations. One in six women in the USA has been a victim of sexual violence (a completed or attempted rape) at some time in her life.

Falls

Falls are a major cause of trauma to face, jaws and teeth in adults and children. Orofacial injuries are common from toddlers falling with a bottle, dummy or sippy cup in their mouth; bottles are most likely to be the source of injury, followed by dummies and sippy cups. Injuries consist mainly of mouth lacerations. Falls may indicate underlying pathology or simple locomotor inadequacy and are especially common after the age of 80 years. In old people, it is important to establish whether they are prone to falls, which may need further investigation. Important individual risk factors include:

- arthritis
- balance or gait deficits
- cognitive impairment
- epilepsy
- depression
- mobility limitation
- muscle weakness
- postural hypotension
- visual impairment.

Road traffic accidents

The effects of RTAs may range from minor and reversible effects to long-term medical, surgical and rehabilitative consequences. Post-traumatic headaches and chronic oral–facial pain is not uncommon. Whiplash-associated disorders (WADs) can lead to temporomandibular pain, predominantly in females. Neuromuscular and glandular damage may cause problems with chewing, swallowing and tearing – or result in facial tics or paralysis.

Craniofacial trauma

In conflicts, assaults and RTAs, injuries often involve multiple organs. Death may result immediately from trauma, especially if there is head injury and brain damage, airway obstruction or damage to the spine and other vital organs (e.g. heart or liver).

HEAD INJURIES

Head injuries are present in about 70% of patients admitted with multiple injuries, and about 3% of multiply injured patients have intracranial haemorrhage. Most head injuries are in previously fit young males because of their risk behaviour: RTAs and assaults are major causes (Fig. 24.4). Children and adolescents can sustain head injuries during sports or fights, and young children, particularly before they have perfected their walking skills, are also uniquely susceptible to head trauma because of higher cranial mass to body ratio.

Head injuries are a major cause of death – almost 50% of which happen before the patient reaches hospital – and most of the remaining deaths follow within the first few hours. Of those with brain injury, 12% die within 2 days. It is important to appreciate that the brain can be fatally damaged without fracture of the skull or even a blemish on the scalp.

IMMEDIATE CARE

Damage to the head, cervical spine, chest, liver or spleen can be immediately life-threatening. In particular, there can be hazards to the airway; damage to the cervical spine; severe haemorrhage; and damage to kidneys or bladder or to other bones. All patients with head injuries must be urgently assessed using the ABC system: *a*irway and cervical spine, *b*reathing and bleeding, and *c*hest injuries (Table 24.1).

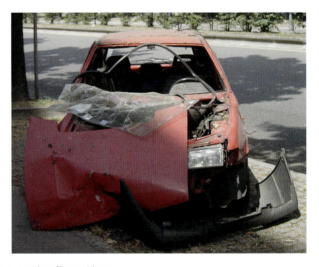

Fig. 24.4 Road traffic accident.

Table 24.1 *Head injuries: initial and early management*

Immediate care (ABC)	General assessment	Assessment of head injury	Assessment for other injuries
Airway and cervical spine	State of consciousness	Skull examination	Neck
Breathing and bleeding	Pulse	Examination for cerebrospinal fluid leak	Spine
Chest injuries	Blood pressure	Neurological assessment	Abdomen
	Respiratory rate	Skull radiography, including computed tomography	Perineum
	Pupil size and reaction	Blood analyses	Limbs

Airway establishment and maintenance has the highest priority. Respiratory obstruction is the most important preventable cause of early death and may be due to several causes, such as those shown in Box 24.1. Many patients have died from neglect of the airway before admission to hospital. Foreign bodies or the tongue can easily fall back to obstruct respiration, especially if there are bilateral fractures or comminution of the mandible, and the patient is unconscious. There is special danger to the airway if there has been trauma to and oedema of the tongue, fauces, pharynx or larynx, or uncontrollable nasoethmoidal haemorrhage.

Severely injured patients must have their airways (mouth and pharynx) cleared of debris and sucked out using direct vision and strong suction; they should be laid semi-prone on their side, face towards the ground, to allow any potential obstruction to fall forwards. Great care must be taken to avoid further neurological damage if a cervical spine injury is suspected. In the case of bilateral mandibular body fractures, a traction suture through the tongue will hold it forward; frequently, however, medial displacement of the posterior fragments prevents the anterior fragment from falling backwards unless the bone is comminuted. Posterior displacement of the maxilla in middle third injuries may cause the soft palate to occlude the airway. Obstruction can then be overcome by manual disimpaction of the maxilla. In the unconscious patient, a cuffed endotracheal tube may be needed to maintain the airway.

Should these non-invasive manoeuvres fail to relieve obstruction immediately, a surgical airway, using endotracheal intubation or cricothyroidotomy, must be made. If there is supraglottic airway obstruction, a temporary airway can be established by laryngotomy using a wide-bore (2–3-mm) needle inserted through the cricothyroid membrane. In certain laryngotracheal crush injuries and other wounds that transect the trachea, it may be necessary to perform emergency tracheostomy (Fig. 24.5) or occasionally submental intubation. Indications for tracheostomy are summarized in Table 24.2.

Chest injuries, particularly those causing tension pneumothorax or flail chest, or those caused by inhalation of toxic or hot gases, further impair respiration (see Burns). Flail chest can be recognized by extreme difficulty in breathing, associated with paradoxical movements of the chest and cyanosis. Intermittent positive-pressure ventilation must be given via a cuffed endotracheal tube.

Cervical spine stabilization is extremely important since injury is possible, especially in patients with injury above the clavicles or head injury resulting in an unconscious state, or any injury produced by high speed. Cervical spine injury is potentially fatal and may be symptomless whilst the patient is conscious due to protective muscle spasm that 'stabilizes' the spine; GA is very dangerous, as this protective muscle spasm is abolished on induction. Features can include neurological deficit and neck pain. Avoid any movement of the spinal column, and establish and maintain proper immobilization with the use of an appropriate neck splint until vertebral fractures or spinal cord injuries have been carefully ruled out with lateral cervical spine radiographs and computed tomography (CT).

Haemorrhage must be controlled. External bleeding is managed by direct pressure over any bleeding site until permanent control can be achieved by clamping and ligation. Shock due to bleeding that has led to hypovolaemia should be prevented or controlled and organ perfusion ensured by using intravenous fluid replacement (Ringer's lactate, normal saline or blood transfusion). Vital signs should be monitored closely.

Severe haemorrhage or shock only rarely results from isolated head injuries or maxillofacial trauma, unless caused by gunshot wounds, so if such a patient is shocked, it is essential to exclude other injuries (damage to internal organs or fractures of the pelvis or limbs). Remember that bleeding may be concealed or occasionally aggravated by disseminated intravascular coagulation (Ch. 8). Severe haemorrhage can lead to cardiac or renal failure or cause fatal cerebral hypoxia. Haemorrhage into the pleural cavity from fractured ribs can embarrass respiration.

Latent haemorrhage may be recognized by rising pulse rate, falling blood pressure, increasing pallor, air hunger or restlessness. If haemorrhage is suspected, a surgical opinion should be sought, a blood sample should be taken for grouping and cross-matching, and the following quarter- or half-hourly observations should be recorded:

- Pulse rate
- Blood pressure

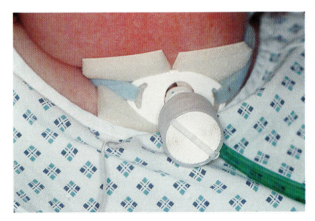

Fig. 24.5 Tracheostomy.

Box 24.1 *Causes of respiratory obstruction*

- Airway obstruction by loose objects, such as broken teeth, dentures or foreign bodies, or by accumulated blood and secretions
- Impaction of the middle third of the facial skeleton
- Injuries to the hyoid and its attached muscles
- Laryngeal spasm or oedema
- Prolapse of the tongue, especially after avulsion of the mandibular symphysis
- Swelling of the tongue and soft palate

Table 24.2 *Indications for tracheostomy*

What is obstructing the airway	Where positive pressure ventilation is needed	Where tracheobronchial suction is needed
Gross retroposition of the middle third of the face	Crushed or flail chest	Chronic obstructive pulmonary disease
Pharyngeal oedema	Prolonged mechanical ventilation	
Uncontrollable nasal haemorrhage		
Loss of tongue control		
Cancer surgery		

■ Respiratory rate
■ Urine output and fluid balance (usually hourly).

Blood transfusion may be indicated but is not needed to replace loss of less than 500 mL in an adult, unless there was pre-existing severe anaemia or deterioration of the general condition warrants transfusion, since there are risks, such as from transfusion reactions, fluid overload and infection. Meanwhile, since time is needed to obtain correctly cross-matched blood, normal saline, plasma or a plasma expander, such as dextran 70 or 110, may be given initially. Dextrans or other plasma expanders, together with tranexamic acid or desmopressin, may be the only possibility for Jehovah's Witnesses. Dextran can interfere with blood-grouping and cross-matching so that blood samples should be collected before a dextran infusion is started (Ch. 8).

Estimation of blood urea and electrolyte levels are needed in case there has been renal failure secondary to loss of blood, and as a baseline to monitor progress and the effects of intravenous fluid replacement. A full blood picture is also needed as a baseline for possible effects of transfusion and for any coincidental haematological disease. Early haemoglobin levels give no useful indication of the amount of blood lost, as haemodilution will not have had time to develop.

Blood and urine samples should be collected for analysis for alcohol, drugs and metabolic disorders, particularly diabetes. However, transient glycosuria unrelated to diabetes may follow the stress of head injuries.

The reader should consult the *Advanced Trauma Life Support Manual* and similar guides for full details on this important topic. A detailed assessment of maxillofacial injuries is only undertaken once the patient has been assessed and stabilized.

GENERAL ASSESSMENT

A good history must be obtained from the patient, if conscious, and witnesses. Reports of loss of consciousness, amnesia, nausea, vomiting or headache must be noted, as well as the medical history, especially use of drugs, including recreational agents or anticoagulants, or any history of epilepsy. A description of the mechanism of injury is useful, as it will give a clue as to what injuries to exclude. Family or friends may help with the patient's medical background.

CONSCIOUS STATE

Many patients are confused, concussed or comatose following head injury, though 30% of those with ultimately fatal head injuries may talk after injury and some are completely lucid for a time. However, the brain is invariably damaged in those who have lost consciousness for however brief a period, and sometimes in those who have not. Amnesia is common. Many are also suffering effects of alcohol or other drugs.

Maintenance of consciousness does not guarantee the absence of brain injury but the extent of retrograde amnesia is a rough measure of its severity.

Concussion, an immediate but transient loss of consciousness, is always associated with a short period of amnesia, and there is some brain damage even if after-effects are not detectable on neurological testing, cerebrospinal fluid (CSF) examination, CT or magnetic resonance imaging (MRI). Although the patient may lose consciousness only transiently, consciousness is almost invariably impaired after diffuse brain damage, and there is usually amnesia for the traumatic event, and afterwards (post-traumatic amnesia) for a period far exceeding that of coma. Consciousness may not be lost if brain damage is local, when, for example, the skull is penetrated by a sharp object.

Table 24.3 *Main cerebral causes of coma*

Brain lesions	Main causes
Cerebral cortex damage	Trauma, haemorrhage, hypoglycaemia, hypoxia, infection
Brainstem compression	Various
Brainstem localized pressure	Cerebellar haemorrhage, abscess, neoplasm
Brainstem reticular activating substance suppression	Drugs (alcohol and others)

Table 24.4 *Glasgow Coma or Responsiveness Scale (GCS)*

Eye opening	E	Motor response	M	Verbal response	V
Spontaneous	4	Obeys	6	Orientated	5
To speech	3	Localizes	5	Confused conversation	4
To pain	2	Withdraws	4	Inappropriate words	3
Nil	1	Abnormal flexion	3	Incomprehensible sounds	2
		Extends	2	Nil	1
		Nil	1		

Prolonged unconsciousness, when there are no complications such as brain haematomas and where there are no focal signs, is often caused by severe brain damage but sometimes by drugs (Table 24.3).

The most essential examination is immediately to assess, record and monitor the level of consciousness using the Glasgow Coma Scale (GCS), which scores points derived from three features: eye opening (E); motor response (M); and verbal response (V) (EMV score; Table 24.4). The degree of brain damage is initially assessed by the level of consciousness as measured by the GCS and, later, by the duration of coma and post-traumatic amnesia. It is important to consider causes of coma other than acute head injury (see Appendix 24.1). The EMV score or responsiveness sum can range from 3 to 15. A fully alert and otherwise well patient with a full and unchanging score of 15 and no neurological signs or symptoms and no skull fracture or intracranial haemorrhage on CT or MRI scan does not need hospital admission for observation, unless for other reasons. All patients who score below 15 points (see Table 24.4) should be admitted to hospital for observation – even if drugs or alcohol are the suspected causes. A score of 7 or less indicates coma in 100%; 9 or more indicates absence of coma. Patients with a GCS score of less than 8 require immediate neurosurgical attention (Table 24.5). About 85% of patients with a score of 3 or 4 succumb within 24 hours.

It is important also to recognize and to treat other factors that can contribute to morbidity and mortality, which can include airway obstruction, hypotension, meningitis, uncontrolled epilepsy, stress-induced gastric bleeding or diabetic ketoacidosis.

Patients who survive with head injuries fall into three main groups. Most are stable neurologically with gradual improvement in consciousness. Some progressively deteriorate in the level of consciousness with localizing signs, often because of intracranial bleeding with or without cerebral oedema, when the bleeding usually needs to be evacuated by craniotomy. Others have rising intracranial pressure (ICP), causing progressive deterioration in consciousness in the absence of localizing signs. ICP should be monitored. Cerebral oedema management remains controversial but general measures include optimal head

Table 24.5 *Indications for neurosurgical attention after head injury*

Immediate neurological attention indicated	Early neurological attention indicated	Admission to hospital for neurological observation
Glasgow Coma Scale score (GCS) < 8	GCS 8–14	GCS <15
Deteriorating consciousness	Convulsions	Minor skull fracture[a]
Neurological lateralization (pupillary inequality and hemiparesis)	Cerebrospinal rhinorrhoea or otorrhoea	Post-traumatic amnesia
Dilated fixed (unreactive to light) pupil	Orbital or retromastoid haematomas	Other serious injuries
Major skull fractures (depressed or compound)	Pneumoencephalocoele	Children
CT signs of compression or obliteration of mesencephalic cisterns, midline hemisphere shift, or one or more surgical masses	Worsening restlessness, headache and vomiting	Patients with psychiatric disease, drug abuse or learning impairment
Uncontrollable bleeding		Patients living alone or without a responsible adult companion
Rising blood pressure with bradycardia		

[a]There is some controversy among neurosurgeons about whether patients with skull fractures with *no* evidence of cerebrospinal fluid leak, cerebral haemorrhage or pneumoencephalocoele should receive observation or operative treatment.

and neck positioning 30° to the horizontal for facilitating intracranial venous outflow, avoidance of dehydration and systemic hypotension, and maintenance of normothermia, while specific therapeutic interventions are controlled hyperventilation, administration of corticosteroids and diuretics, osmotherapy, and pharmacological cerebral metabolic suppression. Ensuring adequate oxygenation, giving furosemide and restricting fluid are common strategies.

Patients must be carefully and regularly observed to detect the development of complications, especially intracranial haematomas, which need immediate neurosurgical attention. The level of consciousness should be charted, as assessed by the GCS and, later, by the duration of coma and of post-traumatic amnesia; this should take place at regular intervals – half-hourly or even more frequently – along with measurements of pulse, blood pressure, respiration, pupil reactivity and temperature.

Deterioration of consciousness is the most important sign, and is sometimes accompanied by worsening restlessness, headache and vomiting. Fixed dilatation of the pupil on the side of the fracture and decerebrate rigidity – late signs caused by raised ICP and brain shift – are soon followed by bilateral pupil dilatation, periodic respiration, respiratory arrest and death, unless there is immediate neurosurgical intervention. Focal signs, such as hemiparesis, dysphasia or focal epilepsy, are uncommon. In deep coma there are no verbal or motor responses, but in less severe cases the eyes may open transiently from time to time and there may be vague or weak responses to stimuli.

Up to 60% of all patients admitted in coma are alcoholics or other drug users who have often had a head injury. Toxic and metabolic disorders cause no focal or localizing neurological signs, although some drug misuse (opiates) can affect pupil reactivity. When there is disease of the central nervous system (CNS) itself, sensory or motor disturbances may indicate the lesion site. In some of these diseases, white cells, bacteria or blood may also appear in the CSF. Intoxications, whether the result of exogenous agents or disorders of metabolism and severe infections, all have essentially similar effects and will not be discussed further.

The level of consciousness is depressed further by sedatives and many analgesics, especially morphine and its analogues, which not only slow respiration but also disguise eye signs of rising intracranial pressure, by causing pupillary constriction. Pentazocine is also contraindicated. If analgesia is essential, codeine, diclofenac or buprenorphine can be used. Benzodiazepines should not be given for controlling fits or to allow suturing, since they cause respiratory depression, which can be fatal unless ventilation is given. If there are repeated fits,

phenytoin by intravenous infusion is less likely to depress respiration. Alcohol must be prohibited.

Pupil size and reaction must be checked for localizing signs of neurological damage. A dilated fixed (unreactive to light) pupil often indicates rising ICP and is usually a serious sign. Severe facial oedema may make examination of the eyes difficult and the eyelids should then be prised open. A fixed dilated pupil may also be caused by local damage to the optic or oculomotor nerves, and must be differentiated by clinical examination, radiographs (usually CT) and MRI, and by the absence of signs associated with brain damage or of rising ICP. Limb reflexes should be tested.

Regular monitoring of blood pressure and pulse rate is essential. A low or falling blood pressure with rising pulse rate is indicative of haemorrhage or shock, which can lead to fatal cerebral anoxia or renal failure. A systolic blood pressure of lower than 60 mmHg brings with it a risk of brain damage. A high or rising blood pressure with bradycardia, by contrast, is indicative of raised ICP secondary to cerebral oedema or haemorrhage as a result of the injury. Respiratory rate, urine output and fluid balance must also be monitored.

ASSESSMENT OF HEAD INJURY

Skull examination

Scalp lacerations may be associated with a fracture; they can cause severe loss of blood and provide a pathway for infection into the cranial cavity. The presence of a skull fracture greatly increases the risk of brain damage and an intracranial haematoma; significant intracranial lesions are found in two-thirds. A depressed skull fracture may be palpable, although it is often concealed by overlying oedema of the soft tissues. About 80% of skull fractures are linear, and many are associated with subepidural or epidural haematomas. Basal skull fractures are usually uncomplicated; they may not be visible on routine radiography but may be revealed by bleeding, which may show as haemotympanum (blood behind the ear drum), as ecchymosis over the mastoid process (Battle's sign), as periorbital ecchymosis (raccoon sign), or by CSF rhinorrhoea or otorrhoea. Alternatively, they may be suggested by cranial nerve lesions involving the olfactory nerve (cribriform plate fracture), optic nerve (sphenoid), facial nerve (petrous) or abducens and facial nerve (sella fracture).

Skull fractures can also cause cranial nerve damage and provide an entry to the CSF for infection or air (pneumocephalus).

Examination for cerebrospinal fluid leak

Particular care must be taken to examine for CSF leaks – rhinorrhoea or otorrhoea – and signs of orbital or retromastoid haematomas (which may indicate fractures with dural tears). In these instances, meningitis is a risk and an early neurosurgical opinion should therefore be obtained. In the early stages, leakage of CSF may be obscured by haemorrhage, but any clear watery discharge from the nose is suspect and should be tested for sugar and protein. CSF, unlike a serous nasal discharge, contains sugar but little protein. However, lacrimal fluid also contains small amounts of glucose, and CSF must therefore be positively identified by protein electrophoresis and accurate measurement of the glucose.

CSF rhinorrhoea is found in about 2% of all head injuries, and in 25% of fractures of the middle third of face and nasoethmoidal complex. CSF leaks usually persist for about a week and the risk of meningitis is greatest within the first fortnight. Post-traumatic CSF leaks will usually resolve without surgical intervention. Successful management in refractory cases often involves a combination of observation, CSF diversion and/or extracranial and intracranial procedures. Occasionally, the fistula may be occluded by herniated brain but the dural tear fails to heal. If there is a dural tear, meningitis may follow after some months or years and therefore dural repair is desirable.

In all patients with ocular or orbital injuries, the orbit should be examined radiologically, usually by CT for fracture; if the latter is suspected, the patient should undergo exploration and receive prophylaxis, as recommended for penetrating intracranial wounds.

Prophylactic antimicrobials are needed if there is a meningitis risk and should therefore be given to all patients with a penetrating brain injury (PBI), where the risk of intracranial infection is high because of contaminating foreign objects, skin, hair and bone fragments driven into the brain. Antimicrobials are also indicated in compound depressed skull fractures, CSF leaks or fractures of the middle third. The infecting agents in meningitis in one study were Gram-positive cocci (*Staphylococcus haemolyticus*, *Staphylococcus warneri*, *Staphylococcus cohnii*, *Staphylococcus epidermidis* and *Streptococcus pneumoniae*) or Gram-negative bacilli (*Escherichia coli*, *Klebsiella pneumoniae* or *Acinetobacter anitratus*). Gram-positive strains were sensitive to vancomycin. All Gram-negative strains appeared resistant to ampicillin and third-generation cephalosporins, but sensitive to imipenem and to ciprofloxacin. Many bacteria causing post-traumatic meningitis are now resistant to sulphonamides. Recommended antimicrobials that readily reach the CSF and are well absorbed when given orally include co-amoxiclav, or cefuroxime with metronidazole, or azithromycin, or vancomycin and ceftazidime. Effective alternatives are rifampicin or minocycline.

Intracranial bleeding

Intracranial haematomas may be *intracerebral* (subarachnoid) haematomas – usually not amenable to surgical intervention; or *epidural* or extradural (between dura mater and skull) – usually due to tearing of the middle meningeal artery after a fracture of the temporal bone and evolving rapidly; these are neurosurgical emergencies requiring burr holes through the skull to drain the clot and ligate the bleeding vessel. The haematoma forms a tumour-like mass, which compresses part of the brain and raises ICP as it expands. Clinically, the typical story is of a heavy blow followed by loss of consciousness. There is usually then a period of apparent recovery (lucid interval), followed by signs of rising ICP. If the clot is not removed, death from respiratory arrest follows. A radiograph showing a fracture line crossing the line of the middle meningeal artery strongly suggests extradural haemorrhage and CT scanning will confirm the diagnosis.

Subdural haematomas – between the dura and leptomeninges – are venous and associated with underlying brain contusion. *Acute subdural* haematoma is often caused by a tear in the arachnoid and may be associated with laceration or contusion of the brain. Clinically, there is a latent interval after the injury, followed by progressive deterioration of consciousness and development of symptoms somewhat similar to those of an extradural haematoma. Once coma has developed, up to 50% die. Early operation to evacuate the clot through burr holes improves survival. *Chronic subdural* haematoma can be caused by a very mild injury but, nevertheless, the veins between the pia and the dura mater get torn and blood leakage into the subdural space is very slow. There is a fibroblastic response and eventually the haematoma becomes enclosed in scar tissue or, occasionally, resorbed. Clinically, the head injury, especially in an elderly person, may be so slight as to have been forgotten but, after several weeks, or even months, symptoms such as headache, dizziness, slowness of thinking, or confusion and disturbance of consciousness develop. There may be localizing signs, such as hemiparesis or aphasia; the patient may have ptosis and be unable to look upwards (pressure on the third nerve).

Neurological assessment

After head injury, approximately 50% of patients have permanent after-effects, such as paralyses, loss of speech, impaired vision, epilepsy, disturbances of personality or severe mental defects, disabling them for life. Delayed effects may result from ischaemia, hypoxia, cerebral oedema, intracranial hypertension and/or abnormalities of cerebral blood flow. Cranial nerve injuries in patients with head injuries may indicate a basal skull fracture or other lesion; cranial nerves I, II, III, V, VII and VIII are most vulnerable (Table 24.6 and Ch. 13). Sense of smell is disturbed or lost (anosmia) in 5–10% of head injuries, since the olfactory nerves are damaged in frontal bone injuries and fractures involving the ethmoid cribriform plate. CSF rhinorrhoea is often associated. Traumatic anosmia improves in only about 10% and perversion of the sense of smell may develop during recovery, effects that are remarkably troublesome or even disabling, but untreatable. The goals of head injury treatment are therefore to detect any damage and prevent or reverse secondary insults to the damaged brain, such as from hypoxaemia, hypotension and intracranial bleeding or haematoma, and to allow recovery of as much damaged brain tissue as possible.

Skull imaging

Radiography should be carried out early before infection can reach the cranial cavity (typically anteroposterior, lateral and Towne's views). CT scans are essential to exclude skull fractures and brain lesions. MRI can provide better brain images but cannot always be used. Imaging may also reveal a depressed fracture involving the paranasal sinuses; this suggests a meningeal tear, which is occasionally confirmed by seeing intracranial air (aerocoele). A linear fracture indicates the possibility of intracranial haematoma but even normal radiographs do not exclude brain damage. About 50% of patients with intracranial injuries have no skull fracture, and approximately 90% of patients with fractures of the skull have no resulting intracranial injury. CT signs, such as compression or obliteration of mesencephalic cisterns, midline hemisphere shift, or one or more surgical masses, correlate with raised ICP and shortened survival.

Table 24.6 *Cranial nerve lesions complicating head injuries*

Nerve lesion	Usual site of injury	Comments
I (olfactory)	Ethmoidal complex (may be no fracture)	Anosmia (usually permanent); apparent loss of taste
II (optic)	Orbit[a] or sphenoid	Pupil dilated and unreactive to light, but consensual reflex retained[b]; partial or complete blindness
III (oculomotor)	Orbit[a]	Affected eye looks down and out. Pupil dilated, unreactive to light. No consensual reflex. Loss of medial and vertical movement of eye. Divergent squint
IV (trochlear)	Orbit[a]	Diplopia only on looking down. Similar features result if superior oblique muscle is entrapped. Pupil reacts normally
V (trigeminal)	Middle fossa, orbit[a], maxilla or mandible	Commonly extracranially. Anaesthesia or paraesthesia in sensory area
VI (abducens)	Orbit[a] or petrous temporal	Diplopia. Loss of lateral movement of eye. Convergent squint. Pupil reacts normally
VII (facial)	Direct trauma to nerve or basal skull fracture (see Facial paralysis)	Facial paralysis, which may be delayed for a few days
VIII (vestibulocochlear)	Petrous temporal	Deafness, vertigo and nystagmus alone or together. Deafness after head injury may also be caused by ruptured ear drum or blood in middle ear
IX–XII	Corticobulbar	Uncommon as a result of head injuries

[a]May be damage to orbital contents with or without fracture. These nerves are often injured together and urgent neurosurgery may be indicated, since nerve dysfunction, if caused by haemorrhage or oedema within the optic canal or other confined space, may be reversible. In the superior orbital fissure syndrome, there may be damage to the lacrimal, frontal, trochlear, abducens and oculomotor nerves with minimal damage to the globe.
[b]Consensual reflex is constriction of the pupil as a normal response when a light is shone into the other eye.

Blood analyses

Sixty percent of coma patients are drug users or alcoholics who have often had a head injury.

ASSESSMENT FOR OTHER INJURIES

Multiply injured patients can be assessed using the revised trauma score (RTS), calculated mainly from the GCS, the blood pressure and the respiratory rate. Injuries can be categorized using the Abbreviated Injury Scale (AIS), which scores from minor (1) to fatal (6) injuries; the injury severity score (ISS) is calculated by the addition of the AIS for the three most severely injured areas of the body.

MEDICAL COMPLICATIONS OF HEAD INJURIES

Medical complications can arise, since the brain, via neurological and hormonal influences, can influence: the cardiovascular system (neurogenic hypertension, myocardial dysfunction, arrhythmias or deep vein thrombosis); the respiratory system (neurogenic pulmonary oedema – a form of acute respiratory distress syndrome [ARDS], infections, embolism); coagulopathy (disseminated intravascular coagulopathy); electrolyte imbalance (hyponatraemia, hypernatraemia or hypokalaemia); the endocrine system (inadequate or inappropriate secretion of antidiuretic hormone; Ch. 6); the gastrointestinal tract (stress gastritis and haemorrhage); fat embolism (mainly where there have been long bone fractures); or infections (of wounds, foreign bodies, CSF, intravenous lines, ICP monitoring devices, sinuses and lungs). Tetanus can be an issue (Ch. 21).

LATE SEQUELAE OF HEAD INJURY

Late sequelae may include: chronic extradural or subdural haematomas; epilepsy (Ch. 13); infection (see earlier); mental or physical disability; compensation neurosis (Ch. 10); or post-traumatic syndrome (which may result from mild brain damage or damage to the cochlear–vestibular apparatus). Complaints include temporary headache, irritability, inability to concentrate, short temper, loss of confidence, vertigo and hyperacusis. If symptoms persist, psychiatric advice should be sought.

MAXILLOFACIAL INJURIES

Most maxillofacial injuries are due to interpersonal violence and the majority are in previously fit young men; alcohol or another drug is frequently a factor. RTAs are also a major cause and produce fractures that often involve the midface, especially in patients who were not wearing seatbelts. Industrial accidents, sports and epilepsy are other causes. Other important sources of facial trauma include abuse (children and older individuals).

High-impact maxillofacial fractures often are associated with head and other bodily injuries that may be life-threatening. Patients are often multiply injured and may have hazards to the airway, head, cervical or thoracolumbar spine, eye, chest, liver, spleen, kidneys, long bones or bladder, and severe haemorrhage from massive midface injuries. Extensive soft-tissue injuries or avulsions and comminuted fractures are difficult to treat and may have poor outcomes. Low-impact maxillofacial fractures rarely result in mortality if proper treatment is administered.

Maxillofacial trauma demands special attention, since it may damage specialized functions, including breathing, sight, hearing, smelling, eating and speech – especially in middle third facial fractures (particularly Le Fort III fractures). The psychological impact of disfigurement can be devastating, and vital structures in the head and neck region are intimately associated.

The bones most commonly fractured are the nasal, zygoma, mandible and maxilla. Many fractures are reduced and fixed with miniplates (Champy plates are rarely used currently) and/or intermaxillary fixation. Closed reduction, open reduction and endoscopic techniques may be employed (see textbooks of maxillofacial surgery).

The management of patients with maxillofacial injuries is similar to that of head and other severe injuries (Box 24.2). Special problems also arise because of mechanical interference with breathing and swallowing. Shock is most unusual in uncomplicated maxillofacial injuries or head injuries, and its presence is often an indication of internal haemorrhage. The possibility of pre-existing disease must always be considered too, as must the possibility that foreign bodies may have been introduced. Management is divided into: emergency, immediate or initial care; early primary care; and reconstructive phases (definitive care and secondary care or revision).

Box 24.2 *Initial management of maxillofacial trauma*

- Maintain airway
- Control haemorrhage
- Reduce fractures
- Prevent infection
- Maintain fluid balance

Table 24.7 *Maxillofacial trauma: immediate and early assessment*

Step	Assess
Immediate care (ABC)	Airway and cervical spine
	Breathing and bleeding
	Chest injuries
General assessment	State of consciousness
	Pulse
	Blood pressure
	Respiratory rate
	Pupil size and reaction
Assessment of head injury	Skull examination
	Examination for cerebrospinal fluid leak
	Neurological assessment
	Skull radiography, including computed tomography
	Blood analyses
Assessment for other injuries	Chest
	Neck
	Spine
	Abdomen
	Perineum
	Limbs

EMERGENCY CARE

Life-threatening injuries must be addressed immediately – airway establishment and maintenance, and control of haemorrhage. A patent airway and an adequate fluid and nutritional intake can be difficult to achieve in maxillofacial injuries because of partial or complete obstruction of the respiratory or alimentary orifices. Altered level of consciousness is the most common cause of upper airway obstruction. Stabilize the cervical spine, which may be fractured, especially in any patient with injury above the clavicle, head injury resulting in unconsciousness, or any injury produced by high speed. Despite the extensive vascularity of the head and neck, massive blood loss due to maxillofacial injuries is uncommon. Penetrating injuries need to be explored. A nasogastric tube may be required for feeding in the immediate postoperative period if there are extensive intraoral wounds. Immediate and early assessment of maxillofacial trauma is summarized in Table 24.7. Consult the *Advanced Trauma Life Support Manual* for full details.

EARLY CARE

The priorities of early management of a patient with maxillofacial and other injuries, especially if in coma, are as follows:

- Maintain a clear airway.
- Establish a neurological baseline.
- Establish baseline blood pressure, pulse and respiratory rates.
- Exclude other serious injuries to the head and neck, thorax and abdomen, other bones and eye, and CSF leak.

- Delay definitive treatment of maxillofacial fractures usually until the patient is out of danger, but stabilize grossly displaced or comminuted facial bone fragments early, as this may facilitate later management and lessen facial deformity. Reduce and immobilize fractures if they threaten the airway or there is severe haemorrhage. Avoid nasotracheal intubation in patients with upper face or upper midface fractures, as it can result in nasocranial intubation or severe nasal haemorrhage. Avoid clamping blind in order to prevent injuries to vital structures.

- Treat soft-tissue injuries early; large open wounds should be checked for foreign material (ultrasound is helpful), debrided and closed in a layered fashion promptly. Wounds that are to be used later for access to repair fractures, or those that are not a priority, may be closed in a temporary manner. In lacerations the skin is crushed and or torn, leading to an irregular skin edge injury, while in incised wounds the skin edges are less irregular; combinations of the two may coexist in the same injury. Nerve injuries in the maxillofacial region primarily affect the sensory (trigeminal) or motor (facial) nerves. In addition, the nerves of the orbit (ophthalmic, oculomotor, trochlear and abducent) may also be injured. Rarely, the other nerves of the head and neck may be injured. Facial fractures may compress or indirectly injure sensory nerves; typically, zygomatico-orbital injuries lead to infraorbital and/or zygomaticotemporal or zygomaticofacial nerve neuropraxias. Mandibular fractures often injure the inferior alveolar nerve along its course, manifesting as mental nerve altered sensation. Facial nerve injuries manifest as weakness or paralysis of the muscles of facial expression. For those injuries that result from transections of the nerve between the facial canal and a line drawn between the lateral canthus and angle of the mouth, early microneural repair is indicated. Salivary gland injuries can lead to fistulas or sialocoeles. Burns, chemical or thermal, also need attention. Appropriate protective dressings are applied and hydration is maintained.

- Prevent infection. Except for facial fractures affecting the ascending ramus, all fractures in which the periosteum is torn are compound and usually communicate with an internal mucous membrane wound and/or the external skin wound. Because of the contiguity of the naso-oral passages and the perforating nature of maxillofacial wounds, they are doubly exposed to contamination. Antibiotic therapy must be started early and maintained until fractures are immobilized (Table 24.8).

- Maintain oral hygiene, with particular attention to the teeth.

The reconstructive phase of care of maxillofacial injuries is discussed in maxillofacial surgery textbooks; a few comments only are included here. The maxillofacial region is divided into the upper face, where fractures involve the nasoethmoidal structures, frontal bone and sinus; the midface; and the lower face, where fractures are isolated to the mandible. Le Fort I fractures are in the lower midface. The upper midface is where Le Fort II and Le Fort III fractures occur and/or where fractures of the nasal bones, nasoethmoidal or zygomaticomaxillary complex, and the orbital floor occur.

A high-impact force is usually required to damage the supraorbital rim, mandible (symphysis and angle) and frontal bones. A low-impact force is all that is required to damage the zygoma and nasal bone.

Pan-facial injuries management is usually by internal rigid fixation using plates and screws.

Table 24.8 *Antimicrobial prophylaxis in facial injuries*

Injuries	Antimicrobial if indicated
Compound fractures	Penicillin or, in penicillin allergy, clindamycin
Contaminated skin lacerations	Cefazolin
Contaminated oral lacerations	Clindamycin
Fractures communicating with antrum	Amoxicillin
Fractures with dural tears or CSF leaks	Co-amoxiclav, or cefuroxime with metronidazole or vancomycin and ceftazidime

COMPLICATIONS OF MAXILLOFACIAL INJURIES

Infective problems

Actinomycosis is discussed in Chapter 21.

Meningitis is an important complication of opening the cranial cavity (shown by leakage of CSF), as discussed above. It can also result from lacerations of the scalp when infection can reach the brain via the emissary veins.

Tetanus is discussed in Chapter 21.

Wound infection and osteomyelitis risks are greater when there is inadequate wound toilet, foreign bodies in the wound, teeth in the fracture line, gross delay in treatment or systemic disease with diminished resistance to infection, particularly alcoholism. Extreme care must be taken to identify foreign material within the tissues; some types of glass and plastic, and all wood, are radiolucent and may be missed unless the wound is systematically probed; they may also be identified on MRI. Gross debris, broken teeth, detached bone and foreign bodies should be removed. After preliminary wound toilet, lacerations can usually be sutured under LA. Larger lacerations can be covered with tulle gras and dry dressings for closure as soon as possible under GA. Teeth in the fracture line may need to be extracted unless required for stabilization of a bone fragment. Intramuscular benzyl penicillin or cefazolin is usually effective antimicrobial prophylaxis.

Ocular or orbital injuries

Zygomatic fractures or isolated orbital injuries may hazard vision. Diplopia (double vision) is common, often because of oedema and haemorrhage within the confined space of the orbit; circumorbital and subconjunctival ecchymoses are usually associated. Occasionally, periorbital emphysema is present. Diplopia sometimes arises from enophthalmos associated with orbital floor or wall fractures, from muscle or nerve injury, or from muscle entrapment. Untreated orbital blowout fractures also depress the level of the eye (this may be concealed initially, as intraorbital oedema maintains the level of the globe) and limit ocular movement, especially upwards.

The superior orbital fissure syndrome of ophthalmoplegia, ptosis, exophthalmos, a fixed dilated pupil or absence of consensual reflex, and some sensory loss over the distribution of the ophthalmic division of the trigeminal nerve, is caused by injury to cranial nerves III, IV, V and VI, where they pass through the orbital fissure. The syndrome may stem from disruption of the bony margins of the superior orbital fissure, haematoma or traumatic aneurysm at this site.

In all patients with ocular or orbital injuries, the orbit should be imaged by CT for fracture; if this is suspected, the individual should undergo exploration and receive prophylaxis, as recommended for penetrating intracranial wounds. If there are ocular injuries, an ophthalmological opinion should be sought, as the eye can be lost or vision impaired.

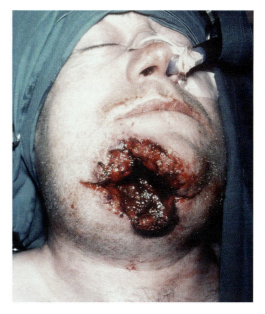

Fig. 24.6 Gunshot wound.

STAB AND OTHER PENETRATING WOUNDS

Stab wounds should always be treated with suspicion, as a small entrance wound can hide injuries to deeper structures or foreign bodies. Ultrasound can be helpful to detect the latter. Radiographs are indicated, especially where the wound is caused by glass, remembering that some glass is radiolucent. The wound may well need to be explored carefully before closure, especially if in the chest, neck, back or abdomen.

Computed tomographic angiography (CTA) has altered the management of patients with penetrating injuries in the neck, with fewer formal neck explorations and virtual elimination of negative exploratory surgery.

GUNSHOT AND EXPLOSIVE WOUNDS

Firearm wounds and deaths have increased dramatically in many countries recently. Gunshot wounds to the head, the most lethal of all firearm injuries, are the leading cause of head injury in many US cities and have a fatality rate of more than 90%, at least two-thirds of the victims dying before reaching a hospital. The management of wounds to the head and neck (Fig. 24.6) is discussed in surgical texts so salient points only are included here.

Bullets inflict tissue damage by laceration and crushing, shock waves and cavitation. Handguns usually inflict low-velocity bullet wounds that damage only the tissues they hit, mainly by laceration; the wounds are managed by conventional surgical methods. Traditionally, civilian injuries were inflicted with low-velocity weapons (90–210 m/s), while military wounds were typically caused by high-velocity weapons (610 m/s and up; Table 24.9). Owing to medium- to high-velocity weapons appearing on the streets, more civilians are suffering from military-type injuries. Such high-velocity missiles (from rifles or explosive blast fragments) can cause extensive tissue damage and contamination, and have a mortality rate 4–5 times higher – thus requiring specialized attention. The entrance wounds may be minute, but can hide extremely severe wounds caused by the cavitation effect of rapid compression and expansion with extensive necrotic tissue contaminated with clostridia spores, other bacteria, clothing and debris. The kinetic energy is directly proportional to the mass of the projectile and proportional to the square of the velocity at which the bullet is travelling. The most efficient missile enters tissues

Table 24.9 *Gunshot wounds*

Type of gun	Comment
Airgun	Can be left *in situ* if deep and not in orbit or causing damage
0.22 rifle	Can be left *in situ* if deep and not in orbit or causing damage
0.410 shotgun	May cause considerable damage at close range
Twelve-bore shotgun	Dangerous, even from a distance; widespread damage
High-velocity bullets	Cause more extensive damage than is initially evident
Explosive bullets	Cause more extensive damage than is initially evident

Table 24.10 *Effects of spinal cord damage*

Early (spinal shock): losses of	Delayed (after 2–3 weeks):
Motor function: quadriplegia if damage in cervical cord, paraplegia if damage in thoracic cord	Motor function may improve if cord not completely transected
Sensation below lesion, leading to skin pressure ulcers	Sensation may improve if cord not completely transected
Reflexes below lesion, with muscle flaccidity	Reflexes: involuntary flexor then extensor spasms below level of lesion
Bladder and bowel sphincter control, leading to urinary or faecal retention	Bladder and bowel sphincter control impaired, causing irregular reflex micturition and defecation

and imparts the majority of its kinetic energy to surrounding structures without exiting the victim.

All patients with gunshot wounds should be imaged to locate the missiles. To avoid gas gangrene, high-velocity wounds must be treated by excision of the damaged tissue and with antibiotics, followed 4–5 days later by delayed primary closure and, if necessary, skin grafts. Consider tetanus risk (Ch. 21).

HUMAN BITES

Human bites are more likely to cause infections than are animal bites (Ch. 33), since the oral flora contains many potentially pathogenic aerobic and anaerobic bacteria; among these are *Staphylococcus*, *Streptococcus*, *Clostridia* (and other anaerobes) and fusiform species, as well as viruses. Tetanus is rarely a concern unless the wound is contaminated by soil. Hepatitis B, hepatitis C and human immunodeficiency virus (HIV) are a concern, since they can be transmitted by bites both from biter to victim and the converse.

Staff working in areas posing a significant risk of biting should not be treated as performing exposure-prone procedures (EPPs). In October 2003, the UK Advisory Panel (UKAP) considered a review of the available literature on the risk of onward transmission from health-care professionals (HCPs) infected with blood-borne viruses to patients. The review showed that the published literature on this subject is very scarce. In follow-up studies of incidents involving infected HCPs working with patients known to be 'regular and predictable' biters, there were no documented cases of transmission from the health-care worker to the biter. However, where biters were infected, there were documented cases of seroconversion in their victims, and the risk of infection was increased in the presence of:

- blood in the oral cavity – risk proportionate to the volume of blood
- broken skin due to the bite
- bite associated with previous injury (i.e. non-intact skin)
- biter deficient in anti-HIV salivary elements (immunoglobulin A-deficient).

Based on the available information, it can only be tentatively concluded that, even though there is a theoretical risk of transmission of a blood-borne virus from an infected HCP to a biting patient, the risk remains negligible. The lack of information may suggest that this has not been perceived to be a problem to date, rather than that there is an absence of risk. UKAP has advised that, despite the theoretical risk, since there is no documented case of transmission from an infected HCP to a biting patient, individuals infected with blood-borne viruses should not be prevented from working in or training for specialties where there is a risk of being bitten.

It is important for biting incidents to be reported and for risk assessments to be conducted in accordance with National Health Service (or equivalent) procedures. Biting poses a much greater risk to HCPs than to patients. Therefore employers should take measures to prevent injury to staff, and HCPs bitten by patients should seek advice and treatment, in the same way as after a needlestick injury.

Patients with hand infections from bite wounds may require hospital admission, antibiotics (co-amoxiclav, most commonly), wound incision and drainage. Any human bite could stem from abuse and therefore should be assessed, preferably by a forensic dentist (http://www.bafo.org.uk/; accessed 30 September 2013). DNA should be retrieved where possible, and serial photographs and casts taken (Ch. 25).

SPINAL CORD INJURIES

Spinal cord injuries (SCIs) are a common result of road traffic or sports injuries. Cord injury is usually the result of vertical compression, sometimes with flexion or extension of the neck, or violent sudden extension of the neck (whiplash injury), as when a vehicle is hit from behind. The possibility of such damage should always be considered in patients involved in road traffic or contact sport accidents, since movement of the neck may then cause serious cord damage, spastic quadriplegia or death. The neck must therefore not be extended or rotated, and a support collar should be fitted prophylactically. Decompression by reduction of any vertebral dislocations should be carried out by the neurosurgeon within 2 hours of injury. Spinal cord damage can be most incapacitating (Table 24.10).

Most vertebral injuries affect the C1–2, C4–7 and T11–L2 vertebrae, the clinical sequelae being determined largely by the level of spinal cord damage, but the result can be fatal or appallingly severe disability (Table 24.11).

Traumatic atlanto-axial dislocation may be fatal. If not, there may only be weakness of the legs or even no immediate neurological sequelae. Transient blackouts, weakness of the limbs, sensory loss, facial paraesthesia, nystagmus, ataxia and dysarthria may be complaints. Atlanto-axial subluxation, or dislocation or fracture of the odontoid peg, may occur in other conditions, such as congenital anomalies of the odontoid process (as in Down syndrome), rheumatoid arthritis or ankylosing spondylitis.

The clinical effects of SCI develop in two main stages: spinal shock and reflex activity (see Table 24.10). If movement can be elicited or any sensation is retained during the first 2–3 days, the prognosis is more favourable. Paraplegia is common but high doses of methylprednisolone given within 8 hours of the injury may minimize cord damage. Any symptoms persisting after 6 months are likely to be permanent.

Most patients with thoracic cord injuries need wheelchairs. Mechanical bracing systems can restore upright mobility following SCI, and can improve bone density, urinary drainage, bowel function, spasticity, respiratory mechanics, contractures and psychological health,

Table 24.11 *Effects of spinal cord injuries at different levels*

Level of spinal cord damage	Features
C1–C5	Quadriplegia (tetraplegia) or death
C5–C6	Paraplegia. Hands paralysed. Arms paralysed, except for abduction and flexion
C6–C7	Paraplegia. Hands but not arms paralysed
T1	Paraplegia. Normal hand function. Patients can perform all functions of a non-injured person, with the exception of standing and walking
T2–T5	Paraplegia. Patients have partial trunk movement and may be able to stand, with long leg braces and a walker, and may be able to walk short distances with assistance
T6–T12	Paraplegia. Patients have partial abdominal muscle strength, and may be able to walk independently for short distances with long leg braces and a walker or crutches
T11–T12	Paraplegia. Sensory loss T12 and below
T12–L1	Legs paralysed below knees
L2	Patients have all movement in the trunk and hips
L3	Patients have knee extension
L4	Patients have ankle dorsiflexion
L5	Patients have extensor hallucis longus function. They are able to walk independently with ankle braces and canes, and may use wheelchairs for long distances
S1–S2	Patients have function of the gastrocnemius and soleus muscles and walk independently on all surfaces, usually without bracing

but are perceived by some to be less safe and more difficult to use than wheelchairs.

Most patients with injuries at or below the lumbar level are wheelchair-independent and may be able to walk independently, with long leg braces and crutches.

General management of paraplegics

Treatment in general is supportive and symptomatic, and mainly directed toward the prevention of complications such as muscle wasting or contractures, pressure sores (bed sores), postural hypotension, urinary infections, constipation or psychological problems.

Physiotherapy is essential to limit muscle-wasting and to maintain function in unparalysed or partly paralysed muscles. Joints must be passively moved on a regular basis, and the position of the patient carefully checked to prevent soft-tissue contractures and pressure sores.

Postural hypotension and autonomic dysreflexia can complicate high-level spinal cord lesions. Intense vasoconstriction below the level of the cord injury follows certain stimuli such as bladder contraction. The vasoconstriction is associated with rapid onset of hypertension, facial sweating and headache.

Urinary retention invariably complicates acute spinal cord lesions, and aseptic catheterization is needed. Infections must be treated promptly. Recurrent urinary infections were previously the main factor in renal disease and amyloidosis complicating paraplegia. Latex allergy commonly develops in such patients.

Dental aspects

Access to health care is a major problem since patients are at least chairbound. Dental management may be uncomplicated, although postural hypotension in the early stages may necessitate treatment in the upright position and latex allergy should be considered (Ch. 17). Quadriplegics

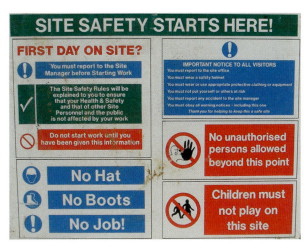

Fig. 24.7 Prevention of occupational trauma.

are at risk from respiratory infections, so that GA should be avoided if possible. Other problems are dealt with in Chapter 13.

TRAUMA PREVENTION

Many of the problems caused by trauma could be avoided by abstention from drug and alcohol use and high-risk behaviour, the use of body protection, and application of health and safety laws and regulations in dangerous occupations, sports and other activities (Fig. 24.7).

BURNS

Burns can be caused by thermal injury, electricity, radiation or chemicals. Chemical burns are caused by exposure to corrosive substances, such as bleach, acids or alkalis, and pesticides.

First-aid care includes:

- airway maintenance
- oxygen administration if there has been exposure to hot air or smoke
- pain reduction by cooling the burn with cold water (not ice) and covering it with clingfilm or other non-adherent protective film. Give analgesics, such as oral paracetamol (acetaminophen), fentanyl (intranasal 1.5 mcg/kg) or morphine (5–15 oral mg for an adult or 0.1 mg/kg i.v.). Burns to the eyes require early copious irrigation with normal saline or water
- removal of any jewellery near the burn and clothing that has absorbed hot water. If clothing is stuck to the wound, do not pull it off; cut around it and remove the rest of the clothing
- ensuring that the electrical source is turned if a casualty has been injured by a household electrical supply (240 volts). A non-conductive object should then be used to move the individual away from the electrical source. If a casualty has been injured by a high-voltage source (1000 volts or more), do not approach them but immediately call the emergency services.

Never:

- put yourself or others in danger
- over-cool an injury, as it can lower the body temperature of a casualty
- apply any oils or creams to burns
- break any blisters that have developed.

Assess the burn severity in terms of depth (Table 24.12). Anyone who has been injured with any of the following should receive immediate treatment in a burns or plastic surgery unit:

- Full-thickness burns
- Chemicals, electricity or explosives
- Large or deep burns – any burn bigger than the affected person's hand – and full-thickness burns of all sizes
- Partial-thickness burns on the face, hands, arms, feet, legs or genitals – these are burns that cause blisters.
- Respiratory or ocular involvement – patients with a raised respiratory rate, abnormal breath sounds (rales) and bilateral diffuse interstitial and intra-alveolar oedema on radiography should be urgently admitted to an intensive care unit.

CLINICAL FEATURES AND MANAGEMENT

Burns are serious injuries, especially where there is airways or circulatory involvement or more than 10% of the body surface area is affected.

Table 24.12 *Burn severity*

Severity	Appearance	Pain	Common causes
Superficial	Dry, red, possibly small blisters, rapid capillary return	+	Sunburn
Partial-thickness, superficial	Moist, red, broken blisters, rapid capillary return	+	Scald
Partial-thickness, deep	Moist, white slough, red mottled, slow capillary return	–	Scald, transient flame contact
Full-thickness	Dry, charred, whitish. No capillary return	–	Flame, electrical or severe scald

Airway and breathing

- Immobilize the cervical spine if there is associated trauma.
- Assess for stridor, hoarseness, black sputum, respiratory distress, singed nasal hairs or facial swelling.
- Intubate immediately if there are oropharyngeal burns and significant neck burns, even if the airway is not yet compromised. If burns have been received in a closed or confined space, a change in voice, hoarseness, dysphonia, stridor and the coughing up of sooty sputum are all signs suggesting inhalation injury; endotracheal intubation or tracheostomy may be indicated. ARDS, sometimes a sequel to burns and other pulmonary injury, is characterized by diffuse alveolar damage, pulmonary oedema and hyaline membrane formation, and may culminate in respiratory failure; mortality is high.

Circulation

- Seek sources of overt or covert bleeding, as early hypovolaemia is rarely caused by the burn injury.
- For circumferential limb burns, check for circulatory obstruction and the need for an escharotomy; elevate the limb.
- For electrical burns, perform electrocardiography (ECG). High-voltage limb burns may require early fasciotomy.

Estimation of body surface area involved

- Calculate body surface area (BSA) involvement (Fig. 24.8).
- Remember that BSA involvement determines the need for fluid resuscitation and admission, as opposed to dressings and potential outpatient management (see below).

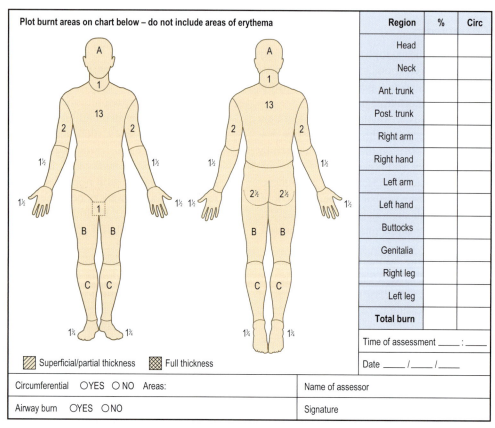

Region	%	Circ
Head		
Neck		
Ant. trunk		
Post. trunk		
Right arm		
Right hand		
Left arm		
Left hand		
Buttocks		
Genitalia		
Right leg		
Left leg		
Total burn		

Plot burnt areas on chart below – do not include areas of erythema

Superficial/partial thickness   Full thickness

Circumferential   ○YES ○NO   Areas:

Airway burn   ○YES ○NO

Name of assessor

Signature

Time of assessment _____ : _____

Date _____ / _____ / _____

Fig. 24.8 Lund and Browder chart used to calculate involvement of body surface area (BSA) after burns.

Documentation

Document:

- time of burn
- extent of burn
- depth of burn
- first aid received
- tetanus status.

Full-thickness burns

Management of major burns (>10% BSA)

Airway and breathing

- If airway burn or lung injury is possible, intubate as soon as possible before airway swelling appears.

Fluids

- Insert an intravenous line through uninvolved skin. Give fluid replacement.
- If the burn covers more than 15% of the BSA or if there is significant perineal burn, insert a urinary catheter.
- If the burn consists of more than 15% deep partial-thickness or full-thickness burns, insert a nasogastric tube and start feeding within 6–18 hours.

Investigations

- Perform haemoglobin, electrolytes, blood glucose, blood group and hold.
- Measure carboxyhaemoglobin levels (if the fire was in a confined space).

Management of minor burns (isolated, <10% BSA)

- Give analgesia.
- Immobilize upper limb burns with a sling and splinting.
- Use closed dressings for partial-thickness burns.
- Remember that the depth of a partial-thickness burn may only be declared after 7–10 days.
- Note that blisters may have a protective function, and reduce pain if left intact for a few days. If they are small, not near a joint and not obstructing the dressing, they should be left intact. If overlying a joint, they should be deroofed, as they may limit function. Deroof if they are large (for assessment) or if blister fluid becomes opaque (suggests infection).

Superficial burns with erythema only

- Treated by exposure, if possible; alternatively, use a protective, low-adherent dressing (e.g. Mepitel™ + Melolin™) with crepe bandage.

Partial-thickness burns

- Cleanse the burn and surrounding area with saline. If the wound is dirty or treatment is delayed, use aqueous chlorhexidine 0.1% then saline.
- For small, superficial, partial-thickness burns, cover with a low-adherent dressing (e.g. Mepitel™ + Melolin™), then a crepe bandage or adhesive paper.
- For more extensive or deeper partial-thickness burns, apply a low-adherent silver dressing (e.g. Acticoat™ or Acticoat 7™).

Facial burns

- Remember that superficial burns only require Vaseline™ to be applied twice daily, whereas partial-thickness burns may need silver dressings. Good education regarding care of the burn is essential.

Care at home

- Clean the face gently with saline or water.
- Apply 1/2 cm thick Vaseline™ to the face by using a large cotton swab, gauze or clean hands.
- Clean and reapply the Vaseline™ twice a day. If it is rubbed off in between, apply more Vaseline.

VULNERABLE PEOPLE

In the UK, the Safeguarding Vulnerable Groups Act 2006 (SVGA; www.legislation.gov.uk/ukpga/2006/47/notes/contents, accessed 30 September 2013) has been amended by the Protection of Freedoms Act 2012 (PoFA). See also http://www.justice.gov.uk/protecting-the-vulnerable/mental-capacity-act; accessed 30 September 2013). These are the salient points:

- A judgment about vulnerability is based on the capacity for self-protection.
- Self-protection refers to being able to demonstrate behaviour that results in defending oneself against threats to one's safety results in successfully meeting one's own basic (safety) needs.
- Vulnerability means being defenceless against threats to one's safety.
- Children and older people may be especially vulnerable to threats to safety. Children from birth to 6 years old, especially infants, are always particularly vulnerable, as are people who are physically handicapped. Individuals who are cognitively limited are also vulnerable.
- A person's vulnerability helps inform what must be done to manage threats and assure protection.

The emotional, mental health or behavioural problems of vulnerable people may irritate and provoke others to act out toward them or to avoid them totally. Regardless of age, intellect and physical capacity, people who are highly dependent and susceptible to others, who are unable to defend themselves against aggression, who cannot or will not seek help and protection, or who are so passive or withdrawn that they are not able to make their basic needs known are vulnerable. Regardless of age, some people who are not visible and not noticed or observed, may have continuing or acute medical problems and needs that make them vulnerable. A 'vulnerable adult' is:

> *a person aged 18 years or over who is, or may be in need of, community care services by reason of mental or other disability, age or illness; and who is, or may be, unable to take care of him or herself, or unable to protect him or herself against significant harm or exploitation.*

The term encompasses those with physical or mental impairments, including dementia and other degenerative illnesses.

Abuse (as defined by the UK Department of Health; Tables 24.13 and 24.14) may be:

- *physical*: hitting, slapping, pushing, kicking, burning or other show of force; misuse of medication; restraint; or inappropriate

Table 24.13 *Features of abuse in a dental practice/domiciliary setting*[a]

General signs	Behaviour of patient	Behaviour of carer	Features of domestic environment
Appointments often missed	Appearing passive or afraid of carer	Attitudes of indifference or anger to vulnerable adult	Lack of amenities, e.g. TV, personal grooming items
Difficulties in arranging appointments/frequent cancellations	Remaining quiet while carer responds to questions	Ignoring of vulnerable adult	Dirty, smelly, unsanitary conditions
Poor compliance with treatment regimens	Withdrawal/detachment	Refusal to allow vulnerable adult to speak	Soiled bed
Injuries inconsistent with explanation given	Anxiety	Inappropriate displays of affection	Indications of unusual confinement, e.g. patient is closed off in a particular room, tied to furniture
Conflicting or vague explanations of injuries	Poor eye contact	Verbal intimidation, berating or use of humiliating language	Obvious absence of assistance or attendance
Delay in presentation for treatment of dental problems/injuries	Closed body position/holding head down	Blame of vulnerable adult (e.g. for bad behaviour, incontinence or forgetfulness)	Obvious absence of protection, e.g. to prevent patient with severe dementia falling out of bed
	Minimization of injuries	Threats of punishment or deprivation	

[a]After Moore and Newton 2012.

Table 24.14 *Type of abuse presenting indicators in general dental practice/domiciliary setting*[a]

Physical abuse	Neglect	Psychological abuse	Financial abuse	Sexual abuse
General signs				
Cuts, lacerations, puncture wounds, open wounds	Impaired skin integrity/ulcers, rashes, sores, lice, unkempt	Helplessness	The vulnerable adult suffers from substandard care in the home	A vulnerable adult telling you that they have been sexually assaulted or raped
Recognizable shape or pattern to bruises, such as slap mark, bite	Soiled clothing or bed	Hesitation to talk openly, fearfulness	Disappearance of a vulnerable adult's possessions in an institutional setting, despite adequate financial resources	Signs of psychological abuse (see left)
Bruises, welts, discoloration, black eyes, burns, bone mark, rope mark	Appearance, body odours	Withdrawal, passive affect		
	Inappropriate clothing	Denial of a situation		
Fractures, concussion	Malnourishment, emaciation or dehydration without an illness-related cause	Confusion or disorientation	Vulnerable adult poorly dressed	
Signs of restraint (visible restraint or bruising, e.g. rope marks)	Lack of appropriate physical aids, such as glasses, hearing aids, assistance with eating and drinking	Anger without apparent cause	Signatures on cheques, etc. that do not resemble the vulnerable adult's	
		Sudden change in behaviour		
		Emotional upset or agitation	The inclusion of additional names on an older person's bank account signature, or signed when the adult cannot write	
Untreated injuries in various stages of healing or not	Failure to provide a safe environment	Depression		
Broken glasses		Unusual behaviour (sucking, biting, rocking)		
A vulnerable adult disclosing an experience of being hit, slapped, kicked or mistreated	A vulnerable adult telling you he/she is left alone for long periods of time	A vulnerable adult telling you they are being verbally or emotionally abused, isolated, or left alone for days on end	Unpaid bills	
			Confusion of a vulnerable adult regarding his/her financial situation	
Overdosing or underdosing of medication			A vulnerable adult telling you that someone has taken their money	
Orofacial signs				
Lip trauma	Poor oral hygiene, halitosis		Lack of dental care	Oral signs of sexually transmitted diseases, e.g. syphilitic or herpetic ulceration
Fractured, subluxated or avulsed teeth	Rampant dental disease		Care-giver questions dentist on necessity of dental work for older person 'at his age'	
	Absence of dentures			
Fractures of the mandible, maxilla or zygomaticomaxillary complex	Glossitis, angular cheilitis other oral infections			
Missing teeth	Xerostomia			
Eye injuries, orbital fractures				
Bruising of the edentulous ridges or the facial tissues				
Unexplained alopecia (from pulling hair)				
Evidence of prior trauma to dental or orofacial structures				

[a]After Moore and Newton 2012.

sanctions. Victims may suffer physical injuries that are minor, like cuts, scratches, bruises and welts, or more serious, such as head injuries or broken bones. Physical injuries can also lead to premature death and aggravate existing health problems.

- *sexual*: including rape and sexual assault or sexual acts to which the vulnerable person has not consented, or could not consent or was pressured into consenting.
- *psychological*: including emotional abuse, threats of harm or abandonment, deprivation of contact, humiliation, blaming, controlling, intimidation, coercion, harassment, verbal abuse, isolation, or withdrawal from services or supportive networks. Such behaviours harm a person's self-worth or emotional well-being (e.g. verbal abuse, name-calling, scaring, embarrassing, refusing access to friends and family).
- *financial or material abuse*: theft, fraud, exploitation, pressure in connection with wills, property or inheritance or financial transactions, or the misuse or misappropriation of property, possessions, assets or benefits.
- *neglect and acts of omission*: ignoring medical or physical care needs, failure to provide access to appropriate health, social care or educational services, withholding of the necessities of life, such as medication, adequate nutrition and heating. Neglect is failure to meet a person's basic needs (e.g. food, housing, clothing and medical care). Abandonment is when a caregiver leaves a person alone, no longer providing care.
- *discriminatory*: including racist, sexist, that based on a person's disability, and other forms of harassment, slurs or similar treatment.

Risk factors in the vulnerable adult person may include:

- social isolation
- dependence on abuser for essential care
- physical and cognitive deterioration
- dementia
- challenging behaviour.

ELDER MALTREATMENT

Elder maltreatment includes violence inflicted upon those aged 60 and older. The violence usually occurs at the hands of a care-giver or a person the elder trusts, and victims are often fearful and anxious. Elder maltreatment can be prevented by:

- listening to elders and their care-givers
- reporting abuse or suspected abuse
- learning how to recognize and report elder abuse and how to differentiate it from the normal aging process.

REPORTING ABUSE

Local social services are the lead agencies to which disclosures of abuse should be made. Telephone referrals to social services should be followed up in writing within 48 hours. Difficulties or concerns should be discussed with a senior colleague and the defence organization. As with all patient information, it is essential that all records are kept entirely confidential.

CONSENT

The patient's consent must first be obtained before disclosing an incident or suspected incident of abuse to social services. The disclosure must be carried out in an appropriate manner so that the patient is not put at increased risk of harm. Details of the discussions and agreement of the patient to disclosure of information to social services should be recorded in the dental records. Disclosure of information can be made without consent in a number of situations where:

- the adult is believed to be at risk of death or serious harm
- the adult is not competent to give consent
- information is required under a court order or another legal obligation.

It is the responsibility of the HCP to 'act at all times in the best interests of the patient based on a risk–benefit assessment, accept final responsibility for his or her actions, and be able to justify them if subsequently challenged'.

RECORDS

Accurate contemporaneous records should be kept of all allegations or suspicions of abuse. Precise factual information of the alleged abuse must be recorded. Details of any discussions and decisions taken and reason for those decisions should be clearly recorded. There should be comprehensive documentation of injuries, including details of site, size, colour, swelling and other distinguishing features. Body maps are recommended and, where appropriate, clinical photos should be taken – with informed consent. In cases where the patient is unable to give informed consent, the dental practitioner should take clinical photos if it is considered to be in the patient's best interest. All injuries should be treated, or a referral made for treatment.

KEY WEBSITES

(Accessed 29 May 2013)
Centers for Disease Control and Prevention. <http://www.cdc.gov/traumacare/>.
Chemical Hazards Emergency Medical Management. <http://www.chemm.nlm.nih.gov/burns.htm>.
MedlinePlus: Burns. <http://www.nlm.nih.gov/medlineplus/burns.html>.
MedlinePlus: Child abuse – physical. <http://www.nlm.nih.gov/medlineplus/ency/article/001552.htm>.
NHS Choices: Burns and scalds. <http://www.nhs.uk/Conditions/Burns-and-scalds/Pages/Treatment.aspx>.
NHS Choices: Major trauma services. <http://www.nhs.uk/NHSEngland/AboutNHSservices/Emergencyandurgentcareservices/Pages/Majortraumaservices.aspx>.

USEFUL WEBSITES

(Accessed 29 May 2013)
Blond McIndoe Research Foundation. <http://www.blondmcindoe.org/skin-burns-and-wounds.html>.
British Red Cross: follow the links from 'Everyday first aid' to 'Burns'. <http://www.redcross.org.uk/What-we-do/First-aid>.
Connecticut Maxillofacial Surgeons, LLC. <http://www.cmsllc.com/toptrm.html>.
Justice. <http://www.justice.gov.uk/protecting-the-vulnerable/mental-capacity-act>.
Merck Manual for Health Care Professionals. <http://www.merckmanuals.com/professional/index.html>.
RehabTeamSite. <http://calder.med.miami.edu/providers/MEDICINE/parap.html>.
Royal Children's Hospital Melbourne. <http://www.rch.org.au/kidsinfo/fact_sheets/Burns_on_the_face/>.
Wikipedia: Stabbing. <http://en.wikipedia.org/wiki/Stabbing>.

FURTHER READING

Andreasen, J.O., et al. 2008. Open or closed repositioning of mandibular fractures: is there a difference in healing outcome? A systematic review. Dent. Traumatol. 24, 17.

Anetzberger, G., 2004. The clinical management of elder abuse. Hawthorne Press, New York.

Assael, L.A., 2003. Managing the trauma pandemic: learning from the past. J. Oral Maxillofac. Surg. 61, 859.

Bagheri, S.C., et al. 2008. Penetrating neck injuries. Oral Maxillofac. Surg. Clin. North Am. 20, 393.

Bell, R.B., et al. 2008. Management of laryngeal trauma. Oral Maxillofac. Surg. Clin. North Am. 20, 415.

Ben-Galim, P.J., et al. 2008. Internal decapitation: survival after head to neck dissociation injuries. Spine 33, 1744.

Bissada, E., et al. 2008. Orbitozygomatic complex fracture reduction under local anesthesia and light oral sedation. J. Oral Maxillofac. Surg. 66, 1378.

Boyd, B.C., 2002. Automobile supplemental restraint system-induced injuries. Oral Surg. Oral Med. Oral Pathol. Oral Radiol. Endod. 94, 143.

Brookes, C.N., 2004. Maxillofacial and ocular injuries in motor vehicle crashes. Ann. R. Coll. Surg. Engl. 86, 149.

Brookes, C., et al. 2003. Maxillofacial injuries in North American vehicle crashes. Eur. J. Emerg. Med. 10, 30.

Cavalcanti, A.L., Melo, T.R., 2008. Facial and oral injuries in Brazilian children aged 5–17 years: 5-year review. Eur. Arch. Paediatr. Dent. 9, 102.

Ceallaigh, P.O., et al. 2006. Diagnosis and management of common maxillofacial injuries in the emergency department. Part 1. Advanced trauma life support. Emerg. Med. J. 23 (10), 796.

Ceallaigh, P.O., et al. 2006. Diagnosis and management of common maxillofacial injuries in the emergency department. Part 2. Mandibular fractures. Emerg. Med. J. 23 (12), 927.

Ceallaigh, P.O., et al. 2007. Diagnosis and management of common maxillofacial injuries in the emergency department. Part 3. Orbitozygomatic complex and zygomatic arch fractures. Emerg. Med. J. 24 (2), 120.

Ceallaigh, P.O., et al. 2007. Diagnosis and management of common maxillofacial injuries in the emergency department. Part 4. Orbital floor and midface fractures. Emerg. Med. J. 24 (4), 292.

Ceallaigh, P.O., et al. 2007. Diagnosis and management of common maxillofacial injuries in the emergency department. Part 5. Dentoalveolar injuries. Emerg. Med. J. 24 (6), 429.

Chen, C.H., et al. 2008. A 162-case review of palatal fracture: management strategy from a 10-year experience. Plast. Reconstr. Surg. 121 (6), 2065.

Cox, D., et al. 2004. Effect of restraint systems on maxillofacial injury in frontal motor vehicle collisions. J. Oral Maxillofac. Surg. 62, 571.

Cunningham, L.L., et al. 2003. Firearm injuries to the maxillofacial region: an overview of current thoughts regarding demographics, pathophysiology, and management. J. Oral Maxillofac. Surg. 61, 932.

Dana, S.E., DiMaio, V.J.M., 2003. Gunshot trauma. In: Payne-James, J. (Ed.), Forensic Medicine: Clinical and Pathological Aspects. Greenwich Medical Media, London, p. 149.

Ducic, Y., 2008. Endoscopic treatment of subcondylar fractures. Laryngoscope 118, 1164.

Ellis III, E., Miles, B.A., 2007. Fractures of the mandible: a technical perspective. Plast. Reconstr. Surg. 120 (7 Suppl. 2), 76S.

Ellis III, E., et al. 2003. Treatment considerations for comminuted mandibular fractures. J. Oral Maxillofac. Surg. 61, 861.

Epstein, J.B., et al. 2010. Orofacial injuries due to trauma following motor vehicle collisions. Part 1. Traumatic dental injuries. J. Can. Dent. Assoc. 76, a171.

Epstein, J.B., et al. 2010. Orofacial injuries due to trauma following motor vehicle collisions. Part 2. Temporomandibular disorders. J. Can. Dent. Assoc. 76, a172.

Espinosa-Aguilar, A., et al. 2008. Design and validation of a critical pathway for hospital management of patients with severe traumatic brain injury. J. Trauma 64, 1327.

Ferreira, P., et al. 2004. Midfacial fractures in children and adolescents: a review of 492 cases. Br. J. Oral Maxillofac. Surg. 42, 501.

Fraioli, R.E., et al. 2004. Facial factures: beyond Le Fort. Otolaryngol. Clin. North Am. 41 51, vi

Francis, D.O., et al. 2006. Air bag-induced orbital blow-out fractures. Laryngoscope 116, 1966.

Frodel Jr., J.L., 2008. Dealing with the difficult trauma and reconstructive surgery patient. Facial Plast. Surg. Clin. North Am. 16 225, vii.

Gasparini, G., et al. 2002. Maxillofacial traumas. J. Craniofac. Surg. 13, 645.

Gibbons, A.J., Patton, D.W., 2003. Ballistic injuries of the face and mouth in war and civil conflict. Dent. Update 30, 272.

Haug, R.H., Brandt, M.T., 2007. Closed reduction, open reduction, and endoscopic assistance: current thoughts on the management of mandibular condyle fractures. Plast. Reconstr. Surg. 120 (7 Suppl. 2), 90S.

Haug, R.H., Foss, J., 2000. Maxillofacial injuries in the pediatric patient. Oral Surg. 90, 126.

Hawkins, S.C., 2003. Saving face: identification and management of facial fractures. J. Emerg. Med. Serv. JEMS 28, 72.

Hermund, N.U., et al. 2008. Effect of early or delayed treatment upon healing of mandibular fractures: a systematic literature review. Dent. Traumatol. 24, 22.

Kim, J.M., et al. 2004. A case of air-bag associated severe ocular injury. Korean J. Ophthalmol. 18, 84.

Krishnan, B., El Sheikh, M.H., 2008. Dental forceps reduction of depressed zygomatic arch fractures. J. Craniofac. Surg. 19, 782.

Krohner, R.G., 2003. Anesthetic considerations and techniques for oral and maxillofacial surgery. Int. Anesthesiol. Clin. 41, 67.

Landes, C.A., et al. 2008. Prospective evaluation of closed treatment of nondisplaced and nondislocated mandibular condyle fractures versus open reposition and rigid fixation of displaced and dislocated fractures in children. J. Oral Maxillofac. Surg. 66, 1184.

Levin, L., et al. 2008. Incidence and severity of maxillofacial injuries during the Second Lebanon War among Israeli soldiers and civilians. J. Oral Maxillofac. Surg. 66, 1630.

Lin, K.C., et al. 2008. The early response of mannitol infusion in traumatic brain injury. Acta Neurol. Taiwan. 17, 26.

Lindbloom, E.J., et al. 2007. Elder mistreatment in the nursing home: a systematic review. J. Am. Med. Dir. Assoc. 8 (9), 610.

Lynham, A.J., et al. 2004. Emergency department management of maxillofacial trauma. Emerg. Med. Australas 16 (1), 7.

Macciocchi, S., et al. 2008. Spinal cord injury and co-occurring traumatic brain injury: assessment and incidence. Arch. Phys. Med. Rehabil. 89, 1350.

Mitchener, T.A., et al. 2008. Air medical evacuations of soldiers due to oral-facial disease and injuries: operations Enduring Freedom/Iraqi Freedom. Mil. Med. 173, 465.

Mitra, B., et al. 2008. Management and hospital outcome of the severely head injured elderly patient. ANZ J. Surg. 78, 588.

Moore, R., Newton, J.T., 2012. The role of the GDP in the management of abuse of vulnerable adults. Dent. Update 39, 556.

Moos, K.F., 2002. Diagnosis of facial bone fractures. Ann. R. Coll. Surg. Engl. 84, 429.

Nemutandani, M.S., et al. 2012. Orofacial injuries among traditional bare-fisted fighters. SADJ 67 (4), 164.

Newlands, S.D., et al. 2003. Surgical treatment of gunshot injuries to the mandible. Otolaryngol. Head Neck Surg. 129, 239.

Nussbaum, M.L., et al. 2008. Closed versus open reduction of mandibular condylar fractures in adults: a meta-analysis. J. Oral Maxillofac. Surg. 66, 1087.

Ocak, G., et al. 2009. Prehospital identification of major trauma patients. Langenbecks Arch. Surg. 394, 285.

Osborn, T.M., et al. 2008. Computed tomographic angiography as an aid to clinical decision making in the selective management of penetrating injuries to the neck: a reduction in the need for operative exploration. J. Trauma 64, 1466.

Plurad, D., et al. 2010. Motor vehicle crashes: the association of alcohol consumption with the type and severity of injuries and outcomes. J. Emerg. Med. 38 (1), 12.10.1016/j.jemermed.2007.09.048 Epub 2008 June 11.

Ramesh, V.G., et al. 2008. A new scale for prognostication in head injury. J. Clin. Neurosci. 15, 1110.

Rezende-Neto, J., et al. 2008. Damage control principles applied to penetrating neck and mandibular injury. J. Trauma 64, 1142.

Rodriguez, E.D., et al. 2007. Microsurgical reconstruction of posttraumatic high-energy maxillary defects: establishing the effectiveness of early reconstruction. Plast. Reconstr. Surg. 120 (7 Suppl. 2), 103S.

Schütz, P., Hamed, H.H., 2008. Submental intubation versus tracheostomy in maxillofacial trauma patients. J. Oral Maxillofac. Surg. 66, 1404.

Thomas, J., et al. 2008. Emergency department imaging: current practice. J. Am. Coll. Radiol. 5 (811), e2.

Undén, J., et al. 2008. Management of minor head injuries with the help of a blood test: S100B analysis can reduce the number of CT examinations and patient admissions. Lakartidningen 105, 1846. [in Swedish]

von Elm, E., et al. 2008. Severe traumatic brain injury in Switzerland – feasibility and first results of a cohort study. Swiss Med. Wkly. 138, 327.

Yokoyama, T., et al. 2006. A retrospective analysis of oral and maxillofacial injuries in motor vehicle accidents. J. Oral Maxillofac. Surg. 64, 1731.

Zaglia, E., et al. 2007. Occipital condyle fracture: an unusual airbag injury. J. Forensic Leg. Med. 14, 231.

APPENDIX 24.1 CAUSES OF COMA

- Acute disseminated encephalomyelitis
- Addison disease
- African sleeping sickness
- Alcohol poisoning
- Asphyxia
- Brain compression
- Brain infection
- Brain inflammation
- Chagas disease
- Concussion
- Creutzfeldt–Jakob disease
- Diabetic ketoacidosis
- Eclampsia
- Ehrlichiosis
- Encephalitis
- Head trauma
- Heatstroke
- Hepatitis
- High-altitude cerebral oedema
- HIV/AIDS
- Hyperparathyroidism
- Hypothermia

- Japanese encephalitis
- Kidney failure
- Lead poisoning
- Liver failure
- Melioidosis
- Meningitis
- Mountain sickness
- Poisoning
- Progressive multifocal leukoencephalopathy
- Pulmonary embolism
- Reye syndrome
- Rift Valley fever
- Rocky Mountain spotted fever
- Shock
- Streptococcal toxic shock syndrome
- Stroke
- Subarachnoid haemorrhage
- Toxoplasmosis
- Typhoid fever
- Viral haemorrhagic fevers
- Yellow fever

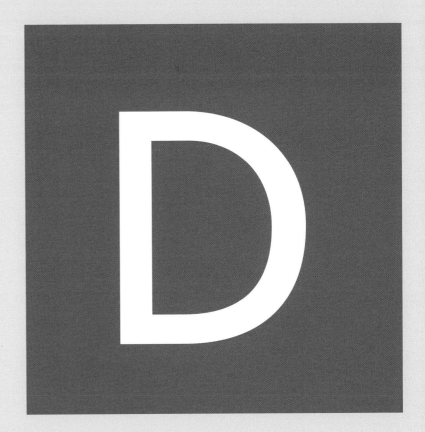

Other health issues

EITHER GENDER

CHILDREN

In the UK, people up to the age of 16 years are regarded as children. It may be necessary to take at least part of the history from a parent.

General aspects

At birth the neonate is classified as premature or preterm (less than 37 weeks' gestation), full-term (37–42 weeks' gestation) or post-dates (born after 42 weeks' gestation). Premature babies are at particular risk from a number of problems.

Premature babies

Up to 10% of all births are preterm, usually with a low birth weight (below 2500 g). Low birth weight may result from intrauterine growth retardation. Causes include multiple pregnancy, infection, maternal smoking, pre-eclampsia, severe anaemia, and heart and renal disease. These babies may go on to have lower IQs and smaller stature. In about 40% the cause is unknown but may be related to maternal issues: that is, elective delivery due to pregnancy complications such as pre-eclampsia (maternal hypertension, fluid retention and proteinuria) or placenta praevia (low-lying placenta). Maternal periodontal infection may possibly be a risk factor. Predictors are shown in Table 25.1.

Preterm babies, depending on the degree of prematurity, may suffer apnoea or irregular breathing, a weak cry, inactivity, ineffective sucking and swallowing (with poor feeding), shiny wrinkled skin with fine body hair (lanugo), soft, flexible ear cartilage, enlarged clitoris (female) or a small scrotum (male). Preterm babies are less able to maintain body temperature and haemostasis, and are prone to several health consequences (Table 25.2). Up to a half suffer long-term sequelae, including low IQ, behavioural disorders, coordination problems, and respiratory and feeding problems.

Neonates

A neonate is a newborn infant up to 1 month old. Neonate behaviour is characterized by six states of consciousness: quiet sleep, active sleep, drowsy waking, quiet alertness, fussing and active crying. The amount a healthy infant cries in the first 3 months varies from 1 to 3 hours a day. Periodic breathing is normal. Temperature control, skin colour, stooling, yawning, gagging, hiccoughing, vomiting and sleep are easily affected by stress and stimulation. Sleep/wake cycles occur in random intervals of 30–50 minutes and gradually increase as the child matures. By 4 months old, most infants will have one long period of uninterrupted sleep and breathing stabilizes. The neonate can see objects within a range of 8–12 inches, has excellent colour vision, can track moving objects up to 180° and sees faces. Infants prefer the frequencies of the human voice. Senses of hearing, touch, taste and smell are mature at birth. Vestibular senses are also mature and the infant responds to rocking and changes of position.

During the neonatal period, most congenital defects (e.g. congenital heart disease) are detected. Congenital infections (e.g. rubella, herpesviruses, toxoplasmosis) may manifest. Immunological immaturity

Table 25.1 *Predictors of preterm birth*

Primary predictors	Secondary predictors
African heritage	Anaemia
Chronic kidney disease	Bacterial vaginosis
Chronic respiratory disease	Chorioamnionitis
Cigarette smoking	Hydramnios
Depression	Inadequate prenatal care
Diabetes mellitus	*In vitro* fertilization (IVF)
Domestic violence	Low maternal weight gain
Family history	Multiple fetuses
Hypertension	Pre-eclampsia
Inflammatory gene polymorphism	Raised fibronectin, alpha-fetoprotein, alkaline phosphatase or granulocyte colony-stimulating factor
Low body mass index	Vaginal bleeding
Low socioeconomic status	
Previous pre-term birth or abortion	
Stress	
Substance abuse	
Young mother	

Table 25.2 *Possible consequences of preterm birth*

Early	Long-term
Bronchopulmonary dysplasia (BPD)	Attention deficit disorder
Hypocalcaemia	Cerebral palsy
Hypoglycaemia	Hearing impairment
Intraventricular brain haemorrhage or periventricular infarction	Learning impairment
Necrotizing enterocolitis	Retinopathy
Neonatal jaundice	
Patent ductus arteriosus	
Respiratory distress syndrome (RDS; hyaline membrane disease)	
Sepsis	

predisposes to candidosis. Infections may be transmitted by parents or carers, or from the environment; even tongue spatulas can be a source of infection.

This is a period of rapid growth and development. Facial, skull, jaw and tooth development can be impaired by radiotherapy, chemotherapy and some immunosuppressants during this time. Oropharyngeal or orogastric intubation may result in palatal grooving, acquired cleft palate and damage to the deciduous dentition. Appliances can be constructed to protect against this damage.

Infants

The first year of life is referred to as infancy. The healthy infant possesses a number of primitive reflexes (Table 25.3). Physical development begins at the head and then progresses to other parts (sucking precedes sitting, which precedes walking). Mental and neurological functions develop, with gross motor (e.g. head control, sitting,

Table 25.3 *Normal infant reflexes*

Reflexes	Composition
Babinski reflex	Toes fan when sole of foot is stroked
Moro reflex	On momentarily releasing head from a supported sitting position, arms abduct, hands open and then arms adduct
Palmar hand grasp	Closure over finger
Plantar grasp	Flexion of toe and forefoot
Rooting and sucking	Turns head in search for nipple when cheek is touched and begins to suck when nipple touches lips
Stepping and walking	Takes brisk steps when both feet placed on a surface, with body supported
Tonic neck response	Leg extends on side of head direction, flexion occurs in opposite arm and leg

Table 25.5 *Developmental milestones in early (pre-school) childhood*

Months	Milestones
14–15	Child is walking well by 14 months and learns to walk backwards and up steps
	Begins to scribble and can place a block in a cup and begin to stack blocks
	Can use 2–3 words (other than mum or dad)
16–18	Able to kick a ball forward; at about 18–24 months is able to throw ball overhand
	Can combine two words
22–24	Can jump
	Can often state their name
	Able to point to named body parts and to name pictures of items and animals

Table 25.4 *Developmental milestones in infancy*

Months	Milestones
0–2	Infant can lift and turn its head when lying on its back
	Cannot support the head upright when held in a sitting position
	Has fisted hands and flexed arms
3–4	Can track objects and discriminate objects from backgrounds with minimal contrast
	Can sit, with support, and keep the head up. Can raise upper torso and head when prone
	Hand and feet actions start to come under willed control and reflexes have disappeared, or are in the process of so doing
5–6	Begins to grasp objects using ulnar–palmar grasp
	Rolls from supine to prone position and starts to sit alone, without support, for short periods
6–9	May pull self into standing position while holding on to furniture; can walk while holding the hand of an adult
	Able to sit steadily without support, for long periods
	Learns to sit down from standing position
9–12	Begins to balance while standing alone
	Takes steps and begins to walk alone
	Says 'mum' and 'dad'

walking), fine motor (e.g. holding a spoon, pincer grasp), sensory, language and social development. There are several recognized 'milestones' in development, as shown in Table 25.4.

Children from 1 year (pre-school children)
Development proceeds with gross motor development recognized by milestones (Table 25.5), as the child becomes able to stand alone, stoop, pick something up and recover to standing (toddler). Young children strive constantly for independence, creating not only special safety concerns, but also discipline challenges.

Children aged 5–12 years (schoolchildren)
School-age children typically have fairly good gross motor skills, but there is wide variance in coordination, endurance, balance, physical tolerance and fine motor skills. They are usually able to use simple, complete, short sentences consistently. Receptive language skills necessary to understand long or complex instructions and the use of increasingly complex sentences develop. Delayed language development may indicate hearing or learning impairment. The attention span increases from about 15 minutes in 5-year-olds to about an hour by the age of 10. By about 10 years old, most children can follow five commands in a row. Reduced attention may herald attention deficiency.

Puberty
Puberty refers to the physical and psychological changes during maturation into an adult capable of reproduction. Manifest by the development of secondary sexual characteristics, it begins between 9 and 16 years of age, but children vary as to exactly when. On average, girls enter puberty 2 years earlier than boys.

The hypothalamus and pituitary gland hormones that control growth and maturation trigger rapid growth at puberty, with increases in height and weight, the appearance of secondary sexual characteristics and increased sexual interest ('sex drive'). Oil glands become more active and acne may appear. Sweat glands become more active and produce more of an odour.

In girls, the ovaries begin to increase oestrogen production (along with other 'female' hormones). Girls experience rapid growth in height and increased hip width, breast enlargement, pubic, axillary and leg hair growth and vaginal secretions, followed by the onset of menstrual periods (menarche). The ovaries begin to release ova that, over 3 or 4 days, travel along Fallopian tubes to the uterus. Meanwhile, the endometrium (uterine lining) thickens by filling with blood and fluid. If the ovum is not fertilized, it dissolves and the endometrium sloughs, causing menstruation (menses). Menstrual cycles occur over about 1 month (28–32 days) and may be irregular initially. There may also be cyclical hormonal and physical changes, such as emotional or depressive reactions – the premenstrual syndrome (PMS) – and cramping menstrual pain. In girls, full physical maturation is usually complete by age 17, but educational and emotional maturity is ongoing.

In boys, the testicles increase testosterone production so that puberty usually occurs between 13 and 15 years of age. The pubescent boy experiences accelerated growth, especially in height, shoulder width and growth of penis and testicles, voice changes and growth of pubic, beard and axillary hair. Sperm is manufactured constantly in the testes (a process termed spermatogenesis) and is stored in the epididymis. This is released following masturbation or sexual intercourse, or during sleep – when it is known as a nocturnal emission or a 'wet dream'.

Adolescence
Adolescence refers to the transition from child to adult, between 13 and 19 years of age. As well as sexual maturation, there are psychological changes resulting in emotional, behavioural and social changes. Specific health concerns for this age group are shown in Box 25.1.

Box 25.1 *Adolescents: health concerns*

- Accidental injuries (leading cause of death [70%] from motor vehicle accidents, drowning or poisoning [usually drug- or alcohol-related])
- Unlawful killing, often gang-related (second leading cause of death)
- Suicide (third leading cause of death)
- Substance abuse
- Stress, depression, eating disorders
- Sexually transmitted diseases
- Pregnancy
- Assaults (gang-related)

Table 25.6 *Drugs that may be contraindicated in children*

Drug contraindicated	Possibility of
Antidepressants	Suicide attempts
Aspirin (salicylates)	Reye syndrome
Codeine	Respiratory depression
Diazepam	Paradoxical reactions
Kaopectate	Reye syndrome
Promethazine	Drowsiness and respiratory depression
Propofol	Propofol syndrome
Tetracyclines	Tooth discolouration

General management

Children rely on parents for protection from harm and for discipline. Accidents are the major cause of morbidity and mortality; children are at increased risk because of a need for strenuous physical activity, a desire for peer approval and increased adventurous behaviour. Continued emphasis upon wearing seatbelts remains the single intervention most capable of preventing major injury or death due to a motor vehicle accident. Children should be taught to play sports in appropriate, safe and supervised areas, with proper equipment and rules, and with safety equipment (such as a bicycle helmet and other safety helmets; knee, elbow, wrist pads/braces, etc.; Chs 24 and 33). Safety instructions regarding contact sports, vehicle use, swimming and water sports, matches, fires, lighters and cooking are important to prevent accidents.

Dental aspects

Care of children is discussed fully in textbooks of paediatric dentistry. Important issues include consent; the treatment of trauma, caries and malocclusion; and issues related to anaesthesia and sedation.

Informed consent can be difficult to ensure in children too young to understand but conversely may be possible in some children under age 16 (Gillick competence). Children may present behavioural challenges in dental treatment; relative analgesia and local anaesthesia (LA) may be difficult or impossible to administer to some. Some drugs are contraindicated in childhood (Table 25.6). Children may also have some unusual reactions to drugs, such as diazepam and intravenous anaesthetics.

Drug doses should be checked in the paediatric *British National Formulary* or equivalent, and adjusted for weight as necessary. Drug doses must be lowered for children and sugar-free preparations used.

After the eruption of the teeth, drugs that cause hyposalivation and procedures such as radiotherapy involving the salivary glands predispose to caries, especially in children. Preventive dental care and dietary counselling are of crucial importance.

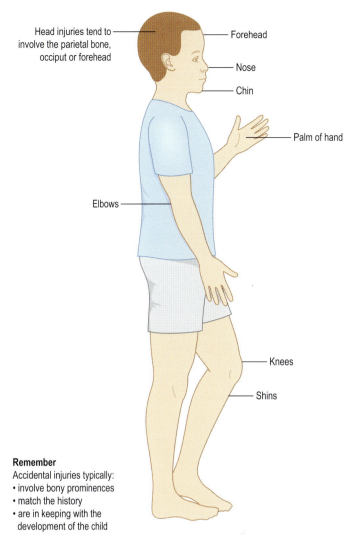

Remember
Accidental injuries typically:
- involve bony prominences
- match the history
- are in keeping with the development of the child

Fig. 25.1 Child non-abuse injuries.

Lengthening survival rates of premature infants have revealed several long-term sequelae, including orofacial defects. Some 20–55% have enamel hypoplasia, compared with 2% of controls, caused by birth trauma, infections and metabolic or nutritional disorders. Calcium disturbances are also common. Laryngoscopy can damage the unerupted maxillary anterior teeth and intubation with an oropharyngeal tube can cause grooving of the anterior maxillary ridge. The latter has few serious consequences.

Disturbed orofacial development can result from a range of causes in childhood, including radiotherapy, chemotherapy, drugs, infections or toxins. Disturbed odontogenesis can have similar causes. Children may also be the subjects of abuse, resulting in orofacial and other injuries.

CHILD ABUSE (BATTERED CHILD SYNDROME; NON-ACCIDENTAL INJURY, NAI)

General aspects of abuse are also discussed in Chapter 24.

General aspects

Up to 50% of children sustain injuries to their mouth by the time they leave school – mostly from accidents. The head and face are also the areas most commonly affected in physical abuse, however; they are involved in 65% of cases (Figs 25.1 and 25.2).

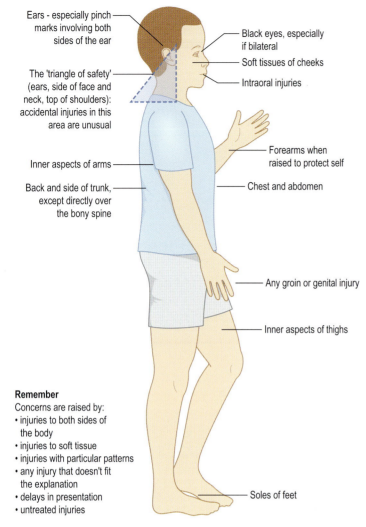

Ears - especially pinch marks involving both sides of the ear

Black eyes, especially if bilateral

Soft tissues of cheeks

The 'triangle of safety' (ears, side of face and neck, top of shoulders): accidental injuries in this area are unusual

Intraoral injuries

Forearms when raised to protect self

Inner aspects of arms

Chest and abdomen

Back and side of trunk, except directly over the bony spine

Any groin or genital injury

Inner aspects of thighs

Soles of feet

Remember
Concerns are raised by:
• injuries to both sides of the body
• injuries to soft tissue
• injuries with particular patterns
• any injury that doesn't fit the explanation
• delays in presentation
• untreated injuries

Fig. 25.2 Child abuse injuries.

Child abuse is any act of omission or commission that endangers or impairs the physical or emotional health or development of a child. The threshold beyond which actions or omissions become abusive or neglectful is, to a certain extent, socially and culturally defined. A child is considered to be abused if he or she is treated in a way that is unacceptable in a given culture at a given time. For example, physical punishment of children has become progressively less acceptable in the UK.

Abuse and neglect are described in four categories, as defined in the UK Department of Health's document 'Working Together to Safeguard Children'; these are physical abuse, emotional abuse, sexual abuse and neglect. Some level of emotional abuse is involved in all types of ill-treatment of a child, though it may occur alone. Physical abuse may involve hitting, shaking, throwing, poisoning, burning or scalding, drowning, suffocating or otherwise causing physical harm to a child. Physical harm may also be caused when a parent or carer fabricates the symptoms of, or deliberately causes, illness in a child.

Abused children are usually below 1 year of age; most are less than 3. The injuries are usually inflicted by an adult, usually a parent, parent's partner or an older sibling, and affected families are predominantly of socioeconomic classes IV and V. Causal factors may be related either to the parent, to social factors or to the child – and often all three (Table 25.7). Young or single parents, parents with learning difficulties, those who themselves have experienced adverse childhoods and those with mental health problems (including drug or alcohol abuse) are all more at risk of abusing their children. The assaulter may be supported by an

Table 25.7 *Non-accidental injury: associated factors*

Parental	Social	Child
Marital disharmony	Poor housing	Abnormal pregnancy or delivery
Emotionally deprived, abused themselves	Poverty	Neonatal separation
Chronic physical illness	Social isolation	Being unwanted
Low intelligence		Hyperactivity, illness or aggression
Young age or single parents		Being a stepchild
Drug/alcohol dependence		Age below 1 year
Mental disorders		

Box 25.2 *Findings suggestive of non-accidental injury*

• Cowed child
• Long interval before attendance for treatment
• Evidence of previous injury (or a previous history of injury)
• Injuries often committed at night
• Multiple injuries incompatible with history at unusual sites

inactive partner. Families living in adverse social environments – for example, due to poverty, social isolation or poor housing – may also find it both materially and socially harder to care for their children.

Children with disabilities are much more at risk of experiencing abuse of all kinds.

Clinical features

Recognition of child abuse is important since there is a very high risk of further assaults on, or death of, the child and of siblings; some 35–60% of physically abused children suffer further injury, with a 5–10% mortality rate. The child who has been subjected to abuse is often cowed, and may also be malnourished and generally neglected; there may be evidence of previous trauma. Psychological trauma from abuse can result in sleep disturbances, eating disorders, developmental growth failure in young children, and nervous habits such as lip- and fingernail-biting and thumb-sucking. Effects may also include chronic underachievement at school and poor peer relationships. In abusive families, physical neglect is commonplace, with inadequate provision of basic needs, including medical and oral health care; there may well be delay in seeking care (Box 25.2). Some suffer significant neurological, intellectual or emotional damage.

The injuries in child abuse can be varied and are often multiple, including bite marks (Ch. 24), bruises, black eyes, torn frenulum, hair loss, laceration, wheals, ligature marks, marks from a gag, burns and scalds, often from cigarettes or demarcated from other objects. Lacerations of the upper labial mucosa and tearing of the lip from the gingiva are found in about 45% of victims but are not diagnostic of child abuse.

Teeth may be devitalized, broken or lost. Bone fractures are common – mainly affecting ribs or long bones – but the skull and jaws can also be fractured. Head injuries are the commonest cause of death in abused children.

General management

After genuine accidents, children are usually taken immediately for medical or dental attention but, when children are abused, there is often considerable delay. Child abuse should also be suspected if any injuries are incompatible with the history and if any of the features in Box 25.2 are noted. Health-care professionals are obliged to know and follow the local child protection procedures (http://www.cpdt.org.uk/; accessed 30 September 2013). Full records must be kept. The child must be examined fully and immediately to exclude serious injury, especially subdural haematomas or intraocular bleeding, and must therefore be admitted to hospital. A skeletal radiographic survey should be undertaken to reveal both new and old injuries (osteogenesis imperfecta may need to be excluded). All injuries, including those to facial and oral tissues, must be carefully recorded, preferably with photographs.

Patients should be kept in hospital until the diagnosis is confirmed, since there is a high risk of further injury, which may be fatal. A paediatrician should be consulted and the general medical practitioner, social services and a child protection agency must be involved early on, but strict confidentiality must be observed. Social services departments keep registers of non-accidental injuries, which help identify known offenders. The child may already be on the 'at-risk' register. Dentists should also inform their medical defence society, as there may later be legal involvement.

Dental aspects

Orofacial lesions are common. Abuse or neglect may present in a number of different ways, such as through a direct allegation (sometimes termed a 'disclosure') made by the child, a parent or some other person; signs and symptoms that are suggestive of physical abuse or neglect; or observations of child behaviour or parent–child interaction.

SEXUAL ABUSE

Sexual abuse can take many forms but, in addition to physical and psychological injury, the victim may also acquire one or more sexually transmitted infection, including human immunodeficiency virus (HIV).

EMOTIONAL ABUSE

Emotional abuse is more difficult to define and prove, but can manifest as development delay, failure to thrive, a watchful 'radar' gaze, behavioural problems and limited attention span.

SELF-INFLICTED (FACTITIOUS) ORAL LESIONS

See Chapter 10.

OLDER PEOPLE

General aspects

Older people now account for some 15% of the UK population and this is set to increase. A growing proportion of the population, especially in developed countries, is over the age of 65 (a chronological criterion of 'elderly'), with a rise in the proportion of older females, a significant number of whom are single (Fig. 25.3).

Many older people enjoy *le troisième âge* but, over the years, they are increasingly likely to need health care (Table 25.8). Up to 75% have one or more chronic diseases (30% have more than three), 11% are housebound, 8% walk with difficulty and some 3% are bedridden. Mobility is one of

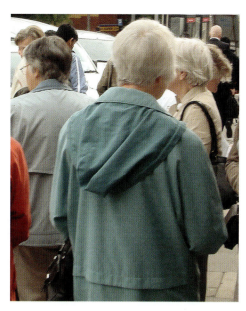

Fig. 25.3 The grey age (le troisieme age).

Table 25.8 *Approximate number of years that older people are likely to be free from disability*

Age group	Men	Women
65–69	9	11
70–74	7	9
75–79	5	7
80–84	3	5
85+	1	3

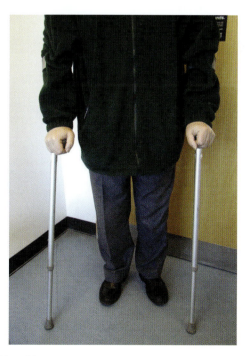

Fig. 25.4 Walking aids.

the major issues, and walking aids such as sticks, crutches and frames are commonly needed (Figs 25.4 and 25.5). Problems may be compounded if older people are from non-dominant populations (Fig. 25.6; see also Ch. 30). In the case of many older individuals, history taking can take considerable time; partners or care-givers may be able to help.

Medical problems

Many older patients have difficulty in accessing health care and some are reluctant to seek attention, especially if they fear consequent hospitalization. There is a greater incidence and severity of many diseases, especially arthritis and cerebrovascular disease, and these may cause ataxia and falls (Table 25.9). Alcohol related problems, mechanical and motor problems are important causes leading to falls among the elderly. Fractures and bruising may result, and senile purpura is common in many older people (Fig. 25.7). Defects of hearing or sight increase the liability to accidents, feelings of isolation and reduction of independence. The eyes may also show an arcus senilis (Fig. 25.8). Common causes of ataxia, faints and falls are visual impairment, transient cerebral ischaemic attacks, parkinsonism, postural hypotension (often drug-related), cardiac arrhythmias or ischaemic heart disease. Cancers are more common at advanced ages.

Atypical symptomatology is common; physical disease may present in a less florid and dramatic way in older people. Temperature regulation may be so disturbed that respiratory, urinary or even more serious infections often fail to cause fever. Older patients also readily become hypothermic, especially if thyroid function is poor. Many disorders in older patients also present with non-specific features, such as general malaise, social incompetence, a tendency to fall and mild amnesia.

Dementia becomes increasingly common with age. If responses are slow, it may be caused by underlying physical disease, especially if the

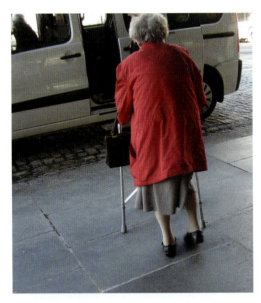

Fig. 25.5 Walking aids: frame.

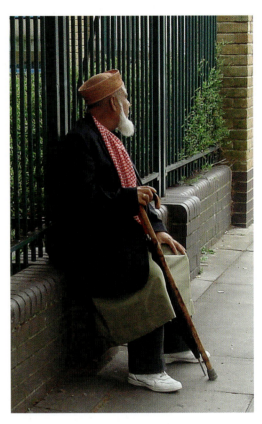

Fig. 25.6 Old age and culture.

Table 25.9 *Diseases especially affecting the older person[a]*

Blood and others	Cardiorespiratory	Genitourinary	Musculoskeletal	Neurological and psychiatric	Oral or predominantly oral
Accidents	Cardiac failure	Prostatic hypertrophy and cancer	Osteoarthritis	Acute confusional states	Atypical facial pain
Anaemia (especially pernicious anaemia)	Chronic bronchitis and emphysema	Renal failure Urinary retention or incontinence	Osteoporosis	Alzheimer disease	Candidosis (denture-induced stomatitis and angular stomatitis)
Cancer	Hypertension Ischaemic heart disease		Paget disease	Ataxia	Carcinoma
Chronic leukaemia	Pneumonia			Dependence on hypnotics	Herpes zoster and post-herpetic neuralgia
Myelodysplasia	Temporal arteritis			Insomnia	Lichen planus
Nutritional deficiencies				Loneliness and depression	Mucous membrane pemphigoid
					Pre-malignant lesions
				Multi-infarct (cerebrovascular) dementia	Sjögren syndrome
				Paranoia	Sore tongue
				Parkinson disease or parkinsonism	Trigeminal neuralgia
				Strokes	
				Visual impairment	

[a]Multiple conditions are common.

symptoms are of acute onset. A confusional state may result acutely from disorders as widely different as minor cerebrovascular accidents, respiratory or urinary tract infections, or left ventricular failure. Confusional states may be more chronic when caused by poorly controlled diabetes mellitus, hypothyroidism, carcinomatosis, anaemia, uraemia or drug therapy.

Social disabilities are common as a result of such causes as loss of the spouse, isolation from family, poverty, and lack of mobility and independence. Old people may need to be thrifty and careful with food purchasing and the heating of their accommodation, contributing to overall self-neglect. Nutrition may also be defective due to apathy, mental disease or dental defects. Malnutrition may, in turn, lead to poor tissue healing and predispose to ill-health. Deterioration in the senses of smell and taste may also result in a poor or unhealthy diet. Psychological disorders, such as loneliness and depression, may follow. Depression may also be a feature in hypothyroidism or a side-effect of medications.

Older people are more likely to be given medication and complications account for about 10% of admissions to geriatric units. Polypharmacy, abnormal reactivity towards many drugs, poor compliance, inappropriate treatment and deteriorating renal and other metabolic pathways affecting drug metabolism can result in toxicity and serious interactions. Older people tend to be more liable to adverse drug reactions, and the reactions tend to be more serious and last longer than in younger people.

Drugs may also precipitate or aggravate physical disorders that are more frequent in the older person. For example, drugs with antimuscarinic activity, such as atropine or antidepressants, may precipitate glaucoma, or may cause dry mouth or, if there is prostatic enlargement,

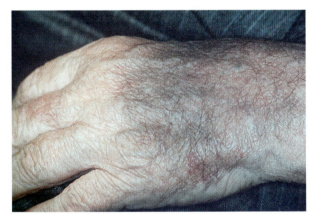
Fig. 25.7 Senile purpura.

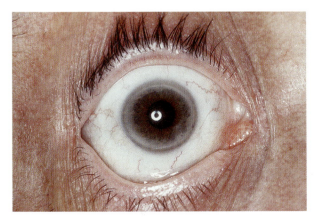
Fig. 25.8 Arcus senilis (corneal arcus).

urinary retention. Phenothiazines may precipitate or aggravate parkinsonism or hypotension, or may cause apathy, hypothermia, excessive sedation or confusion. Drowsiness, excessive sedation or confusional states may also be provoked by the benzodiazepines or tricyclic antidepressants, while depression and postural hypotension not uncommonly follow the use of hypotensive agents. Drugs should therefore be used cautiously (Table 25.10).

The capacity to carry out activities of ordinary life (dressing, eating, bathing, etc.) is assessed with specific tests: for example, the activities of daily living scale (ADLS) or Katz; based on this assessment, the older person is classified as functionally independent or dependent.

General management

Social support is crucial, preserving as much independence and dignity as possible.

Dental aspects

Many older people receive no dental attention whatsoever, despite much evidence of their need. It has been found in one study, for example, that 81% had oral lesions and 20% needed further investigation to exclude serious oral disease. Access to dental care can be a major difficulty for the person who is frail or has limited mobility. Handling of older patients may demand immense patience, but remember always to treat the older patient with sympathy and respect. It can take a long time for a patient in a wheelchair or using a Zimmer frame to get into the surgery and on to the dental chair. Domiciliary care may be more appropriate and avoids the physical and psychological problems of a hospital or clinic visit. Older people are often extremely anxious about treatment and should therefore be sympathetically reassured and, if necessary, sedated.

Mucosal lesions may be present in up to 40% of older people. Most of these are fibrous lumps or ulcers, but a minority are potentially or actually malignant lesions. Oral cancer is mainly a problem of older people and is a further reason for regular oral examination (Ch. 22). Atypical facial pain (often related to depressive illness), migraine, trigeminal neuralgia, zoster and oral dysaesthesias are more common as age advances.

Many older people with remaining teeth have periodontal disease. Dental caries are usually less acute but root caries are more common. Caries may become active if there is hyposalivation, especially if there is overindulgence in sweet foods. Hyposalivation is even more likely with medications such as neuroleptics or antidepressants (Ch. 10). Poor salivation may contribute to a high prevalence of root caries and oral candidiasis, which especially affect hospitalized patients.

Table 25.10 *Drug use in the older person*

	Problems	Possible solutions
Analgesics	Sensitivity to their effects	Restrict dose
Dosage regimens	Difficulties remembering regimens	Simplify regimens and write clear instructions; use dosette boxes
Drug dose	Overdose from sensitivity to agents	Restrict dose
Form of medicine	Difficulty swallowing tablets	Take with water or use liquid preparations
Non-prescribed drugs	Self-medication without medical advice	Restrict drug availability
Psychotropics	Sensitivity to their effects	Restrict dose

Very many older patients are edentulous and some problems of dental management are thereby greatly reduced. It seems, however, that the proportion of edentulous older patients is gradually falling and, as a consequence, more of them need restorative dentistry or surgery of various types. Many edentulous older people have little alveolar bone to support dentures, and have a dry mouth as well as frail, atrophic mucosa. Implants may be helpful. Inability to cope with dentures, or a sore mouth for any reason, or being unable to afford appropriate care readily demoralizes the older patient, and may tip the balance between health and disease.

Food can become tasteless and unappetizing as the result of declining taste and smell perception. Older patients should be encouraged to add seasonings to their food instead of relying on excessive consumption of salt and sugar to provide flavour.

The dentist therefore has an important role in supporting morale and contributing to adequate nutrition. Handling of older patients may demand increased time and patience.

Sound teeth should be conserved if they can serve, at least for a few years, as abutments or retainers for prostheses. It may also be unwise to alter the shape or occlusion of dentures radically when they have been worn for years. It is wise to label the dentures with the name of the patient, particularly for those living in sheltered or other residential accommodation, as dentures can easily be mislaid or mixed up between patients.

Attrition and brittleness of the teeth may complicate treatment, and it may be necessary to provide cuspal coverage in complex or large restorations. Endodontic therapy may be more difficult in view of secondary dentine deposition. Hypercementosis, brittle dentine, low bone elasticity and impaired tissue healing may also complicate surgical procedures.

The major goals of oral health care are preventive and conservative treatment for conditions such as hyposalivation, root caries, secondary caries, periodontal disease and gingival recession, and the elimination/avoidance of pain and oral infections.

Independent people with no serious medical problems may be treated in primary dental care. Dependent people may need domiciliary dental care with portable dental equipment. When significant medical problems are present, the older person may be best seen in a hospital environment, though this raises issues of adequate transportation and availability of escorts.

Prevention is of paramount importance in caring for older adults. Therefore, the most important considerations for dental professionals are how well the patient has compensated for his or her medical problem and the exact dental intervention needed. Non-invasive procedures in patients with minimal incapacity carry less risk than do surgical procedures. Older people tend to be more sensitive to drugs and to trauma. Dental treatment planning may be conditioned by factors such as oral health status, capacity to move, motor and mental skills to follow a preventive programme, survival prognosis and economic resources. The whole range of dental treatments may be considered. Dental implants are not at all contraindicated, and they may help to maintain the remaining alveolar bone.

Appointment times may be conditioned by systemic diseases. Sympathetic reassurance is indicated and, if necessary, sedation, with short-acting benzodiazepines. Treatment is often best carried out with the patient sitting upright, as few like reclining for treatment and some may become breathless and panic. Dentists should recognize that older people, especially women, also heal slowly and bruise readily if tissues are not handled carefully.

To control pain and anxiety, dentists should use LA whenever possible, since the risks of using general anaesthesia (GA) are greater than

---

Box 25.3 *Elder abuse*

- Most abuse is perpetrated against people who are over the age of 70
- Two-thirds of abuse is committed at home
- In nearly a half, two types of abuse occur simultaneously
- In one-third of cases, the abuse is perpetrated by more than one person
- Only rarely is the abuser the main family carer
- 46% of abusers are related to the person they are abusing; a quarter of those who are abusers are sons or daughters
- Staff in care homes or visiting carers may also abuse

---

in younger patients. LA used in recommended dosages has no effect on cardiac arrhythmias in the ambulatory older patient. Intravenous sedation in the dental chair is best avoided if there is any evidence of cerebrovascular disease, as a hypotensive episode may cause cerebral ischaemia. The risks of conscious sedation (CS) or GA are greater than in the young patient, not least because of associated medical problems. Relative analgesia is preferable to benzodiazepines for sedation, and benzodiazepines are preferable to opioids. GA may be necessary for patients unable to cooperate and those with dementia. After long operations, older patients are prone to pulmonary complications, such as atelectasis, deep vein thrombosis and pulmonary embolism; they may also become confused in an unfamiliar environment.

Polypharmacy should be avoided, not only because of the danger of drug interactions but also because of the practical difficulties that the patient may have in taking the correct doses at the correct times. Older people frequently have difficulties in understanding the medication and in remembering to keep to a regimen. Compliance may therefore be lacking. If there is hepatic or renal disease likely to impair drug metabolism or excretion, drug dosage must be reduced appropriately.

ABUSE OF OLDER PEOPLE

Elder abuse occurs when an older person is harmed, mistreated or neglected (see also Ch. 24). There are five types of elder abuse: psychological abuse, physical abuse, financial abuse, sexual abuse and neglect (Box 25.3).

People who are being abused are often scared that they will not be believed. Those who witness or suspect abuse may not want to be seen as 'interfering' or may be scared of 'getting it wrong'. If abuse is suspected, always talk to the 'victim' first and tell them what you want to do. The main charitable and government-sponsored organizations that can offer support to those affected include police, hospitals, general medical practitioners, carer organizations, social services/social work departments, and social care inspection bodies. Be clear about whether the person knows you are reporting your concerns; whether the older person is confused or lacks the capacity to make informed decisions about their life; who you think is being abused (name, address, age); and what you think is happening to that person. Give reasons/examples to illustrate why you think abuse is occurring. It helps if you can provide dates and times of incidents; what has been said; who you believe is responsible; and the relationship of that person with the older person.

See http://www.ageuk.org.uk/ (accessed 30 September 2013).

FACIAL COSMETIC PROCEDURES

Cosmetic facial procedures are increasingly used by both genders and include injections of botulinum toxoid (Ch. 13); removal of unsightly skin lesions; laser resurfacing; chemical peeling; or orthognathic

Table 25.11 *Facial cosmetic procedures other than use of orthognathic surgery or botulinum toxoid*

Common terminology	Alternative terminology	Intended outcomes	Comments
Brow lift	Forehead lift	Eliminate stern or furrowed brows	Multiple incisions within hairline or single incision in upper eyelids. Alternatively a wide incision across top of scalp
Ear surgery	Ear pinning or otoplasty	Correct protruding or deformed ears	–
Eyelid surgery	Blepharoplasty	Eliminate tired or droopy eyelids	Incision within upper eyelid
Face lift	Rhytidectomy	Eliminate facial signs of ageing, including wrinkles and sagging skin	Incisions within hairline, above temple and continued along or just inside ear, ending behind ear. A second incision beneath chin is sometimes necessary
Facial augmentation	Injectable fillers (see Table 25.12)	Change facial contours, lines and creases	Pharmaceutical filler or patient's own fat is injected below skin
Facial implants	–	Used most commonly in the cheek, chin, jaw or nasal region to change facial contours	Polyethylene[a], e- polytetrafluoroethylene (PTFE)[a], silicone[a], hydroxyapatite[a], collagen or injectables used. Incisions, if needed, are placed inside mouth or discreetly externally
Rhinoplasty	Nasal reshaping or nose job	Correct deviated septum, bump on the bridge, wide nostrils, bulbous tip or hooked nose	Incisions at nostril base and/or inside nose

[a]Usually non-resorbable.

surgery – and a range of other procedures, some of which are shown in Table 25.11. These are often performed as outpatient procedures under local anesthesia with or without sedation but general anaesthesia may be used. Outcomes may include pain, swelling, bleeding and bruising and infection. The resultant changes in appearance typically persist for months or sometimes years, notably where non-resorbable materials have been used. More worrying are the do-it-yourself "cosmetic" procedures becoming popular for example in Korea.

Fillers

Injectable fillers are an increasingly popular cosmetic procedure. Results are temporary, lasting a few months with natural products to several years when synthetic materials are used. Complications may include temporary pain, bleeding, bruising, swelling, seromas (fluid collections), infection or allergy; mainly with synthetic materials such as silicone, long-term granulomas/disfigurement are also possible. However, the existence of a so-called silicone immune toxicity syndrome is controversial.

The US Food and Drug Administration (FDA) reviews and approves pharmaceutical fillers in the same manner as medical devices. However, some fillers may be used on an off-label basis and injection of permanent substances (e.g. silicone) in particular poses safety issues such as granuloma formation (Table 25.12).

MEN'S HEALTH

The male genitals include the testes, vas deferens, epididymis and penis, together with accessory structures – the prostate and bulbourethral glands. The testes, located in the scrotum, produce sperm cells and the hormone testosterone, which influences development of body shape and hair, and regulates spermatogenesis. The anatomy of the male genital system is shown in Figure 25.9. Disorders of the gonads are outside the remit of this text.

There are some conditions that affect only men and there are gender differences in regard to patterns of many diseases (Box 25.4). Men generally also access and use health care differently from women (typically less); generally, they are less likely to react to health promotion and are more likely to have lifestyle habits that are detrimental to their health (e.g. alcohol or drug abuse).

Table 25.12 *Some fillers*

Origin	Material	Source
Natural	Collagen	Human or bovine natural skin protein
	Fat (free fat transfer, autologous fat transfer/transplantation, liposculpture, lipostructure micro-lipoinjection)	Human – typically from inner thigh or abdomen
	Hyaluronic acid	Human or animal
	Hydroxyapatite	Mineral suspended in a gel-like formulation
Synthetic[a]	Polyacrylamide	Hydrophilic polyacrylamide gel (HPG)
	Poly-L-lactic acid	
	Polymethylmethacrylate (PMMA)	20–25% PMMA microspheres in collagen gel
	Silicone	Dimethylsiloxane

[a]Usually non-resorbable.

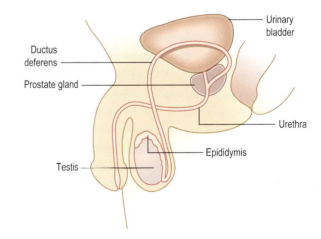

Fig. 25.9 Male genital anatomy.

BALANITIS (BALANOPOSTHITIS)

Balanitis is inflammation of the skin covering the glans penis. The most common cause is neglected hygiene and tight foreskin (phimosis), leading to irritation by smegma, but less common causes are shown in Box 25.5. Treatment depends on the underlying cause.

Box 25.4 *Health problems that are generally more common in men*

- Alcoholism
- Balanitis
- Bladder:
  - Stones
  - Cancer
- Drug abuse and addiction
- Hydrocoele and varicocoele
- Orchitis and epididymitis
- Peyronie disease
- Phimosis and paraphimosis
- Prostate:
  - Prostatitis
  - Benign prostatic hyperplasia
  - Cancer
- Snoring and obstructive sleep apnoea
- Testicular:
  - Torsion
  - Cancer
- Tinea
- Trauma

Box 25.5 *Causes of balanitis*

- Balanitis circinata (Reiter syndrome)
- Candidiasis
- Contact allergy (e.g. to latex)
- Diabetes
- Lichen sclerosis (balanitis xerotica obliterans; BXO)
- Seborrhoeic dermatitis and other skin diseases (e.g. lichen planus, psoriasis, erythema multiforme, erythroplasia of Queyrat – a rare, pre-cancerous skin condition)

BLADDER PROBLEMS

Urine passes from each kidney through the ureter to be stored in the bladder (Ch. 12). An outer muscle layer surrounds the bladder inner lining, which is made up of a uniform transitional epithelium resting on a thin basal lamina. When the bladder is full, the muscles can tighten to allow urination via the urethra.

Bladder stones

General aspects

Bladder stones are common in men, especially in those over 45. They can form in healthy individuals for no apparent reason. Bladder stones can also develop in gout or urinary infections, or if urine stagnates in the bladder as in prostatic hypertrophy. Most are formed of calcium, from excess salt in the urine (or too little water). Most bladder stones form within the bladder, but a few form in the kidneys and then travel to the bladder, causing acute pain or colic *en route* in the ureter.

Clinical features

Bladder stones may be symptomless, or cause frequency and urgency of micturition, pain when urinating or blood in the urine (haematuria). Problems arise when stones become too large to be flushed out during urination, particularly if they become trapped in the urethra, when they cause pain (dysuria) and difficulty passing urine. If left untreated, bladder stones can irritate the muscles of the bladder wall and lead to incontinence.

General management

Diagnosis is confirmed by ultrasound, intravenous urography or cystoscopy. Bladder stones usually need to be broken down during cystoscopy or by lithotripsy in order to flush them out.

Bladder cancer

General aspects

Bladder cancer is the fourth most common cancer in males and incidence is increasing; 90% are transitional cell and 8% are squamous cell carcinomas. Risk factors for bladder cancer include older age, male sex (men are 2–3 times more predisposed than women), a positive family history, and race (Caucasians are twice as frequently affected as Africans, with lowest rates in Asians). Important causes are carcinogens concentrated in the bladder – from cigarette smoking (raises risk by 2–3 times) or occupation (e.g. workers in rubber, chemical, leather, metal, print and textile industries, or hairdressers, machinists, painters or truck drivers), or from treatment with cyclophosphamide or arsenic. Infections – particularly schistosomiasis – may occasionally be implicated (Ch. 21). Factors *not proven* to play a role in the aetiology include coffee, chlorine in drinking water and saccharine, the sweetener that, in large doses, causes bladder cancer in animals.

Clinical features

The most common presentation is painless haematuria, but dysuria, urgency, polyuria and/or urinary obstruction may be seen. Such symptoms are also common in prostatic hyperplasia and carcinoma. Bladder cancer can invade to involve nearby organs such as the prostate (or uterus/vagina) and can metastasize to regional lymph nodes and to lungs, liver or bones.

General management

Malignant cells may be seen on urine cytology; intravenous urography may show a filling defect but cystoscopy and biopsy give the definitive diagnosis. Surgery is the common treatment; other options include transurethral resection (TUR) for superficial cancer, segmental cystectomy for localized cancer and radical cystectomy for more widespread disease. Radiation, intravesical chemotherapy or immunotherapy using intravesical bacille Calmette–Guérin (BCG) may also be used.

Dental aspects

Metastases may involve the jaws. Chemotherapy may cause mucositis.

CIRCUMCISION

Circumcision, a surgical procedure that involves partial or complete removal of the foreskin (prepuce), is a feature of both Judaism and Islam, and many African and New World cultures. About one-fifth of men worldwide have been circumcised, commonly soon after birth or at puberty. Circumcision may also be carried out for medical reasons, such as balanitis, phimosis or paraphimosis (when the foreskin forms a tight tourniquet around the glans, causing pain). Sexually transmitted infections that cause genital ulcers (syphilis, chancroid, herpes simplex) are more common in uncircumcised men. However, penile warts and urethritis are more common in circumcised men. Poor personal hygiene, smoking and exposure to human papillomavirus (HPV) are risk factors for penile cancer and that risk is not reduced by circumcision, but it does appear to reduce the risk of cervical cancer in women. Candidosis is equally common in circumcised and uncircumcised men. Views conflict as to whether circumcision can significantly reduce HIV transmission.

HYDROCOELE

A hydrocoele is an accumulation of fluid around the testis. Diagnosis is confirmed by transillumination and ultrasound. Most hydrocoeles in children resolve spontaneously and rarely cause discomfort. Most hydrocoeles in adults are persistent and therefore are usually managed by draining the fluid under LA, introducing a sclerosing agent to prevent recurrence. Alternatively, the hydrocoele can be removed surgically.

IRRITABLE MALE SYNDROME

Irritable male syndrome (IMS), sometimes called Padam or Del syndrome or late-onset hypogonadism (LOH), is a state of hypersensitivity, anxiety, frustration, and anger that occurs in older males ("grumpy old men"). It appears to be associated with changes in biochemistry, endocrines ("andropause"), stress, and identity. Testosterone substitution may be indicated but lacks controlled clinical trials on efficacy and safety.

ORCHITIS AND EPIDIDYMITIS

Sperm and hormones are produced in the testes and stored in the epididymis before being conveyed to the spermatic ducts (see Fig. 25.9).

Orchitis is an inflammation of testicular tissue. The mumps virus is a common cause. Orchitis causes pain in the scrotum (which may become hot and swollen) and fever; it can also result in infertility. Treatment is bed rest, a suspensory bandage and analgesics. All children are offered mumps vaccination when they are 12–15 months old.

Epididymitis is far more common than orchitis and usually arises from a bacterial urinary infection. Coliforms, pyogenic staphylococci and faecal streptococci are most often responsible, but infection may also be caused by *Chlamydia* or gonorrhoea; in many cases, no organism is identifiable. Symptoms may include fever and a hot, red and painful scrotal swelling; dysuria and frequency may be present. Bed rest, analgesics and antibiotics are indicated.

PEYRONIE DISEASE

This is the slowly progressive development of fibrous plaques around the corpora cavernosa of the penis, which mainly affects young adults and is of unknown aetiology. It causes bending to the affected side on erection. The condition may resolve but otherwise may require surgery.

PROSTATE DISORDERS

Prostatitis

Prostatitis is the most common prostate disease and accounts for up to 25% of all visits to general practitioners by young and middle-aged men with genitourinary symptoms. The types are shown in Table 25.13.

Prostatic hyperplasia

General aspects

The prostate almost invariably enlarges with age (benign prostatic hyperplasia or hypertrophy; BPH), possibly related to oestrogen or dihydrotestosterone (DHT) production, so that at least 50% of men in their sixties and as many as 90% in their seventies and above have symptoms.

Table 25.13 *Prostatitis*

Type	Comments	Therapy
Acute bacterial prostatitis	Fever, pain in the lower back and genital area, urinary frequency and urgency – often at night, burning or painful urination, and urinary infection	Antibiotics
Chronic bacterial prostatitis	Uncommon. Associated with an underlying prostatic defect, forming a focus for infection	Removal of the defect and use of antibiotics
Chronic prostatitis/ chronic pelvic pain syndrome	In the inflammatory form, urine and semen contain leukocytes but no bacteria; in the non-inflammatory form, no evidence of inflammation is found	Antibiotics
Asymptomatic inflammatory prostatitis	Semen contains leukocytes	–

Clinical features

An enlarging prostate constricts the urethra, causing a hesitant, interrupted or weak urine stream. The bladder hypertrophies and then begins to contract, even when it contains little urine, causing urgency, frequency, nocturia and leaking or dribbling. Urinary infections are also more common. The bladder may become distended and atonic, leading to overflow incontinence. Sustained raised intravesical pressure can cause hydronephrosis and renal damage. Acute urinary retention can be precipitated by alcohol, cold temperatures or immobility, and is an emergency.

General management

Investigations indicated may include a prostate-specific antigen (PSA) blood test and digital rectal examination (DRE), mid-stream urine (MSU), urine flow study, and blood urea and electrolytes. Cystoscopy should identify the location and degree of any obstruction and rectal ultrasound with biopsies may be indicated.

The level of PSA can rise in BPH, infection or prostate cancer, so the result should be interpreted with caution, as there is also a high rate of false positives and false negatives. Prostate cancer gene 3 (*PCA3*) is probably a more specific marker for prostate cancer (Ch. 22).

The symptoms of BPH may resolve without treatment in as many as one-third of mild cases, but if BPH causes major inconvenience or complications, treatment is recommended. Drug therapy includes finasteride or dutasteride (5-alpha-reductase inhibitors inhibit DHT production and shrink the prostate), saw palmetto (a herbal remedy possibly as effective as finasteride) or alpha-blockers (e.g. alfuzosin, doxazosin, indoramin, prazosin, tamsulosin or terazosin, which relax the prostate and bladder neck smooth muscle). Surgical treatment includes: transurethral resection of the prostate (TURP); transurethral microwave thermotherapy (TUMT); transurethral needle ablation (TUNA; delivers low-level radiofrequency energy with fewer side-effects compared with TURP); transurethral laser surgery (Nd:YAG lasers); transurethral incision of the prostate (TUIP); or open excisional surgery (prostatectomy).

Prostatic cancer

General aspects

Risk factors for prostate cancer include age (it mainly affects those over 55), family history of prostate cancer, ethnicity (more common in those of African descent), and diet and dietary factors (animal fat may possibly increase the risk, and diets high in fruits and vegetables may lower it; Ch. 22). BPH does *not* seem to raise the chances of contracting prostate cancer.

Clinical features

Early prostate cancer usually causes no symptoms but later features can mimic BPH or infection. These can include: urinary frequency, especially at night; difficulty starting urination or holding back urine; inability to urinate; weak or interrupted urine flow; painful or burning urination; difficulty in having an erection; painful ejaculation; blood in urine or semen; or frequent pain or stiffness in the lower back, hips or upper thighs.

General management

Investigations may include PSA, urinalysis for blood or infection, and a DRE. In some cases, blood prostatic acid phosphatase or PCA3 is helpful, especially if PSA results are positive. All men over 40 should have a DRE once a year to screen for prostate cancer. If results suggest cancer, a prostate biopsy is needed.

Prostate cancer can be managed by watchful waiting, surgery, radiation, chemotherapy or hormone therapy (androgen deprivation therapy [ADT] or androgen suppression therapy). ADT aims to reduce androgens (testosterone and DHT) by: orchidectomy (removal of the testes – the main androgen source); luteinizing hormone-releasing hormone (LHRH) agonists (leuprorelin [leuprolide], goserelin, buserelin, triptorelin), which prevent the testicles from producing testosterone; LHRH antagonists (abarelix); anti-androgens (e.g. flutamide, nilutamide or bicalutamide); or drugs to inhibit adrenal androgen production (e.g. ketoconazole and aminoglutethimide).

Dental aspects

Metastases occasionally involve the jaws and are typically osteosclerotic. Cancer chemotherapy may cause mucositis and immunosuppression.

TESTICULAR PROBLEMS

Torsion

Testicular torsion usually appears in teenage boys. The testicles hang loose in the scrotum and in rare cases they are twisted, obstructing their blood flow. Torsion presents with sudden pain and swelling of the scrotum. Urgent surgery is indicated and, to prevent recurrence, testicular fixation is performed.

Testicular cancer

Testicular cancer affects younger men, particularly those between ages 20 and 40, and is more common in Caucasians than those of African heritage. Most are seminoma, others are non-seminoma – a group which includes choriocarcinoma, embryonal carcinoma, teratoma and yolk sac tumours. Risk factors may include undescended testicle and age.

Clinical features

Testicular cancer usually affects only one testicle, presenting as a swelling, discomfort or feeling of heaviness in the scrotum/testicle, dull ache in the abdomen or groin, sudden collection of fluid in the scrotum, breast enlargement or tenderness, or unexplained fatigue.

General management

Diagnosis is confirmed with ultrasound and biopsy, and staging by computed tomography (CT) scanning. Treatments include radical inguinal orchidectomy, radiotherapy (seminomas respond well) or chemotherapy (the treatment of choice for widespread disease). Chemotherapy may affect sperm production but sperm can be frozen and preserved (cryopreservation) beforehand.

Varicocoele

A varicocoele is enlargement of the veins in the scrotum. It is most common on the left-hand side and may result in scrotal heaviness or pain and impaired fertility. In some cases, an operation can increase fertility.

WOMEN'S HEALTH

The ovaries are a pair of female reproductive organs located in the pelvis, alongside the uterus. They produce ova (eggs) and female hormones (oestrogen and progesterone), which influence the development of breasts, body shape and body hair, and regulate the menstrual cycle and pregnancy. Oestrogen stimulates uterine growth and development at puberty, thickens the endometrium during the first half of the menstrual cycle, and stimulates changes in breast tissue at puberty and childbirth. Progesterone, produced during the last half of the menstrual cycle, prepares the endometrium to receive the ovum. Every month, during the menstrual cycle, an ovum is released from one ovary (ovulation) and travels through the Fallopian tube to the uterus. If the egg is fertilized, progesterone secretion continues, preventing release of additional eggs.

Women generally live longer than men; there are gender differences with regard to patterns of many diseases and some conditions that affect only women (Box 25.6).

Women generally access and use health care differently from men (typically more) and generally react positively to health promotion. There has also been discrimination against women across cultures, and subordination and compromised dignity, and women more frequently suffer the consequences of domestic violence and/or sexual abuse than men.

Certain diseases that can have orofacial manifestations are especially common in women (e.g. anorexia nervosa/bulimia, atypical facial pain, burning mouth syndrome, facial arthromyalgia [temporomandibular joint dysfunction], pemphigus and pemphigoid, rheumatoid arthritis and Sjögren syndrome).

BACTERIAL VAGINOSIS

Bacterial vaginosis (BV) is a common condition due to an imbalance in the normal vaginal bacteria and is not usually a sexually transmitted infection. BV may be symptomless or characterized by a discharge with a fishy smell. It is diagnosed by microbiology and treated with oral metronidazole or with clindamycin vaginal cream.

CANCER

Breast cancer

General aspects

Other than skin cancer, breast cancer is the most common cancer among women and is more frequently found in white women than in those of African or Asian descent. The causes are not clear but most cases are seen over the age of 50, and the risk is especially high over age 60. Risk factors are shown in Box 25.7.

Box 25.6 *Some of the more common problems in women*

- Bacterial vaginosis
- Cancer:
  - Breast
  - Cervical
  - Ovarian
- Cystitis
- Eating disorders
- Endometriosis
- Female genital cutting
- Fibroids
- Osteoporosis
- Pregnancy-related disorders
- Menopausal disorders
- Sexual abuse

Box 25.7 *Risk factors for breast cancer*

- Personal history of breast cancer
- A positive family history: the risk doubles if a woman's mother or sister has had breast cancer, especially at a young age. Genes changes (*BRCA1*, *BRCA2*) increase risk (see Ch. 22)
- A diagnosis of atypical hyperplasia or lobular carcinoma *in situ* (LCIS)
- Oestrogen exposure
- Late childbearing (after about age 30)
- Early menarche
- Breast density
- Radiation therapy
- Alcohol
- A fatty diet
- Long-term use of combined oral contraceptives or hormone replacement therapy (HRT)
- High body mass index (BMI) and taller stature
- Higher social class

Clinical features

Early breast cancer rarely causes pain; more commonly, it may be detected on self-examination as a lump or thickening. Later, cancer may result in a change in breast size or shape, nipple discharge, tenderness or inversion, ridging or pitting (the skin looks like orange skin – *peau d'orange*), or a change in the way the skin of the breast, areola or nipple looks or feels (e.g. warm, swollen, red or scaly; Fig. 25.10).

General management

The current recommendation is 3-yearly screening from the age of 50 but, in cases of increased risk such as positive family history, screening may start earlier, with mammograms (Fig. 25.11). If an area of the breast looks suspicious on screening mammogram, diagnostic mammograms may be needed. Ultrasonography can then often help. Biopsy is generally needed – by needle or open biopsy.

Lobular carcinoma in situ (LCIS) refers to abnormal cells in the lining of a lobule, which seldom become invasive cancer. Tamoxifen, a hormone receptor blocker, is the usual therapy. Occasionally, women with LCIS may decide to have bilateral mastectomy to try to prevent cancer but most just have regular screening.

Ductal carcinoma in situ (DCIS or intraductal carcinoma) refers to abnormal cells in the lining of a duct, which are at greater risk of

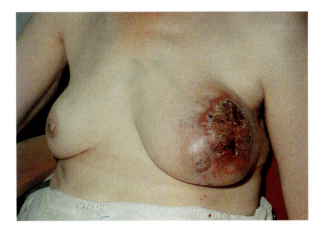

Fig. 25.10 Advanced cancer of the breast.

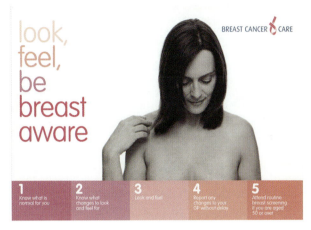

Fig. 25.11 Breast self-awareness.

invasive breast cancer. An association between >10 years of calcium-channel blockers use and a higher risk of ductal breast cancer has been reported. Treatments include breast-sparing surgery followed by radiation therapy or mastectomy, with or without breast reconstruction. Tamoxifen may reduce the risk of developing invasive breast cancer.

Breast carcinoma treatment most commonly involves surgery – usually a wide local excision with axillary node sampling or sentinel node biopsy. Histopathology results then dictate further treatment, which may be more radical surgery, or adjuvant radiotherapy plus or minus chemotherapy. Radiation therapy may lead to ischaemic heart disease and other cardiac conditions, including pericardial disease, peripheral vascular disease, cardiomyopathy, valvular dysfunction and arrhythmias. Treatment may include biological therapy. Hormone (oestrogen and progesterone) receptor tests can help determine whether a tumour is hormone-dependent. Oestrogen receptor (ER) and progesterone receptor (PR) tests help predict response to hormone therapy after surgery. Tamoxifen is the most common hormonal treatment used, usually for 5 years following the main treatment, and may cause hot flushes, vaginal discharge or irritation, nausea and irregular periods. Serious adverse effects are rare but tamoxifen can cause deep vein thrombosis and, in a few women, can increase the risk of uterine cancer or stroke. Anastrozole is a safer alternative in respect of stroke risk.

Human epidermal growth factor receptor-2 or *HER-2* may be associated with a higher risk for cancer recurrence. Trastuzumab – a monoclonal antibody that targets breast cancer cells having excess HER-2 – may be given alone or along with chemotherapy. HER-2 test results help predict response to trastuzumab, other anti-HER-2 treatments and

Table 25.14 *Oestrogen receptors/progesterone receptors and breast cancer*

Breast cancer	Receptor relevance
Newly diagnosed invasive	The cancer is classified as ER-positive (if the tumour has oestrogen receptors) or ER-negative (if the tumour does *not* have oestrogen receptors); PR-positive (if the tumour has progesterone receptors) or PR-negative (if the tumour does *not* have progesterone receptors); and HER-2–positive (if the tumour does have HER-2) or HER-2–negative (if the tumour does *not* have HER-2)
Node-negative	Patients with tumours that do not have urokinase plasminogen activator (uPA) and plasminogen activator inhibitor 1 (PAI-1) have a good prognosis and may not need chemotherapy
Node-negative and ER-positive and/or PR-positive	Oncotype DX test identifies patients who may be successfully treated with tamoxifen alone and may not need chemotherapy
Metastatic	ER and PR tests help predict response to hormone therapy. HER-2 test helps predict response to trastuzumab and other anti–HER-2 treatments. Cancer antigen (CA) 15-3, CA 27.29 and carcinoembryonic antigen (CEA) help monitor patients; these should be used along with the patient's health history, a physical examination, and diagnostic imaging tests such as radiography, bone scans, magnetic resonance imaging and computed tomography
Recurrent	HER-2 test helps predict the response to trastuzumab and other anti–HER-2 treatments, and guides the use of specific chemotherapy

Box 25.8 *Risk factors for ovarian cancer*

- Family history of ovarian, breast or colon cancer (see Ch. 22)
- Personal history of breast or colon cancer
- Age: risk grows as a woman gets older, with the highest risk over 60
- Fertility drugs
- Talc
- Hormone replacement therapy (HRT)
- Endometriosis

some types of chemotherapy (Table 25.14). Such therapy may include anthracyclines, and this and therapies targeting HER-2 can have a cardiotoxic effect. Advanced breast cancer may be treated with vinorelbine; capecitabine may be used for locally advanced or metastatic cancer.

Dental aspects

Metastases occasionally affect the jaws.

Cervical cancer

General aspects

Cancer of the uterine cervix is the most common genitourinary neoplasm and most often affects women over 40 years. It is most frequently found in sexually active persons and recognized to be associated with human papillomaviruses, particularly HPV-16 and HPV-18. Smoking, lower socioeconomic class and HIV disease increase the risk.

A vaccine for HPV-16 and HPV-18 has now been added to the immunization schedule and is given to girls of 12–13 years of age; there will be a catch-up programme for older girls.

Screening for pre-cancerous cells is carried out by a 'cervical smear' test – 3-yearly on women aged 25–50 and then 5-yearly until 64 years of age. The cells from the squamocolumnar junction in the cervical canal are then described as normal; mild dyskaryosis (cervical intraepithelial neoplasia 1 [CIN 1]; this may resolve spontaneously), moderate dyskaryosis (CIN 2) or severe dyskaryosis (CIN 3), sometimes referred to as carcinoma *in situ*.

Clinical features

Pre-cancerous changes of the cervix rarely cause pain. When cancer develops and invades, the most common manifestations are abnormal vaginal bleeding or abnormal vaginal discharge.

General management

Following pelvic examination and liquid-based cytology from brushings at routine screening, women with CIN 2 or 3 then undergo colposcopy and biopsy. Large loop excision of the transformation zone (LLETZ) may be carried out using diathermy, laser ablation or cold coagulation. A cone biopsy removing the entire transformation zone may be carried out and often the entire pre-cancerous area is removed in this way. Staging for cervical cancer includes a pelvic examination, cystoscopy and proctosigmoidoscopy. Other investigations include intravenous pyelography, barium enema, CT scan, ultrasonography and magnetic resonance imaging (MRI). Treatment for a pre-cancerous lesion depends on several factors, such as whether the lesion is low- or high-grade, whether the woman wants to have children, her age and general health, and her preferences. Treatment may be surgery, radiotherapy or chemotherapy, or a combination, depending on the stage. Simple local excision may be all that is required for early disease, whereas for more advanced disease a radical hysterectomy and excision of other involved tissues may be necessary. Radiotherapy may be given alone or with concurrent chemotherapy (e.g. cisplatin).

Dental aspects

Other than the fact that sexual partners and sometimes the patient can have a higher risk of oral cancer, cervical cancer is rarely of direct relevance to oral health. Metastases occasionally involve the jaws and cancer chemotherapy may cause mucositis.

Ovarian cancer

Most ovarian cancer is carcinoma but there are rare germ-cell tumours and cancers that begin in the stroma. The causes are unclear but risk factors are shown in Box 25.8.

Factors that reduce the risk include breast-feeding, use of combined oral contraceptives, a low-fat diet and childbearing (the more children a woman has had, the less likely she is to develop ovarian cancer).

Clinical features

Ovarian cancer often causes no symptoms or only mild symptoms until the disease is advanced but may include abdominal discomfort and/or pain; nausea, diarrhoea, constipation or frequent urination; anorexia; weight gain or loss; and abnormal vaginal bleeding. Fluid in the abdomen (ascites) may be seen when the cancer metastasizes to the peritoneum.

General management

Diagnosis is from pelvic examination together with ultrasound, CA-125 assay, radiography of the lower gastrointestinal tract, or barium enema, CT or MRI and biopsy.

Women at high risk due to a positive family history may consider prophylactic oophorectomy. Treatments for ovarian cancer include surgery (hysterectomy with bilateral salpingo-oophorectomy), chemo-therapy, or external or intraperitoneal radiation therapy.

Dental aspects

Metastases occasionally affect the jaws.

CYSTITIS

Genitourinary tract infections are particularly common in females, often ascending the short urethra from the vulva, frequently as a consequence of intercourse ('honeymoon cystitis'). Cystitis can ascend the ureter to cause pyelonephritis.

Bladder infections usually have little relevance for dental care, although the symptoms of cystitis may cause the patient to defer treatment for a few days. Such infections often suggest that the patient is sexually active and at risk from sexually transmitted diseases (Ch. 32). Cranberry juice (*Vaccinium macrocarpon*), popularly used to prevent cystitis, may enhance warfarin activity.

ENDOMETRIOSIS

General aspects and clinical features

Endometriosis is an enigmatic disease that affects women in their reproductive years, in which endometrium-like tissue is found outside the uterus, where it develops into nodules. Like the endometrium, the nodules usually respond to the menstrual cycle hormones. Tissue accumulates each month, breaks down, and causes bleeding, pain, infertility and other problems. Prostaglandins may cause many of the symptoms. Pregnancy often causes a temporary remission of symptoms, and mild or moderate endometriosis generally ceases after the menopause. About one-third of women with endometriosis are infertile and there is an increased frequency of malignancy in people with endometriosis.

Endometrial nodules occur typically in the abdomen, usually involving the ovaries, Fallopian tubes, outer uterine surface and pelvic lining.

General management

Diagnosis is generally confirmed by laparoscopy. Treatment has varied, with no certain cure. Hormonal treatments for endometriosis aim to suppress ovulation (oestrogen and progestogen, progestogen alone, a testosterone derivative [danazol] and gonadotropin-releasing hormone [GnRH]). Hysterectomy with oophorectomy has been considered a cure but there can be continuation/recurrence. Conservative surgery, either major or laparoscopic, involving removal or destruction of the nodules, can relieve symptoms and allow pregnancy to occur in some cases. Again, recurrences are common.

FEMALE GENITAL CUTTING (CIRCUMSCISION)

Female genital cutting (FGC) is the collective name given to traditional practices involving the partial or total cutting away of, or other injury to, female external genitalia, whether for cultural or other non-therapeutic reasons. FGC is practised predominantly in African, and also in some Middle Eastern cultures, typically being performed on girls between 4 and 12 years old.

FIBROIDS

Fibroids are benign tumours of uterine muscle fibres. Probably 20–50% of women have, or will have, fibroids but they are rare below 20 years

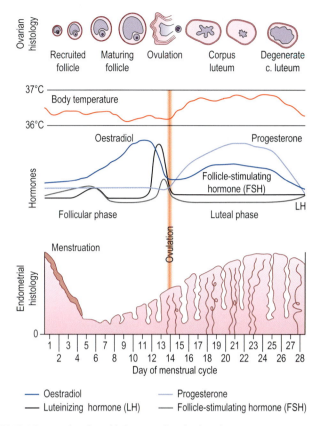

Fig. 25.12 Menstrual cycle, with hormonal and other changes.

of age. Fibroids occur up to nine times more often in black than in white women. The cause is unknown but fibroids seem to be influenced by oestrogen (which might explain why they appear during a woman's middle years, when oestrogen levels are high, and stop growing after the menopause, when oestrogen levels fall). Fibroids are often symptomless but the most common feature is heavy menstrual bleeding. Other symptoms include abdominal pain or pressure, changes in bladder and bowel function, and, in some cases, infertility.

MENSTRUATION AND PREMENSTRUAL ISSUES

Menstruation is the shedding of the endometrium that occurs on a regular basis in females of reproductive age (Fig. 25.12). Plasmin in the endometrium tends to inhibit blood clotting. Normal, regular menstruation lasts for about 3–5 days. The average blood loss during menstruation ranges from 10 to 80 mL and many women experience cramps (dysmenorrhoea) during this time. Premenstrual syndrome (PMS) is a symptom or collection of symptoms that occurs regularly in relation to the menstrual cycle. Usually, symptoms start five to eleven days before the onset of menses and resolve with menses or shortly after. Features may include mood swings, tender breasts, food cravings, fatigue, irritability and depression but can range from bloating to severe cramping and headaches. PMS tends to peak during the late 20s and early 30s and it can affect 75% of women. Treatments and lifestyle adjustments that can help include stress reduction, exercise and:

- Antidepressants
- Nonsteroidal anti-inflammatory drugs (NSAIDs)
- Diuretics
- Oral contraceptives or
- Medroxyprogesterone acetate (http://www.mayoclinic.com/health/premenstrual-syndrome/DS00134).

Table 25.15 *Common complaints in pregnancy*

Main trimester in which complaint occurs		
First	Second	Third
Breast tenderness	Aches and pains	Haemorrhoids
Dizziness	Stretch marks	Heartburn
Frequency of urination	Weight gain	Swelling
Haemorrhoids		Varicose veins
Leg cramps		Dizziness/fainting
Nausea and vomiting		Itching (pruritus of pregnancy or cholestasis of pregnancy)
Nosebleeds, nasal stuffiness		
Tiredness		Shortness of breath
Deepened pigmentation, particularly of the nipples and sometimes the face (chloasma)		Urinary incontinence
		Backache
		Pubic symphysis dysfunction

PREGNANCY

Pregnancy is extremely important to most mothers and families, and this is typically more so if it is the first pregnancy; if there have been previous pregnancy mishaps; if there have been conception difficulties; or if the mother is over about 35 years of age. Pregnancy is often associated with changes in cardiovascular, endocrine, haematological, respiratory, gastrointestinal and genitourinary systems, and can cause features such as nausea, vomiting, nasal congestion, heartburn, changes in taste and food craving, hyperventilation, shortness of breath, fatigue and tiredness. Sex hormones, prolactin and thyroid hormones rise but levels of luteinizing hormone (LH) and follicle-stimulating hormone (FSH) fall. Consequences may include deepened pigmentation, particularly of the nipples and sometimes the face (chloasma), and a rise in both blood volume and cardiac output, associated with tachycardia. Endocrine, cardiovascular, haematological and often mental (attitude, mood or behaviour) changes can be seen.

Variations in hormone levels result in changes that may include those shown in Figure 25.12. Pregnancy may be accompanied by a range of complaints (Table 25.15).

Cardiovascular disorders

Maternal cardiac output increases by 30–50%, with a heart rate increase of 20–30%. Women with high blood pressure values before the 20th week of gestation are assumed to have pre-existing hypertension, but any pregnant woman with a raised blood pressure should be referred to exclude development of pre-eclampsia (hypertension, proteinuria and oedema). Pre-eclampsia affects 5% of all pregnancies.

Blood pressure decreases while the patient is supine, especially in the second and third trimesters, due to decreased venous return to the heart from the compression of the abdominal aorta and inferior vena cava by the gravid uterus; hypotension, bradycardia and syncope characterize this supine hypotension syndrome. It can be relieved by tilting the patient 5–15° on to her left side. If this manœuvre does not work, a full lateral position should be taken.

Hypertension may be asymptomatic but, when associated with oedema and proteinuria (pre-eclampsia), may culminate in eclampsia (hypertension, oedema, proteinuria and convulsions); this, in turn, leads to greater morbidity and mortality in both fetus and mother. Pre-eclampsia or pre-eclamptic toxaemia (PET) may cause intrauterine growth retardation (IUGR), fetal death and extreme prematurity. It rarely occurs before 28 weeks but affects 5–10% of pregnancies. In the mother it can cause haemorrhagic stroke, eclamptic fits, renal or liver failure, or abruption, where the placenta separates from the uterus; this can result in intrauterine death of the fetus. Treatment involves bed rest, antihypertensives, close monitoring of both the mother and fetus, and possible early delivery.

In later pregnancy, up to 10% of patients may become hypotensive if laid supine, when the gravid uterus compresses the inferior vena cava and impedes venous return to the heart (supine hypotension syndrome).

Haematological disorders

Blood hypercoagulability can lead to venous thrombosis, particularly postoperatively, or occasionally to disseminated intravascular coagulopathy. The plasma volume increases significantly, without a corresponding increase in the red cell volume, thereby manifesting as anaemia. The number of white blood cells, erythrocyte sedimentation rate (ESR) and blood coagulation factors VII–X increase, and anti-clotting factors (XI and XIII) decrease, raising the risk of thromboembolism. Thus subcutaneous low-molecular-weight heparin may be indicated; this does not cross the placenta.

Pregnancy may worsen pre-existing anaemias, especially sickle cell anaemia. Deficiency anaemias may develop in about 20%, mainly because of fetal demands for iron and folate. Most pregnant patients are given both of these haematinics. Expansion of the blood volume may cause an apparent anaemia.

Gastrointestinal disorders

Progesterone increases cause nausea and vomiting in about two-thirds of pregnant women, beginning approximately 5 weeks after the last menstrual period and peaking between 8 and 12 weeks. Morning sickness occurs in most pregnant women, and it is best for them to avoid morning dental appointments. Decreased oesophageal sphincter tone, raised gastric pressure and slower gastric emptying may cause gastric reflux, heartburn and regurgitation. The patient should be advised to avoid citrus drinks or fatty foods and to prevent dehydration; frequent sipping of small volumes of liquid may help. Antacids and H_2 antagonists like ranitidine may ease symptoms. If vomiting occurs, procedures should be stopped and the patient repositioned upright.

Gestational glucose metabolism (GDM) disorder

Medical complications can include glycosuria and impaired glucose tolerance, which occasionally cause gestational diabetes. Disturbances of carbohydrate metabolism usually resolve after pregnancy. Diabetic control can be difficult, since insulin requirements rise; pregnant diabetics need specialist monitoring and care.

Gestational diabetes is similar to type 2 diabetes mellitus, in that it involves insulin resistance; oestrogens and progesterone, the hormones of pregnancy, cause insulin resistance in genetically predisposed women. Gestational diabetes occurs in nearly half of these women when pregnant and typically resolves with delivery of the child.

Two criteria, based on a 2-hour 75 g oral glucose tolerance test (OGTT), are used for the diagnosis of GDM: those recommended by the World Health Organization (WHO) and those recommended by the International Association for Diabetes in Pregnancy Study Group (IADPSG). They both identify women at a small increased risk for adverse pregnancy outcomes. Pregnancy hyperglycaemia that does not meet GDM diagnostic criteria affects a significant proportion of pregnant women and is also associated with a range of adverse pregnancy outcomes.

Interventions, including the provision of dietary advice and blood glucose level monitoring for women with pregnancy hyperglycaemia not meeting diagnostic criteria for GDM and type 2 diabetes mellitus, helped reduce the number of macrosomic and large-for-gestational age (LGA) babies without increasing caesarean section and operative vaginal birth rates.

Fetal issues

Fetal development during the first 3 months (trimester) of pregnancy is a complex process of organogenesis and the fetus is then especially at risk from developmental defects. The most critical period is that between the third and eighth weeks (mainly between 18 and 45 days of gestation). All pregnant women have a 3–5% chance of having a baby with a birth defect.

Most fetal developmental defects are of unknown aetiology but, in addition to hereditary influences, infections, alcohol, smoking, drugs (Table 25.16), deficiencies and irradiation can be implicated in some

cases. Folic acid supplements taken pre-conception and for the first trimester may minimize the risk of neural tube defects, such as spina bifida, and of facial clefts.

All drugs should be avoided in pregnancy unless potential benefit outweighs potential risks. Any woman of childbearing age is a potential candidate for pregnancy and may not be aware of pregnancy for 2 months or more, when the fetus is most vulnerable to damage. A total of 10–20% of all pregnancies abort at this time, often because of fetal defects. Alcohol, anticonvulsants, thalidomide and isotretinoin can be teratogenic. Even a single exposure to high alcohol intake can cause significant brain damage; more than 10% of children have been exposed to high levels of alcohol *in utero* and many suffer effects ranging from mild learning disabilities to major physical, mental and intellectual impairment (fetal alcohol syndrome [FAS]; Box 25.9). Nevertheless, very few therapeutic drugs have been proved to be teratogenic.

Table 25.16 *Known risks to the fetus of some drugs used in oral health care[a]*

Category[b]	No risk to fetus in animal model or human studies	Either safe to fetus in animal models without human data, or risk in animal models but safe in human studies	Risk to fetus in animal models but no human studies available, or no human studies support safety	Definitive human data demonstrating risk to fetus
Use systemically unless otherwise stated	*When desired (completely safe)*	*When necessary*	*Only if really essential and after consulting physician*	*Never*
Analgesics	–	Paracetamol (acetaminophen)	Codeine	Aspirin
		Pethidine (meperidine)	Diflunisal	Non-steroidal anti-inflammatory drugs (NSAIDs)[c]
			Mefenamic acid	Opioids
				Pentazocine
Antimicrobials	–	Azithromycin	Aciclovir	Dapsone
		Cefadroxil	Ciprofloxacin	Doxycycline
		Cefalexin	Clarithromycin	Minocycline
		Cefuroxime	Fluconazole	Tetracyclines
		Clindamycin	Itraconazole	
		Erythromycin	Ketoconazole	
		Loracarbef	Miconazole (unless topical)	
		Metronidazole		
		Penciclovir (cream)		
		Penicillins		
Local anaesthetic and vasoconstrictors	–	Lidocaine	Articaine[e]	–
		Felypressin	Bupivacaine	
		Prilocaine[d]	Mepivacaine	
Sedatives	–	Promethazine		Benzodiazepines[e]
				Nitrous oxide[f]
Others	–	–	Corticosteroids (even topical)	Antidepressants
			Epsilon aminocaproic acid	Carbamazepine
			Tranexamic acid	Colchicine
				Danazol
				Gabapentin
				Oxcarbazine
				Phenytoin
				Povidone–iodine
				Retinoids
				Thalidomide
				Warfarin

[a]It is advisable to restrict use to the second or third trimester; see also Appendix 25.1.
[b]US Federal Drug Agency (FDA) pregnancy categories.
[c]May be safer in first and second trimesters.
[d]Prilocaine can cause methaemoglobinaemia.
[e]Sometimes categorized as either safe to fetus in animal models without human data, or risk in animal models but safe in human studies.
[f]Nitrous oxide, though able to interfere with vitamin B_{12} and folate metabolism, does not appear to be teratogenic in normal use, though it is advisable to restrict use to the second or third trimester.

- Asthma
- Attention deficit disorder/attention deficit hyperactivity disorder (ADD/ADHD)
- Autistic traits
- Behavioural problems
- Central auditory processing disorder
- Cerebral palsy
- Cleft palate
- Cognitive perseveration
- Complex seizure disorder
- Deafness
- Death
- Dental abnormalities
- Depression
- Developmental coordination disorder
- Developmental delay
- Developmental speech and language disorder
- Dyslexia
- Echolalia
- Epilepsy
- Extreme impulsiveness
- Heart defects
- Heart failure
- Height and weight deficiencies
- Higher than normal pain tolerance
- Immune defect
- Learning disability
- Little or no capacity for interpersonal empathy
- Little or no capacity for moral judgment
- Little or no retained memory
- Loss of intellectual functioning (IQ)
- Mild to severe vision problems
- Night terrors
- Poor judgment
- Precocious puberty
- Reactive outbursts
- Renal failure
- Rigidity
- Serious maxillofacial deformities
- Severe loss of intellectual potential
- Sleep disorder
- Social problems
- Sociopathic behaviour
- Suicide
- Tourette's traits
- Tremors

Aspirin and other non-steroidal anti-inflammatory drugs (NSAIDs) may cause closure of the ductus arteriosus *in utero* and fetal pulmonary hypertension, as well as delaying or prolonging labour, and therefore are contraindicated in the third trimester. Aspirin, in addition, causes a platelet defect and may induce abortion; it is best avoided throughout pregnancy. Corticosteroids can suppress the fetal adrenals and, if given, steroid cover is needed for labour. Tetracyclines stain developing teeth.

Serious damage to the fetus or child can also be caused by maternal tobacco-smoking during or after pregnancy. Smoking increases the risk of stillbirth, low birth weight and impaired mental and physical development. Smoking by either parent after the child's birth increases the child's risk of respiratory tract infection, asthma and sudden death.

Oral disease

In some pregnant women, gingivitis is aggravated (pregnancy gingivitis) or may even result in a pyogenic granuloma at the gingival margin (pregnancy epulis). These conditions typically arise after the second month and resolve on parturition. Pyogenic granulomas elsewhere may grow rapidly during pregnancy. Chronic periodontal disease in the mother has been linked with babies of low birth weight. About half of pregnant women experience gingivitis due to increased oestrogen and progesterone, which can progress to periodontitis. This typically begins in the second or third month of pregnancy.

In a few women subject to recurrent aphthae, ulcers may stop (or occasionally become more severe) during pregnancy.

Oral health care in pregnancy

There are concerns on the part of patients and health professionals about oral health care in pregnancy but pregnant patients are not medically compromised and should not be denied dental treatment simply because they are pregnant. Performing oral health interventions has not been found to be associated with an increased risk to the developing fetus. A study of 823 pregnant women at 13–21 weeks' gestation found that scaling and root planing for periodontitis, using local anaesthetics as needed, did not increase adverse fetal outcomes; however, it did lower preterm birth rates. Additionally, a randomized controlled trial of 870 women with pregnancy-associated gingivitis found that treatment (i.e. plaque control, scaling, and daily rinsing with chlorhexidine) and maintenance (i.e. oral hygiene instruction and manual supragingival plaque removal every 2–3 weeks until delivery) significantly reduced the rate of preterm births or low birth weight (LBW). Conversely, adverse pregnancy outcomes, such as LBW, preterm birth and pre-eclampsia, may occur in women who have not received oral health care.

Good oral health during pregnancy is important to the overall health of both mothers and their babies. Pregnancy is the ideal opportunity to begin preventive dental education and to advise on fluoride administration to the infant. Prenatal fluorides are not indicated, as there is little evidence of benefit to the fetus. The teeth do not, of course, lose calcium as a result of fetal demands and there is no reason to expect caries to become more active unless the mother develops a capricious desire for sweets.

As much treatment as possible should be postponed until after parturition in those with a history of abortions and those who have achieved pregnancy after years of failure to conceive. During the first trimester, the only safe course of action is to protect the patient as far as possible from infections and to avoid the use of drugs (particularly GA) and radiography. In the second and third trimesters, the fetus is growing and maturing but can still be affected by infections, drugs and possibly other factors. Nevertheless, dental treatment is best carried out during the second trimester, though advanced restorative procedures are probably best postponed until the periodontal state improves after parturition and prolonged sessions of treatment are better tolerated. In the third trimester, the supine hypotension syndrome may result if the patient is laid flat. She should therefore be put on one side to allow venous return to recover. Some pregnant women also have a hypersensitive gag reflex.

Elective dental care should be avoided in the last month of pregnancy, as it is often uncomfortable for the patient. Moreover, premature labour or even abortion may also be ascribed, without justification, to dental treatment. Oral health care under any circumstance should take account of the following cautions.

Table 25.17 *Drug use in pregnancy in dentistry*

Drug	Safe	Unsafe/caution
Anxiolytics	None	Alprazolam
		Diazepam
Local anaesthetics	Articaine	Bupivacaine
	Lidocaine	
	Prilocaine	
Analgesics	Ibuprofen (first and second trimesters)	Aspirin
		Diclofenac
	Paracetamol (acetaminophen; all trimesters)	Ibuprofen (third trimester)
		Mefenamic acid
		Naproxen
Antifungals	Fluconazole	Ketoconazole
	Miconazole	
	Nystatin	
Antibacterials	Azithromycin	Aminoglycosides
	Cephalosporins	Co-trimoxazole
	Clindamycin	Metronidazole
	Erythromycin	Sulphonamides
	Penicillin group	Tetracyclines

analgesics are concerned, paracetamol (acetaminophen) is considered safe in all three trimesters of pregnancy but for short-term usage only. Some NSAIDs are to be avoided in all trimesters of pregnancy, while some are contraindicated in specific trimesters. NSAIDs can also cause gastrointestinal complications in the mother. Ibuprofen is considered a risk in the first trimester and is definitely contraindicated in the last trimester, as it may cause prolonged labour, haemorrhage, premature closure of ductus arteriosus and fetal pulmonary hypertension. Aspirin is safe but there is a risk associated with use of higher doses in the first and third trimesters, and it may cause constriction of ductus arteriosus, prolong gestation and delay labour.

Infections in pregnancy should be treated at the earliest opportunity. Preferred antibacterials are penicillins (amoxicillin and ampicillin) and cephalosporins (oral – cefalexin; parenteral – cefotaxime and ccftriaxone). If the patient is allergic to penicillin, then erythromycin (stearate salt only), azithromycin or clindamycin can be used. Tetracyclines are contraindicated, as they can cause bone and dental staining and anomalies in the fetus, as well as occasional maternal liver toxicity. Metronidazole is contraindicated in the first trimester.

Topical antifungals – nystatin and miconazole – are considered safe in pregnancy, but ketoconazole may cause adrenal insufficiency and hepatotoxicity, and therefore should be avoided. Fluconazole is an alternative but is not safe in the first trimester.

Anaesthesia and sedation

Unnecessary drugs should be avoided (Tables 25.16 and 25.17; Appendix 25.1) and, because of the risk of coincidental mishaps, it is wise to try to avoid giving any potent drugs. LA is probably overall safe, though all LAs cross the placenta to some degree. Highest concentrations in the fetal circulation follow prilocaine injection and the lowest follow bupivacaine, while lidocaine gives intermediate levels. Lidocaine and prilocaine are safe for use in most pregnant women. The vasoconstrictor adrenaline (epinephrine), when used in low concentration in LA, does not cause fetal harm. Felypressin is a vasopressin derivative related to oxytocin and may have the potential to cause uterine contractions, although this is highly unlikely; nevertheless, felypressin is best avoided.

GA, and sedation with midazolam or diazepam, should be avoided in the first trimester and in the last month of the third trimester of pregnancy. Nitrous oxide, though able to interfere with vitamin B_{12} and folate metabolism, does not appear to be teratogenic, though it is advisable to restrict use to the second or third trimester, limit the duration of exposure to below 30 minutes, use 50% oxygen, avoid repeated exposures, and use scavenging in the dental surgery to minimize staff exposure.

When GA is unavoidable and there is a mishap to the fetus, the mother is likely to blame the anaesthetist, even though this may be quite unjustifiable. Yet another hazard is a greater tendency to vomit during induction in the third trimester. Despite such considerations, there is scanty evidence of teratogenic effects in humans from exposure to GA agents. The greater risk is late in pregnancy, when GA may induce respiratory depression in the fetus. As always, GA must be given in hospital. Anxiolytics, such as alprazolam and diazepam, are contraindicated in pregnancy owing to reports of fetal developmental anomalies.

Drugs

Certain drugs can cause miscarriage, teratogenicity and babies of low birth weight. The decision to administer a specific drug requires the benefits to outweigh the potential risks of the drug therapy. As far as

Amalgams

Dental amalgam restorations release mercury vapour when teeth are chewed on or brushed, or the restorations are removed; some of this is inhaled, and some may dissolve in saliva and be swallowed. Most mercury entering the body is excreted, although a small amount accumulates in the kidneys and, to a very much lesser extent, in brain, lungs, liver and gastrointestinal tract. Mercury can cross the placenta to the fetus and the number and surface areas of amalgam fillings in the mother increase mercury concentrations in amniotic fluid; levels are low, however, and there are no proven adverse outcomes in pregnancies or newborns. Mercury can also be detected in breast milk. However, there is no evidence of any link between amalgam use and birth defects or stillbirths. A case-control study of 1117 LBW infants found no association between low birth weight and placement of amalgam during pregnancy. In a database study, there was no association of cumulative amalgam exposure in 1062 births categorized as having 'complications of pregnancy and childbirth'. Study of dental personnel in Norway, a group with possible previous exposure to mercury vapour, showed they had no excess risk of having children with congenital malformations or other adverse pregnancy outcomes compared to the general population.

Hydrogen peroxide, a common bleaching agent, can increase mercury release, so avoidance should be considered.

Generally, it is wise to minimize any health interventions during pregnancy. Although there is no reason to think that the placement or removal of amalgam during pregnancy is harmful, under ideal circumstances amalgams should not, if possible, be placed or removed during pregnancy. This is in spite of the fact that studies and case reports of amalgam exposure during pregnancy have not documented toxicity, including birth defects, neurological sequelae, spontaneous abortions or reduction in fertility.

Imaging

Ultrasound appears to be safe in pregnancy. MRI is probably best avoided during the first trimester. Radiography should also be avoided, especially in the first trimester, even though dental radiography is unlikely to pose a significant risk. Ionizing radiation (X-ray) is composed of high-energy photons that are capable of damaging DNA and generating free radicals. A patient's dose of photons is measured in grays (Gy) and the rem, or in the older and more commonly recognized unit, the rad. The estimated fetal dose from dental radiograph is about 0.0001 rad for about 50 000 examinations. Fetal risk is considered to be negligible at 5 rad or less when compared to the other risks of pregnancy, and the risk of malformations is significantly increased above control levels only at doses above 15 rad. Radiation exposures of greater than 500 mGy are known to cause fetal damage.

Radiation (X-ray) doses of less than 5 rad are not associated with increased congenital malformations; therefore, dental X-rays, which give a fetal dose in a single dental exposure of 0.01 mrad, should not be cause for concern. A UK epidemiological study of a cohort of 7375 mothers did not find a significant association between the use of dental X-ray scans and LBW or preterm delivery. A case-control study found no overall increased risk of childhood brain tumour after exposure to prenatal abdominal X-rays, which produce many times higher radiation exposure than dental X-rays.

The most sensitive period for inducing developmental abnormalities is in the first trimester, and the most vulnerable period for radiation-induced central nervous system damage is 8–15 weeks after conception. Adverse fetal effects associated with radiation exposure include small head size, intellectual deficits or induction of childhood malignancies. Therefore, the radiation risk depends upon gestational age at the time of exposure, fetal cellular repair mechanisms and the absorbed radiation dose level. Even though the exposure dose for full-mouth dental radiographs (0.25 microGy) is negligible and unlikely to cause any abnormalities to the fetus, it is absolutely essential for the dentist to ensure that the pregnant patient avoids the smallest unnecessary dose of radiation.

Dental professionals should have a clear perception of the risks and benefits of performing radiographic studies during pregnancy; radiographs must not be requisitioned unless absolutely necessary and retakes must be avoided. Protective measures, such as high-speed films (E/F speed) and rectangular collimation, should help keep the dose to a minimum. Current guidelines are that exposure must be minimal but a lead apron is unnecessary, unless the beam is directed at the fetus, such as in vertex-occlusal radiography. It has been estimated that two periapical dental X-rays give an exposure less than that which can be ascribed to natural radiation for 1 day.

Hazards to pregnant dental staff

Exposure to infections such as rubella or herpesviruses should be minimized or avoided.

Nitrous oxide scavenging must always be used and some pregnant staff exempt themselves from work involving GA or sedation.

Concern has been expressed, particularly in Sweden, about the risk of placental transfer of mercury as a result of exposure to the metal during pregnancy. However, measurements on female dental personnel, their newborn babies and non-exposed controls have shown no significant differences in plasma mercury levels or in fetal/maternal ratios of mercury levels. Female dental personnel had no observed increased occurrence of:

- congenital malformations (including malformations of the CNS)
- dysplasia of the hip, clubfoot, or malformations of the heart and great vessels

- low birth weight, preterm birth, babies that were small for gestational age, or changed gender ratio
- multiple birth, stillbirth or prenatal death.

On a group level, there was no excess risk of congenital malformations or other adverse pregnancy outcomes among female dental personnel in Norway during 1967–2006 compared to the general population. Experimental and clinical data do not suggest that there should be any restriction on use of amalgams by or work restriction of pregnant dental professionals, provided that work practices are up to accepted standards.

Lactation and breast-feeding

The two main contraindications to breast-feeding are mothers who are HIV-positive or have AIDS, or who are taking drugs/medicines that are contraindicated. Drugs may pass from mother to fetus in the breast milk, and thus care should be taken in their use (see Box 25.9 and Table 25.17). Various drugs can affect infants (see Appendix 25.2).

The National Institute for Health and Care Excellence (NICE) states (2008, www.nice.org.uk/nicemedia/pdf/ph011guidance.pdf; accessed 30 September 2013) that health-care professionals who prescribe or dispense drugs to a breast-feeding mother should consult supplementary sources (e.g. the Drugs and Lactation Database [known as LactMed; http://toxnet.nlm.nih.gov/cgi-bin/sis/htmlgen?LACT; accessed 30 September 2013]) or seek guidance from the UK Drugs in Lactation Advisory Service (www.ukmicentral.nhs.uk/drugpreg/guide.htm; accessed 30 September 2013). They should discuss the benefits and risks associated with the prescribed medication and encourage the mother to continue breast-feeding, if it is reasonable to do so. If drugs are essential, they should preferably be taken by the mother immediately after breast-feeding, so the milk levels of the drug are as low as possible at the next feed. Cefalexin is a useful antimicrobial, as it is not secreted in the milk.

Fluoride passes into breast milk and, if the local water supply contains more than 1 mg/L fluoride, supplements are not indicated for the breast-fed infant.

Drugs contraindicated in breast-feeding

These are shown in Table 25.18.

Infertility

Around one couple in six in the UK is affected by infertility. Main treatments include;

- Artificial insemination (Intrauterine insemination [IUI]); involves directly inserting sperm into a woman's uterus (womb).
- In vitro fertilisation (IVF); an egg is fertilised by sperm outside the body.
- Intra cytoplasmic sperm injection (ICSI); a single sperm is injected into an egg.

However, there are many treatment options as shown in Box 25.10.

THE MENOPAUSE

General aspects and clinical features

The menopause – marked by cessation of menstrual periods – can start at any age between 40 and 55 years. Menopause is the permanent end of menstruation and fertility, defined as occurring 12 months after the last menstrual period, and may give rise to physical and emotional

Table 25.18 *Drugs that may be used in dentistry but are contraindicated in breast-feeding mothers, with alternatives*

Drug group	May be contraindicated	Possible alternatives
Analgesics	Aspirin (high-dose)	Aspirin (low-dose) or paracetamol (acetaminophen)
	Dextropropoxyphene	Codeine or paracetamol (acetaminophen)
	Diflunisal	Diclofenac or paracetamol (acetaminophen)
	Indometacin	Mefenamic acid or paracetamol (acetaminophen)
Antimicrobials	Tetracyclines	Erythromycin
	Aminoglycosides	Cephalosporins
	Co-trimoxazole	Penicillins
	Fluconazole	Nystatin or miconazole topically
	Itraconazole	Nystatin or miconazole topically
		Ganciclovir
	Metronidazole	
	Sulphonamides	
Pre-medication	Atropine	Benzodiazepines (low-dose)
	Chloral hydrate	Phenothiazines (low-dose)
		Beta-blockers
Others	Antidepressants	
	Barbiturates	
	Etretinate	
	Carbamazepine	
	Corticosteroids (high-dose)	
	Povidone–iodine	

Table 25.19 *Marketed herbal alternatives to hormone replacement therapy*

Reported possible benefit		No reported benefit
Herbal alternatives	**Comments**	
Soy and isoflavones (plant oestrogens in beans, particularly soybeans)	Helpful short-term to relieve hot flushes and night sweats. May be harmful to women with oestrogen-dependent breast cancer	Chasteberry (monk's pepper, Indian spice, sage tree hemp or tree wild pepper), dong quai, evening primrose, ginseng, valerian root, wild and Mexican yam
Black cohosh	Helpful short-term (6 months or less) for hot flushes and night sweats	

Box 25.10 *Fertility treatment options*

Assisted hatching
Cycle monitoring
Donor insemination
Egg donation
Embryo cryopreservation
Frozen embryo replacement cycle
Gamete intra fallopian transfer (GIFT)
In-vitro fertilisation (IVF)
Intra cytoplasmic sperm injection (ICSI)
Intra-uterine insemination
Micro epididymal sperm aspiration
Open testicular biopsy with microsurgical techniques
Ovulation Induction – Clomifene Citrate
Parental induction of ovulation
Percutaneous epididymal sperm aspiration
Testicular epididymal sperm extraction
Zygote intra-fallopian transfer (ZIFT)

symptoms. Menopause is a natural process but may be premature if there is hysterectomy/oophorectomy/ovariectomy; radiotherapy; chemotherapy; or primary ovarian dysfunction Although rarely associated with serious physical or other complications, some women in the menopause gain weight, lose muscle tone, develop a few hairs on the chin or upper lip or have hot flushes. These appear to be caused by vasomotor instability, and may sometimes be controlled by hormone replacement therapy (HRT) typically with oestrogens. The menopause is frequently associated with emotional disturbances and stresses, often due to the changes in the pattern of family life around that time. Psychological disorders are not uncommon but are usually mild (e.g. dizziness and insomnia); however, depression or paranoia may develop. CBT and antidepressants may be called for (Ch. 10).

Osteoporosis is more common (Ch. 16); HRT slows its development and reduces the risk of fractures.

General management

HRT is replacement of reduced oestrogen secretion after menopause or oophorectomy, with oestrogens taken orally, via a patch on the skin or implanted; or with oestrogens plus progestogens (progestin). Tibolone, a steroid with oestrogenic, progestogenic and androgenic activities, has the same licensed applications. HRT is used mainly for the benefits it confers for short-term relief of menopausal symptoms and prevention of osteoporosis. There may also be benefits from reduced colorectal cancer. Adverse effects of HRT may include a predisposition to deep vein thrombosis, stroke and coronary heart disease, and an increase in breast, and possibly ovarian and endometrial cancers.

Consideration of the risks and benefits of HRT has concluded that it is beneficial but that the combined HRT involving oestrogen plus progestogen may cause more harm than good. Alternatives to HRT are shown in Table 25.19. Bisphosphonates, along with calcium and vitamin D supplements, can also be used to minimize osteoporosis (Ch. 16).

Dental aspects

LA is satisfactory. CS can be given if required. GA must, as always, be carried out in hospital.

HRT appears to lessen alveolar bone and tooth loss, as well as gingival bleeding, in older women, and improves salivary flow and buffering capacity. Overall, however, HRT appears not to improve complaints such as oral discomfort. Adverse effects from bisphosphonates are discussed in Chapter 16.

Atypical facial pain and oral dysaesthesias are particularly common but there is little evidence of benefit from use of steroid sex hormones.

Dryness of the mouth and desquamative gingivitis are more common in middle-aged or older people, and particularly in females, but are not hormonal – rather immunological – in origin. Sjögren syndrome, lichen planus and mucous membrane pemphigoid are simply more common at this age.

TRANSGENDER

Transgender is the state of gender identity (self-identification) not matching one's 'assigned sex' (identification by others as male or female, based on physical features or genetic make-up) and does not imply any specific form of sexual orientation (http://en.wikipedia.org/wiki/Transgender; accessed 30 September 2013).

IMPLANTS

Antimicrobial prophylaxis for dental treatment is usually unwarranted for people having breast or penile implants/augmentations (http://www.cda-adc.ca/jcda/vol-72/issue-7/619.pdf; accessed 30 September 2013).

KEY WEBSITES

(Accessed 29 May 2013)
Centers for Disease Control and Prevention. <http://www.cdc.gov/aging/disparities/index.htm>
National Institutes of Health: Disability in older adults. <http://report.nih.gov/nihfactsheets/ViewFactSheet.aspx?csid=37>
National Institutes of Health: Men's health. <http://health.nih.gov/category/MensHealth>
National Institutes of Health: Women's health. <http://health.nih.gov/category/WomensHealth>
NHS Choices. <http://www.nhs.uk/NHSEngland/NSF/Pages/Olderpeople.aspx>
NHS Scotland. <http://www.shiftingthebalance.scot.nhs.uk/initiatives/scottish-initiatives/older-people/>

USEFUL WEBSITES

(Accessed 29 May 2013)
American Society for Aesthetic Plastic Surgery. <http://www.surgery.org/>
American Society of Plastic Surgeons. <http://www.plasticsurgery.org/for-medical-professionals.html>
British Association for Forensic Odontology. <http://www.bafo.org.uk/>
Child Protection and the Dental Team. <http://www.cpdt.org.uk/>
DermNet N.Z. <http://dermnetnz.org/contents.html>
lipaugmentation. <http://www.lipaugmentation.com/microimplants.htm>
Monthly Prescribing Reference. <http://www.empr.com/drugs-contraindicated-in-pregnancy/article/125914/>
MOTHERISK. <http://www.motherisk.org/women/index.jsp>
National Cancer Institute. <http://www.cancer.gov/cancertopics/types/prostate>
National Institute for Health and Care Excellence. <http://www.nice.org.uk/CG89>
Organization of Teratology Information Specialists. <http://www.otispregnancy.org/files/miconazole.pdf>
Talksurgery. <http://www.talksurgery.com/>
University of Iowa Hospitals & Clinics. <http://www.uihealthcare.org/Adam/?/HIE+Multimedia/0/200000>
US Food and Drug Administration. <http://www.fda.gov/Safety/MedWatch/SafetyInformation/> (search on 'codeine use in children').
Women's Health. <http://www.womens-health.co.uk/>
womenshealth.gov. <http://www.womenshealth.gov/>

FURTHER READING

Allen, P.F., Whitworth, J.M., 2004. Endodontic considerations in the elderly. Gerodontology 21, 185.

Al-Salehi, S.K., et al. 2007. The effect of hydrogen peroxide concentration on metal ion release from dental amalgam. J. Dent. 35 (2), 172. Epub 2006 Sep 1
Bates, M.N., et al. 2004. Health effects of dental amalgam exposure: a retrospective cohort study. Int. J. Epidemiol. 334, 894–902. Epub 2004 May 20
Chalmers, J.M., 2006. Minimal intervention dentistry. Part 2. Strategies for addressing restorative challenges in older adults. J. Can. Dent. Assoc. 72, 435.
Conde-Agudelo, A., et al. 2008. Maternal infection and risk of preeclampsia: systematic review and metaanalysis. Am. J. Obstet. Gynecol. 198 (1), 7.
Daniels, J.L., et al. 2007. Maternal dental history, child's birth outcome and early cognitive development. Paediatr. Perinat. Epidemiol. 21 (5), 448.
Durso, S.C., 2005. Interaction with other health team members in caring for elderly patients. Dent. Clin. North Am. 49, 377.
Epstein, J.B., et al. 2007. A survey of National Cancer Institute-designated comprehensive cancer centers' oral health supportive care practices and resources in the United States. Support Care Cancer 15, 357.
Ettinger, R.L., 2007. Oral health and older adults. J. Am. Dent. Assoc. 138, 1S.
Fatahzadeh, M., Glick, M., 2006. Stroke: epidemiology, classification, risk factors, complications, diagnosis, prevention, and medical and dental management. Oral Surg. Oral Med. Oral Pathol. Oral Radiol. Endod. 102, 180.
Fayans, E.P., et al. 2010. Local anesthetic use in the pregnant and postpartum patient. Dent. Clin. North Am. 54 (4), 697.
Fiske, J., et al. 2006. Guidelines for the development of local standards of oral health care for people with dementia. Gerodontology 23 (Suppl 1), 5.
Frutos, R., et al. 2002. Oral manifestations and dental treatment in menopause. Med. Oral 7 (26), 31.
Gerodontology Association, 2005. Meeting the challenges of oral health for older people: a strategic review. Gerodontology 22 (Suppl 1), 2.
Gupta, A., et al. 2006. Hyposalivation in elderly patients. J. Can. Dent. Assoc. 72, 841.
Haas, D.A., 2002. An update on local anesthetics in dentistry. J. Can. Dent. Assoc. 68 (9), 546.
Herman, W.W., et al. 2004. New national guidelines on hypertension: a summary for dentistry. J. Am. Dent. Assoc. 135, 576.
Hujoel, P.P., et al. 2005. Mercury exposure from dental filling placement during pregnancy and low birth weight risk. Am. J. Epidemiol. 161 (8), 734.
Hupp, J.R., 2006. Ischemic heart disease: dental management considerations. Dent. Clin. North Am. 50, 483.
Luglie, P.F., et al. 2005 Febb. Effect of amalgam fillings on the mercury concentration in human amniotic fluid. Arch. Gynecol. Obstet. 271 (2), 138.
Mendia, J., et al. 2012. Drug therapy for the pregnant dental patient. Compend. Contin. Educ. Dent. 33 (8) 568, 572, 574; quiz 579, 596
Michalowicz, B.S., et al. 2008. Examining the safety of dental treatment in pregnant women. J. Am. Dent. Assoc. 139 (6), 685.
Michalowicz, B.S., et al. 2006. Treatment of periodontal disease and the risk of preterm birth. N. Engl. J. Med. 355 (18), 1885.
Montandon, A.A., et al. 2006. Quality of life and oral hygiene in older people with manual functional imitations. J. Dent. Educ. 70, 1261.
Muller, F., Schimmel, M., 2007. Management of preventive care for an ageing population. Int. Dent. J. 57, 215.
Nayak, A.G., et al. 2012. Oral healthcare considerations for the pregnant woman. Dent. Update 39 (1), 51.
Ressler-Maerlender, J., et al. 2005. Oral health during pregnancy: current research. J. Womens Health (Larchmt) 14 (10), 880.
Sacco, D., Frost, D.E., 2006. Dental management of patients with stroke or Alzheimer's disease. Dent. Clin. North Am. 50, 625.
Scully, C., Ettinger, R.L., 2007. The influence of systemic diseases on oral health care in older adults. J. Am. Dent. Assoc. 138, 7S.
Scully, C., et al. 2007. Special care in dentistry: handbook of oral healthcare. Elsevier/Churchill Livingstone, Edinburgh.
Shay, K., 2004. The evolving impact of aging America on dental practice. J. Contemp. Dent. Pract. 5, 101.
Siqueira, F.M., et al. 2008. Maternal periodontitis as a potential risk variable for preeclampsia: a case-control study. J. Periodontol. 79 (2), 207.
Tarannum, F., Faizuddin, M., 2007. Effect of periodontal therapy on pregnancy outcome in women affected by periodontitis. J. Periodontol. 78 (11), 2095.
Tosti, A. (Ed.), 2012. Management of complications of cosmetic procedures: handling common and more uncommon problems. Springer, Berlin
Wrzosek, T., Einarson, A., 2009. Dental care during pregnancy. Can. Fam. Physician. 55, 598.
Xiong, X., et al. 2006. Periodontal disease and adverse pregnancy outcomes: a systematic review. BJOG 113 (2), 135.

APPENDIX 25.1 DRUGS CONTRAINDICATED IN PREGNANCY

This chart represents information on select drugs that are contraindicated (pregnancy category X) for women who are pregnant. This is not an inclusive list of products that carry that pregnancy category. Those drugs that are contraindicated at a certain phase of the pregnancy are listed next to the product name. For more information on specific drug monographs, see product entries or consult the manufacturer.

Allergic disorders
Vistaril (hydroxyzine) *Early pregnancy*

Cardiovascular system
Advicor (niacin ext-rel/lovastatin)
Aggrenox (dipyridamole/aspirin) *3rd trimester*
Altoprev (lovastatin)
Bayer (aspirin) *3rd trimester*
Caduet (amlodipine/atorvastatin)
Coumadin (warfarin sodium)
Crestor (rosuvastatin)
Ecotrin (aspirin) *3rd trimester*
Juvisync (sitagliptin/simvastatin)
Lescol (fluvastatin)
Lescol XL (fluvastatin)
Letairis (ambrisentan)
Lipitor (atorvastatin)
Livalo (pitavastatin)
Mevacor (lovastatin)
Multaq (dronedarone)
Pravachol (pravastatin)
Simcor (niacin ext-rel/simvastatin)
Tracleer (bosentan)
Vytorin (ezetimibe/simvastatin)
Zocor (simvastatin)

Central nervous system
Beyaz (drospirenone/ethinyl estradiol)
Doral (quazepam)
Estazolam
Flurazepam
Halcion (triazolam)
Restoril (temazepam)
Vistaril (hydroxyzine) *Early pregnancy*
Yaz (drospirenone/ethinyl estradiol)

Dermatological disorders
Amnesteem (isotretinoin)
Avage (tazarotene)
Beyaz (drospirenone/ethinyl estradiol)
Carac (fluorouracil)
Claravis (isotretinoin)
Efudex (fluorouracil)
Estrostep Fe (norethindrone acetate/ethinyl estradiol)
Fluoroplex (fluorouracil)
Loryna (drospirenone/ethinyl estradiol)
Ortho Tri-Cyclen 28 (norgestimate/ethinyl estradiol)
Propecia (finasteride)
Silvadene (silver sulfadiazine) *Late pregnancy*
Solage (mequinol/tretinoin)
Solaraze (diclofenac sodium) *3rd trimester*

Soriatane (acitretin)
Sotret (isotretinoin)
SSD (silver sulfadiazine) *Late pregnancy*
SSD AF (silver sulfadiazine) *Late pregnancy*
Tazorac (tazarotene)
Tilia Fe (norethindrone acetate/ethinyl estradiol)
Tri-Legest 21 (norethindrone acetate/ethinyl estradiol)
Tri-Legest Fe (norethindrone acetate/ethinyl estradiol)
Tri-previfem (norgestimate/ethinyl estradiol)
Tri-sprintec (norgestimate/ethinyl estradiol)
Yaz (drospirenone/ethinyl estradiol)

Endocrine disorders
Androderm (testosterone)
Androgel (testosterone)
Android (methyltestosterone)
Axiron (testosterone)
Delatestryl (testosterone enanthate)
Depo-testosterone (testosterone cypionate)
Egrifta (tesamorelin)
Fluoxymesterone
Fortesta (testosterone)
Juvisync (sitagliptin/simvastatin)
Lupron (leuprolide acetate)
Methitest (methyltestosterone)
Oxandrin (oxandrolone)
Striant (testosterone)
Supprelin LA (histrelin acetate)
Synarel (nafarelin)
Testim (testosterone)
Testred (methyltestosterone)
Virilon (methyltestosterone)

Gastrointestinal tract
Bellergal-S (phenobarbital/ergotamine tartrate)
Cytotec (misoprostol)

Infections and infestations
Bactrim (sulfamethoxazole/trimethoprim) *3rd trimester*
Copegus (ribavirin)
Flagyl (metronidazole) *1st trimester for trichomoniasis*
Furadantin (nitrofurantoin) *Pregnancy at term*
Gantrisin (sulfisoxazole) *3rd trimester*
Grifulvin V (griseofulvin)
Gris-Peg (griseofulvin)
Macrobid (nitrofurantoin as macrocrystals and monohydrate) *Pregnancy at term*
Macrodantin (nitrofurantoin macrocrystals) *Pregnancy at term*
Rebetol (ribavirin)
Rebetron (ribavirin/interferon alfa-2b)
Septra (sulfamethoxazole/trimethoprim) *3rd trimester*
Sulfadiazine *Pregnancy at term*
Tindamax (tinidazole) *1st trimester*
Urobiotic-250 (oxytetracycline HCl/sulfamethizole/phenazopyridine) *Late pregnancy*
Virazole (ribavirin)

Metabolic disorders
Zavesca (miglustat)

Musculoskeletal disorders
Advil (ibuprofen) *3rd trimester*
Aleve (naproxen sodium) *3rd trimester*
Ansaid (flurbiprofen) *Late pregnancy*

(Continued)

Arava (leflunomide)

Arthrotec (diclofenac sodium/misoprostol)

Bayer (aspirin) *3rd trimester*

BC Arthritis Strength (aspirin/caffeine/salicylamide) *3rd trimester*

Cataflam (diclofenac potassium) *Late pregnancy*

Celebrex (celecoxib) *3rd trimester*

Choline magnesium trisalicylate *Pregnancy at term*

Dantrium (dantrolene)

Daypro (oxaprozin) *3rd trimester*

Diflunisal *3rd trimester*

Duexis (ibuprofen/famotidine) *Late pregnancy (≥30 wks)*

Ecotrin (aspirin) *3rd trimester*

Etodolac *Late pregnancy*

Evista (raloxifene HCl)

Feldene (piroxicam) *Late pregnancy*

Ketoprofen *Late pregnancy*

Mobic (meloxicam) *3rd trimester*

Motrin (ibuprofen) *3rd trimester*

Nabumetone *3rd trimester*

Nalfon (fenoprofen calcium) *3rd trimester*

Naprelan (naproxen) *3rd trimester*

Prevacid Naprapac (lansoprazole/naproxen) *3rd trimester*

Probenecid + Colchicine

Prolia (denosumab)

Rheumatrex (methotrexate sodium)

Salsalate *3rd trimester*

Soma Compound w. Codeine (carisoprodol/aspirin/codeine) *3rd trimester*

Vimovo (naproxen/esomeprazole) *Late pregnancy (≥ 30 wks)*

Voltaren (diclofenac sodium) *Late pregnancy*

Zipsor (diclofenac potassium) *Late pregnancy*

Neoplasms

Bexxar (tositumomab)

Casodex (bicalutamide)

Delestrogen (estradiol valerate)

Efudex (fluorouracil)

Eligard (leuprolide acetate)

Estrace (estradiol)

Evista (raloxifene HCl)

Firmagon (degarelix)

Fluoxymesterone

Menest (esterified estrogens)

Revlimid (lenalidomide)

Targretin (bexarotene)

Thalomid (thalidomide)

Trelstar (triptorelan pamoate)

Trexall (methotrexate)

Vantas (histrelin acetate)

Zytiga (abiraterone acetate)

Nutrition

Didrex (benzphetamine)

Fosteum (genistein/citrated zinc/cholecalciferol)

Megace ES (megestrol acetate)

Megace Suspension (megestrol acetate)

Xenical (orlistat)

Obstetrics/gynaecology

ALL ORAL CONTRACEPTIVES

ALL HORMONE REPLACEMENT THERAPY

Advil (ibuprofen) *3rd trimester*

Aleve (naproxen sodium) *3rd trimester*

Aygestin (norethindrone acetate)

Betadine douche (povidone–iodine)

Bravelle (urofollitropin)

Cataflam (diclofenac potassium) *Late pregnancy*

Celebrex (celecoxib) *3rd trimester*

Cetrotide (cetrorelix)

Clomid (clomiphene citrate)

Depo-subQ provera (medroxyprogesterone acetate)

Endometrin (micronized progesterone) *Ectopic pregnancy*

Flagyl (metronidazole) *1st trimester for trichomoniasis*

Follistim (follitropin beta)

Ganirelex acetate

Gonal-F (follitropin alfa)

Lupron Depot (leuprolide acetate)

Luveris (lutropin alfa)

Menopur (menotropins)

Methergine (methylergonovine)

Midol cramp (ibuprofen) *3rd trimester*

Midol menstrual (acetaminophen/caffeine/pyrilamine) *3rd trimester*

Midol PMS (acetaminophen/pamabrom/pyrilamine) *3rd trimester*

Midol teen (acetaminophen/pamabrom) *3rd trimester*

Mifeprex (mifepristone)

Motrin (ibuprofen) *3rd trimester*

Naprelan (naproxen) *3rd trimester*

Ovidrel (choriogonadotropin alfa)

Ponstel (mefenamic acid) *Late pregnancy*

Repronex 75 IU (follicle-stimulating hormone/luteinizing hormone)

Repronex 150 IU (follicle-stimulating hormone/luteinizing hormone)

Serophene (clomiphene citrate)

Synarel (nafarelin acetate)

Tindamax (tinidazole) *1st trimester*

Zoladex (goserelin)

Pain and pyrexia

Advil (ibuprofen) *3rd trimester*

Advil Migraine (ibuprofen) *3rd trimester*

Aleve (naproxen sodium) *3rd trimester*

Bayer (aspirin) *3rd trimester*

BC Original Formula (aspirin/caffeine/salicylamide) *3rd trimester*

Cafergot (ergotamine tartrate/caffeine)

Caldolor (ibuprofen) *3rd trimester*

Cataflam (diclofenac potassium) *Late pregnancy*

Celebrex (celecoxib) *3rd trimester*

Choline magnesium trisalicylate *Pregnancy at term*

Combunox (oxycodone/ibuprofen) *3rd trimester*

D.H.E. 45 (dihydroergotamine mesylate)

Diflunisal *3rd trimester*

Etodolac *Late pregnancy*

Excedrin Migraine (acetaminophen/aspirin/caffeine) *3rd trimester*

Fiorinal (butalbital/aspirin/caffeine) *3rd trimester*

Fiorinal w. Codeine (butalbital/aspirin/caffeine/codeine phosphate) *3rd trimester*

Ibudone (hydrocodone bitartrate/ibuprofen) *3rd trimester*

Ketorolac *Late pregnancy*

Migranal (dihydroergotamine mesylate)

Motrin Migraine Pain (ibuprofen) *3rd trimester*

Nalfon (fenoprofen calcium) *3rd trimester*

Naprelan (naproxen) *3rd trimester*

Percodan (oxycodone HCl/aspirin) *3rd trimester*

Ponstel (mefenamic acid) *Late pregnancy*

Synalgos-DC (dihydrocodeine bitartrate/aspirin/caffeine) *3rd trimester*

Vicoprofen (hydrocodone bitartrate/ibuprofen) *3rd trimester*

(Continued)

Respiratory tract

None available

Urogenital system

Avodart (dutasteride HCl) *AVOID HANDLING CAPSULES*

Caverject (alprostadil)

Edex (alprostadil)

Jalyn (dutasteride/tamsulosin HCl)

Lithostat (acetohydroxamic acid)

Proscar (finasteride) *AVOID HANDLING CRUSHED/BROKEN TABLETS*

Notes

*Not an inclusive list.
(Rev. 8/2012)

Pregnancy categories

When pregnancy appears as a contraindication or precaution to the use of a drug, it is usually qualified by a category.

Cat. A: Adequate studies in pregnant women have failed to show a risk to the fetus in the first trimester and there is no evidence of risk in later trimesters.

Cat. B: Animal studies have failed to show a risk to the fetus but there are no adequate studies in pregnant women; or animal studies have shown an adverse effect but human studies have not shown a risk to the fetus in the first trimester and there is no evidence of risk in later trimesters.

Cat. C: Animal studies have shown an adverse effect on the fetus but there are no adequate studies in humans, but the benefits may outweigh the risks; or there are no adequate human studies.

Cat. D: Positive evidence of human fetal risk but the benefits may outweigh the risks.

Cat. X: Animal or human studies have shown fetal abnormalities or toxicity and the risk outweighs the benefit

http://www.empr.com/drugs-contraindicated-in-pregnancy/article/125914/ (accessed 30 September 2013).

APPENDIX 25.2 DRUG EFFECTS ON BREAST-FEEDING INFANTS

Drug	Reported outcomes of use
Alcohol (ethanol)	With large amounts, drowsiness, weakness, decrease in linear growth, abnormal weight gain
Aspirin (salicylates)	Metabolic acidosis (rare)
Atenolol	Cyanosis; bradycardia
Bendroflumethiazide	Suppression of lactation
Caffeine	Irritability, poor sleeping pattern, excreted slowly; no effect with moderate intake of caffeinated beverages (2–3 cups per day)
Carbimazole	Goitre
Chloral hydrate	Sleepiness
Contraceptive pill with oestrogen/progestogen	Rare breast enlargement; decrease in milk production and protein content
Danthron	Increased bowel activity
Dexbrompheniramine maleate with D-isoephedrine	Crying, poor sleeping patterns, irritability
Ethosuximide	Appearance of drug in infant blood
Indometacin	Seizure (rare)
Iodides	May affect thyroid activity; goitre
Iodine	Goitre
Iodine (povidone–iodine)	Elevated iodine levels in breast milk, odour of iodine on infant's skin
Nalidixic acid	Haemolysis in glucose-6-phosphate dehydrogenase (G6PD) deficiency
Nitrofurantoin	Haemolysis in infant with G6PD deficiency
Phenobarbital	Sedation; infantile spasms after weaning, methaemoglobinaemia (rare)
Phenytoin	Methaemoglobinaemia (rare)
Sulfapyridine	Caution in jaundice or G6PD deficiency and ill, stressed or premature infant
Sulfisoxazole	Caution in jaundice or G6PD deficiency and ill, stressed or premature infant
Tetracyclines	Tooth discolouration
Theophylline	Irritability
Tolbutamide	Possible jaundice

26 Complementary and alternative medicine

Traditional medicine is widely practised across the world, particularly in Asian and African cultures. In the developed world, therapies that are not currently considered an integral part of conventional allopathic medical practice are termed *complementary* (when used in addition to conventional treatments) and *alternative* (when used instead of conventional treatments). Such therapies (complementary and alternative medicine – or CAM) include, but are not limited to, acupuncture, aromatherapy, chiropractic, colonic irrigation, diet fads (Ch. 27), faith healing, folk medicine, herbal (natural) medicine, homoeopathy, meditation, naturopathy, new-age healing, massage and music therapy.

During 2007, almost 40% of adults in the USA used CAM, the most commonly used therapies being non-vitamin, non-mineral, natural products and deep breathing exercises (http://www.cdc.gov/nchs/data/nhsr/nhsr012.pdf; accessed 30 September 2013). Over the preceding 5 years, there was increased use of acupuncture, deep breathing exercises, hypnotherapy, massage therapy, meditation, naturopathy and yoga, but use for colds showed a marked decrease. However, there is only limited evidence of efficacy for many CAM therapies. For instance, PubMed, the National Library of Medicine journal database, identified 40 systematic reviews involving acupuncture, massage therapy, naturopathy or yoga, only 10 of which (25%) provided sufficient evidence to conclude that a given therapy was effective for a given condition. These were acupuncture for knee pain, insomnia and nausea or vomiting, and acupuncture and yoga for back pain; both acupuncture and massage therapy are included among recommended therapies for back pain. CAM is taken increasingly seriously in the West and there is a National Centre for Complementary and Alternative Medicine (NCCAM) in the USA.

Since there is some evidence of increasing use by the public and of efficacy, this chapter focuses on forms of traditional medicine, acupuncture, herbal medicines and probiotics. Herbal alternatives to hormone replacement therapy are discussed in Chapter 25; omega-3 and omega-6 are discussed in Chapter 27.

TRADITIONAL CHINESE MEDICINE

Traditional Chinese medicine (TCM; http://nccam.nih.gov/health/whatiscam/chinesemed.htm, accessed 30 September 2013) views how the body works, what causes illness and how to treat illness, differently from Western views. TCM is typically delivered by a practitioner who uses acupuncture, herbs and other methods to treat a wide range of conditions. Other TCM practices include cupping, dietary therapy, massage, mind–body therapy and moxibustion (the burning of mugwort, a small herb). Acupuncture has the largest body of evidence and is considered safe if practised correctly. Some Chinese herbal remedies may be safe; others may not be.

ACUPUNCTURE

A limited number of randomized controlled trials (RCTs) support acupuncture as a possible treatment for a range of conditions that include anxiety, cancer and chemotherapy-induced nausea, depression, insomnia, migraine, musculoskeletal pain and postoperative pain. However,

Table 26.1 *Acupuncture in orofacial conditions (benefit proved)*

Probably	Possibly	Inconclusive
Dental pain	Dental local anaesthesia – reduced time to onset	Bell palsy
Postoperative or chemotherapy-induced nausea/vomiting	Gag reflex	Burning mouth sensation
Postoperative pain	Hyposalivation	Mouth ulceration
Temporomandibular joint pain	Neck pain	Sensory loss
		Sinusitis

there is inadequate evidence of benefit in conditions such as asthma, dysphagia, epilepsy, schizophrenia, smoking cessation or stroke.

Dental aspects

There are several publications but few RCTs on acupuncture used for orofacial conditions (Table 26.1). Efforts have been made to clarify mechanisms but consensus has yet to be reached. Any efficacy may be explained by possible release of endogenous opiates (beta-endorphin, enkephalin, endomorphin and dynorphin; Ch. 10) during acupuncture. The serotoninergic descending inhibitory pathway is an alternative suggested mechanism. The autonomic nervous system and resultant inflammatory reflex might be part of antihyperalgesia elicited by acupuncture.

AYURVEDIC MEDICINE

Ayurvedic medicine (Ayurveda; http://nccam.nih.gov/health/ayurveda/introduction.htm; accessed 30 September 2013) originated in India. Its aim is to integrate and balance the body, mind and spirit because it is believed that this helps prevent illness and promote wellness. Many therapies employed in Ayurvedic medicine are also used on their own as CAM – for example, herbs, massage and specialized diets. Some of the products may be harmful (causing adverse effects or interacting with conventional medicines). Different systems used to treat oral diseases, individually or in combinations, include *Acacia chundra* Willd, *Adhatoda vasica* Nees, *Mimusops elengi* L., *Piper nigrum* L., *Pongamia pinnata* (L.) Pierre, *Quercus infectoria* Olivier, *Syzygium aromaticum* L., *Terminalia chebula* Retz and *Zingiber officinale* Roscoe.

CAM IN OTHER CULTURES

Details of African, American Indian, Latin American, Caribbean and other important CAM can be found at: http://www.ncbi.nlm.nih.gov/pmc/journals/970/ and http://americanindianhealth.nlm.nih.gov/ (both accessed 30 September 2013).

HERBAL MEDICINES

Many conventional drugs that have been proven to be effective originated from plant sources. Examples include aspirin (from willow bark), digoxin (foxglove), morphine (opium poppy) and quinine (cinchona bark). However, natural does not signify safe. Some plant products (e.g. opioids, cocaine and peyote) are addictive (Ch. 34) and many are highly toxic; for example, some Chinese weight-loss herbs are nephrotoxic, and kava-kava (*Piper methysticum*) is hepatotoxic. Chamomile, liquorice root, quassia and red clover all contain coumarin derivatives and can provoke a bleeding tendency. Some other herbal products may impair platelet aggregation, thus prolonging bleeding (Table 26.2). Herbals that pose a risk for cardiac patients are shown in Box 26.1.

Some herbal drugs appear to be effective and fairly safe, and there are reliable published data supporting a potential medicinal role for aloe vera, melatonin, saw palmetto and St John's wort (Table 26.3). Reliable published data on efficacy are weaker for gingko biloba and alpha-lipoic acid, and are contradictory for valerian and echinacea. Research into the safety and efficacy of most herbals has been limited because of product variability, lack of controlled studies and few legal controls (Appendices 26.1 and 26.2).

ALOE VERA

Aloe vera, derived from *Aloe barbadensis* Miller, contains many constituents, some of which purportedly have anti-inflammatory, antiseptic and/or analgesic properties. These include:

- vitamins: A (beta-carotene), C, E, B_{12}, folic acid and choline
- enzymes: alkaline phosphatase, amylase, bradykinase, carboxypeptidase, catalase, cellulase, lipase and peroxidase
- minerals: calcium, chromium, copper, selenium, magnesium, manganese, potassium, sodium and zinc
- sugars: monosaccharides (glucose and fructose) and polysaccharides (glucomannans/polymannose)
- anthraquinones
- fatty acids: cholesterol, campesterol, beta-sitosterol and lupeol
- hormones: auxins and gibberellins
- others: amino acids, salicylic acid, lignin and saponins.

Aloe may have healing and protective effects against radiation damage, and anti-inflammatory, antiviral and antiseptic properties. There

Table 26.2 *Herbal products that may inhibit haemostasis*

Herbal	Source
Bilberry	Vaccinium myrtillus
Bromelain	Anas comosus
Cat's claw	Uncaria tomentosa
Devil's claw	Harpagophytum procumbens
Dong quai	Angelica sinensis
Evening primrose	Oenothera biennis
Feverfew	Tanacetum parthenium
Garlic	Allium sativum
Ginger	Zingiber officinale
Ginkgo biloba	Ginkgo biloba
Ginseng	Panax ginseng
Grape seed	Vitis vinifera
Green tea	Camellia sinensis
Horse chestnut	Aesculus hippocastanum
Turmeric	Curcuma longa

Box 26.1 *Herbals that may interact with cardiovascular drugs*

- Liquorice root – contains glycyrrhetinic acid and can increase blood pressure
- Ma huang – contains ephedrine
- Foxglove – source of digitalis
- Hawthorn – contains oligomeric procyanins, with hypocholesterolaemic action, and can enhance digoxin
- Tan shen – may inhibit platelet aggregation and potentiate warfarin
- Willow bark – contains salicin (a source of acetylsalicylic acid [ASA])
- Garlic – antiplatelet activity; high doses may reduce serum thromboxane levels
- Gingko (maidenhair tree) – gingkolides inhibit platelet-activating factor, decrease vascular resistance and improve circulatory flow
- Hellebore – contains alkaloids that may cause bradycardia and hypotension
- Wu-chu-yu (*Evodia rutaecarpa*) – contains rutaecarpine, a vasorelaxant

Table 26.3 *Herbal preparations and supplements of proven efficacy*

Herbal preparation	Effective for treating	Derived from	Possible interactions	Possible adverse effects
Saw palmetto	Benign prostatic hyperplasia	*Serenoa repens*	–	Minimal
Melatonin	Jet lag	Synthetic	Warfarin	–
Aloe vera	Chronic skin issues	*Aloe vera* Linne or *Aloe barbadensis*	Digoxin	Dermatitis
	Lichen planus		Hypoglycaemics	In animals – colon cancer
St John's wort	Mild to moderate depression	A yellow-flowered weed, *Hypericum perforatum*	Induces cytochrome P450 hepatic enzyme system, specifically CYP3A4 isoform, and thus interacts with many drugs (see Box 26.2)	Dry mouth, dizziness, gastrointestinal symptoms, increased sensitivity to sunlight and fatigue
			May also intensify or prolong the effects of some narcotic drugs and anaesthetic agents	
Gingko biloba	Improved memory; stable or slowed deterioration in Alzheimer disease	A flowering tree native to China	Anticoagulant and antiplatelet medicines	Minimal
Echinacea	Increases the 'non-specific' activity of immune system	*Echinacea purpurea*	Anabolic steroids	Should not be used in progressive systemic and autoimmune disorders such as tuberculosis, or connective tissue disorders
	Contradictory reports of efficacy in prevention of upper respiratory infections			

are reports of efficacy in seborrhoeic dermatitis, psoriasis, herpes, burns, wound healing, pressure ulcers, mucositis, radiation dermatitis, acne, lichen planus and aphthous stomatitis.

Aloe may cause redness, burning, a stinging sensation and, rarely, dermatitis. Abdominal cramps, diarrhoea, red urine, hepatitis, dependency or worsening of constipation are also possible. Its laxative effect may cause electrolyte imbalances (low potassium levels). Prolonged use (in animals) has reportedly increased the risk of colorectal cancer.

Oral aloe is not recommended during pregnancy due to theoretical stimulation of uterine contractions, and if taken by breast-feeding mothers it may sometime causes gastrointestinal distress in the nursing infant. Aloe reduces the effectiveness and may increase the adverse effects of digoxin and digitoxin, due to its potassium-lowering effect. It decreases blood sugar levels and thus may interact with hypoglycaemic drugs and insulin. Aloe should not be taken for 2 weeks prior to any surgical procedure, as it may cause increased bleeding.

Further information on aloe is available at: http://umm.edu/health/medical/altmed/ (under 'Herb' and 'Herb Interaction') and http://nccam.nih.gov/health/aloevera (both accessed 30 September 2013).

GINGKO BILOBA

The flavonoids found in ginkgo may help prevent or reduce retinal problems and age-related macular degeneration; they may also enhance neuropsychological/memory processes, and possibly are effective in Alzheimer disease, improving cognitive performance, global function and activities of daily living, and, at least *in vitro*, inhibiting amyloid-beta aggregation and caspase-3 activation (Ch. 13). Meta-analyses comparing ginkgo with acetylcholinesterase inhibitors in Alzheimer disease have shown similar clinical efficacy, with an additional safety benefit for ginkgo. Ginkgo might cause early labour; it might also interfere with diabetes management, provoke seizures or cause a bleeding disorder.

Ginkgo can interact with some medications, including anticonvulsants, antidepressants (SSRIs – may increase the risk of serotonin syndrome), antihypertensives, and drugs such as warfarin, clopidogrel, aspirin and other non-steroidal anti-inflammatory drugs (NSAIDs). It is recommended that ginkgo be stopped at least 2 weeks before surgery.

More information is available at: http://umm.edu/health/medical/altmed/herb/ginkgo-biloba and http://www.nlm.nih.gov/medlineplus/druginformation.html (both accessed 30 September 2013).

MELATONIN

Melatonin taken in the evening in the new time zone will reset the biological clock and alleviate (or prevent) symptoms of jet lag. Melatonin helps determine when a woman starts to menstruate, the frequency and duration of menstrual cycles, and when a woman stops menstruating (menopause). The incidence of adverse effects to melatonin is low. Interactions are possible with anticoagulants, antidepressants, antihypertensives, antipsychotics, benzodiazepines, beta-blockers, corticosteroids or other immunosuppressants, interleukin-2, NSAIDs and tamoxifen.

More information is available at: http://umm.edu/health/medical/altmed/supplement/melatonin (accessed 30 September 2013).

SAW PALMETTO

Saw palmetto, from *Serenoa repens* fruit, can be effective treatment for benign prostatic hypertrophy (BPH), producing similar improvements in urinary symptoms and flow to finasteride – and with fewer adverse effects. However, the long-term effectiveness, safety and ability to prevent BPH complications are unknown. Saw palmetto may interact with anticoagulants, antiplatelets, finasteride, hormonal contraceptives and hormone replacement therapy (HRT).

More information is available at: http://umm.edu/health/medical/altmed/herb/saw-palmetto (accessed 30 September 2013).

ST JOHN'S WORT

St John's wort (*Hypericum perforatum*; SJW) is beneficial in mild to moderate depression. It also induces various drug-metabolizing enzymes (cytochrome P450 isoenzymes, CYP3A4, CYP2C9, CYP1A2, and the transport protein P-glycoprotein), which lowers blood levels and therapeutic effects of some drugs (Box 26.2). It is important also to note that, when patients stop taking SJW, blood levels of interacting

---

Box 26.2 *Drugs to be avoided with St John's wort*

- Anthracycline
- Anticoagulants
- Anticonvulsants
- Antidepressants
- Antiretrovirals
- Azole antifungals
- Benzodiazepines
- Calcium-channel blockers
- Carbamazepine
- Cardiovascular drugs
- Ciclosporin
- Cytotoxic drugs
- Dextromethorphan
- Digoxin
- Docetaxel
- Eszopiclone
- Etoposide
- Hormonal contraceptives
- HRT
- Imatinib
- Immunosuppressants
- Indinavir
- Irinotecan
- Lithium
- Loperamide
- Monoamine oxidase inhibitors (MAOIs)
- Oral contraceptives
- Paclitaxel
- Phenprocoumon
- Protease inhibitors (PIs)
- Ramelteon
- Selective serotonin reuptake inhibitors (SSRIs)
- Statins
- Tamoxifen
- Teniposide
- Theophylline
- Thyroxine
- Tricyclic antidepressants
- Triptans
- Vinca alkaloids
- Warfarin
- Zaleplon
- Zolpidem

medicines may rise, resulting in toxicity. SJW should be stopped at least 5 days or more before surgery.

SJW may worsen symptoms of attention deficit disorder (ADD) and attention deficit hyperactivity disorder (ADHD), increase the risk of psychosis in schizophrenia, and may contribute to dementia in Alzheimer disease.

More information is available at: http://umm.edu/health/medical/altmed/ (under 'Herb' and 'Herb Interaction') and http://nccam.nih.gov/health/stjohnswort (both accessed 30 September 2013).

ALPHA-LIPOIC ACID

Alpha-lipoic acid is found in red meat, liver and yeast, as well as being made by the body, where it is changed into dihydrolipoic acid. Alpha-lipoic acid appears to help lower blood sugar levels and may help people with diabetic peripheral neuropathy. It has been used to treat burning mouth syndrome. Alpha-lipoic acid may interact with hypoglycaemics, chemotherapy or thyroid hormone.

More information is available at: http://umm.edu/health/medical/altmed/ (under 'Supplement' and 'Supplement Interaction'; accessed 30 September 2013).

ECHINACEA

Echinacea was promoted as an immunostimulator, especially for reducing the common cold; however, three of four published studies concluded that taking echinacea to prevent a cold was ineffective. It is also ineffective in combating cancers. People with tuberculosis, leukaemia, diabetes, connective tissue disorders, multiple sclerosis, HIV/AIDS, autoimmune diseases or, possibly, liver disorders should not take echinacea. Echinacea may interact with immunosuppressants. People with asthma and allergies may be at an increased risk for developing adverse reactions. When taken by mouth, echinacea may cause temporary numbing and a tingling tongue. Its safety in pregnancy or breast-feeding is unclear.

More information is available at: http://umm.edu/health/medical/altmed/herb/echinacea (accessed 30 September 2013).

DENTAL ASPECTS OF HERBALS

There are weak data on the possible effects of aloe extracts, berries, chamomile, cocoa, coffee, grapes, honey/propolis, myrtle, polyphenols (stilbenes, flavonoids and proanthocyanidins) and tea on various oral diseases (caries, gingivitis, periodontal disease, candidiasis, aphthae, mucositis, lichen planus, leukoplakia and oral cancer) but no strong evidence (Table 26.4).

Herbals may influence treatment, especially in that they may interact with other drugs (e.g. when benzodiazepine sedation is used; Table 26.5) or produce a bleeding tendency.

PROBIOTICS

Probiotics are live microorganisms, added to food with the intention of benefitting the host by changing intestinal microbial balance. The main probiotics used include *Lactobacillus rhamnosus* GG, *L. reuteri*, bifidobacteria, certain strains of *L. casei* or the *L. acidophilus* group, *Escherichia coli* strain Nissle 1917, certain enterococci (*Enterococcus faecium* SF68) and *Saccharomyces boulardii*.

The underlying mechanisms of probiotic action are unclear but may include strengthening of the non-immunological gut barrier, pathogen

Table 26.4 *Herbals and other preparations and oral disease*

Preparation	Purported effects
Pilocarpine in Brazilian 'slobber plant' (*Pilocarpus jaborandi*)	Helps hyposalivation
Aloe vera	See Table 26.3
Acemannan (an aloe polysaccharide)	Relief in aphthae
B vitamins	
Eupatorium laevigatum Lam.	
Lactobacillus acidophilus and *L. bulgaricus*	
Liquorice with glycyrrhizic acid removed (deglycyrrhizinated liquorice; DGL)	
LongoVital	
Tannins (in agrimony, cranesbill, tormentil, oak, periwinkle and witch hazel)	
Zinc	
Capsaicin	May help in burning mouth syndrome
Lipoic acid	
Zinc	May help in taste disturbances

Table 26.5 *Potential interactions of herbal preparations with benzodiazepines*

Herbal preparation	Potential effect on sedation
Dong quai	Increased
Houpu	Increased
Kava kava	Increased
Passion flower	Increased
St John's wort	Reduced
Tan shen	Increased
Valerian	Reduced

growth inhibition and interference with adhesion, and enhancement of mucosal immune systems, as well as the systemic immune response. Probiotics appear effective in preventing and reducing the severity of a number of conditions, as shown in Box 26.3, but there is insufficient evidence with respect to any suggested benefits from probiotics in prevention or therapy of ischaemic heart diseases, autoimmune disease or cancer.

RCTs on probiotics in oral health are few. Lactic acid-producing bacteria can generate antimicrobial factors (e.g. organic acids, hydrogen peroxide, carbon peroxide, diacetyl, antimicrobial substances, bacteriocins and adhesion inhibitors). *Lactobacillus* and *Bifidobacterium* may inhibit cariogenic streptococci and *Candida* species. Six of seven placebo-controlled studies on the effect of probiotics reported reduced salivary *Streptococcus mutans* and/or yeasts. A study carried out in 3–4-year-old children reported significant caries reduction after 7 months of daily consumption of probiotic milk. The bacteriocin producer *Streptococcus salivarius* K12 may reduce halitosis.

A *prebiotic* is a selectively fermented ingredient that allows specific changes in the composition and/or activity of the gastrointestinal microflora. Only bifidogenic, non-digestible oligosaccharides (particularly inulin, its hydrolysis product oligofructose, and [trans]galacto-oligosaccharides) fulfil criteria for classification as prebiotic; some may help prevent diarrhoea or constipation, and modulate intestinal flora metabolism, and may have positive effects on cancer prevention, lipid metabolism, mineral adsorption and immunity.

Synergistic combinations of probiotics and prebiotics are called *synbiotics*.

Box 26.3 *Conditions that may benefit from use of probiotics*

- Acute diarrhoea in children
- Antibiotic-associated diarrhoea
- Inflammatory bowel disease, especially ulcerative colitis
- Prevention of urogenital tract infection
- Reduction of atopy in children
- Reduction of lactose intolerance
- Reduction of cancer-promoting enzymes and/or gut putrefactive (bacterial) metabolites
- Normalization of passing stool and stool consistency in irritable bowel syndrome
- Prevention of respiratory tract infections (common cold, influenza)

More information on L. acidophilus is available at: http://umm.edu/health/medical/altmed/supplement/lactobacillus-acidophilus (accessed 30 September 2013).

HYPNOTHERAPY

Hypnotherapy is a complementary therapy that uses hypnosis, an altered state of consciousness and, despite there being no strong evidence, is widely promoted as a treatment for breaking certain habits, such as smoking, bruxism, or thumb-sucking, or for various long-term conditions such as anxiety, eczema, gagging, idiopathic facial pain, temporomandibular pain-dysfunction or irritable bowel syndrome.

KEY WEBSITES

(Accessed 29 May 2013)
National Health Statistics Reports: Costs of complementary and alternative medicine (CAM) and frequency of visits to CAM practitioners: United States, 2007. <http://www.cdc.gov/nchs/data/nhsr/nhsr018.pdf>
National Institutes of Health: National Center for Complementary and Alternative Medicine. <http://nccam.nih.gov/>
Patient.co.uk. <http://www.patient.co.uk/doctor/complementary-and-alternative-medicine>

USEFUL WEBSITES

(Accessed 8 July 2013)
About.com. Alternative medicine. <http://altmedicine.about.com/>
Institute for Complementary and Natural Medicine. <http://www.icnm.org.uk/>
National Health Statistics Reports: Complementary and alternative medicine use among adults and children: United States, 2007. <http://www.cdc.gov/nchs/data/nhsr/nhsr012.pdf>

FURTHER READING

Ang-Lee, M.K., et al. 2001. Herbal medicines and perioperative care. JAMA 286, 208.
Armfield, J., Heaton, L.J., 2013. Management of fear and anxiety in the dental clinic: a review. Aust. Dent. J. 58 (4), 390–407. doi: 10.1111/adj.12118 PubMed PMID; 24320894.
Bagan, J., et al. 2012. Topical therapies for oral lichen planus management and their efficacy: a narrative review. Curr. Pharm. Des. 18 (34), 5470. PubMed PMID: 22632394.
Baradari, A.G., et al. 2012. Comparison of antibacterial effects of oral rinses chlorhexidine and herbal mouth wash in patients admitted to intensive care unit. Bratisl. Lek. Listy. 113 (9), 556. PubMed PMID: 22979913.
Bardia, A., et al. 2006. Efficacy of complementary and alternative medicine therapies in relieving cancer pain: a systematic review. J. Clin. Oncol. 24, 5457.
Bergström, I., et al. 2008. A follow-up study of subjective symptoms of temporomandibular disorders in patients who received acupuncture and/or interocclusal appliance therapy 18–20 years earlier. Acta Odontol. Scand. 66, 88.

Bhalang, K., et al. 2013. Acemannan, a polysaccharide extracted from aloe vera, is effective in the treatment of oral aphthous ulceration. J. Altern. Complement Med. 19 (5), 429.10.1089/acm.2012.0164 Epub 2012 Dec 16.
Birch, S., et al. 2004. Clinical research on acupuncture. Part 1. What have reviews of the efficacy and safety of acupuncture told us so far? J. Altern. Complement Med. 10, 468.
Caglar, E., et al. 2005. Bacteriotherapy and probiotics' role on oral health. Oral Dis. 11, 131.
Chen, H.Y., et al. 2007. Auricular acupuncture treatment for insomnia: a systematic review. J. Altern. Complement Med. 13, 669.
Cheuk, D.K., Wong, V., 2006. Acupuncture for epilepsy. Cochrane Database Syst. Rev. 2, CD005062.
Cheuk, D.K., et al. 2007. Acupuncture for insomnia. Cochrane Database Syst. Rev. 3, CD005472.
Dat A.D., et al. Aloe vera for treating acute and chronic wounds. Cochrane Database Syst. Rev. 2012; 2:CD008762. 10.1002/14651858.CD008762.pub2. Review. PubMed PMID: 22336851.
Eitner, S., et al. 2005. A long-term therapeutic treatment for patients with a severe gag reflex. Int. J. Clin. Exp. Hypn. 53, 74.
Endres, H.G., et al. 2007. Role of acupuncture in the treatment of migraine. Expert Rev. Neurother. 7, 1121.
Ezzo, J.M., et al. 2006. Acupuncture-point stimulation for chemotherapy-induced nausea or vomiting. Cochrane Database Syst. Rev. (2), CD002285.
Goddard, G., 2005. Short term pain reduction with acupuncture treatment for chronic orofacial pain patients. Med. Sci. Monit. 11, CR71.
Gordon, D., Heimberg, R.G., Tellez, M., Ismail, A.I., 2013. A critical review of approaches to the treatment of dental anxiety in adults. J. Anxiety Disord. 27 (4), 365–378. doi: 10.1016/j.janxdis.2013.04.002 Epub 2013 Apr 13. PubMed PMID: 2374649.
Hammerschlag, R., 2003. Acupuncture: on what should its evidence base be based? Altern. Ther. Health Med. 9, 34.
He, L., et al. 2007. Acupuncture for Bell's palsy. Cochrane Database Syst. Rev. 4, CD002914.
Holden, A., 2012. The art of suggestion: the use of hypnosis in dentistry. Br. Dent. J. 212 (11), 549–551. doi: 10.1038/sj.bdj.2012.467 PubMed PMID: 22677848.
Jedel, E., 2005. Acupuncture in xerostomia – a systematic review. J. Oral Rehabil. 32, 392.
Jorm, A.F., et al. 2004. Effectiveness of complementary and self-help treatments for anxiety disorders. Med. J. Aust. 181 (7 Suppl), S29.
Ka, L., et al. 2006. Treatment results of acupuncture in inferior alveolar and lingual nerves sensory paralysis after oral surgery. Kokubyo Gakkai Zasshi 73, 40.
Kaye, A.D., et al. 2007. Pharmacology of herbals and their impact in anesthesia. Curr. Opin. Anaesthesiol. 20, 294.
Leo, R.J., Ligot Jr., J.S., 2007. A systematic review of randomized controlled trials of acupuncture in the treatment of depression. J. Affect. Disord. 97, 13.
Lin, J.G., Chen, W.L., 2008. Acupuncture analgesia: a review of its mechanisms of actions. Am. J. Chin. Med. 36, 635.
Little, J.W., 2004. Complementary and alternative medicine: impact on dentistry. Oral Surg. Oral Med. Oral Pathol. Oral Radiol. Endod. 98, 137.
Lu, D.P., Lu, G.P., 2003. Anatomical relevance of some acupuncture points in the head and neck region that dictate medical or dental application depending on depth of needle insertion. Acupunct. Electrother. Res. 28, 145.
McCarney, R.W., et al. 2004. An overview of two Cochrane systematic reviews of complementary treatments for chronic asthma: acupuncture and homeopathy. Respir. Med. 98, 687.
Meurman, J.H., 2005. Probiotics: do they have a role in oral medicine and dentistry? Eur. J. Oral Sci. 113, 188.
Morganstein, W.M., 2005. Acupuncture in the treatment of xerostomia: clinical report. Gen. Dent. 53, 223. quiz 227
Myers, C.D., et al. 2002. A review of complementary and alternative medicine use for treating chronic facial pain. J. Am. Dent. Assoc. 133, 1189. quiz 1259.
Needham, R., Davies, S.J., 2013. Use of the Grindcare® device in the management of nocturnal bruxism: a pilot study. Br. Dent. J. 215 (1), E1. doi: 10.1038/sj.bdj.2013.653 PubMed PMID: 23846087.
Nieuw Amerongen, A.V., Veerman, E.C., 2003. Current therapies for xerostomia and salivary gland hypofunction associated with cancer therapies. Support Care Cancer 11, 226.
Nigenda, G., et al. 2001. Practice of traditional medicine in Latin America and the Caribbean: the dilemma between regulation and tolerance. Salud Publica Mex. 43 (1), 41. In Spanish. PubMed PMID: 11270283.
Pilkington, K., et al. 2007. Acupuncture for anxiety and anxiety disorders – a systematic literature review. Acupunct. Med. 25, 1.
Pirotta, M., 2007. Acupuncture in musculoskeletal disorders – is there a point? Aust. Fam. Physician 36, 447.
Pohodenko-Chudakova, I.O., 2005. Acupuncture analgesia and its application in cranio-maxillofacial surgical procedures. J. Craniomaxillofac. Surg. 33, 118.
Rathbone, J., Xia, J., 2005. Acupuncture for schizophrenia. Cochrane Database Syst. Rev. 4, CD005475.
Robb, K.A., et al. 2008. Transcutaneous electric nerve stimulation (TENS) for cancer pain in adults. Cochrane Database Syst. Rev. 3, CD006276.
Rosted, P., Bundgaard, M., 2003. Can acupuncture reduce the induction time of a local anaesthetic? A pilot study. Acupunct. Med. 21, 92.

Rosted, P., et al. 2006. The use of acupuncture in controlling the gag reflex in patients requiring an upper alginate impression: an audit. Br. Dent. J. 201, 721. discussion 715.

Rosted, P., et al. 2006. The use of acupuncture in the treatment of temporomandibular dysfunction – an audit. Acupunct. Med. 24, 16.

Sari, E., Sari, T., 2010. The role of acupuncture in the treatment of orthodontic patients with a gagging reflex: a pilot study. Br. Dent. J. 208 (10), E19.10.1038/sj.bdj.2010.483 PubMed PMID: 20489741.

Simcock, R., et al. 2013. ARIX: a randomised trial of acupuncture v oral care sessions in patients with chronic xerostomia following treatment of head and neck cancer. Ann. Oncol. 24 (3), 776.10.1093/annonc/mds515 Epub 2012 Oct 25.

Smith, C.A., Hay, P.P., 2005. Acupuncture for depression. Cochrane Database Syst. Rev. 2, CD004046.

Snyder, M., Wieland, J., 2003. Complementary and alternative therapies: what is their place in the management of chronic pain? Nurs. Clin. North Am. 38, 495.

Spanemberg, J.C., et al. 2012. Effect of an herbal compound for treatment of burning mouth syndrome: randomized, controlled, double-blind clinical trial. Oral Surg. Oral Med. Oral Pathol. Oral Radiol. 113 (3), 373.10.1016/j.oooo.2011.09.005 PubMed PMID: 22669143.

Stavem, K., et al. 2008. Health-related quality of life outcomes in a trial of acupuncture, sham acupuncture and conventional treatment for chronic sinusitis. BMC Res. Notes 1, 37.

Sun, Y., et al. 2008. Acupuncture and related techniques for postoperative pain: a systematic review of randomized controlled trials. Br. J. Anaesth. 101, 151.

Surjushe, A., et al. 2008. Aloe vera: a short review. Indian J. Dermatol. 53 (4), 163.10.4103/0019-5154.44785 PMCID: PMC2763764

Thayer, M.L., 2007. The use of acupuncture in dentistry. Dent. Update 34 (244), 249.

Türp, J.C., 2011. Limited evidence that acupuncture is effective for treating temporomandibular disorders. Evid. Based Dent. 12 (3), 89.10.1038/sj.ebd.6400816 PubMed PMID: 21979775

Tweddell, P., Boyle, C., 2009. Potential interactions with herbal medications and midazolam. Dent. Update 36, 175.

Vachiramon, A., et al. 2004. The use of acupuncture in implant dentistry. Implant Dent. 13, 58.

Vicente-Barrero, M., et al. 2012. The efficacy of acupuncture and decompression splints in the treatment of temporomandibular joint pain-dysfunction syndrome. Med. Oral Patol. Oral Cir. Bucal. 17 (6), e1028. PubMed PMID: 22549668. PubMed Central PMCID: PMC3505698.

Wang, H., et al. 2008. Is acupuncture beneficial in depression: a meta-analysis of 8 randomized controlled trials? J. Affect Disord. 111, 125.

Wang, S.M., et al. 2008. Acupuncture analgesia. II. Clinical considerations. Anesth. Analg. 106, 611.

Wang, S.M., et al. 2003. The use of complementary and alternative medicines by surgical patients: a follow-up survey study. Anesth. Analg. 97, 1010.

White, A.R., et al. 2006. Acupuncture and related interventions for smoking cessation. Cochrane Database Syst. Rev. 1, CD000009.

Wong, Y.K., Cheng, J., 2003. A case series of temporomandibular disorders treated with acupuncture, occlusal splint and point injection therapy. Acupunct. Med. 21, 138.

Yan, Z., et al. 2012. A systematic review of acupuncture or acupoint injection for management of burning mouth syndrome. Quintessence Int. 43 (8), 695. PubMed PMID: 23034422.

Zhang, S.H., et al. 2005. Acupuncture for acute stroke. Cochrane Database Syst. Rev. 2, CD003317.

Zheng, L.W., et al. 2011. Traditional Chinese medicine and oral diseases: today and tomorrow. Oral Dis. 17 (1), 7.10.1111/j.1601-0825.2010.01706.x Review. PubMed PMID: 20646230.

Zhuang, L., et al. 2013. The preventive and therapeutic effect of acupuncture for radiation-induced xerostomia in patients with head and neck cancer: a systematic review. Integr. Cancer Ther. 12 (3), 197.10.1177/1534735412451321 Epub 2012 Jul 12.

APPENDIX 26.1 HERBAL PREPARATIONS AND SUPPLEMENTS OF UNPROVEN EFFICACY

Herbal preparation	Purported use for 'treating'	Interactions possible with	Comments
Agnus castus fruit extract	Premenstrual syndrome	–	–
Butterbur (*Petasites hybridus*)	Allergic rhinitis	–	–
Coenzyme Q_{10} (CoQ_{10}, Q_{10}, vitamin Q10, ubiquinone or ubidecarenone)	Breast and other cancer control	Warfarin	–
	Periodontal disease (no proven benefit)	Insulin	
Cranberry–lingonberry juice	Recurrent urinary tract infections	–	Possibly effective
Feverfew (*Chrysanthemum parthenium*)	Migraine prophylaxis	Anticoagulants	–
Garlic	Mildly elevated cholesterol and blood pressure and to help arteries remain elastic. Also has antibacterial properties	Anticoagulants Saquinavir	Has antiplatelet activity
Ginger	Nausea and vomiting	–	May impair platelet activity
Ginseng	Aphrodisiac, antidepressant, increases resistance, and improves both physical and mental performance	–	Possibly effective. Can cause bleeding, hypertension and tachycardia
Glucosamine	Pain control and for improving function in osteoarthritis	–	Possibly effective
Senna	Constipation	–	Possibly effective
Valerian (*Valeriana officinalis*)	Sleep disturbance	Barbiturates	–

APPENDIX 26.2 HERBAL PREPARATIONS AND SUPPLEMENTS OF UNPROVEN EFFICACY HAVING POSSIBLE ADVERSE EFFECTS

Herbal medicine	May also contain	Possible health hazard
Aristolochia plantain	*Digitalis lanata*	Cardiac
Arthrin	Indometacin and alprazolam	Sedation
Chaparral (a traditional American Indian medicine)	–	Liver disease
Comfrey (*Symphytum* species)	–	Hepatic blood flow obstruction
Ephedra, ma huang, Chinese ephedra and epitonin	–	Hypertension, arrhythmia. Nerve damage, insomnia, tremors, headaches, seizures, stroke and death
Germander (*Teucrium* species)	–	Liver disease
Germanium	–	Kidney damage, possibly death
Green leaf tobacco	–	Nicotine poisoning

(Continued)

Herbal medicine	May also contain	Possible health hazard
Hepastat, neutralis, poena, osporo	Indometacin	–
Hua fo	Sildenafil	–
Jin bu huan	–	Liver disease
Kava kava	–	Liver damage
Lobelia (also known as Indian tobacco)	–	Breathing problems. Sweating, hypotension, tachycardia, and possibly coma and death at higher doses
L-Tryptophan	–	Eosinophilia myalgia syndrome
Magnolia–Stephania	–	Renal disease
Neo-melubrina	Metamizole (dipyrone)	–
Niacin	–	Stomach pain, vomiting, bloating, nausea, cramping, diarrhoea, liver disease, muscle disease, cardiac and eye damage
PC-SPES (a formula consisting of a combination of eight herbs that contain a range of plant chemicals including flavonoids, alkanoids, polysaccharides)	Warfarin	Bleeding
Pennyroyal	–	Liver disease
RA Spes	Alprazolam	Sedation
5OA Plus	Indometacin	–
Selenium	–	Tissue damage
Slimming/dieter's teas	–	Nausea, diarrhoea, vomiting, stomach cramps, constipation, fainting
SPES	Alprazolam	Sedation
Vitamin A	–	Birth defects, bone abnormalities, severe liver disease
Vitamin B$_6$	–	Ataxia, nerve injury
Willow bark	Salicylates	Reye syndrome
Wormwood	–	Hypoaesthesia of legs and arms, loss of intellect, delirium and paralyses

DIET AND HEALTH

Dietary factors have been implicated as influencing a range of conditions (Box 27.1; see also Ch. 36).

Minimizing intake of saturated fat (especially from dairy sources) and partially hydrogenated vegetable fats lowers the risk of coronary artery disease and some cancers (Chs 5 and 22). In contrast, consumption of monounsaturated fats, such as olive oil, and omega oils may be beneficial. Generous amounts of vegetables and fruit daily appear to offer some protection against cancers of the stomach, colon and lung, and possibly against cancers of the mouth, larynx, cervix, bladder and breast (Ch. 22). Citrus fruits and juices in excess, however, may cause tooth erosion.

Carbohydrates as wholegrain, unrefined products may offer some protection against colon cancer, diverticulitis and dental caries. A high-fibre diet may offer some protection against hypertension and coronary heart disease (Ch. 5).

MALNUTRITION

Malnutrition is mainly a consequence of lack of resources and education, and results from imbalance between people's needs and their intake of nutrients, which can lead to obesity or to syndromes of deficiency, dependency or toxicity. Overnutrition develops over time from overeating; insufficient exercise; overprescription of therapeutic diets, including parenteral nutrition; excess intake of vitamins, particularly pyridoxine (vitamin B_6), niacin and vitamins A and D; and excess intake of trace minerals. Undernutrition (starvation) usually results from inadequate intake; malabsorption; abnormal systemic loss due to diarrhoea, haemorrhage, renal failure, cancer or excessive sweating; infection; or addiction to drugs. Undernutrition can develop rapidly.

OBESITY

General aspects

To most people, the term 'obesity' means the state of being very overweight; however, 'overweight' is sometimes defined as an excess amount of body weight that includes muscle, bone, fat and water, while 'obesity' specifically refers to excessive body fat. Some people, such as bodybuilders or other athletes with a lot of muscle, can be overweight without being obese. Obesity is the main nutritional problem in developed countries (Fig. 27.1), though some body fat is needed for energy, heat insulation, shock absorption and other functions. As a rule, women have more body fat than men. Men with more than 25% body fat and women with more than 30% body fat are obese.

Almost 25% of North American adults are now clinically obese and obesity is increasing in children. More than 60% of Americans aged 20 years and older are overweight. Europe and Japan follow similar patterns. In 2012 in England, 16% of children and 26% of adults were obese. The prevalence of obesity in England has more than tripled in the last 25 years.

Obesity results from eating more than the body needs – an imbalance between calories in and calories out. Control of eating and weight regulation is complex and involves a range of endocrine and nervous

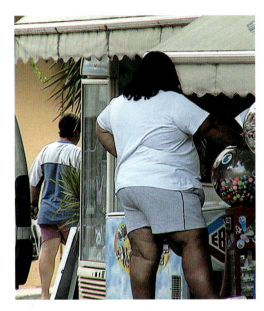

Fig. 27.1 Obesity – the main nutritional problem today.

signals, especially peptide YY, ghrelin, insulin, cholecystokinin and leptin (Table 27.1). The body monitors blood glucose concentration, which contributes to the overall regulation of food intake, via GLUT2 transporters, which mediate glucose entry to the cells, and the glucokinase enzyme. This makes their intracellular adenosine triphosphate (ATP) supply exquisitely sensitive to glucose availability, and forms the basis for their signalling systems by pancreatic beta-cells; portal vein glucose sensor; carotid bodies; the nucleus of the solitary tract; and the hypothalamus – which triggers a massive sympathetic response to hypoglycaemia, with pounding heart, trembling, anxiety, sweating and hunger. However, the effects of hyperglycaemia on feeding and satiation are less obvious, and may even lead to paradoxical overeating. Leptin (from the Greek *leptos*, meaning thin) is a protein hormone released by fat cells that counteracts the effects of neuropeptide Y, a potent feeding stimulant secreted by cells in the gut; it has important effects in regulating metabolism, reproductive function and body weight, acting on the hypothalamic arcuate nucleus to suppress eating behaviour and also to increase energy expenditure. Leptin also acts directly on the liver and skeletal muscle, where it stimulates the oxidation of fatty acids in the mitochondria, reducing the storage of fat in those tissues (but not in adipose tissue). The absence of functional leptin (or its receptor) leads to uncontrolled food intake and resulting

Table 27.1 *Complications of obesity (plus various cancers)*

Cardiovascular	Orthopaedic	Psychosocial	Gastrointestinal	Respiratory	Metabolic and endocrine	Gynaecological
Hypertension	Accidents	Depression	Diverticulitis	Cor pulmonale	Diabetes mellitus	Amenorrhoea
Ischaemic heart disease	Gout	Social effects	Gallstones	Sleep apnoea	Hyperlipoproteinaemias (types II, III and IV)	Menstrual irregularities and infertility
Stroke	Osteoarthritis		Hiatus hernia (and other hernias)			Polycystic ovaries
Varicose veins			Liver disease			Uterine prolapse

obesity. Rarely, mutations in the leptin gene or its receptor are found in obese people but these are only a very uncommon cause of morbid obesity. Recombinant human leptin trials in the hope of reducing obesity in humans have so far had no great benefit.

Many other factors that appear to affect appetite, satiation and obesity include proinflammatory cytokines (tumour necrosis factor alpha [TNFα], interleukin-6 [IL-6] and IL-1); incretins (cholecystokinin, gastric inhibitory peptide [GIP], glucagon-like peptide 1 and glucagon-like peptide 2); the melanocortin receptor system (MCR); cocaine and amphetamine-regulated transcript (CART); thyrotropin-releasing hormone; corticosteroids; and growth hormone (for more information, see http://www.bmb.leeds.ac.uk/teaching/icu3/lecture/26; accessed 30 September 2013).

Environmental factors affecting body weight include lifestyle behaviours, such as what a person eats and their level of physical activity. Psychological factors may play a role; many people eat in response to negative emotions such as boredom, sadness or anger. Some antidepressants can cause weight gain. Genetic factors, hormonal influences, hypothalamic disease (Frohlich, Laurence–Moon–Biedl or Prader–Willi syndromes), endocrinopathies (hypothyroidism, Cushing disease or insulinoma) or drugs (e.g. steroids) can rarely be implicated.

Clinical features

There is about a threefold increase in premature deaths in obese patients because of heart disease, type 2 diabetes, hypertension, stroke and cancer (see Table 27.1; Fig. 27.2). Obese men are more likely than non-obese men to die from cancer of the colon, rectum or prostate. Obese women are more likely to die from cancer of the gallbladder, breast, uterus, cervix or ovaries.

General management

Measuring body fat is not easy. A simple method is to measure the subcutaneous fat thickness in several parts of the body with skin callipers. The most accurate methods are to weigh the person under water or to use dual-energy X-ray absorptiometry (DEXA). Body mass index (BMI), the standard for measuring overweight and obesity, uses a formula based on height and weight: BMI equals weight in kilograms divided by height in metres squared (BMI = kg/m²; Table 27.2). Because measuring body fat is difficult, health-care providers often rely on weight-for-height tables – a range of acceptable weights for a person of a given height. However, these tables do not distinguish between muscle and excess fat.

Bariatric medicine (from the Greek *baros* [weight] and *-iatrics* [medical treatment]) is the term used for the specialty of caring for obese patients. Weight loss is recommended, particularly if there are two or more of the following:

- Family history of heart disease or diabetes
- Pre-existing disorders, such as hypertension, hyperglycaemia or hypercholesterolaemia
- 'Apple' body shape.

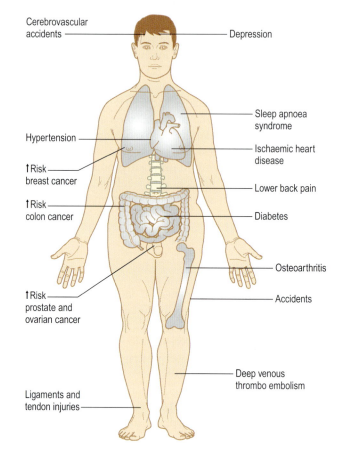

Fig. 27.2 Obesity outcomes.

Table 27.2 *Body mass index (BMI)*

BMI (kg/m²)	Classification
<18.5	Underweight
18.5–24.9	Normal
25.0–29.9	Overweight
30.0–34.9	Obesity class I
35.0–39.9	Obesity class II
≥40	Obesity class III

The method of treatment depends on the degree of obesity, overall health condition and motivation to lose weight. It may include a combination of diet, exercise, behaviour modification and sometimes weight-loss drugs (Table 27.3) or surgery. People who have a BMI of 30 or more can improve their health by weight loss – especially if they are severely obese. A weight loss of 5–10% can do much to improve health by lowering blood pressure and cholesterol levels, and preventing type 2 diabetes in people at high risk for it. Sympathomimetic appetite suppressants are used only in the short-term treatment of obesity since their effect tends to decrease after a few weeks. Tesofensine is a new agent of possible benefit.

Table 27.3 *Drugs used in treatment of obesity*

Drug	Mechanism	Possible adverse effects	Comments
Butabindide	Blocks cholecystokinin breakdown	Not yet in clinical use	Inhibits tripeptidylpeptidase
Cholecystokinin promoters	Increase cholecystokinin receptors	–	–
Glucagon-like peptide 1	Delays gastric emptying, more insulin	–	Used in type 2 diabetes
Orlistat	Blocks pancreatic lipase	Anal leakage	Fatty stools
Sibutramine	Blocks 5-hydroxytryptamine (5HT) uptake/sympathomimetic	Dry mouth, headache	May cause hypertension and tachycardia
(Dex)fenfluramine	Blocks 5HT uptake	Cardiac valve defects	Withdrawn because of adverse effects
Troglitazone	Activates peroxisome proliferator-activated receptor gamma (PPARγ)	Liver damage	Withdrawn because of adverse effects
Topiramate	Central nervous system (CNS) effects	CNS effects	Poor compliance

In severe obesity, bariatric surgery may rarely be recommended. It aims at:

- reducing stomach size:
  vertical banded gastroplasty (Mason procedure, stomach stapling)
  laparoscopic adjustable gastric band (LAGB; REALIZE® band – lap band)
  sleeve gastrectomy
  transoral gastroplasty
- reducing food absorption:
  biliopancreatic diversion (Scopinaro procedure – rare)
- or mixed procedures:
  gastric bypass
  sleeve gastrectomy with duodenal switch
  implantable gastric stimulation.

Severely obese people can encounter many problems relating to health-care access.

Dental aspects

Bariatric surgeries may be associated with an increased risk for gastro-oesophageal reflux and taking a more cariogenic diet, which in turn might account for the higher amount of carious and erosive tooth surface loss seen in bariatric patients. Jaw wiring of obese patients appears to be an effective and safe way of substantially reducing weight in those in whom simpler methods fail, but relapse frequently follows.

Dental treatment of obese patients may be complicated mainly by the sheer size of the patient and difficulties in accessing the dental chair. Bariatric dental chairs suitable for all patient groups up to 454 kg (1000 lb; 71 st) are available, in which large, overweight, obese and bariatric patients can be safely treated (e.g. Diaco, Barico). Respiration is impaired if the patient is laid supine. The total work of breathing is greater and, even at rest, obese patients need to ventilate more than normal. Some 10% of the grossly obese have hypoventilation, cor pulmonale and episodic somnolence (Pickwickian syndrome).

Local anaesthesia (LA) is satisfactory but may prove more difficult because of the thickness of the tissues. Conscious sedation (CS) may be given if required. Cardiac arrhythmias may be produced by the interaction of halogenated anaesthetics and large doses of amphetamines or amphetamine-like appetite suppressants (all controlled drugs), which should be discontinued a week before general anaesthesia (GA).

Treatment may also be complicated by diabetes or, rarely, by an organic cause of the obesity. Sympathomimetic appetite suppressants may interact with a range of drugs (Box 27.2).

Appetite suppressants, including sibutramine and phentermine, and herbal supplements containing ephedrine alkaloids/caffeine (ma huang, kola nut) can produce dry mouth.

Box 27.2 *Drugs that can interact with sympathomimetic appetite suppressants*

- Antidepressants
- Amantadine
- Amphetamines
- Caffeine
- Clofedanol
- Cocaine
- Methylphenidate
- Nabilone
- Pemoline

Table 27.4 *Vegetarianism*

Type of vegetarianism	Dietary habits
Fruitarianism	Eat only fruit products
Veganism	Abstain from all foods from animals, including dairy products
Lacto-vegetarianism	Like vegans, but eat dairy products
Lacto-ovo-vegetarianism	Like vegans, but eat dairy products and eggs
Pesco-vegetarianism	Like vegans, but eat dairy products, eggs and fish
Semi-vegetarianism	Like vegans, but eat dairy products, eggs, fish and poultry

EATING HABITS

Vegetarianism

Vegetarianism includes a range of habits (Table 27.4). *Vegans* are strict vegetarians, avoiding all foods of animal origin, including meat, poultry, fish, dairy products and eggs. This can lead to vitamin B_{12} deficiency (Ch. 8), though this is surprisingly uncommon – vegans typically use yeast extracts and oriental-style fermented foods to provide B_{12}. Calcium, iron and zinc intakes also tend to be low. *Lacto-vegetarians* include dairy products in their diet. *Lacto-ovo-vegetarianism* – whose adherents also eat dairy products and eggs – is the most common form of vegetarianism. *Pesco-vegetarians* eat fish, dairy products and eggs along with plant foods. *Semi-vegetarians* eat some poultry and fish, dairy products and eggs. *Fruitarians* eat only fruit and their diet is thus deficient in protein, salt and many micronutrients; this diet is not recommended.

Vegetarians tend to live longer and develop fewer chronic disabling conditions than their meat-eating peers. However, their lifestyle usually also includes regular exercise and abstention from alcohol and tobacco, which may contribute to their improved health. Vegetarians may have less caries. Disadvantages are few; iron deficiency is the main risk. A fruitarian or prolonged lacto-vegetarian diet may suffer from dental erosion; citrus fruits, vinegar and acidic berries are especially responsible, particularly if ingested just before retiring to sleep.

Fad diets

Many commercial diets claim to enhance well-being or reduce weight but some have resulted in vitamin, mineral and protein deficiency states. Cardiac, renal and metabolic disorders, as well as some deaths, have resulted.

EATING DISORDERS

Eating is controlled by many factors, including appetite; food availability; family, peer and cultural practices; and attempts at voluntary control. Dieting is a common practice in the developed world and heavily promoted by fashion trends, sales campaigns and in some activities (e.g. fashion models). Food fads, selective eating (extreme fussiness) and food avoidance (without any fear of weight gain) are relatively common and usually fairly inconsequential in medical terms. Eating disorders, however, are of concern and are frequent among models, elite performers of certain sports or physical activities, ballet dancers, gymnasium users and bodybuilders.

Dieting to a body weight lower than is needed for health is common; eating disorders are also common and spotting the borderline between the two can be difficult. Eating disorders usually develop during adolescence or early adulthood, most often in females. They often coexist with other mental health issues, such as depression, substance abuse and anxiety disorders; they can disturb growth, lead to endocrine, cardiac and renal disease, and may be fatal. There are probably 90 000 people in UK receiving treatment.

Most people are concerned about their weight, so the early signs of eating disorders may easily be overlooked (Box 27.3). Eating disorders include anorexia nervosa (self-imposed starvation), bulimia nervosa (binge-eating and dieting), binge-eating disorder, and eating disorder not otherwise specified (EDNOS) (Table 27.5). Night-eating syndrome (NES) is also reportedly common – especially in obese people. Nocturnal sleep-related eating disorder (NS-RED) is not strictly an

---

Box 27.3 *Early signs of eating disorders*

- Changes in habits or activities
- Secretive behaviour
- Withdrawal from family or friends
- Weight loss
- Irregular menstruation or amenorrhoea
- Signs of vomiting
- Sudden disappearance of food from kitchen
- Finding of laxatives or diuretics

Table 27.5 *The eating disorders[a]*

Anorexia nervosa	Bulimia nervosa	Binge-eating disorder	Night-eating syndrome	Eating disorder not otherwise specified[b]
Food intake				
Refusal to maintain body weight over a minimal normal for age and height	Recurrent episodes of binge-eating, including eating more than most people in a discrete period of time, and sense of loss of control	Recurrent episodes of binge-eating, including eating more than most people in a discrete period of time, and sense of loss of control	Eating excessively (hyperphagia) at night after retiring to bed	
Behaviour				
Intense fear of gaining weight or of becoming fat, even though underweight	Regular engagement in inappropriate compensatory behaviours	At least three behavioural measures of loss of control during bingeing	Obesity	
Disturbance in body perception	Minimum of at least two bingeing episodes each week for at least 3 months	Rapid eating	Insomnia, anorexia in the mornings	
	Persistent overconcern about body shape and weight	Eating until uncomfortably full	Minimum of at least 2 months	
	May be abuse of medications in order to lose weight	Eating large amounts when not hungry	Eating produces guilt and shame, not enjoyment	
		Eating large amounts outside meal times	Mood lower in mornings	
		Eating alone because of embarrassment at quantities eaten	Depression common	
		Negative feelings about self because of eating		
		Minimum of at least two bingeing episodes each week for at least 6 months		
		Marked distress at bingeing		
		No abuse of medications in order to lose weight		
Others				
Amenorrhoea				

[a]Modified from Diagnostic and Statistical Manual of Disease version 4 (DSM-IV).
[b]Disorders of eating that do not fit criteria for other categories.

eating disorder; rather it is a type of sleep disorder in which people eat while 'sleepwalking', seeming to be sound asleep.

The main disorders that can have life-threatening health complications are anorexia nervosa and bulimia nervosa; they affect mainly females.

Anorexia nervosa

Anorexia nervosa is failure to eat, in the absence of any physical cause, to the extent that more than 15% of body weight is lost. It has several complications and may become life-threatening (Fig. 27.3). Body image may be distorted, so the emaciated patients consider themselves normal or even fat. Intense fear of gaining weight or becoming fat, even though underweight, with resistance to maintaining body weight at or above a minimally normal for age and height, is prominent (Box 27.4). Disturbance in body image, the way in which the body weight or

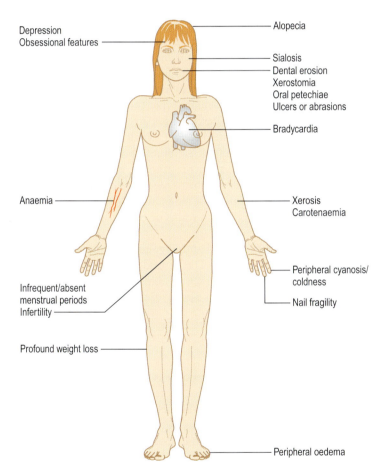

Fig. 27.3 Anorexia nervosa.

shape is perceived, undue influences of body weight or shape on self-evaluation, denial of the seriousness of the current low body weight, obsession in the process of eating and development of unusual habits are common. Examples include avoiding food and meals, picking out a few foods and eating these in small amounts, pushing food around the plate instead of eating, or carefully weighing and portioning food. Anorectics may repeatedly check their body weight, despite severe weight loss (Fig. 27.4). Engaging in techniques to control weight, such as intense and compulsive exercise, purging by means of vomiting, or abuse of laxatives, enemas, appetite suppressants, diuretics and thyroid hormones, is common.

Girls with anorexia often experience a delayed onset of the first menstrual period, since gonadotropin release is impaired. In others, periods may become infrequent or cease. Depression, anxiety, obsessive–compulsive disorder and self-harming are common. Growth may be impaired. Anorexia nervosa may be complicated by anaemia, endocrine disturbances, peripheral oedema and electrolyte depletion (hypokalaemia), peripheral cyanosis and coldness with bradycardia (see Table 27.5).

The course and outcome of anorexia nervosa vary. Some sufferers recover fully after a single episode; some have a fluctuating pattern of weight gain and relapse; and others experience a chronically deteriorating course over many years. The morbidity is high (Table 27.6) and mortality rate is about 12 times increased, cardiac arrest, electrolyte imbalance or suicide being the main causes.

Bulimia nervosa

Bulimia nervosa is recurrent episodes of binge-eating, which may be associated with compensatory behaviours such as self-induced vomiting and purgative abuse. The binge-eating and inappropriate compensatory behaviours are practised, on average, at least twice a week for 3 months. Features include irresistible craving for food, characterized by eating an excessive amount within a discrete period of time and by a sense of lack of control over eating during the episode. Recurrent inappropriate compensatory behaviour in order to prevent weight gain is common, and may include self-induced vomiting or misuse of laxatives, diuretics, enemas or other medications (purging), fasting or excessive exercise. Bulimics often perform their behaviours in secrecy, feeling disgusted and ashamed when binging, and relieved once they purge.

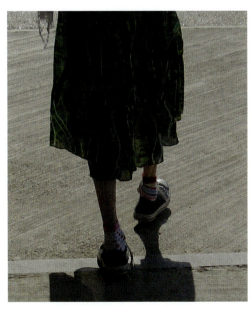

Fig. 27.4 Anorexia nervosa. Severely thin limbs.

Table 27.6 *Medical and oral complications of anorexia nervosa*

Type	Complication
Cardiovascular	Bradycardia
	Hypotension
	Arrhythmias
	Cardiac failure
Endocrinological	Raised cortisol
	Reduced gonadotropins, thyroid and sex hormones
Gastrointestinal	Oesophagitis
	Oesophageal rupture
	Duodenal dilatation
	Constipation
Haematological	Bone marrow hypoplasia
	Pancytopenia
	Lowered plasma protein levels
Metabolic	Dehydration
	Hypothermia
	Hypokalaemia
	Hypercholesterolaemia
	Hypoglycaemia
	Abnormal liver function
Musculoskeletal	Osteoporosis
	Pathological fractures
	Impaired growth
	Myopathies
	Tetany
Neurological	Brain atrophy
	Seizures
Oral	Mucosal atrophy, glossitis and glossodynia
	Dental erosion
	Sialosis
	Hyposalivation
Renal	Low glomerular filtration rate (GFR)
	Hypokalaemic nephropathy

Box 27.5 *Features of bulimia nervosa*

- Recurrent episodes of binge-eating
- Recurrent inappropriate compensatory behaviour in order to prevent weight gain, e.g. self-induced vomiting or misuse of laxatives, diuretics, enemas or other medications (purging)

Bulimics usually weigh within the normal range for their age and height but, like individuals with anorexia, may fear gaining weight, desire to lose weight and feel intensely dissatisfied with their bodies (Box 27.5).

General management of eating disorders

Eating disorders are serious conditions with a high co-morbidity and a poor prognosis: only 30–50% make a full recovery. Acute management of severe weight loss (BMI <13) is usually provided in hospital, where medical care and monitoring are needed to try to restore healthy eating and deal with the underlying emotional/psychological issues (by cognitive behavioural or interpersonal psychotherapy, nutritional counselling and, when appropriate, medication). Selective serotonin reuptake inhibitors (SSRIs) may be helpful for weight maintenance and for resolving mood and anxiety symptoms.

Table 27.7 *Management of patients with tooth erosion*

Minimize tooth exposure to dietary acids	Increase oral pH	Caries protection
Reduce carbonated drinks, fruit juices, vinegar, alcohol	Mouth rinses of water, milk or bicarbonate	Non-cariogenic diet
Use a straw to drink low-pH fluids where feasible	Chewing gum	Fluorides
		Plaque control

Dental aspects of eating disorders

Repeated doses of paracetamol (acetaminophen) may be hepatotoxic in anorexia nervosa; doses should be kept to the minimum. Anaemia and the possibility of hypokalaemia and consequent arrhythmias must be kept in mind if GA is considered necessary.

Oral manifestations (see Table 27.6) can include erosion of teeth (perimylolysis) after repeated vomiting, usually most severe on lingual, palatal and occlusal surfaces. The patient should be counselled about diet and oral hygiene, what drinks and foods to avoid (Table 27.7) and how to reduce further erosion (e.g. by drinking colas and fruit juices through a straw). There is no evidence that tooth-brushing is harmful to eroded teeth, even soon after taking a drink of low pH. Topical bicarbonate after each vomiting incident, combined with daily sodium fluoride gel applications or a 0.05% sodium fluoride mouthwash, may lessen dental damage. Desensitizing toothpaste may also be indicated. Full-coverage plastic splints may be needed to protect the teeth and it may help to fill these splints with magnesium hydroxide. Restorative care may include dentine-bonded resins or composites, crowns or use of a Dahl appliance.

Parotid enlargement (sialosis) and angular stomatitis may develop, as in other forms of starvation. The parotid swellings tend to subside if the patient resumes a normal diet. Oral ulcers or abrasions, particularly in the soft palate, may be caused by fingers or other objects used to induce vomiting.

Pica

Pica is a condition in which the appetite is perverted. It is seen mainly in persons with learning disability or mental health issues, but is sometimes due to pregnancy or iron deficiency. Many unusual objects and substances may be ingested, such as buttons, screws, pins, nails, etc., and some may cause gastrointestinal obstruction or perforation (Fig. 27.5). In the past, children sometimes chewed painted objects and succumbed to lead poisoning, which still occurs in the developing world.

UNDERNUTRITION

General aspects

Severe undernutrition results mainly from poverty, especially in children and older people in the developing world or in war zones. Other causes include eating disorders, abuse (food restriction), oral problems, obstruction to the pharynx or oesophagus, malabsorption and cachexia of malignant disease or HIV/AIDS. Undernutrition is the most common cause of immunodeficiency worldwide.

Infants and children are at particular risk of undernutrition because of a high demand for energy and essential nutrients. Protein-energy malnutrition in children consuming inadequate amounts of protein, calories and other nutrients is a particularly severe form of

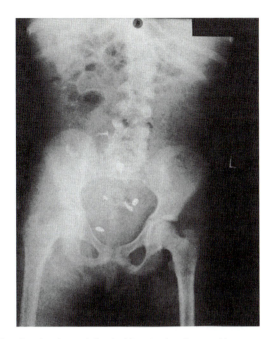

Fig. 27.5 Pica showing intra-abdominal ingested radio-opacities.

undernutrition, which retards growth and development. Deficiencies of iron, folic acid, vitamin C, copper, zinc and vitamin A may develop in inadequately fed infants and children. An exclusively breast-fed infant can develop vitamin B_{12} deficiency if the mother is a vegan.

Adolescents are at risk since nutritional requirements go up as the growth rate increases. Requirements for all nutrients rise during pregnancy and lactation. Anaemia due to folic acid deficiency is common in pregnant women, especially those who have taken oral contraceptives, so folic acid supplements are now recommended to prevent neural tube defects (spina bifida) in their children. Aberrations of diet (rarely including pica) are common in pregnancy. An alcoholic mother may have a handicapped and stunted child with fetal alcohol syndrome. Caffeine has been implicated in miscarriages and underweight babies.

Older people, despite a reduction in physical activity lowering their energy and protein requirements, are at risk of undernutrition because of poverty, apathy or dementia. Diminished senses of taste and smell, poverty (real or perceived), loneliness, physical and mental impairments, immobility and chronic illness can also contribute. Furthermore, absorption may be impaired, contributing to iron deficiency, osteoporosis (also related to calcium deficiency), and osteomalacia due to lack of vitamin D and sunshine exposure (Ch. 25).

Clinical features

Features of undernutrition may include listlessness, emaciation, skin dryness, scaliness, atrophy, petechiae, ecchymoses, spooned nails, depigmentation, loss of hair and orofacial problems (angular stomatitis, glossitis, ulcers and sialosis).

General management

The history may reveal food faddism, lack of variety, inadequate intake of energy-rich and essential nutrients, poor appetite, gastrointestinal disturbance and recent weight loss. Chronic use of alcohol, cocaine, heroin, immunosuppressants or some antibiotics and anticonvulsants raises questions about the adequacy of vitamin and mineral nutrition.

The musculature should be examined for size, strength and tenderness. Neurological examination may detect disorientation, an abnormal gait, altered reflexes, and sensory or motor neuron abnormalities. Painful bones and joints, osteopenia and distortions in the shape or size of bones (e.g. rachitic rosary) may indicate current or past malnutrition.

Nutritional status can be classified on the basis of BMI. The triceps skinfold estimates the amount of body fat within 20% and is therefore useful in determining the body's energy stores. Based on the mid-arm muscle area, muscle mass may be classified as adequate, marginal, depleted or wasted. Imaging (radiography, computed tomography [CT] or magnetic resonance imaging [MRI]) may be needed.

A full blood count and measurement of plasma proteins reflect the adequacy of amino-acid nutrition (albumin, pre-albumin and transferrin). Electrolyte assays may point to a mineral deficiency. Lipids and related lipoproteins should be assayed.

The patient may need hospital treatment, including nasogastric feeding. Refeeding syndrome (see below) must be avoided.

Dental aspects

Undernutrition in children can result in retarded tooth eruption. Latent undernutrition may predispose to burning mouth syndrome, mouth ulcers, glossitis and angular stomatitis. Resulting immunodeficiencies predispose to oral ulceration, angular stomatitis, necrotizing gingivitis and, rarely, gangrenous stomatitis (noma; cancrum oris) or sialosis (Ch. 20).

Whether chronic undernutrition is a significant factor that underlies many oral cancers is unclear, but there is a protective effect of diets rich in fresh fruits and vegetables, and in vitamins A and C. Iron deficiency is seen in the Paterson–Brown-Kelly (Plummer–Vinson) syndrome.

Dental care can be provided under LA. CS may be given in hospital. GA should, as always, be given in hospital.

Protein-energy malnutrition

General aspects

Protein-energy malnutrition (PEM), or protein-calorie malnutrition, is seen mainly in infants and children in some developing nations. Characterized not only by an energy deficit due to a reduction in all macronutrients and a deficit in many micronutrients, PEM is an example of the inadequate protein and/or energy intake that lies between starvation (no food intake) and adequate nourishment.

Clinical features

Clinically, PEM has three forms, which depend on the balance of non-protein and protein sources of energy. Each form can be graded as mild, moderate or severe by calculating weight as a percentage of expected weight for length using international standards (normal, 90–110%; mild, 85–90%; moderate, 75–85%; severe, <75%).

Marasmus (dry, thin, desiccated) is the predominant form of PEM in developing countries, and results from near-starvation with deficiency of protein and non-protein nutrients. The consequence is emaciation due to loss of muscle and body fat. Marasmic infants have hunger, weight loss, growth retardation, and wasting of subcutaneous fat and muscle. Marasmus is associated with the early abandonment or failure of breast-feeding and with consequent infections, notably those causing infantile gastroenteritis.

Kwashiorkor (an African word for 'first child–second child') is characterized by protein deficiency more than energy deficiency, and by oedema. It refers to the observation that the first child develops PEM when the second child is born and takes over at the breast.

Kwashiorkor is confined to areas where staple and weaning foods – such as yam, cassava, sweet potato and green banana – are protein-deficient and excessively starchy (rural Africa, Caribbean and Pacific islands). Generalized oedema, 'flaky paint' skin, thinning, decolouration and reddening of the hair, enlarged fatty liver and apathy are seen, in addition to retarded growth. Pneumonia, diarrhoea, otitis media, genitourinary disease and sepsis are almost invariable.

Marasmic kwashiorkor is a combined form of undernutrition between the two extremes.

General management

Differential diagnosis includes consideration of secondary growth failure due to malabsorption, congenital defects, renal failure, endocrine disease, infections or emotional deprivation.

Fluid and electrolyte abnormalities (hypokalaemia, hypocalcaemia, hypophosphataemia and hypomagnesaemia) must be corrected and infections treated. Macronutrients should be supplied by milk-based formulas. A full-fat desiccated milk product can be fortified with additional corn oil and maltodextrin. After 4 weeks, the formula can be replaced with whole milk plus solid foods, including eggs, fruit, meats, cod liver oil and yeast. In children, mortality varies between 5% and 40%, the lower mortality rates being seen in those receiving intensive care.

Dental aspects

Noma (maxillofacial gangrene; cancrum oris) is a severe, potentially fatal infection common in starving children, particularly in Africa.

Starvation

General aspects

Starvation is the most severe form of malnutrition and may result from famine, fasting, anorexia nervosa, gastrointestinal disease, stroke, cancer or coma. The metabolic response to starvation is conservation of energy and body tissues, but the body mobilizes its tissues, resulting in destruction of organs and muscle, and extreme shrinkage of adipose tissue. Loss of organ weight is greatest in liver and intestines, moderate in heart and kidneys, and least in the nervous system.

Clinical features

Emaciation is most obvious in areas where fat normally deposits. Muscle mass shrinks and bones protrude. The skin becomes thin, dry, inelastic, pale and cold. The hair is dry and sparse, and falls out easily. Most body systems are affected (Box 27.6). Total starvation is fatal in 8–12 weeks.

General management

At first, food repletion must be limited until gastrointestinal function is restored. Food intake is then gradually increased until it is about 5000 kcal/day and weekly weight gain is 1.5–2.0 kg. Non-responsive patients may require nasogastric feeding, and parenteral nutrition is indicated if malabsorption is severe.

Alcohol or drug dependency

Patients with alcohol or drug dependency often have lifestyles in which nourishment is neglected. Nutrient absorption and metabolism are also impaired. For example, alcoholics who consume 1 litre or more

---

Box 27.6 *Features of emaciation*

- Achlorhydria and diarrhoea
- Anaemia
- Apathy and irritability
- Body temperature fall
- Cell-mediated immunity compromised
- Wound-healing impaired
- Fat and muscle loss
- Gonadal atrophy, loss of libido and amenorrhoea
- Heart size and cardiac output fall
- Respiratory rate and vital capacity fall
- Weakness

---

of spirits per day usually lose weight and become undernourished. Alcoholism is the most common cause of thiamine deficiency in the developed world and may also lead to deficiencies of magnesium, zinc, folic acid and other vitamins.

Cachexia

Cachexia is the weakness and emaciation commonly associated with serious illness, such as cancer, HIV/AIDS ('slim disease') and tuberculosis, and seen after burns, major surgery or trauma. Cachexia is mediated by proinflammatory cytokines, such as TNFα (originally termed cachexin), IL-6 and IL-1.

Carnitine deficiency

Carnitine is an amino acid required for the transport of long-chain fatty acyl coenzyme A (CoA) esters into mitochondria. Requirements are met by a combination of dietary intake (mainly animal products) and endogenous biosynthesis. Carnitine deficiency can result from inadequate intake during long-term total parenteral nutrition (TPN), impaired biosynthesis in liver disease, increased requirements in states of ketosis, and high demand for fat oxidation or excess loss of carnitine due to diarrhoea, diuresis or haemodialysis. Although uncommon, carnitine deficiency may cause muscle necrosis, myoglobinuria, lipid-storage myopathy, hypoglycaemia, fatty liver and hyperammonaemia – with muscle aches, fatigue and confusion.

Chronic diseases

In patients with chronic diseases (including those who have undergone major surgery), there may be impaired absorption of fat-soluble vitamins, vitamin B_{12}, calcium and iron. Liver disease impairs the storage of vitamins A and B_{12}, and interferes with protein and energy metabolism. Chronic kidney disease and dialysis lead to deficiencies of protein, iron and vitamin D. Patients receiving long-term home parenteral nutrition, most commonly after total or near-total resection of the gut, tend to develop vitamin and trace mineral deficiencies. Biotin, vitamin K, selenium, molybdenum, manganese and zinc must be adequately supplied.

Essential fatty acid deficiency

Essential fatty acids (EFAs) are those that must be taken in the diet. EFAs are needed for many physiological processes, including maintenance of cell membrane structure, synthesis of prostaglandins and leukotrienes, and skin integrity. EFAs include linolenic acid, eicosa-pentaenoic acid and docosahexaenoic acid (omega-3 fatty acids – largely from fish oils), and linoleic acid and arachidonic acid (omega-6 fatty acids – largely from vegetable oils, such as corn oil, cottonseed oil and soybean oil).

Omega-3 fatty acids are needed for synthesis of prostaglandins and leukotrienes, and tend to reduce inflammation. Eicosapentaenoic acid and docosahexaenoic acid are important components of the brain and retina. Omega-6 fatty acids tend to promote inflammation and cancer, and autoimmune and inflammatory disease. A diet with a high omega-3:omega-6 ratio appears to be the most healthy (Ch. 5).

Deficiency in EFAs may occur in patients with fat malabsorption, serious trauma and burns. EFA deficiency used to be a hazard of long-term fat-free TPN, but fat emulsions prevent this.

Lipodystrophy

Lipodystrophy is a rare condition in which adipose tissue cannot be produced and, in the absence of fat cells, leptin is not produced; as a result, patients cannot become obese but often develop type 2 diabetes. Treatment with recombinant leptin helps.

A rare form of lipodystrophy is facial hemiatrophy of Romberg, starting typically in adolescence and in females; there is progressive disappearance of facial fat unilaterally, mimicking facial paralysis. Patients appear to be otherwise well. Plastic surgery is the only treatment.

Lipodystrophy may also follow active antiretroviral therapy (ART) with protease inhibitors for HIV/AIDS. Clinically, there may be peripheral fat-wasting but central adiposity, with expanding abdominal girth ('protease paunch' or 'Crix belly'), growing dorsicervical fat pads ('buffalo hump'), loss of subcutaneous fat over cheeks and temples (facial thinning), arm, buttock and leg wasting, and growing prominence of leg veins.

Persons with raised blood cholesterol are at greater risk of developing lipodystrophy. Age, use of anabolic steroids and use of psychotropic medications (including antidepressants and benzodiazepines) are also associated with lipodystrophy. Associated adverse metabolic effects include hyperlipidaemia, hypercholesterolaemia, hypertriglyceridaemia, hyperglycaemia, insulin resistance and late-onset diabetes, increasing the risk of cardiovascular and other complications. Parotid lipomatosis can be a complication of ART.

VITAMINS AND THEIR DISORDERS

Vitamins are essential organic dietary factors that cannot be synthesized within the body (Table 27.8). They are required in only small amounts but their deficiency can result in disease (Table 27.9).

Sometimes, vitamin excess can be dangerous (Table 27.10). Vitamin A supplementation has been linked to birth defects and irreversible bone and liver damage. Vitamin D supplementation can cause hypercalcaemia. Other adverse effects include diarrhoea (from vitamin C), neuropathies (long-term use of high doses of vitamin B_6) and flushing (niacin).

VITAMIN A (RETINOL)

Vitamin A is fat-soluble and found in animal fats, milk and liver. It can also be derived from precursors (carotenes or carotenoids) found in plants, particularly green leafy vegetables. Vitamin A is stored in the liver; reserves can last about 1 year.

Table 27.8 *Vitamins*

Fat-soluble	Water-soluble
Vitamin A	Vitamin B_1 (thiamine)
Vitamin D	Vitamin B_2 (riboflavin)
Vitamin E	Vitamin B_6 (pyridoxine)
Vitamin K	Vitamin B_{12}
	Vitamin C (ascorbic acid)
	Folic acid
	Pantothenic acid
	Biotin
	Nicotinic acid (niacin)

Table 27.9 *Vitamin deficiency syndromes*

Vitamin	Deficiency syndrome	Usual causes
A	Night blindness, xerophthalmia	Malabsorption, inadequate diet, protein-energy malnutrition (PEM)
B_1 (thiamine)	Beri-beri, Wernicke encephalopathy	Inadequate diet, alcoholism
B_2 (riboflavin)	Mucosal lesions, corneal opacities	Inadequate diet, drugs, alcoholism
Nicotinic acid (niacin)	Pellagra (dementia, dermatitis, diarrhoea)	Alcoholism, inadequate diet, carcinoid syndrome
B_6 (pyridoxine)	Glossitis, neuropathy, dermatitis	Inadequate diet, drugs (isoniazid, hydralazine)
Folate	Megaloblastosis, villous atrophy, mucosal lesions	Inadequate diet, alcoholism, pregnancy, haemolytic anaemia, drugs
B_{12}	Megaloblastosis, villous atrophy, neuropathies, mucosal lesions	Inadequate diet, pernicious anaemia, Crohn disease
C (ascorbic acid)	Scurvy	Inadequate diet
D	Rickets, osteomalacia	Inadequate exposure to sunlight, malabsorption
E	Spinocerebellar degeneration	Severe fat malabsorption, abetalipoproteinaemia
K	Hypoprothrombinaemia, bleeding	Warfarin, oral antibiotics, biliary obstruction

Table 27.10 *Main consequences of vitamin overdose*

Vitamin	Toxicity
A	Headache, convulsions, hepatotoxicity, bone damage, teratogenicity
B_1 (thiamine)	?
B_2 (riboflavin)	?
Nicotinic acid (niacin)	Vasodilatation, neuropathy
B_6 (pyridoxine)	Peripheral neuropathy
Folate	?
B_{12}	?
C (ascorbic acid)	Increased urinary oxalate
D	Hypercalcaemia, renal failure
E	Nausea, bleeding
K	Hyperbilirubinaemia

Vitamin A deficiency is usually dietary in origin and the eyes are first affected, with night blindness, xerophthalmia and conjunctival ulceration. The skin becomes dry and scaly (follicular hyperkeratosis) and the oral mucosa becomes hyperkeratinized.

Natural derivatives of vitamin A (carotenoids) and synthetic analogues of vitamin A (retinoids) can modulate epithelial cell differentiation, possibly by regulating gene expression, and may have some protective effect against cancers.

In hypervitaminosis A there is alopecia, peeling of the skin, coarsening of the hair and bone pain.

VITAMIN B

There are several B vitamins; all are water-soluble. The most widely recognized deficiencies are of vitamin B_{12} and folic acid.

Vitamin B_{12}

Vitamin B_{12} is found mainly in liver, eggs, meat and milk. Liver stores last for up to 3 years and thus deficiency is rarely of dietary origin, except in vegans.

Vitamin B_{12} deficiency is typically seen in pernicious anaemia, where there is deficiency of the gastric intrinsic factor required for its absorption. Vitamin B_{12} deficiency causes defective cellular uptake of 5-methyltetrahydrofolate and its impaired conversion by the homocysteine methyl transferase reaction, and thus vitamin B_{12} deficiency interferes with development of rapidly dividing cells, including mucosae, erythrocytes, granulocytes and platelets. Impaired erythrocyte production leads to a macrocytic anaemia; haemoglobin synthesis continues relatively normally but cell size remains large, and condensation and extrusion of the nucleus are delayed (megaloblastosis).

Neuropathies (subacute combined degeneration of the cord), glossitis and stomatitis may result from vitamin B_{12} deficiency.

Vitamin B_1 (thiamine, aneurine)

Vitamin B_1 is widely distributed in foods and is necessary in the formation of the coenzyme thiamine pyrophosphate, required for oxidative decarboxylation of pyruvate and alpha-ketoglutarate, and utilization of pentoses.

In vitamin B_1 deficiency, therefore, there is a build-up of lactate and pyruvate that interferes with carbohydrate metabolism. Deficiency of vitamin B_1 is common in alcoholism and leads to beri-beri. This is characterized by polyneuritis, muscular weakness, cardiac failure, mental changes and, in children, growth retardation. Thiamine given intravenously may precipitate anaphylaxis, so caution is advised.

Vitamin B_2 (riboflavin)

Riboflavin is found in leafy vegetables, meat, milk and fish. It acts in the formation of two coenzymes, flavine–adenine dinucleotide and flavine mononucleotide, involved in oxidative metabolism.

Deficiency of vitamin B_2 is commonly dietary and is seen especially in alcoholics. This leads to seborrhoeic dermatitis, corneal vascularization and anaemia, and oral mucosal manifestations similar to those of vitamin B_{12} deficiency.

Vitamin B_6 (pyridoxine)

Vitamin B_6 is found in meat and vegetables. It is involved in the formation of pyridoxal phosphate and pyridoxamine phosphate, coenzymes in amino acid metabolism.

Vitamin B_6 deficiency is found particularly in alcoholism, pregnancy and the use of some drugs (e.g. isoniazid). Deficiency of vitamin B_6 leads to dermatitis and peripheral neuropathy, and oral mucosal manifestations similar to those of vitamin B_{12} deficiency.

Pantothenic acid

Pantothenic acid is needed for the synthesis of coenzyme A, which is necessary for several metabolic pathways.

Biotin

Biotin is a coenzyme in carboxylation reactions. Deficiency is rare.

Nicotinic acid (niacin; nicotinamide)

The active derivative of nicotinic acid, nicotinamide, is necessary for the production of nicotinamide adenine dinucleotide (NAD) and nicotinamide adenine dinucleotide phosphate (NADP) for oxidative metabolism. Wheat, nuts, meat and fish are rich sources of nicotinic acid.

Deficiency of nicotinic acid is seen mainly in alcoholics, and causes pellagra (dermatitis and neurological disturbances), oral mucosal erythema and papillary atrophy of the tongue.

Folic acid

Folic acid (pteroylglutamic acid) is biologically inactive; folates are the active forms. Folate, present in green vegetables, liver and yeast, is converted, after small intestinal absorption, to the active tetrahydrofolate, which is involved in synthesis of purine and pyrimidine bases.

Folate deficiency typically results from a diet deficient in green vegetables and can arise within a relatively short period of time, since body stores last less than 3 months. Alcoholism, phenytoin and some cytotoxic drugs (e.g. methotrexate), are other relatively common causes of folate deficiency.

Folate deficiency leads to impaired synthesis and repair of DNA with megaloblastic change in haemopoietic and other cells. The oral effects of folate deficiency in humans are virtually indistinguishable from those of vitamin B_{12} deficiency.

VITAMIN C (ASCORBIC ACID)

Vitamin C is water-soluble, and found especially in fresh fruits (mainly in citrus fruits) and vegetables, including potatoes. It is involved in the hydroxylation of proline in collagen synthesis.

Deficiency results from a dietary lack of vitamin C, and leads to defective collagen with capillary fragility, a haemorrhagic state, anaemia, and follicular hyperkeratosis and gingival changes (scurvy) of swelling and haemorrhage.

VITAMIN D

Vitamin D is the general name for a group of fat-soluble sterols (cholecalciferol) found in fish, eggs and milk products. Cholecalciferol from the diet is converted into 25-hydroxycholecalciferol in the liver and this is converted in the kidneys to the active form, 1,25-dihydroxycholecalciferol. Ultraviolet light converts a skin precursor, 7-dehydrocholesterol, to vitamin D.

Vitamin D affects immunity, and calcium and phosphate metabolism; deficiency leads to rickets or osteomalacia. This is increasing in communities where sun exposure is limited. Vitamin D can modulate both innate and adaptive immune responses and deficiency in vitamin D is associated with increased susceptibility to infection and increased autoimmunity. The vitamin D receptor is expressed on immunocytes such as antigen presenting cells and B and T lymphocytes, cells also capable of synthesizing active vitamin D. The extrarenal

1-α-hydroxylase enzyme in macrophages differs from the renal enzyme as it is not regulated by PTH, but is dependent upon circulating levels of active vitamin D or it may be induced by proinflammatory cytokines such as IFN-γ, IL-1 or TNF-α.

VITAMIN E

Vitamin E is the general name for a group of fat-soluble tocopherols that are found particularly in asparagus, avocado, nuts, olives and vegetable oils. Vitamin E is important in erythropoiesis and helps the body to use vitamin K. It has been claimed that alpha-tocopherol is the most important lipid-soluble antioxidant. It may have some protective effect against some leukoplakias and carcinomas.

Deficiency is rare, except in premature infants, people with fat malabsorption and rare genetic abnormalities in the alpha-tocopherol transfer protein (ataxia and vitamin E deficiency; AVED). Neuropathies may result. There is no good evidence that vitamin E is cardioprotective.

VITAMIN K

Vitamin K is a fat-soluble naphthaquinone derivative found in green vegetables.

Malabsorption, parenteral nutrition and warfarin cause deficiency, the manifestations of which can include gingival bleeding and postoperative haemorrhage.

OXIDATIVE DAMAGE AND ANTIOXIDANTS

In humans, oxidation by oxides and peroxides from atmospheric pollution, cigarette smoke and some normal bodily processes can cause DNA mutations (and hence cancer risk), oxidize polyunsaturated fatty acids (and thus contribute towards heart disease and strokes), and damage proteins (e.g. eye proteins are particularly vulnerable because light also assists oxidation). Considerable evidence indicates that oxidative damage is associated with and may contribute to most major age-related degenerative diseases (e.g. cancer, heart disease, strokes, diabetes, cataracts, Parkinson disease and Alzheimer disease). In fats and oils, oxidation is the prime cause of rancidity, causing them to become unpleasant to eat and potentially dangerous.

Antioxidants are chemicals that slow oxidation reactions, which can otherwise produce the damaging 'free radicals' or 'reactive oxygen species'. All fats and oils will become rancid, given enough exposure to air, sunlight and heat, but antioxidants will combat this, and offer huge economic and environmental benefits in preventing wastage of food. It is not clear which antioxidants are the most effective. Many foods, particularly pecan nuts, walnuts and various beans, contain high levels of various antioxidants (Table 27.11). Flavonoids, typical examples of which are quercetin in onions and apples, and epigallocatechin in tea, are other antioxidants. Fruits are high in antioxidants, the purple, blue, red and orange fruits being the most antioxidant-rich. Good sources of flavonoids include citrus fruits (hesperidin, quercetin, rutin) and berries (due to their dark colour, purple berries are as much as 50% higher in antioxidants than some of the more common berry varieties). Both red and white wine contain flavonoids but, since red wine is produced by fermentation in the presence of grape skins, red wine has higher levels of flavonoids and other polyphenolics, such as resveratol. Green plants or herbs contain antioxidants, as do green tea (contains catechins), jiaogulan (southern ginseng or xiancao – the 'immortality herb'– contains gypenosides), tomatoes (lycopene), chocolate (relatively high amounts of epicatechin) and grape seeds (resveratol).

Table 27.11 *Antioxidant-containing foods*

Food	High in antioxidants	Very high in antioxidants
Beans	Various beans	Cacao (including chocolate)
Beverages	Beer, cider, coffee, tea	Green tea, red wine
Cereals	Barley, hops, maize, millet	–
Fruits	Apples, cherries, lemons, mangos, melons, oranges, peaches, pineapples, plums, tangerines	Blackberries, blackcurrants, blueberries, cranberries, elderberries, pomegranates, raspberries, strawberries
Nuts	Almonds, pistachios	Hazelnuts, pecans, walnuts
Vegetables	Artichokes, mushrooms, onions, parsley, peppers, spinach	–

Vitamins A, C and E, and plant polyphenols (including flavonoids) and carotenoids (including beta-carotene and lycopene) are amongst the most powerful antioxidants. Vitamin C (E300) and vitamin E (E306) are found in fruit and vegetables, and are also widely used as supplementary additives. They are amongst the safest chemicals known; 'ACES' products contain pro-vitamin *A* (beta-carotene), vitamin *C*, vitamin *E* and selenium.

Heart disease, strokes, diabetes, cataracts, Parkinson disease and Alzheimer disease seem to occur less frequently in people who eat antioxidant-rich diets, but it is a moot point whether or not the effect is due to some other lifestyle factor. Some dietary antioxidant vitamins are required for good health, and antioxidant-containing foods are recommended. However, although some foods are high in antioxidants, not all are absorbed because of variable absorption or metabolism (bioavailability) in the gut. There is considerable doubt as to whether antioxidant *supplementation* is beneficial. Some studies have suggested that antioxidant supplementation benefits health, but several large clinical trials have failed to demonstrate definite benefit, and excess supplementation may even be harmful. The most common synthetic antioxidants are butylated hydroxyanisole (E320) and butylated hydroxytoluene (BHT; E321). BHT has been controversial; it has produced adverse reactions in dogs but, like all antioxidants, is anticarcinogenic.

POLYPHENOLS

Polyphenols (PPs) are derived from L-phenylalanine. The most important PP classes are phenolic acids, flavonoids, lignans and stilbenes. Flavonoids are divided into flavonols (e.g. quercetin and kaempferol, the most ubiquitous flavonoids in foods), flavones, isoflavones, flavanones, anthocyanidins (pigments responsible for the colour of fruits) and flavanols (catechins, monomers and proanthocyanidins). The PPs that are best absorbed are isoflavones and gallic acid (a phenolic acid), followed by flavanones, catechins and quercetin glucosides. The least well absorbed are proanthocyanidins, anthocyanins and galloylated catechins. All PPs are excreted chiefly in the urine and bile.

PPs have powerful antioxidant activities *in vitro* and are capable of scavenging a range of reactive oxygen, nitrogen and chlorine species, such as superoxide, hydroxyl radical, peroxyl radicals, hypochlorous acid and peroxynitrous acid.

PPs have been proposed to have beneficial effects in cancers, cardiovascular diseases and neurodegenerative disorders but, although there are many epidemiological studies, comprehensive data are

Table 27.12 *Food additives that may present health risks*

Additive[a]	Possible associations	Possible carcinogenicity
Aluminium sulphide, aluminium phosphate, sodium phosphate, aluminium chloride – common leavening agents in baked goods	Possible link to Alzheimer disease	–
Artificial sweeteners (aspartame, acesulphame K and saccharin)	Behavioural problems, hyperactivity, allergies	+
Artificial food colours	Allergies, asthma, hyperactivity	+
Artificial flavours	Allergic or behavioural reactions	–
Bromates (usually potassium bromate)	?	Carcinogenic in animals
Caffeine	Promotes stomach acid secretion, temporarily raises blood pressure, and dilates some blood vessels while constricting others. Excessive caffeine intake results in 'caffeinism', with symptoms ranging from nervousness to insomnia	–
Carbonated beverages	Tooth erosion; obesity, metabolic syndrome, chronic kidney disease, pancreatic carcinoma; rarely, hyponatraemia	–
Food waxes (protective coating of produce, as in cucumbers, peppers and apples)	May trigger allergies, can contain pesticides, fungicide sprays or animal by-products	–
Hydrogenated fats	Cardiovascular disease, obesity	–
Monosodium glutamate (MSG)	Common allergic and behavioural reactions, including headaches, dizziness, chest pains, depression and mood swings; also a possible neurotoxin	–
Nitrites and nitrates	Headaches	Can develop into nitrosamines in body, which can be carcinogenic
Olestra (an artificial fat)	Diarrhoea and digestive disturbances. Olestra inhibits the absorption of some vitamins and other nutrients	–
Phosphorous compounds, which make soft drinks bubbly (phosphoric acid), as well as keeping canned vegetables firm (calcium phosphate) and dried instant oatmeals and soup mixes easy to hydrate (sodium phosphate)	Might possibly interfere with calcium absorption and predispose to osteoporosis	–
Plastic packaging	Immune reactions, lung shock	+ (vinyl chloride)
Preservatives – butylated hydroxyanisole (BHA) and butylated hydroxytoluene (BHT), etc.	Allergic reactions, hyperactivity; BHT may be toxic to the nervous system and the liver	+
Refined flour	Low-nutrient calories, carbohydrate imbalances, altered insulin production	–
Salt (excessive)	Fluid retention and blood pressure increases	–
Sugar and sweeteners	Obesity, dental caries, diabetes and hypoglycaemia, increased triglycerides or candidiasis	–
Sulphites (sulphur dioxide, metabisulphites and others) can keep cut fruits and vegetables looking fresh – they also prevent discolouration in apricots, raisins and other dried fruits; control 'black spot' in freshly caught shrimp; and prevent discolouration, bacterial growth and fermentation in wine	Allergic and asthmatic reactions	–

[a]Some are naturally present in some foods.

available only for flavonoids, specifically flavonols, flavones and catechins – indicating that flavonoids reduce coronary artery disease risk. In contrast, the association between flavonoid intake and cancer protection is controversial.

There is also some alleged antimicrobial activity of PPs against some infectious diseases but high dietary PP intake could potentially be more of an oxidative risk than a benefit – a concern corroborated by an epidemiological study reporting an association between flavonoid intake and colon cancer. This suggests that dietary supplementation with large amounts of a single antioxidant might be *deleterious* to human health.

FOOD ADDITIVES

The main reasons for adding chemicals to foods include to improve shelf-life or storage time; make food convenient and easy to prepare; increase nutritional value (e.g. added vitamins); improve flavour and enhance attractiveness; and improve consumer acceptance. For decades,

the food industry has created new chemicals to manipulate, preserve and transform food, and has produced altered versions of breads, fruits, vegetables, meats, dairy products and many more commonly used foods; now there are even 'foods', such as coffee creamers, sugar substitutes and confectionery, that consist almost entirely of artificial ingredients.

Some additives have undoubted health benefits, such as antioxidants. Other food additives may actually cause disease – such as benzoates, tartrazine and cinnamonaldehyde, implicated, for example, in orofacial granulomatosis (Table 27.12). Some are dangerous; the recent adulteration of milk in China with melamine and the subsequent renal or bladder stones, or cancer, is a prime example. Appendix 27.1 outlines E numbers.

NUTRITIONAL INTERVENTIONS

Most conventional nutritional interventions ('diets') recommend recognized 'healthy' patterns of eating (reduction or elimination of fat, sugar, alcohol and coffee, and an increase in fresh vegetables and fibre) that most people with normal digestion can tolerate without adverse effects. These are generally to be recommended.

Unconventional nutritional interventions include nutritional supplements, dietary modification and 'therapeutic' systems. Some supplements are taken to improve general health and performance, whereas others are purported to be for specific clinical indications, not always with evidence for efficacy. Vitamin D supplementation is discussed above. High doses of single minerals or amino acids may induce deficiencies in nutrients that share similar metabolic pathways. Some trace mineral supplements have had toxic effects; excessive doses of zinc and selenium can cause immune suppression, and evening primrose oil may exacerbate temporal lobe epilepsy.

Dietary modifications, such as many commercial fad diets, are claimed to enhance well-being or reduce weight but some have resulted in frank vitamin, mineral and protein deficiency states. Cardiac, renal and metabolic disorders, as well as some deaths, have resulted. Many diets, such as vegetarianism and veganism, originated as 'movements' characterized by political and/or ecological concerns, a moral stance toward food, and a view of diet as inseparable from lifestyle. Very low-calorie diets (below 400 kcal/day) cannot sustain health for long, and high-dose nutritional supplementation can sometimes lead to adverse effects. Many diets are based on theoretical considerations rather than empirical data. For example, the rationale for the Hay diet is that starch and protein should not be eaten together since each type of food requires a different pH for optimum digestion. The principle of the Stone Age diet is that humans are not adapted by evolution to eat grains and legumes. The Zone diet advocates consuming calories from carbohydrates, protein and fat in a balanced ratio.

'Therapeutic' systems include techniques such as elimination dieting and naturopathy. Elimination dieting is based on the principle that foods particular to each patient may contribute to chronic symptoms or disease when eaten in normal quantities. Exclusion dieting definitely appears to benefit conditions including coeliac disease, orofacial granulomatosis, rheumatoid arthritis, hyperactivity and migraine. Unlike classic allergies, these 'food intolerances' do not involve a conventionally understood immune mechanism or have a rapid onset. Diagnosis consists of eliminating all but a few foods from the diet and then reintroducing foods one by one to see if they provoke symptoms. After a period of complete exclusion, the problem substances can usually be reintroduced gradually without recurrence of symptoms. Although practitioners commonly diagnose wheat and dairy 'intolerance', each patient is said to be sensitive to a different set of foods.

Less evidence-based 'therapeutic' diets are also promoted. In 'Vega' or electrodermal testing, an electrical circuit is made that includes both the patient and the food suspected of causing disease. In applied kinesiology, practitioners claim to be able to diagnose allergy or deficiency on the basis of changes in muscle function. Naturopathy emphasizes the philosophy of 'nature cure' and incorporating dietary intervention among other practices such as hydrotherapy and exercise. For example, a naturopath might advise a patient with vaginal candidosis to undertake a fast, reduce foods containing sugar and yeast, and take herbal and probiotic preparations. Another therapeutic system tests patients for 'subclinical' nutritional deficiencies – thought to arise where systems of food intake, digestion or absorption are not fully functional – and gives appropriate supplementation. Tests include biochemical assays of the vitamin and mineral content of blood or hair. The evidence for the effectiveness of many of these unconventional nutritional interventions in treating disease is often doubtful.

Box 27.7 *Foods that might influence drug absorption*

- Antacids
- Citrus fruits (mainly grapefruit)
- Garlic
- Minerals (mainly calcium and iron)
- Phytates
- Vitamin K

Box 27.8 *Drugs whose absorption is reduced by antacids*

- Angiotensin-converting enzyme inhibitors (ACEIs)
- Antimicrobials – azithromycin, ciprofloxacin, isoniazid, nitrofurantoin, norfloxacin, pivampicillin, rifampicin, some tetracyclines (doxycycline, demeclocycline), antimalarials, itraconazole, ketoconazole
- Bisphosphonates
- Digoxin
- Gabapentin
- Lithium
- Penicillamine
- Phenothiazines
- Phenytoin

EFFECTS OF FOODS ON DRUG ABSORPTION

Foods and drugs can affect the absorption or activity of various drugs (Box 27.7). Monoamine oxidase inhibitors, such as phenelzine or tranylcypromine, and eating chocolate could be dangerous, causing a sharp rise in blood pressure. The caffeine in chocolate can also interact with stimulant drugs and increase the effect of methylphenidate, or decrease the effect of sedative-hypnotics such as zolpidem. Other foods that should be avoided when taking MAO inhibitors include bologna, aged cheese, pepperoni, salami and sausage. Licorice may cause digoxin toxicity or reduce the effects of antihypertensive drugs or diuretics, including hydrochlorothiazide and spironolactone.

Minerals may influence drug absorption. Iron can reduce absorption of quinolones (e.g. ciprofloxacin). Calcium in dairy foods and in supplements chelates tetracyclines. Avoiding high-calcium foods within 2 hours of taking the medication minimizes this problem.

Phytates in chapattis bind calcium and impair its absorption.

Antacids can cause early release of drugs from enteric-coated capsules, and can reduce absorption of antimicrobials and drugs, such as those listed in Box 27.8.

Citrus fruit acids may cause some medications to dissolve prematurely in the stomach rather than in the intestine and, therefore, taking drugs with acid fruit juices (and carbonated sodas) is usually not recommended. Citrus juice, however, improves the absorption of iron.

Grapefruit – fresh, canned or frozen, grapefruit juice or drinks that contain grapefruit juice can affect the metabolism of several drugs (Box 27.9 and Table 27.13), typically enhancing their activity. Sour orange juice (e.g. from Seville oranges), real lime juice, pomelos and tangelos (a hybrid of grapefruit) may possibly have this effect too. Furthermore, other fruits and juices, including cranberry, Goji berry and apple, contain other active moieties that can affect different P450 isoforms and transporters, and interact with different drugs. The effect appears to last for at least 3 days but may vary, depending on brand, juice fraction and time of year. It results from irreversible inhibition of certain intestinal drug-metabolizing cytochrome P450 enzymes

- Antiarrhythmics (amiodarone, propafenone, dronedarone)
- Anticoagulants (apixaban, rivoraxaban)
- Artemether
- Astemizole
- Caffeine
- Calcium-channel blockers (verapamil, amlodipine, felodipine, nifedipine, nicardipine)
- Cisapride
- Colchicine
- Cytotoxics (nilotinib, sunitinib, lapatanib)
- Diazepam
- Dihydropyridine calcium antagonists
- Diltiazem
- Drugs that act on the central nervous system (buspirone, carbamazepine, pimozide, quetiapine, sertraline, triazolam)
- HIV-protease inhibitors (e.g. efavirenz, saquinavir)
- HMG-CoA reductase inhibitors
- Immunosuppressants (ciclosporin, tacrolimus, sirolimus)
- Ivabradine
- Lovastatin
- Methadone
- Midazolam
- Nisoldipine
- Ranolazine
- Rupatadine
- Sildenafil
- Statins (atorvastatin, simvastatin)
- Tadalafil
- Terfenadine
- Tolvaptan
- Vardenafil

[a]Actions of aliskiren and bilastine are reduced.

Table 27.13 *Effects of grapefruit juice on some relevant drugs*

Drug(s)	Effect of grapefruit juice	Implications
Benzodiazepines	Increases blood drug concentrations	Increased sedation. Clinical significance of effect on cognitive function unclear
Carbamazepine	Increases blood drug concentrations	Toxicity (e.g. dizziness, poor balance and coordination, drowsiness, nausea, vomiting, tremor and agitation)
Ciclosporin	Increases blood drug concentrations	Toxicity, such as kidney and liver damage, and immune suppression
Corticosteroids	Increases blood drug concentrations	Consumption of large amounts of grapefruit might increase the risk of adverse effects
Itraconazole	Impairs drug absorption	The clinical significance of this interaction is unclear; theoretically, it could decrease efficacy of itraconazole

(CYP3A4) by furanocoumarins (such as 6′,7′-dihydroxybergamottin). CYP3A4 is involved in the metabolism of around 50% of drugs, so a wide variety of drugs can be affected by the consumption of grapefruit juice. The consequence is a large rise in the effects of these drugs. Impaired metabolism of various cardiac drugs after ingestion of grapefruit juice has led to an increase in QT interval and torsades de pointes (Ch. 5). Statins are also affected, leading to rhabdomyolysis.

A second mechanism involves the inhibition by grapefruit of an influx transporter protein family (organic anion transporter polypeptide; OATP) due to flavonoids such as naringin and hesperidin. The effect is reduced bioavailability of the drug and a decreased efficacy lasting about 4 hours. Drugs affected via this mechanism include aliskiren, celiprolol, ciprofloxacin, fexofenadine and talinolol. Grapefruit juice constituents, including flavonoids (naringin and naringenin, along with the furanocoumarins, bergapten and 6′,7′-dihydroxybergamottin), have also been implicated in activating P-glycoprotein, an intestinal-wall drug efflux mechanism.

Dental aspects

In dentistry, the main problem is with drugs that act on the central nervous system (benzodiazepines, buspirone, carbamazepine, pimozide, quetiapine). For example, one glass of grapefruit juice more than triples the bioavailability of diazepam, with more drowsiness. The bioavailability of oral midazolam and triazolam is also increased. Patients about to be given benzodiazepines, therefore, should avoid grapefruit (see Table 27.13). Anticoagulants, antiarrhythmics, calcium-channel blockers, cytotoxics immunosuppressants (ciclosporin, tacrolimus, sirolimus) and statins (atorvastatin, simvastatin) are the other main problems.

Most other citrus fruits, such as lemons, naturally sweet oranges and tangerines, are considered safe in this respect.

Cranberry juice (*Vaccinium macrocarpon*) may enhance warfarin.

Garlic supplements appear to enhance anticoagulants.

Pomegranate may inhibit cytochrome P450 and increase the effects and adverse effects of codeine, carbamazepine, diclofenac, midazolam, tramadol and other drugs (Box 27.10)

Vitamin K in foods (e.g. liver, cabbage, spinach, cauliflower, green tea and broccoli), in contrast, can substantially reduce the effectiveness of warfarin.

Medications such as itraconazole, ketoconazole, ciclosporin, diltiazem and erythromycin may inhibit both intestinal CYNA4 and hepatic CYP3A4.

NUTRITIONAL SUPPORT

Methods to improve or maintain nutritional intake are known as nutrition support and include:

- oral nutrition support – e.g. fortified foods, additional snacks and/or sip feeds
- enteral tube feeding – delivery of a nutritionally complete feed into the gut directly via a tube (nasogastric [NG] or per-enteric gastrostomy [PEG])
- (total) parenteral nutrition ([T]PN) – delivery of nutrition intravenously.

Nutrition support should be considered in people who are malnourished, as defined by any of the following:

- a BMI of less than 18.5 kg/m^2
- unintentional weight loss of more than 10% within the past 3–6 months
- a BMI of less than 20 kg/m^2 plus unintentional weight loss of more than 5% within the last 3–6 months.

- Alfentanil
- Amitriptyline
- Amlodipine
- Captopril
- Carbamazepine
- Celecoxib
- Codeine
- Desipramine
- Diclofenac
- Diltiazem
- Enalapril
- Fentanyl
- Flecainide
- Fluoxetine
- Fluvastatin
- Glipizide
- Ibuprofen
- Indinavir
- Irbesartan
- Lisinopril
- Losartan
- Midazolam
- Nelfinavir
- Ondansetron
- Phenytoin
- Piroxicam
- Propranolol
- Ramipril
- Ritonavir
- Rosuvastatin
- Saquinavir
- Tamoxifen
- Tolbutamide
- Torsemide
- Tramadol
- Verapamil
- Warfarin

Nutrition support should also be considered in people at risk of malnutrition, defined as those who have:

- eaten little or nothing for more than 5 days and/or are likely to eat little or nothing for 5 days or longer
- a poor absorptive capacity and/or high nutrient losses and/or increased catabolism.

ENTERAL TUBE FEEDING

Enteral tube feeding may be appropriate for people who are malnourished or at risk of malnutrition and if:

- they have an inadequate or unsafe oral intake
- they have a functional, accessible gastrointestinal tract
- they have been admitted to intensive care – these patients should be fed via a tube into the stomach, unless there is upper gastrointestinal dysfunction
- they have upper gastrointestinal dysfunction (or an inaccessible upper gastrointestinal tract) – these patients should be considered for post-pyloric (duodenal or jejunal) feeding

- they have long-term (4 weeks or more) needs – gastrostomy should be considered
- PEG tubes have been placed without apparent complications – these can be used for enteral tube feeding 4 hours after insertion)
- they have an inability to swallow safely or take sufficient energy and nutrients orally – these patients should have a 2–4-week trial of NG enteral tube feeding).

The position of all NG tubes should be confirmed after placement and before each use by aspiration and pH-graded paper (with X-ray if necessary), with repeat checks of the tube position. Enteral tube feeding should be stopped when the patient is established on adequate oral intake.

PARENTERAL NUTRITION

PN provides formulae that contain nutrients such as glucose, amino acids and lipids, plus vitamins and minerals. It is termed *total parenteral nutrition* (TPN) or *total nutrient admixture* (TNA) when no significant nutrition is obtained by other routes.

TPN is mainly used in gastrointestinal diseases that cause malabsorption, such as inflammatory bowel disease (Crohn disease), surgical bowel removal (short bowel syndrome) and abnormal bowel function (motility problems due to surgical adhesions, radiation enteritis, neurological disorders, etc.).

PN may be called *total peripheral nutrition* (also TPN) when administered through a limb vein rather than through a central vein. When PN is done at home, it is called *home parenteral nutrition* (HPN).

Two types of catheter can be used for TPN/HPN. Both are inserted into a large vein – most commonly, a soft silicone tube with a segment exiting the chest, or an implantable venous access device or port. Tunnelling subclavian lines is recommended for long-term use (more than 30 days). Catheters do not have to be tunnelled for short-term use (less than 30 days).

Continuous administration of PN is the preferred method of infusion in severely ill people. Cyclical delivery of PN should be considered when using peripheral venous cannulae with planned routine catheter change. A gradual change from continuous to cyclical delivery should be considered in patients requiring PN for more than 2 weeks.

Dental aspects

There are no indications for giving antimicrobial prophylaxis for dental care in people with central catheters (http://www.cda-adc.ca/jcda/vol-72/issue-7/619.pdf; accessed 30 September 2013).

Complications

PN may occasionally lead to complications related to catheter insertion, including pneumothorax, accidental arterial puncture and:

- infection – with a mortality rate of approximately 15% per infection
- blood clots
- hepatic steatosis and liver failure
- acute cholecystitis
- cholelithiasis
- hyperglycaemia
- refeeding syndrome (hypokalaemia, hypophosphataemia, hypomagnesaemia) (Box 27.11).

Box 27.11 *Criteria for determining people at high risk of developing refeeding problems[a]*

Patient has one or more of the following

- BMI <16 kg/m^2
- Unintentional weight loss >15% within the last 3–6 months
- Little or no nutritional intake for >10 days
- Low levels of potassium, phosphate or magnesium prior to feeding

Or patient has two or more of the following

- BMI <18.5 kg/m^2
- Unintentional weight loss >10% within the last 3–6 months
- Little or no nutritional intake for >5 days
- A history of alcohol abuse or drugs, including insulin, chemotherapy, antacids or diuretics

[a]NICE. *Nutrition support in adults: oral nutrition support, enteral tube feeding and parenteral nutrition. Clinical Guideline 32.* February 2006.

Refeeding syndrome

Refeeding syndrome can be defined as the potentially fatal shifts in fluids and electrolytes that may occur in malnourished patients receiving artificial refeeding and that result from hormonal and metabolic changes. The main feature is hypophosphataemia but there can be abnormal sodium and fluid balance; changes in glucose, protein and fat metabolism; thiamine deficiency; hypokalaemia; and hypomagnesaemia. If the syndrome is detected, the feeding rate should be slowed down and essential electrolytes replenished, and the hospital specialist dietetics team should be involved.

For people at high risk of developing refeeding problems, consider:

- starting nutrition support at a maximum of 10 kcal/kg/day, increasing levels slowly to meet or exceed full needs by 4–7 days
- using only 5 kcal/kg/day in extreme cases (e.g. BMI less than 14 kg/m^2 or negligible intake for more than 15 days) and monitoring cardiac rhythm continually in these people and any others who already have or develop any cardiac arrhythmias
- restoring circulatory volume and monitoring fluid balance and overall clinical status closely
- providing immediately before and during the first 10 days of feeding: oral thiamine 200–300 mg daily, vitamin B compound strong 1 or 2 tablets, three times a day (or full-dose daily intravenous vitamin B preparation, if necessary), and a balanced multivitamin/trace element supplement once daily
- providing oral, enteral or intravenous supplements of potassium (likely requirement 2–4 mmol/kg/day), phosphate (likely requirement 0.3–0.6 mmol/kg/day) and magnesium (likely requirement 0.2 mmol/kg/day intravenous, 0.4 mmol/kg/day oral) unless pre-feeding plasma levels are high. Pre-feeding correction of low plasma levels is unnecessary.

KEY WEBSITES

(Accessed 30 September 2013)
Centers for Disease Control and Prevention. <http://www.cdc.gov/healthyyouth/nutrition/facts.htm>.
Patient.co.uk. <http://www.patient.co.uk/health/Healthy-Eating.htm>.
US Department of Agriculture. <http://fnic.nal.usda.gov/diet-and-disease>.

USEFUL WEBSITES

(Accessed 30 September 2013)
Beat (beating eating disorders). <http://www.b-eat.co.uk/>.
Eating Disorders Resources. <http://www.edr.org.uk/>.
Food Standards Agency. <http://collections.europarchive.org/tna/20100927130941/http://food.gov.uk/healthiereating/>.
National Institute for Health and Care Excellence. <http://www.nice.org.uk/CG9> and <http://www.nice.org.uk/nicemedia/live/10978/29978/29978.pdf>.
National Institutes of Health: National Institute of Mental Health. <http://www.nimh.nih.gov/health/topics/eating-disorders/index.shtml>.
Obesity Society. <http://www.obesity.org/education/>.

FURTHER READING

Ashcroft, A., Milosevic, A., 2007. The eating disorders. 1. Current scientific understanding and dental implications. Dent. Update 34, 544.
Ashcroft, A., Milosevic, A., 2007. The eating disorders. 2. Behavioural and dental management. Dent. Update 34, 612.
Barbosa, C.S., et al. 2009. Dental manifestations in bariatric patients – review of literature. J. Appl. Oral Sci. 17 (sp. issue), 1.
Dhingra, R., et al. 2007. Soft drink consumption and risk of developing cardiometabolic risk factors and the metabolic syndrome in middle-aged adults in the community. Circulation 116, 480. [Erratum in *Circulation* 2007; 116:e557].
Dubois, L., et al. 2007. Regular sugar-sweetened beverage consumption between meals increases risk of overweight among preschool-aged children. J. Am. Diet. Assoc. 107, 924. discussion 934.
Faine, M.P., 2007. Recognition and management of eating disorders in the dental office. Dent. Clin. North Am. 47, 395.
Harris, R., et al. 2003. Dietary effects on drug metabolism and transport. Clin. Pharmacokinet. 42, 1071.
Hoek, H.W., Van Hoeken, D., 2003. Review of the prevalence and incidence of eating disorders. Int. J. Eat. Disord. 34, 383.
Holick, M.F., 2007. Vitamin D deficiency. N. Engl. J. Med. 357 (3), 266–281.
Kitchens, M., Owens, B.M., 2007. Effect of carbonated beverages, coffee, sports and high energy drinks, and bottled water on the in vitro erosion characteristics of dental enamel. J. Clin. Pediatr. Dent. 31, 153.
Larsson, S.C., et al. 2006. Consumption of sugar and sugar-sweetened foods and the risk of pancreatic cancer in a prospective study. Am. J. Clin. Nutr. 84, 1171.
Lo Russo, L., et al. 2008. Oral manifestations of eating disorders: a critical review. Oral Dis. 14, 479.
Mehanna, H.M., et al. 2008. Refeeding syndrome: what it is, and how to prevent and treat it. BMJ 336 (7659), 1495. doi:10.1136/bmj.a301 Review. PubMed PMID: 18583681; PubMed Central PMCID: PMC2440847.
Milosevic, A., et al. 2003. Satisfaction with dento-facial appearance in the eating disorders. Eur. J. Prosthodont. Restor. Dent. 11, 125.
Mortelmans, L.J., et al. 2008. Seizures and hyponatremia after excessive intake of diet coke. Eur. J. Emerg. Med. 15, 51.
Petti, S., Scully, C., 2009. Polyphenols, oral health and disease. J. Dent. 37, 413.
Pirmohamed, M., 2013. Drug–grapefruit juice interactions. BMJ 346, f1. doi:10.1136/bmj.f1.
Ravaldi, C., et al. 2003. Eating disorders and body image disturbances among ballet dancers, gymnasium users and body builders. Psychopathology 36, 247.
Saldana, T.M., et al. 2007. Carbonated beverages and chronic kidney disease. Epidemiology 18, 501.
Yellowlees, W., 2002. Marine fat and human health. Nutr. Health 16, 345.

APPENDIX 27.1 E-NUMBERS: REFERENCE NUMBERS USED BY THE EUROPEAN UNION TO HELP IDENTIFICATION OF FOOD ADDITIVES

- All food additives allowed and used in the European Union (EU) are identified by an E-number.
- 'E' stands for 'Europe' or 'European Union'.
- Normally, each food additive is assigned a unique number, though occasionally, related additives are designated by an extension (e.g. a, b, i or ii, etc.) to another E-number.
- The Commission of the European Union assigns E-numbers after the additive is cleared by the Scientific Committee on Food

(SCF), the body responsible for the safety evaluation of food additives in the EU. A summary is given below:

- E100–199: food colours
- E200–299: preservatives
- E300–399: antioxidants, phosphates and complexing agents
- E400–499: thickeners, gelling agents, phosphates, emulsifiers
- E500–599: salts and related compounds
- E600–699: flavourings
- E700–899: not used for human food additives (used for animal feed additives!)
- E900–999: surface coating agents, gases, sweeteners
- E1000–1399: miscellaneous additives
- E1400–1499: starch derivatives.

■ E-numbers are only used for substances added directly to food products, so contaminants, enzymes and processing aids, which may be classified as additives in the USA, are not included in the E-number system.

■ There is an EU directive on food labelling that requires food additives to be listed in the product ingredients whenever they are added for technological purposes. This includes colouring, sweetening and flavour enhancement, as well as for preservation, thickening, emulsifying and the like.

■ Ingredients must be listed in descending order of weight, which means that they are generally found close to the end of the list of ingredients.

■ Substances used in the protection of plants and plant products, flavourings and substances added as nutrients (e.g. minerals, trace elements or vitamins) do not need to be included in the ingredient list. Because of this, some substances that are regulated as food additives in other countries may be exempt from the food additive definition in the EU.

The International Classification (ICIDH) system, distinguishes impairment (I) from disability (D) and handicap (H; Table 28.1). Terminology related to disability varies in different countries. For example, the term 'mental retardation', as used in the USA, is not used in UK, where 'learning disability' and 'learning, intellectual or cognitive impairment' are accepted terms. The UK Disability Discrimination Act 1995 (DDA) considers a person as disabled if they have a mental or physical impairment that interferes with their ability to carry out everyday activities. Barriers that can create disability from impairment are shown in Table 28.2. The DDA, the Americans with Disabilities Act 1990 and similar acts in other developed countries make it unlawful to treat disabled people less favourably for reasons related to their disability, and thus service providers need to ensure that the physical features of their premises overcome any barriers to access.

The main conditions causing disability are shown in Table 28.3. Only patients with physical or mental impairment and some specific conditions will be considered here. Patients with other important specific diseases that can prove disabling, such as haemophilia, neurological disorders and muscular dystrophies, as well as children and older people, are discussed in other chapters.

PHYSICAL IMPAIRMENTS

General aspects and clinical features

Physical disabilities include orthopaedic, neuromuscular, cardiovascular and pulmonary disorders. The disability may be either congenital or acquired – typically the result of injury or disease. People with disabilities often rely for mobility upon devices such as wheelchairs, crutches, frames (e.g. Zimmer), walking sticks and artificial limbs. Some people may have additional hidden (non-visible) disabilities, which include epilepsy or respiratory and other disorders.

General management

Limited access to transport and buildings or reluctance of staff to provide care are the major barriers to health care. Decreased physical stamina and endurance, impaired eye–hand coordination or impaired verbal communication may complicate care.

Accept the fact that a disability exists and approach the patient with sensitivity (Box 28.1). When it appears that a person needs assistance, ask if help can be given. Assistance, if requested, should be provided. If a person's speech is difficult to understand, do not hesitate to ask them to repeat. Sensitivity to using words like 'walking' or 'running' is inappropriate; people who are handicapped use such words. Always ask first while facing a person who uses a wheelchair; never come up from behind and push them. Try to have conversations at the same eye level by sitting, kneeling or squatting where appropriate. However, a wheelchair is part of the person's body space, so do not hang or lean on it.

Some who have to use wheelchairs can achieve amazing feats, such as in the Para-Olympic Games (Fig. 28.1), and can walk with the aid of canes, braces, crutches or walkers. Others cope with extraordinary impairments and perform amazing feats.

Table 28.1 *International Classification system*

Term	Definition
Impairment	The functional limitation caused by physical, mental or sensory impairment (i.e. it is organ-based)
Disability	The loss or limitations of opportunities to participate in the normal life of the community on an equal level with others, due to physical or social barriers (i.e. it is person-based)
Handicap	The disadvantage suffered as a consequence of impairment and disability (i.e. it is socially based)

Table 28.2 *Barriers that can create disability from impairment*[a]

Barriers	Main problems	Possible consequences
Discrimination	Access to:	Difficulties with stairs
	premises	Inappropriate toilets
	facilities	Inadequately trained staff
	health care	Often lower wages
	education	
	employment	
	recreation	
Prejudice	Denial of anonymity	Being stared at
	Deal of respect	Being regarded as a 'burden'
	Hostility	Intolerance
	Patronization	
	Lowered expectations of achievements	
Ignorance	Fear of people with disabilities	Fear of aggression or being bitten
	Inadequate education of carers or professionals	Lack or scarcity of undergraduate training

[a]Reproduced from Scully C, et al. (2007).

Table 28.3 *Important conditions with impairments*

Mental impairment	Visual defects and hearing defects	Physical disorders
Autism disorders	Various	Cardiac disease
Chromosomal anomalies, especially Down syndrome		Cerebral palsy
Dyslexia		Cleft deformities
Learning impairments		Cystic fibrosis
		Hydrocephalus
		Juvenile arthritis
		Muscle diseases
		Spinal cord damage (especially paraplegia) and spina bifida
		Thalidomide deformities

Dental aspects

Guidelines for care are available at http://www.bsdh.org.uk/guidelines/physical.pdf (accessed 30 September 2013).

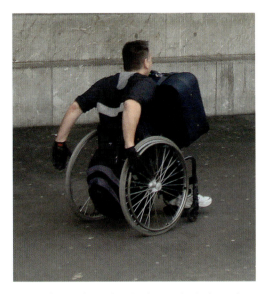

Fig. 28.1 A person with paraplegia showing impressive independence.

CEREBRAL PALSY

Cerebral palsy (CP) is the most common congenital physical handicap. It is caused by brain damage early in development, either during fetal life, during the birth process or during the first few months of infancy. Brain damage is caused mainly by hypoxia, trauma, infection or hyperbilirubinaemia, but genetic or other biochemical factors may be involved. Risk factors are shown in Box 28.2.

Clinical features

People with CP have abnormalities of motor control that can cause abnormalities of movement and posture in various parts of the body. CP shows no uniform pattern because of the many variations in brain damage (Table 28.4), but features may include delays in motor skills development, poor control over hand and arm movement, weakness, abnormal walking with one foot or leg dragging, and excessive drooling or difficulties in swallowing. Many patients are highly intelligent but may have such severely impaired speech as to *appear* to have learning impairment. Up to 50% do have additional challenges, such as epilepsy, defects of hearing, vision or speech, learning impairment or emotional disturbances.

Box 28.2 *Risk factors for cerebral palsy*

- Breech presentation
- Low birth weight
- Maternal infection
- Meconium staining of amniotic fluid – caused by stool passed by the fetus *in utero*
- Vaginal bleeding during pregnancy

Table 28.4 *Types of cerebral palsy*

Type	Subtype	Involves
Spastic	Monoplegic	Only one limb
	Paraplegic	Lower extremities
	Hemiplegic	One upper and lower limb on same side
	Double hemiplegic	All limbs but mainly the arms
	Diplegic	All limbs but mainly the legs
	Quadriplegic (tetraplegic)	All limbs equally
Athetoid	Athetosis	All limbs equally
	Chorea	
	Choreoathetosis	
Ataxic		
Rigid		
Mixed		

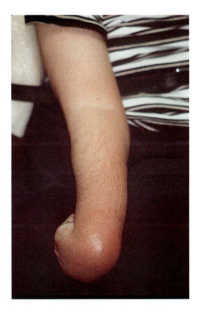

Fig. 28.2 Cerebral palsy showing contractures in spasticity.

Spastic cerebral palsy is the most common type, and CP patients were sometimes loosely referred to as 'spastics'. It is an upper motor neuron lesion that manifests with excessive muscle tone and contractures, pathological reflexes and hyperactive tendon reflexes (Fig. 28.2). Many people with CP may need to use wheelchairs (Fig. 28.3). Hemiplegia is a common subtype, often associated with neurological disorders such as epilepsy, or sensory or visual field defects. Quadriplegics may more frequently have learning impairment but are less often epileptic. Paraplegics and diplegics have an intelligence quotient (IQ) intermediate in level between quadriplegics and hemiplegics, but are the least likely to have epilepsy.

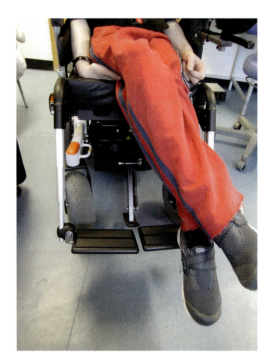

Fig. 28.3 Cerebral palsy – wheelchair user.

Athetoid cerebral palsy accounts for 15% of CP. It is caused by extrapyramidal damage, usually in the basal ganglia, giving rise to smooth worm-like movements that become exaggerated under stress. There is excessive muscle tone of the 'lead-pipe' type: the limb, when flexed, moves like a lead pipe that is being bent, but there are normal tendon reflexes and no contractures. Athetoid CP is mainly caused by intrauterine rubella and by hyperbilirubinaemia (kernicterus as in rhesus incompatibility). It usually involves the arms especially but all four limbs are affected; it is often accompanied by high-tone deafness. Epilepsy can be associated but learning impairment is less common than in spastic CP.

Ataxic cerebral palsy, caused by a cerebellar lesion, accounts for about 10% of all CP, and is characterized by disturbed balance.

General management

CP brain damage is unfortunately irreversible, but muscle training and exercises help the child's strength, balance and mobility, and increase independence. Muscle relaxants ease stiffness and anticonvulsants reduce seizures. Support from occupational therapists, speech therapists, audiologists, ophthalmic specialists, orthopaedic specialists and dieticians is invaluable.

Dental aspects

Patients restricted to wheelchairs can sometimes be treated in their wheelchair or using a double-articulating headrest, but otherwise it is often better to transfer them to the dental chair by carrying them, using a hoist or sliding them across a 'banana' transfer board placed between the wheelchair and dental chair, or to tilt their wheelchair. Ataxic and some other patients may need the wheelchair to be tilted backwards. Many, however, become apprehensive when this is done. If not, some clinics provide a wheelchair-tilting device such as Versatilt®, Safari® or Diaco®.

Uncontrollable movements, especially in athetosis, bruxism, abnormal attrition and spontaneous dislocation or subluxation of the temporomandibular joint (TMJ), are common.

Communication difficulties, along with concentration, which is often poor, may give a misleading impression of low intelligence.

Epilepsy may be seen. Abnormal swallowing and drooling are common due to poor control of the oral tissues and head posture. Anxiety may worsen athetosis or spasticity, so that anxiolytic drugs such as diazepam are useful as pre-medication.

Preventive dental care is important. Parental counselling about diet, oral hygiene procedures and the use of fluorides should be started early. Manual dexterity is usually poor but favourable results are often achievable with an electric toothbrush or a modified handle on a normal brush. Most dental disease is more common when the arms are severely affected. Periodontal disease is frequently found, especially in the older child, because soft-tissue movement is abnormal and oral cleansing is impaired. Mouth-breathing worsens the periodontal state, and papillary hyperplastic gingivitis may be seen, even in the absence of treatment with phenytoin.

There may be delayed eruption of the primary dentition and enamel hypoplasia is common. Caries activity appears normal, unless there is overindulgence by carers or others, but lack of treatment frequently leads to premature loss of primary teeth and earlier eruption of premolars and permanent canines. Malocclusion is common, probably caused by abnormal muscle behaviour. The maxillary arch is frequently tapered or ovoid, with a high palate. The upper teeth are often labially inclined, due to the pressure of the tongue against the anterior teeth during abnormal swallowing. Most, however, have skeletal patterns within normal limits.

CLEFT LIP AND PALATE

See Chapter 14.

HYDROCEPHALUS

General aspects

Hydrocephalus (*hydro* from the Greek for water and *cephalus* from the Greek for head) is a neurological disorder that affects approximately 1 in 1000 children. It is caused by raised intracranial pressure (ICP), usually due to an abnormal accumulation of cerebrospinal fluid (CSF) within the ventricles and/or subarachnoid space. CSF is overproduced, its flow is obstructed, or there is a failure to reabsorb it. In *normal pressure* hydrocephalus, the ventricles are enlarged but there is little or no rise in ICP.

Hydrocephalus is considered *congenital* when X-linked, or its origin can be traced to a birth defect or brain malformation that impairs drainage of CSF. Congenital hydrocephalus can be caused by TORCH syndrome from intrauterine infection, usually with *t*oxoplasmosis, *o*ther infections, *r*ubella, *c*ytomegalovirus or *h*erpes. Congenital hydrocephalus may be seen in spina bifida with myelomeningocoele, or as a part of other neurological conditions and congenital malformations (e.g. Dandy–Walker syndrome, neural tube defects, Chiari malformations, vein of Galen malformations, craniosynostosis, schizencephaly and tracheo-oesophageal fistula).

Hydrocephalus can be *acquired* later in life if there is a rise in resistance to CSF drainage, such as by obstruction from a brain tumour, arachnoid cyst, intracranial or intraventricular haemorrhage (IVH), trauma, or infection such as meningitis.

The term 'communicating hydrocephalus' means that the site of raised resistance to CSF drainage is outside the ventricular system in the subarachnoid space. Non-communicating, or *obstructive*, hydrocephalus is caused by a CSF obstruction within the ventricular system, especially in the aqueduct of Sylvius, at outlets of the fourth ventricle (foramina of Luschke and Magendie) or from the lateral ventricles into the third ventricle at the foramina of Monro.

Table 28.5 *Hydrocephalus*

Signs	Complications
Large head and bulging fontanelles in children	Epilepsy
	Spasticity
Headache, vomiting, mental changes, papilloedema	Learning impairment or dementia
	Visual impairment

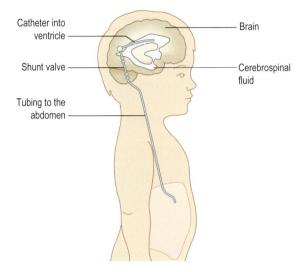

Fig. 28.4 Hydrocephalic shunt.

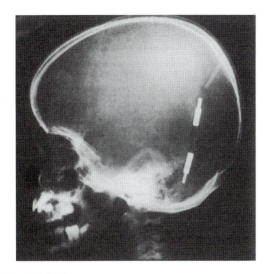

Fig. 28.5 Hydrocephalic shunt.

Clinical features

The main features of hydrocephalus are outlined in Table 28.5.

General management

Hydrocephalus can be treated directly, by removing the cause of CSF obstruction or overproduction, or indirectly, by diverting the CSF build-up to somewhere else. Diuretics (acetazolamide and furosemide) may help reduce CSF production. Endoscopic third ventriculostomy (ETV) may relieve CSF pressure. However, in many cases, CSF has to be redirected. Initially, such 'shunts' were into the right atrium (Spitz–Holter shunt, ventriculo-atrial [VA] shunt; Fig. 28.4) but now they are typically into another body cavity (usually the peritoneal cavity – ventriculo-peritoneal [VP] shunt) via an implanted silastic device (Fig. 28.5). Shunt-lengthening surgery may be needed as the child grows.

Dental aspects

The weight of the hydrocephalic head may cause difficulties, especially in the anaesthetized patient, and there may be other management challenges, including shunt infection, or frequently associated spina bifida, latex allergy, epilepsy, or learning or visual impairment.

The consequences of infection can be so devastating that antibiotic cover may occasionally need to be given before oral procedures that might produce bacteraemia in patients with a VA shunt. There is probably no indication for antimicrobial prophylaxis for patients with a VP shunt. The risk of CSF shunt infection following dental procedures appears to be almost negligible and there are no reported cases. There is no evidence that *Streptococcus viridans* isolated from CSF shunt infections has been of oral origin (https://www.evidence.nhs.uk – search

on 'hydrocephalus shunts and antibiotic prophylaxis'; accessed 30 September 2013).

SPINA BIFIDA

General aspects

Spina bifida is failure of fusion of the vertebral arches; it is an important cause of spinal cord disease and severe physical handicap. Deficiency of folic acid in pregnancy may predispose but most cases are of unknown aetiology.

Clinical features

There is a range of impairments in spina bifida (Table 28.6) but patients with myelomeningocoele are most severely handicapped and tend to suffer from an inability to walk, liability to develop pressure sores, urinary incontinence, faecal retention and other problems, such as hydrocephalus, epilepsy or learning impairment, and other vertebral or renal anomalies.

General management

Surgical closure of myelomeningocoele and decompression of hydrocephalus are often carried out in early infancy. Patients require specialist attention to manage urinary tract, bowel and locomotion disabilities.

Dental aspects

Bowel and bladder are best emptied before dental treatment. Postural hypotension is likely, and thus the patient is best not treated supine. In any event, many are chair-bound (see above).

Care must be taken not to traumatize the patient who is unable to respond protectively. There is a very high prevalence of latex allergy in these people (Ch. 17) and some are on anticoagulants or other medication.

THALIDOMIDE SYNDROME

General aspects

In 1957, the hypnotic thalidomide was marketed for morning sickness and soon became the 'drug of choice to help pregnant women'.

Table 28.6 *Types of spina bifida*

Type	Features
Spina bifida occulta	Rarely any obvious clinical or neurological disorder but may be detected by a small naevus or tuft of hair over the lumbar spine in some patients, and radiographically in about 50% of apparently healthy children
Spina bifida cystica	Extensive vertebral defect through which the spinal cord or its coverings protrude
Meningocoele	Protrusion of the meninges as a sac covered by skin, rarely causing neurological defect, but 20% have hydrocephalus
Myelomeningocoele	Characterized by meninges and nerve tissue protruded and exposed, and liable to infection, particularly meningitis. Causes severe neurological defects, typically complete paralysis of, and loss of sensation and reflexes in, the lower limbs (paraplegia)

Table 28.7 *Causes of learning impairment*

Cause	Examples
Genetic conditions	
Chromosomal anomalies	Autosomal trisomies (Edward, Patau and Down syndromes). Deletions (chromosome 5, short arm – *cri du chat* syndrome; chromosome 4, short arm – Wolf syndrome)Sex chromosome anomalies (XO Turner syndrome; XXX superfemale; XXY Klinefelter syndrome; XYY syndromes). Fragile X syndrome
Inborn errors of metabolism	Hypothyroidism (cretinism), phenylketonuria, homocystinuria, Wilson disease, galactosaemia, mucopolysaccharidosis, Tay–Sachs disease, Gaucher disease, Lesch–Nyhan syndrome
Phakomatoses	Neurofibromatosis (von Recklinghausen disease), encephalofacial angiomatosis (Sturge–Weber syndrome), tuberous sclerosis (epiloia)
Microcephaly	Angelman syndrome
Pregnancy problems	
Drugs	Fetal alcohol syndrome, fetal anticonvulsant syndrome
Infections	Herpes simplex virus, cytomegalovirus, human immunodeficiency virus (HIV), rubella, syphilis, toxoplasmosis
Hypoxia	
Prematurity	
Birth problems	
Hypoxia	
Metabolic/toxins	Rhesus incompatibility, kernicterus, hypoglycaemia
Postnatal problems	
Infections	Pertussis, measles, meningitis, encephalitis, HIV
Metabolic/toxins	Hypoglycaemia, extreme malnutrition, lead or mercury
Trauma	Accidents or assaults with head trauma
Hypoxia	
Radiation	
Alzheimer disease	

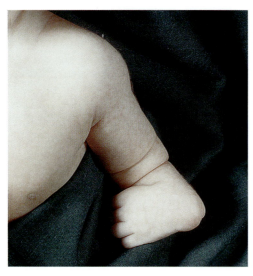

Fig. 28.6 Thalidomide phocomelia.

It was widely prescribed. The years that followed witnessed a dramatic increase in babies born with birth defects, which included deafness, blindness, cleft palate, malformed internal organs and phocomelia (seal-like limbs). Thalidomide did not affect normal intelligence. Since the withdrawal of thalidomide, those affected are now adults.

Thalidomide has activity against tumour necrosis factor (TNF) and is therefore now being used sometimes to treat leprosy, cancers, Behçet disease and major aphthae, on a named-patient basis.

Clinical features

The severe limb deformities (phocomelia) manifest as trunks lacking either arms or legs or both, or sometimes flippers extended from the shoulders, or toes extended directly from the hips (Fig. 28.6).

Dental aspects

Many thalidomide victims have a globular head with hypertelorism (widely spaced eyes), depressed nasal bridge and a central facial naevus extending from the forehead down to the nose. Oral effects include enamel hypoplasia, cleft palate and abnormalities in tongue morphology.

LEARNING IMPAIRMENT

General aspects

Learning impairment or disability is a term used for limitations in mental functioning and in skills such as communicating, self-care and social skills. In the USA, this same term is usually used to denote specific learning impairments, such as dyslexia, rather than impaired cognition.

The average intelligence quotient (IQ) score in the general population is 100. An IQ of less than 70 is the arbitrary dividing line that defines learning disability. Learning impairment affects as many as 3 out of every 100 people and is frequently the result of brain damage, often of unknown reason; defined causes are shown in Table 28.7.

Clinical features

Most patients have an IQ between 50 and 75, and often live at home. However, patients with severe learning impairment (IQ below 50) are often totally dependent on others. Brain damage may cause not only mental but also physical impairment and epilepsy; visual defects, hearing, speech or behavioural disorders, facial deformities or cardiac defects are often associated. The limitations cause children to learn and develop more slowly than normal children. They typically take longer to learn to speak, walk and take care of their personal needs, such as dressing or

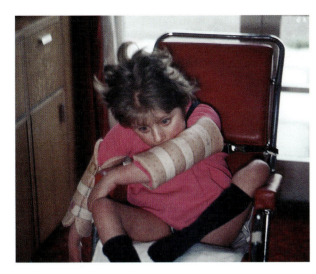

Fig. 28.7 Self-harm in a person with learning impairment.

eating, and often have trouble learning. They may sit up, crawl, walk or talk late, or have difficulty speaking. They may find it hard to remember things, and have trouble solving problems or thinking logically. They may also find it difficult to understand social rules and how to pay for things and can have trouble seeing the consequences of their actions.

Other problems may include psychiatric disorders (symptoms are often modified by poor language development and other defects), hyperkinesis and stereotyped movements (body-rocking and self-mutilation are common; Fig. 28.7). Feeding difficulties may be present. Pica (the ingestion of inedible substances) is also fairly common.

General management

Learning impairment is diagnosed by the ability to learn, think, solve problems and make sense of the world, and whether the person has the skills needed to live independently (adaptive behaviour or adaptive functioning). Adaptive behaviour skills include skills of daily living (getting dressed, going to the bathroom and feeding), communication skills (understanding what is said and being able to answer) and social skills (with peers, family members, adults and others).

Learning impairment is so varied in severity and character that generalizations about care cannot be made. Many people learn to live independently as adults in community housing. Others can be cared for adequately by committed parents or guardians.

Limited access to buildings and reluctance of staff to provide care are major barriers. Complications may result from prolonged medication (e.g. sedatives, tranquillizers or anticonvulsants); overindulgence (with consequent obesity and its sequelae); or infections (viral hepatitis, gastrointestinal infections or infestations, and tuberculosis – particularly a problem in institutionalized persons in the past).

Access and informed consent to treatment can be difficult issues for people with learning impairment. Some individuals may not be able to give informed consent themselves and, in many countries, relatives and staff have no legal right to give consent on the patient's behalf. If a person is not capable of giving or refusing consent, and has not validly refused such care in advance, treatment may often still be given lawfully if it is deemed to be in the patient's best interests. However, this should happen only after full consideration of its potential benefits and unwanted effects, and after consultation with the carer(s), relatives and other people close to the patient. See Chapter 2 and the Mental Capacity Act (http://www.justice.gov.uk/protecting-the-vulnerable/mental-capacity-act; accessed 30 September 2013).

Dental aspects

Diet make-up, maintenance of good oral hygiene, and prevention of caries and periodontal disease can be significant challenges. People with learning disability tend to have the same pattern of caries as the general population of similar age but with more teeth decayed and missing, and fewer filled teeth. Age-adjusted community periodontal index of treatment need (CPITN) scores differ significantly. Those people with severe physical and learning disability have the highest CPITN 3 category mean score. It is frequently impossible for these patients to improve their level of plaque control because of impaired cognition, mobility and manual dexterity. Powered toothbrushes may be easier and more effective for these people to use, or they may need help.

Many people with learning disability are amenable to treatment in the dental surgery, but more time may be required and they may require special facilities or an escort. Regular routine scaling usually improves the oral health considerably. Routine conservative dental treatment should be carried out wherever possible to preserve the teeth. Local anaesthesia (LA), if necessary with inhalational or intravenous sedation, is preferable and usually satisfactory. Up to one-third require sedation or general anaesthesia (GA) for dental treatment, sometimes because they are unable to understand and cooperate. GA may also be used to carry out more complex procedures and save time. GA must be performed in hospital with advanced life support facilities. Intraoperative complications are uncommon but may include non-fatal ventricular arrhythmias, slight falls in blood pressure or hypertension (more than 20% of the preoperative value), laryngospasm and minor airway problems resulting in a desaturation of oxygen to a level below 85%.

Restoring the dentition and preventing further dental disease avoids the situation of loss of teeth and the need to manage dentures. Clinical prosthetic work can be very difficult. Impression-taking is facilitated by using a viscous composition or a putty-type material. If the patient objects violently, it can be readily removed without leaving unset material in the oropharynx. If patients will not keep their mouths open, a mouth prop on alternate sides and sectional impressions may overcome the difficulty. In severely handicapped patients with severe cerebral palsy, stridor can be caused by a bite block. Those people who are more severely handicapped tend to have a deterioration of breathing function when using a bite block. Registration of occlusal records can be very difficult.

Prostheses may also be contraindicated in severe epileptics, who may inhale foreign bodies during a convulsion. Any prosthesis for an epileptic should be constructed of radio-opaque material and marked with the patient's name on a strip added to the fitting surface at flasking and covered with clear acrylic before processing. Those patients incapable of managing full dentures become dental cripples in addition to their other disabilities.

Self-mutilation may involve the oral or orofacial tissues, as in those with severe mental health problems or Lesch–Nyhan syndrome (Ch. 23), in which the lips or tongue may be chewed severely. Rarely, oral self-mutilation is accidental in patients with congenital indifference to pain, including Riley–Day syndrome (familial dysautonomia; Ch. 23).

AUTISM SPECTRUM DISORDERS

Autism spectrum disorders (ASDs) include:

- classic autism
- Asperger syndrome
- Rett syndrome
- childhood disintegrative disorder

Table 28.8 *Differences in behaviour of young children with and without autism*

Autism	Non-autism
Avoid eye contact	Study mother's face
May appear deaf	Are easily stimulated by sounds
Start developing language, then abruptly stop talking altogether	Keep adding to vocabulary and expanding grammatical usage
Social relationships	
Act as if unaware of others	Recognize familiar faces and smile
Physically attack and injure others without provocation	Cry when mother leaves room
	Become anxious with strangers
Are inaccessible	Become upset when hungry or frustrated
Exploration of environment	
Remain fixated on single item or activity	Move from one object or activity to another
Display habitual rocking or hand-flapping	Reach out to acquire objects
Sniff or lick toys	Explore and play with toys
Appear to have no sensitivity to burns or bruises	Seek pleasure
	Avoid pain
May engage in self-mutilation	

- pervasive developmental disorder not otherwise specified (usually referred to as PDD-NOS).

This is a distinct group of developmental neurological conditions characterized by a greater or lesser degree of impairment in language and communication skills, as well as repetitive or restrictive patterns of thought and behaviour.

Autism

General aspects

Autism is a spectrum of disorders with three cardinal clinical features: onset within the first 2–3 years of life, autism (profound aloneness) and an obsessional desire for maintaining an unchanging environment. Autism affects about 1 or 2 in every thousand and is 3–4 times more common in boys; it is seen mainly in first-born males and a genetic basis is possible. Genes on chromosomes 5 and 7, which affect synapses, are implicated. The genes involved appear to include: *NLGN1*, *ASTN2*, *CDH9* and *CDH10* – which code for nerve cell surface proteins that facilitate adhesion between neurons; and *DOCK4* and *IMMP2L* – which affect dendrite development.

Clinical features

Autists seem to live in isolated worlds of their own (Table 28.8), apparently indifferent and remote, unable to form emotional bonds, and incapable of understanding other people's thoughts, feelings and needs. They appear to have severe difficulties in communicating and in forming relationships with other people, in developing language, and in having repetitive and limited patterns of behaviour and obsessive resistance to any changes in familiar surroundings.

Children with autism reject people, act strangely, and lose language and social skills already acquired. They seem to have difficulty learning to engage in the give-and-take of human interaction. They appear to fail to respond to any stimuli, even to being lifted by their parents. They show complete lack of interest in other humans but are often fascinated by inanimate objects. They seem to prefer being alone, may resist attention and affection or passively accept hugs and cuddling, and seldom seek comfort or respond to anger or affection. They rarely become upset when the parent leaves or show pleasure when they return. There is ritualistic or compulsive behaviour. Autists typically demand consistency in their environment – eating the same foods, at the same time, sitting at precisely the same place. They may become annoyed with any minor change in their routine (e.g. if their toothbrush has been moved). Many engage in repetitive activities, such as rocking or banging their heads, or rigidly following familiar patterns in their routines. Most characteristic are finger-flicking near the eyes, hand-flapping, facial grimaces, jumping and toe-walking, and all such mannerisms are exaggerated if the person becomes anxious or excited. Some autists are especially sensitive to sound, touch, sight or smell, but some seem oblivious to cold or pain. Rages, tantrums and self-directed aggression are common.

The autistic child rarely employs the pronoun 'I' and frequently uses meaningless words or phrases in a generally immature speech. Language and intelligence often fail to develop fully, making communication and social relationships difficult; delayed or immediate echolalia (repetition of words heard) may develop. Some autistics are highly intelligent but 70% have an IQ of less than 70. Temporal lobe epilepsy develops in about 30%.

It is essential to rule out other disorders, including hearing loss, speech problems, learning disability, neurological problems and Rett syndrome (a progressive brain disease that affects only girls and causes repetitive hand movements, bruxism and loss of language and social skills).

General management

Medications used to treat certain symptoms of autism include clomipramine and selective serotonin reuptake inhibitors (SSRIs).

Dental aspects

It is essential to ensure that the child is not kept waiting and has a short, quiet visit with a routine that includes always seeing the same dental staff. Patients with autism may be disturbed by noise, such as a high-speed aspirator or air rotor, and it may be necessary to avoid their use. Autists may be unable to accept dental treatment under LA. GA may be needed but some patients may be on medication, such as antidepressants, which can complicate treatment.

Asperger syndrome

Asperger syndrome (AS) is an ASD. AS is considerably more common than classic autism; however, in AS features typically appear later in childhood. Indeed, the diagnosis is not usually suspected or made until school age, and patients often go on to have the capacity to live an independent adult life. The sex ratio of AS is about 8 boys to 1 girl and the prevalence among schoolboys is about 0.3%.

Unlike with autism, children with AS retain their early language skills. The most distinguishing symptom of AS is a child's obsessive interest in a single object or topic to the exclusion of any other. Children with AS want to know everything about their topic of interest and their conversations with others will be about little else. Their expertise, high level of vocabulary, and formal speech patterns make them seem like little professors. Other characteristics of AS include repetitive routines or rituals; peculiarities in speech and language; socially and emotionally inappropriate behaviour and the inability to interact successfully with peers; problems with non-verbal communication; and clumsy and uncoordinated motor movements.

Children with AS become isolated because of their poor social skills and narrow interests. They may approach other people but make normal conversation impossible by inappropriate or eccentric behaviour, or by wanting only to talk about their singular interest. Children with AS usually have a history of developmental delays in motor skills and are often awkward and poorly coordinated, with a walk that can appear either stilted or bouncy.

Positron emission tomography (PET) scan studies in AS have shown an absence of the normal task-related activity in the left medial prefrontal cortex region, although normal activity is observed in the areas immediately adjacent.

Treatment for AS may include social skills training, cognitive behavioural therapy and medication for coexisting conditions.

SPECIFIC TYPES OF LIMITED LEARNING DISABILITY

Dyslexia (reading disability)

Dyslexia is a commonly known learning disability: an impairment in the ability to translate written images into meaningful language. It is primarily used to describe difficulty with language processing and its impact on reading, writing and spelling. People with dyslexia have normal intelligence and normal speech, but often have difficulty interpreting spoken language and writing, and read at levels lower than expected. There is often a family history.

Clinical features

Common signs are delay in speaking; delay in learning the alphabet, numbers, days of the week, months, colours and shapes; reduced reading achievement; lack of awareness of phonemes (sounds that make up words); difficulty in spelling and difficulty with sequences of letters in words; and problems in understanding language subtleties (such as jokes). Inability to recognize words and letters on a printed page; reading ability level much below that expected; problems processing and understanding; difficulty with rapid instructions, more than one command at a time or remembering the sequence of things; and reversals of letters (e g b for d) and words (e.g. saw for was) are common. Untreated, dyslexia may lead to low self-esteem, behavioural problems, delinquency, aggression, and withdrawal or alienation from friends, parents and teachers.

General management

Treatment is by remedial education.

Dysgraphia

Dysgraphia involves difficulty with writing but there are also issues with spelling and the formulation of written composition. The common signs include problems involving the steps of putting together a written document, bad handwriting, awkward pen grip, avoidance of tasks that involve writing, difficulty fleshing out ideas on paper in contrast to the ability to discuss such ideas verbally, and inconsistency in the way letters and words look. People with dysgraphia can benefit from explicit instruction in the skills required to produce written work. Computers can help enormously.

Dyscalculia

Dyscalculia involves difficulty with mathematical skills (addition, subtraction, multiplication) and concepts (sequencing of numbers). Memory of mathematical facts, concepts of time, money and musical concepts can be affected. Language and other skills, however, may be advanced, and visual memory for the printed word is good. There may be a poor sense of direction, as well as trouble reading maps, telling the time, grappling with mechanical processes, handling abstract concepts of time and direction, dealing with schedules, keeping track of time, and knowing the sequence of past and future events. Individuals with dyscalculia need help in organizing and processing information related to numbers and mathematical concepts. Again, computers can help.

Dyspraxia

Dyspraxia (apraxia) is difficulty with motor planning, affecting a person's ability to coordinate appropriate body movements. It results in various problems such as:

- *ideomotor dyspraxia* (inability to perform single motor tasks, such as combing hair or waving goodbye)
- *ideational dyspraxia* (difficulty with multilevel tasks, such as taking the proper sequence of steps for brushing teeth)
- *dressing dyspraxia* (difficulty with dressing and putting clothes on in order)
- *oromotor dyspraxia* (difficulty with speech)
- *constructional dyspraxia* (difficulty with spatial relations).

Features may include: coordination problems, including awkwardness in walking, clumsiness or trouble with hopping, skipping, throwing and catching a ball, or riding a bicycle; confusion about which hand to use for tasks; inability to hold a pen or pencil properly; sensitivity to touch; poor short-term memory; trouble with reading and writing; poor sense of direction; speech problems; phobias or obsessive behaviour; and impatience.

CHROMOSOMAL ANOMALIES

Chromosomal anomalies may sometimes be associated with physical and/or mental impairments. Most human cells contain 46 chromosomes (23 pairs), half of which are inherited from each parent. Only the reproductive cells (the sperm cells in males and the ova in females) have 23 *individual* chromosomes, not pairs. When the sperm and ovum combine at fertilization, the fertilized egg that results contains 23 chromosome pairs. A fertilized egg that will develop into a female contains chromosome pairs 1–22 and the XX pair. A fertilized egg that will develop into a male contains chromosome pairs 1–22 and the XY pair.

Chromosomal anomalies affect sex chromosomes and autosomes equally. Sex chromosome anomalies are usually compatible with life and are rarely associated with severe physical disability. Autosomal anomalies affecting the larger chromosomes commonly cause spontaneous abortions and natal and early neonatal deaths. However, anomalies of the smaller chromosomes may be compatible with life, though they can cause multiple impairments, as in Down syndrome.

The most common source of major chromosomal anomalies is an error in meiosis (non-disjunction). One chromosome too few, or one too many, enters a gamete and subsequently the zygote. Most of the chromosomal anomalies are rare and many affected individuals survive for only a few years. Chromosomal deletions may also cause learning disability.

The most common chromosomal anomalies of significance in dentistry are Down syndrome and fragile X syndrome. Medical problems and the main oral manifestations of other chromosomal anomalies are summarized in Appendix 28.1.

Table 28.9 *Genes implicated in Down syndrome*

Gene	Gene product	Possible sequelae
APP	Amyloid beta A4 precursor protein	Cognitive difficulties
COL6A1	Collagen type 1	Cardiac defects
CRYA1	Crystallin, alpha-A	Cataracts
DSCR1	Down syndrome critical region gene 1	Defect in signal transduction pathway involving both heart and brain
DYRK	Tyrosine phosphorylation-regulated kinase 1A	Poor mental development
ETS2	Avian erythroblastosis virus E26 oncogene homologue 2	Lymphocyte and thymus abnormalities
IFNAR	Interferon receptor	Impaired interferon expression; immune defect
SOD1	Superoxide dismutase	Dementia; immune defect

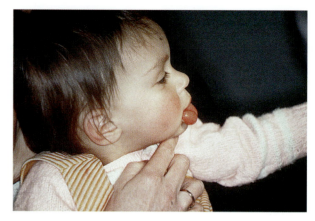

Fig. 28.8 Down syndrome facies.

Down syndrome (mongolism or trisomy 21)

General aspects

Down syndrome is the most frequent genetic cause of learning impairment, appearing in 1 in 800 live births. It is caused by an error in cell division that results in the presence of an additional third chromosome 21 (trisomy 21), derived from the mother in 88%. The resultant range of physical disabilities varies, depending on the proportion of cells carrying the additional chromosome 21.

In 92%, there is an extra chromosome 21 in all cells (*trisomy 21*). In 2–4% there is a *mosaic trisomy 21* – the extra chromosome 21 is present in some cells only. In approximately 3–4%, material from one chromosome 21 is translocated on to another chromosome (*translocation trisomy 21*); cells then have two normal chromosomes 21, but also have additional chromosome 21 material on the translocated chromosome, usually chromosome 14 or 15. There may be an increased likelihood of Down syndrome in future pregnancies when the mother has had a child with translocation trisomy 21. An older mother is more likely to have a baby with Down syndrome but, since older mothers have fewer babies, about 75% of babies with Down syndrome are born to younger women. A range of chromosome 21 genes is implicated in Down syndrome features (Table 28.9).

Clinical features

The characteristic features are short stature, learning disability, and a typical facies with brachycephaly, widely spaced eyes, Brushfield spots in the iris and epicanthic folds (Fig. 28.8). The hands show clinodactyly (short fifth finger) and simian (single) palmar creases. However, Down syndrome also affects many, if not most, organs, and some patients succumb in their first few years (Fig. 28.9). Approximately 50% have congenital cardiac disorders (atrial septal defect, mitral valve prolapse or, less often, atrioventricular and ventricular septal defect) and associated early onset of pulmonary hypertension (Fig. 28.10). Mitral valve prolapse can lead to arrhythmias, embolism or sudden death. If it causes a systolic murmur, it can predispose to infective endocarditis, particularly in older persons.

Seizure disorders affect between 5% and 13%, a tenfold greater incidence than in the general population. Dementia, or memory loss and impaired judgment similar to that in Alzheimer disease patients, may develop. There is susceptibility to transient myelodysplasia or defective development of the spinal cord. Atlantoaxial instability can cause spinal cord compression if the neck is not handled gently. The external

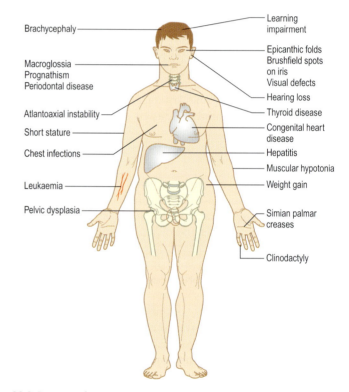

Brachycephaly

Macroglossia
Prognathism
Periodontal disease

Atlantoaxial instability

Short stature

Chest infections

Leukaemia

Pelvic dysplasia

Learning impairment

Epicanthic folds
Brushfield spots on iris
Visual defects

Hearing loss

Thyroid disease

Congenital heart disease

Hepatitis

Muscular hypotonia

Weight gain

Simian palmar creases

Clinodactyly

Fig. 28.9 Down syndrome.

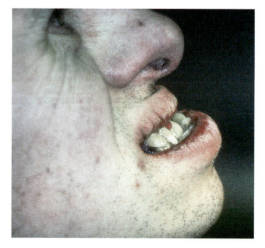

Fig. 28.10 Down syndrome: cyanosis and prognathism.

ear and the bones of the middle and inner ear may develop differently and thus up to 90% have hearing loss of greater than 15–20 decibels in at least one ear. Cataracts appear in approximately 3%. Children with Down syndrome are 10–15 times more likely than other children to develop leukaemia.

Multiple immune defects mean that infections of the skin and gastrointestinal and respiratory tracts, and periodontal disease are common; superoxide dismutase has been shown to increase in Down syndrome and may be implicated in the immune defect. Chronic respiratory infections include tuberculosis and recurrent middle ear, tonsil, nasal and sinus infections. Institutionalized patients are also liable to be hepatitis B carriers. There is a 12-fold higher mortality rate from infectious diseases, particularly pneumonia.

The life expectancy for people with Down syndrome, though low, has increased substantially to age 50 and beyond, particularly because infections are now more readily controlled.

General management

Many specialists recommend that women who become pregnant at age 35 or older undergo prenatal testing for Down syndrome. After counselling, this includes the following:

- blood screening for maternal serum alpha-fetoprotein (MSAFP – low in Down syndrome), human chorionic gonadotropin (hCG – raised in Down syndrome) and unconjugated oestriol (uE3 – low in Down syndrome)
- amniocentesis – analysis of a small sample of fetal cells from the amniotic fluid (generally safe but cannot be done until the 14–18th weeks of pregnancy, and it usually takes more time to determine whether cells contain extra material from chromosome 21)
- chorionic villus sampling (CVS), conducted at 9–11 weeks of pregnancy; involves testing a small amount of chorionic villi, obtained through the abdomen or cervix, for extra material from chromosome 21
- percutaneous umbilical blood sampling (PUBS), the most accurate method and used to confirm the results of CVS or amniocentesis; cannot be performed until later in the pregnancy (during the 8th–22nd weeks) and carries the greatest risk of miscarriage.

With assistance from family and carers, many adults with Down syndrome develop the skills required to hold jobs and to live semi-independently.

Dental aspects

People with Down syndrome are usually amiable and cooperative, and generally more easily managed than many other types of patient with learning disability.

Most can be treated under LA with sedation if necessary. GA must be administered by a specialist anaesthetist in hospital or is best avoided where possible, in view of other management difficulties; the latter may include cardiac defects, anaemia, possible atlantoaxial subluxation (care needed when extending the neck) or respiratory disease. There may also be difficulty in intubation because of the hypoplastic midface, congenital respiratory anomalies and the increased susceptibility to chest infections.

The tongue may be absolutely or relatively large and is often scrotal, especially after the age of about 4 years (Table 28.10). The circumvallate papillae enlarge but filiform papillae may be absent. The lips tend to be thick, dry and fissured. Poor anterior oral seal and also a strong tongue thrust may be seen.

Table 28.10 *Orofacial abnormalities in Down syndrome*

Hard tissue	Soft tissue
Omega-shaped palate	Macroglossia
Midface hypoplasia	Tongue fissuring
Hypodontia	Lip fissuring
Microdontia	Cheilitis
Delayed eruption in both dentitions	Drooling
Bruxism	

Anterior open bite, posterior cross-bite and other malocclusions are common. The maxillae and molars are small and the mandible is relatively protrusive. Class III malocclusion is common, but 46% of cases are class I. The orthodontic prognosis may be poor because of learning disability, parafunctional habits and severe periodontal disease. The palate often appears to be high, with horizontal palatal shelves (the omega palate), but a short palate is more characteristic. There is also a higher incidence of bifid uvula, cleft lip and cleft palate.

The first dentition may begin to appear only after 9 months and may take 5 years to complete, if ever. The deciduous molars may erupt before the deciduous incisors, and deciduous lateral incisors are absent in about 15%. The eruption of the permanent teeth is frequently also irregular. Missing teeth are common; the third molars and lateral incisors are most often absent. Up to 30% have morphological abnormalities in both dentitions, particularly teeth with short small crowns and roots. The occlusal surfaces of the deciduous molars may be hypoplastic and both dentitions may be hypocalcified. Caries activity is usually low in both dentitions.

Severe early-onset periodontal disease may be partly due to poor oral hygiene, but may be the result of impaired cell-mediated and humoral immunity and a deficient phagocytic system. Acute ulcerative gingivitis may also be seen. Short roots and poor manual dexterity and oral hygiene often complicate the situation.

A well-planned preventive dental health programme, started early, can lead to some success in the prevention of dental diseases.

Fragile X syndrome

General aspects

Fragile X syndrome affects 1 in 1500 of the population and is, after Down syndrome, the second most common chromosomal defect associated with learning impairment. Fragile X syndrome is so named because the tip of the X chromosome is susceptible to breakage. Fragile X syndrome is a sex-linked dominant trinucleotide repeat disorder (other trinucleotide repeat disorders include Huntington chorea, spinocerebellar ataxia, myotonic dystrophy and Friedreich ataxia).

Clinical features

Fragile X syndrome affects males and manifests with learning impairment, long face, prominent ears, large testes and seizures.

Dental aspects

Hyperactivity, a short attention span and behavioural disorders similar to those of autism often make dental management difficult. Cross-bite and open bite are abnormally frequent.

ATTENTION DEFICIT (HYPERACTIVITY) DISORDER

Attention deficit (hyperactivity) disorder (ADD/ADHD) may be associated with learning difficulties (Ch. 10).

OTHER HANDICAPPING SYNDROMES

See Appendices 28.1 and 23.1 for inborn errors of metabolism.

KEY WEBSITES

(Accessed 11 June 2013)
British Society for Disability and Oral Health. <http://www.bsdh.org.uk/index.php>.
GOV.UK. <https://www.gov.uk/browse/disabilities>.
National Institutes of Health. <http://health.nih.gov/topic/DisabilitiesGeneral>.

USEFUL WEBSITES

(Accessed 11 June 2013)
ADA.gov. Information and Technical Assistance on the Americans with Disabilities Act. <http://www.ada.gov/>.
British Society for Disability and Oral Health. <http://www.bsdh.org.uk/guidelines/physical.pdf>.
FACES: The National Craniofacial Association. <http://www.faces-cranio.org/>.
MedlinePlus. <http://www.nlm.nih.gov/medlineplus/cleftlipandpalate.html>.
Hydrocephalus Center. <http://www.patientcenters.com/hydrocephalus>.

National Institutes of Health: National Institute of Neurological Disorders and Stroke. <http://www.ninds.nih.gov/disorders/cerebral_palsy/cerebral_palsy.htm>.
National Institutes of Health: Down syndrome. <http://health.nih.gov/topic/DownSyndrome>.
National Organization for Rare Disorders. <http://www.rarediseases.org/> (under the 'Rare Disease Information' tab, search on 'TORCH syndrome').
Succeeding Together: People with Disabilities in the Workplace: online publication. <http://www.neads.ca/en/about/projects/student_leadership/access_to_success/access_resources.php>.

FURTHER READING

Acs, N., et al. 2006. Population-based case-control study of the common cold during pregnancy and congenital abnormalities. Eur. J. Epidemiol. 21, 65.
Chew, L.C.T., 2006. Special care. Autism: the aetiology, management and implications for treatment modalities from the dental perspective. Dent. Update 33, 70.
Garg, A., et al. 2012. Neural tube defects and their significance in clinical dentistry: a mini review. J. Investig. Clin. Dent. doi:10.1111/j.2041-1626.2012.00141.x.
Mahoney, E.K., et al. 2008. Effect of visual impairment upon oral health care: a review. Br. Dent. J. 204, 63.
Proctor, R., et al. 2004. Cerebrospinal fluid shunts and dentistry: a short review of relevant literature. J. Disabil. Oral Health 5, 27.
Rosenberg, G.A., 2008. Brain edema and disorders of cerebrospinal fluid circulation. In: Bradley, W.G. (Ed.), Neurology in clinical practice (5th edn.). Butterworth–Heinemann, Philadelphia.
Scully, C., et al. 2002. Down syndrome: lip lesions (angular stomatitis and fissures) and Candida albicans. Br. J. Dermatol. 147, 37.
Scully, C., et al. 2007. Special care in dentistry: handbook of oral healthcare. Churchill Livingstone/Elsevier, Edinburgh.
Stanfield, M., et al. 2003. The oral health of clients with learning disability: changes following relocation from hospital to community. Br. Dent. J. 194, 271.

APPENDIX 28.1 CHROMOSOMAL ANOMALIES ADDITIONAL TO THOSE DISCUSSED IN THE TEXT

Syndrome	Anomaly	Features and possible management problems	Orofacial manifestations
Angelman syndrome	Chromosome 15 deletion	'Happy puppet' – laughs and claps, learning impairment, ataxia, seizures	Microcephaly
Cri du chat syndrome	Chromosome 5 short arm deletion	Learning impairment, cardiac defects, respiratory infections	Cranial abnormalities Malocclusions
DiGeorge syndrome	Chromosome 22 microdeletion	Hypoparathyroidism, thymic hypoplasia, T-cell defect, major cardiac anomalies, learning disability	Cleft palate Candidosis Dental hypoplasia
Edwards syndrome	Trisomy 18	Learning impairment, cardiac defects, renal disease	Cranial abnormalities Microstomia Hypoplastic parotids Gingival cysts
Klinefelter syndrome	47,XXY	Tall stature, personality defects, diabetes, asthma	Taurodontism
Patau syndrome	Trisomy 13	Rarely survive infancy, learning impairment, cardiac defects in 80%, deafness, epilepsy	Cranial abnormalitiesCleft lip or palate in 75%
Superfemale	Trisomy X (47,XXX)	Tall females, learning impairment, early menopause	–
Turner syndrome	Monosomy X (45,X)	Females only, normal intelligence, infertility, short stature, webbed neck, renal anomalies, cardiac defects, diabetes, keloid formation, lymphoedema	Small mandible Malocclusions
Williams syndrome	Microdeletion of elastin gene on chromosome 7	Supravalvular aortic stenosis, hypercalcaemia, learning impairment	Elfin facies Dental anomalies
Wolf syndrome	Short arm of chromosome 4 deletion	Learning impairment	Hypodontia
XYY	47,XYY	Tall males, normal intelligence, behavioural abnormalities	–

Few of the dental materials or drugs commonly used cause significant interactions or adverse reactions (see Appendices). The main concern is allergies (e.g. especially to latex [Ch. 17] and some drugs). Other issues include adverse reactions to dental materials (especially amalgam/mercury, chlorhexidine, nickel, iodides and radiocontrast media, resins, titanium), fluorides and anaesthetics – and other drug adverse effects, oral adverse effects, drug interactions and the effects of foods on drugs.

DENTAL MATERIALS

Allergies are discussed in Chapter 17 and also below, alphabetically. Possible toxic effects of mercury on the nervous system are discussed here and in Chapter 17; fluoride is also discussed in this chapter.

ALLERGIES

Latex allergy

Latex allergy (see also Ch. 17) is one of the most important factors to be elicited from the medical history. People with severe latex allergy can react with anaphylaxis as they enter a health-care facility where latex is present in the environment!

Chlorhexidine allergy

Chlorhexidine is a cationic chlorophenyl-biguanide antiseptic and disinfectant, commonly used as the diacetate or digluconate salt, and has excellent antimicrobial properties. Chlorhexidine allergy must be rare but is important, since chlorhexidine is present in many antiseptic preparations, including some mouth rinses, disinfectants and cosmetics. Medical devices that incorporate chlorhexidine include: intravenous catheters, topical dressings and implanted surgical mesh.

Chlorhexidine used topically, intra-urethrally as catheter lubricant, as a mouthwash and with impregnated catheters has been associated with hypersensitivity reactions and some deaths. Chlorhexidine has been used in the UK since 1954 and reactions have been reported since 1962, ranging from contact dermatitis, to urticaria to anaphylactic shock with cardiac arrest. Fatal cases of anaphylaxis prompted the FDA in 1998 to issue an alert to the medical community. Patients with suspected allergies should be investigated for evidence of chlorhexidine-specific IgE by skin or blood tests.

Management is along the lines for latex allergy (Ch. 17), essentially avoiding exposure, and using povidone-iodine as an alternate skin preparation or hexetidine mouthwash as an alternate for oral use.

Patch testing using chlorhexidine has revealed positive reactions in more than 2% of patients tested. In eczema patients, the rate may be as high as 5%.

Reactions to other dental materials

Dental materials such as alloys, bonding, cements, plastics, primers, resins and other materials can cause allergies leading to dermatitis, rashes, blistering, itching or burning – though these features are usually seen only in people highly sensitive to epoxy resins. Illustrative of the difference between skin and mucosa in response to sensitizing agents is the fact that a substance, to which the patient is sensitized when it is put in the mouth, can occasionally induce the typical skin rash. This has been reported, for example, in the case of nickel sensitivity when a nickel-containing denture caused a rash but no oral reaction.

Alloys

With few exceptions, metals used in dentistry are alloys – solid mixtures of two or more metals.

'Gold allergies'

Gold alloys may occasionally be used for dental restorations or prostheses. Pure gold, because of its softness, is not indicated for use in the mouth except as gold foil – rarely used now. The basic alloys used are casting gold, gold solder, wrought gold and gold plate, and these may contain silver, copper, platinum, palladium or zinc. Lichenoid oral reactions to gold alloys are rare.

'Mercury allergy'

Dental amalgam is a combination of mercury mainly with a silver–tin alloy. The American Dental Association (ADA) specifies that the alloy must include a minimum of 65% silver, and maximums of 29% tin, 6–13% copper and 2% zinc by weight. Alloys with high copper content usually have lower creep values than conventional silver–tin alloys. Some alloys are completely zinc-free and can therefore be used more successfully in a moisture-contaminated environment. Dental amalgam may cause mucosal reactions such as lichenoid lesions, but the evidence is controversial and mercury absorbed from amalgams into the mucosa frequently causes no histological reaction.

Mercury and its salts are potential sensitizing agents; exposure to them can occasionally lead to contact dermatitis, and the frequency of positive patch tests increases as dental students progress through their course. Also, a few patients have genuine contact sensitivity to mercury, though they can generally tolerate the placement of amalgam restorations, provided that none is spilt on to the skin. 'Baboon syndrome' is a special form of systemic contact-type dermatitis manifesting with bright red buttocks and flexural eczema that occurs after ingestion or systemic absorption of a contact allergen in individuals previously sensitized by topical exposure to the same allergen in the same areas; it has been reported as a reaction to mercury.

Another group of patients appear to have symptoms such as headache, lassitude or a general feeling of ill-health that they ascribe to mercury toxicity, although there is no reliable evidence that mercury underlies these problems. Such patients may also suffer more frequently from other unrelated complaints, such as chronic craniofacial pain, than do controls.

Nickel allergy

Nickel-containing alloys are widely used, especially in orthodontics. The highest nickel content is in nickel–titanium, especially in flexible wires, but even stainless steel contains almost 10% nickel; most of this is bound, however, and unlikely to cause allergy – so can safely be used in nickel-allergic people. Nickel allergy often arises from jewellery and the prevalence appears to have increased with the advent of body piercing. Safe alternatives to nickel wires include stainless steel, composites, titanium and gold-plated wires. Wires of nickel–titanium that are 'altered' or coated with plastics or resin might be safe. Brackets of stainless steel, titanium, ceramics or polycarbonates are safe. Plastic-coated studs on headgear will avoid the issue with nickel studs.

'Titanium allergy'

Degradation of metallic biomaterials may result in products leading to metal hypersensitivity reactions. Titanium has been considered an inert material but it has been suggested that it can rarely induce toxicity or allergic type I or IV reactions in susceptible patients. In a systematic review it has been shown that titanium allergy develops among patients at any age, the most common clinical manifestations being dermal inflammatory conditions and gingival swelling. A significantly higher risk of positive allergic reactions was found in patients showing allergic symptoms after implant placement or unexplained implant failures. The risk of an allergy to titanium is increased in patients who are allergic to other metals. Alternative materials (e.g. zirconium oxide) are available.

Cements

Dental cements include zinc phosphate, zinc oxide and eugenol, poly-carboxylate (zinc oxide powder mixed with polyacrylic acid) and glass ionomer cements (GICs). Allergic reactions to most dental cements are rare but GICs contain a polyalkenoic acid such as polyacrylic acid plus a fluoride-containing silicate glass (fluoroaluminosilicate) powder, and do occasionally cause reactions. Resin-modified glass ionomer cements (RMGICs) usually contain HEMA (hydrophilic monomer) plus a fluoride-containing glass and polyacrylic acid. Tri-cure GICs also incorporate a chemical curing tertiary amine-peroxide reaction to polymerize the methacrylate, along with the photo-initiation and acid–base ionic reaction. These resins may cause reactions.

Plastics and resins

Some chemicals in resins may cause reactions. Polymethyl methacrylate (PMMA), polystyrene, polyvinylchloride (PVC) and so on contain potential allergens such as long hydrocarbon-based chains produced from small monomer units (e.g. methyl methacrylate [MMA], styrene, vinyl chloride, etc.). A few individuals may react to the potential allergens shown in Box 29.1 and some reactive materials may leach from set material at least for a few days, as may degradation products (e.g. formaldehyde).

PMMA (acrylic) is used for clothing, plastic items or dentures and is itself probably inert, but dental MMA contains a wide range of components that are potentially sensitizing (Table 29.1). There are rare cases, particularly in dental health-care professionals (HCPs), of allergic reactions to MMA monomer and associated chemicals. Affected persons should avoid exposure. Surgical rubber, latex or vinyl gloves offer little, if any, protection, as they are quickly penetrated by the chemicals, but commercial laminated disposable protective gloves are available.

Resins are also used in dentistry as bonding agents, composite resins, pit and fissure sealants, and resin-based cements. Often referred to as direct-filling resins, they are of several types; the older type was an unfilled polymethacrylate, while the more recent type is a composite resin based mainly on dimethacrylates plus silanated glass. Acid-modified composites (compomers) consist of methacrylate monomers such as urethane dimethacrylate (UDMA) and fluoride-containing glass. The monomers most commonly used are UDMA and 2,2,-bis(4(2-hydroxyl-3-methacryloxyloxypropoxy)-phenyl) propane – bisphenol A glycidal methacrylate (BPA; BIS-GMA) – combined with lower-molecular-weight monomers such as triethylene glycol dimethacrylate

---

Box 29.1 *Potential allergens in dental resins*

- 1,4-Butanediol dimethacrylate (BUDMA)
- 1,7,7-Trimethylbicyclo-2,2,1-heptane
- 2-Hydroxyethyl methacrylate (2-HEMA)
- 2-Hydroxypropyl methacrylate (2-HPMA)
- 2,2-Dimethoxy-1,2-diphenyletanone (DMBZ)
- 4-Dimethylaminobenzoic acid ethyl ester (DMABEE)
- Acrylated epoxy oligomer
- DL-Camphorquinone
- Ethylene glycol dimethacrylate (EGDMA)
- Methyl methacrylate (MMA)
- Triethylene glycol dimethacrylate (TEGDMA)
- Urethane dimethacrylate (UDMA)

Table 29.1 *Typical components of dental methyl methacrylate*

Liquid	Powder
Dimethacrylate (cross-linker)	Organic peroxides (initiators)
Hydroquinone (inhibitor)	Pigments
Methyl methacrylate (monomer)	Polymethyl methacrylate
Organic amines (accelerator)	Titanium dioxide
Ultraviolet absorber	

(TEGDMA). Photo-initiators such as camphoroquinone facilitate polymerization via light curing.

The major sensitizers appear to be EGDMA, 2-HEMA, 2-hydroxy-propyl methacrylate (2-HPMA), MMA and acrylated epoxy oligomer. 1,4-Butanediol dimethacrylate (BUDMA) and UDMA seem to be only weak sensitizers.

Allergic reactions in the mouth are typically lichenoid but occasionally urticarial or anaphylactoid, and dermatological reactions in HCPs are usually contact dermatitis or eczema – so direct skin contact is best avoided. Allergic reactions may be produced by the catalyst methyldi-chlorobenzene sulphonate in dibenzyltoluol present in *Impregum* and by the catalyst methyl *p*-toluene sulphonate in dibenzyltoluol present in *Scutan*. Some people are sensitive to colophony resins, found in wound sticking plasters, periodontal dressings, impression materials, cements, fix adhesives and some fluoride varnishes (e.g. Duraphat). Eugenol in periodontal dressings can also be a contact allergen.

Apart from allergic reactions, there are few data to indicate significant toxicity from most resin components, though BPA may have some oestrogenic activity *in vitro*. BPA has also been implicated in heart disease and diabetes, though only minuscule amounts are found in dental resin restorations, and much more is present in other items such as plastic bottles and can linings. BPA leaches out from food and beverage containers, as well as from dental resins. Indeed, a recent survey by the Centers for Disease Control and Prevention (CDC) found bisphenol in the urine of 95% of people in USA. High levels of BPA have been correlated with obesity, diabetes, cardiovascular diseases, polycystic ovaries or low sperm count. In 2008, the ADA stated:

There is also evidence that some dental sealants, and to a lesser extent dental composites, may contribute to very low-level BPA exposure. The ADA fully supports continued research into the safety of BPA but, based on current evidence, the ADA does not believe there is a basis for health concerns relative to BPA exposure from any dental material.

CONCERNS ABOUT DENTURE FIXATIVES

Some denture fixatives contain zinc, which may be absorbed and cause copper deficiency, myelopathy and 'human swayback disease' with polyneuropathies.

CONCERNS ABOUT FLUORIDE

Some studies, now criticized for their analyses, suggested associations of bladder cancer with occupational fluoride exposure and of osteosarcoma with water fluoridation. A recent systematic review confirmed the benefit of fluoride in protection against dental caries, and found that water fluoride to a concentration of 1 ppm had no proven adverse effects on bone strength, bone mineral density, fracture incidence (protective or deleterious), cancer incidence or mortality, or on other conditions such as prevalence of Down syndrome, congenital abnormalities or stillbirths. For details, see http://www.nhmrc.gov.au/guidelines/publications/eh41 (accessed 30 September 3013).

Another recent systematic review and meta-analysis, however, produced results that supported the possibility of an adverse effect of high fluoride exposure on child neurodevelopment.

CONCERNS ABOUT MERCURY

Mercury is a well-known neurotoxin and nephrotoxin. There also may be an association between mercury exposures over time and coronary artery disease, including myocardial infarction. There are three kinds of mercury involved in exposure (and poisoning): organomercury, inorganic mercury and elemental (metallic) mercury poisoning.

Organic mercury poisoning from methylmercury is the most common type; it is well recognized and, except in rare cases (e.g. exposure to laboratory reagents), is exclusively associated with fish ingestion. Mercury in the environment, especially that released into the air through industrial pollution, falls into and can accumulate in rivers and oceans, where it is turned into methylmercury. Fish absorb the methylmercury as they feed and so it accumulates in them. Shark, swordfish, king mackerel and tilefish contain high mercury levels, and white tuna can have fairly high levels. The most commonly eaten fish that are low in mercury are shrimp, canned light tuna, salmon, pollock and catfish. The US Food and Drug Administration (FDA) outlines pregnancy concerns and fish mercury levels at http://www.fda.gov/Food/FoodborneIllnessContaminants/Metals/default.htm (accessed 30 September 2013).

The most infamous example of methylmercury poisoning was at Minamata Bay and Nigata, Japan, in the 1950s. Many people suffered neurological damage, some died and there was a high incidence of cerebral palsy in neonates (Minamata disease) as a result of eating fish contaminated by mercury in industrial discharge found in the sea. Mercury poisoning of this type continues as a problem in parts of China, Brazil, Peru, Philippines, Suriname and Venezuela, and is associated mainly with occupations such as mining activities. Examples of gold mining-associated mercury pollution (often with cyanide and arsenic) are known in Africa, Canada, China, Philippines, Siberia, South America and USA. For further information, see http://www.nrdc.org/health/effects/mercury/medical.asp (accessed 30 September 2013).

Inorganic mercury salts poisoning, now rare, caused acrodynia (pink disease), a condition seen mainly at the end of the nineteenth century in children and others who used calomel (a mercury salt) in teething powders and gastrointestinal medications; it was also caused by inorganic mercurials used as disinfectants in detergents and baby powders. Inorganic mercury poisoning is still occasionally seen in people using mercuric chloride in skin creams available in the developing world, in some traditional Chinese and herbal preparations, in some ritual spiritual or 'medical' practices, in suicide attempts and in forensic science, as well as in bizarre accidents. Poisoning can cause:

- acrodynia – skin peeling, salivation, hypotonia, swelling of extremities
- gastrointestinal ulceration and necrosis
- renal failure.

Metallic mercury poisoning is an issue with dental amalgam but is actually confined almost exclusively to the occupational setting. Dental amalgam is a mixture of 50% metallic mercury with other metals, and there is concern that mercury can be released as vapour, ions or fine particles, which can be inhaled or ingested. Studies of amalgam exposure, even during pregnancy, have not documented any toxicity, including birth defects, neurologic sequelae, spontaneous abortions or reduction in fertility. Poisoning was, however, well recognized in the past among people working with metallic mercury (e.g. thermometer makers and makers of felt hats – hence, 'mad as a hatter'). Poisoning has more recently been reported among people who use mercury for activities such as gold mining, where mercury is added to the pan to amalgamate the gold and is subsequently boiled off. Metallic mercury is also used in Santería – a Caribbean religious practice in which mercury may be sprinkled inside a home and can cause serious overexposure. Accidents also continue to occur, metallic mercury still being found in some older equipment such as thermometers, fluorescent lights and computers. Mercury can be absorbed by inhalation of its vapour or through skin and mucous membranes (and mercury salts can be absorbed after their ingestion). There are even some who inject it intravenously in suicide attempts! Mercury is highly lipid-soluble, rapidly penetrates the blood–brain barrier and infiltrates neurons.

Acute poisoning by massive inhalation of mercury vapour is rare but can cause potentially fatal pneumonitis and neurological symptoms, particularly tremor and excitability. Chronic poisoning by mercury vapour inhalation primarily causes lassitude, gastrointestinal disturbances, anorexia and weight loss, and affects the central nervous system (CNS) with tremor, memory loss and excitability (erethism). Other effects include hypersalivation, accelerated periodontitis and a black gingival line due to deposition of mercury sulphides (like the lead line). Rarely, jaw necrosis follows.

Mercury hazards to dental health workers

Amalgam use may be associated with occupational exposure of dental health workers (DHWs) to metallic mercury if personnel fail to follow good work practices. On average, up to 1.5 kg of mercury are used by a dental practice annually; in the past, when less attention was paid to occupational hazards, mercury vapour in the surgery atmosphere and its levels in the blood, hair, nails and urine of DHWs were frequently above controls. Droplets of mercury could also accumulate in significant amounts in surgery carpeting or crevices in the floor. Mercury is also absorbed during the outmoded practice of hand trituration of amalgam or during other skin contact. In the past, after decades of practice, a few DHWs suffered chronic mercury toxicity with tremor, incoordination, polyneuropathies and accelerated senility. Autopsy studies have also shown mercury deposits, particularly in the pituitary glands and occipital lobes. Rarely, deaths have been reported after prolonged heavy exposure.

In a study of female DHWs, a history of reproductive failures, menstrual disorders and spina bifida in their children was suggested to be related to mercury levels in hair, but this has not been widely confirmed – and other larger studies have shown no such correlation. Indeed, the perinatal death and birth defect rate for infants born to dentists is currently *lower* than average. Further, urinary mercury levels appeared to be falling in studies of dentists in the 1990s, and more recent studies of DHWs have not shown excessively high urinary mercury levels where good mercury hygiene was practised. Another study found no consistent association between either urinary mercury or chronic mercury exposure and any category of self-reported symptoms of depression, anxiety and memory loss. Exposure of DHWs to mercury is currently now very low – probably as a result of increased awareness of mercury toxicity and improved methods of preparing amalgam – especially the use of encapsulated mercury amalgam. Thus it seems unlikely that there is now a significant risk to DHWs who work in practices where adequate standards of mercury hygiene appertain. Indeed, mercury levels in DHWs are highest in those who eat fish, indicating that at least part of their mercury burden was from dietary – not dental – sources.

Risks from dental amalgam restorations

Dental amalgam restorative materials continually emit mercury vapour, which is increased by chewing, eating, brushing and drinking hot liquids. The World Health Organization's maximum recommended mercury intake is 2 micrograms/kg/day; release of mercury from dental amalgam is around 10 micrograms/day. Hydrogen peroxide can increase mercury release, so should be avoided. Removal of old amalgams from teeth with an air-rotor produces traces of mercury vapour – but not if adequate water-cooling and aspiration are used. The responses of official bodies to public concerns about mercury toxicity are shown in Appendix 29.1, and suggest a very low risk of toxicity. In one large study, children who received dental restorative treatment with amalgam did not, on average, have statistically significant differences in neurobehavioural assessments or in nerve conduction velocity, compared with children who received resin composite materials only. In the New England Children's Amalgam Trial, a randomized study involving children, the hypothesis that restorations using amalgam resulted in worse psychosocial outcomes than restorations using composite resin over a 5-year period following initial placement was not supported by the results. These findings, combined with the trend of higher treatment need later among those receiving composite restorations, suggested that amalgam should remain a viable dental restorative option for children.

Thus, according to present scientific evidence, the use of amalgam is not a proven health hazard and, to date, there is no dental material that can fully substitute for amalgam as a restorative material. More recent studies and reviews have also found little to no correlation between systemic or local diseases and amalgam restorations, although extensive amalgam restorations in pregnant or nursing women are not recommended. Nevertheless, the state governments of California, Connecticut, Maine and Vermont, and the federal governments of Denmark, Finland, Norway and Sweden have legislation requiring that dental patients receive informed consent information about the restorative material that will be used. Apart from Norway, Denmark and Sweden, dental amalgam has not been banned in any European Union country. A European Commission report by the BIO Intelligence Service (BIOIS), however, recommends the phasing-out of amalgam, and of mercury in button cell batteries (http://ec.europa.eu/environment/chemicals/mercury/pdf/review_mercury_strategy2010.pdf; accessed 30 September 2013).

Mercury disposal

The greatest hazard from inhalation of mercury vapour is as a result of any spillage. Dentists should use dental amalgam separators to trap excess amalgam waste coming from surgeries and avoid release into the sewers; separators generally have a removal efficiency of approximately 95%. Captured amalgam solid waste should be appropriately recycled or retorted. Amalgam in waste waters proceeds to publicly owned treatment works (POTWs), most of which have more than 90% efficiency at removing amalgam waste. The rest is discharged from POTWs as a component of sewage sludge, which may then be disposed of:

- in landfills – where mercury may be released into the groundwater or air
- through incineration – when mercury may be emitted into the air
- through use on agricultural land as fertilizer – when mercury may be released into the groundwater or atmosphere.

Mercury waste from dental surgeries thus contributes significantly to the overall mercury contamination in wastewater, and may be the source of about 50% of all mercury entering POTWs – far exceeding pollution from all other commercial and residential sources. Other amalgam constituents (e.g. silver, tin, copper and zinc) have not been reported in dental clinics' wastewater.

Cremation and burial can also be responsible for mercury pollution. Cremation has recently gained in popularity due to the shedding of negative religious connotations but it releases quantities of atmospheric mercury from amalgams. Burial is important for many cultures, such as Catholics and Muslims; it also releases mercury and might reach drinking water sources. This issue is being addressed (http://www.epa.gov/hg/dentalamalgam.html and http://ec.europa.eu/environment/chemicals/mercury/pdf/review_mercury_strategy2010.pdf; both accessed 30 September 2013). The United Nations Environmental Programme (UNEP) has expressed concerns and also outlined the action required (http://www.unep.org/hazardoussubstances/mercury/tabid/434/default.aspx; accessed 30 September 2013).

CONCERNS ABOUT TOOTH-WHITENING PRODUCTS

Tooth-whitening products are widely available for sale over the counter (OTC) or ARE dispensed by dentists for patients' use at home. Most products release hydrogen peroxide (H_2O_2). Self-applied bleaching agents either contain or generate H_2O_2, as gel in trays, paint-on films or whitening strips. A nightguard bleach typically uses 10% carbamide peroxide (which contains approximately 3% H_2O_2) and OTC whitening strips contain approximately 6% H_2O_2, while in-surgery bleach uses 25–35% H_2O_2. These can all potentially produce comparable whitening but strips are slightly more effective at whitening than is a gel in a tray. In the UK, Cosmetic Product (Safety) Regulations apply to products that contain or release more than 0.1% H_2O_2.

Recently, attention has focused on dentist-prescribed home bleaching, in which the teeth and oral soft tissues can be in contact with peroxide-type agents for long periods; this creates a different situation from the use of in-surgery bleaching or home oral health-care products, such as peroxide-containing toothpastes and mouthwashes, from the standpoint of both dose and time. Hydrogen peroxide is a highly reactive substance that can damage oral soft and hard tissues when employed at high concentrations and with prolonged exposures. Direct exposure of mucosae, skin or eyes to 30% H_2O_2 may cause severe irritation, burns, blistering and ulceration. The much lower concentrations used in dental whitening products do not appear to produce such adverse effects, but tooth sensitivity and gingival irritation are common.

CONCERNS ABOUT ORAL HEALTH-CARE PRODUCTS

Contact dermatitis can occasionally be precipitated on the lip vermilion or, more frequently, the perioral skin by components of toothpastes, lipsticks and some foods (notably mangoes and oranges) or by dental impression materials. Toothpastes or chewing gum components, especially cinnamon, can also cause plasma cell gingivitis or inflammation of other parts of the oral mucosa. Gingivitis, cheilitis, perioral dermatitis and other lesions have been described in patients using tartar-control toothpastes that contain cinnamonaldehyde or pyrophosphates. Some substances (e.g. zirconium) occasionally cause granulomatous oral reactions, and allergic reactions may underlie orofacial granulomatosis.

DRUGS

Relatively few drugs are used in general dentistry, and the rarity of hypersensitivity reactions and lack of evidence of significant interactions of local anaesthesia (LA) with drugs must be stressed. The many relative and absolute drug contraindications, as well as drug interactions, are discussed in Chapter 3 and its appendices. Drugs used in the practice of oral medicine and surgery may also produce adverse reactions or interactions.

However, children need lower doses of virtually all drugs. Older people tend to be more liable to adverse drug reactions, and the reactions tend to be more serious and last longer than in younger people. Older people are also more likely to be given drugs.

Sedative techniques are more likely and general anaesthesia (GA) is much more likely to produce adverse reactions.

DRUG REACTIONS AND ALLERGIES

Any suggestion of a previous drug adverse reaction or allergy, and particularly any adverse reaction during anaesthesia or imaging, must be taken seriously. Drug allergy or hypersensitivity results from interactions between a drug and the immune system, mediated by immunoglobulin E (IgE), but some reactions involve additional, poorly understood mechanisms. Identifiable risk factors for drug reactions include:

- advancing age
- female gender
- concurrent illnesses
- previous hypersensitivity to related drugs.

Furthermore, patients with allergy to one drug, and individuals with Sjögren syndrome or human immunodeficiency virus (HIV) disease may be particularly liable to drug allergies.

Drug hypersensitivity is usually a clinical diagnosis made on the basis of a rash or anaphylaxis. Laboratory testing may be useful, with skin testing providing the greatest specificity. Treatment includes discontinuation of the offending agent, symptomatic treatment and patient education.

Drug-induced hypersensitivity syndrome (DIHS) is a glandular fever-like syndrome (fever, rash, cervical lymphadenopathy, raised white cell count with atypical lymphocytes, and liver dysfunction) that follows the use of certain drugs – especially anticonvulsants such as carbamazepine and phenytoin, isoniazid and sulphonamides. Many cases also appear to be associated with the reactivation of human herpesvirus 6 (HHV-6) or other herpesviruses.

Many drug reactions could not be predicted and it is only by recording suspected adverse drug reactions to an appropriate authority (Figs 29.1 and 29.2) that serious adverse reactions of apparently safe drugs can be elicited (e.g. the cardiotoxicity of cyclo-oxygenase-2 inhibitors). Drug interactions are possible and it is also important to bear in mind that OTC and herbal preparations, foods and other substances can

sometimes interact by affecting drug absorption or efficacy, or by causing other interactions (Ch. 27 and Appendix 3.3).

DRUG ADVERSE EFFECTS

Many adverse drug reactions are probably not, at present, recognized. A full medical history should always be taken, asking specifically about adverse drug reactions. Certain conditions increase the risk of adverse reactions (Table 29.2) and can influence the choice of drugs. The excessive use of virtually any drug can cause harm. Patients should be warned if serious adverse reactions are likely, and provided with the appropriate warning card.

Anaesthetics and related agents

The use of excessive amounts of LA agents can be dangerous. Lidocaine with adrenaline (epinephrine), the most widely used drugs in dentistry, have proved to be remarkably safe in practice over very many years but gross overdose can be dangerous. One dentist has been found guilty of manslaughter, having given 16 cartridges of lidocaine with adrenaline to an elderly patient, who subsequently died.

Intravenous anaesthetic agents can cause anaphylactic-type reactions, either because of hypersensitivity or by directly inducing histamine release (the term 'anaphylactoid' may then be more appropriate). Tachycardia, vascular collapse and skin reactions (flushing, oedema or urticaria) are the most frequent signs, but reactions can range from minor symptoms to bronchospasm and a sharp fall in blood pressure. Treatment is as for anaphylaxis.

Anaphylactoid reactions have been reported particularly for thiopental. Such reactions have sometimes been fatal, probably because of failure to recognize their nature, since the loss of consciousness that results must be distinguished from the onset of anaesthesia; many intravenous agents have been discontinued because of this.

Suxamethonium, the muscle relaxant, may also cause an anaphylactoid reaction but alcuronium, tubocurarine and other relaxants are sometimes implicated; as there does not need to be previous exposure to the agent, cross-reacting antigens are presumably implicated.

Halothane hypersensitivity may be a cause of 'halothane hepatitis' (Ch. 9). LA agents have been routinely used since the late nineteenth century but adverse reactions and allergy are not common (Ch. 3). True IgE-mediated LA allergy must be very low indeed; one recent paper reviewed 23 case series involving 2978 patients with reactions and found only 29 patients with true IgE-mediated allergy to LA (less than 1%).

Hypersensitivity to the ester-type LA agents, which used to be commonly employed, is low and esters such as amethocaine and benzocaine are now restricted mainly to use in surface anaesthetics. The risk with amide LAs, such as articaine, lidocaine, mepivacaine or prilocaine, is probably lower. Lidocaine rarely causes reactions. The most sensitizing component of LA solutions has been the preservative: initially, methylparabens was used (parabens are now rarely used). There may be allergies to sulphite antioxidants or to latex in the LA cartridge diaphragm or bung (Ch. 17).

Attempts to confirm putative allergy to LAs by skin testing (prick tests or intracutaneous tests) are time-consuming and usually uninformative; they can provoke anaphylaxis in the uncommon instances of true allergy and are therefore rarely justified. Challenge tests are also typically negative. Where there are multiple supposed allergies, it may be best to administer sterile saline subcutaneously first to demonstrate any non-allergic response, and then give rising concentrations of diluted LA at 30-minute intervals (resuscitation facilities must be at hand). Clearly, it is of great importance to avoid labelling patients

In Confidence

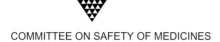

COMMITTEE ON SAFETY OF MEDICINES

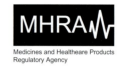

Medicines and Healthcare Products
Regulatory Agency

SUSPECTED ADVERSE DRUG REACTIONS

If you are suspicious that an adverse reaction may be related to a drug or combination of drugs please complete this Yellow Card. For reporting advice please see over. Do not be put off reporting because some details are not known.

PATIENT DETAILS   Patient Initials: _____   Sex: M / F   Weight if known (kg): _____

Age (at time of reaction): _____   Identification number (Your Practice / Hospital Ref.)*: _____

SUSPECTED DRUG(S)
Give brand name of drug and
batch number if known

	Route	Dosage	Date started	Date stopped	Prescribed for
_____	_____	_____	_____	_____	_____
_____	_____	_____	_____	_____	_____

SUSPECTED REACTION(S)
Please describe the reaction(s) and any treatment given:

Outcome

Recovered ☐
Recovering ☐
Continuing ☐
Other ☐

Date reaction(s) started: _____   Date reaction(s) stopped:_____

Do you consider the reaction to be serious?   Yes / No

If yes, please indicate why the reaction is considered to be serious (please tick all that apply):

Patient died due to reaction ☐   Involved or prolonged inpatient hospitalisation ☐

Life threatening ☐   Involved persistent or significant disability or incapacity ☐

Congenital abnormality ☐   Medically significant; please give details:_____

OTHERS DRUGS (including self-medication & herbal remedies)
Did the patient take any other drugs in the last 3 months prior to the reaction?   Yes / No

If yes, please give the following information if known:

Drug (Brand, if known)	Route	Dosage	Date started	Date stopped	Prescribed for
_____	_____	_____	_____	_____	_____
_____	_____	_____	_____	_____	_____
_____	_____	_____	_____	_____	_____
_____	_____	_____	_____	_____	_____
_____	_____	_____	_____	_____	_____

Additional relevant information   e.g, medical history, test results, known allergies, rechallenge (if performed), suspected drug interactions. For congenital abnormalities please state all other drugs taken during pregnancy and the last menstrual period.

REPORTER DETAILS
Name and Professional Address: _____
_____
_____

Post code: _____   Tel No: _____
Speciality: _____
Signature: _____   Date: _____

CLINICIAN (if not the reporter)
Name and professional Address: _____
_____
_____   Post code: _____
Tel No: _____   Speciality: _____

If you would like information about other adverse reactions associated with the suspected drug, please tick this box ☐

---

* This is to enable you to identify the patient in any future correspondence concerning this report

Please attach additional pages if necessary

Fig. 29.1 Form for reporting serious adverse drug reactions in the UK.

Postage will be paid by licensee	Do not affix Postage Stamps if posted in Gt. Britain, Channel Islands, N. Ireland or the Isle of Man

BUSINESS REPLY SERVICE
Licence No. SW 2991

Medicines and Healthcare products Regulatory Agency
151 Buckingham Palace Road
London
SW1W 9SZ

SECOND FOLD HERE

Remember if in Doubt - Report

SUSPECTED ADVERSE DRUG REACTIONS REPORTING ADVICE

New Black triangle (▼) Drugs - report ALL suspected adverse reactions
(New medicinal drugs can be indentified by the presence of a black triangle(▼)
both on the product information for the drug and BNF and MIMS)

Other Drugs - only report SERIOUS suspected adverse reactions
For instance those which are:
- Fatal
- Life threatening
- Involves or prolongs inpatient hospitalisation
- Involves persistent or significant disability or incapacity
- Congenital abnormality
- Medically significant (please exercise your judgement)

Please remember the areas of particular concern– delayed drug effects, the elderly, congenital abnormalities, children (including offlabel use of medications) and any herbal remdies

For more information contact:
- The National Yellow Card Information Service on Freephone 0800-7316789
- The MHRA website http://medicines.mhra.gov.uk
- Reporters can send suspected adverse drug reaction reports by electronic Yellow Card, via the MHRA Website.
- More detailed guidelines are given in the BNF

DO NOT BE PUT OFF REPORTING BECAUSE SOME DETAILS ARE NOT KNOWN

FIRST FOLD HERE

Fig. 29.2 Form for reporting serious adverse drug reactions in UK. (See http://yellowcard.mhra.gov.uk; accessed 30 September 2013).

Table 29.2 *Risk factors for adverse drug reactions[a]*

Factors	Non-immune reaction (majority)	Hypersensitivity (minority)
Female gender	+	+
Infections: herpes, human immunodeficiency virus (HIV)	+	+
Systemic lupus	+	+
Others	Alcoholism	Adult
	Chronic kidney disease	Asthma
	Liver disease	Beta-blocker use
	Polypharmacy	Previous hypersensitivity to chemically related drug
	Serious illness	

[a]Adapted from Riedl MA, Casillas AM. Adverse drug reactions: types and treatment options. *Am Fam Physician* 2003; 68:1781.

inappropriately as allergic to LAs in the first place. If a patient claims to be allergic to an LA, then a non-cross-reacting agent should be used; alternatively, a GA may be required.

Analgesics

Non-steroidal anti-inflammatory drugs (NSAIDs) may, rarely, induce allergic reactions. Aspirin can provoke allergic reactions but, in relation to the scale of its use, these are almost negligible. Aspirin-induced asthma is a rare possibility, seen mainly in patients with nasal polyps ('triad asthma' – asthma, nasal polyps and aspirin sensitivity). Other NSAIDs may, even more rarely, induce allergic reactions. If there is a history of allergy to a drug, it should not be given.

NSAIDs should not be used in patients taking anticoagulants, alcohol or high-dose methotrexate. They should also be avoided in older or renally impaired patients on digoxin, and avoided over the long term in those taking other NSAIDs. It is possible, but unconfirmed, that NSAIDs should not be given to patients taking lithium. NSAIDs are probably appropriate in the short term for patients taking anti-hypertensives, unless they have severe congestive heart disease or renal function is compromised.

Aspirin is a safe analgesic but readily causes platelet dysfunction, and excessive doses have led to post-extraction bleeding. It should also not be given to patients taking oral hypoglycaemics, valproic acid or carbonic anhydrase inhibitors.

Paracetamol (acetaminophen) is also safe but, when given in repeated doses, can cause severe liver damage. It may be used in the short term for any patient with a healthy liver, but should not be given to heavy drinkers or to persons who have recently stopped alcohol after chronic intake.

Opioids should not be given to heavy alcohol drinkers.

Antibiotics

Some antimicrobials (erythromycin, clarithromycin, metronidazole, ketoconazole and itraconazole) give rise to potentially life-threatening interactions with a host of other drugs, whose metabolism is impaired by them.

Antibiotics may also interfere with the effects of warfarin via sup-pression of gut bacteria that produce vitamin K. Commonly employed antibiotics may also impair the effectiveness of oral contraceptive agents, though the evidence for this is not strong (Fig. 29.3).

Anaphylaxis to antibiotics is a real possibility and has been esti-mated to have caused approximately 300 deaths annually in USA. Hypersensitivity reactions to beta-lactams (in penicillin and cephalo-sporins) are the most common reactions and are more likely to follow parenteral than oral administration. Patients allergic to penicillin usually react to any other penicillin except aztreonam. Individuals with penicillin allergy should avoid carbapenems and use caution with cephalosporins. About 10% of those sensitized to penicillin are said also to react to the cephalosporins. However, some allergic reactions can be selective for certain semi-synthetic penicillins, and some patients tolerant of benzylpenicillin can show delayed reactions to aminopeni-cillins. The causal antigen appears to be the penicilloyl group, which forms from metabolic cleavage of the beta-lactam ring and acts as a hapten, binding to body proteins to become antigenic. Specific IgE antibodies to penicillin are the cause of the anaphylactic reactions by binding to mast cells and triggering mediator release. There appears to be *no* association between penicillin anaphylaxis and atopic disease, despite both being mediated by the same mechanism. The most com-mon drug allergic reactions, apart from anaphylaxis, are urticarial and irritating rashes or sometimes a serum sickness type of reaction (joint pains and fever follow days or weeks after administration).

A history of previous reactions to penicillin suggests a greater risk of acute anaphylaxis – but there is no completely reliable method of pre-diction. Unfortunately, the first manifestation of sensitivity can occa-sionally be anaphylaxis and, rarely, a patient who has had penicillins on several occasions without ill effect can suddenly develop anaphylaxis. A negative history therefore reduces the chances but does not exclude the possibility of anaphylaxis when the patient claims to be allergic to peni-cillin. From the practical and medicolegal viewpoints, therefore, reliance has to be placed on the history and an alternative antimicrobial should be used – but never any penicillin derivatives (except aztreonam). Since a negative history of penicillin allergy does not totally exclude the pos-sibility of anaphylaxis, it is arguable that penicillin should not be given immediately before a GA, since recognition under such circumstances can be difficult. If penicillin has to be given, 30 minutes should be allowed to elapse before induction of GA; after such a period, a severe reaction is unlikely. Depot penicillins, which are slowly excreted, can maintain the antigenic challenge so that treatment of an allergic reaction may have to be continued until all the antigen is used up. Occasionally, procaine penicillin can additionally cause vertigo, hallucinations and acute anxiety reactions if given intravenously (or if it accidentally enters a vein) – reactions that may be mistaken for anaphylaxis.

A patient should, of course, be lying down when any injections are given, as fainting after injections is common and may be confused with anaphylaxis.

Anticonvulsants

Anticonvulsants are used to treat epilepsy and trigeminal neuralgia. Anticonvulsant hypersensitivity syndrome (AHS) is a potentially fatal, drug-induced, multiorgan syndrome reported with carbamazepine, phenytoin, phenobarbital and lamotrigine. The exact mechanism of AHS is unclear but it may have three components: deficiency or abnor-mality of the epoxide hydroxylase enzyme that detoxifies metabolites of aromatic amine anticonvulsants; reactivation of herpesviruses; and ethnic predisposition, especially an association with human leukocyte antigen (HLA)-B*1502 (HLA BFNx011502 allele) in some Asian but not in Caucasian and Japanese patients.

Whilst up to 1 in 5 patients on phenytoin may develop skin erup-tions, only a small proportion will progress to AHS – with urticaria, purpura, erythema multiforme and exfoliative dermatitis. Toxic epi-dermal necrolysis is uncommon, and usually occurs in patients who are re-exposed or who continue to receive anticonvulsants after hypersensitivity has developed. AHS is a clinical diagnosis; fever, rash and hepatitis are common features. Treatment is symptomatic. The offending drug should be immediately discontinued. Topical steroids and antihistamines are helpful in controlling symptoms. Systemic cor-ticosteroids are often used.

Radiocontrast media (RCM) reactions

Intravascular iodinated RCM agents are based on a tri-iodinated ben-zene ring and can cause adverse reactions. These can be:

- anaphylactoid
- non-anaphylactoid

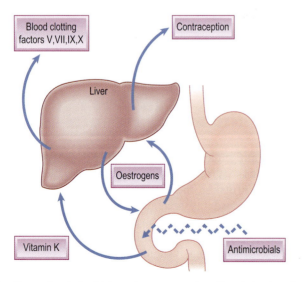

Fig. 29.3 Effects of antimicrobials on the contraceptive pill and vitamin K (hence on warfarin).

- chemotoxic – organ-specific:
  cardiovascular toxicity
  nephrotoxicity
  neurotoxicity
- vasovagal.

RCM usually act by directly releasing histamine from mast cells rather than provoking an allergic response. High-osmolar contrast media (HOCM) are the oldest but have largely been superseded by less toxic non-ionic compounds – low-osmolar contrast media (LOCM). Additional modifications to reduce toxicity further include: adding calcium ions (reduces cardiotoxicity), having a neutral pH (low pH predisposes to vasodilatation), and altering number and distribution of OH ions (decreases neurotoxicity).

People at higher risk for reactions to RCM include those who:

- have had past reactions to RCM (up to 40% chance of repeat reaction)
- have asthma
- have a history of allergies
- have a history of heart disease
- have a history of kidney disease
- are taking beta-blockers
- are female
- are older.

Reactions to RCM are relatively quite common – 5–8% of people receiving an intravenous dye. Most reactions are mild: a feeling of warmth, nausea and vomiting, lasting only briefly and requiring no treatment. Moderate reactions, including severe vomiting, hives and swelling, occur in 1% of people receiving RCM, and may need treatment. Severe, life-threatening reactions, including anaphylaxis, occur in 0.1% of people receiving RCM and occasionally are fatal. Delayed contrast reactions can occur anywhere from 3 hours to 7 days following the administration of contrast. Non-ionic low-osmolality contrast media LOCM are the preferred form, given their better safety record, although they are far more expensive than HOCM. Unfortunately, there is no test available to diagnose RCM allergy, and even 'test doses' can be fatal.

Iodine and iodides are also present in some antiseptics such as povidone–iodine, and can provoke dangerous reactions. Povidone–iodine is a commonly used antibacterial agent used in other products such as foods, drugs (e.g. antihistamines, diuretics and analgesics), hair products and toothpastes. Allergic contact reactions to povidone–iodine preparations are rare and do not necessarily indicate reactivity to RCM; anaphylaxis to povidone–iodine is thought to be caused by povidone, and cross-reactivity between these antiseptics and iodinated contrast media has not been demonstrated. Reactions to RCM can be limited by prophylaxis with a systemic steroid, diphenhydramine, and ephedrine or a histamine H_2-receptor antagonist.

Monoclonal antibodies

Monoclonal antibodies (see also Ch. 19) specifically bind to a substance and can serve to detect or purify that substance or act as a therapeutic medicine. When used as medications, the generic name ends in -*mab*. Monoclonal antibodies are available to treat cancer, cardiovascular disease, inflammatory diseases, transplant rejection, multiple sclerosis and viral infections (Table 29.3).

Table 29.3 *Some therapeutic monoclonal antibodies (mAb)/fusion proteins*[a]

mAb/fusion protein	Brand names	Target	Applications
Abatacept	Orencia	Cluster of differentiation 80 (CD80) and CD86	Transplant rejection, rheumatoid arthritis
Abciximab	ReoPro	Glycoprotein II/IIIa	Coronary interventions
Adalimumab	Humira	Tumour necrosis factor alpha (TNFα)	Crohn disease, rheumatoid arthritis, psoriasis
Alefacept	Amevive	CD2	Psoriasis
Alemtuzumab	Campath	CD52	Chronic lymphoid leukaemia, rheumatoid arthritis
Anakinra	Kineret	Interleukin (IL)-1R	Rheumatoid arthritis
Basiliximab	Simulect	IL-2R	Transplant rejection
Belatacept	Nulojix	CD80 and CD86	Transplant rejection
Bevacizumab	Avastin	Vascular endothelial growth factor (VEGF)	Cancers (various)
Bortezomib	Velcade	Proteasome	Multiple myeloma
Canakinumab	Ilaris	IL-1beta	Juvenile arthritis
Catumaxomab	Removab	Epithelial cell adhesion molecule	Cancers
Certolizumab	Cimzia	TNFα	Crohn disease, rheumatoid arthritis, psoriasis
Cetuximab	Erbitux	Epidermal growth factor receptor (EGFR)	Head and neck cancer
Daclizumab	Zenapax	IL-2R	Transplant rejection
Denosumab	Prolia	Receptor activator of nuclear factor kappa-B ligand (RANKL)	Osteoporosis
Eculizumab	Soliris	C5	Paroxysmal nocturnal haemoglobinuria
Efalizumab	Raptiva	CD11a	Psoriasis
Etanercept	Enbrel	TNFα	Crohn disease, rheumatoid arthritis, psoriasis, sarcoid
Gemtuzumab	Mylotarg	CD33	Acute myeloid leukaemia
Golimumab	Simponi	TNFα	Crohn disease, rheumatoid arthritis, psoriasis
Ibritumomab	Zevalin	CD20	Non-Hodgkin lymphoma (NHL)
Infliximab	Remicade	TNFα	Crohn disease, rheumatoid arthritis, psoriasis, sarcoid
Muromonab	Orthoclone OKT3	CD3	Transplant rejection
Natalizumab	Tysabri	Integrin receptor antagonist	Multiple sclerosis, Crohn disease
Omalizumab	Xolair	Immunoglobulin E (IgE)	Asthma
Palivizumab	Synagis	Respiratory syncytial virus	Respiratory syncytial virus

(Continued)

Table 29.3 (Continued)

mAb/fusion protein	Brand names	Target	Applications
Panitumumab	Vectibix	EGFR	Cancers
Ranibizumab	Lucentis	VEGF	Age-related macular degeneration
Raxibacumab	ACthrax	*Bacillus anthracis*	Anthrax
Rilonacept	Arcalyst	IL-1	Autoinflammatory disease
Rituximab	Rituxan or MabThera	CD20	NHL, rheumatoid arthritis
Sunitinib	Sutent	Tyrosine kinase	Cancers (renal)
Tocilizumab	Actemra	IL-6R	Rheumatoid arthritis
Tofacitinib	Xeljanz	Janus kinases	Rheumatoid arthritis
Tositumomab	Bexxar	CD20	NHL
Trastuzumab	Herceptin	ErbB2 (Her 2)	Breast cancer
Ustekinumab	Stelara	IL-12 and IL-23	Psoriasis

[a]See also http://en.wikipedia.org/wiki/List_of_monoclonal_antibodies (accessed 30 September 2013).

Immunomodulator agents

An immunomodulator (see also Ch. 19) is a substance (e.g. a drug) that has an effect on the immune response (Table 29.4), which may be stimulatory or suppressive. Immunostimulatory agents include, for example, vaccines and colony-stimulating factors. Immunosuppressive agents (see Chs 16, 18 and 35) can be classified into:

- glucocorticosteroids
- cytostatic agents
- antibodies
- drugs acting on immunophilins
- others (e.g. interferons, tumour necrosis factor [TNF]-binding agents, mycophenolate).

Hyperbaric oxygen therapy (HBO)

Hyperbaric oxygen therapy is the medical use of oxygen at a level higher than atmospheric pressure. Indications, contraindications and possible adverse effects are summarized in Table 29.5.

Other agents

Other medicines, such as sulphonamides, sulphones and allopurinol, have also caused a multiorgan hypersensitivity syndrome. Starch glove powder can cause direct skin irritation, interfere with wound healing and impair implant osseo-integration and composite bonding.

DRUG INTERACTIONS

Almost any drug may cause interactions, so no drug should be given unless there are good indications (Table 29.6). Drug metabolism can be affected by other drugs. Polypharmacy should be avoided and dentists should only use drugs with which they are familiar. Possible drug interactions are more likely when GA is used (Ch. 3), in older people and in patients with learning disability.

Drug absorption can be impaired by other drugs; for example, iron, magnesium and aluminium in drugs can impair absorption of tetracyclines. Aluminium can impair absorption of azole antifungals. Metoclopramide enhances absorption of paracetamol (acetaminophen) and aspirin.

DRUG CONTRAINDICATIONS

Possible contraindications to the main drugs prescribable by the dental surgeon are tabulated in Chapter 3.

Table 29.4 *Immunomodulators*[a]

Group	Mechanisms	Examples
Antimetabolites	Purine synthesis inhibitor	Azathioprine
		Mycophenolic acid
	Pyrimidine synthesis inhibitor	Leflunomide
		Teriflunomide
	Antifolate	Methotrexate
Interleukin-1 (IL-1) receptor antagonists	Block IL-1	Anakinra
IL-2 inhibitors	FK506 binding protein (FKBP)/ cyclophilin/calcineurin	Abetimus
		Ciclosporin
		Gusperimus
		Pimecrolimus
		Tacrolimus
Inhibitors of (*m*ammalian *t*arget *o*f *r*apamycin mTOR)	Inhibit mTOR – a serine/ threonine protein kinase that regulates cell growth, proliferation, motility, survival, protein synthesis and transcription	Ridaforolimus (deforolimus)
		Everolimus
		Sirolimus
		Temsirolimus
		Zotarolimus
Tumour necrosis factor alpha (TNF-α) inhibitors	Inhibit TNF	Lenalidomide
		Thalidomide

[a]See Chapter 19.

Table 29.5 *Hyperbaric oxygen therapy*

Possible indications	Contraindications	Possible adverse effects
Air embolism	Pneumothorax	Oxygen toxicity
Carbon monoxide poisoning	Upper respiratory infections	Barotrauma affecting sinuses, middle ear or teeth
Crush injuries or gas gangrene	Middle ear barotrauma	Possible ocular complications
Burns	Chest surgery	
Skin flaps that are compromised	Emphysema	
Intractable soft-tissue infections	Malignant disease	
Bone disorders such as osteomyelitis or osteoradionecrosis	Medication with disulfiram, doxorubicin, mafenide acetate or cisplatin	

ORAL ADVERSE EFFECTS OF DRUGS

Oral adverse effects caused by drugs are relatively uncommon but may be important. Drugs that may occasionally cause oral complications are listed in Appendices 29.2–29.23.

Table 29.6 *Antimicrobial interactions*

Drug	May interact with	Symptoms	Consequences
Ampicillin, amoxicillin	Beta-blockers	Hypertension	Lowered antihypertensive levels. Greater severity of anaphylactic reactions
Erythromycin	Benzodiazepines	Anxiety states	High benzodiazepine levels
	Carbamazepine	Epilepsy, trigeminal neuralgia	Carbamazepine toxicity
	Ciclosporin	Immunosuppression	Ciclosporin toxicity
	Digoxin	Cardiac failure	Digitalis toxicity
	Statins	Hyperlipidaemia	Muscle damage
	Terfenadine	Allergies	Arrhythmias
	Theophylline	Asthma	Theophylline toxicity
	Warfarin	Anticoagulation	Increased bleeding tendency
Metronidazole	Ethanol (alcohol)	Abuse	Disulfiram-type reaction
	Lithium	Manic depression	Lithium toxicity
	Warfarin	Anticoagulation	Increased bleeding tendency
Tetracyclines	Antacids	Gastric disease	Reduced tetracycline absorption
	Digoxin	Cardiac failure	Digitalis toxicity
Fluconazole	Statins	Hyperlipidaemia	Muscle damage
	Warfarin	Anticoagulation	Increased bleeding tendency
Miconazole	Statins	Hyperlipidaemia	Muscle damage
	Warfarin	Anticoagulation	Increased bleeding tendency

Some drugs almost invariably cause oral adverse effects; for example, the most common drug-induced oral disorders are dry mouth (caused by many drugs with an atropinic action), ulcers (from cytotoxic drugs and others), candidosis (usually caused by tetracyclines, ampicillin or corticosteroids), gingival swelling (usually caused by phenytoin, ciclosporin and calcium-channel blockers) and lichenoid reactions (from NSAIDs and many others). Some habits, such as the use of oral snuff (smokeless tobacco), can cause gingival recession and leukoplakia, and possibly predisposes to oral cancer; oral use of cocaine can cause gingival ulceration or desquamation.

Drug-related cheilitis

Cheilitis is commonly caused by contact reactions to cosmetics or foods, but drugs may be implicated.

Drug-related contact stomatitis (stomatitis venenata)

Fixed drug eruptions comprise repeated ulceration at the same site in response to a particular drug. However, intraoral contact stomatitis is a dubious entity. In any such reactions, the lips or perioral skin are far more likely to be affected.

Drug-related erythema multiforme

A wide range of drugs may give rise to erythema multiforme, and it may be impossible to distinguish drug-induced erythema multiforme clinically from disease with other causes.

Drug-related infections

Opportunistic infection secondary to cytotoxic chemotherapy can cause oral ulceration. In particular, herpes simplex virus 1, varicella zoster and cytomegalovirus give rise to oral ulceration. Less commonly, ulceration may be due to Gram-negative bacterial infections.

Candidosis arises secondary to treatment with broad-spectrum antibiotics, corticosteroids (both systemic and inhaled preparations) and other immunosuppressive regimens (e.g. ciclosporin) and cytotoxic drugs. More rarely, mucormycosis and aspergillosis may cause thrush-like areas in patients on long-term immunosuppressive treatment.

Human papillomavirus infection manifesting as wart-like growths may develop in patients on long-term immunosuppressive therapy. Oral hairy leukoplakia, usually affecting the dorsum and lateral borders of the tongue and floor of the mouth, may be a consequence of Epstein–Barr virus infection in patients on corticosteroids (topical and systemic), ciclosporin or other long-term immunosuppressive regimens.

Drug-related leukoplakia

Tobacco and alcohol use are important risk factors for leukoplakia and oral cancer. A greater frequency of lesions with epithelial dysplasia of the lips (but not oral mucosa) has also been observed in some iatrogenically immunosuppressed patients. Sanguinarine, the principal alkaloid of the bloodroot plant (*Sanguinaria canadensis*), which is used in some mouthwashes and dentifrices for its antiplaque activity, may be associated with the development of oral leukoplakia.

Drug-related lichenoid reactions

Since these were noticed as an adverse effect of antimalarial therapy, there has been an ever-growing list of drugs that may give rise to mucocutaneous lichen planus-like eruptions (lichenoid reactions). The drugs now most commonly implicated are the NSAIDs and the angiotensin-converting enzyme inhibitors (ACEIs).

Drug-related lupus-like disorders

Systemic lupus erythematosus (SLE) may be induced by a wide variety of different drugs.

Drug-related malodour (halitosis)

Oral malodour may be related to treatment with isosorbide dinitrate, dimethyl sulfoxide or disulfiram, although drugs causing xerostomia can indirectly lead to, or aggravate this problem.

Drug-related movement disorders

Several different drug-induced movements can affect the mouth and face, particularly tardive dyskinesia (secondary to antipsychotics) and dystonias (e.g. with metoclopramide). Although these disorders principally affect the face, there can be abnormal movements of the tongue, e.g. dystonia secondary to carbamazepine therapy.

Drug-related neoplasms

Non-Hodgkin lymphoma, usually manifesting as ulceration of the gingivae, fauces or palate, and Kaposi sarcoma (see later) are rare complications of long-term immunosuppressive therapy.

Drug-related neuropathies

Facial or oral paraesthesia, hypoaesthesia or anaesthesia can be due to interferon-alpha, acetazolamide, labetalol, sultiame, vincristine and occasionally some other agents, such as hepatitis B vaccination and some of the protease inhibitors.

Drug-related pain and dysaesthesia

Captopril and lisinopril may very rarely cause a scalded-type sensation of the mouth.

Drug-related pemphigoid and other bullous disorders

Drug-induced pemphigoid may be due to drugs acting as haptens or drug-induced immunological dysfunction.

Drug-related pemphigus

Pemphigus-like reactions may occasionally be associated with drugs with active thiol groups in the molecule, such as penicillamine and captopril, or by rifampicin or diclofenac.

Drug-related pigmentation

Superficial transient discoloration of the dorsum of the tongue, other soft tissues and teeth, which may be of various colours (typically yellowish or brown), may be caused by some foods and beverages (coffee and tea), habits (tobacco, betel and crack cocaine use) and some drugs (iron salts, bismuth, chlorhexidine or antibiotics), especially if these also induce hyposalivation.

Localized areas of pigmentation of the mucosa may be due to amalgam, while gingival pigmentation may be secondary to the gold or metal alloys of crowns. Heavy metal salts, used in the past, caused pigmentation, particularly of the gingival margin.

Blue, blue–grey or brown mucosal pigmentation can be an adverse effect of antimalarials, phenothiazines and phenytoin or amiodarone. Minocycline frequently causes widespread brown pigmentation of the gingivae and mucosae.

Discolouration of saliva may be caused by rifampicin, rifabutin and a few other drugs.

Drug-related salivary gland pain

Salivary gland pain can be an adverse effect of some drugs, such as bethanidine, bretylium, clonidine, methyldopa and some cytotoxics.

Drug-related sialorrhoea

Anticholinesterases are the main cause of sialorrhoea.

Others

Drug-related swelling

Gingival enlargement is a well-recognized oral adverse effect of treatment with phenytoin, ciclosporin and the calcium-channel blockers.

Drug-induced mucosal swelling predominantly affects the lips and floor of the mouth (although rare isolated swelling of the uvula is possible). It is typically due to type I hypersensitivity reactions.

Many drugs, particularly penicillins, ACEIs and aspirin, can cause angioedema.

Drug-related taste disturbance

Drugs commonly impair taste because they cause a loss of acuity (hypogeusia) or distortion of function (dysgeusia), either by interfering in the chemical composition or flow of saliva or, more specifically, affecting taste receptor function or signal transduction. Hyposalivation also disturbs taste.

Drug-related ulceration

Oral ulceration may follow burns from the local application of aspirin or toothache preparations, potassium tablets, pancreatic supplements and other agents, such as trichloroacetic acid or hydrogen peroxide.

Mucositis and ulceration are caused by many chemotherapy regimens, particularly those involving methotrexate, 5-fluorouracil, doxorubicin, melphalan, mercaptopurine or bleomycin.

Aphthous-like ulcers can be caused by NSAIDs and beta-blockers, and possibly by nicorandil, alendronate and everolimus.

Drug-related xerostomia

Common habits, such as tobacco smoking, alcohol use (including in mouthwashes) and use of beverages containing caffeine (coffee, some soft drinks), can cause some oral dryness.

Drugs are the most common cause of reduced salivation. Those most often implicated in dry mouth are the tricyclic antidepressants, antipsychotics, atropinics and antihistamines. The complaint of dry mouth is therefore particularly common in patients treated for hypertensive, psychiatric or urinary problems.

The cause for which the drug is being taken may also be important. Patients with anxiety or depression may complain of dry mouth even in the absence of drug therapy or evidence of diminished salivary flow.

KEY WEBSITES

(Accessed 11 June 2013)
Scottish Dental Clinical Effectiveness Programme. <http://www.sdcep.org.uk/index.aspx?o=2334>.
WebMD: Medicines & Treatments Centre. <http://drugs.webmd.boots.com/drugs/>.
WebMD: Oral Care. <http://www.webmd.com/oral-health/medications-used-dentistry>.
Wikipedia: Dental restorative materials. <http://en.wikipedia.org/wiki/Dental_restorative_materials>.

USEFUL WEBSITES

(Accessed 11 June 2013)
American Academy of Family Physicians. <http://www.aafp.org/online/en/home.html>.
American Dental Association. Bisphenol A and dental materials. <http://www.ada.org/1766.aspx>.

American Dental Association. Statement on dental amalgam. <http://www.ada.org/1741.aspx>.

Australian and New Zealand College of Anaesthetists and Royal Australasian College of Dental Surgeons. Guidelines on conscious sedation for dental procedures. <http://www.ada.org.au/app_cmslib/media/lib/0703/m52386_v1_consedps21_2003.pdf>.

Australian Prescriber. <http://www.australianprescriber.com/magazine/30/4/98/101/>.

British National Formulary. <http://www.bnf.org/bnf/index.htm>.

Canadian Dental Association. <www.cda-adc.ca/_files/position_statements/amalgam.pdf>.

Health Canada. <http://www.hc-sc.gc.ca/dhp-mps/pubs/md-im/dent_amalgam-eng.php>.

National Institutes of Health: National Center for Complementary and Alternative Medicine. <http://nccam.nih.gov/>.

UK Medicines Information. <http://www.ukmi.nhs.uk>.

US Food and Drug Administration. <http://www.fda.gov/Drugs>.

Wikipedia. List of therapeutic monoclonal antibodies. <http://en.wikipedia.org/wiki/List_of_monoclonal_antibodies>.

World Health Organization: Exposure to mercury: a major public health concern. <www.who.int/phe/news/Mercury-flyer.pdf>.

FURTHER READING

Bae, Y.J., et al., 2008. A case of anaphylaxis to chlorhexidine during digital rectal examination. J. Korean Med. Sci. 23, 526.

Bassin, E.B., et al., 2006. Age-specific fluoride exposure in drinking water and osteosarcoma (United States). Cancer Causes Control 17, 421.

Beatty, P., et al., 2011. A complicated case of chlorhexidine-associated anaphylaxis. Anaesthesia 66 (1), 60. doi: 10.1111/j.1365-2044.2010.06573.x PubMed ID: 21198508.

Bellinger, D.C., et al., 2006. Neuropsychological and renal effects of dental amalgam in children: a randomized clinical trial. JAMA 295, 1775.

Bellinger, D.C., et al., 2007. Dental amalgam restorations and children's neuropsychological function: the New England Children's Amalgam Trial. Environ. Health Perspect. 115 (3), 440. doi:10.1289/ehp.9497 Published online 2006 October 30.

Bellinger, D.C., et al., 2008. Dental amalgam and psychosocial status: the New England Children's Amalgam Trial. J. Dent. Res. 87, 470.

Bjerrum, L., et al., 2003. Exposure to potential drug interactions in primary health care. Scand. J. Prim. Health Care 21, 153.

Brownawell, A.M., et al., 2005. The potential adverse health effects of dental amalgam. Toxicol. Rev. 24, 1.

Choi, A.L., et al., 2012. Developmental fluoride neurotoxicity: a systematic review and meta-analysis. Environ. Health Perspect. 120 (10), 1362. doi:10.1289/ehp.1104912 Epub 2012 Jul 20.

Clarkson, T.W., Magos, L., 2006. The toxicology of mercury and its chemical compounds. Crit. Rev. Toxicol. 36, 609.

Clarkson, T.W., et al., 2003. The toxicology of mercury – current exposures and clinical manifestations. N. Engl. J. Med. 349, 1731.

Corbett, C.E., et al., 2007. Health evaluation of gold miners living in a mercury-contaminated village in Serra Pelada, Pará, Brazil. Arch. Environ. Occup. Health 62, 121.

Davydov, L., Botts, S.R., 2000. Clozapine-induced hypersalivation. Ann. Pharmacother. 34, 662.

DeRouen, T.A., et al., 2006. Neurobehavioral effects of dental amalgam in children: a randomized clinical trial. JAMA 295, 1784.

Diz Dios, P., Scully, C., 2002. Adverse effects of antiretroviral therapy: focus on orofacial effects. Expert Opin. Drug Saf. 1, 307.

Douglass, C.W., Joshipura, K., 2006. Caution needed in fluoride and osteosarcoma study. Cancer Causes Control 17, 481.

Edlich, R.F., et al., 2007. Need for informed consent for dentists who use mercury amalgam restorative material as well as technical considerations in removal of dental amalgam restorations. J. Environ. Pathol. Toxicol. Oncol. 26, 305.

Eilers, H., Niemann, C., 2003. Clinically important drug interactions with intravenous anaesthetics in older patients. Drugs Aging 20, 969.

Eramo, S., et al., 2010. Estrogenicity of bisphenol A released from sealants and composites: a review of the literature. Ann. Stomatol. (Roma) 1 (3–4), 14. Epub 2011 Feb 13. PubMed ID: 22238710; PubMed Central PMCID: PMC3254379.

Garvey, L.H., et al., 2007. IgE-mediated allergy to chlorhexidine. J. Allergy Clin. Immunol. 120, 409.

Göhring, T.N., et al., 2008. Is amalgam a health hazard? Ther. Umsch. 65, 103.

Guleri, A., et al., 2012. Anaphylaxis to chlorhexidine-coated central venous catheters: a case series and review of the literature. Surg. Infect. (Larchmt) 13 (3), 171. Epub 2012 May 8. Review. PubMed ID: 22568873.

Halbach, S., et al., 2008. Blood and urine mercury levels in adult amalgam patients of a randomized controlled trial: interaction of Hg species in erythrocytes. Environ. Res. 107, 69.

Hasson, H., et al., 2006. Home-based chemically-induced whitening of teeth in adults. Cochrane Database Syst. Rev. (4), CD006202.

Heyer, N.J., et al., 2008. The association between serotonin transporter gene promoter polymorphism (5-HTTLPR), self-reported symptoms, and dental mercury exposure. J. Toxicol. Environ. Health A 71, 1318.

Hidaka, M., et al., 2005. Effects of pomegranate juice on human cytochrome p450 3A (CYP3A) and carbamazepine pharmacokinetics in rats. Drug Metab. Dispos. 33 (5), 644.

Jones, D.W., 2004. Putting dental mercury pollution into perspective. Br. Dent. J. 197, 175.

Khan, R.A., et al., 2011. Near fatal intra-operative anaphylaxis to chlorhexidine – is it time to change practice? BMJ Case Rep. doi: 10.1136/ bcr.09.2009.2300 PubMed ID: 22715203.

Kim, H., et al., 2006. Inhibitory effects of fruit juices on CYP3A activity. Drug Metab. Dispos. 34 (4), 521.

Li, Y., 2003. The safety of peroxide-containing at-home tooth whiteners. Compend. Contin. Educ. Dent. 24, 384.

Little, J.W., et al., 2002. Dental Management of the Medically Compromised Patient, sixth ed. Mosby, St Louis.

Magos, L., Clarkson, T.W., 2006. Overview of the clinical toxicity of mercury. Ann. Clin. Biochem. 43, 257.

McDonagh, M.S., et al., 2000. Systematic review of water fluoridation. BMJ 321 (7265), 855.

Melchart, D., et al., 2008. Biomonitoring of mercury in patients with complaints attributed to dental amalgam, healthy amalgam bearers, and amalgam-free subjects: a diagnostic study. Clin. Toxicol. (Phila) 46, 133.

Metz, M.J., et al., 2007. Clinical evaluation of 15% carbamide peroxide on the surface microhardness and shear bond strength of human enamel. Oper. Dent. 32, 427.

Mohundro, M., Ramsey, L.A., 2003. Pharmacologic considerations in geriatric patients. Adv. Nurse Pract. 11 21, 25.

Nagendran, V., et al., 2009. IgE-mediated chlorhexidine allergy: a new occupational hazard? Occup. Med. (Lond) 59 (4), 270. Epub 2009 Mar 26. PubMed ID: 19325161.

Naik, S., et al., 2006. Hydrogen peroxide tooth-whitening (bleaching): review of safety in relation to possible carcinogenesis. Oral Oncol. 42, 668.

Nations, S.P., et al., 2008. Denture cream: an unusual source of excess zinc, leading to hypocupremia and neurologic disease. Neurology 71 (9), 639. doi:10.1212/01.wnl.0000312375.79881.94 Epub 2008 Jun 4. PubMed ID: 18525032.

Noel, J., et al., 2012. A case report of anaphylaxis to chlorhexidine during urinary catheterisation. Ann. R. Coll. Surg. Engl. 94 (4), e159–e160. PubMed ID: 22613287.

Olea, N., et al., 1996. Estrogenicity of resin-based composites and sealants used in dentistry. Environ. Health Perspect. 104 (3), 298. PubMed ID: 8919768; PubMed Central PMCID: PMC1469315.

Olver, I.N., 2006. Xerostomia: a common adverse effect of drugs and radiation. Aust. Prescr. 29, 97.

Parkes, A.W., et al., 2009. Anaphylaxis to the chlorhexidine component of instillagel: a case series. Br. J. Anaesth. 102, 65.

Pemberton, M.N., et al., 2004. Miconazole oral gel and drug interactions. Br. Dent. J. 196, 529.

Pollick, H.F., 2006. Concerns about water fluoridation, IQ, and osteosarcoma lack credible evidence. Int. J. Occup. Environ. Health 12, 91.

Rahilly, G., Price, N., 2003. Current products and practice: nickel allergy and orthodontics. J. Orthodont. 30, 171.

Rode, D., 2006. Are mercury amalgam fillings safe for children? An evaluation of recent research results. Altern. Ther. Health Med. 12, 16.

Scully, C., 2003. Drug effects on salivary glands: dry mouth. Oral Dis. 9, 165.

Scully, C., Bagan, J.V., 2004. Adverse drug reactions in the orofacial region. Crit. Rev. Oral Biol. Med. 15, 221.

Scully, C., et al., 2008. Over-the-counter remedies for oral soreness. Periodontology 2000 48, 76.

Sharma, A., Chopra, H., 2009. Chlorhexidine urticaria: a rare occurrence with a common mouthwash. Indian J. Dent. Res 20, 377.

Sijbesma, T., et al., 2011. Severe anaphylactic reaction to chlorhexidine during total hip arthroplasty surgery: a case report. Hip Int. 21 (5), 630. doi: 10.5301/HIP.2011.8644 PubMed ID: 21948038.

Sivathasan, N., Goodfellow, P.B., 2011. Skin cleansers: the risks of chlorhexidine. J. Clin. Pharmacol. 51 (5), 785. Epub 2011 Mar 7. PubMed ID: 21383335.

Söderholm, K.J., Mariotti, A., 1999. BIS-GMA–based resins in dentistry: are they safe? J. Am. Dent. Assoc. 130 (2), 201. Review. PubMed ID: 10036843

Sorokin, A.V., et al., 2006. Rhabdomyolysis associated with pomegranate juice consumption. Am. J. Cardiol. 98 (5), 705.

Stålenheim, G., et al., 2010. Chlorhexidine caused anaphylactic reaction. Not only drugs should be considered in the investigation of allergy, according to a case report. Lakartidningen 107 (1–2), 37. Swedish. PubMed ID: 20184271.

Stockley, I.H. (Ed.), 2002. Stockley's Drug Interactions (sixth ed.). Pharmaceutical Press, London

Tillberg, A., et al., 2008. Risks with dental materials. Dent. Mater. 24 (7), 940. doi:10.1016/j.dental.2007.11.009 Epub 2008 Mar 4. PubMed ID: 18164381.

Tredwin, C., et al., 2006. Hydrogen peroxide tooth-whitening (bleaching) products: review of adverse effects and safety issues. Br. Dent. J. 200, 371.

Yorifuji, T., et al., 2008. Long-term exposure to methylmercury and neurologic signs in Minamata and neighboring communities. Epidemiology 19, 3.

Wills, A., 2009. Chlorhexidine anaphylaxis in auckland. Br. J. Anaesth. 102 (5), 722. PubMed ID: 19359402.

APPENDIX 29.1 SUMMARY OF OFFICIAL BODY COMMENTS ON DENTAL AMALGAM SAFETY

In 2004, an expert panel reviewed the peer-reviewed, scientific literature published from 1996 to December 2003 on potential adverse human health effects caused by dental amalgam and published a report. The review, conducted by the Life Sciences Research Office (LSRO) and funded by the National Institutes of Dental and Craniofacial Research, National Institutes of Health and Centers for Devices and Radiological Health, US Food and Drug Administration (FDA) states that:

The current data are insufficient to support an association between mercury release from dental amalgam and the various complaints that have been attributed to this restoration material. These complaints are broad and nonspecific compared to the well-defined set of effects that have been documented for occupational and accidental elemental mercury exposures. Individuals with dental amalgam-attributed complaints had neither elevated urinary mercury nor increased prevalence of hypersensitivity to dental amalgam or mercury when compared with controls. (www.lsro.org)

In 2006, the *Journal of the American Medical Association* (JAMA) and *Environmental Health Perspectives* published the results of two independent clinical trials designed to examine the effects of mercury release from amalgam on the central and peripheral nervous systems and kidney function, concluding that:

there were no statistically significant differences in adverse neuropsychological or renal effects observed over the 5-year period in children whose caries are restored using dental amalgam or composite materials

and

children who received dental restorative treatment with amalgam did not, on average, have statistically significant differences in neurobehavioral assessments or in nerve conduction velocity when compared with children who received resin composite materials without amalgam. These findings, combined with the trend of higher treatment need later among those receiving composite, suggest that amalgam should remain a viable dental restorative option for children.

In May 2008, a Scientific Committee of the European Commission addressed safety concerns for patients and professionals, and the use of alternative restorative materials, concluding that dental amalgams are effective and safe for both patients and dental personnel, and also noted that alternative materials are not without clinical limitations and toxicological hazards.

The American Dental Association (ADA) Council on Scientific Affairs prepared a comprehensive literature review that summarized the state of the evidence for amalgam safety (from January 2004 to April 2009). Based on the results of this review, the Council reaffirmed at its July 2009 meeting that the scientific evidence supports the position that amalgam is a valuable, viable and safe choice for dental patients.

On 28 July 2009, the FDA issued its final rule on encapsulated dental amalgam, classifying amalgam and its component parts, elemental mercury and powder alloy, as a class II medical device. Previously there was no classification for encapsulated amalgam, and dental mercury (class I) and alloy (class II) were classified separately. This new regulation places encapsulated amalgam in the same class of devices as most other restorative materials, including composite and gold fillings. At the same time, the FDA also reaffirmed the agency's position that the material is a safe and effective restorative option for patients.

The situation has been summarized by one author as follows:

Amalgam fillings release mercury (mercury vapour or inorganic ions) at a low level (about 2–5 micrograms/day in an adult). Evidence on the health effect of dental amalgams comes from studies of the association between their presence and signs or symptoms of adverse effects or health changes after removal of dental amalgam fillings. More formal risk assessment studies focus on occupational exposure to mercury and health effects. Numerous methodological issues make their interpretation difficult but new research will continue to challenge policymakers. Policy will also reflect prudent and cautious approaches, encouraging minimization of exposure to mercury in potentially more sensitive population groups. Wider environmental concerns and decreasing tolerance of exposure to other mercury compounds (for example, methylmercury in seafoods) will ensure the use of mercury in dentistry remains an issue, necessitating dentists keep their patients informed of health risks and respect their choices. (Spencer AJ. Dental amalgam and mercury in dentistry. Aust Dent J 2000; 45:224)

APPENDIX 29.2 DRUGS IMPLICATED IN DRY MOUTH

• Alfuzosin	• Chlormezanone	• Diazepam	• Ephedrine
• Amiloride	• Chlorpromazine	• Dicycloverine (dicyclomine)	• Fenfluramine
• Amitriptyline	• Citalopram	• Didanosine (dideoxyinosine)	• Fluoxetine
• Amoxapine	• Clemastine	• Dihydrocodeine	• Furosemide
• Benzhexol	• Clomipramine	• Disopyramide	• Guanfacine
• Benztropine	• Clonidine	• Donepezil	• Hyoscine
• Biperiden	• Clozapine	• Dosulepin	• Imipramine
• Bupropion	• Cyclizine	• Doxepin	• Indoramin
• Buspirone	• Cyclobenzaprine	• Duloxetine	• Interferon-alpha
• Cannabis	• Desipramine	• Ecstasy	• Interleukin-2
• Cetirizine	• Dexamfetamine	• Elliptinium	• Ipratropium

(Continued)

- Iprindole
- Isocarboxazid
- Isotretinoin
- Ketorolac
- Ketotifen
- Lansoprazole
- L-Dopa
- Lithium
- Lofepramine
- Lofexidine
- Loratadine
- Maprotiline
- Mepenzolate
- Methyldopa
- Mianserin
- Mirtazapine
- Morphine
- Moxonidine
- Nabilone
- Nefopam
- Nortriptyline
- Olanzapine
- Omeprazole
- Orphenadrine
- Oxitropium
- Oxybutynin
- Paroxetine
- Phenelzine
- Pipamperone
- Pipenzolate
- Pirenzipine
- Poldine
- Procyclidine
- Propafenone
- Propantheline
- Propiverine
- Pseudoephedrine
- Quetiapine
- Reboxetine
- Rilmenidine
- Risperidone
- Rizatriptan
- Selegiline
- Sertraline
- Sibutramine
- Sucralfate
- Tamsulosin
- Terazosin
- Tiabendazole
- Tiapride
- Tiotropium
- Tizanidine
- Tolterodine
- Tramadol
- Tranylcypromine
- Trazodone
- Triamterene
- Trimipramine
- Trospium chloride
- Venlafaxine
- Viloxazine
- Zopiclone

APPENDIX 29.3 DRUGS IMPLICATED IN SALIVARY GLAND PAIN OR SWELLING

- Bethanidine
- Bretylium
- Cimetidine
- Clonidine
- Clozapine
- Deoxycycline
- Famotidine
- Guanethidine
- Insulin
- Interferon
- Isoprenaline
- Methyldopa
- Naproxen
- Nicardipine
- Nifedipine
- Nitrofurantoin
- Oxyphenbutazone
- Phenylbutazone
- Phenytoin
- Ranitidine
- Ritodrine
- Trimepramine

APPENDIX 29.4 DRUGS IMPLICATED IN HYPERSALIVATION

- Alprazolam
- Amiodarone
- Buprenorphine
- Buspirone
- Clonazepam
- Diazoxide
- Ethionamide
- Gentamicin
- Guanethidine
- Haloperidol
- Imipenem/cilastatin
- Iodides
- Kanamycin
- Ketamine
- Lamotrigine
- L-Dopa
- Mefenamic acid
- Mercurials
- Nicardipine
- Niridazole
- Pentoxifylline
- Remoxipride
- Risperidone
- Rivastigmine
- Tacrine
- Tobramycin
- Triptorelin
- Venlafaxine
- Zaleplon

APPENDIX 29.5 DRUGS IMPLICATED IN DISCOLOURATION OF SALIVA

- Clofazimine
- L-Dopa
- Rifabutin
- Rifampicin

APPENDIX 29.6 DRUGS IMPLICATED IN DISTURBED TASTE

- Acarbose
- Acetazolamide
- Albuterol
- Alcohol
- Allopurinol
- Amiloride
- Amitriptyline
- Amphetamines
- Amphotericin
- Amrinone
- Anticholinergics
- Aspirin
- Atorvastatin
- Auranofin
- Aurothiomalate
- Azathioprine
- Azelastine
- Aztreonam
- Baclofen
- Biguanides
- Bisphosphonates
- Bleomycin
- Bretylium
- Calcitonin
- Captopril
- Carbamazepine
- Carbimazole
- Carboplatin
- Celecoxib
- Cetirizine
- Chlorhexidine
- Chlormezanone
- Choline magnesium trisalicylate
- Cilazapril
- Cisplatin
- Clarithromycin

(Continued)

- Clidinium
- Clofibrate
- Clomipramine
- Cocaine
- Colestyramine
- Diazoxide
- Dicycloverine (dicyclomine)
- Diltiazem
- Dipyridamole
- Disodium etidronate
- Dorzolamide
- Emelastine
- Enalapril
- Esomeprazole
- Eszopiclone
- Ethambutol
- Ethionamide
- Etoposide
- Famotidine
- Flunisolide
- Fluoxetine
- Flurazepam
- 5-Fluorouracil
- Fluvoxamine
- Glycopyrrolate
- Gold
- Griseofulvin
- Hexetidine
- Hydrochlorothiazide
- Hydrocortisone
- Hyoscyamine
- Imipenem
- Imipramine
- Indometacin
- Interferon-gamma
- Iodine
- Isotretinoin
- L-Dopa
- Levamisole
- Lincomycin
- Lisinopril
- Lithium
- Lomefloxacin
- Losartan
- Lovastatin
- Metformin
- Methimazole
- Methotrexate
- Methyl methacrylate
- Methylthiouracil
- Metronidazole
- Nifedipine
- Niridazole
- Nitroglycerin
- Ofloxacin
- Omeprazole
- Palifermin
- Penicillamine
- Pentamidine
- Pergolide
- Perindopril
- Phenformin
- Phenindione
- Phenylbutazone
- Phenytoin
- Procaine penicillin
- Propafenone
- Propantheline
- Propranolol
- Propylthiouracil
- Quinapril
- Ramipril
- Rifabutin
- Rivastigmine
- Selegiline
- Sodium lauryl sulfate
- Spironolactone
- Sulfasalazine
- Terbinafine
- Tetracycline
- Tocainide
- Topiramate
- Trandolapril
- Triazolam
- Venlafaxine
- Zopiclone

APPENDIX 29.7 DRUGS IMPLICATED IN ORAL ULCERATION

- Adalimumab
- Alendronate
- Allopurinol
- Aurothiomalate
- Aztreonam
- Captopril
- Carbamazepine
- Clarithromycin
- Diclofenac
- Emepronium
- Everolimus
- Flunisolide
- Gold
- Indometacin
- Interferons
- Interleukin-2
- Isoprenaline
- Ketorolac
- Losartan
- Molgramostim
- Naproxen
- Nicorandil
- Non-steroidal anti-inflammatory drugs (NSAIDs)
- Olanzapine
- Pancreatin
- Penicillamine
- Phenindione
- Phenylbutazone
- Phenytoin
- Potassium chloride
- Proguanil
- Sertraline
- Sulindac
- Tacrolimus
- Vancomycin
- Zalcitabine (dideoxycytidine

APPENDIX 29.8 DRUGS IMPLICATED IN LICHENOID REACTIONS

- Allopurinol
- Amiphenazole
- Bacille Calmette–Guérin (BCG) vaccine
- Barbiturate
- Captopril
- Carbamazepine
- Carbimazole
- Chloral hydrate
- Chloroquine
- Chlorpropamide
- Cholera vaccine
- Cinnarizine
- Clofibrate
- Colchicine
- Dapsone
- Dipyridamole
- Ethionamide
- Flunarizine
- Gaunoclor
- Gold
- Griseofulvin
- Hepatitis B vaccine
- Hydroxychloroquine
- Interferon-alpha
- Ketoconazole
- Labetalol
- Levamisole
- Lincomycin
- Lithium
- Lorazepam
- Mepacrine
- Mercury (amalgam)
- Metformin
- Methyldopa
- Metronidazole
- Niridazole
- Oral contraceptives
- Oxprenolol
- Para-aminosalicylate
- Penicillamine
- Penicillins
- Phenindione
- Phenothiazines
- Phenylbutazone
- Phenytoin
- Piroxicam
- Practolol
- Prazosin
- Procainamide
- Propranolol
- Propylthiouracil
- Prothionamide
- Quinidine
- Quinine
- Rifampicin
- Rofecoxib
- Streptomycin
- Tetracycline
- Tocainide
- Tolbutamide
- Triprolidine

APPENDIX 29.9 DRUGS IMPLICATED IN ORAL CANDIDOSIS

- Broad-spectrum antimicrobials
- Corticosteroids
- Drugs causing xerostomia
- Immunosuppressives

APPENDIX 29.10 DRUGS IMPLICATED IN PEMPHIGOID-LIKE REACTIONS

- Amoxicillin
- Azapropazone
- Clonidine
- Furosemide
- Ibuprofen
- Isoniazid
- Mefenamic acid
- Nadolol
- Penicillamine
- Penicillin V
- Phenacetin
- Practolol
- Salicylic acid
- Sulfasalazine
- Sulphonamides

APPENDIX 29.11 DRUGS IMPLICATED IN PEMPHIGUS-LIKE REACTIONS

- Ampicillin
- Arsenic
- Benzylpenicillin
- Captopril
- Cefadroxil
- Cefalexin
- Diclofenac
- Gold
- Interferon-beta
- Interleukin-2
- Oxyphenbutazone
- Penicillamine
- Phenobarbital
- Phenylbutazone
- Piroxicam
- Probenecid
- Procaine penicillin
- Rifampicin

APPENDIX 29.12 DRUGS IMPLICATED IN ERYTHEMA MULTIFORME (AND STEVENS–JOHNSON SYNDROME AND TOXIC EPIDERMAL NECROLYSIS)[a]

- Acetylsalicylic acid
- Allopurinol
- Amlodipine
- Arsenic
- Atropine
- Busulfan
- Carbamazepine
- Chloral hydrate
- Chloramphenicol
- Chlorpropamide
- Clindamycin
- Codeine
- Co-trimoxazole
- Diclofenac
- Diflunisal
- Digitalis
- Diltiazem
- Ethambutol
- Ethyl alcohol
- Fluconazole
- Fluorouracil
- Furosemide
- Gold
- Griseofulvin
- Hydantoin
- Hydrochlorothiazide
- Indapamide
- Measles/mumps/rubella (MMR) vaccine
- Meclofenamic acid
- Mercury
- Mesterolone
- Minoxidil
- Nifedipine
- Omeprazole
- Oxyphenbutazone
- Penicillin derivatives
- Phenolphthalein
- Phenylbutazone
- Phenytoin
- Piroxicam
- Progesterone
- Pyrazolone derivatives
- Quinine
- Retinol
- Rifampicin
- Streptomycin
- Sulfasalazine
- Sulindac
- Tenoxicam
- Tetracyclines
- Theophylline
- Tocainide
- Tolbutamide
- Trimethadione
- Vancomycin
- Verapamil
- Zidovudine

[a]For antiretrovirals see Chapter 20.

APPENDIX 29.13 DRUGS IMPLICATED IN LUPOID REACTIONS

- Ethosuximide
- Gold
- Griseofulvin
- Hydralazine
- Isoniazid
- Methyldopa
- Para-aminosalicylate
- Penicillin
- Phenothiazines
- Phenytoin
- Procainamide
- Streptomycin
- Sulphonamides
- Tetracyclines

APPENDIX 29.14 DRUGS IMPLICATED IN CHEILITIS

- Actinomycin
- Atorvastatin
- Busulfan
- Clofazimine
- Clomipramine
- Cyancobalamin
- Ethyl alcohol
- Etretinate
- Gold
- Indinavir
- Isoniazid
- Isotretinoin
- Lithium
- Menthol
- Methyldopa
- Penicillamine
- Selegiline
- Streptomycin
- Sulfasalazine
- Tetracycline
- Vitamin A

APPENDIX 29.15 DRUGS APART FROM SMOKING IMPLICATED IN ORAL MUCOSAL HYPERPIGMENTATION

- Adrenocorticotropic hormone (ACTH)
- Amodiaquine
- Anticonvulsants
- Arsenic
- Betel
- Bismuth
- Bromine
- Busulfan
- Chlorhexidine
- Chloroquine
- Clofazimine
- Copper
- Cyclophosphamide
- Doxorubicin
- Gold
- Heroin
- Iron
- Lead
- Manganese
- Mepacrine
- Methyldopa
- Minocycline
- Oral contraceptives
- Phenolphthalein
- Phenothiazines
- Quinacrine
- Quinidine
- Silver
- Thallium
- Tin
- Vanadium
- Zidovudine

APPENDIX 29.16 DRUGS IMPLICATED IN ORAL MUCOSAL COLOURATION: DIFFERENT COLOURS

Black	Blue	Brown (hypermelanosis)	Green	Grey	White
Amiodiaquine	Amiodarone	Aminophenazone	Copper	Amodiaquine	Palifermin (keratinocyte growth factor)
Betel nut	Antimalarials	Betel nut		Chloroquine	Sanguinarine
Bismuth	Bismuth	Bismuth		Fluoxetine	
Methyldopa	Mepacrine	Busulfan		Hydroxychloroquinine	
Minocycline	Minocycline	Clofazimine		Lead	
	Phenazopyridine	Contraceptives		Silver	
	Quinidine	Cyclophosphamide		Tin/zinc	
	Silver	Diethylstilbestrol			
	Sulfasalazine	Doxorubicin			
		Doxycycline			
		Fluorouracil			
		Heroin			
		Hormone replacement therapy			
		Ketoconazole			
		Menthol			
		Methaqualone			
		Minocycline			
		Phenolphthalein			
		Propranolol			
		Smoking			
		Zidovudine			

APPENDIX 29.17 DRUGS IMPLICATED IN GINGIVAL SWELLING

Drugs most commonly implicated	Drugs occasionally implicated
Amlodipine	Basiliximab
Ciclosporin	Co-trimoxazole
Diltiazem	Diphenoxylate
Felodipine	Erythromycin
Lacidipine	Ethosuximide
Nifedipine	Interferon-alpha
Oral contraceptives	Ketoconazole
Phenytoin	Lamotrigine
Verapamil	Lithium
	Mephenytoin
	Nitrendipine
	Norethisterone + mestranol
	Phenobarbital
	Primidone
	Sertraline
	Topiramate
	Valproate
	Vigabatrin

APPENDIX 29.18 DRUGS IMPLICATED IN ANGIOEDEMA

- Angiotensin-converting enzyme inhibitors (ACEIs)
- Asparaginase
- Carbamazepine
- Clindamycin
- Clonidine
- Co-trimoxazole
- Disulfite sodium
- Droperidol
- Enalapril
- Epoetin alfa
- Ibruprofen
- Indometacin
- Ketoconazole
- Mianserin
- Miconazole
- Naproxen
- Nitrofurantoin
- Penicillamine
- Penicillin derivatives
- Pyrazolone derivatives
- Quinine
- Streptomycin
- Sulphonamides
- Thiouracil

APPENDIX 29.19 DRUGS IMPLICATED IN TRIGEMINAL PARAESTHESIA OR HYPOAESTHESIA

- Acetazolamide
- Amitryptiline
- Articaine
- Chlorpropamide
- Colistin
- Ergotamine
- Gonadotropin-releasing hormone analogues
- Hydralazine
- Interferon-alpha
- Isoniazid
- Labetalol
- Mefloquine
- Methysergide
- Monoamine oxidase inhibitors
- Nalidixic acid
- Nicotinic acid
- Nitrofurantoin
- Pentamidine
- Phenytoin
- Prilocaine
- Propofol
- Propranolol
- Prothionamide
- Stilbamidine
- Streptomycin
- Sulphonylureas
- Sultiame
- Tolbutamide
- Tricyclics
- Trilostane
- Vincristine

APPENDIX 29.20 DRUGS IMPLICATED IN INVOLUNTARY FACIAL MOVEMENTS

- Carbamazepine
- L-Dopa
- Lithium
- Methyldopa
- Metoclopramide
- Metirosine
- Phenytoin
- Tetrabenazine
- Trifluoroperazine

APPENDIX 29.21 DRUGS IMPLICATED IN HALITOSIS

- Dimethyl sulfoxide (DMSO)
- Disulfiram
- Isosorbide dinitrate

APPENDIX 29.22 DRUGS IMPLICATED IN OROFACIAL PAIN

- Benztropine
- Biperiden
- Griseofulvin
- Lithium
- Penicillins
- Phenothiazines
- Stilbamidine
- Ticarcillin
- Vinca alkaloids
- Vitamin A

APPENDIX 29.23 DRUGS IMPLICATED IN TOOTH DISCOLOURATION

- Antibiotics
- Clarithromycin
- Enalapril
- Essential oil
- Etidronate
- Fosinopril
- Imipenem
- Lisinopril
- Metronidazole
- Penicillin
- Pentamidine
- Perindopril
- Propafenone
- Quinapril
- Ramipril
- Terbinafine
- Tetracyclines
- Trandolapril
- Zopiclone

This chapter focuses (alphabetically) mainly on medical issues related to ethnic and cultural groups, homeless people, immigrants, people in custodial institutions, refugees and asylees, Roma, sexual minorities and socioeconomically deprived people. The importance of 'protected characteristics' as defined by the Equalities and Human Rights Commission are noted in Chapter 2 (http://www.equalityhumanrights.com/advice-and-guidance/new-equality-act-guidance/protected-characteristics-definitions/).

ETHNIC AND CULTURAL GROUPS

This section tabulates some of the main aspects (Table 30.1). Population mobility increases inexorably, leading to enormous changes in the structure of many populations across the world. This is especially evident in the developed world and as a consequence of conflicts and climate change.

For example, by 2011 almost 1 in 8 people living in the UK were foreign-born. The proportion of the UK population born outside Europe reached 10% overall, with large regional variations from, for example, 3% in the far south-west to 30% in East London. Ongoing expansion of the European Union is producing major changes, as are conflicts and economic issues worldwide. Some of these people fall into one or more of the groups below.

It is difficult to characterize all the different faiths and cultures, since differences exist according to social class, background, ethnicity and other factors, but Table 30.2 attempts to highlight some relevant aspects.

Communication is crucial between dental professionals and patients from different faiths, cultures and countries. Professional interpreters may therefore be required.

HOMELESS PEOPLE

Homeless people and those who live in poor accommodation tend to have more illness, mainly due to exposure, inadequate diet, inadequate hygiene, stress, violence, accidents and exposure to communicable

Table 30.1 *Ethnic and cultural groups: languages, religions, habits and medical aspects*[a]

Ethnic group	Main language(s)	Main religion(s)	Common diet, habits and medical aspects
Albanians (Kosovars)	Albanian	Islam	Alcohol use and smoking endemic, and younger generation uses narcotics at an increasing rate
		Christianity	
Afro-Caribbeans	English	Christianity	Seventh Day Adventists consume no pork, tea, coffee or alcohol. Rastafarians often use marijuana but may be vegan or eat no pork. Crack and cocaine use is common in Jamaicans
	French		
	Spanish		
Arabs	Arabic	Islam	See Table 30.2
Armenians	Armenian	Christianity	–
Bangladeshi	Bengali	Islam	Healthy diet. Dislike oral medication. Females prefer female health-care workers. Often smoke or use paan
	Urdu		
Bosnian	Serbo-Croat	Islam	Healthy diet. Dislike oral medication. Females prefer female health-care workers
Cambodian	Khmer	Buddhist	Traditional medicine may be preferred
Chinese	Cantonese	Taoism	Traditional Chinese medicine may be used. Doctor-shopping common. Often eat rice diet and smoke heavily. May not like venepuncture
	Mandarin	Confucianism	
		Buddhism	
Eritreans	Tigrinya	Christianity	Coptic Christians do not consume meat or dairy products for more than half of each year
	Arabic	Islam	
Ethiopians	Amharic	Christianity	Coptic Christians do not consume meat or dairy products for more than half of each year
		Islam	
Ghanaian	Twi	Islam	Traditional medicine may be used
		Christianity	
Greeks	Greek	Christianity	Healthy diet. High tobacco use
Gujaratis	Gujarati	Hinduism	Often eat no meat, eggs or fish
Indian	Hindi	Hinduism (mainly)	Traditional (Ayurvedic) medicine. Often vegetarian or vegan. High tobacco and betel use. Rarely, vitamin B_{12}-deficient from veganism
	Punjabi	Islam	
	English	Christianity	
		Sikhism	
		Zoroastrianism	
Iranian	Farsi	Islam	–
Iraqi	Arabic	Islam	–
Irish	English	Christianity	May have high alcohol intake

(Continued)

Table 30.1 (Continued)

Ethnic group	Main language(s)	Main religion(s)	Common diet, habits and medical aspects
Japanese	Japanese	Buddhism Shintoism	Diet often of rice, raw fish and eggs
Koreans	Korean (Han-gul)	Confucianism Shamanism Taoism Buddhism	Traditional medicine commonly used. Be aware of communication styles and patterns, such as no eye contact, smiling at inopportune times represents lack of respect and intelligence
Kurds (a diverse ethnic group from Kurdistan, encompassing parts of Turkey, Iran, Iraq, Syria)	Kurdish	Islam	–
Laotians	Laotian	Buddhism	–
Latin Americans	Spanish Portuguese	Christianity	–
Liberians	English		Traditional medicine may be used
Nigerians	Four peoples/languages: Hausa, Yoruba, Ibo and Fulani	Islam Christianity	Traditional medicine may be used
Pakistanis	Punjabi	Islam	See Table 30.2
Portuguese	Portuguese	Christianity	High tobacco use
Russian Federation	Russian	Christianity	–
Somalis	Somali Arabic	Islam	May have qat habit
South Africans (whites)	English Afrikaans	Christianity	–
Sudanese	Arabic English	Islam Christianity	Traditional medicine may be used
Tamils	Tamil	Hinduism	Vegetarian
Tibetans	Tibetan Chinese	Buddhism	Ayurvedic tradition
Turks	Turkish	Islam	See Table 30.2
Vietnamese	Vietnamese Cantonese	Buddhism Christianity	Vegetarian

[a]Adapted with permission from Scully C, Wilson N (2006).

diseases and drug abuse (Fig. 30.2). Mental health problems, including psychotic illness, depression and anxiety, alcohol addiction or injecting drug use, are common. There are high rates of blood-borne and other infections, such as hepatitis B and C, and human immunodeficiency virus (HIV), all of which can be associated mainly with drug use and neglect of health. Tuberculosis is common (Ch. 15). Most report negative oral health impacts, having caries and inflammatory periodontal disease; over half have current orofacial pain. Additional oral health impacts include difficulty with eating, smiling, concentrating and talking. Dental anxiety status is related to dental disease experience, which impacts negatively on quality of life. Various studies have confirmed that few had dental care in the previous year.

The problems, summarized in Table 30.3, serve to perpetuate homelessness and impede access to health care. There is a need to provide more accessible and affordable health services to homeless people.

IMMIGRANTS

Immigrants and refugees can arrive from diverse social, economic, educational, cultural, religious and ethnic backgrounds for a variety of reasons: to seek work, education or economic advantage; flee war,

political upheaval or persecution; or join families from which they have been separated. Many arrive with inadequate resources and suffer social exclusion and inequality of health-care provision. The acute phase following immigration, particularly from the developing world, war zones and tropical regions, attracts most concern (Table 30.4), and is particularly at this time that health can be neglected.

Many come from health-care systems that differ from traditional Western medicine and may involve traditional remedies. Lifestyle factors predispose some to specific diseases (e.g. areca nut use and oral submucous fibrosis). Hereditary factors are sometimes important too, as in sickle cell disease, thalassaemia and glucose-6-phosphate dehydrogenase deficiency.

Other problems may include malnutrition, intestinal parasites (*Enterobius*, *Trichuris*, *Strongyloides* and *Ascaris*), filariasis, leishmaniasis, hepatitis A, B and C, tuberculosis, low immunization rate, typhoid fever, yellow fever, malaria, trachoma, syphilis, dengue fever, HIV infection, diarrhoeal illnesses, leprosy, hypertension, coronary disease, gastrointestinal problems, diabetes, depression, lactose intolerance, carcinomas of cervix, breast and mouth, vitamin D deficiency, alcoholism and substance abuse.

The second phase, transition, typically takes at least 5 years, with acculturation and modification of social norms, attitudes, values, behaviours and diet, bringing changes not least in the use of

Table 30.2 *Main faiths/religions and their medical relevance*[a]

Faith/ religion	Main festival or religious occasion(s)	Dietary aspects	Possible main medical problems	Other comments
Buddhism	Wesak	Often vegetarian	–	–
Jehovah's Witnesses	Christmas, Easter	–	Firmly believe that blood has sacred meaning and that it should not be removed from the body and stored; nor should donor blood be taken in during a transfusion. Often refuse blood transfusions and organ transplants, and human blood products like platelets (Ch. 8)	Jehovah's Witness Watchtower Society places a biblical ban on the storage/use of animal blood (see also Appendix 30.1 and Fig. 30.1)
Hinduism	Diwali, Maha Shivaratri, Ram Navami, Janmashtami	Often eat no meat (particularly beef) or meat products, eggs or fish Some drink no tea, coffee or alcohol, and eat no garlic or onions	Vitamin B_{12}-deficient from veganism	–
Islam (Muslim)	Ramadan, Mawlid, al-Nabi	Eat no pork, drink no alcohol. Eat only Halal meat. During Ramadan, between sunrise and sunset, eat and drink nothing (including water), and smoke nothing, unless ill, young, old or pregnant	May be non-compliant with oral medication during fasts such as Ramadan. Alcohol-free oral products should be used. Meningitis vaccination indicated at Haj and Umra	Often cover much of the body and head/face. Right hand is considered clean, and used for eating and shaking hands. Handshakes are appropriate only between men or between women. It is not acceptable for a man to shake the hand of a Shiite woman Women are not permitted to be alone with a man who is not her husband or relative. At public events, women are segregated from men
Judaism	Rosh Hashanah, Yom Kippur, Pesach	Eat no pork or shellfish, and only kosher meat Fast for 25 h from eve of Yom Kippur	Orthodox Jews may refuse organ transplants. Liable to Tay–Sachs disease (inherited neurological defects), Canavan disease (inherited brain disorder), Fanconi anaemia, pemphigus	No work on Sabbath (Saturday)
Sikhism	Vaisakhi, Diwali, Hola	Eat no fish or eggs, and usually no beef or pork Often vegetarian	Vitamin B_{12}-deficient from veganism	Invariably cover head

[a]It is impossible to generalize; always consider the individual and their wishes and needs. See also Table 30.1.

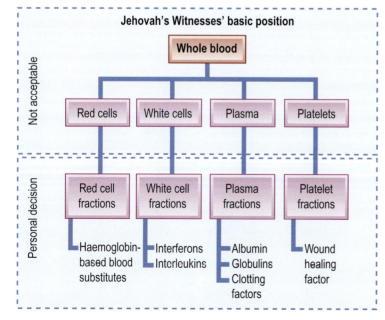

Fig. 30.1 Jehovah's Witnesses' acceptance of various procedures/substances.

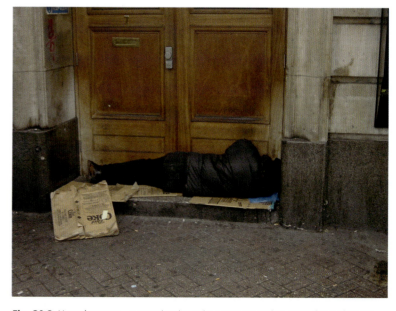

Fig. 30.2 Homelessness – a growing issue in many countries, even those that are resource-rich.

health-care services. Most younger people become well integrated into the community.

The third phase, 10 or more years after arrival, is typified by the resettled refugee suffering a variety of chronic conditions, seen at least partly as a consequence of resettlement, but many have acculturated and others continue to live and often work in their own communities, in a multicultural society.

PEOPLE IN CUSTODIAL CARE

Prisoners' general health is compromised by lifestyle behaviours, such as the use of tobacco, alcohol and drugs of abuse, high-sugar diets and homosexual practices. In particular, there are high levels of violence, mental illness and infectious disease, such as hepatitis virus infections and HIV. Prisoners' oral health status often includes high levels of caries and relatively high levels of both missing and filled teeth; oral health is poor, and remains poor in comparison with non-institutionalized individuals where appropriate comparisons have been made. The main barriers to health care are cost, anxiety and access.

Table 30.3 *Medical problems prevalent in homeless people*[a]

Type	Detail
Assaults	Physical
	Psychological
	Sexual
Cardiovascular	Hypertension
	Peripheral vascular disease
Exposure	Hypothermia
Gastrointestinal	Vomiting and diarrhoea
Infections	Infestations (lice, fleas, scabies)
	Lower respiratory infections, e.g. influenza, pneumonia, tuberculosis
	Sexually shared infections
	Upper respiratory viral infections
	Viral hepatitis
Mental	Depression
	Schizophrenia
	Stress, anxiety, substance abuse
Nutritional	Malnutrition
Substance abuse	Alcohol
	Illegal drugs and volatile substance abuse
	Tobacco

[a]Often multiple or complex problems, over and above the problems afflicting others, and poor access to health-care services.

REFUGEES AND ASYLEES

A *refugee* is someone who, 'owing to a well-founded fear of being persecuted for reasons of race, religion, nationality, membership of a particular social group, or political opinion, is outside the country of his nationality, and is unable to or, owing to such fear, is unwilling to avail himself of the protection of that country' (United Nations Refugee Convention 1951). *Asylees* (asylum-seekers) have submitted a claim for refugee status. Refugees and asylees comprise most displaced persons resettled to the developed world or from country to country within the developed or developing worlds. The current main countries of refugee origin are shown in Table 30.5.

ROMA

Roma (or Romanies) is the preferred term for people commonly but incorrectly known as gypsies. Most Roma refer to themselves as *rom* or *rrom*. Worldwide there is an estimated population of at least 15 million Roma but many are not registered for fear of discrimination. Most Roma are from Eastern Europe (Romania, Bosnia, Bulgaria, Czech Republic, Kosovo and Slovakia), southern Europe (Greece, Portugal, Spain) or America. 'New Age travellers' are *not* Roma.

Roma are generally a nomadic people with an alternative lifestyle and refusal to conform; they speak Romani – derived primarily from Sanskrit. There is no separate Romani religion; they traditionally adopt the dominant religion of the country in which they live, and are usually Hindu, Christian, Protestant or Muslim (Sufis).

Traditional Roma place a high value on the extended family. At the top of the family is the oldest man or grandfather, and men generally have much more authority than women. Virginity is essential in

Table 30.5 *Countries of origin of refugees and asylees (2012–13, UK)*

Refugees	Asylees
Afghanistan	Chad
Angola	China
Burundi	Iran
Democratic Republic of Congo	Pakistan
Iraq	Syria
Myanmar	Tanzania
Somalia	
Sudan	
Turkey	
Vietnam	

Table 30.4 *The phases of acculturation*[a]

Phase	Possible medical and social problems	Barriers to care	Possible outcomes
Acute	Communicable illnesses (tuberculosis, hepatitis B virus, human immunodeficiency virus) and tropical diseases, malnutrition, trauma, conflict intergenerationally and with other cultures, domestic violence, gambling and substance abuse	Lack of language fluency and understanding of health-care system	Linguistic and cultural isolation; help-seeking behaviour becomes one of emergency care only
Transition	Hypertension, diabetes, psychological disorders and other post-traumatic stress	Lack of language fluency and understanding of health-care system by older generation	Younger generations integrate into host health-care system; continued isolation of older generations
Integration	Hypertension, coronary heart disease and diabetes are the most common disorders. Morbidity and mortality from cancers, particularly cervical, are high	Emotional difficulties as family structures break down	Intergenerational conflicts can arise and there can be heavy alcohol consumption

[a]From Scully C, Wilson N (2006).

unmarried women, and both women and men tend to marry young; there may even be child marriage.

Roma often suffer from unemployment, socioeconomic deprivation and discrimination; they are frequently accused of petty crime and can be faced with barriers to education. Dietary habits include high fat and salt content in foods, and a large percentage of Roma smoke and are obese. These factors can put Roma at increased risk for hypertension, diabetes, occlusive vascular disease, strokes and myocardial infarction. Crowded living conditions can lead to an increase incidence of gastro-intestinal infections and respiratory infections. Nutritional deficits, hepatitis B, tuberculosis and post-traumatic stress disorder may be increased in Roma populations. Social (or societal) isolation also leads to an increase in consanguineous marriages, and thus an increased risk for birth defects.

In the health-care setting, only the elder males of some groups are likely to communicate with health-care personnel. Women are not permitted to interrupt men or to be alone with a man who is not their husband or relative. Washing hands before touching the upper body is required after touching the lower body. Separate soap and towels are used on the upper and lower parts of the body and they must not be allowed to mix. When a clan member must enter a hospital, family members are expected to remain with that person day and night to watch over, protect and perform caring and curing rituals for them. Roma are especially fearful of any surgical procedure that requires general anaesthesia (GA) because of their belief that a person under GA undergoes a 'little death'. It is especially important for the family to gather around the person recovering from GA.

SEXUAL MINORITIES

Sexual minorities are those who identify as lesbian, gay, bisexual or transgender (LGBT), or who have sexual contact with persons of the same or both sexes. Many sexual minority youth successfully transition to adulthood but others struggle to cope because of increased risk for certain health issues. For example, health risks for which the prevalence is higher for gay, lesbian or bisexual students than for heterosexual students include binge drinking. Young gay and bisexual males have disproportionately high rates of HIV, syphilis and other sexually shared infections (SSIs), and lesbian and bisexual females are more likely to have been pregnant than their heterosexual peers.

Lesbians can suffer the same conditions as heterosexual women but additional issues of concern may include:

- breast cancer – lesbians are more likely to have risk factors for breast cancer yet less likely to undergo screening examinations
- depression/anxiety
- heart health – smoking and obesity are the biggest risk factors for heart disease among lesbians
- gynaecological cancer – lesbians have higher risks for certain types of gynaecological cancers compared to heterosexual women
- fitness – lesbians are more likely to be overweight or obese compared to heterosexual women
- tobacco – lesbians use tobacco more often than heterosexual women do
- alcohol – heavy drinking and binge drinking are more common among lesbians compared to other women
- substance use – lesbians may use drugs more often than heterosexual women
- intimate partner violence – some lesbians experience violence in their intimate relationships

- sexual health – lesbians can contract the same SSIs as heterosexual women.

Sexually active bisexuals and gays have a high rate of SSIs, including chlamydia, gonorrhoea, hepatitis viruses, herpesviruses, HIV, human papillomaviruses, pubic lice and syphilis. Men who have sex with men may be at an increased risk of SSIs but safe sex reduces the risk of receiving or transmitting infection. Women who have sex with women have lower rates of infections, but if they have sex with gay or bisexual men (who have increased rates), they may be at risk. Sex with multiple partners (of any gender) increases risk of infection.

Immunizations are available to prevent hepatitis A virus and hepatitis B virus infection. Safe sex is effective at reducing the risk and is currently the most reliable means of preventing HIV and hepatitis C virus infections.

Bisexuals may have problems with body image and are much more likely to experience an eating disorder. The use of substances such as anabolic steroids and certain supplements can be dangerous.

Bisexuals and gays appear to suffer depression and anxiety at a higher rate than the general population. They may also use substances at a higher rate than the general population, and these range from tobacco and amyl nitrate ('poppers'), to marijuana, Ecstasy and amphetamines.

Bisexuals and gays may be at risk for prostate, testicular, breast, cervical and colon cancer.

Sexual minorities may have behaviours that:

- contribute to violence
- relate to attempted suicide
- contribute to unintentional injuries
- result in adverse lifestyles (substance use, sexual risk) and adverse dietary habits, physical activity and weight management.

Sexual minorities may also face stigma, discrimination, family and social disapproval or rejection, and violence. These factors can:

- limit ability to access quality health care
- affect income, employment and the ability to get and keep health insurance
- contribute to poor mental health and suicide attempts
- affect ability to establish and maintain long-term sex relationships that reduce HIV and SSI risk
- make it difficult to be open about sex behaviours with others, which can increase stress, limit social support and negatively affect health
- increase risk of being bullied and/or of being rejected by their families and, as a result, increase risk of homelessness.

SOCIOECONOMICALLY DEPRIVED PEOPLE

Socioeconomic status is considered to be a major social basis for inequalities and an important predictor of health at all ages. Socioeconomic deprivation appears to predispose to a wide range of health issues, from disease to access to provision of and outcomes of health care. Examples are shown in Box 30.1.

Socioeconomically disadvantaged men and women have higher overall mortality rates than persons with a higher socioeconomic status. Moreover, relationships between class and mortality are consistent for almost every cause of death, with only a few exceptions – notably certain cancers. In almost all countries, rates of death due to common causes (e.g. cardiovascular disease and cancer), causes related to smoking, causes related to alcohol use and causes amenable to medical

Centers for Disease Control and Prevention: Sexual identity, sex of sexual contacts, and health-risk behaviors among students in grades 9–12. <http://www.cdc.gov/mmwr/> (search on 'Sexual identity').
Health & Social Care Information Centre: JSNA best practice – Islington. <http://www.ic.nhs.uk/article/1872/JSNA-best-practice---Islington>.

FURTHER READING

Allard, S.W., et al., 2003. Proximity to service providers and service utilization among welfare recipients: the interaction of place and race. J. Policy Anal. Manage. 22, 599.
Berkman, L., Epstein, A.M., 2008. Beyond health care – socioeconomic status and health. N. Engl. J. Med. 358, 2509.
Bezrucha, S., 2005. Review of: the status syndrome: how social standing affects our health and longevity. N. Engl. J. Med. 352, 1159.
British Dental Association, 2003. Dental Care for Homeless People. BDA, London.
Bunt, G.R. (Ed.), 2005. Faith Guides for Higher Education. Higher Education Authority. Centre for Philosophical and Religious Studies, Leeds.
Bussey-Jones, J., Genao, I., 2003. Impact of culture on health care. J. Natl. Med. Assoc. 95, 732.
Ciaranello, A.L., et al., 2006. Providing health care services to the formerly homeless: a quasi-experimental evaluation. J. Health Care Poor Underserved 17, 441.
Cohen, D.A., et al., 2003. Why is poverty unhealthy? Social and physical mediators. Soc. Sci. Med. 57, 1631.
Collins, J., Freeman, R., 2007. Homeless in North and West Belfast: an oral health needs assessment. Br. Dent. J. 202, E31.
Conte, M., et al., 2006. Oral health, related behaviors and oral health impacts among homeless adults. J. Public Health Dent. 66, 276.
Conway, D.I., et al., 2008. Socioeconomic factors influence selection and participation in a population-based case-control study of head and neck cancer in Scotland. J. Clin. Epidemiol. 61, 1187.
Cortellazzi, K.L., et al., 2008. Risk indicators of gingivitis in 5-year-old Brazilian children. Oral Health Prev. Dent. 6, 131.
De Palma, P., Nordenram, G., 2005. The perceptions of homeless people in Stockholm concerning oral health and consequences of dental treatment: a qualitative study. Spec. Care Dent. 25, 289.
De Palma, P., et al., 2005. Oral health of homeless adults in Stockholm, Sweden. Acta Odontol. Scand. 63, 50.
Demakakos, P., et al., 2008. Socioeconomic status and health: the role of subjective social status. Soc. Sci. Med. 67, 330.
Department of Health, 2003. Strategy for Modernizing Dental Services for Prisoners in England. Department of Health, London.
Dogan, M.C., et al., 2006. The oral health status of street children in Adana, Turkey. Int. Dent. J. 56, 92.
Eaton, D.K., et al., 2010. Youth risk behavior surveillance – United States, 2009. MMWR Surveill Summ. 59 (5), 1, PubMed PMID: 20520591.
Eaton, D.K., et al., 2011. Associations between risk behaviors and suicidal ideation and suicide attempts: do racial/ethnic variations in associations account for increased risk of suicidal behaviors among Hispanic/Latina 9th- to 12th-grade female students? Arch. Suicide Res. 15 (2), 113. doi:10.1080/13811118.2011.565268 PubMed PMID: 21541858.
Eaton, D.K., et al., 2012. Youth risk behavior surveillance – United States, 2011. MMWR Surveill Summ. 61 (4), 1. PubMed PMID: 22673000.
Epstein, A.M., 2004. Health care in America – still too separate, not yet equal. N. Engl. J. Med. 351, 603.
Fan, J., et al., 2006. Tooth retention, tooth loss and use of dental care among long-term narcotics abusers. Subst. Abus. 27, 25.
Gibson, G., et al., 2008. Dental treatment improves self-rated oral health in homeless veterans – a brief communication. J. Public Health Dent. 68, 111.
Haugejorden, O., et al., 2008. Socio-economic inequality in the self-reported number of natural teeth among Norwegian adults – an analytical study. Community Dent. Oral Epidemiol. 36, 269.
Heidari, E., et al., 2008. An investigation into the oral health status of male prisoners in the UK. J. Disabil. Oral Health 9, 3.
Hunter, D.J., Richards, T., 2008. Health and wealth in Europe. BMJ 336, 1390.
Irwin, A., et al., 2006. The Commission on Social Determinants of Health: tackling the social roots of health inequities. PLoS Med. 3, e106.
Kahabuka, F.K., Mbawalla, H.S., 2006. Oral health knowledge and practices among Dar es Salaam institutionalized former street children aged 7–16 years. Int. J. Dent. Hyg. 4, 174.
Kanli, A., et al., 2008. Effects of oral health behaviors and socioeconomic factors on a group of Turkish adolescents. Quintessence Int. 39, e26.
Kann, L., et al., 2011. Sexual identity, sex of sexual contacts, and health-risk behaviors among students in grades 9–12 – youth risk behavior surveillance, selected sites, United States, 2001–2009. MMWR Surveill Summ. 60 (7), 1. PubMed PMID: 21659985
King, T.B., Gibson, G., 2003. Oral health needs and access to dental care of homeless adults in the United States: a review. Spec. Care Dent. 23, 143.

Box 30.1 *Some health issues that are more prevalent in lower socioeconomic groups*

- Arthritis
- Assaults
- Asthma
- Cancers
- Coronary heart disease, and death from first infarcts
- Obesity
- Oral health issues
- Malnutrition
- Mental health problems
- Physical health problems
- Psychiatric referral, admission rates and length of stay
- Substance abuse
- Surgical outcomes – unsatisfactory
- Uptake of blood pressure and medical checks

intervention (e.g. tuberculosis and hypertension), as well as poorer self-assessments of health, are substantially higher in groups of lower socioeconomic status.

Socioeconomic factors also influence oral health in terms of, for example, hygiene practices, diet, gingivitis and dental caries. Attending a state school, being female and having parents with low educational attainment were identified as risk factors both for having dental caries and for having a high level of caries. Lack of oral health care may lead to periapical abscesses and other odontogenic infections, which have caused morbidity and even mortality.

Such inequalities in health care might be reduced by improving educational opportunities, income distribution, health-related behaviour and access to health care. Policies related to preventive social, economic and behavioural interventions in areas such as poverty and income, education, unemployment, housing, transportation, the environment (including pollution) and nutrition may well have a much greater effect on reducing health disparities than would traditional medical interventions.

DENTAL ASPECTS IN MINORITIES

Dental issues related to ethnic and cultural groups, homeless people, immigrants, people in custodial institutions, refugees and asylees, Roma, sexual minorities and socioeconomically deprived people have much in common. Generally speaking, there is more oral disease in most groups, and often multiple barriers to care.

KEY WEBSITES

(Accessed 11 June 2013)
Centers for Disease Control and Prevention. <http://www.cdc.gov/minorityhealth/>.
Office of Minority Health: US Department of Health and Human Services. <http://minorityhealth.hhs.gov/templates/browse.aspx> (follow the links under 'Health Topics' and 'Oral Health').
Public Health England. Ethnic minority health. <http://www.apho.org.uk/resource/view.aspx?RID=78571>.

USEFUL WEBSITES

(Accessed 11 June 2013)
Centers for Disease Control and Prevention: Health risks among sexual minority youth. <http://www.cdc.gov/healthyyouth/disparities/smy.htm>.

Kuthy, R.A., et al., 2005. Students' comfort level in treating vulnerable populations and future willingness to treat: results prior to extramural participation. J. Dent. Educ. 69, 1307.

Lang, I.A., et al., 2008. Neighbourhood deprivation and dental service use: a cross-sectional analysis of older people in England. J. Public Health (Oxf) 30 (4), 472.

Lee, J.W., 2005. Public health is a social issue. Lancet 365, 1005.

London Health Commission, 2007. Health in London: Looking Back, Looking Forward. London Health Commission, London.

Lunn, H., et al., 2003. The oral health of a group of prison inmates. Dent. Update 30, 135.

Mackenbach, J.P., et al., 2008. Socioeconomic inequalities in health in 22 European countries. N. Engl. J. Med. 358, 2468.

Mautino, K.S., 2003. Immigration and ancillary health care providers. J. Immigr. Health 5, 45.

Mello, T., et al., 2008. Prevalence and severity of dental caries in schoolchildren of Porto, Portugal. Community Dent. Health 25, 119.

Nahouraii, H., et al., 2008. Social support and dental utilization among children of Latina immigrants. J. Health Care Poor Underserved 19, 428.

Palinkas, L.A., et al., 2003. The journey to wellness: stages of refugee health promotion and disease prevention. J. Immigr. Health 5, 19.

Pikhart, H., et al., 2007. Obesity and education in three countries of the Central and Eastern Europe: the HAPIEE study. Cent. Eur. J. Public Health 15, 140.

Price, J.H., Khubchandani, J., McKinney, M., Braun, R., 2013. Racial/ethnic disparities in chronic diseases of youths and access to health care in the United States. Biomed. Res. Int. 2013, 787616. doi: 10.1155/2013/787616 Epub 2013 Sep 23. PubMed PMID: 24175301; PubMed Central PMCID: PMC3794652.

Raimer, B.G., Stobo, J.D., 2004. Health care delivery in the Texas prison system: the role of academic medicine. JAMA 292, 485.

Reifel, N., 2005. Federal role in dental public health: dental care for special populations. J. Calif. Dent. Assoc. 33, 553.

Sabbah, W., et al., 2007. Social gradients in oral and general health. J. Dent. Res. 86, 992.

Sabbah, W., et al., 2008. Effects of allostatic load on the social gradient in ischaemic heart disease and periodontal disease: evidence from the Third National Health and Nutrition Examination Survey. J. Epidemiol. Community Health 62, 415.

Scully, C., Wilson, N., 2006. Culturally Sensitive Oral Healthcare. Quintessence, London.

Thomas, S.J., et al., 2008. Is there an epidemic of admissions for surgical treatment of dental abscesses in the UK? BMJ 336, 1219.

Vallejos-Sánchez, A.A., et al., 2008. Sociobehavioral factors influencing toothbrushing frequency among schoolchildren. J. Am. Dent. Assoc. 139, 743.

Walsh, T., et al., 2008. An investigation of the nature of research into dental health in prisons: a systematic review. Br. Dent. J. 204, 683. discussion 667.

Webb, E., et al., 2008. Childhood socioeconomic circumstances and adult height and leg length in Central and Eastern Europe. J. Epidemiol. Community Health 62, 351.

Wides, C.D., Brody, H.A., Alexander, C.J., Gansky, S.A., Mertz, E.A., 2013. Long-term outcomes of a dental postbaccalaureate program: increasing dental student diversity and oral health care access. J. Dent. Educ. 77 (5), 537–547. PubMed PMID: 23658398; PubMed Central PMCID: PMC3718543.

Wilmoth, J.M., Chen, P.C., 2003. Immigrant status, living arrangements, and depressive symptoms among middle-aged and older adults. J. Gerontol. B Psychol. Sci. Soc. Sci. 58, S305.

APPENDIX 30.1 ACCEPTABLE ALTERNATIVE PRODUCTS SUITABLE FOR JEHOVAH'S WITNESSES[a]

Blood-oxygen monitoring devices
- Transcutaneous pulse oximeter
- Paediatric ultra-microsampling equipment
- Multiple tests per blood draw

Haemopoietic agents
- Intravenous iron
- Folic acid
- Vitamin B_{12}
- Vitamin C
- Granulocyte colony-stimulating factor
- Interleukin-11
- Recombinant stem-cell factor

Operative and anaesthetic techniques
- Hypotensive anaesthesia
- Induced hypothermia
- Mechanical occlusion of bleeding vessel

Haemostatic agents
- Avitene
- Gelfoam
- Oxygel
- Surgicel
- Desmopressin (DDAVP)
- Epsilon-aminocaproic acid (Amicar)
- Tranexamic acid (Cyklokapron)
- Vasopressin (Pitressin)
- Aprotinin (Trasylol)
- Vincristine (Oncovin)
- Conjugated oestrogens
- Vitamin K
- Recombinant factor VIIa
- Recombinant factor IX

Volume expanders: crystalloids
- Ringer's lactate
- Saline

Volume expanders: colloids
- Dextran
- Gelatin
- Hetastarch
- Pentastarch

Oxygen therapy
- Hyberbaric oxygen therapy
- Perfluorocarbon solutions

Surgical devices and techniques
- Electrocautery
- Ligature vessel

Personal decisions
Medical products and therapy
- Albumin
- Any drug buffered with albumin
- Immunoglobulins
- Natural clotting factors
- Cryoprecipitate
- Plasma protein fractions
- Tissue adhesives
- Natural interferons
- Haemoglobin-based blood substitutes
- Platelet-derived wound healing factors

Medical tests
- Red or white blood cell tagging

Surgical procedures
- Dialysis and heart–lung equipment
- Blood salvage without blood storage

[a]Adapted with permission from http://www.ajwrb.org (accessed 30 September 2013).

This chapter discusses the health of dental health workers (DHWs; dental professionals). Many occupations, especially the construction industry and armed services, are far more dangerous. The chapter also covers hazards to patients from some physical or chemical agents.

HEALTH OF DHWS

The standardized mortality ratio (SMR) – the ratio of observed deaths in an occupation or from any disease to the national average death rate for the same age and sex – is lower in dentists than in the general population. The main causes of death among dentists in UK, USA and other industrialized countries are cardiovascular disease, cancer and suicides, as in non-dental groups of similar socioeconomic status.

The risks in male dentists from liver cirrhosis and suicide are somewhat higher than in the general population, and dentists are also a risk group for malignant melanoma – presumably a consequence of sun exposure on holiday. Dentists, however, have a lower SMR for cancers, ischaemic heart disease, cerebrovascular disease and chronic lung diseases (bronchitis, emphysema and asthma).

Infections and physical, chemical and radiation hazards are the main occupational problems for DHWs. Nearly half of DHWs report sharp instrument injury at some time while treating patients. There are also risks from other accidents, and damage to eyes, hearing, mental health, musculoskeletal system, the fetus in pregnancy, respiratory systems and the skin (Table 31.1). Significantly greater numbers of female DHWs seem to experience musculoskeletal disorders and allergy to latex than males. The most prevalent preventive measure reported by DHWs is changing gloves between patients and using a face mask. Also, most DHWs have undergone hepatitis B virus and other vaccinations.

In the UK, governmental concern and the defining of safe work practices have brought the question of occupational hazards into sharper focus, as have the measures for implementing safe practices enshrined in the Health and Safety at Work etc. Act (1974) and regulations such as the Ionizing Radiations Regulations (1988) and Control of Substances Hazardous to Health Regulations (1988). In the USA, the Department of Labor Occupational Safety and Health Administration (OSHA) has extensive legislation, which may be found at http://www.osha.gov/SLTC/dentistry/standards.html (accessed 30 September 2013).

INFECTIONS (SEE ALSO CH. 21)

Overall, the major infectious hazards are respiratory and hepatitis B (HBV) and C virus (HCV) infections, and, to a very much lesser extent, human immunodeficiency virus (HIV), prions and health-care-associated infections (HCAIs), such as meticillin-resistant *Staphylococcus aureus*, *Clostridium difficile*, tuberculosis and *Legionella*.

Blood, serum and saliva are the sources most likely to transmit serious infection, as well as dental instruments that are often contaminated after use, and also bites. The transmission of blood-borne viruses is determined by the dose and viral concentration of an

Table 31.1 *Known occupational hazards in dentistry*

Hazard	Examples
Infections	
Bacteria	Legionellosis
	Syphilis
	Tuberculosis
Viruses	Common cold and other respiratory viruses
	Hand, foot and mouth disease
	Hepatitis viruses
	Herpangina
	Herpesviruses
	HIV/AIDS and other retroviruses
	Human papillomavirus
	Parvoviruses
Prions	
Physical and chemical	
Accidents and assaults	
Burns (chemical heat/cold/radiation)	
Chemical sterilizers	
Disinfectants	
Electrical accidents	
Fires and explosions	
Flammable or explosive agents	
Formaldehyde	
Inhalational anaesthetic agents	
Mercury	
Minerals	
Non-anaesthetic agents	
Poisons	
'Sick building syndrome'	
Solvents	
Vibration injury	
X-ray processing chemicals	
Radiation	
Ionizing radiation	X-rays
Non-ionizing radiation	Electromagnetic radiation
	Light (ultraviolet, blue, white)
	Lasers
Video display units (VDUs or monitors)	
Pacemaker cardioverter and hearing aid interference	
To specific body systems	
Eyes	
Hearing	
Mental health	Reaction of staff to stress
	Adapting to stress
Musculoskeletal complaints	
Pregnancy	General anaesthetic agents
	Infectious agents
	Ionizing radiation
	Mercury

(Continued)

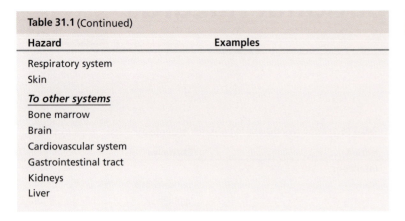

Table 31.1 (Continued)

Hazard	Examples
Respiratory system	
Skin	
To other systems	
Bone marrow	
Brain	
Cardiovascular system	
Gastrointestinal tract	
Kidneys	
Liver	

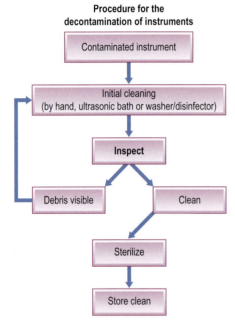

Procedure for the
decontamination of instruments

Contaminated instrument

↓

Initial cleaning
(by hand, ultrasonic bath or washer/disinfector)

↓

Inspect

Debris visible   Clean

↓

Sterilize

↓

Store clean

Fig. 31.1 Instrument decontamination.

Box 31.1 *Ten main points to minimize cross-infection in the dental surgery*

1. Avoid needlestick or other sharps injuries
2. Use effective sterilization, decontamination and disinfection procedures
3. Have clinical staff immunized, particularly against hepatitis B
4. Ask patients to use 0.2% chlorhexidine mouth rinse preoperatively to decrease the number of oral microbes present
5. Use a rubber dam to isolate the tooth or treatment area; use high-speed evacuation
6. Avoid causing oral bleeding wherever possible
7. Wear protective gloves, masks, eyewear and/or face shields, and follow good hygiene procedures
8. Wear clean clinical attire; change clothes before leaving the clinic; disinfect hands with an alcohol-based disinfectant (containing 1–3% glycerol to avoid skin dehydration)
9. Minimize the working area; use a tray system, or cover surfaces and equipment with disposable plastic, paper or foil wraps. Uncovered surfaces and equipment should be wiped with absorbent towelling and then disinfected following work activities
10. Take especial care with patients in high-risk groups for blood-borne infections

exposure. Whereas HBV transmission can be prevented by immunization of DHWs, controlling HCV and HIV requires efforts to reduce the incidence and dosage of exposures to blood and body fluids. Such strategies include the design and use of safe devices, targeted interventions, the use of gloves and other barriers, and ongoing surveillance and analysis of exposures.

Since there is a potential for transmission of various infections, dental equipment should, where at all possible, be single-use and all reusable instruments must be sterilized or at least decontaminated (Fig. 31.1). DHWs should pay considerable attention to avoidance of needlestick (percutaneous inoculation; sharps) infections/injuries and bites.

Standard (universal) infection control must be implemented; infection control guidelines can be found at http://www.bda.org/dentists/advice/ba/ic.aspx (accessed 30 September 2013).

The main points to remember in order to minimize cross-infection are shown in Box 31.1.

NEEDLESTICK/OCCUPATIONAL EXPOSURE TO INFECTIONS

Exposure-prone procedures (EPPs) are defined by the UK Department of Health as those where there is a risk that injury to the worker may result in exposure of the patient's open tissues to the blood of the worker. These procedures include those where the worker's gloved hands may be in contact with sharp instruments, needle tips or sharp tissues (spicules of bone or teeth) inside a patient's open body cavity, wound or confined anatomical space where the hands or fingertips may not be completely visible at all times. Most procedures in dentistry are defined as EPPs, with the exception of:

■ examination using a mouth mirror only
■ extra-oral radiography
■ visual and digital examination of the head and neck
■ visual and digital examination of the edentulous mouth
■ impressions of edentulous patients
■ the construction and fitting of full dentures.

However, taking impressions from dentate or partially dentate patients would be considered exposure-prone, as would the fitting of partial dentures and fixed or removable orthodontic appliances, where clasps and other pieces of metal could result in injury to the dentist.

DHWs need not refrain from performing EPPs pending follow-up of occupational exposure to an HIV-infected source. The combined risks of contracting HIV infection from the source patient and then transmitting this to another patient during an EPP are so low as to be considered negligible.

Blood-borne microorganisms that can be transmitted via blood exposure include:

■ viruses:
  HBV
  HCV
  HIV
  cytomegalovirus (CMV)
  Epstein–Barr virus (EBV)
  parvovirus
■ bacteria:
  Treponema pallidum (syphilis)
  Yersinia
■ parasites:
  Plasmodium.

Accidental exposure to blood caused by needle injuries or injuries following, cutting, biting or splashing incidents carries the risk of infection, particularly by blood-borne viruses though risks vary (Table 31.2).

Table 31.2 *Blood-borne viruses*

	Hepatitis C virus	Hepatitis B virus	Human immunodeficiency virus
Risk of transmission by needlestick injury	3% (3–10%)	30% (5–40%)	0.3% (0.2–0.5%)
Prevalence is higher than average in people who:	have had multiple blood transfusions; are dialysis patients or intravenous drug users	are intravenous drug users or men who have sex with men; are from developing countries	are men who have sex with men or intravenous drug users; are from areas where the condition is endemic

Preventing needlestick injury and avoiding infection

The single most important measure that will help to prevent needlestick injury is to avoid recapping and resheathing. Keep a rigid puncture-proof container close to hand for used needles to avoid the temptation of recapping. It is equally important to use proper protective clothing such as gloves, mouth mask and goggles.

Every DHW at risk from accidental exposure to blood should be trained in infection control and vaccinated against HBV (there are no preventive vaccines available for HCV or HIV).

Action after exposure to potentially contaminated material includes (Fig. 31.2) the following measures:

- If there is a wound, let it bleed for a moment and then cleanse thoroughly using an ample amount of soap and water followed by 70% alcohol.
- In case of contact with mucous membranes, it is important to rinse immediately and thoroughly, using water or a saline solution only, *not* alcohol.

Under the Reporting of Injuries, Diseases and Dangerous Occurrences Regulations (1995), it is not usually necessary to tell the Health and Safety Executive (HSE) about an occupational exposure to blood or saliva; however, if the occupational exposure involves a known carrier of a blood-borne disease, this is classified as a dangerous occurrence and reporting then becomes mandatory – as it is when acute ill health has resulted from exposure to, or transference of, a biological pathogen. Recording of occupational exposure to blood or saliva in an accident report book is strongly advised and the incident should be reported immediately to the department dealing with occupational accidents.

Post-exposure prophylaxis (PEP) against HIV has been estimated to reduce the risk of transmission by 75%; it should be carried out within 1 hour for maximum effect, so an initial assessment must be performed as soon as possible. Even if there is a delay, it is still worth considering PEP within 24 hours of the exposure. A blood sample should be taken from the exposed person as soon as possible after the injury to act as a baseline value in case infection does arise. Further blood samples to test for HBV, HCV and HIV are collected after 1, 3, 6 and 12 months. If the source of the blood is known, the patient must be asked for permission to take a sample of blood for an HCV and HIV test. If the patient refuses, then they must be assumed to be a carrier. If the origin of the blood is unknown, then any blood present on the needle can be used for a serological examination.

Management is based on determining the level of risk of contracting HBV, HCV or HIV, depending on whether or not the injured person is non-immune, partially immune or fully immune for HBV (from vaccination or otherwise). If there is only limited immunity to HBV, then 5 mL intramuscular hepatitis B immunoglobulin (HBIG) should be given within 48 hours of the injury. After a potential HCV infection, combination treatment of pegylated interferon and ribavirin is the treatment of choice. A liver specialist should be consulted.

No PEP is currently available for hepatitis C. However, early treatment of acute hepatitis C infection may prevent chronic hepatitis C infection. Follow-up of exposed patients should be as that described in management for occupational exposure to hepatitis C.

A course of hepatitis B vaccination with or without immunoglobulin may be recommended as PEP following exposure to hepatitis B.

Post-exposure prophylaxis for HIV infection

After a potential HIV infection, the actual risk depends on the type of contact and on the amount of virus in the contaminated material. The risk of an HIV infection following exposure to blood is very small but factors associated with a higher risk are:

- deep wounds (e.g. needlesticks, scalpel wounds)
- visible blood on the instrument
- needlestick injury from using hollow-bore needles containing blood
- intravenous or intramuscular injection of contaminated blood
- blood from a patient with a high virus level (e.g. untreated or terminal AIDS patients).

Decision 1: What is the level of risk of HIV transmission?

Level of risk is classed as low or negligible, which does not require PEP, or as a significant injury with a higher risk of transmission, which may require PEP. In the latter case, the source should be informed that the injury is significant enough to carry a risk of transmission and their permission should be obtained for a review of their social and medical histories. In the case of a splash, the volume of exposure should be assessed, as both HIV and HCV are reported to have been transmitted through only 0.5 mL of blood to the conjunctiva. In the unlikely event of a splash to a mucous membrane, then the exposure would be classed as a significant injury.

Decision 2: Is your patient at risk of carrying HIV?

A social and medical history can help determine whether HIV transmission is likely to have occurred and the associated degree of risk of that happening. Questions will relate to the patient's sexuality and lifestyle; ideally, questioning should take place in a private room and the patient needs to be reassured that the discussion will remain confidential. The recipient of the injury should not ask the questions because he or she may be too anxious. When assessing the risk factors for acquiring HIV, the operator should concentrate on high-risk activities (Box 31.2) that increase the potential for transmission of the infection rather than concentrating on the main risk groups. The patient should be informed that guidelines are laid down by the UK health departments for the management of occupational exposures to blood or saliva, and that some questions need to be asked that relate to the risk of the patient having acquired HIV.

Low risk

If it is decided that the patient is in the low-risk category for HIV, then the procedure outlined under mild injury is followed.

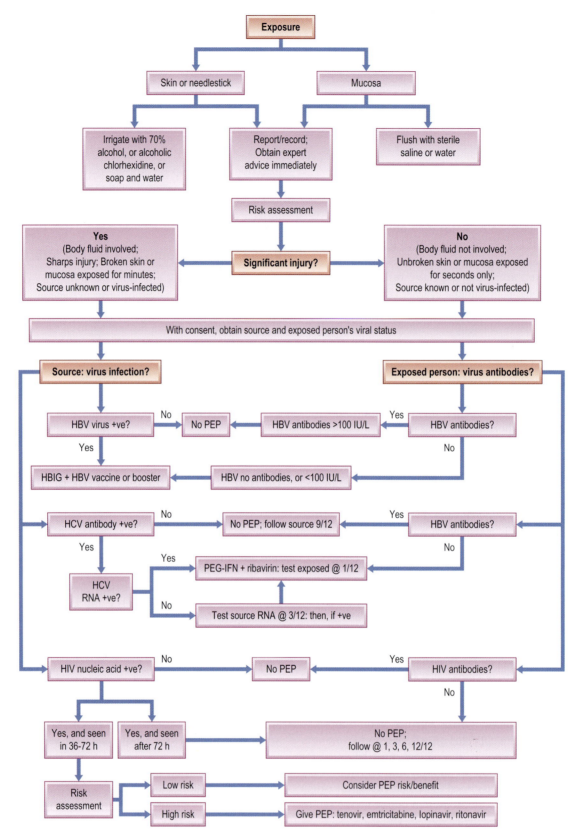

Fig. 31.2 Algorithm for post-exposure prophylaxis (PEP). HBIG = hepatitis B immunoglobulin; HBV/HCV = hepatitis B/C virus; HIV = human immunodeficiency virus; PEG-IFN = pegylated interferon; RNA = ribonucleic acid. After Samaranayake and Scully 2013.

High risk

If the patient admits to having participated in a high-risk activity, in an area with a high prevalence of HIV, then the specialist may recommend an HIV test. The test must *not* be carried out until trained health-care advisors have counselled the patient about the consequences of such a test. This takes more than an hour to carry out and the specialist may advise the recipient to attend a local hospital to be given initial doses of PEP drugs. Once the initial doses have been taken, a formal risk assessment for HIV may be carried out and a decision made as to whether to continue PEP until the HIV test result is known. If the injury occurs outside normal working hours, an alternative source of advice must be found and, if necessary, the first few doses of PEP

- Do you donate blood?
- Have you ever had sex with a partner from abroad?
- Have you ever had a partner who is bisexual or uses intravenous drugs?
- Have you ever had sex with anyone that you did not know well?
- Have you ever exchanged money or drugs for sex?
- Have you ever injected non-prescription drugs (recreational drugs like heroin, cocaine, speed, etc.) or used injectable steroids?
- Have you ever lived in or visited Africa?
- Have you ever had tattoos or body piercings?
- Have you attended a clinic for sexually shared diseases?
- Have you been tested for HIV?

Box 31.3 *Checklist for assessing the need for post-exposure prophylaxis and the most suitable drug regimen*

- Is the person generally well?
- Do they know their CD4 (T-helper cell) count and/or viral load, when it was taken and if the level has changed recently?
- Are they on any medication? If so, what?
- Has their medication changed recently and why?
- What is the name of their general medical practitioner, and the address and telephone number of the HIV clinic they are attending?

Box 31.4 *Decontamination in general dental practice*

Use a dedicated decontamination area, separated from the patient treatment area and preferably in another room or rooms, with:

- a separate hand-washing facility
- a setting-down area for dirty instruments
- a washing sink with detergent for cleaning instruments
- a setting-down area for washed instruments
- an ultrasonic cleaner (35–55 kHz), if appropriate
- a rinsing sink
- a setting-down area for rinsed instruments
- an automated washer–disinfector includes drying cycle; thermodisinfectors fulfilling requirements in EN 15883 are the safest and most reliable)
- a setting-down area with task lighting and magnifier for inspection of all instruments (to check instruments for visible contamination and functionality or damage, and to ensure instruments are dry)
- an area for packing instruments (only if a benchtop vacuum sterilizer is to be used)
- a steam sterilizer (in accordance with EN 13060)
- an area for setting down and wrapping instruments sterilized in a benchtop non-vacuum (bowl and instrument) sterilizer
- clean, orderly, enclosed storage for instruments prior to use (not open shelving)
- a dedicated, clean, rigid, labelled box with a lid to transport instruments to the clinical area safely and securely

obtained. The designated specialist can give guidance on this and the local accident and emergency department would probably be the first contact for advice and PEP.

What happens if the patient refuses to be tested?

A patient cannot be forced to give consent for the taking and testing of blood. The designated specialist can evaluate the history taken and give advice on whether the patient is at risk of a blood-borne disease. The patient can be asked to give permission for the practitioner to consult with the patient's general medical practitioner for additional information. The incident should be recorded in detail in an accident report book.

What happens if the source patient is not known?

Exposure may occur while cleaning instruments from several patients. In this case, the patients should be identified and their medical histories reviewed. If the injury can be assessed as constituting a low risk for the transmission of HIV, the immediate administration of PEP against HIV is not necessary. The procedure outlined under mild injury should be followed, with the patients being contacted and asked to give blood for a hepatitis screen. If the injury is significant, then the designated specialist should be asked for advice as to whether PEP is necessary until the patients' medical histories can be reviewed.

Immediate action after high-risk exposure

If PEP is advisable (Box 31.3), then it is important to discuss:

- the advantages and disadvantages of PEP
- the necessary follow-up examinations (of liver and kidneys) after 2 weeks and at 1, 3 and 6 months
- follow-up examination for HIV infection (after 1, 3 and 6 months)

- the importance of avoiding transmission to sexual partner(s) (use of condoms).

Start PEP as soon as possible after this. PEP for cases constituting a high risk of HIV infection is a three-drug combination consisting of two reverse transcriptase inhibitors and at least one protease inhibitor. The current regimen is:

- one Truvada tablet (245 mg tenofovir and 200 mg emtricitabine [FTC]) once a day

plus

- two Kaletra film-coated tablets (200 mg lopinavir and 50 mg ritonavir) twice a day.

The risk of acquiring HIV infection following occupational exposure is *low* – less than 3 per 1000 injuries.

Guidance on HIV PEP from the UK Chief Medical Officers' Expert Advisory Group on AIDS (EAGA; 2008) is given in Appendix 31.1.

Current CDC guidance is similar. Nelfinavir, which was once used, is no longer recommended, since some preparations contain ethyl methane mesylate (EMS), a known animal carcinogen, mutagen and teratogen. This might be relevant to the choice of drugs included in an HIV PEP regimen because many health-care personnel are female and many are of child-bearing age.

INFECTION CONTROL MEASURES

The four UK Health Departments' decontamination policies are generally driven by the European Union's Medical Devices Directive (MDD) 93/42/EEC and the Medical Device Regulations (MDR) 2005 (Box 31.4). 'HTM 01-05', published by the UK Department of Health in 2008 as 'Health Technical Memorandum 01-05: Decontamination in primary care dental practices' and superseded by a new edition published in April 2009 (http://www.dh.gov.uk/en/Publicationsandstatistics/Publications/PublicationsPolicyAndGuidance/DH_089245; accessed 30 September 2013), sets the standards for decontamination.

Infection control includes the safe disposal of sharps and disposable items, and the cleaning and sterilization of reusable dental instruments and devices. Care must be taken to ensure that all instruments are cleaned prior to sterilization, in a safe manner to avoid injury. Use of closed-system cassettes reduces the risk to the DHW during the execution of infection control. When using ultrasonic cleaners, washers and sterilizers, it is important always to follow the manufacturer's instructions. Assurance of sterility of instruments and devices can be obtained through the use of one of several tests; these tests must be performed regularly to ensure that the sterilizer is cleaning all instruments and devices and that these are safe for use on patients. Disinfection after cleaning reduces the number of viable microorganisms on instruments, making them safer to handle; it is not acceptable to use chemical disinfectants (unless this is specifically recommended by the manufacturer), however, and therefore thermal disinfection is necessary.

Thermal disinfection is best achieved by using an automated washer–disinfector (WD), which precedes the use of autoclaves (sterilizers). The high temperature of the water and chemical additives in these devices clean and disinfect the instruments.

Two types of sterilizer are found in primary care dentistry:

- The *vacuum benchtop sterilizer type B* is suitable for wrapped and unwrapped solid items, hollow items and porous loads, and as such is particularly valuable for sterilizing dental handpieces. It is the standard for use in dental practice, since wrapped items can be readily transported, remain sterile up to the point of use, and can be stored for use at a later date, minimizing the risk of cross-contamination.
- The *type N benchtop sterilizer* is an unwrapped instrument and utensil sterilizer suitable for solid devices that are not wrapped. Provided that the proper irrigation and cleaning of lumens and internals of handpieces has been achieved in combination with a WD, handpieces may also be processed in a type N sterilizer. Where remaining hollow items used in the practice are single-use, a type N sterilizer may be the appropriate solution, although this type of technology is being increasingly overtaken by the vacuum-type sterilizer (type B). Instruments processed in a type N sterilizer should ideally be used directly from the sterilizer, as transportation and storage of sterilized items may pose a risk of re-contamination, and should be risk-assessed and controlled to minimize the risk.

Some instruments cannot be steam sterilized and must then be decontaminated according to the manufacturer's instructions. If sending instruments for repair or disposal, decontaminate first.

HEALTH-CARE–ASSOCIATED INFECTIONS

Health-care facilities, particularly hospitals, are well-recognized reservoirs of infection and may be responsible for a wide range of nosocomial (hospital) infections (Ch. 21).

DENTAL UNIT WATER LINES

The main routes of spread for prions, viruses, bacteria, fungi and protozoa in dental environments are via blood, infected equipment, saliva and water droplets, and direct patient contact. The dental unit structure favours the formation of aquatic microbial biofilms in dental unit waterlines (DUWLs), the small-bore flexible plastic tubing that conveys water to handpieces.

Biofilms are well-organized microorganism communities, and active biofilms are a source of microbial contamination of delivered water.

Water delivered to a dental unit is by the so-called independent water system, the microbiological quality of which is extremely important for the water quality flowing from dental handpieces. In one study, over half of the water samples did not comply with the norms for potable water, though no *Enterococcus* or *Legionella* species were detected.

DHWs and patients can be exposed to direct contact with contaminated water both as splatter and as aerosol emitted by handpieces, including rotating and ultrasonic instruments. The most intensive aerosol and splatter emission occurs from an ultrasonic scaler tip or a high-speed handpiece.

Contamination of water in DUWLs is commonplace and the microbes isolated are various (Table 31.3). In one national survey (in Italy), for example, there was water microbial contamination in all dental surgeries examined, and 33% contained *Legionella* species.

Legionella are common in DUWL, as are *Legionella* antibodies in DHWs. One 82-year-old patient appears to have contracted and died from *Legionella* infection emanating from her dental practice, and another case of fatal legionellosis in a dental surgeon concluded that the DUWL was the likely source of the infection. Although there are reports of unusual microbes, such as fungi (*Exophiala mesophila*) or non-tuberculous mycobacteria (NTM; *Mycobacterium simiae* and *M. mucogenicum*), in DUWL, other serious sequelae appear to be reported rarely. DUWL water in one study was only weakly contaminated by *Legionella* species and NTM, leading the authors to conclude that their aerosolization during dental treatment was not significant. The proportion of water samples with microbial levels above those recommended decreases during working or following attempts at disinfection.

Similar microbial contamination is also found in the operatory air, particularly close to the patient and DHW. Nevertheless, the number of published cases of infection resulting from exposure to water from contaminated DUWL is limited.

There is, however, a medico-legal requirement to comply with potable water standards and to conform to public perceptions of water safety. Despite the lack of evidence of a significant level of infection risk, few patients (or DHWs) would choose to be treated in a dental unit where any infection might be present.

Reservoirs and DUWLs should be subject to an effective protocol to eliminate microbial contamination, and routine monitoring to guarantee uncontaminated water for use in dental treatment. Though most of the microorganisms isolated are of low pathogenicity, effective decontamination should be ensured, especially in view of the ever-increasing number of immunocompromised patients treated. It is not the mere presence of microorganisms that is important in DUWL contamination monitoring, but their number, the presence of potential pathogens, and patients' oral cavity microflora. There are challenges in biofilm removal and prevention of regrowth in DUWLs but strategies to reduce the level of contamination are shown in Box 31.5.

PHYSICAL AND CHEMICAL HAZARDS

BURNS

In dentistry, an obvious but avoidable cause of heat burns is instruments just removed from disinfectors/sterilizers; these burns are often caused by the difficulty in gauging the instruments' temperature through the rubber gloves worn by all staff. Autoclaves, WDs and laboratory and surgery compressors can also present explosive risks.

Provided the water-cooling is working efficiently, high-speed handpieces cannot cause burns; if not cooled, they can overheat and burn

Table 31.3 *Microbes isolated in studies from dental unit water lines*[a]

Bacteria	Fungi
Achromobacter xylosoxidans	*Alternaria alternata*
Acinetobacter spp.	*Aspergillus (= Eurotium herbariorum) repens*
Actinomyces spp.	*Aspergillus amstelodami*
Alcaligenes denitificans	*Aspergillus fumigatus*
Bacillus spp.	*Aspergillus glaucus* group
Brevibacterium spp.	*Aspergillus repens*
Brevundimonas vesicularis	*Aspergillus terreus*
Burkholderiaceae	*Candida albicans*
Flavobacterium indologenes	*Candida curvata*
Klebsiella pneumoniae	*Citromyces* spp.
Legionella spp.	*Cladosporium cladosporioides*
Micrococcus luteus	*Geotrichum candidum*
Micrococcus lylae	*Penicillium (glabrum) frequentans*
Moraxella lacunata	*Penicillium aspergilliforme*
Nocardia spp.	*Penicillium diversum*
Ochromobacterum anthropi	*Penicillium herquei*
Pasteurella haemolytica	*Penicillium pusillum*
Pseudomonas acidovorans	*Penicillium roseopurpureum*
Pseudomonas aeruginosa	*Penicillium turolense*
Pseudomonas cepacia	*Rhizopus nigricans*
Pseudomonas fluorescens	*Sclerotium sclerotiorum (Sclerotinia sclerotiorum)*
Pseudomonas pickettii	
Pseudomonas paucimobilis	
Pseudomonas stutzeri	
Pseudomonas testosteroni	
Pseudomonas vesicularis	
Ralstonia pickettii	
Serratia marcescens	
Sphingomonas paucimobilis	
Stenotrophomonas maltophilia	
Staphylococcus capitis	
Staphylococcus cohnii	
Staphylococcus hominis ss. *Novobiosepticus*	
Staphylococcus saprophyticus	
Staphylococcus warneri	
Streptococcus spp.	
Streptomyces albus	
Xanthomonas maltophilia	

[a]Many are also identified in operatory air.

Box 31.5 *Strategies to minimize water-line contamination*

- Flushing water lines for several minutes at the beginning of the day and after periods of disuse
- Using an independent water reservoir system separate from the municipal water source (sterile water)
- Using an independent water reservoir system combined with periodic or continuous application of chemical germicides such as sodium hypochlorite
- Using water purification systems: carbon filtration, reverse osmosis and distillation

---

the patient's mouth. Other possible causes of thermal burns include hot gutta percha, hot dental composition, hot wax, boiling water, steam, naked flames, flammable or explosive fluids, lasers or diathermy, and even operating lights. Fluids heated in a microwave oven may be hotter than they appear, as the container remains cooler. Diathermy is a form of high-frequency electrical energy used either for local tissue warming or for cutting, which can cause burns. Accidents have resulted from metallic parts of the dental chair becoming involved in the electric current path. The localized increase in current density can then cause superficial burns of the skin. Some serious accidents of this nature have also resulted from the use of diathermy units in operating theatres, where higher powers are used and the current path is normally completed by a large area electrode to reduce the current density, which is placed under the patient. Diathermy can cause superficial burning, should the current be misdirected, but any part of the body can be involved if the current density is high enough.

Burns are more likely to occur in the laboratory. Bunsen burners are often causes of burns, and long hair and gloves or clothing can catch light in a Bunsen flame. Burns from the melting and casting of alloys can be more severe. Hot wax knives can cause burns.

CHEMICAL AND MATERIAL HAZARDS

Where work practices are poor, staff can be exposed to a wide range of noxious chemical substances in the dental environment, including gases, vapours, liquids, fumes, dusts and solids. The UK Control of Substances Hazardous to Health (COSHH) Regulations (1988 S1 No. 1657) place specific obligations on employers and the self-employed to control hazardous substances. Such a substance is 'any natural or artificial substance whether it is in solid or liquid form or in the form of a gas or vapour (including micro-organisms) which can constitute a hazard'. In summary, employers are required to:

- assess health risks created by work involving substances hazardous to health
- prevent or control exposure to substances hazardous to health
- provide and use control measures, personal protective equipment, etc., and take all reasonable steps to ensure these are properly used or applied
- maintain control measures in an efficient state and in good working order and repair
- monitor exposure to substances hazardous to health
- provide suitable health surveillance, where appropriate, for the protection of all employees exposed to substances hazardous to health.

All employees and, so far as is reasonably possible, persons on the premises where the work is being carried out, who may be exposed to substances hazardous to health, must be properly informed, instructed and trained. Employees must take steps to protect themselves and others, make full use of control measures and report any defect immediately. COSHH is enforced in the same way as the Health and Safety at Work. Act or any other regulations made under it. Part IA1 of the Approved List for the Classification Packaging and Labelling of Dangerous Substances Regulations (1984; ISBN 011 8839012) lists very toxic, corrosive, harmful or irritant substances hazardous to health.

Most of the chemicals used in dentistry are currently listed on either the OSHA website at http://www.osha.gov/SLTC/laboratories/hazard_recognition.html (accessed 30 September 2013) or the European Union dangerous substances list – Annex 1 of the 67/548/EEC Directive, or are designated as sensitizers by the relevant agencies or institutions, such as the American Conference of Governmental Industrial Hygienists (ACGIH) or the German Senate Commission of the Deutsche Forschungsgemeinschaft (DFG).

Occupational exposure should be minimized wherever possible and it should be a fundamental principle to do this via safe work practices, particularly by storing material in correctly labelled, appropriate and preferably unbreakable containers; avoiding spills and splatter; avoiding contact with eyes and skin; and washing away spilt material with running tap water (see later).

It is better still to consider whether a potentially hazardous substance can be substituted with an innocuous one – as is the case with dental amalgams.

Amalgams and mercury

Mercury hazards are discussed in Chapter 29. Global production and consumption of mercury is decreasing, and the use of amalgam has fallen in many countries. In general, the mercury body burden of DHWs can be kept below the normally accepted toxicological limits and reproductive effects have not been proven, provided a proper mercury hygiene regimen is adopted. Also it is possible to reduce the environmental burden of mercury from dental clinics still further. Mercury levels in saliva do not correlate with the concentrations in blood and urine, but rather with the number of amalgam fillings or of the filling surfaces; mercury in saliva is therefore not recommended for biological monitoring.

Acids and chemicals

Generally, the primary issue for the DHW, as far as acids and chemicals are concerned, is the skin and the eyes (allergic and irritative dermatitis, ocular irritative diseases); acute effects, sensitive effects and inhalation may all be important. Volatile organic compounds (VOCs) in the dental environment include aldehydes (formaldehyde, acetaldehyde, glutaraldehyde propionaldehyde and benzaldehyde), benzene, chloroform, ethylbenzene, methyl methacrylate, toluene and xylenes. Inhalation of these should be avoided as far as possible. One study of chloroform reported no negative health effects on the dentist or assistant, with air vapour levels well below Health and Safety maximum levels.

Chemical burns are all too common. Acids used clinically, such as phosphoric, chromic and trichloracetic, can cause burns. Many stronger acids and corrosives are used in the laboratory; hydrofluoric, sulphuric and nitric acids, as well as caustic soda, are especially dangerous. Such acids and pickling solutions must be stored safely in appropriate and clearly labelled containers and with proper safety precautions (see later).

Anaesthetic gases

Dental clinical personnel may be chronically exposed to anaesthetic gases and vapours, especially if the anaesthetic or relative analgesia equipment is faulty, poorly maintained or used without an effective scavenging system, or if the agents are abused. Nitrous oxide and halothane have known adverse effects but there are as yet few data on any possible adverse occupational effects of isoflurane, enflurane or other agents, apart from occasional asthma (Ch. 15). However, such pollutants are inhaled and absorbed, and appear in the blood and secretions such as breast milk. Headache is common, especially where halothane is used, and there are rare confirmed cases of occupationally acquired halothane hepatitis. However, occupational exposure does not appear to give rise to neuropsychiatric disorders. Mental and neurological performance is not significantly impaired by exposure to inhalational anaesthetic agents under normal working conditions; however, they are, not surprisingly, impaired after exposure to excessive amounts of inhalational anaesthetics – to a greater degree by nitrous oxide than by halothane.

Abuse of nitrous oxide, however, is a well-recognized hazard and can produce neurological damage, a myeloneuropathy caused by nitrous oxide, interfering with vitamin B_{12} metabolism and subsequent DNA production, similar to that of subacute combined degeneration of the spinal cord. Nitrous oxide impairs the enzyme methionine synthetase, which normally catalyses the conversion of homocysteine to methionine. There is early sensory impairment, L'Hermitte's sign (shooting pains when the neck is flexed), leg weakness, ataxia, impotence and loss of sphincter control. Fortunately, the myeloneuropathy improves after exposure to the gas is stopped, though some damage remains, especially in the central nervous system (CNS). Interference with vitamin B_{12} metabolism probably also underlies the bone marrow damage, leading to megaloblastosis seen in bone marrow biopsies of dentists chronically overexposed to nitrous oxide but, surprisingly, macrocytic anaemia does not seem to result. Nitrous oxide appears to be the agent most frequently responsible for occupational exposure.

It has been suggested that DHWs exposed to inhalational general anaesthesia (GA) may be predisposed to disorders of health and reproduction, but the evidence is equivocal. Male dentists have been reported to have more liver, kidney and neurological disorders than controls, while their partners have been reported to have an increased rate of spontaneous abortions. Female dentists exposed to inhalational GA agents have been reported to have an increased risk of spontaneous abortion, congenital abnormalities in children and higher rates of cancer, renal and hepatic diseases. Dental nurses chronically exposed to GA agents may suffer from similar problems and (it has been suggested) may have an increased incidence of cancer of the cervix.

A recent critical review of the available evidence indicates that none of the criteria for the demonstration of toxicity by trace concentrations of GA agents has been adequately fulfilled, and that anxieties over occupational exposure may have been unjustifiably exaggerated. The consensus of data from animal experiments at subanaesthetic concentrations has not yielded convincing evidence of toxicity. Epidemiological studies have also provided no convincing evidence of any effect of chronic exposure to anaesthetic agents on mental performance, cancer or fetal disorders such as low birth weight, stillbirth or malformation. In contrast to anaesthetic personnel, exposure of DHWs to inhalational GA agents is usually for short periods, except where relative analgesia is frequently used.

Though there is little evidence of any significant hazard from gases in the surgery atmosphere, the following precautions should be taken where GA or relative analgesia (inhalational sedation) is used. To reduce contamination of the surgery atmosphere by gases, relative analgesia should not be overused, the machine should be carefully used, adequate surgery ventilation should be provided and, most importantly, a scavenger system should be used. Scavenging systems reduce air pollution by inhalational GA agents but, even when used, nitrous oxide levels in dental surgeries using relative analgesia can still exceed 150 ppm.

Occupational exposure to nitrous oxide can be minimized by the use of scavenging systems, local exhaust systems, careful sedation technique and equipment management. To provide a safer workplace, the following preventive measures should be implemented:

- Reduction of exposure levels to minimum
- Monitoring of levels in the surgery
- Use of effective scavenging equipment and monitoring devices
- Use of an effective delivery system, including a readily visible and accurate flow meter, and a vacuum pump with the capacity for up to 45 L of air per minute per workstation

- Regular inspection of administration equipment for leaks
- Regular maintenance and servicing of equipment
- Direction of waste gas away from windows, ventilators, air-conditioning inlets, or other areas that might allow gases back into the area
- Venting of exhaust gases to the exterior
- Maintenance of adequate ventilation (the general ventilation should provide good room air mixing)
- Use of an airsweep fan
- Minimization of conversation with patients and control of mouth breathing during the use of nitrous oxide
- Shutting off and securing the equipment after each day's use
- Fitting the nasal mask on the patient as well as possible.

Additional recommendations are as follows:

- Improvement of circulation in the surgery by opening a window or using a non-recycling air conditioning system
- Use of a variety of mask sizes to ensure a proper fit for individual patients.

Health-care personnel who should avoid exposure to nitrous oxide (Schumann 1990) include:

- women in the first trimester of pregnancy
- infertile individuals using *in vitro* fertilization procedures
- individuals with neurological complaints
- immunocompromised individuals who are at risk from bone marrow suppression.

Pregnant staff, or staff likely to become pregnant, should not work in a contaminated environment unless there is an effective scavenging system.

Antiseptics

DHWs and patients may also be exposed to chemical agents that are used as topical antiseptics in the dental practice. For example, carbol camphor, eugenol, guaiacol and thymol are endodontic medicaments used as pulp sedatives; zinc oxide as a pulp-capping agent and a root canal antiseptic; hydrogen peroxide and hypochlorite as root canal irrigants; m-cresol, formaldehyde and glutaraldehyde as root canal antiseptics; and chloroform and iodoform may be used during root canal filling. Benzalkonium chloride, benzethonium chloride, chlorhexidine and iodine are antiseptics directly administered to the oral mucosa.

Disinfectants

DHWs may be exposed to disinfectants (such as hydrogen peroxide, sodium hypochlorite, chlorhexidine, formalin, etc.), organic solvents and active (antibacterial) ingredients of disinfectants when they clean surfaces or instruments (with solvent-based disinfectants or water-based agents). Other workers commonly exposed include radiographers, X-ray technicians and cleaners. Reducing workplace exposure to its lowest possible level represents the most important hazard reduction strategy, achieved by keeping containers tightly sealed when not in use, maintaining adequate ventilation levels and adhering rigidly to the use of appropriate personal protective equipment.

Examples of active ingredients in the disinfectants used in the dental environment are o-phenylphenol, benzoyl-p-chlorophenol and n-alkyl-n-benzyl-n,n-dimethylammonium chloride, as well as many others (Box 31.6). Alcohols (ethyl and isopropyl alcohol) are rapidly bactericidal, tuberculocidal, fungicidal and virucidal, but not sporicidal.

Box 31.6 *Disinfectants*

Inorganic

- Acids: boric acid, hydrochloric acid, sulphochromic acid, tartaric acid
- Alkalis: calcium hydrate, potassium hydroxide, sodium carbonate, sodium hydroxide
- Oxidants: peroxide, potassium permanganate
- Inorganic halogens: calcium chloride, chlorine derivates (chloramines, chlorate, hypochlorites), iodine
- Heavy metal salts: mercuric bichloride, mercuric ossicyanide

Organic

- Alcohols: ethyl alcohol, isopropyl alcohol
- Aldehydes/phenols: chlorine cresol, chlorine xylenol, cresol; dichlorine, formaldehyde, glutaraldehyde, hexachlorophene, phenol, polyphenols; xylenol
- Mercury organic compounds: mercurochrome, mercuric phenyl nitrate
- Chlorine/iodine organic compounds: chloramine, dichloramine iodine, povidone/betadine
- Quaternary ammonium derivates: benzalkonium, benzoxonium, benzetonium chloride, cetrimide

---

Sodium hypochlorite has broad-spectrum antimicrobial activity but is inactivated in the presence of organic matter, and hypochlorite solutions may bleach and damage the texture of fabrics and corrode or damage materials such as stainless steel instruments. Hypochlorite solutions are unstable; they need to be prepared fresh for use and to be used within 24 hours. Antiseptics or disinfectants that have raised most concern have included formaldehyde and glutaraldehyde.

Formaldehyde is bactericidal, tuberculocidal, fungicidal, virucidal and sporicidal. However, its irritant and carcinogenic properties limit its use. Glutaraldehyde is an effective disinfectant but is irritant to eyes, skin and lungs, so gloves of material impermeable to glutaraldehyde, full facial shield and waterproof gowns or aprons are necessary for personal protection wherever glutaraldehyde preparations are used. It has been withdrawn or banned in many countries.

Methyl methacrylate

Acrylic monomer is the most common organic solution used in dentistry; the main component is methyl methacrylate, but it may also contain other monomers such as N-butylmethacrylate, isobutyl-methacrylate, laurylmethacrylate, 1,4-butanediol dimethacrylate or ethylene glycol dimethacrylate. Polymerization inhibitors such as hydroquinone, p-methoxyphenol or butylated cresols; plasticizers such as dibutyl phthalate; ultraviolet light absorbers such as benzophenone; and activators such as dimethyl-p-toluidine may also be found.

Methyl methacrylate and cyanoacrylate may be used for solvent abuse but, in the absence of abuse, there is little evidence of a serious hazard if reasonable care is taken. Chemical hepatitis due to overexposure to methyl methacrylate monomer has been rarely reported, as have methyl methacrylate and cyanoacrylate-induced occupational asthma or dermatitis. Methyl methacrylate monomer may cause transient nausea if inhaled in large quantities, possibly by central depression of gastric motor function; *rarely*, monomer has caused dyspnoea and hypertension. It may also soften soft contact lenses.

In technicians using methyl methacrylate, the monomer is absorbed through skin, even to some extent where 'protective' creams are used. Unfortunately, many gloves are permeable to monomer, and barrier creams may impede the setting of acrylic. Urine analysis shows low methacrylate levels in the morning but clear evidence of percutaneous absorption throughout the working day. Handling of methyl methacrylate may occasionally cause transient finger and palmar paraesthesia, pain and whitening of the fingers in the cold, local neurotoxicity and an eczema-like reaction. Contact dermatitis as a result of handling methyl methacrylate monomer is also a possibility but is surprisingly rare.

Methyl methacrylate is embryotoxic and fetotoxic to rats (as is toluene). Though there is no evidence of such a danger to humans from methyl methacrylate, this should be borne in mind as a hazard, but probably no more than a theoretical one, in the case of female dental technicians.

There is no evidence of any permanent toxic effects from methyl methacrylate monomer under conditions of normal use.

Volatile, highly flammable chemicals

Methyl methacrylate monomer and gases such as oxygen are commonly used in dentistry. These must be stored properly in a correctly labelled strong container and not used near flames, or a fire or explosion could result. Many alcohols, acetone, and solvents and thinners are toxic and may be flammable (Box 31.7). Some can also cause dermatitis and damage the eyes and respiratory tract; chronic exposure may cause renal or liver damage; and some, such as toluene, are teratogenic.

X-ray developers

Developers for radiographs contain hydroquinone; fixatives contain acetic acid and sodium thiosulphate. These solutions may cause

---

Box 31.7 *Especially hazardous flammable fluids that may be used in dentistry*

- Acetone
- Alcohols (ethyl alcohol, methyl alcohol, isopropyl alcohol)
- Benzene[a]
- Butane
- Ethers
- Ethylene oxide[a]
- Methyl methacrylate monomer
- Propane
- Toluene
- Xylene

Acids

- Chromic
- Hydrochloric
- Hydrofluoric
- Nitric
- Phosphoric
- Sulphuric
- Trichloracetic

Alkalis

- Ammonium hydroxide
- Sodium hydroxide
- Sodium hypochlorite

Other dangerous fluids

- Carbon tetrachloride[a]
- Chloroform[a]
- Methylene chloride

[a] Possible carcinogens.

---

dermatitis, conjunctivitis or bronchitis, and so should be handled carefully and with rubber gloves, avoiding contact with the eyes (it is best to wear protective eyewear) and avoiding excessive inhalation.

'Sick building syndrome'

The term 'sick building syndrome' refers to vague symptoms that develop in some office workers during the working week but abate at weekends and during holidays. The cause is unclear.

'Darkroom disease'

There have been reports of an unexplained medical syndrome, 'darkroom disease', among radiographers or medical radiation technologists. Several of the symptom clusters reported are similar to those of other medically unexplained syndromes with overlapping features, such as sick building syndrome. These workers have potential exposure to processing chemicals involved in developing and fixing films, including sensitizers and irritants, such as glutaraldehyde, formaldehyde, sulphur dioxide (SO_2) and acetic acid.

RADIATION HAZARDS

Radiation hazards in dental practice are mainly from ionizing radiation, as in X-rays, but there may also be hazards from the light sources used for curing composite materials and occasionally from other sources, such as lasers.

IONIZING RADIATION

Ionizing radiation has a wavelength shorter than 10 nm, and can be artificial (such as X-rays) or come from natural sources. Exposure can induce mutations in the germinal tissues (teratogenic effect) or malignant tumours in other tissues (oncogenic effect). Exposure to ionizing radiation must therefore be kept to the absolute minimum. It is a hazard especially to the fetus or young child, or where cells are proliferating rapidly, as in the gonads and bone marrow.

Acute high-level overexposure may cause radiation sickness and gastrointestinal and haematological damage, but most occupational exposure is at a lower level and is prolonged; radiosensitive, rapidly dividing cells (such as in the fetus, skin or bone marrow) are then at risk. Additional and possibly more important radiation hazards are those from accidents (e.g. Fukushima, Chernobyl), nuclear explosions, and domestic radon exposure in buildings situated over uranium-bearing strata, in such areas as parts of Cornwall, Devon, Somerset and Aberdeen, and also in some areas of Cumbria, Staffordshire, the West Midlands and Mid-Glamorgan. More than 75% of the annual exposure of the UK population to ionizing radiation is from such natural sources from radon (an alpha-emitting gas) – a hazard that might equal in magnitude that posed by cigarette smoking and toxic waste.

Therapeutic radiation may also predispose later to malignant tumours but there has really been concern only about diagnostic radiation in this respect. The use of dental diagnostic radiographs has been implicated as a risk for meningioma. Patients receiving bitewing or panorex dental X-ray examinations annually or more frequently were more than twice as likely to develop meningioma (in children the risk was greater). There may also be an increased risk of thyroid cancer.

Long-term follow-up studies of patients who have had radiation treatment have also shown significant risk for tumours to develop in the radiation field. For example, radiotherapy for Hodgkin disease may lead to breast cancer later; patients irradiated for breast carcinoma, particularly smokers, may develop lung cancer.

There is an increased risk of salivary tumours in patients who have received radiation to the tonsils and nasopharynx. More worryingly, radiotherapy in the past for benign diseases of the skin (acne, tinea capitis, haemangiomas) and for tonsillitis led to substantially increased risks of thyroid cancer and parotid, parathyroid and CNS tumours. Radiation treatment for benign conditions has increased with the advent of stereotactic delivery and, in particular, single high-dose gamma-knife therapy. This is used for benign CNS tumours (e.g. vestibular schwannoma, meningioma, pituitary adenoma and haemangioblastoma). There are concerns regarding the use of radiotherapy in childhood and in tumour-predisposing syndromes. Intensity-modulated radiation therapy (IMRT) may reduce the adverse effects of radiation on normal tissues but this is controversial. Proton therapy may offer further improvement in dose localization over photons (X-rays) and reduce the risk of second malignancies.

NON-IONIZING RADIATION

Non-ionizing radiation has many forms.

Electromagnetic (radiofrequency) radiation is emitted by a variety of sources ranging from transmitter towers to electric power lines, computer terminals, electric clocks, microwave ovens and electric blankets. The public has become concerned about possible adverse effects from electromagnetic fields emanating from power transmission lines but the evidence indicates that there is little, if any, reliable evidence for a health risk; in any event, there is more exposure to electromagnetic radiation from household appliances and wiring than from power lines. Moreover, *natural* electromagnetic radiation is at least 100 times as intense as that induced by power lines. There is no evidence that exposure to electromagnetic radiation at these radiofrequencies and power levels poses any other health hazard to normal persons but some individuals fitted with cardiac pacemakers could be at risk (Ch. 5).

Ultraviolet (UV) light is emitted especially by the sun and the universally recognized consequence of overexposure is sunburn, but there are also hazards to the eyes mainly (cataracts) and skin (predisposition to melanoma and squamous or basal cell carcinoma). UV and other lights may be used in dentistry (Table 31.4). The eyes are at risk from acute and cumulative effects, mainly due to back-reflection of the blue light. Furthermore, phototoxic and photoallergic reactions originating from absorbed radiation in endogenous or exogenous substances accumulated in the DHW's eyes and skin, as well as the patients' oral mucosa, must also be taken into consideration. Prevent problems by reading the manufacturers' instructions and using radiation-filtering protection goggles.

UVB (wavelengths between 286 and 320 nm) is responsible for most sunburn and also snow blindness (actinic retinitis). UVA (wavelengths between 320 and 400 nm) is the most dangerous and causes chronic damage to the eye, cataracts and damage to the retina. UVA light sources in dentistry include UV sources for curing of restorative resins and fissure sealants and UV plaque lights (320–365 nm), but these have largely been replaced by blue light sources. Protective eyewear should be worn to absorb the wavelengths of any light sources used.

Blue light (400–500 nm) sources were developed to overcome the dangers of UV radiation and activate diketones in dental composite materials. However, blue light is not entirely safe, since it contains high-energy photons with the potential to form reactive free radicals in the eye, and these produce peroxides that denature photoreceptors in the retina. Blue light may be up to 30 times more damaging than UV light to the retina and may possibly also predispose to cataract.

White (visible) light (400–700 nm) is much safer but also emits minute amounts of both UV and blue light, and green light (490–600 nm), so protective eyewear that absorbs these wavelengths should still be worn.

Laser is the acronym for *l*ight *a*mplification by *s*timulated *e*mission of *r*adiation. In general, lasers rapidly heat and acoustically shock tissues; all are potentially hazardous, particularly because of eye damage, burns and the risks of fire or electric shock. There is also concern that microorganisms might be transmissible in laser smoke. *All* lasers should therefore always be used with great care and *never* shone into the eyes, in unintended directions or on to brightly plated instruments that reflect the laser. Protective eyewear and facemasks should be worn.

The effect of a laser on target tissue depends on the wavelength, beam power, degree of focus, duration of exposure and distance to target, as well as the absorption by the tissue. The wavelength of the photons (radiation) is controlled by the type of laser and the lasing medium. There are hundreds of different lasers in use but the main ones used in health care are the carbon dioxide (CO_2), Nd:YAG (neodymium, yttrium, aluminium, garnet) and argon-ion lasers (Table 31.5).

The CO_2 *laser* emits infrared light (wavelength 10.6 micrometres), which is invisible but absorbed by water-containing tissues. It damages tissue by heat and can be used to cut soft and hard tissues. Because the CO_2 laser is invisible, it is used co-axially with a helium–neon laser to produce a visible red beam. CO_2 lasers are expensive and potentially very dangerous.

Table 31.4 *Light hazards*

Radiation	Based on	Applications
Conventional blue or white light	Light-emitting diode (LED) or tungsten quartz halogen	Bonding, composite resin sealants and restorative materials, luting agents
Plasma arc lamps	430–490 nm	Rapid-cure resins
Intense pulsed light (IPL)	Xenon lamp	Aesthetic surgery

Table 31.5 *Lasers*

Laser	Based on	Applications
Argon	488 nm	Tooth whitening
		Increase of resin adhesion, polymerization and reduction of microleakage
	514.5 nm	Soft-tissue surgery
Carbon dioxide	10 600 nm	Soft-tissue surgery
Diode	800–830 nm	Soft-tissue surgery
	980 nm gallium aluminium arsenide (GaAlAs)	Bleaching
Erbium	2940 nm and 2780 nm	Hard- and soft-tissue procedures
Nd:YAG (neodymium, yttrium, aluminium, garnet)	1064 nm	Soft-tissue surgery
Potassium titanyl phosphate (KTP)	532 nm	Aesthetic surgery

The *Nd:YAG laser* (wavelength 1.06 micrometres) and krypton lasers are also used clinically and have the great advantage that they can be transmitted down a fibreoptic path. The Nd:YAG (near-infrared) laser is invisible and therefore used with a helium–neon laser. It is employed in dentistry for cutting dentine and soft tissues, and also for photocoagulation.

The *argon laser* produces a blue–green light of 0.5-micrometre wavelength and can be transmitted by fibreoptics. It is used in dentistry mainly for polymerizing some composite materials. It is also used for photocoagulation.

Soft lasers include the helium–neon (He–Ne) laser, which produces light of 0.63-micrometre wavelength, and the diode laser (0.90-micrometre wavelength), which emits light in the near-infrared or visible part of the spectrum and, if restricted to only milliwatt powers, produces little if any heating or a direct photochemical effect on tissues. The beam of a soft laser penetrates directly only to a depth of about 0.8 mm and is less damaging than others, but still must be used with care as there is some hazard to the retina.

Video display units (VDUs or monitors) operate in the same way as television receivers, emitting light that forms the image on the screen, but excitation of the phosphors by the electron beam also causes emission of minute amounts of UV and infrared rays, and low-energy X-rays. Very low-frequency (VLF) and extremely low-frequency (ELF) electromagnetic radiation is also emitted but the levels are exceedingly low – often lower than those from domestic appliances.

The evidence indicates that VDUs are not responsible for cataracts, reproductive disorders, fetal congenital abnormalities or facial dermatitis. Musculoskeletal disorders and stress may be induced by VDUs. There is some evidence that these can be genuine problems, and that pains and stiffness in the neck, shoulders, back and wrists, along with carpal tunnel syndrome – repetitive strain injury (RSI), are not uncommon; however, this is related more to poor posture and the elimination of tasks that once required office workers to get up and move around once in a while, rather than concentrating on the VDU itself. Prolonged work at VDUs is fatiguing, particularly for those with minor visual defects, as correction for middle-distance viewing is rarely carried out adequately, and it is possible that the resulting eyestrain may lead to blurred vision, tension and headaches. This, in turn, can lead to depression and some of the other symptoms sometimes ascribed to working with VDUs. A further concern has been that the flickering of the VDU display might provoke epileptic attacks but there is no good evidence.

HAZARDS TO SPECIFIC BODY SYSTEMS

EYES

Care should be taken to avoid eye infections and damage from projected particles when using the air rotor, grinding metals or cutting wire. Penetrating wounds can cause deep injuries and even loss of sight. Chemicals such as chromic acid, hydrofluoric acid, phosphoric acid, sodium hypochlorite and trichloracetic acid can also cause serious eye damage. Radiation is an eye hazard.

Blue and UV light sources with wavelengths shorter than 400–500 nm (this is mainly a UV danger) cause cumulative eye damage; the shortest wavelengths are most damaging. Protective glasses should be worn to filter out all light under about 500 nm; glasses with red-, orange- or yellow-coloured lenses of sufficient optical density are therefore indicated when using blue or UV light. Ordinary dark glasses do *not* filter

out these offending wavelengths; indeed, by absorbing visible light, they can cause pupil dilatation and therefore aggravate the problem.

HEARING

Loud noise (85 dB or more) can irreversibly damage the inner ear hair receptor cells of the organ of Corti in the cochlea. Ultrasonic scalers may produce slight tinnitus after prolonged use but this rarely appears to be clinically significantly either to patients or to staff. Otherwise, the overall evidence suggests that hearing is not impaired in clinical DHWs compared with age-matched controls, provided modern well-maintained equipment (such as air rotors) is used.

MENTAL HEALTH

Despite the low risks in dentistry, DHWs clearly perceive that occupationally related diseases, especially stress, are common. Dentistry, even for students, appears to be somewhat stressful but perhaps less so than medicine and some other professions. Dentists and dental hygienists complain particularly of musculoskeletal discomfort and of stress; dental nurses complain mainly about allergies and respiratory infections.

Drug abuse in dentistry and medicine is increasing, and the incidence of alcohol and other drug abuse (including nitrous oxide or other inhalational anaesthetics) by doctors and dentists is higher than for comparable groups.

MUSCULOSKELETAL COMPLAINTS

Probably as a result of poor working positions and possibly stress, DHWs tend to develop musculoskeletal complaints. Although there appear to be few reliable objective studies of postural and skeletal problems in DHWs, one radiograph survey in Finland showed cervical spondylosis in about 50% of dentists, compared with about 20% of farmers of the same age. Dentists also had somewhat more radiographic changes in the shoulder joint but less lumbar spondylosis than farmers.

Activities involving repetitive wrist and hand movements, especially in women, may result in oedema beneath the transverse carpal ligament at the wrist. This can lead to compression of the median nerve and subsequent pain (especially at night), paraesthesia, hypoaesthesia and weakness in the wrist and hand (carpal tunnel syndrome). Though this is a common consequence of a variety of activities and is predisposed to by, for example, pregnancy or hypothyroidism, carpal tunnel syndrome has been reported in hygienists and endodontists in particular. Symptoms and signs consistent with partial carpal tunnel syndrome have been noted in one-quarter or more of hygienists in some surveys, but the diagnosis is far less frequent. Typists may also suffer the same symptoms.

Rest and analgesics usually provide adequate relief but, occasionally, splinting or corticosteroid injections are required. Surgical decompression may be indicated for recalcitrant cases.

PREGNANCY

Hazards from exposure to anaesthetic gases, mercury, ionizing radiation and infections have caused concern among female dental staff, but most evidence suggests that there is little if any specific occupational risk to the outcome of pregnancy. Pregnant female staff may, understandably, be concerned about possible risks to their fetus from ionizing radiation but, provided the rules of radiation protection are carefully followed, even female radiography or radiology staff appear to be at no significant risk. However, non-immune or immunocompromised female staff and their fetus may be at risk from various infections, notably rubella, cytomegalovirus and varicella zoster virus. Pre-conception immunization and universal cross-infection control procedures should obviate this risk.

One study of 558 female dental surgeons and 450 high-school teachers who had given birth to at least 1 living child examined the effects of practising dentistry and of workplace exposure on fertility. Most of the female dental surgeons were using amalgam for fillings during the period they tried to conceive; 33% placed more than 50 fillings a week; 75% of the dental surgeons reported handling chloroform-based root-canal sealers; and 40% were exposed to disinfectants (containing ethanol and benzene) on a daily basis. No difference in fertility was found between the dental surgeons and the high-school teachers. Exposure to mercury, chloroform and benzene was not associated with decreased fertility.

RESPIRATORY SYSTEM

DHWs should position patients properly and use barriers (e.g. face shields, surgical masks, gowns), rubber dams and high-volume evacuators to prevent contact with splashes and splatter; these tend not to pass to the lungs but may settle on the conjunctiva or nasal mucosa, or on the nearby surfaces or equipment. Aerosols are suspensions of fine particles less than 50 micrometres in size; most of them are smaller than 5 micrometres. They remain airborne for extended periods of time – 24 hours or more, are dispersed widely by air currents and may be inhaled. Aerosols and splatter can contain microorganisms arising from the dental unit water or the patient, and readily contaminate the operating area. Infections of most concern, owing to their high morbidity or mortality, are hepatitis viruses and HIV, though the evidence discounts a risk (http://www.cdc.gov/oralhealth/infectioncontrol/faq/aerosols.htm; accessed 30 September 2013). However, respiratory viruses such as those causing avian flu, and bacteria such as those causing tuberculosis and legionellosis (Ch. 15), have been transmitted to dental staff, as have adenoviruses and a variety of agents, including *Chlamydia trachomatis* – but these incidents are rare.

Dusts can also damage the respiratory system. They can be created during various dental procedures and can constitute a hazard where work practices are poor, especially in the dental laboratory (Table 31.6).

There is little evidence of occupational lung disease among clinical dental staff but the drilling of teeth and old amalgams creates dust (and mercury vapour) if there is inadequate water-cooling. There has also been concern about the increased microbial counts and silica particles of the aerosols and dusts produced during procedures such as orthodontic debonding. Mixing alginate impression materials can also create dust from alginate salts and calcium sulphate, silica compounds and diatomaceous earth, fluoride salts, zinc oxide or barium sulphate and various filler particles. These materials may produce a hazard because of either the lead content or the siliceous fibres, though objective evidence for injury from these is weak.

In the laboratory, there are a number of possible sources of dust, ranging from pumice to various metals. The possible consequences of inhalation of these dusts are unclear but there are reports of mild dyspnoea, respiratory infections, pneumoconioses and possibly lung cancer in dental laboratory technicians. To date, most reports of pneumoconiosis in dental technicians relate to silica dust inhalation from polishing and sandblasting using outdated equipment. Cancer may be due to tobacco use rather than dust inhalation.

Chemicals can also damage the respiratory system, directly or via allergic reactions. Clinical staff have occasionally developed asthma after exposure to enflurane. Dental laboratory technicians may be exposed to a number of toxic materials, including metal alloys such as Vitallium, Wisil, Duralium and Vironite, which are used in the production of crowns, bridges and dental prostheses; the most common constituents are chromium, cobalt, molybdenum, nickel, silica, tantalum and other metals. Occupational asthma has been precipitated in nurses and dental technicians by methyl cyanoacrylates and methacrylate. Beryllium, chlorhexidine, chromium, cobalt, formaldehyde, glutaraldehyde and nickel are other potential causes.

Electrostatic or high-efficiency particulate air (HEPA) filters significantly reduce aerosols containing microorganisms or dusts. Face masks rarely filter particles smaller than 5 micrometres in diameter and their filtering efficiency varies from 14% to 99%. Nevertheless, face masks do filter a great deal of debris. They should preferably be changed every hour. In the laboratory, local lathe ventilation is mandatory; a plexiglass shield will reduce splatter and dust extraction is vital.

SKIN

The main skin problems in dentistry are maceration (water-logging) and dermatitis from repeated hand-washing, candidosis secondary to maceration, and infections such as herpetic whitlow and contact dermatitis. It has been suggested that as many as one-third of dental staff suffer from contact allergies.

Dermatitis can result from direct chemical irritation of the skin or, in a susceptible individual, from an allergic response (contact allergy), which is a type 4 (delayed hypersensitivity) reaction (Table 31.7). Hand dermatitis is seen particularly frequently in dental technicians, of whom up to one-third may suffer; the most common causes are direct irritation and a reaction to acrylic monomer.

DHWs may be at increased risk of developing occupational allergic diseases, especially to methacrylates in acrylic resins, or dental bonding products that can permeate many disposable gloves. DHWs may develop dermatitis from chemicals or latex gloves, or mainly from repeated hand-washing.

Using adequate personal protective equipment, like nitrile rubber or neoprene gloves, is the most important preventive measure.

Table 31.6 *Possibly hazardous mineral dusts in dentistry*

Mineral	Found in some
Albite	Porcelain veneers
Andalusite	Silicate cement powders
Calcium sulphate	Gypsum products
Chrysolite	Asbestos ring liners
Cristobalite	Casting investments
Diatomite	Alginates
Labradorite	Porcelain veneers
Metals (various)	See text
Microcline	Porcelain veneers
Orthoclase	Porcelain veneers
Quartz	Casting investments
Sillimanite	Silicate cement powders
Spinelles	Cement powders

Table 31.7 *Some skin irritants and allergens used in dentistry*

Irritants	Recognized allergens	Rarely allergic
Abrasives (pumice, silica, calcium carbonate)	p-Chloro-m-xylenol	Acrylic monomer
	Epoxy resin	Balsam of Peru
Adhesives (epoxy and cyanoacrylates)	Ethylenediamine dihydrochloride	Beeswax
		Benzalkonium chloride
	Formaldehyde	Benzocaine
Amalgam	Lanolin	Benzophenone
Detergents	Latex	Benzoyl peroxide
Essential oils (eugenol)	Mercaptobenzothiazole (rubber gloves, rubber bands and dams, Band-Aids)	Bronopol
Etching compounds (phosphoric acid, 38%)		Camphor (plasticizer in acrylics)
Germicidal solutions	Neomycin	Chlorhexidine
		Chlorocresol
Resins and catalysts	Nickel	Chlorothymol
Soaps	Parabens (medications, toothpaste)	Cinnamon oil
Solvents		Cobalt
	Potassium dichromate	Eugenol
	Rosin (colophony)	Glutaraldehyde
	Thiomersal (disinfectants)	Gold
		Hexachlorophane
		Hexylresorcinol
		Hydroquinone (inhibitor for acrylic resin systems)
		N-Isopropyl-N-phenyl-p-phenylenediamine (IPPD; rubber)
		Menthol
		Methyl dichlorobenzene sulphonate
		Methyl ethyl ketone (MEK) peroxide (catalyst for acrylic resin systems)
		Methyl-p-toluene sulphonate
		Methyl salicylate (toothpastes)
		Nickel
		Penicillin
		Povidone–iodine
		Procaine
		Resorcinol monobenzoate (ultraviolet inhibitor in clear plastics)
		Tetracaine (amethocaine)
		Triethylenetetramine (catalyst for epoxy resins)
		Zirconium (e.g. polishing paste)

KEY WEBSITES

(Accessed 11 June 2013)

Centers for Disease Control and Prevention. <http://www.cdc.gov/niosh/topics/dentistry/>.

Health and Safety Executive. <http://www.hse.gov.uk/pubns/ohindex.htm>.

NHS Scotland. <http://www.scotland.gov.uk/Resource/Doc/158730/0043080.pdf>.

USEFUL WEBSITES

(Accessed 11 June 2013)

American Academy of Family Physicians. <http://www.aafp.org/>.

Centers for Disease Control and Prevention. <http://www.cdc.gov/niosh/topics>.

Medicines and Healthcare Products Regulatory Agency: A–Z index. <http://www.mhra.gov.uk/SearchHelp/A-Zindex/index.htm>.

Medicines and Healthcare Products Regulatory Agency: Guidance on the safe use of lasers, IPL systems and LEDs – DB 2008(03). <http://www.mhra.gov.uk/Publications/Safetyguidance/DeviceBulletins/CON014775>.

RDH. <http://www.rdhmag.com/articles/print/volume-27/issue-4/feature/instrument-sterilization-in-dentistry.html>.

FURTHER READING

Ajami, B., et al., 2012. Contamination of a dental unit water line system by Legionella pneumophila in the Mashhad School of Dentistry in 2009. Iran. Red Crescent Med. J. 14 (6), 376. Epub 2012 Jun 30. PubMed PMID: 22924117; PubMed Central PMCID: PMC3420029.

American Academy on Pediatric Dentistry Clinical Affairs Committee; American Academy on Pediatric Dentistry Council on Clinical Affairs, 2008–2009. Policy on minimizing occupational health hazards associated with nitrous oxide. Pediatr. Dent. 30 (Suppl. 7), 64.

Brown, P.N., 2004. What's ailing us? Prevalence and type of long-term disabilities among an insured cohort of orthodontists. Am. J. Orthod. Dentofacial Orthop. 125, 3.

Bruzell Roll, E.M., et al., 2004. Health hazards associated with curing light in the dental clinic. Clin. Oral Investig. 8, 113.

Castiglia, P., et al., 2008. Italian multicenter study on infection hazards during dental practice: control of environmental microbial contamination in public dental surgeries. BMC Public Health 8, 187. doi:10.1186/1471-2458-8-187.

Claus, E.B., et al., 2012. Dental x-rays and risk of meningioma. Cancer 118 (18), 4530. doi:10.1002/cncr.26625 Epub 2012 Apr 10. PubMed PMID: 22492363; PubMed Central PMCID: PMC3396782.

Corrocher, P.A., Presoto, C.D., Campos, J.A., Garcia, P.P., 2013. The association between restorative pre-clinical activities and musculoskeletal disorders. Eur. J. Dent. Educ.10.1111/eje.12070 [Epub ahead of print] PubMed PMID: 24266890.

Dutil, S., et al., 2007. Aerosolization of mycobacteria and legionellae during dental treatment: low exposure despite dental unit contamination. Environ. Microbiol. 9 (11), 2836. PubMed PMID: 17922766.

Fasunloro, A., Owotade, F.J., 2004. Occupational hazards among clinical dental staff. J. Contemp. Dent. Pract. 5, 134.

Godwin, C.C., et al., 2003. Indoor environment quality in dental clinics: potential concerns from particulate matter. Am. J. Dent. 16, 260.

Harrel, S., Molinari, J., 2004. Aerosols and splatter in dentistry: a brief review of the literature and infection control implications. J. Am. Dent. Assoc. 135, 429.

Helmis, C.G., et al., 2007. Indoor air quality in a dentistry clinic. Sci. Total Environ. 377, 349.

Hörsted-Bindslev, P., 2004. Amalgam toxicity – environmental and occupational hazards. J. Dent. 32, 359.

Hylander, L.D., et al., 2006. High mercury emissions from dental clinics despite amalgam separators. Sci. Total Environ. 362, 74.

Iyer, R., Jhingran, A., 2006. Radiation injury: imaging findings in the chest, abdomen and pelvis after therapeutic radiation. Cancer Imaging 6 (Spec No A), S131.

Khan, S.A., Chew, K.Y., 2013. Effect of working characteristics and taught ergonomics on the prevalence of musculoskeletal disorders amongst dental students. BMC Musculoskelet Disord 14, 118.10.1186/1471-2474-14-118. PubMed PMID: 23547959; PubMed Central PMCID: PMC3626888.

Kumar, S., et al., 2010. Dental unit waterlines: source of contamination and cross-infection. J. Hosp. Infect. 74 (2), 99.10.1016/j.jhin.2009.03.027 Review. PubMed PMID: 20113847.

Labrie, D., et al., 2011. Evaluation of ocular hazards from 4 types of curing lights. J. Can. Dent. Assoc. 77, b116.

Leggat, P.A., et al., 2007. Occupational health problems in modern dentistry: a review. Ind. Health 45, 611.

Longstreth Jr., W.T., et al., 2004. Dental X-rays and the risk of intracranial meningioma: a population-based case-control study. Cancer 100 (5), 1026. PubMed PMID: 14983499.

Memon, A., et al., 2010. Dental X-rays and the risk of thyroid cancer: a case-control study. Acta Oncol. 49 (4), 447. doi:10.3109/02841861003705778 PubMed PMID: 20397774.

Mikov, I., et al., 2011. Occupational contact allergic dermatitis in dentistry. Vojnosanit. Pregl. 68 (6), 523.

Nermin, Y., 2006. Musculoskeletal disorders (MSDs) and dental practice. Part 1. General information terminology, aetiology, work-relatedness, magnitude of the problem, and prevention. Int. Dent. J. 56 (6), 359.

Ozcan, M., et al., 2012. Possible hazardous effects of hydrofluoric acid and recommendations for treatment approach: a review. Clin. Oral Investig. 16 (1), 15. doi:10.1007/s00784-011-0636-6 Epub 2011 Nov 9.

Palenik, C.J., 2012. Legionella pneumonia and dental unit waterlines. Dent. Update 39 (4), 237. PubMed PMID: 22774685.

Palenik, C.J., 2012. Mandatory influenza vaccination. Dent. Update 39 (7), 454. PubMed PMID: 23094566.

Pandis, N., et al., 2007. Occupational hazards in orthodontics: a review of risks and associated pathology. Am. J. Orthod. Dentofacial Orthop. 132, 280.

Pankhurst, C.L., Coulter, W.A., 2007. Do contaminated dental unit waterlines pose a risk of infection? J. Dent. 35 (9), 712. Epub 2007 Aug 6. Review. PubMed PMID: 17689168.

Porteous, N.B., et al., 2003. Isolation of an unusual fungus in treated dental unit waterlines. J. Am. Dent. Assoc. 134 (7), 853. PubMed PMID: 12892442.

Porteous, N.B., et al., 2004. Isolation of non-tuberculosis mycobacteria in treated dental unit waterlines. Oral Surg. Oral Med. Oral Pathol. Oral Radiol. Endod. 98 (1), 40. PubMed PMID: 15243469.

Puriene, A., et al., 2007. Occupational hazards of dental profession to psychological wellbeing. Stomatologija 9, 72.

Ricci, M.L., et al., 2012. Pneumonia associated with a dental unit waterline. Lancet 379 (9816), 684. doi:10.1016/S0140-6736(12)60074-9 PubMed PMID: 22340301.

Samaranayake, L., Scully, C., 2013. Needlestick and occupational exposure to infections: a compendium of current guidelines. Br. Dent. J. 215 (4), 163.10.1038/sj.bdj.2013.791 PubMed PMID: 23969653.

Schumann, D., 1990. Nitrous oxide anaesthesia: risks to health personnel. Int. Nurs. Rev. 37 (1), 214.

Scully, C., et al., 1990. Occupational hazards to dental staff. B. Dent. J., London.

Shorman, H.A., et al., 2002. Management of dental unit water lines. Dent. Update 29, 292.

Szymańska, J., 2001. Environmental health risk of chronic exposure to nitrous oxide in dental practice. Ann. Agric. Environ. Med. 8, 119.

Szymańska, J., 2004. Risk of exposure to Legionella in dental practice. Ann. Agric. Environ. Med. 11, 9–12.

Szymańska, J., 2005. Evaluation of mycological contamination of dental unit waterlines. Ann. Agric. Environ. Med. 12 (1), 153. PubMed PMID: 16028882.

Szymańska, J., 2005. Microbiological risk factors in dentistry. Current status of knowledge. Ann. Agric. Environ. Med. 12, 157.

Szymańska, J., Sitkowska, J., 2013. Bacterial contamination of dental unit waterlines. Environ. Monit. Assess. 185 (5), 3603. doi:10.1007/s10661-012-2812-9 Epub 2012 Aug 17.

Tadakamadla, J., et al., 2012. Occupational hazards and preventive practices among students and faculty at a private dental institution in India. Stomatologija 14 (1), 28.

Takigawa, T., Endo, Y., 2006. Effects of glutaraldehyde exposure on human health. J. Occup. Health 48 (2), 75.

Toroglu, M.S., et al., 2003. Possibility of blood and hepatitis B contamination through aerosols generated during debonding procedures. Angle Orthod. 73, 571.

Veronesi, L., et al., 2004. Health hazard evaluation in private dental practices: a survey in a province of northern Italy. Acta Biomed. 75, 50.

Zimmer, H., et al. 2002. Determination of mercury in blood, urine and saliva for the biological monitoring of an exposure from amalgam fillings in a group with self-reported adverse health effects. Int. J. Hyg. Environ. Health 205, 205.

APPENDIX 31.1 GUIDANCE ON HIV PEP FROM THE UK CHIEF MEDICAL OFFICERS' EXPERT ADVISORY GROUP ON AIDS (EAGA; 2008)

All health-care workers (HCWs) should be informed and educated about possible risks from occupational exposure, and should be aware of the importance of seeking urgent advice following occupational exposure.

Any significant exposure to blood and some other body fluids or tissues has the potential to transmit blood-borne infections. Many exposures result from failure to follow recommended safe handling and disposal of needles and syringes, or wearing personal protective eyewear.

An integrated approach to post-exposure management with respect to HIV, HBV and HCV is recommended. Employers should have a policy on the management of exposures, which should specify the local arrangements for risk assessment, advice and the provision of PEP. The policy must ensure that adequate 24-hour cover is available and should designate one or more doctors to whom exposed persons may be referred urgently for advice.

HIV AND SIGNIFICANT OCCUPATIONAL EXPOSURE

The risk of acquiring HIV infection following occupational exposure is *low* – less than 3 per 1000 injuries. There is no risk of HIV transmission where intact skin is exposed to HIV-infected blood.

Administration of zidovudine prophylaxis to HCWs occupationally exposed to HIV has been associated with an 81% reduction in risk for HIV infection.

Four factors are associated with increased risk of occupationally acquired HIV infection:

- Deep injury
- Visible blood on the device that caused the injury
- Injury with a needle that has been placed in a source patient's artery or vein
- Terminal HIV-related illness in the source patient.

IMMEDIATE ACTION

Immediately following *any* exposure – whether or not the source is known to pose a risk of infection – the site of exposure, e.g. wound or non-intact skin, should be washed liberally with soap and water without scrubbing. Antiseptics and skin washes should not be used – there is no evidence of their efficacy, and their effect on local defences is unknown. Free bleeding of puncture wounds should be encouraged gently but wounds should not be sucked. Exposed mucous membranes, including mouth or conjunctivae, should be irrigated copiously with water.

Prompt reporting of injuries is a necessary first step to enabling appropriate and rapid prescribing of PEP.

A risk assessment needs to be carried out urgently by an appropriately trained doctor to determine the appropriateness of starting PEP; this should be done by a person who is *not* the exposed HCW.

CIRCUMSTANCES OF EXPOSURE

PEP should be considered after an exposure with the potential to transmit HIV, based on the type of body fluid or substance involved, and on the route and severity of the exposure. Exposures associated with significant risk include:

- percutaneous injury (from needles, instruments, bone fragments, significant bites that break the skin, etc.)
- exposure of broken skin (abrasions, cuts, eczema, etc.)
- exposure of mucous membranes, including the eye.

Some HCWs may have had occupational exposures that, after careful assessment, are not considered to have the potential for HIV transmission. Such workers should be advised that the potential side-effects and toxicity of taking PEP outweigh the negligible risk of transmission posed by this type of exposure because it is considered insignificant, whether or not the source patient is known or considered likely to be HIV-infected.

ASSESSMENT AND TESTING OF THE SOURCE PATIENT

If initial assessment indicates that an exposure has been *significant*, consideration should then be given to the HIV status of the source patient. Since HIV PEP is most likely to be efficacious if started within the hour, an urgent preliminary risk assessment should assess whether it is appropriate to recommend taking the first dose of PEP. A more thorough risk assessment should then be undertaken to inform a decision about whether to continue the PEP regimen.

The designated doctor should ensure that appropriate arrangements are made to approach a source patient whose HIV status is not known and to ask for their informed agreement to HIV testing. *This approach should not be undertaken by the exposed worker*. A universal approach to asking source patients to agree to have an HIV test avoids the need to make difficult judgments, simplifies and normalizes the process, and avoids potential discrimination.

It is good practice for all hospitals to have the capacity to obtain an HIV test result within 8 hours ideally, and not more than 24 hours, after source blood is taken.

Starting PEP, where appropriate, should not be delayed while the result of source patient testing is being awaited.

EXPOSURE TO DISCARDED NEEDLE/UNKNOWN SOURCE

Where it is not possible to identify the source patient (e.g. needlestick injury caused by a discarded needle), a risk assessment should be conducted to determine whether the exposure was significant. PEP is unlikely to be justified in most exposures of this type.

WHEN TO PRESCRIBE PEP

PEP should be recommended to HCWs if they have had a significant occupational exposure to blood or another high-risk body fluid from a patient or other source either known to be HIV-infected or considered to be at high risk of HIV infection, but where the result of an HIV test has not or cannot be obtained.

PEP should not be offered:

- after exposure through any route with low-risk materials (e.g. urine, vomit, saliva, faeces) unless they are visibly blood-stained (e.g. saliva in association with dentistry)
- where testing has shown that the source is HIV-negative
- where risk assessment has concluded that HIV infection of the source is highly unlikely.

When offering PEP, it is important to take into account any views of the exposed HCW. Depending on the outcome of the preliminary risk assessment, if the exposure was significant, the exposed HCW may wish to consider starting PEP until further information is available about the source patient. In this way, the option of possible benefit from prompt PEP will have been kept open. Changes can be made to the PEP regimen, including cessation, if further information becomes available.

If the HIV status of the source cannot be established, the exposed HCW should have the opportunity to consider whether or not to continue PEP. The decision should be informed by all that is known about the source patient in terms of past exposure to risk of HIV infection and also the nature and severity of the exposure. These aspects should be considered, together with the potential for unpleasant short-term adverse effects and unknown long-term effects of taking PEP drugs.

The relative risk of HIV transmission may be increased considerably if the source patient has a high plasma viral load (e.g. at the time of seroconversion or in the later stages of HIV disease).

FURTHER MANAGEMENT ISSUES

All exposed HCWs should be encouraged to provide a baseline blood sample for storage and a follow-up sample for testing.

PEP is not a licensed indication for any antiretroviral drugs, which are therefore prescribed on an 'off-label' basis.

PEP is most likely to be effective when it is initiated as soon as possible after exposure (within hours, and certainly within 48–72 hours), and continued for at least 28 days. All HCWs occupationally exposed to HIV should have follow-up counselling, post-exposure testing and medical evaluation, *whether or not* they have received PEP.

EAGA now recommends, as a minimum, that follow-up should be for at least 12 weeks after the exposure or, if PEP was taken, for at least 12 weeks from when PEP was stopped, for the following reasons:

- A negative test at 12 weeks provides a very high level of confidence of freedom from infection.
- It minimizes the period of anxiety suffered by exposed HCWs waiting for the 'all clear'.
- In the majority of cases where seroconversion has occurred following occupational exposure, despite the use of triple PEP, seroconversion has been detected within 12 weeks of exposure.

Employers and medical, dental and nursing schools should consider making 7-day starter packs of PEP drugs available to workers/students travelling to countries where antiretroviral therapy is not commonly available.

BODY FLUIDS AND MATERIALS THAT MAY POSE A RISK OF HIV TRANSMISSION IF SIGNIFICANT OCCUPATIONAL EXPOSURE OCCURS

- Amniotic fluid
- Blood
- Cerebrospinal fluid
- Exudative or other tissue fluid from burns or skin lesions
- Human breast milk
- Pericardial fluid
- Peritoneal fluid
- Pleural fluid
- Saliva in association with dentistry (likely to be contaminated with blood, even when it is not obviously so)
- Semen
- Synovial fluid
- Unfixed human tissues and organs
- Vaginal secretions
- Any other body fluid if visibly blood-stained.

PEP DRUGS

Antiretroviral agents from three classes of drug are currently licensed for first-line treatment of HIV infection, namely:

- nucleoside/nucleotide analogue reverse transcriptase inhibitors (NRTIs)
- non-nucleoside reverse transcriptase inhibitors (NNRTIs)
- protease inhibitors (PIs).

Zidovudine (an NRTI) is the only drug to date that has been studied and for which there is evidence of a reduction in risk of HIV transmission following occupational exposure.

In HIV-infected patients, triple therapy has proved more effective than monotherapy or dual therapy in suppressing HIV replication and avoiding the emergence of viral resistance. US guidelines recommend two-drug PEP regimens following lower-risk incidents and three-drug regimens only for higher risks. This two-tier approach adds to the complexity of the risk assessment process, at the expense of greater potency and protection for the exposed worker, and is not recommended. A potent three-drug PEP regimen is preferred because resistance to antiretroviral drugs is found at significant levels in both treated and untreated infected individuals in the UK.

PEP STARTER PACKS

Zidovudine is no longer recommended for PEP starter packs, preference being given to newer drugs with better tolerability.

Starter packs should provide a generic regimen of two NRTIs plus boosted PI – recommended for PEP following non-occupational exposure. For occupational exposure, the regimen is:

- one Truvada tablet (245 mg tenofovir and 200 mg emtricitabine [FTC]) once a day

  plus

- two Kaletra film-coated tablets (200 mg lopinavir and 50 mg ritonavir) twice a day.

Truvada plus Kaletra is the preferred regimen, but Combivir plus Kaletra may be considered as an option if there are difficulties sourcing starter packs containing Truvada. Due to concerns about long-term stability outside the original container, some prepacking units may be unable to supply starter packs containing Truvada.

ADVERSE EFFECTS

Side-effects of the NRTIs (e.g. tenofovir and emtricitabine) include gastrointestinal effects (e.g. nausea, diarrhoea), as well as dizziness and headache. In clinical trials of Kaletra, the most commonly reported side-effect was diarrhoea, followed by other gastrointestinal disturbances, asthenia, headache and rash. Inclusion of an NNRTI (nevirapine and efavirenz) in PEP regimens is not recommended; nevirapine has the potential to cause severe rashes (which may be confused with the rash associated with HIV seroconversion) and sometimes Stevens–Johnson syndrome, while efavirenz is associated with neurological side-effects and is also contraindicated in pregnancy. Serious adverse events (including life-threatening hepatotoxicity) have been reported in HCWs taking nevirapine as part of PEP.

Pregnancy is discussed in Chapter 25. This chapter deals with contraception and sexually shared infections, though others, especially those that are also bloodborne, such as hepatitis viruses are discussed in Chapter 9 and HIV in Chapter 20, and others in Chapter 21.

CONTRACEPTION

Different methods of contraception vary in effectiveness (Table 32.1). The most widely used and effective forms are the oral contraceptive pill (OCP; 'the Pill') and the male condom. The latter also confers protection against transmission of infections and, in the face of the increase in many sexually shared (transmitted) infections (SSIs), is therefore recommended. Contraception is best guaranteed by planned regular use of OCPs plus barrier precautions such as a condom.

EFFECTIVE CONTRACEPTION

Hormonal contraception is not completely effective in preventing pregnancy and provides no protection against SSIs.

Oral contraceptive pill

General aspects

OCPs act by inhibiting ovulation via their action on the hypothalamic–pituitary axis; by altering uterine cervical mucus composition; and by impeding ovum implantation. Emergency contraception may prevent pregnancy when taken within 72 hours of intercourse but is not reliable. OCPs are usually combinations of synthetic oestrogens and progestogens; the mini-pill contains only a progestogen and is less effective than the combination pill. Two types of synthetic oestrogen are used in OCPs – ethinylestradiol and mestranol. The synthetic progesterone is progestogen. Norethindrone and levonorgestrel are other examples.

OCP adverse effects are thought to be caused by the oestrogen component, which is now only 50 mg or less. The major risk is the higher incidence of thromboembolic disease (thrombosis of deep veins and coronary or cerebral thrombosis), but the incidence of cardiovascular or cerebrovascular disease is normally so low in young women that, even with a four- or fivefold increase in incidence, these complications are still uncommon. Hypertension, diabetes, jaundice and liver tumours, usually benign, are also increased in those taking OCPs (Table 32.2; see also Ch. 29). Long-term OCP use may increase the risk of cervical cancer and possibly of breast cancer, but OCPs appear to lower the risk of ovarian cancer by 40% and may also reduce the risk of endometrial cancer. *However, any risks from adverse effects of OCPs are low compared with the health risks associated with pregnancy.*

OCPs are absorbed from the intestine, but their effect may be impaired by: excessive intestinal motility, as in diarrhoea; antimicrobials, such as amoxicillin, ampicillin or tetracycline, which suppress the gut flora that deconjugate bile salts, thereby interrupting the enterohepatic recycling of the oestrogen; or drugs such as carbamazepine that enhance the liver enzymes that metabolize the OCPs. As a result, these drugs may, at least theoretically, increase the pregnancy risk; the risk

Table 32.1 *Methods of contraception*

Contraceptive methods	Efficacy (%)
Majority use	
Oral contraceptive pill (OCP), including the mini-pill	99
Male condom	98
Minority use	
Contraceptive coil (intrauterine contraceptive device)	95
Contraceptive patch	99
Contraceptive injection	99
Contraceptive implants	99
Intrauterine system (Mirena)	99
Cap or diaphragm	95
Female condom	95
Withdrawal method	? (low)
Natural family planning (the rhythm method)	? (low)

Table 32.2 *Possible adverse effects of oral contraceptives*

Minor	Moderate	Serious
Nausea	Intermenstrual bleeding	Thromboembolic disease[a]
Depression		Hypertension[a]
Loss of libido		Myocardial infarction[a]
Breast pain		Gallstones
Fluid retention		Liver benign tumours
Weight gain		Cancer of cervix and breast

[a]More frequent in smokers and older women.

Table 32.3 *Some drugs interacting with oral contraceptives pills (OCPs) to reduce their effect and predispose to pregnancy*

Significantly interfering with OCPs	Slightly interfering with OCPs
Antibiotics:	Oral antibiotics:
Rifampicin (rifabutin)	Amoxicillin
Anticonvulsants:	Ampicillin
Barbiturates	Metronidazole
Carbamazepine	Tetracyclines
Dichloralphenazone	
Phenytoin	
Primidone	

is minimal for most antimicrobials, though rifampicin (rifabutin) is an exception (Table 32.3; see also Ch. 29). Rifampicin can interfere with:

- combined OCP
- progestogen-only OCP
- implant
- patch
- vaginal ring.

If antibiotics, or the illness the antibiotics are required for, cause diarrhoea or vomiting, the OCP may be affected.

Women on OCPs and prescribed antimicrobials are best advised to use additional contraceptive measures whilst taking the antimicrobial and for at least 7 days afterwards (4 weeks in the case of rifampicin). This is not an issue with other forms of contraception.

Carbamazepine and some anti-human immunodeficiency virus (HIV) agents may interfere with the OCP.

Contraceptive injections, implants and patches

Progestogen injections are available as two types: Depo-Provera (medroxyprogesterone), which protects from pregnancy for 12 weeks, and Noristerat (norethisterone), which protects for 8 weeks. They act by inhibiting ovulation, thickening cervical mucus, inhibiting the progress of sperm and thinning the endometrium.

A *progestogen implant* is a small flexible rod placed under the skin in the upper left arm. It works for up to 3 years. It contains etonorgestrel (Implanon). Some medicines render an implant less effective; these include drugs to treat HIV, epilepsy and tuberculosis, and St John's wort.

Contraceptive patches (Evra) provide progestogens and oestrogens, and work for about 1 week, so new patches are used each week for 3 weeks, followed by a week's break – just like the OCP.

Dental aspects of contraception

OCPs can interact with anticoagulants to disturb anticoagulant control and can impair the effect of tricyclic antidepressants. The significance of drug interactions for dental antibiotics with the OCP is probably low.

The predisposition to thromboembolic disease and hypertension theoretically necessitates precautions for operations under general anaesthesia (GA). However, if the patient is otherwise well, GA – in hospital of course – is not contraindicated. Despite the risk of thromboembolism, the disadvantages of discontinuing OCPs before GA outweigh any advantages.

OCPs may worsen gingivitis and possibly periodontitis and may increase the risk of dry sockets; jaw radio-opacities or altered trabecular patterns may appear.

Condoms

Male and female latex rubber condoms are available; they are inexpensive, have a high success rate approaching 100%, have virtually no side-effects and also protect against SSIs.

Other contraception that is more than 90% effective

- *Intrauterine contraceptive device (IUCD)*: originally termed the coil or loop because early devices took those shapes, IUCDs are now often T-shaped. They contain some copper (to increase efficacy). The IUCD acts by inhibiting sperm movement through the uterus, altering the mucus and affecting the endometrium.
- *Intrauterine system (Mirena)*: this intrauterine system contains a reservoir of progestogen steadily released for up to 5 years.
- *Cap or diaphragm*: this mechanically impedes sperm entry into the uterus.

UNRELIABLE FORMS OF CONTRACEPTION

- *Withdrawal method*: coitus interruptus (Latin for 'interrupted intercourse')

Table 32.4 *The most important sexually transmitted diseases and their causal agents*

Class of agent	Microorganism	Diseases
Bacteria	*Treponema pallidum*	Syphilis
	Mycoplasma genitalium	Non-specific urethritis
	Ureaplasma urealyticum	Non-specific urethritis
	Neisseria gonorrhoeae	Gonorrhoea
	Chlamydia trachomatis	Chlamydia
		Lymphogranuloma venereum
	Haemophilus ducreyi	Chancroid
	Calymmatobacterium granulomatis	Granuloma inguinale
	Staphylococcus aureus	Meticillin-resistant *Staph. aureus* (MRSA) in men who have sex with men
Viruses	Herpes simplex viruses (human [alpha] herpesvirus)	Genital herpes
	Human papillomaviruses	Genital warts (condyloma acuminatum)
	Hepatitis B and C viruses	Hepatitis
	Human immunodeficiency virus	HIV/AIDS
Fungi	*Candida*	Thrush
Parasites	*Phthirus pubis* (crab lice)	Pubic lice
	Sarcoptes scabiei	Scabies
	Trichomonas vaginalis	Trichomoniasis

- *Natural family planning (the rhythm method)*: avoidance of intercourse when ovulation is probable, as assessed by the calendar method, temperature method or mucus test.

SEXUALLY SHARED INFECTIONS SEEN WORLDWIDE

Sexually shared infections (SSIs), or sexually transmitted diseases (STDs) or infections (STIs), include bacterial, viral and fungal infections, and infestations (Table 32.4); they were formerly termed venereal diseases (VDs). Non-specific urethritis (NSU) and *Chlamydia* are probably the most common. There can be infection with more than one SSI, and SSIs generally increase the liability to transmission of viruses such as HIV, especially if there is mucosal or cutaneous ulceration. The group of the most common serious SSIs has been given the acronym SHAG (syphilis, herpes, anogenital warts and gonorrhoea).

Young people (age 16–24 years) now account for half of all SSI cases, and the incidence of virtually all of these infections is increasing. In the UK in 2008, nearly half a million people attended clinics for SSIs. Sexually promiscuous people can be the source of transmission to literally hundreds of others (Fig. 32.1). The risk of infection is highest in sex workers.

Prevention

SSIs are passed from person to person by direct contact, mainly via the external genitals, vagina, anus or rectum, or on the lips and in the mouth. Transmission of the microorganism occurs during vaginal, anal or oral sex. Pregnant women can sometimes pass infection to the fetus.

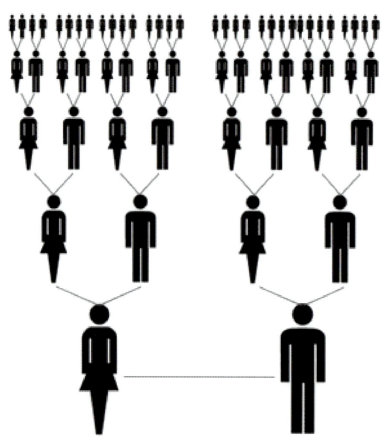

When you have sex with someone, you are having sex With everyone they have had sex with, and with Everyone they have had sex with, and with Everyone they have had sex with, and with Everyone they have had sex with, and with Everyone they have had sex with, and with Everyone they have had sex with, and with Everyone they have had sex with, and with

Fig. 32.1 Chart demonstrating the spread of sexually shared infections to other partners. (From www.positive-choice.org; accessed 30 September 2013).

- Promiscuous heterosexuals
- Gay or bisexual people
- Prostitutes
- Drug addicts
- Alcoholics
- Armed forces personnel
- Merchant seamen
- Aircrew
- People in custodial institutions
- Frequent business travellers
- People with learning impairment
- Sexual partners of the above groups

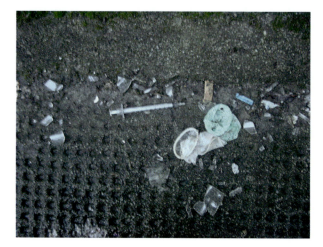

Fig. 32.2 The outfall from street prostitution: heroin syringe and condoms

Oral, anal, vaginal or penile ulcers or other lesions make it easier to transmit and acquire SSIs. However, because SSI lesions can be hidden in the vagina or anus, under the foreskin or in the mouth, it may not be obvious that a sex partner is infected. Unless a person knows that their sex partners have been tested and treated, they may be at risk of reinfection from an untreated sex partner.

Since SSIs are passed from person to person through unsafe sexual practices, the risk of infection can be reduced by avoiding casual and unprotected sexual intercourse via:

- *a*bstinence
- *b*eing monogamous
- *c*ondom use always.

The surest way to avoid transmission of SSIs is to abstain from sexual intercourse, or to be in a long-term mutually monogamous relationship with an uninfected partner who remains so. A man should always use a condom during sexual intercourse, each time, from start to finish, and a woman should make sure that her partner uses one. A woman can also protect herself from SSIs by using a female condom. Dental dams have been advocated for protection against transmission of SSIs during cunnilingus or oroanal contacts.

Although any person can be at risk of contracting SSIs, members of certain groups can be at especially high risk; some sell sex to underpin their drug habits (Box 32.1 and Fig. 32.2). Close contact is essential to SSI transmission; they cannot be spread through social contact or via toilet seats, doorknobs, swimming pools, hot tubs, bathtubs, shared clothing or eating utensils.

It is important to refer all sexual partners of infected people to be checked to prevent spread of SSIs and to prevent the patient from becoming re-infected. Providers should routinely test persons who:

- are men who have sex with men (MSM)
- have HIV infection
- have partner(s) who have tested positive
- are pregnant.

Persons should abstain from sexual contact with new partners until the situation is clarified and treatment effective. Persons must notify their sex partners so that they also can be tested and treated.

Multiple infections are not uncommon and substance abuse may be seen. Vaccination against hepatitis B is to be considered. Preventive vaccines against oncogenic human papillomaviruses are available in some countries. When accidental exposure occurs, post-exposure prophylaxis (PEP) may be available for hepatitis B and HIV. Pre-exposure prophylaxis for HIV (PREP) is also available.

UK law on intentional or reckless transmission of sexual infection can be found under the alphabetical list at: http://www.cps.gov.uk/legal/ (accessed 30 September 2013).

ALPHABETICAL LIST OF SEXUALLY SHARED INFECTIONS

This section discusses SSIs that are not discussed elsewhere; for viruses (herpesviruses, papillomaviruses, HIV), fungi (candidosis) and parasites (crab lice and scabies), see Chapters 20 and 21.

Chlamydia

General aspects

Chlamydia trachomatis, the most frequently reported bacterial SSI in the USA and UK in women, initially infects the cervix and urethra, or rectum. In men, infection is urethral or rectal. *Chlamydia* can be found in the pharynx of women and men who have oral sex with an infected sex partner.

Clinical features

About three-quarters of *Chlamydia*-infected women and half of infected men have no symptoms. If symptoms do occur, they usually appear within 1–3 weeks after exposure. Women may develop vaginal discharge or dysuria (a burning sensation when urinating). Some have lower abdominal pain, low back pain, nausea, fever, dyspareunia (pain during intercourse) or intermenstrual bleeding (between periods). *Chlamydia* can cause pelvic inflammatory disease (PID), which can permanently damage the fallopian tubes, uterus and surrounding tissues, or cause ectopic pregnancies. Rectal *Chlamydia* may cause pain, discharge or bleeding. Men may have a urethral discharge or dysuria. Complications among men are rare but include epididymitis with pain, fever and, rarely, sterility. Chlamydial infections in pregnancy can lead to premature delivery, and babies born to infected mothers can suffer chlamydial pneumonia and conjunctivitis (pink eye).

Rarely, genital chlamydial infection in adults can cause arthritis accompanied by skin lesions and inflammation of the eye and urethra (Reiter syndrome). *Chlamydia* may also cause lymphogranuloma venereum (LGV; see below).

General management

Culture, direct immunofluorescence, enzyme immunoassay (EIA), nucleic acid amplification tests (NAATs) and nucleic acid hybridization tests are available for *C. trachomatis* detection. The Centers for Disease Control and Prevention (CDC) recommends annual screening of all sexually active women aged 25 years or below, and those older women with risk factors (e.g. those with a new sex partner or multiple partners). Treatment is with azithromycin (single dose), doxycycline (twice daily for a week), erythromycin, ofloxacin or levofloxacin.

Gonorrhoea

General aspects

Gonorrhoea (meaning 'flow of seed') is caused by the bacterium *Neisseria gonorrhoeae*. Infection predominantly involves the urethra, endocervix, rectum, pharynx and conjunctivae. Transmission is by genital–genital, genital–anorectal, oro–genital or oro–anal contact, or by mother-to-child transmission at birth. Gonorrhoea is less common than most other SSIs but is about 15 times more common than syphilis. The highest incidence of gonorrhoea is in young adults with a disproportionate prevalence in ethnic minority groups and MSM.

Clinical features

Gonorrhoea in all sites is often asymptomatic, a fact that increases the chances of transmission. Rectal and pharyngeal infections in either gender are mostly asymptomatic. Some 50% genital tract infections in women (up to 10% in men) are asymptomatic. In males, acute urethritis is the main symptomatic presentation, with urethral discharge and dysuria; in females, endocervical and urethral infection causes increased or altered vaginal discharge, intermenstrual bleeding, dysuria and menorrhagia. In neonates of infected women, gonorrhoea can cause blindness.

An important complication of genital gonorrhoea is urethral stenosis. Infection can ascend the genital tract to cause PID and epididymoorchitis or disseminate in bacteraemia.

General management

The diagnosis of gonorrhoea is established by identification of *N. gonorrhoeae* in secretions. Microscopy using Gram or methylene blue staining has high sensitivity and specificity where there is discharge but poor sensitivity in asymptomatic men and in the identification of endocervical or rectal infection. Culture allows confirmatory identification and antimicrobial susceptibility testing. NAATs are generally more sensitive than culture and can be used on urine, vaginal swabs, and swabs from the endocervix and urethra, and are significantly more sensitive than are cultures from pharyngeal and rectal swabs. Serological tests are uninformative. Demonstration of *N. gonorrhoeae* in a clinical specimen by detection of antigen or detection of nucleic acid via nucleic acid amplification (e.g., PCR) or hybridization with a nucleic acid probe, is most specific.

The level of tetracycline resistance in *N. gonorrhoeae* is high, so tetracyclines and penicillin are usually ineffective. Current treatment now uses single doses of:

- ceftriaxone 250 mg i.m.

  or

- cefixime 400 mg oral

  or

- spectinomycin 2 g i.m.

The fluoroquinolones (ciprofloxacin, ofloxacin, levofloxacin) cannot be used in pregnancy. Since co-infection with *Chlamydia trachomatis* is common in young heterosexuals with gonorrhoea, this should also be treated – with ceftriaxone plus doxycycline or azithromycin.

Dental aspects

Oropharyngeal infection appears uncommon, except in MSM. Fellatio is probably the main cause but normally saliva strongly inhibits *N. gonorrhoeae*. Gonococcal stomatitis may be suspected when there is severe but ill-defined inflammation or painful ulceration, red swollen tonsils with a greyish slough and regional lymphadenitis in a young adult, especially when there is a history of recent oro–genital or oro–anal contact. However, the infection can be asymptomatic and the throat may appear normal. There is no evidence that oral gonococcal infections can be transmitted to the dentist by coughing and droplet infection, or by saliva. Furthermore, dental procedures on an infected patient will not produce haematogenous spread or deep infection.

Hepatitis virus infection

See Chapter 9.

Herpesvirus infections

See Chapter 11.

HIV infection

See Chapter 20.

Human papillomavirus (HPV) infections

See Chapter 21.

Non-specific urethritis

Non-specific urethritis (NSU) is urethritis not caused by *Chlamydia* or gonorrhoea; it manifests with dysuria and stains on underwear. *Mycoplasma genitalium* or *Ureaplasma urealyticum* may be implicated. Diagnosis is from a smear showing numerous polymorphonuclear leukocytes. Treatment is doxycycline or azithromycin. Frequently, no cause for cervicitis is found and it is then referred to as 'non-specific'. Fewer than half are infected with *Chlamydia*; others have gonorrhoea, and a few have other bacterial or herpes simplex virus infections.

Pelvic inflammatory disease

Pelvic inflammatory disease (PID) refers to infection of the uterus, fallopian tubes and other reproductive organs. It is a serious complication of some SSIs, especially chlamydia and gonorrhoea. Sexually active women in their childbearing years are most at risk. The more sex partners a woman or her partners have, the greater her risk of developing PID. A prior episode of PID increases the risk of another episode Women who have an IUD may be at slightly increased risk.

Clinical features

Features of PID vary from mild to severe and include fever, vaginal discharge, painful intercourse, painful urination, irregular menstrual bleeding and pain in the right upper abdomen. PID can lead to infertility (in 10%), ectopic pregnancy, abscess formation and chronic pelvic pain.

General management

Pelvic ultrasound is helpful to see whether the fallopian tubes are enlarged or an abscess is present. In some cases, a laparoscopy may be necessary to confirm the diagnosis.

PID is usually treated with at least two broad-spectrum antibiotics, and sex partner(s) should also be treated to decrease the risk of re-infection, even if the partner(s) is symptomless.

Syphilis

Syphilis is an SSI caused by *Treponema pallidum*, a bacterium that may damage cardiovascular and nervous systems, and can also be fatal. The incidence of syphilis, though low, is currently rising and over 80% of cases are in MSM. More than 60% of reported primary and secondary syphilis cases are among MSM, and 20–70% have HIV. In HIV, syphilis can be atypical and severe (lues maligna).

Syphilis is transmitted from person to person by direct contact with syphilis lesions via vaginal, anal or oral sexual contact. Infected pregnant women can pass it to their fetus. The average time between infection with syphilis and appearance of the first symptom is 21 days, but this can range from 10 to 90 days.

Other treponemal infections (*non-venereal* [endemic] treponematoses) can be acquired where poverty, overcrowding and unhygienic practices facilitate infection transmission (Appendix 32.1).

Primary syphilis

Over 80% of syphilis cases are in MSM. The incubation is about 3 weeks (range 10–90 days).

Clinical features

T. pallidum causes a chancre (primary or Hunterian chancre), which begins as a small, firm, pink and typically single macule (usually on the glans penis or vulva). This changes to a papule and then ulcerates to form a painless round ulcer with a raised margin and indurated base. Primary chancres occasionally involve the lips or tongue. Untreated chancres heal in 3–8 weeks, but are highly infectious and are associated with enlarged painless regional lymph nodes.

If the infected person does not receive adequate treatment, the infection progresses to the secondary stage.

Management of primary syphilis

Diagnosis is by microscopy of lesional exudate and serology. In oral lesions, the diagnosis can be confused by oral commensal treponemes, so specific fluoresceinated antibodies should be used or lesions should be thoroughly swabbed with sterile gauze or cotton wool to remove as many contaminating bacteria as possible, then gently but thoroughly scraped with an instrument such as a sterile plastic spatula. The scraping is then transferred to a slide and examined as quickly as possible by dark-ground microscopy. If the lesion is a chancre, many large but slender, regular, helical forms with a leisurely rotational movement across the field are seen. A negative test does not rule out syphilis. Biopsy may be suggestive, and diagnostic if specific antibodies are used. Demonstration of *T. pallidum* in clinical specimens by polymerase chain reaction (PCR) or equivalent direct molecular methods is specific.

Serology is required but often negative at this stage. *Non-specific (reaginic) serological tests*, useful for screening such, include the Venereal Disease Research Laboratory (VDRL) test, rapid plasma reagin (RPR) card test, automated reagin test (ART) and toluidine red-treated serum test (TRUST). Treponemal EIAs are an appropriate alternative but another treponemal assay, such as the *T. pallidum* haemagglutination test (TPHA), should be used for confirmation. The VDRL test appears positive towards the end of primary syphilis and usually becomes negative 1–2 years after treatment; but it remains positive in untreated secondary or tertiary syphilis. False-positive VDRL results may be seen after immunizations, in autoimmune disease and in some other infections (treponematoses, HIV, viral pneumonia, tuberculosis, malaria or leptospirosis). *Specific serological tests*, such as the fluorescent treponemal antibody absorbed (FTA-Abs) test, TPHA and the treponemal immobilization (TPI) test, overcome the problem of false-positive VDRL results but cannot differentiate syphilis from other treponematoses. The FTA-Abs is probably best reserved for specimens giving discrepant results. Specific tests become positive during primary disease and remain positive through untreated secondary or tertiary syphilis but, in contrast to VDRL, remain positive even in treated syphilis.

Primary syphilis is treated with procaine penicillin, doxycycline or erythromycin. Patients must be followed up clinically and serologically for 2 years and contacts traced.

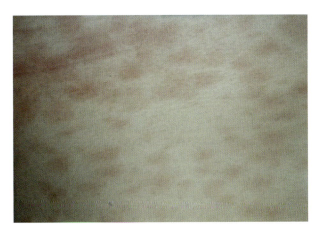

Fig. 32.3 Rash of secondary syphilis. This SSI has increased enormously in many countries.

Secondary syphilis

Secondary syphilis follows the primary stage after 6–8 weeks.

Clinical features

Syphilis is the great mimic. Skin rashes (Fig. 32.3) and/or sores in the mouth, vagina or anus mark this stage. Features may often be non-specific, with malaise, weight loss, fever, headache, rash (symmetrically distributed, coppery maculopapules on the palms and soles, characteristically), patchy hair loss and generalized painless lymph node enlargement with unusual enlargement of epitrochlear nodes. Large, raised, grey or white lesions (condylomas) may develop in warm, moist areas such as the mouth, axilla or groin. Oral lesions are seen in only about one-third of patients and include painless ulcers (mucous patches and snailtrack ulcers), split papules and condyloma lata. The mucosal lesions are highly infectious.

The features of secondary syphilis resolve with or without treatment. Without treatment, syphilis will progress to the latent and possibly late stages.

Management of secondary syphilis

Mucosal lesions should be examined for *T. pallidum* as above and blood should be taken for serological examination. Treatment is as for primary syphilis (see below for the Jarisch–Herxheimer reaction).

Late and latent stages

The latent (hidden) stage of syphilis begins when primary and secondary symptoms disappear and can last years; although the person remains infected, they exhibit no signs or symptoms.

Tertiary syphilis

About 15% of people not treated develop late-stage syphilis, up to 10–30 years after infection.

Clinical features

Features include difficulty coordinating muscle movements, paralysis, numbness, gradual blindness and dementia. Syphilis damages the brain, nerves, eyes, heart, blood vessels, liver, bones and joints, and can result in death. The main feature is a localized non-infectious granuloma (termed a gumma), varying in size from a pinhead to several centimetres, which breaks down to form a deep punched-out ulcer. Skin gummas heal with depressed shiny scars (tissue-paper scars). Bone gummas may affect the long bones (especially the tibia – 'sabre tibia') or

skull, producing lytic lesions and periostitis with new bone formation. Mucosal gummas may destroy bone, particularly the palate, or involve the tongue. The other main oral manifestation is leukoplakia, particularly of the tongue dorsum, with a high potential for malignant change.

Cardiovascular syphilis (aortitis, coronary arterial stenosis or aortic aneurysms) affects about 10% of patients as a late complication.

Neurosyphilis, sometimes with sensorineural deafness, also affects about 10%. *Meningovascular neurosyphilis* has highly variable early symptoms but late effects may be hydrocephalus or lesions of the second, third and eighth cranial nerves, and the pupils are also unequal and unresponsive to light (Argyll Robertson pupils). *Paretic neurosyphilis* begins insidiously with subtle mental disturbance, going on to severe personality changes, complete dementia and widespread paralyses (general paresis of the insane; GPI). *Tabes dorsalis* (*locomotor ataxia*) is characterized by atrophy of lumbar posterior nerve roots and sometimes the optic nerves, and characterized by sudden attacks of lightning-like pain and paraesthesiae of leg or trunk, with loss of normal pain sensation and of deep proprioceptive reflexes. These latter cause a tabetic gait in which the feet are slapped on the ground as a result of loss of sense of their position, and the neuropathic joints then become disorganized (Charcot joints). Neurosyphilis is a rare cause of atypical trigeminal neuralgia.

Management of tertiary syphilis

The patients are serologically reactive and diagnosis is confirmed by serology. Treatment is procaine penicillin, 600 000 units daily for 3 weeks, and lifelong follow-up. Systemic corticosteroids are given at the start of antibiotic therapy to reduce the possibility of a Jarisch–Herxheimer reaction (febrile reaction often with exacerbation of the local syphilitic lesions).

Syphilis associated with HIV infection may take an atypical accelerated course with rapid progress to the tertiary stage; gummas may develop while the secondary stage is still active (lues maligna). The antibody response is atypical and unpredictable. Relapse is common, despite treatment, or the response to penicillin may be poor.

Congenital syphilis

A pregnant woman with syphilis can, after the fifth month, pass the infection to her fetus, with resultant low birth weight, premature delivery or stillbirth. An infected baby may be born without features of disease but, if not treated immediately, may develop serious problems within a few weeks (such as cataracts, deafness or seizures) and can die. Syphilis in the fetus may cause learning disability, deafness and blindness, and typically results in frontal bossing, a saddle nose and Hutchinson's teeth – screwdriver-shaped incisors. A classic mucocutaneous sign is depressed linear scars radiating from the orifice of the mouth; these are termed rhagades (parrot lines). Affected children are highly infectious until about 2 years of age. To protect their babies, pregnant women at risk should be tested for syphilis regularly during the pregnancy and at delivery; if positive, they should receive immediate treatment, usually with penicillin.

Trichomoniasis

General aspects

The parasite *Trichomonas vaginalis* causes trichomoniasis (TV) – a common SSI. Women can acquire the disease from infected sex partners, but men usually contract it only from infected women. The vagina is the most common site of infection in women, and the urethra is the most common site of infection in men. Transmission is via penis-to-vagina intercourse or vulva-to-vulva contact. Rarely, it is caught by sharing towels or washcloths with an infected person.

Clinical features

Symptoms are more common in women. TV usually causes an odiferous vaginal discharge, with vulval pruritus and erythema. In males, TV is usually symptomless but may cause dysuria.

General management

Metronidazole and tinidazole are usually effective.

SSIs SEEN MAINLY IN PEOPLE FROM THE DEVELOPING WORLD

Chancroid

Chancroid, caused by the Gram-negative bacterial rod, *Haemophilus ducreyi*, is a frequent cause of genital ulcers in developing countries but is uncommon in industrialized nations.

Clinical features

After an incubation of 2–10 days, a papule or pustule erupts and erodes to form a painful deep ulcer with ragged margins. More than one-half of patients have multiple ulcers. Painful regional lymphadenopathy is common.

General management

Azithromycin, ceftriaxone, erythromycin or ciprofloxacin is used.

Granuloma inguinale (donovanosis)

Calymmatobacterium granulomatis, a Gram-negative bacillus seen in people from the Americas, Far East and Africa, causes this chronic, ulcerative, granulomatous disease.

Clinical features

After an incubation of 1–4 weeks, a papule or nodule appears, usually in the inguinal or anogenital region, and progresses to a locally destructive granulomatous lesion. Three main types of donovanosis have been described: ulcerative, exuberant and cicatricial.

General management

Direct examination of a piece of granulation tissue compressed between two slides and stained by Giemsa for the presence of Donovan bodies (clusters of bacilli lying within leukocytes) is the best diagnostic method.

Tetracycline, ampicillin or trimethoprim–sulfamethoxazole is the first-line therapy.

Lymphogranuloma venereum

Lymphogranuloma venereum (LGV) or lymphogranuloma inguinale, caused by *Chlamydia trachomatis*, is seen worldwide but is particularly common in Latin America, India, Indonesia and Africa.

Table 32.5 *Possible complications from body art*

Procedure	Complications
Dental grillz	Can impair oral hygiene, cause tooth movement or surface loss
Piercings	Pain, oedema, haemorrhage, infection
	Staphylococcus aureus infections, osteomyelitis, toxic shock syndrome and endocarditis, *Pseudomonas aeruginosa* infection and HIV transmission, Ludwig angina, bleeding into the pharynx and airways, and acute hypotension
	Oral piercings can impair speech and mastication, cause mucosal or gingival trauma, chipped or fractured teeth, hypersalivation, calculus accumulation, and foreign body granulomas or allergies
Tattooing	Pain, oedema, haemorrhage, infection
	Staphylococcus aureus infections, and transmission of hepatitis B and C viruses, and HIV
	Foreign body granulomas or allergies, or scarring
Tongue-splitting	Pain, oedema, haemorrhage, infection

Clinical features

LGV primarily affects the external genitalia, inguinal lymph nodes and lymphatics. About 10 days after exposure, a small vesicle appears, which ruptures and heals without scarring. About 1 week to 2 months later, there may be swelling and tenderness of the regional lymph nodes and suppuration. Healing involves scarring, which blocks lymphatic channels and causes oedema (elephantiasis).

General management

Diagnosis is by isolation of *C. trachomatis* and serological tests. A non-specific skin test (Frei test) is available. LGV is treated with sulphonamides, tetracycline, erythromycin or rifampicin.

BODY ART

Tattooing and more invasive procedures, with distortion or mutilation of body parts, have been commonplace in many cultures for centuries and often have sexual connotations. For example, facial scarification and female circumcision are common in some African cultures. In some East African groups, the uvula is removed in children in the belief that health will be improved. In some Amazonian tribes and in the Surma tribe of Ethiopia, large plates are worn in the lower lip.

In the developed world, the expression of individualism through body art such as tattooing and body piercing, and the wearing of jewellery in 'unconventional' sites is popular. Oral piercings, tongue splitting and 'dental grills' (also termed bling, tooth jewellery, grillz or fronts) are increasingly seen. Grillz are generally removable and made from metal (silver, gold or platinum), some being encrusted with expensive precious stones and jewels.

Complications possible from body art are shown in Table 32.5.

KEY WEBSITES

(Accessed 11 June 2013)
Centers for Disease Control and Prevention. <http://www.cdc.gov/sexualhealth/>.
Family Planning Association. <http://www.fpa.org.uk/>.
MedlinePlus. <http://www.nlm.nih.gov/medlineplus/sexualhealthissues.html>.

NHS Choices. <http://www.nhs.uk/Livewell/Sexualhealthtopics/Pages/Sexual-health-hub.aspx>.

USEFUL WEBSITES

(Accessed 11 June 2013)
Centers for Disease Control and Prevention. Sexually transmitted diseases (STDs). <http://www.cdc.gov/std>.
GOV.UK. <http://www.dh.gov.uk/health/category/policy-areas/public-health/>.
National Institutes of Health. <http://health.nih.gov/topic/SexualHealthGeneral>.
Public Health England. <http://www.hpa.org.uk>.

FURTHER READING

Antonio, A.G., et al., 2005. Premature loss of primary teeth associated with congenital syphilis: a case report. J. Clin. Pediatr. Dent. 29, 273.

Bignell, C., 2009. European (IUSTI/WHO) Guideline on the diagnosis and treatment of gonorrhoea in adults. Int. J. STD & AIDS 20, 453.
Bruce, A.J., Rogers 3rd, R.S., 2004. Oral manifestations of sexually transmitted diseases. Clin. Dermatol. 22, 520.
Cliffe, S.J., et al., 2008. Chlamydia in the Pacific region, the silent epidemic. Sex. Transm. Dis. 35, 801.
Dalmau, J., et al., 2006. Nodules on the tongue in an HIV-positive patient. Scand. J. Infect. Dis. 38, 822.
Dan, M., et al., 2006. Pharyngeal gonorrhea in female sex workers: response to a single 2-g dose of azithromycin. Sex. Transm. Dis. 33, 512.
Eccleston, K., et al., 2008. Primary syphilis. Int. J. STD AIDS 19, 145.
Gurlek, A., et al., 2005. The continuing scourge of congenital syphilis in 21st century: a case report. Int. J. Pediatr. Otorhinolaryngol. 69, 1117.
Leão, J.C., et al., 2006. Oral manifestations of syphilis. Clinics 61, 161.
Lewis, D.A., et al., 2004. The 374 clinic: an outreach sexual health clinic for young men. Sex. Transm. Infect. 80, 480.
Menni, S., 2007. Acquired primary syphilis on a child's lip. Acta Derm. Venereol. 87, 284.
Platt, L., et al., 2007. Effects of sex work on the prevalence of syphilis among injection drug users in 3 Russian cities. Am. J. Public Health 97, 478.
Scully, C., 2001. Oral piercing in adolescents. CPD Dent. 2, 79.

APPENDIX 32.1 NON-VENEREAL TREPONEMATOSES (ENDEMIC TREPONEMATOSES)

Aetiology/epidemiology	Clinical features	Management
Bejel (endemic syphilis) Caused by *Treponema pallidum*; prevalent among nomads in the Arabian peninsula and sub-Saharan Africa	No obvious primary stage. Secondary and tertiary stages are encountered, mainly manifesting on skin and mucosae; mucous patches, angular stomatitis, rashes, pigmentary changes and tenderness of long bones may be seen. About one-third of patients develop lesions of the late or tertiary stage of the disease, which are mainly gummatous. Skin lesions are usually extensive, chronic and destructive, healing with scarring and depigmentation. Gummatous destruction of the nasal septum, lips, soft palate and nasopharynx may lead to facial deformity (rhinopharyngitis mutilans)	Dark-ground microscopy and serology are needed to confirm the diagnosis. Penicillin is the drug of choice; tetracycline and erythromycin are alternatives
Pinta Caused by *T. carateum*; almost exclusively confined to Central and South America; transmitted by either direct or indirect contact	Incubation period is usually 2–3 weeks. The primary lesion is a slowly developing subcutaneous granulomatous lesion on the trunk, leg or face, usually in young adults of 15–30 years of age. Secondary lesions (pintides) are papules that develop into plaques with scaly and centrally pigmented areas, tending eventually to become depigmented and atrophic. Hyperkeratosis of the palms and soles may be seen and facial skin is extensively affected	Dark-ground microscopy and serology are needed for the diagnosis. Penicillin is the treatment of choice
Yaws (framboesia; pian; bouba) Caused by *T. pertenue*; seen throughout Equatorial Africa, Asia, Central and South America, the South Pacific Islands and Australia; transmitted either by contact with the early infectious lesions or via contaminated utensils or possibly insects	Incubation period is between 9 and 90 days. The primary papular stage may be of very short duration. One to three months later, painless papillomas or framboesial granulomas appear in the axilla or groin, or around the body orifices. Skin lesions may spontaneously heal in about 3–6 months. Most patients then have a stage of latency, which may last a lifetime but in some, about 5 years after the primary infection, gummatous nodular ulcerative lesions may develop. Bone and cartilage lesions are frequently found, including osteitis, periostitis and dactylitis. In infected growing children, 'sabre tibia' may develop. Bone involvement may result in thickening of the face on either side of the nose, giving rise to a characteristic facial appearance called 'goundou'. The other type of lesion is a destructive lesion of the palate, eventually destroying parts of the nose (gangosa) and causing a 'saddle-nose' defect	Dark-field microscopy, biopsy and serology are useful. Treatment is with penicillin, erythromycin or tetracycline

SPORTS

Exercise has clear benefits to both health and quality of life (Ch. 36). However, there are occasional sudden deaths (Table 33.1) and there may be risks from trauma, such as in sports, sometimes from other issues such as travel, and occasionally from associated disordered eating, menstrual disturbances and supplement use.

TRAUMA

See also Chapter 24 and http://www.aans.org/ (Sports-related head injury is under the Patient information/Conditions and Treatments tabs; accessed 30 September 2013).

Head, orofacial, ocular and other injuries are a risk in many sports; therefore the wearing of helmets and eye, face, jaw and mouth protection is often indicated, along with other protection.

Motion sports

Head injuries and maxillofacial and dental trauma are all too common in any sport involving fast movement, including those involving vehicles, roller-blading, skateboarding, snowboarding and skiing. Indeed, trauma is possible in all motion sports and as new types of sports become popular, the injuries associated with them also increase. Helmets are mandatory and, in some instances, protection for eyes, jaws, hands, knees, elbows and wrists is indicated.

Contact sports

Contact sports include football (soccer and rugby), boxing, martial arts (e.g. wrestling, karate and judo), gymnastics and hockey; to a degree, there is contact in some other sports such as baseball and basketball. Injuries to the teeth and orofacial soft tissues are common, particularly in football, boxing, martial arts and hockey.

Most sports injuries affect the maxillary incisors and involve young males. In soccer and rugby, players have about a 10% chance of injury per season. This may include head injury, cerebral concussion and neck injuries, which can be fatal or lead to paraplegia. Maxillofacial and dental injuries account for about 13% of the costs of all soccer injuries.

Prevention and adequate preparation are the key elements in minimizing injuries from such sports. Teaching skills such as tackling, use of appropriate equipment, safe playing areas and the wearing and utilization of properly fitted protective equipment like helmets and mouthguards are essential. A properly fitted mouthguard may also reduce the chances of sustaining a concussion from a blow to the jaw. Mouthguards are usually made of vinyl or acrylic, and three main types are available (Box 33.1).

Non-contact sports

Non-contact sports, such as tennis and volleyball, can also be dangerous. Custom-made protectors could offer the best protection against dental damage.

Box 33.1 *Mouthguards*

- Custom-made protectors – offer the best protection (vacuum custom-made and pressure laminated custom-made, ethylene vinyl acetate [EVA])
- Mouth-formed protectors – moulded on to the teeth ('boil and bite'); give variable protection but are useful where orthodontic appliances are worn
- Stock protectors – cheap and easily adjusted but less comfortable, protective or retentive

---

Water sports

Athletes who swim more than 6 hours per week in pools chemically treated to maintain safe water quality standards may develop tooth stains mistermed 'swimmer's calculus' and/or tooth erosion. The stains can usually be removed with professional cleaning.

Scuba divers depend on air in the form of compressed air from a tank, transmitted to the mouth by way of a regulator held in the mouth by the teeth, so that there is an airtight seal between the teeth and lips. Inability to hold the mouthpiece because of missing teeth poses a contraindication to scuba diving. Dental concerns in divers include temporomandibular joint (TMJ) and muscle pain from holding the regulator ('diver's mouth syndrome'), barotrauma and barodontalgia (from the effects of pressure changes), and the management of prostheses. Many divers experience TMJ and/or facial muscle pain or headache from the continuous jaw clenching. Mouthpieces are usually made of neoprene or silicone rubber and are held in place by bite tabs that fit into the dentition at the canine and premolar area. The average dive lasts 30–60 minutes and requires constant jaw muscle effort. Extending the bite tabs to cover the molar teeth balances the weight of the regulator and can relieve stress on the TMJ.

Barodontalgia (pain in the tooth caused by pressure changes) can arise in divers (or people in aircraft or at high altitude) if there are pulp lesions, abscesses or sinusitis. Antral pain may have a similar cause. Teeth that have been opened for endodontic treatment and temporarily sealed have been known to explode from air trapping and expansion on surfacing – mainly in deep divers using a helium–oxygen mixture. Full porcelain crowns can also shatter from relatively shallow dives of 65 feet. Raised pressure in the middle ear can occasionally cause facial palsy (baroparesis) but this typically resolves spontaneously over a few hours.

Divers cannot wear full or partial dental prostheses while diving, as they may be dislodged and aspirated. To eliminate the possibility of dislodgment completely, a custom mouthpiece to obviate the chance of aspiration of the prosthesis can be made. Full arch impressions are taken with the patient holding silicone putty in the roof of the mouth until it is set; they are then mounted in a hinge articulator and sent to the laboratory with the silicone putty impression.

DRUG USE IN SPORTS

Further information is available at: http://sportsanddrugs.procon.org/ (accessed 30 September 2013).

Table 33.1 *Endogenous causes of sudden death in athletes*

Cardiac causes	Other causes
Anomalous origin of coronary artery	Alcohol
Aortic rupture (Marfan syndrome)	Amphetamine
Aortic stenosis	Cocaine
Coronary artery disease	Erythropoietin (EPO)
Electrical conduction system abnormalities	Head trauma
Hypertrophic cardiomyopathy	Vascular event
Long QT syndrome	
Myocarditis	
Obstructive cardiomyopathy	
Right ventricular dysplasia	

Table 33.2 *Substances and methods not permitted for use by athletes[a]*

Prohibited at all times	Prohibited in competition	Prohibited in certain sports
S1 Anabolic agents	S6 Stimulants	Alcohol
S2 Peptide hormones, growth factors and related substances	S7 Narcotics	Beta-blockers
	S8 Cannabinoids	
S3 Beta agonists	S9 Glucocorticosteroids	
S4 Hormone and metabolic modulators		
S5 Diuretics and other masking agents		
M1 Manipulation of blood and blood components		
M2 Chemical and physical manipulations		
M3 Gene doping		

[a]The World Anti-Doping Agency (WADA) is responsible for maintaining and updating this list. See http://www.wada-ama.org/en/World-Anti-Doping-Program/ (under 'International Standards/Prohibited List'; accessed 30 September 2013).

Table 33.3 *Examples of agents permitted for use by athletes for certain complaints[a]*

Complaints	Drugs permitted
Allergies	Astemizole, cetirizine, chlorphenamine, loratadine, terfenadine
Diarrhoea	Diphenoxylate, loperamide
Bacterial infections	Antibiotics (all)
Fungal infections	Amphotericin, fluconazole, nystatin, miconazole, terbinafine
Viral infections	Aciclovir, idoxuridine
Asthma	Cromoglicate, theophylline, fluticasone (under specific conditions), beclometasone, salbutamol, formoterol, terbutaline, salmeterol
Coughs and colds	Antihistamines, dextromethorphan, guaifenesin, pholcodine
Oral or ear, nose and throat problems	Sprays or drops containing: betamethasone, dexamethasone, docusate, hydrocortisone, beclometasone, fluticasone, tramazoline
Eye problems	Ointments or drops containing: antazoline, betamethasone, hydrocortisone, beclometasone, chloramphenicol
Hay fever	Antihistamines
Pain and inflammation	Aspirin, paracetamol (acetaminophen), non-steroidal anti-inflammatory drugs (NSAIDs), codeine, dextropropoxyphene
Nausea and vomiting	Cimetidine, cinnarizine, domperidone, metoclopramide, prochlorperazine

[a]Check with governing bodies, as regulations may vary, or apply under specific circumstances/conditions.

Sports people may wish to take drugs as medication for disease; to improve their performance (performance-enhancing drugs; PEDs) and, in doing so, to gain an unfair advantage; or for 'recreational' reasons. Some substances are banned only during competition, while others depend on the method of administration (e.g. inhalation versus tablet or injection form). The list of prohibited substances is updated annually to keep up with advances in science and technology, a new list being issued on 1 January. A substance is added to the list if it meets two of the three criteria listed:

- The potential for enhanced performance
- The potential for being detrimental to health
- Violation of the spirit of sport.

The International Olympic Committee permits or prohibits the use of various drugs (Table 33.2). A comprehensive list of banned substances from the World Anti-Doping Agency (WADA) is available at: http://www.wada-ama.org/en/World-Anti-Doping-Program/ (under 'International Standards/Prohibited List'; accessed 30 September 2013).

Some drugs are banned at all times; others are permissible when not competing but not during competition; and some are banned in some sports but not others. Banned substances can include alcohol and caffeine above a certain level. Some agents are permitted for use for certain complaints (Table 33.3). In some cases, an athlete may have a pre-existing medical condition that requires them to take medication

that is listed. In this case, the athlete can apply to their international federation for a Therapeutic Use Exemption (TUE), which must be verified by their physician. In order for their request to be accepted, the following must be true:

- The athlete would suffer significant health problems if they do not take the medication
- There is no suitable alternative that is not listed
- There are no considerable performance-enhancing benefits.

Anabolic steroids

Anabolic steroids are available legally by prescription only, for conditions in which the body produces abnormally low amounts of testosterone, such as delayed puberty and some types of impotence. They are also used to treat body wasting in, for example, patients with human immunodeficiency virus/acquired immunodeficiency syndrome (HIV/AIDS). Athletes (and others) may misuse anabolic (androgenic) steroids (AAS) – synthetic substances related to male sex hormones – to enhance performance (and also to improve physical appearance); these are taken orally or injected, typically in cycles of weeks or months ('cycling'), rather than continuously. There are two types of AAS:

- *Exogenous*: synthetic versions of testosterone. Common examples include nandrolone and danazol.
- *Endogenous*: naturally occurring substances involved in the metabolic pathways of testosterone. For testing of drug use, all endogenous steroids have a normal range. Results outside of this normal range are deemed positive.

Due to the enhancement of testing procedures in the detection of anabolic steroids, 'designer steroids' such as tetrahydrogestrinone (THG) have been developed. THG breaks down during the preparation method used for normal steroid testing procedures. A test specifically for the detection of THG has since been developed.

Anabolic steroids given to adolescents may accelerate pubertal changes and cause premature skeletal maturation, halting growth. The major toxic effects include kidney and liver tumours (and jaundice), fluid retention and hypertension, increases in low-density lipoprotein (LDL) and decreases in high-density lipoprotein (HDL), severe acne, trembling, hostility and aggression, and other psychiatric effects. Gender-specific adverse effects include: for men – testicular atrophy, low sperm count, infertility, baldness, breast development and prostate cancer; and for women – facial hair growth, baldness, menstrual changes, clitoris enlargement and deepened voice. Injecting anabolic steroids is also associated with the risk of contracting or transmitting HIV or viral hepatitis.

Blood doping

Blood doping is the process of artificially increasing the amount of erythrocytes in an attempt to improve athletic performance. In the past this was accomplished by autologous transfusion, a practice now outlawed. Erythropoietin (EPO) stimulates erythrocyte production and is also illegal. It increases blood viscosity, may lead to thromboses and is one of the causes of the 'sudden death syndrome' seen in occasional athletes (see Table 33.1 and www.uksport.gov.uk; accessed 30 September 2013).

There are major side-effects associated with erythropoietin use, which have proven to be fatal in previous cases:

- Increased blood viscosity (which increases the risk of heart attack and stroke)
- Fever
- Seizures
- Nausea
- Headache
- Anxiety.

Human growth hormone

Human growth hormone (hGH), sometimes known as somatotropic hormone or somatotropin, is credited with having the following effects:

- Increased muscle mass
- Decreased fat stores
- Accelerated muscle recovery

Many small studies, however, have shown no increases in muscle size or strength following injection with hGH. A common practice among body-builders and weightlifters is to combine hGH and anabolic steroids, with recent research demonstrating beneficial effects.

The side-effects of hGH are vast and some are serious:

- Gigantism (pituitary gigantism or giantism) in younger athletes (abnormally excessive growth in height, considerably above average)
- Acromegaly in adult athletes (a condition in which the pituitary gland produces too much hGH, resulting in the growth and swelling of body parts, typically hands, feet, nose but possibly progressing to brow and jaw protrusion and swelling of internal organs)
- Hypothyroidism (low production of thyroid hormone, which disrupts metabolic rate and protein production)
- Cardiomyopathy (disease of the cardiac muscle, increasing the risk of arrhythmia and sudden cardiac death)
- Cardiac failure
- Hypercholesterolaemia (presence of high levels of cholesterol in the blood)

- Ischaemic heart disease (a lack of blood to the heart, often due to coronary artery disease)
- Myopathies (neuromuscular diseases affecting the function of muscle fibres)
- Arthritis
- Diabetes
- Impotence
- Osteoporosis
- Menstrual irregularities in women
- Creutzfeldt–Jakob disease (CJD or mad cow disease; transmission is possible when hGH is obtained from cadavers).

Insulin-like growth factor

Due to its perceived anabolic effects, athletes use insulin-like growth factor (IGF)-1 to increase muscle mass and strength, although clinical studies have not proven that it does so. It is thought that it is actually IGF binding protein-3 that is responsible for growth, rather than the growth factor itself. IGF-1 does, however, inhibit cell death and so may have a role in reducing recovery times.

Side-effects of IGF include:

- acromegaly in adult athletes
- organomegaly (the abnormal enlargement of organs)
- hypoglycaemia (lower than normal levels of glucose in the blood)
- cancer (prostate, lung and colorectal cancers have all been reported).

Human chorionic gonadotrophin

hCG is mainly used by male athletes, as it increases the production of both testosterone and epitestosterone, so keeping the testosterone-to-epitestosterone ratio unchanged from normal values (vital in avoiding detection of the presence of other prohibited substances). It is also used to maintain testicular volume in males who are using anabolic steroids. However, it is now thought that it is follicle-stimulating hormone (FSH) that is responsible for maintaining testicular volume and so hCG use would be entirely ineffective; in females there would be no beneficial effect at all.

Side-effects associated with hCG use are rare and non-serious:

- Gynaecomastia (the development of abnormally large mammary glands in males due to increased levels of the oestrogen).

The combination of hCG and anabolic steroids can cause:

- headaches
- depression
- oedema (swelling caused by fluid within the body's tissues).

Other substances

Gamma hydroxybutyrate (GHB) is also used by some body-builders. Drugs such as modanifil have been used to help alertness. Other banned substances not described above include:

- adrenocorticotropic hormone (ACTH)
- beta$_2$ agonists
- hormone antagonists and modulators
- diuretics
- artificial oxygen carriers
- gene doping
- amphetamines
- ephedra

- cocaine
- caffeine
- narcotics
- cannabinoids
- glucocorticosteroids.

Smokeless tobacco

Smokeless tobacco is associated with some sports in the USA, and is potentially dangerous in terms of oral keratoses and malignant change.

EATING DISORDERS IN SPORTS

Some athletes, mainly women, in cross-country, track and field, gymnastics, dancing, figure skating, volleyball and basketball, may be prone to develop eating disorders (Ch. 27). Tooth erosion may then be seen.

In endurance sports, such as long-distance running, triathlons or cycling, athletes may consume a high amount of refined carbohydrates ('carbo-load'), as well as carbohydrate gels or drinks (sports drinks – often containing carbohydrates, electrolytes, B vitamins and an acid such as citric, malic, tartaric or phosphoric).

Further information is available at: http://www.uksport.gov.uk/publications/eating-disorders-in-sport (accessed 30 September 2013).

DENTAL ASPECTS IN SPORTS

Preventive dental care and prevention of caries and erosion are important. Operative care for athletes under local anaesthesia (LA) is permitted. Analgesics such as aspirin, NSAIDs and paracetamol (acetaminophen) are permitted but opioids are banned and opiate-related analgesics are problematical. Codeine is not on the WADA list of banned substances, and combinations such as co-codamol and co-proxamol appear acceptable, but as screening does not always differentiate adequately between the various narcotic or codeine-related compounds, they are best avoided.

Anxiolytics may sometimes be banned. Alcohol and beta-blockers are illegal in certain sports, and therefore alcohol-containing oral health-care products are also best avoided. Some vitamin, herbal and nutritional supplements are banned.

Antimicrobials of all types are generally permitted. Therapeutic preparations used for topical oral use are also generally permitted; for example, topical corticosteroids are permitted but systemic corticosteroids are best avoided, or a TUE is required.

TRAVEL AND LEISURE

International travel is undertaken by ever-growing numbers of people for social, recreational, professional and humanitarian purposes, and can result in a variety of health risks in unfamiliar environments that present variable levels of risk and standards of health care, as well as the transmission of infectious agents and the appearance globally of diseases hitherto confined to certain areas. Most problems can be minimized by common sense, with suitable precautions taken before, during and after travel (see UK Department of Health booklet *Health advice for travellers* [T7.1], Fig. 33.1; available at http://www.dh.gov.uk/en/Publicationsandstatistics/Publications/PublicationsPolicyAndGuidance/DH_4123441, accessed 30 September 2013).

The countries to be visited and the duration of the visit are important in determining the likelihood of exposure to many problems, such as violence and infectious agents, and will influence decisions on the

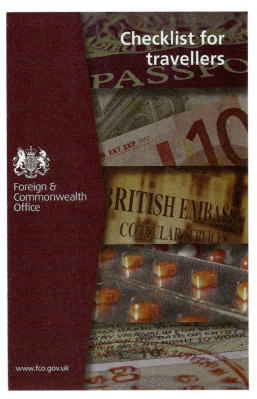

Fig. 33.1 *Health advice for travellers* – a sensible read.

need for protection and certain vaccinations or antimalarial or other medication. The behaviour of the traveller is also important: exposure to the risk of assault or accidents, or to insects, rodents or other animals, infectious agents and contaminated food and water, is often a lifestyle choice. A business trip to a city in the high-income world, for instance, typically involves far fewer risks than a visit to remote rural areas in the tropics. For example, going outdoors in the evenings in a malaria-endemic area without using precautions, such as wearing protective clothing, applying repellents and taking antimalarials, is highly risky. The duration of the visit may also determine whether the traveller may be subjected to wide changes in temperature and humidity, or to other environmental factors.

Travellers are far more likely to be killed or injured in accidents or through violence than to be struck down by an exotic infectious disease. Assaults are common in some areas and lone travellers are particularly vulnerable. Accidents and injuries are common at mass gatherings (where in addition, infections can spread) in mountain sports and other outdoor adventures. Accidents, injuries and infections are also possible in recreational waters in association with swimming, diving, sailing and other activities.

HIGH ALTITUDES

At high altitude, atmospheric pressure is lowered and the fall in oxygen pressure can lead to hypoxia, as discussed below. At 1500–3500 m, exercise tolerance is impaired and ventilation is stimulated. At 3500–5500 m, there is hypoxia and altitude sickness is possible.

Rapid ascent may lead to acute hypoxia; the affected person becomes faint and may lose consciousness. Acute mountain sickness may develop after 1–6 hours at high altitudes; headache is followed by anorexia, nausea and vomiting, insomnia, fatigue, lassitude and irritability. The outcome is sometimes fatal due to the development of pulmonary and cerebral oedema.

Travellers making a rapid ascent to high altitude (over 3000 m) can consider prophylactic medication (acetazolamide). Those planning to climb or trek at high altitude benefit from a period of gradual adaptation.

FLYING

Flight phobia (fear of flying) is common, particularly since 11 September 2001. There also appears to be an increase in the use of alcohol on flights, with air rage – a form of disruptive behaviour – linked to high levels of stress and frequently precipitated by alcohol.

Dehydration is common. Cabin humidity is low, usually less than 20%, and may cause discomfort of the eyes, mouth and nose, especially in Sjögren syndrome. Fluid should be taken to prevent dehydration – non-alcoholic beverages (water and fruit juices) rather than alcohol, which contributes to dehydration.

Deep vein thrombosis (DVT; Ch. 8) can develop from prolonged immobility leading to pooling of blood, which is probably aggravated by dehydration. Most DVTs are in the calves and cause no symptoms; some cause swelling, stiffness and discomfort. They are usually reabsorbed but, occasionally, pulmonary embolism may follow, with serious consequences including chest pain, dyspnoea and even death, sometimes many hours or days later. Exercise and properly fitted, graduated compression stockings specially designed for air travel may be helpful. Aspirin is often advised prophylactically for its antiplatelet activity for long-distance flights, along with ample fluids and exercise in-flight.

Jet lag – the disruption of sleep patterns and other circadian rhythms (the body's internal clock) caused by crossing multiple time zones in a short period of time – is commonplace. The adverse effects of jet lag may lead to indigestion, general malaise, insomnia, and reduced physical and mental performance. Melatonin may help resynchronize the body's internal clock.

Hypoxia may be experienced because cabin air pressure is relatively low; the blood oxygen saturation is therefore slightly reduced, leading to mild hypoxia. Travellers with pre-existing cardiovascular or pulmonary disease or anaemia (especially sickle cell disease) are highly sensitive to hypoxia, which can be dangerous and even life-threatening.

In people with *ear, nose and sinus or dental infections, or after recent surgery* or injury, there may be pain if air or gas trapped in air-filled body cavities expands. This occurs especially after abdominal trauma and gastrointestinal surgery, craniofacial and ocular injuries, brain operations, and eye operations involving penetration of the eyeball.

Dental issues include head and facial barotraumas (barotrauma-related headache, external otitic barotrauma, barosinusitis and barotitis media), dental barotrauma (barometric pressure-related tooth injury) and barodontalgia (barometric pressure-related oro-dental pain). Special considerations may be required when planning restorative, endodontic, prosthodontic and surgical treatment to aircrew. Prevention is crucial, as is periodic examination, good restorative dentistry and flight restriction (grounding) if there are pulpal issues. Dental documentation is important for forensic purposes.

Infections can occasionally be transmitted in aircraft, as in any confined space, and even influenza and tuberculosis have been transmitted between passengers on long-haul flights. Modern aircraft recirculate up to 50% of cabin air by passing it through high-efficiency particulate air (HEPA) filters, which clean recirculated cabin air, but incompletely. Viruses in particular can be recirculated. Passengers may occasionally also be infected by *insects* in the aircraft and there have been outbreaks of malaria in the vicinity of airports, due to the escape of transported mosquitoes ('airport malaria').

Contraindications to air travel are shown in Box 33.2.

Box 33.2 *Contraindications for air travel*

- Infants under 7 days old
- Women in the last 4 weeks of pregnancy (8 weeks for multiple pregnancies) and until 7 days after delivery
- People with serious medical/surgical conditions:
  - Angina pectoris, recent myocardial infarction or stroke
  - Acute contagious disease
  - Decompression sickness after diving
  - Raised intracranial pressure
  - Recent surgery or injury where trapped air or gas may be present
  - Chronic respiratory disease, breathlessness at rest or unresolved pneumothorax
  - Sickle cell disease
  - Uncontrolled hypertension of more than 200 mmHg (27 kPa) systolic pressure
- Recent psychiatric illness.

HOT OR HUMID CLIMATES

Exposure to hot, dry, dusty air may cause irritation and infection of the eyes and respiratory tract, and may lead to heat exhaustion and heat stroke. Dehydration is particularly likely unless care is taken to maintain adequate fluid intake. Consumption of salt-containing food and drink helps to replenish the electrolytes in case of heat exhaustion and after excessive sweating.

Fungal skin infections (e.g. tinea) can be aggravated by heat and humidity, and taking a daily shower, wearing loose cotton clothing and applying talcum powder to sensitive skin areas help control their development or spread. Many other infections are also more prevalent in such climes (Appendix 21.9 and Ch. 21).

SUN EXPOSURE

Ultraviolet (UV) radiation from the sun includes both UVA (wavelength 315–400 nm) and UVB (280–315 nm) radiation. Radiation may penetrate clear water to a depth of 1 m or more. UVB radiation is particularly intense in summer and in the 4-hour period around solar noon. Both forms of UV radiation are damaging to skin and eyes. Adverse acute effects include sunburn, particularly in light-skinned people, acute keratitis ('snow blindness') and actinic cheilitis (solar keratosis). Long-term adverse effects can include accelerated skin ageing, skin cancers (melanoma, basal cell carcinoma and squamous carcinoma), lip cancer (squamous carcinoma), cataracts, photosensitization (to drugs such as oral contraceptives, antimalarials and antimicrobials, and to perfumes containing oil of bergamot or other citrus oils) and immune suppression, increasing the risk of infectious disease and limiting the efficacy of vaccinations.

INFECTIONS PREVALENT IN THE DEVELOPING WORLD

See Appendix 21.9, and also Chapters 21 and 32.

Some infections are acquired mainly in the tropics but can appear elsewhere, particularly in areas bordering the tropics and subtropics, war zones or places where there are other disasters that lead to poor water and food hygiene, and the proliferation of rodents and other pests. Such infections are increasingly found and imported into high-income countries (e.g. airport malaria, severe acute respiratory syndrome [SARS], bird flu and swine flu) with global warming and the spread of vectors, and with increasing global travel and migration.

Box 33.3 *Main infective hazards associated with travel to developing countries*

- Cholera
- Dengue fever
- Dysentery
- Hepatitis viruses (particularly A)
- HIV and other sexually shared infections
- Infective (travellers') diarrhoea (the most common hazard)
- Malaria (the most important hazard) – a significant health risk in the developing world, especially West Africa; in severe falciparum malaria, mortality is ~30% despite appropriate treatment
- Rabies
- Respiratory viruses
- Tuberculosis
- Yellow fever

The main infective hazards are shown in Box 33.3 but there are many others. Some are potentially lethal, such as dengue fever, which is mosquito-transmitted. Ebola fever, Lassa fever and Marburg disease are highly contagious from human–human contact and are lethal.

BLOOD-BORNE INFECTIONS

Hepatitis B and C, HIV and other agents can be transmitted by direct contact with infected blood or other body fluids, especially by inoculation.

SEXUALLY SHARED INFECTIONS

See Chapter 32.

FOOD-BORNE AND WATER-BORNE HEALTH RISKS

More information on food safety and the prevention of food- and water-borne diseases can be found at: http://www.cdc.gov/food-safety/diseases/ and http://www.nathnac.org/pro/factsheets/food.htm (accessed 30 September 2013).

Food spoilage

Spoilage bacteria cause food to deteriorate and develop unpleasant odours, tastes and textures, but rarely cause food poisoning. There are different spoilage bacteria and each reproduces at specific temperatures: some at low temperatures in refrigerators or freezers, others at room temperature, and most where they have access to nutrients and water. Some of the conditions that accelerate spoilage also encourage growth of pathogenic microorganisms. Food-borne infections are seen worldwide, especially from shellfish, poultry and milk.

Food poisoning

A range of microorganisms can enter the body in food in any country if the food is inadequately cooked, or on the food – for example, if the person preparing the food fails to wash their hands before handling it. *Campylobacter* infection in milk and poultry is the most common cause of food poisoning but other common causes include *Salmonella*, *Listeria*, *Shigella* and *Clostridia*. *Escherichia coli* infections can be serious but are uncommon (Ch. 21). Some infections take a few hours to cause symptoms, others a few days. Contaminated food may also spread a wide range of other infections or infestations, occasionally even worms, such as cysticercosis and echinococcosis (Ch. 21).

Travellers' diarrhoea

Infections transmitted by ingesting contaminated food and water include 'travellers' diarrhoea' (caused by a wide range of viruses and bacteria); this may affect up to 80% of travellers to high-risk destinations. This is essentially food poisoning, and *E. coli* bacteria are the most common culprit.

Most diarrhoeal attacks are self-limiting, with recovery in a few days. It is important, especially for children, to avoid becoming dehydrated, so fluids (e.g. bottled, boiled or treated water, or weak tea) should be taken. If diarrhoea continues for more than 1 day, oral rehydration salt (ORS) solution should be taken. Antidiarrhoeal medicines (e.g. loperamide) are not generally recommended but may be used exceptionally. If the stools contain blood, medical help should be obtained or a course of antibiotics may be taken (for children and pregnant women, azithromycin; for other adults, ciprofloxacin).

Norovirus

Noroviruses are a group of viruses that cause gastroenteritis and an acute onset of pain, nausea, and severe vomiting and diarrhoea. Norovirus illness is usually brief in people who are otherwise healthy but can be serious, especially in young children, the elderly, and people with other medical illnesses, who are most at risk for more severe or prolonged infection.

Norovirus can be found early on in the faeces and for 2 or more weeks after recovery. Being infected with one type of norovirus may not protect against other types. Norovirus is a highly contagious virus transmitted from an infected person, contaminated food or water, or contact with contaminated surfaces. Norovirus infection is preventable by proper hand-washing and general cleanliness. It can spread quickly in closed places like restaurants, daycare centres, nursing homes, schools and cruise ships.

Foods implicated include

- leafy greens (such as lettuce)
- fresh fruits
- shellfish (such as oysters).

Recreational water illnesses

Chlorine is used to decontaminate recreational water but does not kill all microorganisms instantly; some are very tolerant to chlorine and were not known to cause human disease until recently. Recreational water illnesses (RWIs) are increasing, and include gastrointestinal, skin, ear, respiratory, eye, neurological and wound infections. RWIs are spread by swallowing, breathing in mists or aerosols of, or contact with contaminated water in swimming pools, hot tubs, water parks, water play areas, interactive fountains, lakes, rivers or oceans. RWIs can also be caused by chemicals in the water or chemicals that evaporate from the water and cause indoor air quality problems.

Legionellosis is sometimes an RWI. The most common ones, however, are cryptosporidiosis (diarrhoea caused by *Cryptosporidium*) and *Giardia*, *Shigella*, norovirus and *E. coli* O157:H7. The most common causes of gastroenteritis are certain viruses. In children rotavirus is frequently found to be the culprit, but in adults norovirus is more common. All such organisms are contagious, being transmitted by the faeco-oral route and also by vomiting. Rotavirus is the leading cause of severe diarrhoea in infants and young children worldwide. Rotavirus causes severe watery diarrhoea, often with vomiting, fever and abdominal pain; in babies and young children, it can lead to dehydration.

Contamination of spas and whirlpools can lead to infection by *Legionella*, *Pseudomonas aeruginosa* and non-tuberculous mycobacteria. Otitis externa and infections of the urinary tract, respiratory tract, wounds and cornea have also been linked to spas.

Swimming or paddling in water in the developing world may lead to schistosomiasis or other infections such as leptospirosis. Other hazards may include cholera, cryptosporidiosis, giardiasis, hepatitis A and E, legionellosis, leptospirosis, listeriosis and typhoid fever. Direct person-to-person contact or physical contact with contaminated surfaces in the vicinity of swimming pools and spas anywhere may spread the viruses that cause molluscum contagiosum and warts (human papillomaviruses), and fungal infections of the hair, fingernails and skin, especially tinea pedis (athlete's foot).

Other issues

See Chapter 21 for other infections.

Illness can also be caused by biological toxins found in seafood, which may be paralytic, neurotoxic or amnesic (e.g. shellfish; ciguatera toxin; scombroid or puffer fish). 'Red tides' are harmful algal blooms in water that result in the production of potentially lethal neurotoxic brevetoxins, mainly domoic acid and saxitoxins. Brevetoxins cause neurotoxic shellfish poisoning (NSP); domoic acid is a neurotoxin that causes amnesic shellfish poisoning (ASP); and saxitoxin causes paralytic shellfish poisoning (PSP).

DISEASES TRANSMITTED FROM SOIL

Soil-transmitted diseases include those caused by spores, such as anthrax, tetanus and deep mycoses. Some intestinal parasites, such as ascariasis and trichuriasis, are transmitted via soil and infections may result from consumption of soil-contaminated vegetables.

ZOONOSES (DISEASES TRANSMITTED FROM ANIMALS)

A zoonosis is an infection seen in wild or domestic animals that can be transmitted to humans. Infections can be caused by bacteria, viruses, fungi, prions or parasites, which include protozoa and helminths. A partial list of animals that can carry infectious organisms that may be zoonotic is shown in Box 33.4. Rats can, for example, transmit rat-bite fever – infection by bacteria (*Streptobacillus moniliformis* [Haverhill fever] or *Spirillum minus* [sodoku]) – and a wide range of other diseases ranging from typhus to leptospirosis.

Zoonoses include a wide range of infections (such as malaria, dengue fever, Chagas disease, rabies, brucellosis, leptospirosis and certain viral haemorrhagic fevers), which can be transmitted to humans through animal bites or from parasites such as fleas or ticks; via contact with contaminated body fluids or faeces from animals; or by consumption of foods of animal origin, particularly meat and milk products. A partial list of important zoonoses is shown in Box 33.5.

Glanders and SARS (possibly, civet cats may spread the disease, or may catch the disease from humans) might also be zoonoses.

The risk of infection can be reduced by avoiding close contact with any insects or animals – including wild, captive and domestic animals – in places where infection is likely to be present. Pets are no exception and, apart from the dangers from bites (Ch. 24), various infections can

Box 33.4 *Main animals apart from humans that can transmit zoonoses*
• Bats
• Birds
• Cats
• Cattle
• Chickens
• Chimpanzees
• Dogs
• Ducks
• Fish
• Fleas
• Geese
• Goats
• Hamsters
• Horses
• Insects
• Monkeys
• Opossums
• Pigs
• Rabbits and hares
• Raccoons
• Rats
• Rodents
• Sheep
• Sloths
• Snails

be contracted. Particular care should be taken to prevent children from approaching and handling any animals.

INFESTATIONS

See also Chapter 21.

Fleas

General aspects and clinical features

Fleas are parasites of humans and other animals, and are transmitted to those in close proximity. They live mainly on the hairy parts of the body, depositing eggs that can cause an itchy rash. Rodent fleas in particular can act as vectors of life-threatening infections, such as typhus (*Rickettsia prowazekii*; Ch. 21) and plague (*Yersinia pestis*), and have been responsible for recent outbreaks of plague in India and other areas.

General management

Improved hygiene and malathion are indicated.

Lice

General aspects and clinical features

Lice infestations, which are increasing in many areas, especially in vagrants, can be of three main types:

■ Head lice (*Pediculosis humanus* var. *capitis*) infest hair and are particularly common in schoolchildren.
■ *Pediculosis corporis* infests the body and clothes.

- Anthrax
- Avian influenza (bird flu)
- Bolivian haemorrhagic fever
- Borreliosis (Lyme disease and others)
- Borna virus infection
- Bovine tuberculosis
- Brucellosis
- Campylobacteriosis
- Chagas disease
- Creutzfeldt–Jakob disease (variant CJD)
- Crimean–Congo haemorrhagic fever
- Cryptosporidiosis
- Cutaneous larva migrans
- Dengue fever
- Ebola virus infection
- Echinococcosis
- Hantavirus infection
- Hendra virus infection
- Henipavirus infection
- Korean haemorrhagic fever
- Lábrea fever
- Lassa fever
- Leishmaniasis
- Leptospirosis
- Listeriosis
- Lyme disease
- Lymphocytic choriomeningitis virus
- Malaria
- Marburg virus infection
- Monkey B virus
- Nipah virus
- Ocular larva migrans
- Orf
- Ornithosis (psittacosis)
- Oropouche fever
- Plague
- Psittacosis ('parrot fever')
- Q fever
- Rabies
- Rift Valley fever
- Ringworms (*Tinea canis*, mainly)
- Salmonellosis
- Sodoku
- Swine flu
- Toxoplasmosis
- Trichinosis
- Tuberculosis (badgers, cows, elephants)
- Tularaemia ('rabbit fever')
- Typhus and other rickettsial diseases
- Venezuelan haemorrhagic fever
- Visceral larva migrans
- Yellow fever

■ *Phthirus pubis* (crab lice) infests the pubic hair area and is sexually transmitted.

Lice are transmitted by close contact or via discarded clothing and feed off the host's blood; the puncture wounds can become itchy and bleed. Lice can also, under appropriate circumstances,

transmit diseases such as typhus (*Rickettsia prowazekii*), relapsing fever (*Borrelia recurrentis*) and trench fever (*R. quintana*; Ch. 21).

General management

Treatment of lice infestation is with improved hygiene and the use of malathion and carbaryl.

Bedbugs

Bedbugs (*Cimex lectularius*) are small insects that live in cracks and crevices around some beds. Attracted by body heat and carbon dioxide, they bite exposed skin and feed on blood. There has been an explosion in bedbug infestations around the world, particularly in America. Increasing tourism and a growing resistance to insecticides are to blame. Bedbugs feed on blood to mature, but they are resilient and can survive for up to a year without feeding. They can also be found in other furniture, carpets and elsewhere, and spread easily from room to room, not by flying or jumping but by crawling. They can soon invade blocks of flats, hotels, hospitals or other buildings. The bugs can be transported in luggage, clothing, furniture and bedding. Bedbugs do not transmit human diseases. Skin reactions to bedbug bites are typically pruritic red bites, often in straight lines; they appear after 1–9 days, usually on the face, neck, hands or arms.

Treatment is to:

■ wash infected materials at 60° or clean in a dryer on a hot setting for 30 minutes to kill the bugs
■ dismantle bed and furniture and inspect every seam, crevice and joint
■ vacuum to remove any bugs
■ use insecticide spray specially designed for bedbugs; ordinary insect repellent for mosquitoes and ticks does not seem to be effective
■ throw away a mattress if it appears to be heavily infested.

Ticks

General aspects and clinical features

Ticks are parasitic on various animals (Table 33.4) and have the following characteristics:

■ They are arachnids, relatives of spiders.
■ They live in wooded areas mainly.
■ They survive by eating host blood.
■ They can transmit infections from one host to the next, including humans.

Diseases that can be transmitted to humans include the following:

■ 364D rickettsiosis (*Rickettsia phillipi*) is transmitted to humans by the US Pacific Coast tick (*Dermacentor occidentalis*).
■ Anaplasmosis is transmitted to humans by the black-legged tick (*Ixodes scapularis*) in the north-eastern and upper mid-western USA, and by the western black-legged tick (*Ixodes pacificus*) along the Pacific coast.
■ Babesiosis is caused by parasites that infect erythrocytes. In most cases, *Babesia microti* is transmitted by the black-legged tick (*I. scapularis*) and is found primarily in the north-east and upper mid-western USA.
■ Crimean–Congo haemorrhagic fever is found in Eastern Europe, particularly in the former Soviet Union, and in north-western

Table 33.4 *Tick-borne diseases of humans*

Human disease	Microorganism	Main tick implicated	Main host	Clinical features	Treatment: remove tick and use
Babesiosis	*Babesia microti*	*Ixodes scapularis*	Mice	Malaria-like illness. Fatal in elderly or asplenia	Quinine Clindamycin Atovaquone Azithromycin
Colorado tick fever	Coltivirus	*Dermacentor andersoni* or *D. variabilis*	Deer Dog	Acute high fever	Tetracycline
Human monocyte ehrlichiosis	*Erhlichia chaffeensis*	*Amblyomma americanum*	Deer	Fever, myalgia, leukopenia, malaise, nausea	Doxycycline
Human granulocyte ehrlichiosis	*Anaplasma phagocytophila*	*I. scapularis*	Deer Mice	Fever, myalgia, leukopenia, malaise, nausea	Doxycycline
Lyme disease	*Borrelia burgdorferi*	*I. scapularis*	Deer	Rash, arthropathy, neuropathy	Tetracyclines, penicillins, cephalosporins
Powassan virus	Powassan virus	*Ixodes* spp.	Foxes, skunks, racoons	Encephalitis	–
Relapsing fever	*Borrelia* spp.	*Ornithodorus* spp.	Rodents	Fever	Tetracycline
Spotted fever (many different types worldwide)	*Rickettsia rickettsiae* in USA (Rocky mountain spotted fever), other species worldwide	*D. andersoni* or *D. variabilis* in USA	Deer Dog	Fever, myalgia, rash, malaise, nausea Severe disease in glucose-6-phosphate dehydrogenase (G6PD) deficiency	Tetracycline
Tick paralysis	No organism – tick toxin only	*D. andersoni*	Dog	Paralysis, including facial, leading to respiratory paralysis	–
Tularaemia, or rabbit fever	*Franciscella tularensis*	*A. americanum*, *D. andersoni* or *D. variabilis*	Rabbit Dog	Ulcer, lymphadenopathy, fever	Streptomycin, gentamicin

China, Central Asia, southern Europe, Africa, the Middle East and the Indian subcontinent.

- Ehrlichiosis is transmitted to humans by the lone star tick (*Amblyomma americanum*), found primarily in the south–central and eastern USA.
- Imported tick-borne spotted fevers (rickettsial infections) have caused infection in returning travellers. In the USA, the culprit is usually *Rickettsia africae* (the agent of African spotted fever).
- Lyme disease can be caused by several different species of *Borrelia burgdorferi*. It is transmitted by the black-legged tick (*I. scapularis*) in the north-eastern and upper mid-western USA, and by the western black-legged tick (*I. pacificus*) along the Pacific coast.
- *Rickettsia parkeri* causes a rickettsiosis that is transmitted to humans by the Gulf Coast tick (*Amblyomma maculatum*).
- Rocky Mountain spotted fever (RMSF) is transmitted by the American dog tick (*Dermacentor variabilis*), Rocky Mountain wood tick (*Dermacentor andersoni*) and the brown dog tick (*Rhipicephalus sanguineus*) in the USA. The brown dog tick and other tick species are associated with RMSF in Central and South America.
- Southern tick-associated rash illness (STARI) transmitted via bites from the lone star tick (*A. americanum*), found in the south-eastern and eastern USA.
- Tick-borne encephalitis (TBE) is caused by three virus subtypes: European or western tick-borne encephalitis virus, Siberian tick-borne encephalitis virus and Far eastern tick-borne encephalitis virus (formerly Russian spring/summer encephalitis virus).
- Tick-borne relapsing fever (TBRF) is transmitted to humans through the bite of infected soft ticks.
- Tularaemia is transmitted to humans by the dog tick (*D. variabilis*), the wood tick (*D. andersoni*), and the lone star tick (*A. americanum*).

General management

Prevention is by wearing long trousers and long-sleeved shirts in rural areas.

SPIDERS

In the UK, spiders are not normally hazardous to health but a dozen or more species are capable of causing a significant bite. There are more hazards in the developing world, and even in some high-income countries. Some produce neurotoxins and other poisons, and so should be avoided.

More information is available at: http://www.nhm.ac.uk/nature-online/life/insects-spiders/identification-guides-and-keys/spider-bites/, http://www.findaspider.org.au/info/hazards.htm and http://www.cdc.gov/niosh/topics/spiders/ (accessed 30 September 2013).

SNAKES

Not all snakes are poisonous but some are, and some bites are lethal. Remember that snakes may be swimming in water, as well as hiding under objects. If you see a snake, back away slowly and never touch it.

Signs and symptoms of snakebite may include:

- a pair of puncture marks
- redness and swelling around the bite
- severe pain
- nausea and vomiting
- laboured breathing
- disturbed vision
- increased salivation and sweating
- numbness or tingling around face and/or limbs

If a person is bitten, try to see and remember the colour and shape of the snake, and:

- keep the bitten person still in order to slow the venom spread
- seek medical attention
- apply first aid:
  Lay or sit the person down with the bite below the heart level
  Tell them to stay calm and still
  Cover the bite with a clean, dry dressing.

Do not interfere in any way with the bite, or let the victim drink alcohol or caffeine.

More information is available at: http://www.bt.cdc.gov/disasters/pdf/snakebite.pdf (accessed 30 September 2013).

TRAVEL PRECAUTIONS

Comprehensive travel and medical insurance should be obtained before travelling, checking any exclusions and cover for all intended activities.

Before travelling

Since trauma is the greatest danger, travellers should always avoid areas of conflict, violence or natural disasters. Before travel it is advisable to consult: https://www.gov.uk/foreign-travel-advice (accessed 30 September 2013). Infections such as malaria, dengue fever or MERV or H5N7 may need to be considered in the potential traveller's risk-benefit analysis.

Travellers should also consult a travel medicine clinic or medical practitioner at least 4–6 weeks before the journey, particularly if vaccinations or antimalarials may be required, or if they intend to visit a developing country, especially if they intend to be in rural areas for prolonged periods (Box 33.6). Awareness of risk is important and precautionary behaviour indicated. For example, hepatitis, yellow fever, cholera and typhoid immunisation may be prudent or essential before visits to the tropics. Meningitis vaccination may be indicated before hajj or similar gatherings (see Mass Gathering Medicine).

Infants and young children, pregnant women, older people, the disabled and those who have pre-existing health problems may need to take special precautions.

While travelling

Preventing contact with disease-producing organisms is best achieved by: avoiding their habitat (e.g. swamps, jungles); avoiding contact with animals; using barrier precautions (e.g. wearing long sleeves and trousers); avoiding insect bites (e.g. using insect repellents); avoiding exposure to animal excreta; and maintaining high levels of food, water and personal hygiene. Do not consume food that could be contaminated; this is best achieved by drinking and using bottled water, and by eating freshly cooked meat or fish. Use of chlorine and other disinfectants controls most viruses and bacteria in water, though parasites such as *Giardia* and *Cryptosporidium* are highly resistant to routine disinfection; they are, however, inactivated by ozone or eliminated by filtration. Antimicrobial prophylaxis against diarrhoeal disease is not recommended; precautions are shown in Box 33.7.

Avoid direct contact with blood and body fluids by not using potentially contaminated needles and syringes for injection or any other medical or cosmetic procedure that penetrates the skin (including acupuncture, body piercing and tattooing), and by avoiding transfusion of unsafe blood.

Box 33.6 *Vaccines for travellers*

Routine vaccination

- Diphtheria/tetanus/pertussis (DTP)
- *Haemophilus influenzae* type b (Hib)
- Hepatitis B (HBV)
- Measles (measles/mumps/rubella; MMR)
- Poliomyelitis (oral or inactivated poliomyelitis vaccine [OPV or IPV])

Mandatory vaccination

- Meningococcal meningitis (for Haj, Umra)
- Yellow fever (certain countries)

Selective use[a]

- Cholera
- Hepatitis A (HAV)
- Influenza
- Japanese B encephalitis
- Lyme disease
- Meningococcal meningitis
- Pneumococcal disease
- Rabies
- Tick-borne encephalitis
- Tuberculosis (bacilli Calmette–Guérin; BCG)
- Typhoid fever
- Yellow fever

[a]Check for country to be visited.

Box 33.7 *Prophylaxis against diarrhoeal disease*

Eat

- Only food that has been cooked thoroughly and is still hot

Boil

- Unpasteurized (raw) milk before consumption
- Drinking water, if its safety is doubtful; a certified, well-maintained filter and/or a disinfectant agent can also be used

Avoid

- Cooked food kept at room temperature for several hours
- Uncooked food, apart from fruit and vegetables that can be peeled or shelled
- Fruits with damaged skins
- Dishes containing raw or undercooked eggs
- Food or ice cream bought from street vendors
- Ice, unless it has been made from safe water
- Brushing teeth with unsafe water; bottled or packaged cold drinks are usually safe, provided that they are sealed
- Contaminated recreational water, particularly sewage-polluted sea water or fresh water in lakes and rivers, as well as water in swimming pools and spas

On return

On return, travellers should have a medical examination if they: suffer from a chronic illness, such as cardiovascular disease, diabetes mellitus or chronic respiratory disease; experience illness, particularly fever, persistent diarrhoea, vomiting, jaundice, urinary disorders, skin disease or genital infection; consider that they have been exposed to a serious infectious disease; or have spent more than 3 months in a developing country.

MASS GATHERING MEDICINE

Mass gatherings are occasions such as sports events, music festivals or religious celebrations that attract a large number of people: for example, the annual Muslim Hajj pilgrimage to Saudi Arabia and Mecca, or the Hindu Magh Mela in India and Allahabad. Mass gatherings may be defined as public events attended by in excess of 1000–25 000 people. Such events can give rise to disasters such as stampedes with physical injuries and deaths, and to eventualities ranging from infectious disease outbreaks to terrorist attacks – with implications beyond the scope of typical public health provision. Factors influencing demand for the health care at mass gatherings may include:

■ alcohol/drugs
■ crowd containment (fenced/contained or not)
■ crowd density
■ crowd movement
■ event duration
■ communicable disease spread
■ weather.

See Chapter 21.

PETS

Bites, scratches and infections are discussed above and in Chapters 21 and 24.

KEY WEBSITES

(Accessed 8 July 2013)
Centers for Disease Control and Prevention. <http://wwwnc.cdc.gov/travel/>.
GOV.UK. Foreign travel advice. <https://www.gov.uk/foreign-travel-advice>.
National Institute of Arthritis and Musculoskeletal and Skin Diseases. <http://www.niams.nih.gov/health_info/sports_injuries/>. <http://www.who.int/csr/mass_gatherings/en/>.

USEFUL WEBSITES

(Accessed 11 June 2013)
British Association of Sport & Exercise Medicine. <http://www.basem.co.uk/>.
Medscape Reference. <http://www.emedicine.com/sports/index.shtml>.
Peak Performance. <http://www.pponline.co.uk/>.
Sports Medicine Online. <http://www.sportsmedicine.com/>.
Travax. <http://www.travax.nhs.uk>.

Travel Doctor. <http://www.traveldoctor.co.uk>.
UK Sport. <http://www.uksport.gov.uk>.
World Anti-Doping Code (under 'International Standards/Prohibited List'). <http://www.wada-ama.org/en/World-Anti-Doping-Program/>.
World Health Organization: Disease Outbreak News (DONs). <http://www.who.int/csr/don/en>.

FURTHER READING

Antoun, J.S., Lee, K.H., 2008. Sports-related maxillofacial fractures over an 11-year period. J. Oral Maxillofac. Surg. 66, 504.
Barnett, F., 2003. Prevention of sports-related dental trauma: the role of mouthguards. Pract. Proced. Aesthet. Dent. 15, 391.
Brewer, P.A., Barry, M., 2002. Survey of Web-based health care information for prospective cruise line passengers. J. Travel Med. 9, 194.
Cossar, J.H., et al., 2003. A comparison of travel related ID admissions in Glasgow (1985; 1998/99). Scott. Med. J. 48, 49.
Foster, M., Readman, P., 2009. Sports dentistry – what's it all about. Dent. Update 36, 135.
Gassner, R., et al., 2003. Cranio-maxillofacial trauma: a 10 year review of 9,543 cases with 21,067 injuries. J. Craniomaxillofac. Surg. 31, 51.
Horvath, L.L., et al., 2003. Travel health information at commercial travel websites. J. Travel Med. 10, 272.
Kirkpatrick, B.D., Alston, W.K., 2003. Current immunizations for travel. Curr. Opin. Infect. Dis. 16, 369.
Kolars, J.C., 2002. Rules of the road: a consumer's guide for travelers seeking health care in foreign lands. J. Travel Med. 9, 198.
Lang, B., et al., 2002. Knowledge and prevention of dental trauma in team handball in Switzerland and Germany. Dent. Traumatol. 18, 329.
Lee, K.H., Steenberg, L.J., 2008. Equine-related facial fractures. Int. J. Oral Maxillofac. Surg. 37, 999.
Lo Re III, V., Gluckman, S.J., 2003. Fever in the returned traveller. Am. Fam. Physician 68, 1343.
Macpherson, A., Spinks, A., 2008. Bicycle helmet legislation for the uptake of helmet use and prevention of head injuries. Cochrane Database Syst. Rev. (3) CD005401
McInnes, R.J., et al., 2002. Unintentional injury during foreign travel: a review. J. Travel Med. 9, 297.
McIntosh, A.S., Janda, D., 2003. Evaluation of cricket helmet performance and comparison with baseball and ice hockey helmets. Br. J. Sports Med. 37, 325.
Memish, Z.A., et al., 2012. Mass gatherings medicine. Lancet Infect. Dis. 12 (1), 10. doi:10.1016/S1473-3099(11)70319.
Muller-Bolla, M., et al., 2003. Orofacial trauma and rugby in France: epidemiological survey. Dent. Traumatol. 19, 183.
Newsome, P.R.H., et al., 2001. The role of the mouthguard in the prevention of sports-related dental injuries: a review. Int. J. Paediat. Dent. 11, 396.
Papakosta, V., et al., 2008. Maxillofacial injuries sustained during soccer: incidence, severity and risk factors. Dent. Traumatol. 24, 193.
Solomon, T., 2003. Exotic and emerging viral encephalitides. Curr. Opin. Neurol. 16, 411.
Spira, A.M., 2003. Assessment of travellers who return home ill. Lancet 361, 1459.
Spira, A.M., 2003. Preparing the traveller. Lancet 361, 1368.
Zadik, Y., 2009. Aviation dentistry: current concepts and practice. Br. Dent. J. 206 (1), 11. doi:10.1038/sj.bdj.2008.1121.
Zazryn, T.R., et al., 2003. 16 year study of injuries to professional boxers in the state of Victoria, Australia. Br. J. Sports Med. 37, 321.

Dependence or addiction is characterized by impaired control over drug use, compulsive use, continued use despite harm, and/or craving. Substance or chemical dependence or abuse (misuse) covers a range of mind-altering substances and is present when at least three of the conditions listed in Box 34.1 apply. Most addictive substances directly or indirectly stimulate the brain's reward centre by increasing release of dopamine – the neurotransmitter involved in the regulation of emotion, cognition, movement, motivation and pleasure. Brain stimulation with dopamine produces intense euphoria, a pleasurable sensation reinforced by continued drug use.

Drug abuse causes central nervous system (CNS) effects that produce changes in the mind, behaviour, thoughts and mood, levels of awareness or perceptions and sensations. It is defined as self-administration without any medical indication and despite adverse medical and social consequences, in a manner that deviates from the cultural norm and is harmful. Social, mental and physical sequelae are common and discussed below.

Use of some of these drugs is illegal, and being found in possession of them can lead to criminal charges, particularly, if there is any intention of dealing (supplying; Table 34.1). In the UK, illegal drugs are classified under the Misuse of Drugs Act 1971 as A, B and C, depending on how dangerous they are to health; this classification can only be changed and added to by the Home Secretary. In some countries, use or possession may result in more serious punishments – even execution.

RISK FACTORS FOR DRUG ABUSE

Addiction is a primary, chronic, neurobiological condition, influenced by genetic, psychosocial and environmental factors. Men are twice as likely as women to experience drug problems. Factors that may contribute to drug use include:

- genetic factors
- environmental factors, such as:
  home and family, friends and acquaintances who use drugs
  time of drug use
  personality (low self-esteem, stress)
  availability of drugs
  method of drug administration
  coexisting mental problems.

PERSONS WHO USE DRUGS (PWUD)

Substance abuse is increasingly common in many parts of the world. The pattern of drug use in the British Crime Survey by 2012 is shown in Box 34.2.

The 2012/13 Crime Survey for England and Wales showed that in the past year:

- Cannabis was the most commonly used drug
- The next most commonly used were powder cocaine and ecstasy.
- Young adults (aged 16 to 24) were more likely to use drugs.
- Around 1 in 12 adults had taken an illicit drug.

In the USA, the highest rates of illicit drug use are: in males – in entertainment, food preparation and service, cleaning services and construction; and in females – in food preparation and service, social work and legal professions, including lawyers and legal assistants. Abuse of alcohol is highest among construction workers, car mechanics, food preparation workers, light truck drivers and labourers. Unmarried workers or those having three or more jobs in the previous 5 years report about twice the rate of illicit drug and heavy alcohol use as married workers or those who had two or fewer jobs.

The lowest rates of illicit drug use are in workers in occupations that require public trust, such as health-care professions (HCPs), police officers, teachers and child-care workers. Between 10 and 15% of HCPs misuse drugs or alcohol at some time during their life – rates similar to those seen in the general population. Alcohol abuse is relatively common among doctors and dentists, and one study of USA medical personnel found that over half had tried marijuana or cocaine recreationally, or opioids or tranquillizers for self-treatment. HCPs have higher rates of abuse with benzodiazepines and opiates, and abuse drugs for performance enhancement and as self-treatment for various reasons, such as pain, anxiety or depression. Those in anaesthesia, emergency medicine and psychiatry have the highest rates of drug abuse.

Drugs and alcohol used by medical and dental students are mostly for 'recreational' purposes. More than a half of UK dental students in 2003 had used cannabis and over one-third admitted other illicit drug use. Some 6–10% of dentists may abuse drugs, but there is limited evidence to suggest that they are at a greater risk for abusing alcohol or other drugs than the public. Alcohol and tobacco are the substances abused most frequently by dentists, followed by opiates (mainly hydrocodone and oxycodone) and nitrous oxide. Other substances abused include marijuana; opiates (e.g. morphine, fentanyl, pethidine (meperidine),

---

Box 34.1 *Features suggesting substance dependence*

- Some symptoms of the disturbance must have persisted for at least 1 month or have recurred repeatedly over a longer period
- Substances are often taken in larger amounts or over longer periods than intended
- There is a persistent desire or one or more unsuccessful efforts to reduce or control substance use
- Excessive time is spent in activities that lead to obtaining the substance (e.g. theft), taking the substance (e.g. chain smoking) or recovering from its effects
- Important social, occupational or recreational activities are reduced or abandoned because of substance misuse
- There is continued substance use, despite the knowledge that it produces persistent or recurrent social, psychological or physical problems
- There is growing tolerance – greatly increased amounts of the substance are needed to achieve the desired effect, or greatly diminished effect is produced by continued use of the same amount
- There are characteristic withdrawal symptoms
- Substances are often taken to relieve or avoid withdrawal symptoms

Table 34.1 *Main drug classes and penalties for possession and supply*

	Class under the UK Misuse of Drugs Act		
	A	**B**	**C**
Considered a danger to health	Most dangerous	Dangerous	Least harmful
Drugs	Cocaine (including crack; nicknamed charlie, coke, snow)	Amphetamine (an ingredient of ecstasy; nicknamed speed, whizz, dexies)	Anabolic steroids (nicknamed roids)
	Diconal	Barbiturates	Benzodiazepines, including valium and Rohypnol (flunitrazepam) (nicknamed roofies and sometimes referred to as date-rape drugs)
	Heroin (nicknamed smack, H, gear, skag, brown)	Cannabis, cannabis resin and cannabinol	GHB (gamma-hydroxybutrate; nicknamed liquid ecstasy and sometimes referred to as date-rape drugs)
	LSD (lysergic acid diethylamide; nicknamed acid, trips, blotters, tabs)	Codeine (in concentrations above 2.5%)	Ketamine (nicknamed special K, vitamin K, green)
	Magic mushrooms	DF118 (dihydrocodeine)	Methaqualone
	MDMA ((3,4-methylenedioxy-*N*-methylamphetamine)	Cathinones (mephedrone, naphyrone)	
	Mescaline	Methoxetamine	
	Methadone	Ritalin	
	Methylamphetamine		
	Morphine		
	Opium		
	PCP (phencyclidine; nicknamed angel dust)		
	Pethidine		
	Poppy straw		
	Psilocybin		
	STP (amphetamine; nicknamed serenity, tranquillity and peace)		
Maximum penalties			
Possession	7 years in prison and/or a fine	5 years in prison and/or a fine	2 years in prison and/or a fine
Supply	Life in prison and/or a fine	14 years in prison and/or a fine	5 years in prison and/or a fine

---

Box 34.2 *UK drug use in 2011–2012[a]*

- 1 in 3 adults (36.5%) had taken an illicit drug in their lifetime
- 15.6% of adults had taken a class A drug in their lifetime
- 8.9% per cent of adults had used an illicit drug in the last year (this remains around the lowest level since measurement began in 1996)
- Among 16- to 59-year-olds, 3.0% had used a class A drug in the last year (similar to levels in the 2010/11 [3.0%] and 2009/10 [3.1%] surveys)
- Cannabis was the most commonly used type of drug in the last year (6.9% of adults), followed by powder cocaine (2.2%)
- The other main drugs used included ecstasy, amyl nitrite, amphetamines and ketamine

[a]Does not cover groups like the homeless or those living in institutions such as prisons, who have potentially high rates of drug use, and problematic drug users who are unable to take part in an interview. From http://www.homeoffice.gov.uk/publications/science-research-statistics/research-statistics/crime-research/drugs-misuse-dec-1112/extent-adults (accessed 30 September 2013).

hydromorphone and oxycodone); minor opiates (e.g. hydrocodone and codeine); and anxiolytics (e.g. alprazolam and diazepam). Interpersonal and life circumstances that contribute to dentists misusing drugs and alcohol include career choice dissatisfaction, domestic breakdown, low professional or self-esteem, obsessive–compulsive and perfectionist behaviour, interpersonal relationship difficulties, and stress at work.

Dentists who become aware and are sure of a colleague's chemical dependency have professional and ethical responsibilities to intervene in a constructive manner. All dentists have an ethical obligation to urge chemically impaired colleagues to seek treatment. Interventions involve discussing the issue with the addicted dentist, offering help if possible, and reporting the dentist to a wellness committee. Once a person with an addiction accepts the presence of the issue and expresses a desire to change, treatment can begin, but it should be individually designed by professionals experienced in treating drug and alcohol abuse. Clinicians in the UK who have such issues can receive support from the Practitioner Health Programme, initiated by the National Clinical Assessment Service (NCAS; http://www.php.nhs.uk/, accessed 30 September 2013).

RECOGNIZING AND DETECTING SUBSTANCE ABUSE

Behavioural traits that should increase the level of concern include loss of reliability, mood changes, impaired driving, and the self-prescribing of mood-altering medications. Care should be taken with any patient who has subjective symptoms with no objective evidence of the disorder; makes a self-diagnosis and requests a specific drug, especially a psychoactive agent; appears to have a dramatic but unexpected complaint, such as trigeminal neuralgia, requiring potent analgesics; firmly rejects treatments that exclude psychoactive drugs; and has no interest in the diagnosis or investigations, or refuses a second opinion.

To help a friend/colleague address such problems, it is important to document the dates and times when people have expressed concern and when the signs of substance abuse were noted. These may include the smell of alcohol, tremor, slurred speech, ataxic gait and sloppy appearance. It is important to monitor and document incidents so that this information will be available when discussing concerns with a friend or colleague. The user's first response is typically denial – and a person in denial will often try to convince others that their assessments are wrong or misguided. Recognition of abuse in an HCP may include, in addition to the above, patient and staff complaints about deteriorating attitude and behaviour, worsening personal and professional isolation, excessive amounts of time spent near a drug supply, heavy 'wastage' of drugs, sloppy record-keeping, suspect ledger entries and drug shortages, inappropriate prescriptions, or insistence on the personal administration of injected narcotics to patients.

MEDICAL AND SOCIAL COMPLICATIONS OF DRUG ABUSE

There may be intense drug dependence (or psychological addiction; Table 34.2) and physical effects (physical addiction) in people who use drugs (PWUD) or if a drug of abuse is stopped (withdrawal syndrome) (Fig. 34.1).

Use of illicit drugs is associated with increased rates of infections (e.g. tuberculosis and sexually shared infections [SSIs]), and health and social issues related to alcohol, tobacco and other drugs. Injection drug use is an important route of transmission of blood-borne infections, particularly HIV and viral hepatitis B and C.

Drugs bought on the street are especially hazardous, as they are not necessarily pure and are frequently adulterated or falsely labelled, often with unknown ingredients that may be dangerous in their own right. For example, PWUD who think they are purchasing a drug such as MDMA (ecstasy; 3,4-methylenedioxy-N-methylamphetamine) may be in danger of receiving synthetic cathinones instead; mephedrone has been found as a substitute for MDMA in pills sold as ecstasy in some countries. Intravenous use and the mixing of drugs (polydrug use) are particularly hazardous; those who misuse drugs not uncommonly

misuse several substances, including alcohol and tobacco, and may well neglect their health – general and oral. Heroin and cocaine are especially dangerous. Tobacco and alcohol also cause significant harm, but cannabis appears to be less harmful in general.

Almost every month, new synthetic drugs, opiate painkillers and other substances emerge as popular among partygoers and drug addicts. Recently appearing new drugs include:

- *Molly* – the most-refined, crystalline form of MDMA, blamed for lethal drug overdoses
- *Crocodile* or 'krokodil' – previously used in Russia and former Soviet Bloc nations. Cases have started appearing in the USA and other countries. It is desomorphine, a cheap codeine derivative mixed with gasoline, oil, alcohol or paint thinner. Addicts shoot the mixture directly into their skin with a needle, resulting in dark, scaly patches of necrotic skin. Users are often severely disfigured for life, suffering serious scarring, bone damage, amputated limbs, speech impediments, poor motor skills and varying degrees of brain damage
- *Butane hash oil* (BHO), also known as amber, honey, wax and ear wax – a highly concentrated form of tetrahydrocannabinol (THC). The BHO high is nothing like regular marijuana and users may lose consciousness after inhaling it
- *2C-P* – a long-lasting and very potent psychedelic drug whose effects begin only after a few hours but can last for 10–20 hours
- *Suboxone* (buprenorphine) – an opiate analgesic used to wean addicts off powerful opiates like heroin and hydrocodone; it is also abused.

See also "LEGAL HIGHS" and "EMERGING DRUGS".

Table 34.2 *Drug dependence*[a]

Drug	Psychological dependence	Physical dependence
Heroin	++++++	++++++
Cocaine	+++++	+++
Alcohol	++++	+++
Tobacco	+++++	++++
Barbiturates	++++	++++
Benzodiazepines	++++	++++
Amphetamine	+++	++
LSD	++	+
Cannabis	+++	+
Ecstasy	++	+

[a]Adapted from: Nutt D, et al. Development of a rational scale to assess the harm of drugs of potential misuse. *Lancet* 2007; 369 (9566): 1047.

CLINICAL FEATURES

Signs and symptoms that may indicate drug addiction include behavioural and social features, as well as health aspects (Table 34.3). There can be serious medical and behavioural consequences affecting both user (and any fetus) and others in the community, not least because of assaults, theft and prostitution used to fund the drug habit. Maxillofacial injuries and sexually shared and other infectious diseases are thus common consequences. Intravenous injection is common in drug misuse, often with filthy injection technique, sharing of needles or syringes (with the risk of blood-borne infections) and even use of water from a lavatory pan to dissolve the drug. Viral hepatitis (particularly B, C, D and others), chronic liver disease, human immunodeficiency virus (HIV) and other blood-borne agents are common consequences of intravenous drug abuse or drug 'snorting'. Infective endocarditis and consequent cardiac lesions may stem from infected injections. Venous thromboses are common, making intravenous injection difficult.

GENERAL MANAGEMENT

Common management difficulties are behavioural problems, including irregular health care, poor attendance and compliance, effects of trauma and the frequent risk of maxillofacial and other injuries during assaults or fights, and hazards of cross-infection with hepatitis viruses, HIV and, increasingly, tuberculosis. PWUDs who collapse or become hyperthermic, drowsy or panicky may well need emergency care (Table 34.4). Many drugs of abuse can alter behaviour or interact with drugs used for medical or dental purposes (Ch. 29). There can therefore be substantial difficulties in interactions between HCPs and

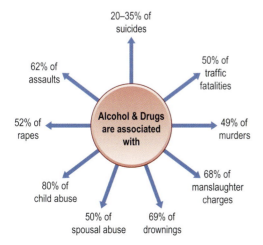

Fig. 34.1 Outcomes from substance abuse.

Table 34.3 *Features possibly suggesting drug misuse (recognition of persons who use drugs)*

Presentation	Features	Behaviour	Social history
Specific requests for drugs of misuse No fixed abode	Progressive deterioration in personal appearance and hygiene, deterioration of handwriting, alcohol on the breath, nicotine on fingers, smell of marijuana, tremors, avoidance of eye contact, constricted or dilated pupils, a history of liver disease, wearing long sleeves when inappropriate Puncture marks, scars or pigmentation over veins Jaundice	Personality change – mood swings, anxiety, depression, lack of impulse control, suicidal thoughts or gestures, and deteriorating interpersonal relations with rare admittance or acceptance of blame for errors or oversights. Unusually elated, drowsy or restless	Frequent changes of health carers Family disruption Frequent changes in or loss of employment Self-discharge from health care History of offences to obtain money Work absenteeism, frequent disappearances from work, improbable excuses and frequent or long trips to the lavatory or stockroom where drugs are kept Unreliability in keeping appointments, meeting deadlines and work performance

Table 34.4 *Emergency care of people who use drugs*

Patient problem	Possible causal drugs	Steps		
		1	2	3
Consciousness lost	Alcohol, heroin, tranquillizers, solvent abuse, ecstasy	Place in recovery position. Call ambulance	Cardiopulmonary resuscitation	
Dehydrated and hot	Ecstasy, methedrone, speed	Reassure and calm person. Give non-alcoholic drinks (1 pint/h). Move to cool area. Remove hot clothing	Call ambulance	Cardiopulmonary resuscitation
Drowsy	Heroin, tranquillizers, solvent abuse	Reassure	Place in recovery position Avoid coffee	Call ambulance
Panicky	Ecstasy, LSD, methedrone, magic mushrooms, speed	Reassure and calm the person	Keep in quiet area, accompanied	Call ambulance

drug users. However, it is unethical to withhold treatment from any patient on the basis of a moral judgment that the patient's activities or lifestyle might have contributed to the condition for which treatment was being sought.

MAIN GROUPS OF DRUGS ABUSED

Patterns of drug misuse change rapidly, depending on fashion and cultural factors, availability and cost. New agents are constantly appearing, often in an attempt to circumnavigate the law and frequently under a variety of names, and may have adverse effects. For example, benzylpiperazine (BZP; A2, legal E, legal XTC, legal high, Jax, London Underground, Pep twisted or Pep love) appeared as an alternative to ecstasy but caused serious adverse effects (see http://www.justice.gov/dea/druginfo/factsheets.shtml and http://www.talkto-frank.com/home_html.aspx; accessed 30 September 2013).

The main groups of drugs abused are stimulants (uppers), depressants (hypnotics/sedatives/downers), hallucinogens (psychedelics) and anabolic steroids (Table 34.5). Alcohol, tobacco, solvents, cannabis and ecstasy have been popular for many years; apart from these, heroin is the main drug of misuse, followed closely by mephedrone, methadone and cocaine (Tables 34.5 and 34.6). Other drugs commonly abused include amphetamines, barbiturates, benzodiazepines, methaqualone and opium alkaloids. Drugs abused may be obtained legally from a doctor or chemist, or may be illicitly obtained. They may be taken orally, inhaled, or injected into the skin, muscle or a vein.

Prescription drugs are commonly abused – notably stimulants, CNS depressants, analgesics and opioids.

Club drugs are those used by teenagers and young adults who are part of a nightclub, bar, trance or rave scene – night-long dances, often

Table 34.5 *Common drugs of misuse and the possible consequences*

Drug type	Risks from misuse	Examples	Intravenous use and possible consequent blood-borne virus infection transmission, endocarditis or septicaemia
Stimulants	Behavioural disturbances and psychoses	Amphetamines	+
		Cocaine	+
		Crack cocaine	−
		MDMA (ecstasy)	+
Sedatives	Fatal overdose	Alcohol	−
	Seizures on withdrawal	Barbiturates	+
		Benzodiazepines	+
Opioids	Respiratory arrest in overdose	Buprenorphine	+
		Dipipanone	+
		Heroin	+
		Methadone	+

held in warehouses (Table 34.7). In high doses, club drugs can cause a sharp rise in body temperature (malignant hyperthermia) leading to muscle breakdown and renal and cardiovascular system failure.

Date-rape drugs, such as gamma-hydroxybutyric acid (GHB), Rohypnol (flunitrazepam) and ketamine, are used because they lack colour, taste and odour, and thus can be added to beverages to be ingested unknowingly by the victim. They are CNS depressants that cause loss of inhibitions and memory. They can also readily cause unconsciousness.

Table 34.6 *Main groups of substances abused*

Stimulants (uppers)	Depressants (hypnotic/sedatives/downers)	Hallucinogens (psychedelics)	Analgesics	Anabolic steroids
Actions				
Speed brain activity	Slow brain activity	Distort brain activity	Decrease pain	Promote growth and muscle
Examples				
Amphetamine, caffeine, cocaine, crack, dextroamphetamine, diethylpropion, mephedrone, methylphenidate, naphyrone, nicotine, phenmetrazine, tobacco	*Anxiolytics*: alprazolam, benzodiazepines, clorazepate, meprobamate *Barbiturate* *Ethanol (alcohol)* *Inhalants*: amyl nitrite, butyl nitrite, enflurane, ether, halothane, isoflurane, nitrous oxide, petrol, solvents (various)	Lysergic acid diethylamide (LSD), mephedrone, mescaline (peyote), methyl-dimethoxy amphetamine (STP; DOM), methylene dioxyamphetamine (MDA), 3,4-methylenedioxy-methamphetamine (MDMA; ecstasy), phencyclidine (PCP), psilocybin *Cannabinoids*: marijuana	*Opioids*: codeine, fentanyl, heroin, hydrocodone, lomotil, pethidine (meperidine), methyl-phenyl-tetra-hydropyridine (MPTP), morphine, oxycodone, propoxyphene	Nandrolone (Deca-Durabolin), Sustanon 250, Dianabol, Anavar, stanozolol
Main CNS and adverse effects				
Exhilaration, energy, reduced appetite, weight loss, alertness; rapid or irregular heart beat; raised heart rate, blood pressure, metabolism	Feeling of well-being; lowered inhibitions; slowed pulse and breathing; lowered blood pressure; poor concentration, confusion, fatigue; impaired coordination, memory, judgment; respiratory depression and arrest	Altered states of perception and feeling; nausea, psychoses, persisting perception disorder (flashbacks)	Pain relief, euphoria, drowsiness, nausea, confusion, constipation, sedation, respiratory depression and arrest, unconsciousness, coma	No intoxication effects

Table 34.7 *Currently popular club drugs*

Street name	Constituents	Effects	Comments
Cat	Methcathinone	Produces a cocaine-like high with hallucinations similar to mescaline	Analogue of methamphetamine
China white	Beta-hydroxy methylfentanyl	6000 times the potency of natural heroin. Responsible for many narcotic overdose deaths	Analogue of fentanyl
Double stack or PMA	Paramethoxyamphetamine	Does not produce the pleasurable MDMA effects, so users take more drug. Dramatic rise in body temperature in excess of 109°F. Death from hyperthermia	Analogue of methamphetamine
DXM	Dextromethorphan	Hallucinations and a heavy 'stoned' feeling in users but no desirable ecstasy effects	Often passed off as ecstasy. Found in over-the-counter cold remedies
Ecstasy	3,4-Methylenedioxy-methamphetamine (MDMA)	Resembles methamphetamine, but also produces mild hallucinations and a feeling of emotional closeness to other people	The most sought-after club drug
Eve	3,4-Methylenedioxymethamphetamine (MDE)	Does *not* produce the ecstasy feeling of emotional closeness	Analogue of ecstasy
GBL (gamma-butyrolactone and 1,4-butanediol)	Gamma-butyrolactone and 1,4-butanediol. Together they convert to GHB	Taken alone, or especially when mixed or with alcohol, produces stupor, vomiting and coma	Related to GHB. Sold over the Internet to avoid laws against GHB
GHB, super-G, liquid G, liquid ecstasy	Gamma-hydroxybutyric acid	Taken alone, or especially when mixed with alcohol, produces stupor, vomiting and coma	A clear, odourless liquid with a slightly salty taste. Originally thought to be a human growth hormone, it was abused by body-builders until banned in 1991 by the Food and Drug Administration (FDA)
Ice	Methamphetamine	Produces a 10-h high	A smokable form of recrystallized methamphetamine similar to crack
Meow meow (see also Cat)	Mephedrone	Feelings of euphoria, alertness, talkativeness, empathy, anxiety, paranoia and overstimulation of the heart and circulatory system. Over-excitation of the nervous system, which can cause seizures	Was sold over the Internet as a 'legal high', often described as a plant food, research chemicals or bath salts
Naphyrone		Similar to mephedrone	
Nexus or 2C-B	4-Bromo-2, 5-dimethoxyphenethylamine	Produces strong, ecstasy-like feelings of closeness and sexual enhancement	Phenylethylamine analogue of powerful hallucinatory drug 4-bromo-2, 5-dimethoxyamphetamine (DOB)
Rohypnol	Flunitrazepam	Mixed with alcohol, as a 'date-rape' drug	Analogue of diazepam but ten times as powerful
Special K	Ketamine	Produces hallucinations and stupor and is highly addictive	Analogue of phencyclidine (PCP)
YABA	Methamphetamine	Produces a 10-h high	Ultrapure form of methamphetamine often combined with caffeine

Table 34.8 *Common stimulants*

Main stimulant groups	Street names[a]	Comments
Adrenaline (epinephrine) derivatives ephedrine and pseudoephedrine	Bennies, black beauties, crosses, hearts, LA turnaround, speed, truck drivers, uppers	Raised heart rate, blood pressure, metabolism, feelings of exhilaration, energy, increased mental alertness, rapid or irregular heart beat, reduced appetite, weight loss, heart failure, rapid breathing
Phentermine		Hallucinations/tremor, loss of coordination, irritability, anxiousness, restlessness,
Amphetamine		delirium, panic, paranoia, impulsive behaviour, aggressiveness, tolerance, addiction
Caffeine	Found in tea and coffee, cola and a number of energy drinks	Energy, increased mental alertness, rapid or irregular heart beat
Cocaine	Blow, bump, C, candy, charlie, coke, crack, flake, rock, snow, toot, white	Raised temperature, chest pain, respiratory failure, nausea, abdominal pain, strokes, seizures, headaches, malnutrition
Cocaine hydrochloride		
Methylenedioxy-methamphetamine (MDMA)	DOB, DOM, MDA, adam, clarity, ecstasy, eve, lover's speed, peace, STP, X, XTC, E, pills, XTC, disco biscuits, Mitsubishis, Rolexs, dolphins	Mild hallucinogenic effects, increased tactile sensitivity, empathic feelings, hyperthermia, impaired memory and learning
Methamphetamine	Chalk, crank, crystal, fire, glass, go fast, ice, meth, speed	Aggression, violence, psychotic behaviour, memory loss, cardiac and neurological damage, impaired memory and learning, tolerance, addiction
Mephedrone	White magic, miaow, meph, meow meow, MC, M-CAT, drone, charge, bubble, bounce, 4-MMC	Feelings of euphoria, alertness, talkativeness, empathy, anxiety, paranoia and overstimulation of the heart and circulatory system. Over-excitation of the nervous system, which can cause seizures
Methylphenidate	Ritalin, JIF, MPH, R-ball, skippy, the smart drug, vitamin R	Increase or decrease in blood pressure, psychotic episodes, digestive problems, loss of appetite, weight loss
Naphyrone	NRG, O-2482 or naphthylpyrovalerone	Similar to mephedrone. Was sold over the Internet as a 'legal high', often described as a plant food, research chemicals or bath salts. Feelings of euphoria, alertness, talkativeness, empathy, anxiety, paranoia and overstimulation of the heart and circulatory system. Over-excitation of the nervous system, which can cause seizures
Nicotine	Bidis, chew, cigars, cigarettes, smokeless tobacco, snuff, spit tobacco	Tolerance, addiction, additional effects attributable to tobacco exposure – adverse pregnancy outcomes, chronic lung disease, cardiovascular disease, stroke, cancer

[a] See Appendix 34.1.

STIMULANTS

Stimulants are substances that cause excitement and euphoria (a 'high'), which may last several hours. Withdrawal symptoms (restlessness, agitation, sleeplessness and depression) may follow. Heavy use of strong stimulants for weeks may cause paranoia and auditory hallucinations – effects that may be irreversible (Table 34.8).

Stimulants cause moderate to severe psychological addiction. Withdrawal is purely psychological and psychosomatic. They include:

- amphetamine and methamphetamine
- caffeine
- cocaine
- mephedrone
- nicotine.

Stimulants used in various cultures include betel, caffeine, cocaine, kava, khat, kratom, marijuana, salvia and tobacco (Table 34.9). Common herbal sources of psychedelics include *Psilocybe* mushrooms ('magic mushrooms'), seeds of *morning glory* (from the *Convolvulus* family), *peyote* (from a cactus in the south-west USA), various *ayahuasca* preparations (from the *Banisteriopsis* species of vine from Amazonia), *San Pedro cactus* (from a cactus found in Peru, Bolivia, Chile and Ecuador) and *Hawaiian baby woodrose* (a vine from India, the Caribbean, Hawaii and Africa).

Inhalants are stimulants that are volatile chemical vapours that produce psychoactive effects. Many are available over the counter, including solvents (paint thinners, gasoline, glues), gases (butane, propane, aerosol propellants, nitrous oxide), nitrites (isoamyl, isobutyl, cyclohexyl – used to enhance sexual arousal) and sprays (e.g. deodorants; Table 34.10). 'Laughing gas', 'poppers', 'snappers' and 'whippets' are commonly used terms. Sniffing inhalants produces psychotomimetic effects somewhere between those of alcohol and general anaesthesia (GA), in that initially users may feel slightly stimulated; with successive inhalations, they may feel less inhibited and less in control. Users may appear drunk and giggling with slurred speech and unsteadiness. Adverse effects include headache, nausea or vomiting, wheezing, unconsciousness, cramps, weight loss, muscle weakness, depression, memory impairment, damage to cardiovascular and nervous systems, and unconsciousness. Inhalant misuse is increasingly common in children and young adults, and has led to many deaths. Sniffing highly concentrated chemicals such as fluorocarbons and butane-type gases can damage liver and CNS, or cause delusions, hypoxia, arrhythmias and sometimes sudden death. Deliberately inhaling from an attached paper or plastic bag, or in a closed area, greatly increases the chances of suffocation. Users can also choke on their own vomit. Chronic solvent misuse can impair memory and concentration, and permanent damage to the brain, liver or kidneys has been reported. Respiratory damage, anaemia, lead poisoning and cranial nerve palsies can follow chronic misuse of petrol. A syndrome of learning disability, hypotonia, scaphocephaly and high malar bones has also been reported in children of mothers who inhaled petrol during pregnancy (fetal gasoline syndrome). Specific chemicals may also have additional adverse effects (Table 34.11). Signs of solvent misuse include slurred speech, euphoria, anorexia and a circumoral (glue sniffers') rash. Jaundice may be seen and the pulse may be irregular.

DEPRESSANTS

Depressants (including alcohol) depress the CNS, causing drowsiness; poor concentration, judgment and memory; disorientation; ataxia; and, in severe cases, unconsciousness (Table 34.12). Sedatives and hypnotics may cause mild to severe psychological addiction, and severe physiological addiction; abrupt withdrawal may be fatal. They include:

- alcohol
- barbiturates
- benzodiazepines, particularly alprazolam, Rohypnol (flunitrazepam), triazolam, temazepam and nimetazepam; z-drugs (e.g. zimovane) have a similar effect

Table 34.9 *Stimulants used in various cultures*

Stimulant	Sources	Comments
Betel	See text	
Caffeine	See text	
Cocaine	See text	
Kava	Kava (ava, intoxicating pepper, kawa kawa, kew, sakau, tonga, yangona) from *Piper methysticum* (intoxicating pepper), a shrub native to the South Pacific Islands, including Hawaii. The term kava also refers to the non-fermented, psychoactive beverage prepared from the rootstock. Kava-containing dietary supplements are marketed for the treatment of anxiety and insomnia	Pacific Island societies have long used kava beverages for social, ceremonial and medical purposes. The pharmacologically active compounds are kavalactones. Effects include euphoria, muscle relaxation, sedation and analgesia. High doses can have transient central nervous system (CNS) depressant effects (e.g. sedation and muscle weakness). Individuals may experience a numbness or tingling of the mouth upon drinking kava due to its local anaesthetic activity. Liver damage (hepatitis and cirrhosis) and failure have been associated with commercial extracts of kava. Kava inhibits cytochrome P450 enzymes and has potential for drug interactions
Khat	Khat (qat, kat, chat, miraa, quaadka), the leaves of *Catha edulis*, a shrub native to East Africa and the Arabian Peninsula, widely used as a recreational drug by indigenous people from Somalia, Ethiopia, Yemen and the Middle East	Khat has amphetamine-like effects from cathinone and cathine. Cathinone (alpha-aminopropiophenone), the principal active stimulant, is structurally similar to D-amphetamine and almost as potent as a CNS stimulant. Cathine (D-norpseudoephedrine) is about ten times less potent than cathinone as a CNS stimulant. Mephedrone (dimethylmethcathinone) and naphyrone (naphthylpyrovalerone) are cathinones found in khat
Kratom	Kratom (*Mitragyna speciosa* Korth, thang, kakuam, thom, ketum, biak) – a tree indigenous to Thailand, Malaysia and Myanmar	Used as a herbal drug. Mitragynine (9-methoxy-corynantheidine) is the primary active alkaloid and has opioid-like activity
Marijuana	See text	
Salvia	*Salvia divinorum* (Maria Pastora, sage of the seers, diviner's sage, salvia, Sally-D, magic mint) – a perennial herb native to the Sierra Mazateca region of Oaxaca, Mexico	Salvinorin A (divinorin A) is believed to be the ingredient responsible for hallucinogenic effects
Tobacco	See text	

Table 34.10 *Inhalants: solvents and gases*

Solvents	Gases
Industrial or household solvents	Butane and propane in household or commercial products
Art or office supply solvents	Aerosol propellants
Paint thinners or solvents, degreasers (dry-cleaning fluids), petrol and glues	Anaesthetics
Correction fluids, felt-tip-marker fluid and electronic contact cleaners	Whipping cream aerosols or dispensers (whippets) and refrigerant gases
	Spray paints, hair or deodorant sprays, and fabric protector sprays
	Nitrous oxide, halothane, ether and chloroform

Table 34.11 *Adverse effects from inhalants*

Chemical	Found in	Effects
Benzene	Petrol	Bone marrow damage
Chlorinated hydrocarbons	Correction fluids, dry-cleaning fluids	Liver and kidney damage
Hexane	Glues, petrol	Peripheral neuropathies or limb spasms
Methylene chloride	Varnish removers, paint thinners	Blood oxygen depletion
Nitrites	'Poppers', 'bold' and 'rush'	Blood oxygen depletion
Nitrous oxide	Whipping cream, gas cylinders	Peripheral neuropathies or limb spasms
Toluene	Paint sprays, glues, dewaxers	Liver, kidney and central nervous system damage, hearing loss
Trichloroethylene	Cleaning fluids, correction fluids	Hearing loss

Table 34.12 *Main depressants*

Main groups	Chemical names	Street name(s)[a]	Comments
Alcohol	Ethanol	Booze	Reduced pain and anxiety, feeling of well-being, lowered inhibitions, slowed pulse and breathing, lowered blood pressure, poor concentration, confusion, fatigue, impaired coordination, memory, judgment, respiratory depression and arrest, addiction
Barbiturates	Amobarbital, pentobarbital, secobarbital, phenobarbital	Barbs, reds, red birds, phennies, tooies, yellows, yellow jackets	Sedation, drowsiness, depression, unusual excitement, fever, irritability, poor judgment, slurred speech, dizziness
Benzodiazepines	Various	Ativan, Halcion, Librium, Valium, Xanax; candy, downers, sleeping pills, tranks	Sedation, drowsiness, dizziness
	Flunitrazepam	Rohypnol; forget-me pill, Mexican valium, R2, Roche, roofies, roofinol, rope, rophies	Visual and gastrointestinal disturbances, urinary retention, memory loss while under the drug's effects
GHB	Gamma-hydroxybutyrate	G, Georgia home boy, grievous bodily harm, liquid ecstasy	Drowsiness, nausea/vomiting, headache, loss of consciousness, loss of reflexes, seizures, coma, death
Methaqualone	Methaqualone	Mandrax, quaaludes	Euphoria, depression, poor reflexes, slurred speech, coma

[a]See Appendix 34.1.

Table 34.13 *Main hallucinogens*

Main hallucinogen groups	Chemical names	Street names[a]	Comments
Ketamine	Ketamine	Ketalar SV; cat, K, special K, vitamin K	Altered states of perception and feeling, nausea, temporary blindness, aggression, chronic mental disorders, persisting perception disorder (flashbacks) plus, at high doses, delirium, depression, respiratory depression and arrest
LSD	Lysergic acid diethylamide	Acid, blotter, boomers, cubes, microdot, yellow sunshines	Increased body temperature, heart rate, blood pressure, loss of appetite, sleeplessness, numbness, weakness, tremors
MDMA	Methylenedioxy-methamphetamine	Ecstasy	Increased body temperature, heart rate, blood pressure, loss of appetite, sleeplessness, numbness, weakness, tremors
Mephedrone	Mephedrone	White magic, miaow, meph, meow meow, MC, M-CAT, drone, charge, bubble, bounce, 4-MMC	Feelings of euphoria, alertness, talkativeness, empathy, anxiety, paranoia and overstimulation of the heart and circulatory system. Over-excitation of the nervous system, which can cause seizures
Naphyrone	Naphyrone	NRG, O-2482 or naphthylpyrovalerone	Similar to mephedrone. Was sold over the Internet as a 'legal high', often described as a plant food, research chemicals or bath salts. Feelings of euphoria, alertness, talkativeness, empathy, anxiety, paranoia and overstimulation of the heart and circulatory system. Over-excitation of the nervous system, which can cause seizures
Mescaline	Trimethoxy-phenethylamine	Buttons, cactus, mesc, peyote	Increased body temperature, heart rate, blood pressure, loss of appetite, sleeplessness, numbness, weakness, tremors
PCP and analogues	Phenylcyclidine	Phencyclidine; angel dust, boat, hog, love boat, peace pill	Possible decrease in blood pressure and heart rate, panic, aggression, violence, loss of appetite, depression
Psilocybin	Psilocybin	Magic mushroom, purple passion, shrooms	Nervousness, paranoia
THC compounds (tetrahydrocannabinoids; cannabis)	Marijuana	Hashish, boom, chronic, gangster, hash, hash oil, hemp, blunt, dope, ganja, grass, herb, joints, Mary Jane, pot, reefer, sinsemilla, skunk, weed	Euphoria, slowed thinking and reaction time, confusion, impaired balance and coordination, cough, frequent respiratory infections, impaired memory and learning, increased heart rate, anxiety, panic attacks; tolerance, addiction

[a]See Appendix 34.1.

- methaqualone and the related quinazolinone sedative-hypnotics
- opiate and opioid analgesics (mild to severe psychological addiction, mild to severe physiological addiction; abrupt withdrawal is unlikely to be fatal):
  morphine and codeine (two naturally occurring opiate analgesics) semi-synthetic opiates, e.g. heroin (diacetylmorphine; morphine diacetate), oxycodone, buprenorphine and hydromorphone synthetic opioids, e.g. fentanyl, pethidine (meperidine) and methadone.

HALLUCINOGENS

Hallucinogenic drugs cause sensory distortions, including mood changes, feelings of disassociation, auditory and visual disturbances, and changes to taste or smell. Hallucinations are quite dangerous, as sufferers may present extreme danger either to themselves or to others (Table 34.13).

ANABOLIC STEROIDS

See Chapter 33.

ALPHABET OF DRUGS OF MISUSE

Appendix 34.1 gives the main street names for the most important drugs of abuse but there are many others (see http://www.drugrehab.co.uk/street-drug-names.htm).

ALCOHOL

Alcohol (ethanol) is the most common drug of abuse. It accounts for about as much of the burden of world disease as tobacco and hypertension, is exceeded only by the burdens caused by malnutrition and unsafe sex (Fig. 34.2), and consumption is rising across the globe. Alcohol in drinks is generally measured in units (Table 34.14): 1 alcohol unit (AU) equates to 10–12 mL of pure ethanol, contained in a standard bottle or a can of regular beer, a glass of dinner wine (125 mL), a small glass (30 mL) of spirits and a measure (60 mL) of aperitif. Moderate alcohol use is defined as 1 AU daily for women and 2 for men. A safe maximum daily alcohol consumption is generally regarded as 3 units for a man and 2 for a woman. Alcohol misuse, defined as a daily intake in excess of 5 units, is the most common form of drug misuse. The World Health Organization estimates that there are almost 80 million people worldwide with diagnosable alcohol misuse disorders. Over 25% of the UK population appear to drink to excess (44% of men in Scotland also drink to excess). There seems to be a genetic predilection to alcoholism.

The term 'alcohol', as used in medicine and by the lay public, typically applies to ethanol (CH_3CH_2OH), which is produced by yeast fermentation of carbohydrates, such as in fruit and starch. Fermentation is incomplete in beer but complete in wine, with resulting alcohol contents of 3–8% and 7–18% by volume, respectively. Spirits (e.g. whisky, brandy and vodka) are produced by distillation of fermented products, and are 30% or greater alcohol by volume.

A cocktail is a mixed drink usually containing one or more alcoholic beverages, flavourings and one or more fruit juices, sauces, honey, milk, cream or spices, etc. A subgroup of cocktails are pre-mixed and bottled cocktails, generally known as alcopops, RTDs (ready to drink) or FABs (flavoured alcoholic beverages); they are usually made from vodka, beer, whisky or rum, to reach an alcohol concentration of 4–7% by volume, and are sweet and fruit-flavoured because they are mixed with cola, lemonade, ginger ale, etc.

Ethanol is rapidly absorbed through the gastric and duodenal mucosae, and metabolized by the liver, with a small fraction metabolized by oral and upper digestive tract mucosa. Alcohol dehydrogenase

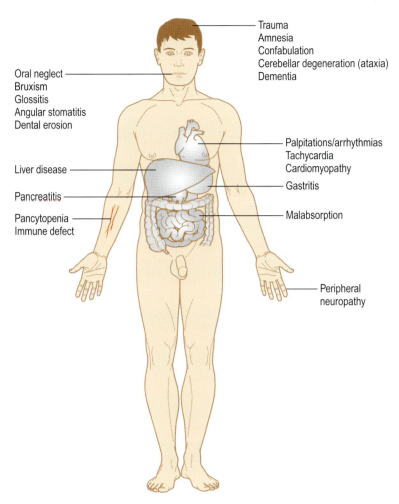

Trauma
Amnesia
Confabulation
Cerebellar degeneration (ataxia)
Dementia

Oral neglect
Bruxism
Glossitis
Angular stomatitis
Dental erosion

Liver disease

Pancreatitis

Pancytopenia
Immune defect

Palpitations/arrhythmias
Tachycardia
Cardiomyopathy

Gastritis

Malabsorption

Peripheral
neuropathy

Fig. 34.2 Alcoholism.

Table 34.14 *Alcohol in various alcoholic beverages*

Beverage	Strength of alcohol	Amount	Units of alcohol
Beer, cider, lager	3.5%	Half-pint	1
	3.5%	Pint	2
	Export strength 5%	Pint	2.5–3
	8%	Pint	4.5
Alcopop	5%	330 mL	1.7
Wine	10%	One glass	1
	10%	750 mL	7.5
	12%	750 mL	9
	Fortified (e.g. sherry) 15–20%	700 mL	16
Spirits	40%	One measure	1
	40%	700 mL	32

catalyses ethanol oxidation to acetaldehyde, which is oxidized into non-toxic acetate by aldehyde dehydrogenase. In turn, acetate is oxidized into fatty acids, carbon dioxide and water. Ethanol blocks nitrosamine metabolism in the liver, thus allowing nitrosamines to circulate to other organs, such as the kidneys and oesophagus, where they can be activated into carcinogens. Alcoholic beverages also contain polyphenols – plant secondary metabolites, which play an important protective role via their potent antioxidant activity; resveratrol in red wine is one example. In contrast, the diet of alcoholics is often B-vitamin–deficient.

Box 34.3 *Mental effects of alcohol*

- Acute intoxication
- Amnesic syndrome
- Dependence syndrome
- Psychotic disorder
- Withdrawal state

Table 34.15 *Acute effects of alcohol (blood alcohol level in mg/dL)*

<100	100–200	200–300	300–400	400–500	>500
Dry and decent	Delighted and devilish	Delinquent and disgusting	Dizzy and delirious	Dazed and dejected	Dead drunk

Clinical features

Alcohol is a CNS depressant and can have a range of mental effects (Box 34.3). Acute effects are mainly on judgment, concentration and coordination, individuals becoming aggressive and failing to comply with instructions. Effects are dose-related; they eventually interfere with cerebellar function, causing ataxia and motor incoordination, and ultimately unconsciousness (Table 34.15). After a large alcoholic binge, suppression of the cough reflex can result in inhalation of vomit and death.

Alcohol misuse (alcoholism) is consumption of alcohol to such a degree as to cause deterioration in social behaviour or physical illness and the development of dependence, from which withdrawal is difficult or causes adverse effects. The mortality rate in alcoholism is significantly raised and over 15 years may be about 300% above the norm. Alcohol interferes with CNS function and is causally related to more than 60 different medical conditions; some, such as suicide, homicide and different forms of accidents (e.g. falls, poisoning, accidents caused by flames or by motor vehicles), are acute consequences of alcohol use. Alcohol is an important, if not the main, causal factor in over 25% of road traffic accidents and also in many other accidents or assaults. Acute alcoholic hepatitis may follow binge-drinking; cirrhosis commonly results from chronic alcoholism. Alcohol contributes to the spread of SSIs (including HIV), and to impaired wound-healing and predisposition to respiratory infections, especially pneumonia and tuberculosis.

The probability of developing alcoholism is greater in several groups, especially those to whom alcohol is freely available (Table 34.16). Late signs or symptoms of chronic excessive alcohol drinking include palpitations and tachycardia, cardiomyopathy, liver disease, chronic pancreatitis, malnutrition, peripheral neuropathy, amnesia and confabulation (in Wernicke and Korsakoff CNS syndromes). Cerebellar degeneration and ataxia, dementia, haemorrhagic stroke and various forms of cancer are consequences of chronic alcohol use (Table 34.17).

A diet poor in fruits and vegetables is typical of heavy drinkers and can cause nutritional defects, leading in turn to immune defects and peripheral polyneuropathies (burning hands and feet), pellagra, amblyopia (visual defects) and organic brain disorders (Wernicke encephalopathy and Korsakoff psychosis).

Alcohol is now the most common teratogen apart from smoking, and drinking during pregnancy has a detrimental effect on fetal development. It can lead to spontaneous abortion or the fetal alcohol syndrome (FAS), the prevalence of which is similar to that of Down syndrome. FAS affects growth, the CNS and orofacial features. Most affected children are of short stature; microcephaly is common and

Table 34.16 *Alcoholism*

Risk factors	Suggestive findings	Outcomes
Armed forces	Absenteeism	Brain damage and epilepsy
Bachelors over 40	Accidents	Cancers
Bored housewives	Assaults	Fetal alcohol syndrome
Commercial travellers	Cirrhosis	Gastrointestinal disease: gastritis and peptic ulcer
Doctors	Family history of alcoholism	Heart disease: cardiomyopathy
Entertainers	Frequent job changes	Inadequate diet leading to immune defects, peripheral polyneuropathies and organic brain disorders
Publicans and other workers in the drinks industry	Gamma-glutamyl transpeptidase raised	Impaired haemostasis
	Macrocytosis	Impaired wound healing
	Marital disharmony	Infections, especially pneumonia and tuberculosis
	Medical history	Injuries (including maxillofacial), from accidents or assaults
	Social history	Liver disease: alcoholic hepatitis and cirrhosis
	Violence	Muscle disease: myopathy
		Nutritional defects
		Pancreatic disease; pancreatitis

Table 34.17 *Effects of chronic alcohol use*

System	Possible effects	Biochemical changes
Cardiac	Cardiomyopathy, hypertension, arrhythmias	–
CNS	Intoxication, dependency, dementia	Raised blood alcohol
	Wernicke–Korsakoff syndrome	Decreased thiamine levels
Gastric	Gastritis, ulceration, carcinoma	–
Haematological	Pancytopenia	Macrocytosis, anaemia
	Folate deficiency	Thrombocytopenia, leukopenia
	Thiamine deficiency	Reduced blood-clotting factors: II, VII, IX, X
	Immune defect	
Hepatic	Hepatitis, fatty liver (steatosis), cirrhosis, liver cancer	Raised gamma-glutamyl transpeptidase, carbohydrate-deficient transferrin (CDT), liver enzymes, bilirubin
Intestinal	Glucose and vitamin malabsorption	Reduced folate, thiamine and vitamins B_{12}, A, D, E and K
Musculoskeletal	Myopathy, gout	–
Oesophageal	Gastro-oesophageal reflux disease (GORD), Mallory–Weiss syndrome, carcinoma	–
Pancreatic	Pancreatitis	Raised serum amylase
Reproductive	Impotence, dysmenorrhoea, low-birth-weight babies, fetal alcohol syndrome	–

individuals may have a low IQ, difficulties in eating and speech, and muscular incoordination. The FAS patient is irritable as an infant, hyperactive as a child and highly unsociable as an adult. Facial features include hypoplastic maxillae, a low nasal bridge, an indistinct philtrum with a hypoplastic upper lip, and other features, including small teeth with dysplastic enamel.

Alcohol should only be drunk in moderation, with meals, and when consumption cannot put others at risk. It should not be consumed by: children; women trying to conceive or already pregnant; anyone about to drive a motor vehicle, fly a plane or take on any other skilled activity; HCPs about to treat patients; and anyone taking prescription or over-the-counter medicines that affect CNS or respiratory function.

General management

Recognition of the alcoholic is notoriously difficult and the history unreliable. Findings that suggest alcoholism may arise from the social or medical history (Table 34.18). The CAGE questionnaire may be helpful and a positive response to any of the following questions suggests a diagnosis of alcoholism:

- Have you ever felt the need to *c*ut down on drink?
- Have you ever felt *a*nnoyed by criticism of your drinking?

Table 34.18 *Findings suggesting alcoholism*

Social history	Medical history
Absenteeism	Accidents
Assaults	Cirrhosis
Violence	Macrocytosis
Frequent job changes	Folate deficiency or raised carbohydrate-deficient transferrin (CDT) or gamma-glutamyl transpeptidase
Marital disharmony	Family history of alcoholism

- Have you ever felt *g*uilty about drinking?
- Do you drink a morning *e*ye opener?

Two or more affirmative answers indicate probable alcoholism. A five-shot questionnaire suggests alcoholism if it produces scores over 5 (Table 34.19). The NHS has a useful questionnaire (Appendix 34.2).

Signs may include discovery of used bottles at home, at work or elsewhere. Signs or symptoms of chronic excessive alcohol intake include: slurred speech; alcohol on the breath; self-neglect (whether of the mouth or shabbiness of clothes); an evasive, truculent, over-boisterous or facetious manner; indigestion (particularly heartburn); anxiety (often with insomnia); or tremor. Later signs or symptoms

Table 34.19 *Five-shot questionnaire for detecting alcoholism*

Question	Scores				
	0	0.5	1.0	1.5	2.0
How often do you have a drink containing alcohol?	Never	<Monthly	2–4 times/month	2–3 times/week	≥4 times/week
How many drinks containing alcohol do you have on a typical day when you are drinking?	1 or 2	3 or 4	5 or 6	7 or 8	10 or more
Have people annoyed you by criticizing your drinking?	No	No	Yes	Yes	Yes
Have you ever felt bad or guilty about drinking?	No	No	Yes	Yes	Yes
Have you ever had a drink first thing in the morning to steady your nerves or get rid of a hangover?	No	No	Yes	Yes	Yes

include palpitations and tachycardia, cardiomyopathy and signs of malnutrition.

Blood investigations that may be diagnostically helpful may detect macrocytosis, raised levels of alcohol, gamma-glutamyl transpeptidase (gamma-GT or GGT) and other hepatic enzymes, levels above 1.3% of carbohydrate-deficient transferrin isoforms (% CDT), and folate deficiency of no obvious cause.

Treatment of alcoholism is by encouraging the patient to drink in a less damaging way and to accept help to deal with the crises and the physical, behavioural and social damage that result, or to learn to abstain from alcohol. Admission to manage rehabilitation and ensure abstinence, nutritional replacement of thiamine and folate, and drugs that reduce dependence (naltrexone, acamprosate or clomethiazole) or that cause unpleasant side-effects if alcohol is taken (disulfiram [Antabuse]) may help.

If the alcohol supply is reduced or cut off, or if blood alcohol levels fall sharply, the abstinence or alcohol withdrawal syndrome (AWS) may appear, with morning 'shakes' – typically trembling of the hands but possibly involving the whole body. Morning nausea and vomiting are sometimes called 'toothbrush heaves'. Other withdrawal symptoms are diarrhoea, sweating, rapid pulse and raised blood pressure, confusion, agitation, fits, illusions, misperceptions, hallucinations or delusions. The full-blown syndrome is called 'delirium tremens' or 'DTs'. The whole withdrawal syndrome lasts about a week and requires medical supervision and use of benzodiazepines or clomethiazole.

Dental aspects

Many alcoholics present no dental management problems, though there may be issues related to informed consent if the person is inebriated. Challenges may also include erratic attendance for dental treatment and aggressive behaviour. Alcoholics are best given an early morning appointment, if that is when they are least likely to be under the influence of alcohol.

The main relevant medical complications stem from the fact that cirrhosis delays the metabolism of many drugs and may cause a bleeding tendency. Chronic alcoholism may also depress the bone marrow to cause anaemia and thrombocytopenia. Other problems may include cardiomyopathy, poly-substance misuse, smoking and drug interactions. Alcohol can interact with other drugs, sometimes inducing the cytochrome P450 enzyme system to accelerate their metabolism, in others depressing their metabolism. Warfarin, paracetamol (acetaminophen) and benzodiazepines may be affected.

GA is best avoided, especially if patients have pre-medicated themselves with alcohol, and increased the risk of vomiting and inhalation of vomit. Alcoholics are especially prone to aspiration lung abscess. Alcoholic heart disease is also a contraindication.

Alcoholics are also notoriously resistant to GA. Once liver disease develops, the position is reversed: drug metabolism is then impaired

(Ch. 9) and drugs have a disproportionately greater effect. Sedatives (including benzodiazepines and antihistamines) or hypnotics generally have an additive effect with alcohol, although these interactions are not entirely predictable. Heavy drinkers, however, become tolerant not only of alcohol but also of other sedatives.

Aspirin and non-steroidal anti-inflammatory drugs (NSAIDs) should be avoided; in the alcoholic patient they are more likely to cause gastric erosions and precipitate bleeding. Opioids may enhance sedation. The hepatotoxic effects of paracetamol (acetaminophen) are enhanced, though it is probably the safest analgesic.

Alcohol-containing preparations, such as some mouthwashes, should be avoided in patients given metronidazole within the last 48 hours. Metronidazole inhibits the liver breakdown of acetaldehyde, which accumulates to cause widespread vasodilatation, nausea, vomiting, sweating, headache and palpitations similar to the disulfiram (Antabuse) reaction. The effects of penicillins and erythromycin may be reduced by alcohol.

Wound healing may also be impaired in the severely chronic alcoholic, and alcoholism may be a common factor in patients with osteomyelitis following jaw fractures. The most common oral effect of alcoholism is neglect, leading to advanced caries and periodontal disease, and there is sometimes tooth surface loss from caries, dental erosion from regurgitation (or from the beverage low pH) and/or attrition from bruxism.

Alcohol may be a cause of leukoplakia and oral cancer. There may be folate deficiency or other anaemia causing glossitis and sometimes angular stomatitis or recurrent aphthae. A rare manifestation is bilateral painless swelling of the parotids or other major salivary glands (sialosis).

Other orofacial features include a smell of alcohol on the breath, telangiectases and possibly rhinophyma ('grog blossom').

AMPHETAMINES

Amphetamines stimulate alpha- and beta-adrenergic receptors in the CNS and peripheral nervous system, essentially producing similar effects to cocaine. They are used for euphoriant effect, for staving off fatigue in order to continue work or for slimming. Amphetamines are usually taken orally but can also be injected, snorted or smoked (ice; crystal).

Amphetamines raise the blood pressure and sometimes temperature, and cause sleeplessness and anorexia. Acute amphetamine toxicity causes dry mouth, dilated pupils, tachycardia, aggression, talkativeness, tachypnoea and hallucinations, leading to seizures, hyperpyrexia, arrhythmias and collapse. High doses can cause mood swings and psychoses – including hallucinations and paranoia – and can cause respiratory failure and death. Chronic amphetamine toxicity causes restlessness, hyperactivity, loss of appetite and weight, tremor, repetitive movements, picking at the face and extremities, and bruxism, and there can be hyposalivation and increased caries incidence.

Amphetamines have no true withdrawal syndrome and, in this respect, addiction is quite different from opioid or barbiturate dependence. Unfortunately, psychoses can persist after the drug has been stopped. Addicts may be remarkably resistant to GA and, if taking drugs intravenously, may have many of the infective problems of opioid addicts. If GA is required, intravenous barbiturates may induce convulsions, respiratory distress or coma, and should be avoided. Opioids are also contraindicated. Amphetamines enhance the sympathomimetic effects of adrenaline (epinephrine) and thus vasoconstrictors are best avoided, since hypertension and cardiotoxicity can result. Monoamine oxidase inhibitors are contraindicated.

BARBITURATES

Barbiturates are depressant drugs used mainly to treat anxiety, tension and sleep disorders; they cause sedation and depress respiration and heart rate, as well as impairing thought processes and memory, and causing incoordination and ataxia. With chronic use, addicts begin to think slowly and to have increasing emotional lability; concentration and judgment are increasingly impaired, and the barbiturate addict becomes irritable and shows signs of self-neglect.

Although tolerance to barbiturates develops, the lethal dose remains the same, with only a small gap between relatively safe and lethal levels. Accidental overdose is a comparatively common cause of death from respiratory failure and CNS depression, especially if alcohol is also taken. Barbiturates are also often used to adulterate more expensive drugs such as heroin and are responsible for many of the fatal overdoses. There is no antidote to overdose; artificial ventilation is used until respiratory function recovers.

Two main types of barbiturate addict are recognized and either may also misuse other drugs. Middle-aged women, often living alone, taking large quantities of barbiturates orally and living in a dream world, form the largest group; chronic toxicity, such as rashes and ataxia, often develops. Young addicts, who take barbiturates ('sleepers') for immediate effect by injection, are at risk of complications from filthy injection technique, including multiple abscesses, gangrene, hepatitis, HIV infection, infective endocarditis or occasionally tetanus.

Should barbiturates be withdrawn, the addict initially improves and any ataxia disappears but, within 12–16 hours, a dangerous withdrawal syndrome can develop. Nausea, anxiety, tremor, insomnia, tachycardia, weakness and postural hypotension are followed by abdominal pain. After 36–48 hours, in heavy users, there may be loss of consciousness, often fits and sometimes death. The syndrome has a slower onset in those who have been using long-acting barbiturates.

Dental management may be complicated by barbiturates enhancing the sedative effects of some drugs, or inducing liver drug-metabolizing enzymes and causing resistance to anaesthetics. Other problems may include hepatitis B and C, HIV infection and SSI, epilepsy, maxillofacial injuries and tetanus.

Oral complications of barbiturate misuse are rare. A bullous mucosal reaction has been reported but manifestations such as idiopathic facial pain, related to the underlying condition for which the drug was prescribed, are more common.

BENZODIAZEPINES

Benzodiazepines are prescribed to treat anxiety, acute stress reactions and panic attacks. Memory loss is a major feature. Psychological dependence on benzodiazepines is common but the effects are considerably less severe than with most other sedatives. Physical dependence can develop fairly quickly – sometimes within 1 month. Withdrawal symptoms are frequently delayed in onset compared with the barbiturates but may last 8–10 days. Typical effects include insomnia, anxiety (which may be incorrectly attributed to the return of the original anxiety state), loss of appetite, tremor, perspiration and perceptual disturbances, and occasionally fits or psychoses. Sudden withdrawal, particularly of short-acting benzodiazepines, is dangerous since it can cause confusion, fits, toxic psychosis or a condition resembling delirium tremens.

BETEL

Betel quid or paan chewing is widely used and is claimed to produce a sense of well-being, euphoria, sweating, salivation, palpitation, heightened alertness and increased capacity to work. Betel quid is a mixture of areca (betel) nut and slaked lime, to which tobacco can be added, all wrapped in betel leaf. Arecoline (methyl-1-methyl-1,2,5,6-tetrahydropyridine-3-carboxylate) is the primary active ingredient of areca nut and is responsible for CNS stimulant effects, comparable to those of nicotine. Arecoline is an agonist of acetylcholine muscarinic M_1, M_2 and M_3 receptors, causing pupillary constriction, bronchial constriction and so on. Plasma noradrenaline (norepinephrine) and adrenaline (epinephrine) levels also rise during betel quid chewing. The specific quid components vary between communities and individuals where it is used, having a major social and cultural role in communities throughout the Indian subcontinent, South-East Asia and locations in the western Pacific. Betel use is well recognized by tooth and soft-tissue staining (Fig. 34.3) and can have a number of health consequences (Table 34.20), especially oral submucous fibrosis (OSMF). Though not regarded as a connective tissue disease, OSMF has pathological changes very similar to those of scleroderma. It is a chronic disease and is almost entirely confined to Asians, related to the use of areca nut in gutkha or paan masala, or in other chewables (kharra, chewable tobacco). OSMF causes severe and often disabling fibrosis, characterized by fibrous bands beneath the oral mucosa that progressively contract so that mouth-opening is increasingly severely limited. As many as 10% of OSMF patients develop oral carcinoma. Intralesional corticosteroids and regular stretching of the oral soft tissues with an interdental screw may delay fixation in the closed position. Failing this, operative treatment may become necessary.

CAFFEINE

Caffeine is an alkaloid stimulant widely used in many cultures. Found in over 60 plants, it is most commonly derived from coffee or tea plants. Other sources include kola, cocoa, guarana and yerba mate. Chocolate contains a small amount. Caffeine is called guaranine when found in *guarana*, mateine when found in *mate* and theine when found in *tea*. There is far more caffeine in coffees than in teas. Significant amounts of caffeine are also added to some soft and 'energy' drinks (e.g. Red Bull, Relentless, Cocaine; the amount of caffeine has to be stated on the label where it contains more than 150 mg caffeine/L). Some of these 'energy drinks' are banned in some countries.

Caffeine is diuretic and psychoactive, leading to a rise in brain dopamine, serotonin and catecholamines. Caffeine metabolites include theobromine (increases the blood flow to the brain and muscles), theophylline (relaxes bronchioles and increases heart rate and efficiency) and paraxanthine (increases lipolysis, releasing glycerol and fatty acids for use as a muscle energy source). Coffee and tea also contain other xanthine alkaloids: for example, cardiac stimulants theophylline and

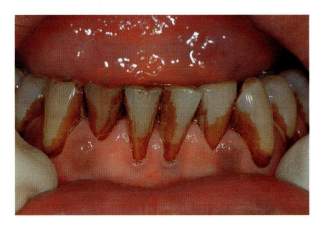

Fig. 34.3 Betel staining.

Table 34.20 *Possible adverse health effects from betel chewing*

Health effect	Examples
Cancer and potentially malignant conditions	Hepatocellular cancer
	Oesophageal cancer
	Oral cancer
	Oral submucous fibrosis
	Pancreatic cancer
Cardiovascular and diabetes	Hypertension
	Metabolic syndrome
Adverse birth outcomes	Lower birth weight
	Lower male-to-female sex ratio
	Reduced birth length
Others	Contact dermatitis
	Chronic kidney disease
	Liver cirrhosis
	Periodontitis
	Urinary calculi (related to use of calcium hydroxide 'chuna' in the betel quid)

theobromine (tea only) and other substances such as polyphenols, which can complex insolubly with caffeine and alter its activity.

Caffeine tolerance develops very quickly, especially among heavy coffee and energy drink consumers; when caffeine use is stopped, the falling serotonin levels can cause anxiety, irritability, inability to concentrate and diminished motivation or depression. Excess caffeine can lead to caffeine intoxication, caffeine-induced anxiety disorder or caffeine-induced sleep disorder.

Studies suggesting caffeine intake is associated with a risk of miscarriage or a reduced risk of developing Parkinsonism or cardiovascular disease are inconclusive. Some Latter-day Saints (Mormons), Christian Scientists and Gaudiya Vaishnava Hindus do not consume caffeine.

COCAINE

Cocaine is widely used worldwide and in all levels of society. Cocaine hydrochloride, from the plant *Erythroxylon coca*, is one of the most widely abused drugs and is powerfully addictive. Having once tried cocaine, individuals may not be able to control the extent to which they will continue to use it. 'Crack' is the street name given to cocaine processed with ammonia or sodium bicarbonate (baking soda) and water, and heated to remove the hydrochloride (producing a crackling sound) to a free base for smoking. Cocaine is often snorted – inhaled through the nose, where it is rapidly absorbed into the blood – giving a 'high' lasting 15–30 minutes. It may also be injected or smoked.

Cocaine has profound and almost immediate CNS effects, potentiating catecholamines and interfering with dopamine reabsorption. Euphoric effects appear in less than 5 minutes and include hyperstimulation and diminished fatigue and appetite. Extremely high doses reach the brain quickly and bring an intense and immediate high, which can last 5–10 minutes. Physical effects of cocaine mimic those of catecholamines, and include dilated pupils, constricted peripheral blood vessels, and raised temperature, pulse rate and blood pressure. Cocaine causes feelings of well-being and heightened mental activity; the cocaine addict is garrulous, witty and the life and soul of the party – aptly described as a 'sexed-up extrovert with dilated pupils'. High doses of cocaine and/or prolonged use can, however, trigger paranoia, visual hallucinations (snow lights) and tactile hallucinations. The latter are typically of insects crawling over the skin (formication, 'cocaine bugs'). Toxic reactions include angina, coronary spasm, ventricular arrhythmias, myocardial infarction, cerebrovascular accidents, convulsions and respiratory depression. Cocaine-related deaths are often a result of cardiac arrest, cerebrovascular accidents or seizures followed by respiratory arrest. Prolonged cocaine snorting can result in ischaemic necrosis with ulceration of the nasal mucous membrane and nasal septum collapse, ulceration of the palate, and sphenoidal sinusitis. It occasionally leads to brain abscess.

As a constituent of Brompton cocktail (cocaine, heroin or morphine, and alcohol), cocaine is also sometimes used to make terminal disease more tolerable. However, when people choose to mix cocaine and alcohol, they are also compounding the dangers, since the liver combines them, manufacturing cocaethylene, which intensifies the euphoric effects and increases the risk of sudden death. Use of cocaine plus heroin intravenously ('speedballing') is also highly dangerous.

When cocaine is stopped, symptoms proceed through a crash phase of depression and craving for sleep, a withdrawal phase of lack of energy, and then an extinction phase of recurrence of craving evoked by various external stimuli but of lesser intensity. Depression, fatigue, bradycardia and psychoses may be seen. Behavioural interventions, particularly cognitive behavioural therapy, can be effective in reducing cocaine misuse.

Behavioural problems or drug interactions may interfere with dental treatment. Injected cocaine brings the risk of the same blood-borne infections as in other addicts. It is important to avoid local anaesthesia (LA) containing adrenaline (epinephrine) in persons using cocaine until at least 2 hours have elapsed because of enhanced sympathomimetic action and subsequent arrhythmias, acute hypertension or cardiac failure. Therefore, it is best not to give dental treatment until 6 hours after the last dose of cocaine has been taken. When GA is needed, isoflurane and sevoflurane are preferred to halothane, which may induce arrhythmias. Ketamine and suxamethonium (scoline) are also best avoided.

Oral use of cocaine temporarily numbs the lips and tongue, and can cause gingival or mucosal erosions (Fig. 34.4). The main oral effects of cocaine addiction may be a dry mouth and bruxism or dental erosion. Caries and periodontal disease, especially acute necrotizing gingivitis, are more frequent. Cocaine may precipitate cluster headaches. Children born to cocaine-using mothers are more prone to have ankyloglossia.

DEXTROPROPOXYPHENE

Co-proxamole (because of the dextropropoxyphene, a weak opioid) is also abused.

DIPIPANONE

Dipipanone is sometimes abused in tablet form and in combination with an anti-emetic (Diconal). It is less sedating than morphine.

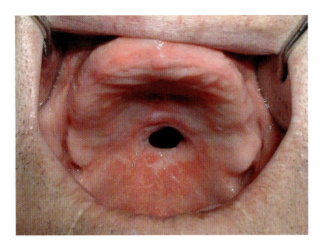

Fig. 34.4 Cocaine damage in palate.

ECSTASY (3,4-METHYLENEDIOXY-METHAMPHETAMINE; MDMA)

Ecstasy is a synthetic, psychoactive, amphetamine-like drug with sympathomimetic activity, and both stimulant and hallucinogenic properties. Like other amphetamines, it produces euphoria and appetite suppression, but is more potently hallucinogenic.

Ecstasy is usually taken orally, giving effects after 20–60 minutes. Unfortunately, the tablets may contain other amphetamine derivatives, caffeine, ketamine or salicyclic acid, or ecstasy may be used along with cannabis, alcohol, amphetamine or cocaine (increasing the hazards of use). Adverse effects from ecstasy include neurological effects (e.g. ataxia and seizures), psychiatric sequelae (e.g. agitation or paranoia) and cardiovascular effects (e.g. tachycardia, arrhythmias or infarction), as well as renal or hepatic failure or other effects – unrelated to the dose. Ecstasy causes brain injury, affecting dopamine-containing neurons that use serotonin to communicate with other neurons. The serotonin system plays a direct role in regulating mood, aggression, sexual activity, sleep and sensitivity to pain. Ecstasy users face risks similar to those caused by cocaine and amphetamine – psychological difficulties, including confusion, depression, sleep problems, drug craving, severe anxiety and paranoia, during and sometimes weeks after taking it, and physical symptoms such as muscle tension, involuntary teeth-clenching, nausea, blurred vision, rapid eye movement, faintness, and chills or sweating.

Ecstasy can cause a sharp, potentially fatal rise in body temperature (malignant hyperthermia), leading to muscle breakdown and kidney and cardiovascular system failure. Ecstasy users need to take water or non-alcoholic drinks frequently and in large amounts to avoid hyperthermia ('chill-out'). Deaths are rare but usually caused by high temperatures, raised heart rate and blood pressure, and myocardial infarcts, hyponatraemia or asthma. At special risk are people with circulatory or heart disease. Individuals who develop a rash resembling acne after using ecstasy may be risking severe liver damage if they continue to use the drug. After long-term use, tolerance develops but there is no physical dependence or withdrawal symptoms.

Teeth-clenching and bruxism appear to be common; temporomandibular joint dysfunction, dry mouth, attrition, erosion, mucosal burns or ulceration, circumoral paraesthesiae and periodontitis have been reported. Ecstasy can interact with adrenaline (epinephrine) and with tricyclic or selective serotonin reuptake inhibitor (SSRI) antidepressants.

GHB (GAMMA-HYDROXYBUTYRATE)

GHB is abused for euphoric, sedative and anabolic (body-building) effects. GHB and two of its precursors, gamma-butyrolactone (GBL) and 1,4-butanediol (BD), have been involved in poisonings, overdoses, date rapes and deaths. Coma and seizures can follow misuse of GHB and, when combined with methamphetamine, there appears to be an increased risk of seizure. Combining use with other drugs such as alcohol can result in nausea, difficulty in breathing and unconsciousness. GHB may also produce withdrawal effects, including insomnia, anxiety, tremors and sweating.

HEROIN

See Opiates and opioids.

KETAMINE

Ketamine is a GA agent related to phencyclidine (PCP), which can cause a dream-like state and hallucinations; it has been used as a date-rape drug. Ketamine effects come on and recede faster than those of LSD but include aggression (as with PCP) and temporary blindness; the drug can also cause delirium, amnesia, impaired motor function, hypertension, depression and potentially fatal respiratory problems.

KHAT (QAT)

Khat is from a shrub that has been chewed for centuries by people from the Horn of Africa and Arabian peninsula, including the UK, particularly from countries such as Somalia, Ethiopia and Yemen. It is a stimulant like amphetamine and the active ingredients, cathinone and cathine, are Class C drugs. Khat chewing causes oral white lesions on the chewing side and a correlation between khat chewing and oral cancer has been suggested. There is weak evidence for khat chewing influencing the incidence of myocardial infarction, cardiomyopathy, hypertension, cerebrovascular disease, diabetes, sexual dysfunction, duodenal ulcer and hepatitis.

LEGAL HIGHS

New psychoactive (NPS) substances include "legal highs" – substances used like illegal drugs but not covered by current misuse of drugs laws – and so it is legal to possess or to use – though temporary laws are being introduced for some. Examples include

- a new range of synthetic cannabinoids, methoxetamine and other related compounds and O-desmethyltramadol
- desoxypipradrol (2-DPMP), its related compounds and phenazepam
- naphyrone and other synthetic cathinones, tapentadol and amineptine
- NBOMe and benzofuran (Benzofury) compounds
- para-methyl derivative of 4-methylaminorex ('Speckled Red' or 'Brown Cherries').

LSD (LYSERGIC ACID DIETHYLAMIDE)

LSD (acid) is a major hallucinogen; it is manufactured from lysergic acid, found in ergot, a fungus that grows on rye and other grains. Within 30–90 minutes of taking LSD orally, several different emotions appear at once or swinging rapidly from one to another (a 'trip'). Synaesthesia, the overflow from one sense to another when, for example, colours are heard, is common. These effects can last up to 12 hours and, even months after such a 'trip', many LSD users experience flashbacks – recurrence of certain aspects of a person's experience – without the user having taken the drug again. There is often lability of mood, panic ('bad trip') and delusions of magical powers, such as being able to fly. If taken in a large enough dose, LSD causes delusions, visual hallucinations and paranoia. The sense of time and self becomes distorted. LSD intoxication can cause severe, terrifying thoughts and feelings, as well as despair; fatal accidents have been precipitated. Taking LSD is especially risky because each tablet can contain very different amounts of drug – from as little as 25 micrograms to as much as 250 micrograms – enough to cause serious side-effects. The physical effects from LSD are similar to those of catecholamines – dilated pupils; raised temperature, heart rate and blood pressure; sweating; loss of appetite; sleeplessness; dry mouth; and tremors. The effects of LSD are not only unpredictable but also prolonged, often lasting up to about 12 hours, depending on the amount taken, the user's personality, mood and expectations, and the surroundings in which the drug is used. However, LSD is not considered an addictive drug since it does not produce the compulsive drug-seeking type of behaviour as shown by users of drugs such as cocaine, amphetamine, heroin, alcohol and nicotine. Most users of LSD voluntarily limit or stop its use over time.

MARIJUANA (CANNABIS)

Marijuana is the most commonly abused illicit drug in the developed world, aside from alcohol, and is used religiously in Rastafarianism. A dry, shredded, green/brown mix of flowers, stems, seeds and leaves of the hemp plant *Cannabis sativa* or *Cannabis indica*, it is usually smoked as a cigarette (joint, nail) or in a pipe (bong). It is also smoked in blunts – cigars that have been emptied of tobacco and refilled with marijuana – often in combination with another drug. Use also might include mixing marijuana in food or brewing it as a tea. As a more concentrated, resinous form it is called hashish and, as a sticky black liquid, hash oil.

The main active chemical in marijuana is delta-9-tetrahydrocannabinol (THC), which binds to brain receptors that influence pleasure, memory, thought, concentration, sensory and time perception, and coordinated movement. The marijuana currently used is many times more potent than that taken in the 1950s. The short-term adverse effects of marijuana use can include difficulties with memory and learning, distorted perception, difficulty in thinking and problem-solving, and loss of coordination. Critical skills related to attention, memory and learning are significantly impaired; students who smoke marijuana obtain lower examination grades and are less likely to graduate compared with non-smoking peers. Marijuana use is associated with depression, anxiety and personality disturbances; schizophrenia may be triggered in some.

Marijuana affects blood pressure and heart rate, and lowers the blood oxygen-carrying capacity. Smoking marijuana may more than quadruple the risk of myocardial infarction in the first hour, and frequently leads to respiratory illnesses such as infections, daily cough and sputum production, and obstructed airways. Marijuana smoke contains 50–70% more carcinogenic hydrocarbons than tobacco smoke and THC impairs immune function. Marijuana has been implicated in lung and oral cancer, as well as some other malignant disease, but the evidence is equivocal and could be related to concurrent tobacco use or other factors. Babies born to women who used marijuana during pregnancies display abnormal responses to visual stimuli, tremulousness and a high-pitched cry, features that may indicate neurological maldevelopment. Later there may be behavioural problems and poor performance on tasks of visual perception, language comprehension, sustained attention and memory. No medications are currently available for treating marijuana misuse.

There are no specific aspects of addiction that influence dental management in most patients, but there is a tendency to a dry mouth and increased cravings for certain foods ('the munchies'), hyposalivation, increased *Candida* carriage and oral white lesions.

MEPHEDRONE (MEOW MEOW)

Mephedrone (dimethylmethcathinone, 4-methylmethcathinone or 4-methylephedrone) and naphyrone (naphthylpyrovalerone) are cathinones, synthetic stimulants closely related to amphetamines and found in the African plant khat. Other cathinones include methadrone, methylone and related compounds. Slang names include drone, meph, MC, 4-MMC, MCAT, miaow, bath salts, white magic, plant feeder, just plant, charge, bounce and Bubbles.

Mephedrone is sold as an inexpensive white powder that is usually snorted in a similar way to cocaine. It is also found in capsules and pills or can be dissolved in a liquid. In very rare cases it can be injected. Mephedrone initially was not controlled under the UK Misuse of Drugs Act and therefore was sometimes called a 'legal high', but in 2010 mephedrone and MDPV (methylenedioxy-pyrovalerone) were reclassified as illegal group B drugs.

The main effects and risks of mephedrone include euphoria, alertness and feelings of affection towards the people around, as well as feelings of anxiety and paranoia. Mephedrone has physical effects: for example, on the cardiovascular system, with tachycardia and arterial constriction leading to cold, blue hands and feet. Excessive CNS stimulation may cause headaches, insomnia, agitation and hallucinations, as well as seizures, which may be fatal. Snorting mephedrone can damage the nose, causing nosebleeds. Other adverse effects include bruxism, nausea and vomiting, appetite suppression, sweating and changes in body temperature. Most of those adverse effects are like those of ecstasy and cocaine. Anecdotal reports suggest that heavy use can lead to paranoia, hallucinations and serious panic attacks.

METHAMPHETAMINE

Methamphetamine is an addictive stimulant with stronger CNS effects than amphetamine, releasing high levels of dopamine, which enhance mood and body movement. Unlike amphetamine, methamphetamine users may become quickly addicted. Methamphetamine is also neurotoxic, damaging brain cells that contain dopamine and serotonin and, over time, lowering levels of dopamine, which can result in Parkinsonism. Methamphetamine also raises heart rate and blood pressure, and can cause cardiovascular collapse, strokes, hyperthermia and convulsions, which can be fatal. 'Meth mouth' is the term given to the neglect and poor oral hygiene seen in methamphetamine users.

METHOXETAMINE

Methoxetamine (also known as roflcoptr, rhino ket, MXE, moxy, MKET, mexy and mexxy) is a newly reported 'legal high', chemically related to 'dissociative anaesthetics' like ketamine and PCP, and having similar effects. It produces feelings of euphoria, warmth, 'enlightenment' and detachment from the world around, as well as hallucinations, restlessness and a feeling of being on edge, insomnia, tremors and sweating. Some people feel as if they have extra energy.

Table 34.21 *Main types of tobacco smoking in different cultures*

African	Arabic	South Asian	Western
Cigarettes	Cigarettes, hookah (shisha – water pipe)	Cigarettes, bidi (cheerot), chuta (reverse smoking) kreteks, hookah	Cigarettes, cigars, pipe

Table 34.22 *Diseases associated with cigarette smoking*

System	Diseases
Cardiovascular	Ischaemic heart disease
	Peripheral vascular disease
	Buerger disease
Respiratory	Sinusitis
	Chronic obstructive pulmonary disease
Carcinomas	Oropharyngeal and oral
	Bronchial
	Bladder
	Breast
	Colorectal
	Laryngeal
	Pancreatic
Fetus	Higher prevalence of abortion
	Low birth weight
	Higher risk of perinatal and sudden infant deaths
Gastrointestinal	Periodontal disease
	Peptic ulcer
Central nervous system	Alcoholism
	Cerebrovascular disease
	Dementia

METHYLPHENIDATE (RITALIN)

Methylphenidate is a CNS stimulant often prescribed for children with attention deficit hyperactivity disorder (ADHD). It may amplify dopamine release, thereby improving attention and focus. It has effects similar to, but more potent than, caffeine but less potent than amphetamine. Some individuals misuse it for stimulant effects, appetite suppression, euphoria, wakefulness and enhanced focus/attentiveness.

NAPHYRONE

Naphyrone is a white crystalline powder that is snorted, or swallowed as 'bombs'. It may also be known as, or found mixed with other drugs in, NRG-1, Energy1 or O-2482. Naphyrone is much more potent than mephedrone, perhaps even 10 times more so, and this could lead to a greater risk of overdose as the temptation is to use it in amounts similar to mephedrone. There is also a possible risk of naphyrone causing cancer – the naphthyl part of the compound is known to be carcinogenic. Naphyrone has physical effects: for example, on the cardiovascular system – it may cause tachycardia and arterial constriction leading to cold, blue hands and feet. Excessive CNS stimulation may cause headaches, insomnia, agitation and hallucinations, and seizures, which may be fatal.

NICOTINE AND TOBACCO

Tobacco is one of the most common lifestyle habits worldwide. It is frequently smoked in cigarettes but there are several other forms used in different cultures (Table 34.21).

Derived from plants of the genus *Nicotiana*, tobacco releases nicotine, one of the most heavily used and highly addictive stimulant drugs. Nicotine binds to a CNS receptor and, like cocaine, heroin and marijuana, raises the level of dopamine as well as opioids and glucose, and activates the nucleus accumbens. The type of nicotine cholinergic receptor and the enzyme CYP2A6 influence the chances of addiction. Nicotine also causes a discharge of adrenaline (epinephrine) from the adrenals, which stimulates the CNS and other endocrine glands, and a sudden release of glucose. Nicotine is absorbed readily from tobacco smoke in the lungs, acting in seconds on the brain but affecting the body for up to 30 minutes. Stimulation is followed by depression and fatigue, leading the abuser to seek more nicotine. If a person tries to stop smoking, withdrawal symptoms may appear, with excessive anger, hostility and aggression.

Tobacco smoking is a major health hazard, the smoke also containing a dozen gases (mainly carbon monoxide) and tar, which varies from about 15 mg for a regular cigarette to 7 mg in a low-tar cigarette. About 4000 compounds, including 40 known carcinogens such as nitrosamines and aromatic amines, are present, and promote many diseases including cancers (Table 34.22 and Fig. 34.5). There is also now suspicion that nicotine itself may also be carcinogenic. Cigarette smoking is particularly linked to cancers of lung, oesophagus, mouth and bladder, and to increased risk of cardiovascular disease, chronic obstructive pulmonary disease, hypertension and stroke – and thus is a leading cause of death. If women smokers also take oral contraceptives, they

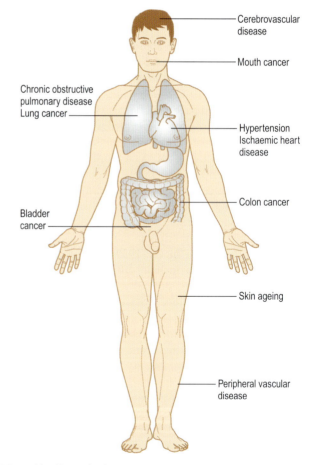

Fig. 34.5 Health effects of tobacco use.

are more prone to cardiovascular and cerebrovascular diseases than are other smokers; this is especially true for women older than 30. Pregnant women who smoke cigarettes run a greater risk of having stillborn or premature infants or infants with low birth weight, and the children have a raised risk for developing conduct disorders. Women who smoke generally have an earlier menopause. Second-hand smoke

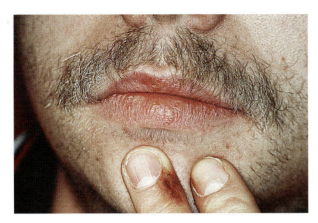

Fig. 34.6 Tar staining on lips and fingers in a tobacco smoker.

Table 34.24 *Nicotine replacement therapies (NRTs)*

Type of NRT	Delivery system	Possible adverse effects
Chewing gum	Chewed gently to release nicotine	Jaw ache Gastric irritation Unsuitability for denture wearers
Inhalor/inhalator	Puffed steadily for about 20 min/h	–
Lozenges	Sucked until dissolution	–
Nasal spray	1–2 doses per hour taken for 2 months	Irritation of nasal mucosa
Sublingual tablets	4 mg hourly taken for 3 months	–
Transdermal patches	Worn during waking hours	Local skin irritation

Table 34.23 *Smoking history*

	Smoker		
Questions	Current	Former	Never
What smoked?			
How many per day?			
Age starting?			
How many years?			
Quit attempt?			
Quit success?			
Exposed to passive smoke?			

(passive smoking) causes lung cancer in adults and greatly increases the risk of respiratory illnesses in children and of sudden infant death.

Tobacco smoking may be recognized from the odour, or staining of fingers, teeth and even lips (Fig. 34.6), but a smoking history should be taken (Table 34.23).

Smoking cessation

Smoking cessation should be a gradual process, because withdrawal symptoms are less severe in those who quit gradually than in those who quit quickly. Rates of relapse are highest in the first few weeks and months, and diminish considerably after 3 months. There are five crucial steps in advising people to stop smoking, known as the 'five As':

- Ask
- Assess
- Advise
- Assist
- Arrange.

Ask

It is important that every patient who is seen by a health professional has their tobacco use noted on clinic records and that the information is kept as up to date as possible. Such a record should cover the frequency of smoking and how long the person has smoked. If the patient uses other forms of tobacco, this should be noted.

Assess

The HCP should inquire whether the patient is keen to quit, and ideally should elicit more detailed information on whether they have ever tried to give up. Any aids used in smoking cessation in the past should be noted.

Advise

Every smoker must be told of the value that stopping smoking will have for them and of the dangers in continuing. Particularly if a risk lesion, such as an oral white or red patch was found, it is important to discuss the sequelae of continuing smoking – give plain, precise and personalized advice. Other reasons for quitting (e.g. the benefits for preventing heart disease) should be included in the advice. Pharmacological treatments combined with psychological treatment result in some of the highest long-term abstinence rates, so the advice, where appropriate, should include directions to use nicotine replacement therapy (NRT). There is little difference in effect between the different types of NRT (Table 34.24). Bupropion is as effective as NRT but can cause dry mouth, headache and gastrointestinal symptoms, and is contraindicated in pregnancy, people who have seizures, the under-18s, people with eating disorders, people with a CNS tumour, people on epileptogenic medications and the very old. Varenicline is more effective than NRT, and has a better efficacy and fewer adverse effects than bupropion; it may cause some nausea and depression, however, and interfere with driving. Electronic cigarettes (e-cigarettes) are becoming popular as a smoking cessation aid. The efficacy of e-cigarettes, as evaluated in preliminary studies, suggests success. Studies on nicotine craving when using e-cigarettes have had mixed results. A few studies have examined the effects of e-cigarettes on plasma nicotine levels and heart rate, and found negligible effects. Surveys have shown only minor side-effects, such as mouth and throat irritation, headache, vertigo and/or nausea. However, the Food and Drug Administration (FDA) has expressed concerns about manufacturing practices and the presence of carcinogens in products tested.

Assist

Other clinic staff should be encouraged to help any smoker who wishes to stop. Setting a date for quitting and arranging to remind a smoker through reception staff may be helpful. In the UK, the patient could be provided with the telephone number of the NHS smoking helpline or advised on how to visit an appropriate website. Useful leaflets should be available in the surgery for distribution.

Arrange

Arranging a follow-up is important, preferably within 1 week of quitting. Heavy smokers may also be referred to local smoking cessation services and helplines. This is important since studies show that people are twice as likely to quit successfully with intensive counselling.

Table 34.25 *Non-smoking tobacco use in different cultures*

African	Arabic	South Asian	Western
Toombak	Shama/ shammaah Nass/ naswar	Paan (pan; betel quid) ingredients can be used alone (e.g. mishri, zarda and kiwan)	Chewing tobacco (plug, loose leaf and twist)
	Zarda	Khaini	Snuff
		Gutkah	Snuss
		Oral cleaning products (e.g. gudakha)	
		Bajar and creamy snuff	

Table 34.26 *Main opiate and opioid analgesics that are abused*

Chemical names	Street names	Comments
Codeine	Captain Cody, Cody, schoolboy; (with glutethimide) doors and fours, loads, pancakes and syrup	Less analgesia, sedation and respiratory depression than morphine
Fentanyl	Apache, China girl, China white, dance fever, friend, goodfella, jackpot, murder 8, TNT, tango and cash	100 times more potent analgesic than morphine
Heroin (diacetylmorphine)	Rock, harry, brown sugar, dope, H, horse, junk, skag, skunk, smack, white horse	Staggering gait, constipation, miosis
Methadone	The done	
Opium	Laudanum, paregoric; big O, black stuff, block, gum, hop	

Fortunately, smoking is increasingly being banned in public places in many countries.

Smokeless tobacco

Tobacco use in other forms is also deleterious to health (Table 34.25); nicotine is also absorbed readily when tobacco is chewed.

Dental aspects of nicotine and tobacco use

Difficulties in dental management of tobacco users may include associated disorders such as chronic obstructive pulmonary disease, ischaemic heart disease, alcoholism or peptic ulcer. Smokers metabolize some other drugs more rapidly and require, for example, higher doses of benzodiazepines than non-smokers. Smoking may cause mucosal keratinization and pigmentary incompetence, and is linked to oral cancer. Smoker keratosis, in which there is diffuse hyperkeratosis of the palate, is typically caused by pipe smoking; it is benign and rapidly reversible, even after years of pipe smoking. Oral snuff dipping and chewing tobacco predispose to leukoplakia and oral cancer. Up to 46% of regular users develop leukoplakia. Currently there is particular concern over the mucosal reactions and the carcinogenic potential of smokeless tobacco by children and adolescents, which is widespread, especially in the USA. Smoking also predisposes to periodontal disease, particularly necrotizing gingivitis, and to implant failure, dry socket, candidosis and xerostomia. Cigarette smoking is the most common cause of extrinsic staining of teeth.

Stopping smoking reduces the risk of oral cancer so that, by 5 years, it is down to that of a non-smoker. However, smoking cessation not only is difficult but also may bring other problems. Aggravation or the onset of recurrent aphthae is noted by some, while others take to eating sweets as a substitute for smoking and may then have more caries activity or put on weight. Use of nicotine-containing chewing gum may reduce the risk of aphthae but may cause hypersalivation. Bupropion may cause dry mouth.

NITRITES

Aliphatic nitrites, including amyl, butyl and cyclohexyl nitrite (used as 'poppers' to enhance sexual activity), may be inhaled. They are dangerous if ingested.

NITROUS OXIDE

Nitrous oxide induces impaired consciousness with a sense of dissociation and often of exhilaration (laughing gas). Addiction to nitrous oxide is an occupational hazard of anaesthetists and others who have access, such as dental staff. Cases of nitrous oxide misuse have been reported in the USA among dental and medical students who stole large hospital cylinders. The reason that it has not become a widely abused drug is simply the practical problem of carrying such heavy cylinders around.

Chronic misuse of nitrous oxide can lead to interference with vitamin B_{12} metabolism and neuropathy. Vague neurological symptoms have also been reported by dental staff working in environments contaminated by nitrous oxide.

Other GA agents that may be misused include halothane (liver damage can result; Ch. 9), methoxyflurane (fluorosis, hypertension and renal damage) and ketamine. Ether and chloroform were widely abused in the past but now rarely so, as other agents are more readily available.

OPIATES AND OPIOIDS

General aspects

Opiate analgesics (morphine and heroin [diacetylmorphine]) are narcotics derived from the opium poppy. These, and synthetic compounds (opioids) such as methadone, dipipanone, dihydrocodeine and pethidine, are widely used and potent analgesics that act by mimicking the natural brain peptides enkephalins and endorphins. They can produce pain relief and euphoria, but also drowsiness/respiratory depression and arrest, nausea, confusion, constipation, sedation, unconsciousness, coma, tolerance and addiction (Table 34.26). Misuse is widespread, mainly in urban areas, and particularly in new towns and major cities amongst adolescents and young adults. Opiates and opioids can be abused orally and are sometimes smoked, sniffed or injected subcutaneously (skin popping), but the maximum effect is obtained by intravenous injection. Many addicts also misuse alcohol, cocaine or other drugs. Misuse leads to tolerance at an early stage and dependence after some months.

Heroin is highly addictive and differs from morphine mainly in the difficulty in overcoming addiction; indeed, heroin is probably the most addictive drug known. Heroin users will do almost anything to fund their addiction, which is why heroin use is often associated with antisocial and criminal behaviour, such as burglary. Heroin can be sniffed, smoked from a tin-foil ('chasing the dragon') or injected.

Clinical features

The short-term effects of heroin misuse appear soon after a single dose, with a surge of euphoria ('rush') accompanied by a warm flushing of the skin, a dry mouth and heavy extremities – probably due to histamine release – that can last up to 4 hours. Mental functioning then becomes clouded due to the depression of the CNS, and the heroin user goes into an alternately wakeful and drowsy state ('on the nod'). The addict is said to be 'a depressed introvert with constricted pupils'. Loss of weight, emaciation, pupil constriction, lack of concentration, poor work performance, irritability, a desire to be left alone, absences from home or self-neglect may be indicators. Constipation, respiratory depression, orthostatic hypotension, infections, neglect of general health and hygiene, and poor diet are common. Early signs of misuse can be difficult or impossible to detect but may be suspected if needle marks are seen, syringes are found or medical complications develop. Needle marks or venous thromboses, particularly in the forearms and legs, are common, but addicts are remarkably adept at finding veins that escape casual inspection, such as lingual or penile veins.

Syringes and needles are often reused or shared by others; therefore, infective complications such as viral hepatitis B, C and D, HIV, septicaemia and pneumonia are common. Acute right-sided staphylococcal endocarditis, from injection of skin bacteria, can be rapidly fatal or leave substantial cardiac damage. Sexually shared infections are also widespread.

Heroin is a respiratory depressant and its use also predisposes to pneumonia, lung abscesses and fibrosis, and other health disorders, including spontaneous abortion. Long-term effects include collapsed veins, infective endocarditis, abscesses and cellulitis. 'Street' heroin may contain only about 10% heroin – most is filler such as lactose, flour, fruit sugars or powdered milk, substances that do not readily dissolve and result in infection or infarction in lungs, liver, kidneys or brain, thromboses, abscesses and gangrene. Drugs such as ecstasy may also have been added.

With regular heroin use, tolerance develops so that, as progressively higher doses are taken over time, physical dependence and addiction ensue. With physical dependence, the body has adapted to the presence of the drug, and withdrawal symptoms result if the drug is reduced or stopped.

The mortality rate among addicts is 2–6% per annum; deaths are usually from overdose, suicide, assaults and HIV/AIDS.

General management

Opiate or opioid withdrawal is unpleasant but not usually dangerous. Early features include lacrimation, rhinorrhoea, sweating and persistent yawning. After about 12 hours, a phase develops of restless tossing sleep (yen) with pupil dilatation, tremor, gooseflesh ('cold turkey'), anorexia, nausea, vomiting, muscle spasms with kicking movements ('kicking the habit'), orgasms, diarrhoea and abdominal pains. Pulse rate and blood pressure also rise. Once the main features have subsided, there may be weakness and insomnia for weeks or months. Sudden withdrawal in heavily dependent users who are in poor health is occasionally fatal.

Medical supervision and opioid agonists such as methadone (a synthetic medication taken orally as a syrup that blocks the effects of heroin for about 24 hours), buprenorphine, naltrexone or LAAM (synthetics that can block heroin effects for up to 72 hours) are used.

Dental aspects

Dental treatment for narcotic addicts can often be given without fear of complications. In the established addict, non-narcotic analgesics may be ineffective in controlling dental pain, so that large doses of opioids may have to be used. However, opioids should not be given or prescribed without first seeking expert advice and their only indication in dentistry is for severe postoperative pain. Pentazocine, being a narcotic antagonist, should not be used for opiate addicts, as it may precipitate withdrawal. Many addicts tolerate pain poorly and complain that LA is insufficient for operative procedures. Those under treatment for addiction have a period of several weeks during which they are particularly hypersensitive to pain and stress. In such patients, opioids must be avoided. Although the withdrawal syndrome subsides within about a week, the addict is, for a few weeks thereafter, intolerant of stress and pain. Simulation of pain is a common manoeuvre to obtain analgesics. Prescription pads may be stolen or drug cabinets raided. Dental drugs that may attract the opiate addict include pethidine (meperidine), codeine, pentazocine and dextropropoxyphene (in co-proxamol).

Other management aspects include behavioural disturbances and withdrawal symptoms, cardiac lesions, maxillofacial injuries, hepatitis or chronic liver disease, infective endocarditis, SSIs including HIV infection, venous thromboses – making intravenous injection difficult, tetanus and drug interactions. Opioids may enhance the sedation of conscious sedation agents and GA. Methadone can affect the P450 drug metabolism system. GA requires admission to hospital. Nausea and vomiting are common if the narcotics are stopped preoperatively.

There are no specific oral effects of opiate dependence but there is often oral neglect, advanced periodontal disease and caries. Diet and sometimes the medications predispose to caries because they contain sugar and/or they cause hyposalivation. Opiate addicts also tend to adopt a cariogenic diet. Caries is often left untreated by the patient who, because of the opioid, may be undisturbed by the pain.

Adverse effects relevant to dentistry include impaired ability to metabolize drugs, hypertension, arrhythmias, hypercoagulability and disturbed behaviour, such as aggression, irritability, paranoia, headache and psychoses. In relation to the use of GA, gastrointestinal inflammation may predispose to vomiting, and there may be suxamethonium (scoline) sensitivity. Low plasma cortisol levels might be an indication for corticosteroid cover before operation. Bleeding tendency or drug intolerance may influence dental care.

Lofexidine and methadone can cause hyposalivation. Preventive oral health care is indicated. Sugar-free preparations should be used but they are acidic and may predispose to tooth erosion.

PARAMETHOXYAMPHETAMINE

Paramethoxyamphetamine (PMA) is an MDMA (ecstasy)-like substance that has been involved in the deaths of some people who mistakenly thought they were using MDMA. Deaths were mainly due to complications from hyperthermia.

PCP (PHENCYCLIDINE; ANGEL DUST)

PCP was developed as an intravenous anaesthetic but discontinued because patients often became agitated, delusional and irrational. PCP has a reputation for causing unpleasant psychological effects, users often becoming violent or suicidal, and a danger to themselves and to others. Many people, therefore, after using the drug once, will not knowingly use it again.

PCP is addictive and snorted, smoked or eaten. Low to moderate doses of PCP cause a slight rise in breathing rate, a pronounced rise in blood pressure and pulse rate, flushing and profuse sweating. Generalized numbness of the extremities and muscular incoordination may also occur.

High doses of PCP cause a fall in blood pressure, pulse rate and respiration, which may be accompanied by nausea, vomiting, blurred vision, flicking up and down of the eyes, drooling, loss of balance, and dizziness, and sometimes a syndrome closely resembling schizophrenia and manic depressive psychosis. Speech is often sparse and garbled. PCP can also cause seizures, illusions and hallucinations, coma and death. Long-term PCP use can lead to memory loss, difficulties with speech and thinking, depression and weight loss. PCP may cause facial grimacing and flushing, hypersalivation and jaw clenching.

PENTAZOCIN

Pentazocine, despite its dysphoric effects, is also used as a drug of dependence, particularly amongst medical and paramedical personnel in the USA. Pentazocine tablets together with an antihistamine (Ts and blues) have been used intravenously as an alternative to the more expensive heroin.

ROHYPNOL (FLUNITRAZEPAM)

Rohypnol is a benzodiazepine that has been used by perpetrators to commit rapes, especially when mixed with alcohol, as it can incapacitate victims and prevent them from resisting sexual assault; since it causes 'anterograde amnesia', individuals may not remember such events. Rohypnol may be lethal when mixed with alcohol and/or other depressants.

EMERGING DRUGS

Designer drugs, created to avoid drug laws, appear at a remarkable pace. '*Spice*' refers to designer cannabinoids such as JWH-018, JWH-073, JWH-200 and (C8)-CP 47,497, initially found in 'herbal smoking blends'; these are sold under many names, including K2, fake weed, Yucatan fire, skunk, moon rocks and others. Synthetic cannabinoid agonists, including RCS-4, RCS-8 and AB-001, are also available. Spice abusers report tachycardia, vomiting, agitation, confusion and hallucinations. Spice can raise blood pressure and cause myocardial ischaemia, and has occasionally been associated with heart attacks. Regular users may experience withdrawal and addiction symptoms. One concern is that there may be harmful heavy metal residues in spice mixtures.

'*Bath salts*' contain synthetic substituted cathinones related to amphetamines such as mephedrone, methylenedioxypyrovalerone (MDPV) and methylone – all highly addictive. Sometimes marketed as 'plant food', 'jewellery cleaner' or 'phone screen cleaner', they are sold online under a variety of names, such as K4 rage, cloud nine, ocean snow, ivory wave, sextacy ultra, white rush, white lightning, bloom, lunar wave, vanilla sky and scarface. Bath salts are typically taken orally, smoked, inhaled or injected – the worst outcomes being after snorting or injection. Users experience euphoria followed by paranoia, depression, agitation and intense craving for more, and some display psychotic and violent behaviour. Bath salts produce an intense high, extreme energy, tachycardia, excessive sweating and insomnia reported to last up to 8 hours, but with redosing the symptoms are prolonged, even for several days. Patients with the 'excited delirium' syndrome from taking bath salts may become dehydrated, with skeletal muscle breakdown, renal failure and even death. K2 can induce a limitless high the more a user smokes, and effects can be up to 10 times more intense than those of marijuana.

Salvia (*Salvia divinorum*) is an herb from Mexico and Central and South America that contains salvinorin A, a potent activator of brain kappa opioid receptors. Salvia users may chew leaves, drink extracted juices or use dried leaves smoked as a joint, consumed in water pipes, or vaporized and inhaled. People who abuse salvia generally have hallucinations or 'psychotomimetic' episodes (a transient psychosis).

Designer stimulants include geranamine, mephedrone, MDPV and desoxypipradrol. Designer sedatives include methylmethaqualone and premazepam.

Another novel development is the use of agents for cosmetic rather than recreational purposes, such as the non-approved alpha-melanocyte-stimulating hormone tanning drugs known as melanotan peptides. Designer analogues of sildenafil (Viagra) have been used as active compounds in 'herbal' aphrodisiac products.

DENTAL ASPECTS OF DRUG ABUSE

Drug abuse may be associated with:

- rampant caries
- periodontal disease
- tooth grinding and tooth surface loss (and masseteric hypertrophy)
- oral mucosal lesions.

Rampant caries is seen in opioid abuse including methadone treatment, stimulant abuse including methamphetamines ('meth mouth'), cocaine and ecstasy, and barbiturate abuse. Rapidly progressing caries affects all tooth surfaces and may involve surfaces that are usually caries-free. The following may predispose to rapidly progressing caries:

- drug-induced hyposalivation; stimulants (e.g. methamphetamine) may lead to dehydration hyposalivation
- poor oral hygiene
- consumption of large amounts of carbonated sugary drinks; opiates and amphetamines often lead to sugar craving
- use of methadone in a sugar syrup form.

Addicts tend to have poor oral hygiene, and many also smoke tobacco – another risk factor in periodontal disease.

Tooth surface loss may be caused by:

- bruxism and clenching – reported mainly with opioid and stimulant use
- hyposalivation
- erosive (acidic) drinks taken in an effort to relieve xerostomia
- regurgitation, bulimia and vomiting, as in alcoholism – may induce erosion, particularly of palatal surfaces of maxillary anterior teeth.

Candida infection is common in drug abusers due to:

- dry mouth
- compromised immune responses
- poor denture hygiene.

Premalignant and malignant mucosal lesions are particularly associated with alcohol, tobacco and betel, and marijuana use.

Management issues include:

- behavioural problems
- compliance with treatment
- viral hepatitis (C and/or B), HIV or other SSIs
- liver damage causing a bleeding tendency and impaired drug metabolism
- malnourishment
- immune defects
- acute anxiety, dysphoria and paranoid thoughts.

LA with adrenaline (epinephrine) may prolong the acute tachycardia already induced by cannabis.

Pain management may be challenging for several reasons:

- Resistance to LA
- Anxiety
- Dental pain from carious teeth – may become evident when a patient stops heroin and starts a methadone maintenance programme
- Potentially addictive analgesics – NSAIDs are best for pain control
- GA or sedation – can trigger a relapse to drug abuse
- Methadone – if prescribed by the physician, this should be maintained during treatment.

Dental management should include:

- attention to oral hygiene
- attention to diet, reducing frequency of sugar intake
- sugar-free chewing gum to stimulate salivary flow
- treatment that is kept as simple as possible
- use of simple excavation of gross caries and glass ionomer cement (ART)
- application of fluoride varnish to saveable carious lesions
- extraction of grossly carious and painful teeth
- treatment of candidal infections with sugar-free topical antifungals.

KEY WEBSITES

(Accessed 11 June 2013)
Centers for Disease Control and Prevention. <http://www.cdc.gov/pwud/addiction.html>.
National Institutes of Health: Drug abuse. <http://health.nih.gov/topic/DrugAbuse>.
National Institutes of Health: Substance abuse. <http://health.nih.gov/category/SubstanceAbuse>.
Public Health England. <http://www.nta.nhs.uk/>.

USEFUL WEBSITES

(Accessed 8 July 2013)
emedicinehealth. <http://www.emedicinehealth.com/drug_dependence_and_abuse/article_em.htm>.
National Institute on Drug Abuse: Commonly abused drugs. <http://www.drugabuse.gov/sites/default/files/cadchart.pdf>.
National Institute on Drug Abuse: Drugs of abuse. <http://www.drugabuse.gov/drugs-abuse>.
White House: Office of National Drug Control Policy. <http://www.whitehouse.gov/ondcp/prescription-drug-abuse>.
NHS – The Education Centre for Health and Social Care: Smoking, drinking and drug use among young people in England in 2011 . <http://www.hscic.gov.uk/catalogue/PUB11334>.

FURTHER READING

Akhter, R., et al. 2008. Relationship between betel quid additives and established periodontitis among Bangladeshi subjects. J. Clin. Periodontol. 35, 9.
Allen, S.E., et al. 2006. The increased risk of urinary stone disease in betel quid chewers. Urol. Res. 34, 239.
Araujo, M.W., et al. 2004. Oral and dental health among inpatients in treatment for alcohol use disorders: a pilot study. J. Int. Acad. Periodontol. 6, 125.
Autti-Rämö, I., et al. 2006. Fetal alcohol spectrum disorders in Finland: clinical delineation of 77 older children and adolescents. Am. J. Med. Genet. A 140, 137.
Avon, S.L., 2004. Oral mucosal lesions associated with use of quid. J. Can. Dent. Assoc. 70, 244.
Baldisseri, M.R., 2007. Impaired healthcare professional. Crit. Care. Med. 35 (2 Suppl), S106.
Brand, H.S., et al. 2008. Ecstasy (MDMA) and oral health. Br. Dent. J. 204, 77.

Brazier, W.J., et al. 2003. Ecstasy related periodontitis and mucosal ulceration – a case report. Br. Dent. J. 194, 197.
Brown, R.E., Morisky, D.E., Silverstein, S.J., 2013. Meth mouth severity in response to drug-use patterns and dental access in methamphetamine users. J. Calif. Dent. Assoc. 41 (6), 421–428. PubMed PMID: 23875434.
Calhoun, F., et al. 2006. National Institute on Alcohol Abuse and Alcoholism and the study of fetal alcohol spectrum disorders. Int. Consort. Ann. Ist Super Sanitá 42, 4.
Carda, C., et al. 2004. Alcoholic parotid sialosis: a structural and ultrastructural study. Med. Oral 9, 24.
Carpenter, J.M., et al. 2005. Oral carcinoma associated with betel nut chewing in the Pacific: an impending crisis? Pac. Health Dialog. 12, 158.
Carretero Pelaez, M.A., et al. 2004. Alcohol-containing mouthwashes and oral cancer: critical analysis of literature. Med. Oral 9, 120.
Chaloupka, F.J., et al. 2002. The effect of price on alcohol consumption and alcohol-related problems. Alcohol. Res. Health 26, 22.
Chen, C.C., et al. 2008. Association among cigarette smoking, metabolic syndrome, and its individual components: the metabolic syndrome study in Taiwan. Metabolism 57, 544.
Chikte, U.M., et al. 2005. Patterns of tooth surface loss among winemakers. South Afr. Dent. J. 60, 370.
Cho, C.M., et al. 2005. General and oral health implications of cannabis use. Austral. Dent. J. 50, 70.
Chung, F.M., et al. 2006. Areca nut chewing is associated with metabolic syndrome: role of tumor necrosis factor-alpha, leptin, and white blood cell count in betel nut chewing-related metabolic derangements. Diabetes Care 29, 1714.
Cole, P., et al. 2003. Alcohol-containing mouthwash and oropharyngeal cancer: a review of the epidemiology. J. Am. Dent. Assoc. 134, 1079.
Ezzati, M., et al. 2002. Comparative Risk Assessment Collaborating Group: selected major risk factors and global and regional burden of disease. Lancet 360, 1347.
Fasanmade, A., et al. 2007. Oral squamous cell carcinoma associated with khat chewing. Oral Surg. Oral Med. Oral Pathol. Oral Radiol. Endod. 104, e53.
Foxcroft, D.R., et al. 2003. Longer-term primary prevention for alcohol misuse in young people: a systematic review. Addiction 98, 397.
Fung, E.Y., Lange, B.M., 2011. Impact of drug abuse/dependence on dentists. Gen. Dent. 59, 356.
Furr, A.M., et al. 2006. Factors associated with long-term complications after repair of mandibular fractures. Laryngoscope 116, 427.
García-Algar, O., et al. 2005. Prenatal exposure to arecoline (areca nut alkaloid) and birth outcomes. Arch. Dis. Child. Fetal Neonatal Ed. 90, F276.
Goodisson, D., et al. 2004. Head injury and associated maxillofacial injuries. N. Z. Med. J. 117, U1045.
Graham, C.H., Meecham, J.G., 2005. Dental management of patients taking methadone. Dent. Update 32, 477.
Guh, J.Y., et al. 2007. Betel-quid use is associated with heart disease in women. Am. J. Clin. Nutr. 85, 1229.
Hashibe, M., et al. 2005. Epidemiologic review of marijuana use and cancer risk. Alcohol 35, 265.
Hornecker, E., et al. 2003. A pilot study on the oral conditions of severely alcohol addicted persons. J. Contemp. Dent. Pract. 4, 51.
Hoyme, H.E., et al. 2005. A practical clinical approach to diagnosis of fetal alcohol spectrum disorders: clarification of the 1996 Institute of Medicine criteria. Pediatrics 115, 39.
Hsiao, T.J., et al. 2007. Risk of betel quid chewing on the development of liver cirrhosis: a community-based case-control study. Ann. Epidemiol. 17 (6), 479.
Hsu, S.D., et al. 2002. Chemoprevention of oral cancer by green tea. Gen. Dent. 50, 140.
IARC Working Group on the Evaluation of Carcinogenic Risks to Humans., 2004. Betel-quid and areca-nut chewing and some areca-nut derived nitrosamines. IARC Monogr. Eval. Carcinog. Risks. Hum. 85, 1.
Jang, Y.C., et al. 2006. Face burns caused by flambé drinks. J. Burn. Care. Res. 27, 93.
Jones, L., et al. 2002. Studies on dental erosion: an in vivo-in vitro model of endogenous dental erosion – its application to testing protection by fluoride gel application. Aust. Dent. J. 47, 304.
Kamisawa, T., et al. 2003. Salivary gland involvement in chronic pancreatitis of various etiologies. Am. J. Gastroenterol. 98, 323.
Kenna, G.A., Lewis, D.C., 2008. Risk factors for alcohol and other drug use by healthcare professionals. Subst. Abuse. Treat. Prev. Policy 3, 3.
Kenna, G.A., Wood, M.D., 2004. Prevalence of substance use by pharmacists and other health professionals. J. Am. Pharm. Assoc. 44 (6), 684.
Kenna, G.A., Wood, M.D., 2005. The prevalence of alcohol, cigarette and illicit drug use and problems among dentists. J. Am. Dent. Assoc. 136 (7), 1023.
Klasser, G.D., Epstein, J.B., 2006. The metamphetamine epidemic and dentistry. Gen. Dent. 54, 431.
Kwasnicki, A., et al. 2008. The significance of alcohol misuse in the dental patient. Dent. Update 35, 7.
Lin, C.F., et al. 2008. Prevalence and determinants of biochemical dysfunction of the liver in Atayal Aboriginal community of Taiwan: is betel nut chewing a risk factor? BMC Gastroenterol. 8, 13.
Lugasi, A., Hovari, J., 2003. Antioxidant properties of commercial alcoholic and nonalcoholic beverages. Nahrung. 47, 79.
Lussi, A., et al. 2004. The role of diet in the aetiology of dental erosion. Caries. Res. 38 (Suppl 1), 34.

Mack, F., et al. 2003. Study of health in Pomerania (SHIP): relationship among socioeconomic and general health factors and dental status among elderly adults in Pomerania. Quintessence Int. 34, 772.

Mandel, L., 2005. Dental erosion due to wine consumption. JADA 136, 71.

Mandic, R., et al. 2005. Sialadenosis of the major salivary glands in a patient with central diabetes insipidus – implications of aquaporin water channels in the pathomechanism of sialadenosis. Exp. Clin. Endocrinol. Diabetes 113, 205.

McGrath, C., Chan, B., 2005. Oral health sensations associated with illicit drug abuse. Br. Dent. J. 198, 159.

McLellan, A.T., et al. 2000. Drug dependence, a chronic medical illness: implications for treatment, insurance, and outcomes evaluation. JAMA 284 (13), 1689.

Molin, S., Plewig, G., 2007. Betel quid chewing: traditional habit with side effects. MMW Fortschr. Med. 149, 46.

Mutsvangwa, T., Douglas, T.S., 2007. Morphometric analysis of facial landmark data to characterize the facial phenotype associated with fetal alcohol syndrome. J. Anat. 210, 209.

Naidoo, S., et al. 2005. Fetal alcohol syndrome: anthropometric and oral health status. J. Contemp. Dent. Pract. 6, 101.

Naidoo, S., et al. 2006. Foetal alcohol syndrome: a cephalometric analysis of patients and controls. Eur. J. Orthod. 28, 254.

Naidoo, S., et al. 2006. Foetal alcohol syndrome: a dental and skeletal age analysis of patients and controls. Eur. J. Orthod. 28, 247.

Nathwani, N.S., Gallagher, J.E., 2008. Methadone: dental risks and preventive action. Dent. Update 35 (542), 547.

Odum, L.E., et al. 2012. Electronic cigarettes: do they have a role in smoking cessation? J. Pharm. Pract. 25 (6), 611.10.1177/0897190012451909 Epub 2012 Jul 13

O'Sullivan, E.M., 2012. Dental health of Irish alcohol/drug abuse treatment centre residents. Community Dent. Health 29 (4), 263–267. PubMed PMID: 23488206.

Petti, S., Scully, C., 2005. The role of the dental team in preventing and diagnosing cancer. 5. Alcohol and the role of the dentist in alcohol cessation. Dent. Update 32, 454.

Rafeek, R.N., et al. 2006. Tooth surface loss in adult subjects attending a university dental clinic in Trinidad. Int. J. Dent. 56, 181.

Reece, A.S., 2007. Dentition of addiction in Queensland: poor dental status and major contributing drugs. Aust. Dent. J. 52, 144.

Rehm, J., et al. 2003. The relationship of average volume of alcohol consumption and patterns of drinking to burden of disease – an overview. Addiction 98, 1209.

Room, R., et al. 2005. Alcohol and public health. Lancet 365, 519.

Saini, G.K., Gupta, N.D., Prabhat, K.C., 2013. Drug addiction and periodontal diseases. J. Indian Soc Periodontol. 17 (5), 587–591. Review. PubMed PMID: 24174750; PubMed Central PMCID: PMC3808011.

Sant'Anna, L.B., Tosello, D.O., 2006. Fetal alcohol syndrome and developing craniofacial and dental structures – a review. Orthod. Craniofac. Res. 9, 172.

Scheutz, F., 1984. Five-year evaluation of a dental care delivery system for drug addicts in Denmark. Community. Dent. Oral Epidemiol. 12, 29.

Scully, C., 2007. Aspects of human disease. 34. Alcoholism. Dent. Update 36, 317.

Scully, C., 2007. Cannabis: adverse effects from an oromucosal spray. Br. Dent. J. 203, 336.

Scully, C., Bagán, J.V., 2004. Adverse drug reaction in the orofacial region. Crit. Rev. Oral Biol. Med. 15, 221.

Scully, C., et al. 2008. Sialosis: 35 cases of persistent parotid swelling from two countries. Br. J. Oral. Maxillofac. Surg. 46, 468.

Shekarchizadeh, H., Khami, M.R., Mohebbi, S.Z., Virtanen, J.I., 2013. Oral health behavior of drug addicts in withdrawal treatment. BMC Oral. Health 13, 11. doi: 10.1186/1472-6831-13-11 PubMed PMID: 23368406; PubMed Central PMCID: PMC3583702.

Shepherd, J.P., et al. 2006. Relations between alcohol, violence and victimization in adolescence. J. Adolesc. 29, 539.

Smith, A.J., et al. 2003. A randomized controlled trial of a brief intervention after alcohol-related facial injury. Addiction 98, 43.

Substance Abuse and Mental Health Services Administration. Results from the 2008 national survey on drug use and health: national findings. Rockville, MD, 2009, Office of Applied Studies. NSDUH Series H-36, HHS Publication No. SMA 09-4434.

Tilakaratne, W.M., et al. 2006. Oral submucous fibrosis: review on aetiology and pathogenesis. Oral Oncol. 42, 561.

Titas, A., Ferguson, M.M., 2002. Impact of opioid use on dentistry. Austral. Dent. J. 47, 94.

Tredwin, C., et al. 2005. Drug-induced dental disorders. Adverse. Drug. React. Bull. 232, 891.

Tredwin, C., et al. 2005. Drug-induced disorders of teeth. J. Dent. Res. 84, 596.

Tsai, J.F., et al. 2001. Betel quid chewing as a risk factor for hepatocellular carcinoma: a case-control study. Br. J. Cancer 84, 709.

Tsai, J.F., et al. 2004. Habitual betel quid chewing and risk for hepatocellular carcinoma complicating cirrhosis. Medicine (Baltimore) 83, 176.

Versteeg, P.A., et al. 2008. Effect of cannabis usage on the oral environment: a review. Int. J. Dent. Hyg. 6, 315.

Warburton, A.L., Shepherd, J.P., 2002. Alcohol-related violence and the role of oral and maxillofacial surgeons in multi-agency prevention. Int. J. Oral Maxillofac. Surg. 31, 657.

Warburton, A.L., Shepherd, J.P., 2006. Tackling alcohol related violence in city centres: effect of emergency medicine and police intervention. Emerg. Med. J. 23, 12.

World Health Organization (WHO), 2004. Department of Mental Health and Substance Abuse Global status report on alcohol 2004. WHO, Geneva.

World Health Organization (WHO) (2002). World Health Report 2002: reducing risks, promoting healthy life. WHO, Geneva.

Yang, M.S., et al. 2008. The effect of maternal betel quid exposure during pregnancy on adverse birth outcomes among aborigines in Taiwan. Drug. Alcohol. Depend. 95, 134.

Young, W.G., 2005. Tooth wear: diet analysis and advice. Int. Dent. J. 55, 68.

Zero, D.T., Lussi, A., 2006. Behavioral factors. Monogr. Oral Sci. 20, 100.

Zero, D.T., Lussi, A., 2005. Erosion – chemical and biological factors of importance to the dental practitioner. Int. Dent. J. 55 (4 Suppl 1), 285.

APPENDIX 34.1 SOME STREET NAMES AND OTHER TERMS FOR DRUGS OF MISUSE

Street names	Drugs
Acapulco gold	Cannabis
Acid	LSD
Angel dust/mist	Phencyclidine
Animal tranquillizer	Phencyclidine
Base	Cocaine
Bath salts	Mephedrone
Beans	Amphetamine
Bennies	Amphetamine
Bhang[a]	Cannabis
Billy	Amphetamine
Biscuits	Ecstasy
Black tar	Heroin
Blanco	Heroin
Blow	Cannabis
Blue angel/devil/heaven	Amylobarbital
Bolivian	Cocaine

Street names	Drugs
Booze	Alcohol
Bounce	Mephedrone
Bubble	Mephedrone
C	Cocaine
Cadillac	Cocaine
Candy	Barbiturates
Charas	Cannabis
Charlies	Cocaine
Chip	Heroin
Christmas trees	Barbiturates
Coke	Cocaine
Co-pilot	Methamphetamine
Crack	Cocaine free base
Crystal	Methamphetamine
Crystal joints	Phencyclidine
Cubes	LSD
Dagga[a]	Cannabis
Dennis the Menace	Ecstasy

(Continued)

Street names	Drugs
Dexies	Dexamphetamine
Disco (disco biscuit)	Ecstasy
Doe	Methamphetamine
Dope	Heroin
Dot	LSD
Downers	Barbiturates
Drinamyl	Amphetamine
Drone	Mephedrone
E	Ecstasy
Ecstasy	Methylenedeoxy-methamphetamine
Edwards	Ecstasy
Elephant	Phencyclidine
Freebase	Cocaine
Ganga[a]	Cannabis
GHB	Gamma-hydroxybutyrate
Girl	Cocaine
Gold dust	Cocaine
Goofballs	Barbiturates
Goon	Phencyclidine
Grass	Cannabis
Gunk	Morphine
H	Heroin
Hash (hashish[a])	Cannabis
Hocus	Morphine
Hog	Phencyclidine
Horse	Heroin
Horse tranquillizer	Phencyclidine
Ice	Methamphetamine
Jack up	Amylobarbital
Jellies	Tranquillizers
Junk	Cocaine
K (special K)	Ketamine
KJ	Phencyclidine
Lady	Cocaine
Lilly	Secobarbital
Love drug/dove	Methamphetamine or ecstasy
Ludes	Methaqualone
(Marihuana)[a] marijuana	Cannabis
Meow meow	Mephedrone
Meph	Mephedrone
Mesc	Mescaline
Microdot	LSD
Mist	Phencyclidine
Monkey	Morphine
Mushroom	Psilocybin

Street names	Drugs
Nebbies	Pentobarbital
Panama gold	Cannabis
Paris	Methaqualone
PCP	Phencyclidine
Peace pills	Phencyclidine
Peaches	Amphetamine
Pink	Morphine
Plant feeder	Mephedrone
Poppers	Amyl nitrite
Pot	Cannabis
Purple haze	LSD
Purple hearts	Dexamphetamine and amylobarbital
Quads	Methaqualone
Red devils	Secobarbital
Reefer	Cannabis
Rhubarb and custard	Ecstasy
Rock	Cocaine
Rocket fuel	Phencyclidine
Scuffle	Phencyclidine
Sensi	Cannabis
Shit	Heroin
Silly putty	Psilocybin
Skunk	Cannabis
Smack	Heroin
Snow	Cocaine
Soapers	Methaqualone
Soma	Phencyclidine
Speed	Amphetamine (intravenously)
Speedball	Opioids and amphetamine (or cocaine and heroin)
Spliff	Cannabis
Strawberry	LSD
Sulfate	Amphetamine
T	Phencyclidine
Tea	Cannabis
Tic tac	Phencyclidine
Ts and blues	Pentazocine and tripelennamine
Vitamins	Ecstasy
Wash	Cocaine
Weed	Cannabis
White lightning	LSD
White magic	Mephedrone
Yellow jackets	Pentobarbital

[a]Correct name in country of origin.

APPENDIX 34.2 NHS ALCOHOL SELF-ASSESSMENT

From: http://www.nhs.uk/Tools/Documents/Alcohol%20self%20assessment.htm (accessed 30 September 2013).

ARE YOU DRINKING TOO MUCH?

If you're not really sure about the amount you are drinking, take this short test.

It'll help you to assess the effects of your drinking and if it suggests you're drinking too much you'll get advice on how to cut down or seek further help.

QUESTIONS

1. How often do you have a drink containing alcohol?

a) Never (0 points)
b) Once a month or less (1 point)
c) 2 to 4 times a month (2 points)
d) 2 to 3 times a week (3 points)
e) 4 or more times a week (4 points)

2. How many units of alcohol do you have on a typical day when you are drinking?

1–2 (0 points)
3–4 (1 point)
5–6 (2 points)
7–9 (3 points)
10 + (4 points)

What is a unit?

You can't just count each drink as a unit of alcohol. The number of units depends on the different strength and size of each drink, so it can vary a lot.

Here's some examples:

- Pint of beer, 4%, is 2.3 units
- 500 ml can of strong lager, 6%, 3 units
- 250 ml glass of wine, 11%, 2.8 units
- 330 ml can of cider, 5%, 1.7 units
- Single (25 ml) measure of spirits (e.g. vodka or gin), 1 unit

3. How often do you have six or more units on one occasion?

a) Never (0 points)
b) Less than monthly (1 point)
c) Monthly (2 points)
d) Weekly (3 points)
e) Daily or almost daily (4 points)

What's binge drinking?

Binge drinking usually refers to drinking lots of alcohol in a short space of time or drinking to get drunk.

There is no consistently agreed measure of binge drinking but drinking more than eight units on any day for men, and more than six units for women, is the measure normally used.

The vital thing is to avoid drinking heavily in one session or drinking to intoxication.

Binge drinking is a major factor in accidents, violence and anti-social behaviour.

4. How often during the last year have you failed to do what was normally expected from you because of your drinking?

a) Never (0 points)
b) Less than monthly (1 point)
c) Monthly (2 points)
d) Weekly (3 points)
e) Daily or almost daily (4 points)

5. How often during the last year have you found that you were not able to stop drinking once you had started?

a) Never (0 points)
b) Less than monthly (1 point)
c) Monthly (2 points)
d) Weekly (3 points)
e) Daily or almost daily (4 points)

6. How often during the last year have you needed an alcoholic drink in the morning to get yourself going after a heavy drinking session?

a) Never (0 points)
b) Less than monthly (1 point)
c) Monthly (2 points)
d) Weekly (3 points)
e) Daily or almost daily (4 points)

7. How often during the last year have you had a feeling of guilt or remorse after drinking?

a) Never (0 points)
b) Less than monthly (1 point)
c) Monthly (2 points)
d) Weekly (3 points)
e) Daily or almost daily (4 points)

8. How often during the last year have you been unable to remember what happened the night before because you had been drinking?

a) Never (0 points)
b) Occasionally (1 point)
c) Monthly (2 points)
d) Weekly (3 points)
e) Daily (4 points)

9. Have you or somebody else been injured as a result of your drinking?

a) No, this has never happened (0 points)
b) Yes, but not in the past year (2 points)
c) Yes, during the past year (4 points)

10. Has a relative, friend, doctor or health worker been concerned about your drinking or suggested you cut down?

a) No, never (0 points)
b) Yes, but not in the past year (2 points)
c) Yes, during the past year (4 points)

RESULTS

0–8 points

Based on your answers today you're drinking in a way that is sociable and is unlikely to harm your health.

As long as your drinking does remain within recommended levels, there is only a low risk that the way you drink will contribute to future health problems.

The NHS recommends that women should not regularly drink more than 2–3 units a day and men should not regularly drink more than 3–4 units a day.

Remember, there can be risks from one-off episodes of heavy drinking too.

8–20 points

Based on your answers today your drinking does appear to be putting you at increased risk of developing health problems, so you might want to think about cutting down.

The following can help you cut down:

- Work out a daily limit and stick to it.
- Do more activities that don't involve drinking.
- Eat before and while you're drinking.
- Don't let anyone top up your drinks.
- Tell your friends you're cutting down.
- Count your units.

The NHS recommends that women should not regularly drink more than 2–3 units a day and men should not regularly drink more than 3–4 units a day.

20–100 points

Based on your answers today your drinking is already causing you problems.

The NHS recommends that women should not regularly drink more than 2–3 units a day and men should not regularly drink more than 3–4 units a day.

You may want help to reduce your drinking. You can find local alcohol services through the 'Find services' section of NHS Choices or your GP will be able to help you find them. You can also contact the National Drinkline 0800 917 8282 open 24 hours, seven days a week.

USEFUL LINKS

NHS Choices:

Alcohol Support. Where to get help if you need it. http://www.nhs.uk/Livewell/alcohol/Pages/Alcoholsupport.aspx
Binge drinking. http://www.nhs.uk/Livewell/alcohol/Pages/Bingedrinking.aspx
'I used to drink all day'. Real story: how I stopped drinking. http://www.nhs.uk/Livewell/alcohol/Pages/Alldaydrinker.aspx
'Social drinking': the hidden risks http://www.nhs.uk/Livewell/alcohol/Pages/Socialdrinking.aspx

35 | Transplantation and tissue regeneration

TRANSPLANTS

Transplantation of organs and tissues has developed rapidly alongside enormous advances in immunology, immunosuppressive therapy (Ch. 19) and medical and surgical technology. Organs and tissues currently transplanted are shown in Table 35.1.

INDICATIONS

Transplantation is frequently a life-saving procedure. Solid organ transplants (SOTs) of kidney, liver, heart, lung, pancreas and small bowel are now the treatments of choice for end-stage organ failure with substantial limitation of daily activities and limited life expectancy.

Autografts (autologous transplants) refer to cells that are collected from an individual and given back to that same person (e.g. veins used for coronary artery bypass grafting, skin used for grafts or blood). Autografts are the most common type of transplant used to treat patients with haemopoietic stem-cell transplantation (HSCT; or bone marrow transplantation [BMT]).

Allografts (allogeneic transplants) refers to cells that come from another individual, who may be a relative or not, but the donor's blood must be closely matched to the recipient's (more likely when the donor is a sibling).

Isografts are allografts in which organs or tissues are transplanted from a donor to a genetically identical recipient (e.g. an identical twin). Most human tissue and organ transplants are allografts that are not so closely matched, which means that the recipient needs to be immunosuppressed to prevent transplant rejection. Organ donation is crucial to provide adequate material.

HSCT is the transfer of haemopoietic stem cells from one individual to another (allogeneic HSCT), or the return of previously harvested cells to the same individual (autologous HSCT) after manipulation of the cells and/or the recipient. It developed from the infusion of bone marrow cells into patients after prior radio- or chemotherapy and is also widely employed in many neoplastic and autoimmune conditions (Fig. 35.1). *Allogeneic* HSCT can cure or improve outcomes in a variety of conditions, including leukaemias, lymphomas, myeloproliferative disorders, myelodysplastic syndromes, bone marrow failure syndromes, congenital immunodeficiencies, enzyme deficiencies and haemoglobinopathies.

Best transplant results are in ambulatory patients with rehabilitation potential, who have no other significant co-morbidity, a satisfactory psychosocial profile, an emotional support system and nutritional status. Transplantation may be refused by some Jehovah's Witnesses and Orthodox Jews.

Peripheral blood stem-cell transplantation (PBSCT) and umbilical cord blood transplantation are also used as sources of haemopoietic stem cells for transplants.

SOLID ORGAN SOURCES

Transplants can be from live or dead ('cadaveric') donors, or from donors who are living but 'brain-dead' – a state defined by an irreversible cessation of all brain and brainstem functions; this is determined on clinical criteria during two separate examinations performed 24 hours apart, or by ancillary studies to assess brain activities. An absence of drugs, hypothermia or metabolic derangements must be confirmed. Brain death criteria are shown in Box 35.1. One of the main obstacles to transplantation is the lack of donors (Fig. 35.2).

TRANSPLANTATION OUTCOMES

Success for different types of organ transplanted can, in some instances, approach 90% at 1 year, the major barrier to success being immunological rejection. Except for transplants between identical twins, all transplant donors and recipients are immunologically incompatible and host cells attempt to destroy or reject the transplanted organ, which, with time, can lead to graft failure or patient death. The other main cause of graft rejection is patients' failure to continue taking their immunosuppressive drugs.

To try to avoid transplant rejection, transplant recipients and donors are tissue-typed to determine the human leukocyte antigen (HLA) class I and class II loci; the degree of incompatibility is defined by the number of antigens mismatched at each HLA locus. The degree of humoral sensitization to HLA antigens is also determined; sensitization happens when the recipient has received multiple blood

Table 35.1 *Transplantation*

Organs/tissues	Source	Type
Thoracic organs	Heart	Deceased donor only
	Lung	Deceased donor and living donor
	Heart/lung	Deceased donor and domino transplant
Abdominal organs	Kidney	Deceased donor and living donor
	Liver	Deceased donor and living donor
	Pancreas	Deceased donor only
	Small intestine	Deceased donor and living donor
Tissues, cells, fluids	Blood transfusion/blood parts transfusion	Living donor and autograft
	Blood vessels	Autograft and deceased donor
	Bone	Deceased donor, living donor and autograft
	Bone marrow/adult stem cell	Living donor and autograft
	Cornea	Deceased donor only
	Face replant	Autograft
	Face transplant (rare)	Deceased donor only
	Hand	Deceased donor only
	Heart valve	Deceased donor, living donor and xenograft (porcine/bovine)
	Pancreas islet cells	Deceased donor and living donor
	Penis	Deceased donor only
	Skin	Deceased donor, living donor and autograft
	Trachea	Autograft

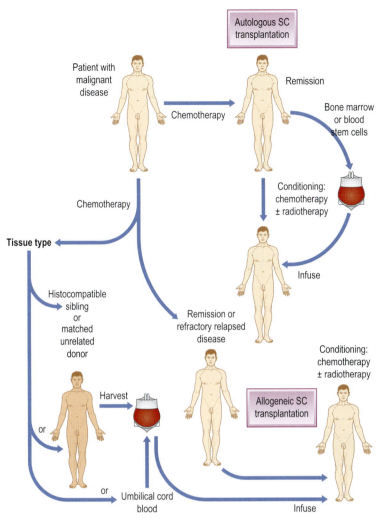

Fig. 35.1 Stem cell (SC) transplantation for lymphoproliferative disease.

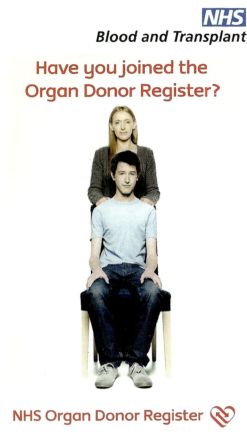

Fig. 35.2 Organ donation is crucial to transplantation programmes.

Box 35.1 *Criteria for brain death*

- Known cause of condition
- Temperature higher than 95°F
- No drug intoxication or neuromuscular blocking agent
- No significant metabolic derangement
- No gag, cough or corneal reflexes
- Absence of dull-eye reflex
- Pupils fixed and dilated
- No spontaneous respirations or movements
- Negative results on apnoea test
- Isoelectric electroencephalogram (EEG)
- Computed tomographic evidence of brain herniation
- Negative results on cerebral blood flow studies (i.e. brain scan or intracranial angiography)

---

transfusions from a previous organ transplant or during pregnancy. Cross-matching is an *in vitro* assay to determine whether a potential transplant recipient has preformed anti-HLA class I antibodies against those of the organ donor. A negative cross-match must be obtained before accepting an organ for transplantation. Transplantation of an organ into a recipient sensitized against donor class I HLA antigens puts the recipient at high risk of hyperacute antibody-mediated rejection. ABO blood group determination is used to establish whether the

patient is a potential target of recipient circulating preformed cytotoxic anti-ABO antibody. Transplantation across incompatible blood groups may result in a humorally mediated hyperacute rejection.

PREVENTION OF REJECTION

Following transplantation, all patients need treatment with immunosuppressive drugs for life, to prevent T-cell alloimmune rejection. These are discussed in Chapter 19.

Treatment goals are to achieve the highest rates of patient and graft survival, and to minimize toxicity, infections and malignancy. The current high graft survival rate is due to increasingly effective immunosuppression. There is no consensus as to the single best protocol, and each transplant programme uses slightly different regimens.

Induction immunosuppression immediately after transplantation is a short course of intensive treatment to almost abolish the circulating lymphoid cells critical to rejection. Induction agents are given less often if the graft functions immediately, as in recipients of living kidney donors, especially HLA-ID grafts. *Maintenance immunosuppression* usually uses corticosteroid-sparing agents, such as calcineurin inhibitors (e.g. ciclosporin or tacrolimus) and/or corticosteroids, sometimes along with antiproliferative agents (e.g. azathioprine, mycophenolate mofetil or rapamycin; Table 35.2), inhibitors of *m*echanistic *t*arget *o*f *r*apamycin (mTOR; e.g. temsirolimus, everolimus, sirolimus or deforolimus), anti-T cytotoxic (anti-Tc; abatacept, belatacept) or anti-interleukin-2 (basiliximab, daclizumab) agents, or other biological therapies. Many new agents are being trialled, such as eculizumab and bortezomib for treatment of antibody-mediated rejection; these and the more commonly used immunosuppressive drugs and agents, along with their adverse effects, are discussed more fully in Chapter 19. Transplantation regimens used in children may affect the developing dentition.

Table 35.2 *Immunosuppressive agents commonly used in transplantation*

Drug	Mode of action	Main adverse effects	Main drug interactions with
Azathioprine	Metabolized by thiopurine methyl transferase (TPMT) to the active mercaptopurine, which reduces DNA synthesis and inhibits lymphocyte division	Myelosuppression Leucopenia Thrombocytopenia Increases risk of myelosuppression with low TPMT Hepatotoxicity	Allopurinol, cytostatic drugs, muscle relaxants, warfarin
Basiliximab	Antibody against cluster of differentiation 25 (CD25) T cells	Hypersensitivity reactions	–
Ciclosporin	Highly lipid-soluble and metabolized in the liver by cytochrome P450 (CYP3A4). Ciclosporin binds to cyclophilins (cytosolic receptors) and inhibits calcineurin. Ciclosporin prevents dephosphorylation of NFAT (nuclear translocation of nuclear factor of activated T cells), and thus blocks interleukin-2 (IL-2)	Neurotoxicity, hypertension, tremulousness, hypertrichosis, gingival swelling, hepatotoxicity, nephrotoxicity with hyperkalemia and/or renal tubular acidosis No bone marrow effect	Carbamazepine, phenytoin, isoniazid, rifampicin, phenobarbital and other drugs that induce CYP3A4 may lower ciclosporin levels. Drugs that inhibit CYP3A4 may raise ciclosporin levels (see Table 35.4) Acute renal failure, rhabdomyolysis, myositis and myalgias when taken concurrently with statin
Corticosteroids	May reduce inflammation by reversing increased capillary permeability and suppressing polymorphonuclear neutrophilic leukocytes (PMNs)	Hypertension, diabetes, osteoporosis and fractures, hip necrosis, cataracts, acne and obesity	–
Daclizumab	Antibody against IL-2 receptors	Hypersensitivity reactions	–
Mycophenolate mofetil	Inhibits inosine monophosphate dehydrogenase to impair cytotoxic T cells	Bone marrow suppression	Aciclovir, antacids, ganciclovir, colestyramine
Rapamycin	Cytotoxic	Cytopenias and hyperlipidaemia	–
Sirolimus	A non-calcineurin inhibitor. Inhibits lymphocyte proliferation and impairs cytotoxic T cells	Hyperlipidaemia	See Table 35.4
Tacrolimus	A calcineurin inhibitor macrolide antibiotic similar to ciclosporin. Inhibits IL-2, interferon-gamma and IL-3 production; transferrin and IL-2 receptor expression; mixed lymphocyte reactions; and cytotoxic T-cell generation through an immunophilin protein – the FK-binding protein (FKBP) that inhibits NFAT. Tacrolimus is metabolized by the same P450 system as ciclosporin	Hyperglycaemia, neurotoxicity and nephrotoxicity Cardiomyopathy if given with ciclosporin to children	Aciclovir, antacids, azathioprine, colestyramine, probenecid See Table 35.4

Adverse effects may include the following:

- *Ciclosporin*: liver/kidney dysfunction, hypertension, bleeding tendency and poor wound healing. Gingival overgrowth incidence varies and is dependent on each patient and their drug regimen. Calcium-channel blockers may exacerbate the problem. Children tend to be more susceptible to gingival overgrowth than adults.
- *Tacrolimus*: less gingival overgrowth but associated with oral ulceration and numbness or tingling, especially around the mouth.
- *Azathioprine*: bone marrow suppression and related complications, such as stomatitis and opportunistic infections.
- *Mycophenolate mofetil*: decreased white cell counts, opportunistic infections, and gastrointestinal problems.
- *Corticosteroids*: hypertension and high blood glucose (steroid-induced diabetes), increased risk for infection, poor wound healing, peptic ulceration, depression and adrenal suppression. Corticosteroids may also mask the early signs of oral infection.
- *Sirolimus*: hypertension, joint pain, low white-cell count, hypercholesterolaemia and oral ulceration.

A number of drugs can interfere with immunosuppressive agents (see Tables 35.4, 29.1 and 29.2).

TRANSPLANTATION COMPLICATIONS

Patients who survive transplant surgery are liable to infection, multi-organ failure and acute allograft rejection; in the long term, malignant neoplasms may possibly supervene.

INFECTIONS

Immunosuppressive therapy is designed to suppress T-lymphocyte–mediated transplant rejection but leads to liability to infections especially with mycobacteria, fungi and viruses (Table 35.3). Infections may spread rapidly, may be opportunistic and may be clinically silent or atypical. Even mild infections can be a serious threat and, as an adjunct to anti-infective therapy, immunosuppression may need to be reduced or even stopped temporarily. Antimicrobial prophylaxis may be appropriate. Bacterial sepsis is better tolerated with ciclosporin than with azathioprine but still must be treated aggressively, as it is the most common cause of death during the first postoperative months. *Legionella* infections are increased in immunosuppressed patients, and often cause dyspnoea and hypoxaemia before the chest radiograph shows any significant infiltrate; a patient who develops such symptoms or a pulmonary infiltrate of unknown aetiology should be treated early with erythromycin.

Table 35.3 *Main possible post-transplantation infections*

Infection	Month post-transplantation		
	1	2	>2
Fungal	Candidosis	Candidosis	Candidosis
		Deep mycoses	Deep mycoses
Viral	Hepatitis	Hepatitis	Hepatitis
	Herpesviruses	Herpesviruses	Herpesviruses
Bacterial	Wound	Wound	Tuberculosis
	Urinary tract	Urinary tract	Pneumonia
	Pneumonia	Tuberculosis	
		Pneumonia	

Viral infections also account for substantial morbidity and mortality. Herpes simplex virus (HSV) infections are common and usually treated with a 10–14-day course of aciclovir or famciclovir. Varicella zoster virus (VZV) infections may appear, especially herpes zoster, and should be treated with similar antivirals. Cytomegalovirus (CMV) infection is one of the other most common viral infections; it usually appears 3 weeks or more after transplantation, presenting with fever, leukopenia and malaise. The CMV status of the donor must therefore be recorded and the CMV titre assessed as part of the pre-transplant evaluation, so that the results are available immediately after transplantation. A tissue diagnosis of CMV should be sought, either by the histological findings or by biopsy cultures. Patients with systemic CMV infections are treated with ganciclovir.

Fungi commonly cause severe local or even systemically invasive infections in transplant patients, and infections in sputum, blood, urine, bile or drains are an indication for systemic antifungal therapy. Candida species are behind the most common fungal infections; as a general rule, if *Candida* grows from two or more sites (e.g. urine, wound), even if not from blood, the patient should be treated and managed as having systemic candidosis. Intravenous amphotericin, or fluconazole intravenously or orally, is usually used. *Aspergillus niger*, *A. flavus* or *A. fumigatus* infections may infect the lungs, upper respiratory tract, skin, soft tissues or central nervous system (CNS), most frequently causing diffuse pneumonia with patchy infiltrates. Amphotericin should be initiated; a long course of systemic therapy is indicated. Development of a brain abscess is insidious and cure rare. *Cryptococcus neoformans* infections may cause pulmonary, CNS and disseminated disease, diagnosed by examination of the cerebrospinal fluid (CSF; lumbar puncture), staining with traditional India ink stains and testing for CSF cryptococcal antigen. Systemic amphotericin treatment is indicated. *Mucor* and *Rhizopus* infections (phycomycoses) are rare but can cause destructive CNS or soft-tissue infections. Treatment includes local excision and a long course of systemic amphotericin. *Pneumocystis* infections are frequently found, and a patient who develops a pulmonary infiltrate of unknown aetiology should be treated early with co-trimoxazole for *Pneumocystis* infections; these commonly cause dyspnoea and hypoxaemia before chest radiography shows any significant infiltrate.

MALIGNANCIES

Transplant recipients are at increased risk from some malignant neoplasms – including melanoma, basal cell carcinoma, Kaposi sarcoma, lymphoma, squamous cell carcinoma of skin and lip, and carcinoma of cervix, external genitalia and perineum. There may be a recurrence of pre-existing cancers in recipients, or donor-transmitted neoplasms or *de novo* malignancies.

Skin cancers affect more than half of organ-transplant recipients and those who develop cutaneous squamous cell carcinomas are at high risk (up to 80%) for multiple subsequent skin cancers. Skin cancers are up to 20 times more frequent in transplant recipients than in the general population and tend to be aggressive. Transplant recipients should therefore avoid sun exposure and undergo routine skin evaluations, with aggressive management of any suspect lesions.

Malignancies are often virally induced. Carcinoma of the skin, lip and cervix may be associated with human papillomaviruses (HPV). Kaposi sarcoma is associated with human herpesvirus-8 (HHV-8; KSHV); it may affect the skin, oropharynx, lungs or other viscera, and treatment involves lowering immunosuppression and then often chemotherapy or radiotherapy. Lymphomas and post-transplant lymphoproliferative disease may be associated with Epstein–Barr virus (EBV).

Some malignancies are seen more frequently in certain subpopulations, according to pre-existing risk factors or behaviours, such as oropharyngeal and lung cancer in those who smoke, or colon cancer in patients with pre-existing inflammatory bowel disease. Directed screening in these patients is desirable, by regular oropharyngeal examinations, chest radiographs and colonoscopies.

Post-transplant lymphoproliferative disorders

General aspects

Post-transplant lymphoproliferative disorders (PTLDs) are a heterogeneous group of potentially, and frequently, fatal B-cell proliferations, associated with EBV infection (from either virus reactivation or primary post-transplant infection); they range from B-cell hyperplasia to malignant immunoblastic lymphoma. The more intense the immunosuppression, the higher the incidence of PTLD, and the earlier it appears. In cardiac transplantation, the incidence ranges from 5% to 13%, reflecting the greater immunosuppression used. PTLDs are relatively uncommon after solid organ and allogeneic bone marrow transplantation (about 2%), but about ten times higher if the patient receives mismatched T cell-depleted bone marrow or anti-T-cell monoclonal antibodies for graft-versus-host disease (GVHD).

Clinical features

PTLDs typically develop within 1 year of transplantation (range 1 month to 14 years). Clinical presentation varies from aggressive diffuse disease appearing early in the post-transplantation period and with polyclonal lesions developing over days or weeks, to localized indolent lesions growing slowly over months. Whether localized or disseminated, PTLD tumours are progressive, with mortality rates as high as 60–100%.

Features include fever, weight loss, an infectious mononucleosis-like syndrome (anorexia, lethargy, sore throat, lymphadenopathy), gastrointestinal symptoms (diarrhoea, abdominal pain), pulmonary symptoms (dyspnoea) and CNS or neurological symptoms. Sites most commonly involved are lymph nodes (59%), liver (31%), lung (29%), kidney (25%), bone marrow (25%), small intestine (22%), spleen (21%), CNS (19%), large bowel (14%), tonsils (10%) and salivary glands (4%).

General management

PTLDs are diagnosed by having a high index of suspicion. A patient who has recently undergone transplantation and presents with unexplained fever, weight loss, lymphadenopathy, hepatosplenomegaly and positive histopathology, and with EBV-DNA, RNA or viral protein on biopsy, is likely to have PTLD.

Treatment is ganciclovir for EBV and reduction or withdrawal of immunosuppression but, since this carries the risk of allograft dysfunction or loss, additional treatment modalities are indicated. These may include rituximab, interferon-alpha (IFNα), intravenous immunoglobulin, cytotoxic T lymphocytes, surgical excision, localized radiation or combination chemotherapy.

T-cell PTLD not associated with EBV infection tends to affect extranodal sites.

MULTIORGAN FAILURE

Transplant patients may also develop recurrent organ and multiorgan disease; for example, they have a 10–20 times increased risk of coronary heart disease. HSCT in particular may be complicated by GVHD.

IMMUNE RECONSTITUTION SYNDROME (IRIS OR IRS)

Restoration of immunity during treatment of infections, particularly if restoration is abrupt and rapid, has the potential to promote excessive inflammatory pathology and tissue damage and an immune reconstitution syndrome (IRIS or IRS). IRIS is more commonly seen in HIV/AIDS therapy but can occur after transplantation. It probably is mediated by anti-inflammatory (Tregs and Th2 cells) and proinflammatory (Th17 and Th1 cells) responses. Pathogens activate naive CD41 cells (Th0) to differentiate into Th1 and Th2 cells. IRIS is mainly an antigen-driven Th1-cell response; Th1 cells produce IFN-c, activate macrophages, promote natural killer (NK) cell-induced cytotoxicity, and elicit proinflammatory responses. Th2 cells secrete interleukin (IL)-4 and IL-10, leading to anti-inflammatory responses. Th17 cells, which produce IL-17 and IL-22, promote potent proinflammatory responses and induce chemokines and metalloproteinases, which recruit neutrophils. Tregs limit the inflammation and subsequent tissue damage.

Antimicrobial agents (e.g. antimycotics) may contribute to the pathogenesis and post-transplant IRIS has been observed with infection with various fungi, *Mycobacterium tuberculosis*, cytomegalovirus and polyoma virus.

Treatments include corticosteroids, intravenous immunoglobulins, non-steroidal anti-inflammatory drugs (NSAIDs) and infliximab.

DENTAL ASPECTS

BEFORE ORGAN TRANSPLANTATION

There should be a full oral and dental evaluation, and careful attention to oral and dental disease, bearing in mind that after transplantation the patient will be chronically immunosuppressed and at high risk from infection. A full oral health care programme should be instituted, and oral hygiene and preventive care must be maintained at a high standard throughout and following transplantation.

Where possible, active dental disease should be treated before transplantation:

- Eliminate oral infections.
- Extract unrestorable teeth.
- Consider removing orthodontic bands or adjusting prostheses for patients expected to receive ciclosporin to obviate gingival overgrowth.
- Carry out treatment on days that the patient with end-stage renal disease does not undergo haemodialysis.
- Educate patients about effective oral health care.
- Consider anxiety and pain tolerance in organ transplant patients.

The timing of treatment, need for antibiotic prophylaxis, precautions to prevent excessive bleeding, and appropriate medication and dose should be taken into account. Some patients are only suitable for treatment in a hospital setting and factors that should be considered include:

- antibiotic prophylaxis
- infection: active infections should treated
- excessive bleeding: take precautions to limit bleeding
- medication: transplantation patients are usually on multiple medications such as anticoagulants, beta-blockers, calcium-channel blockers, diuretics and others. Their adverse effects and drug interactions must be borne in mind
- other medical problems: patients with end-stage organ failure may have co-morbidities.

AFTER ORGAN TRANSPLANTATION

Immunosuppressive therapy can lead to liability to infections and to a bleeding tendency. After transplantation, elective dental care is best deferred for at least 3 months, to avoid unnecessary complications. Infection is most likely at this time – the period of intense immunosuppression. During the immediate post-transplant and chronic rejection phases, only emergency dental care is recommended and should be undertaken in a hospital. Any invasive dental treatment should only be carried out after consultation with the responsible physician and with due consideration to the liability to infection, bleeding tendency related to anticoagulation, risk of adrenal crisis in relation to steroid therapy and impaired drug metabolism; this applies probably for at least 2 years post-transplantation. Dental treatment guidelines include attention to prevent infection – use of antiseptic mouthwashes (e.g. chlorhexidine gluconate) – before treatment. Antibiotic prophylaxis is indicated for invasive dental procedures, particularly if provided within 6 months post-transplantation. In addition, steroid cover may be indicated. Macrolide antibiotics and azole antifungal drugs should be avoided because they may alter serum levels of some immunosuppressive drugs, thus increasing their toxicity. Pre-existing illnesses of transplant candidates often need to be considered, as they can influence oral health care.

GA should be avoided, but, if essential, must only be given in hospital with appropriate expertise and facilities.

Drugs that should be used with caution include aspirin and NSAIDs; these should be avoided since they potentiate the nephrotoxicity of ciclosporin and tacrolimus, may cause a bleeding tendency, and exacerbate peptic ulcer if the patient is on corticosteroids. Sedatives and paracetamol (acetaminophen) are also best avoided. Erythromycin and azole antifungals may affect ciclosporin levels (Table 35.4). There may also be a greater risk from nephrotoxicity with co-trimoxazole, aminoglycosides and quinolones. Drugs used in transplant patients, such as ciclosporin, nifedipine and basiliximab, may induce gingival overgrowth, impaired healing and infections, and may interact with prescribed drugs.

Patients may need steroid supplementation and cover during dental treatment (Ch. 6), probably for at least 2 years post-transplantation. Viral hepatitis B and C infections may be present, especially in older patients who have received blood transfusions before blood was routinely screened. Oral infections, such as HSV, VZV, CMV or EBV, to which the immunosuppressed patient is prone, are discussed in Chapter 20. Several other complications associated with marked immunosuppression manifest in the mouth, including herpes zoster, hairy leukoplakia and aphthous ulcers. Progressive periodontal disease, delayed wound healing and excessive bleeding may also become problems.

Table 35.4 *Drug use in transplanted patients that may change blood levels of immunosuppressants and affect treatment or health*

Drugs that may change blood levels of immunosuppressants			Drugs that increase nephrotoxicity	Drugs that increase hepatotoxicity
Ciclosporin	Tacrolimus	Sirolimus		
Raise levels				
Amphotericin	Clarithromycin	Ciclosporin	Amphotericin	Aminoglycosides
Clarithromycin	Diltiazem	Diltiazem	Clarithromycin	Co-trimoxazole
Erythromycin	Erythromycin	Grapefruit juice	Diclofenac	Erythromycin
Grapefruit juice	Fluconazole	Itraconazole	Erythromycin	Halothane
Ketoconazole	Grapefruit juice	Ketoconazole	Indometacin	Quinolones
Norfloxacin	Itraconazole	Miconazole	NSAIDs	Tetracyclines
	Ketoconazole	Telithromycin	Sulfamethoxazole	
	Miconazole	Voriconazole	Vancomycin	
	Nelfinavir			
	Nifedipine			
	NSAIDs			
	Omeprazole			
	Quinupristin			
	Ritonavir			
	Telithromycin			
Lower levels				
Carbamazepine	Rifampicin (rifampin)	Rifampicin (rifampin)		
Phenytoin				
Sulfamethoxazole				

Oral HSV and VZV infections can be prevented, deferred or ameliorated by prophylactic low-dose oral aciclovir.

Spontaneous bacterial peritonitis and endarteritis are possible peri- and post-transplantation, particularly after liver transplantation, and may necessitate antimicrobial prophylaxis; however, there is no evidence that, after the first 3 months following transplantation, there is any routine need for antimicrobial cover for dental interventions. Some patients carry enterococci in plaque. Rarely, oral or dental infections may spread, with serious complications such as cavernous sinus thrombosis or metastatic infections, and oral bacteria are an important source of bacteraemias.

Oral candidosis may be persistent or mixed bacterial plaques may develop on the oral mucosa. Oral candidosis can usually be managed with topical nystatin, amphotericin or miconazole (Fig. 35.3).

Routine cancer surveillance is mandatory to assure rapid diagnosis and treatment of any malignancy, since patients on immunosuppressive treatment after organ transplantation have a greatly raised incidence of malignant disease, as discussed above (Fig. 35.4). This may be the case especially in those with a history of tobacco or alcohol use and is often so in adults needing liver transplants. Kaposi sarcoma, lymphoma and squamous cell carcinoma are among the oral malignancies that sometimes occur in organ transplant patients.

ORGAN REJECTION

If there is organ rejection, only emergency dental care should be provided.

HAEMOPOIETIC STEM-CELL TRANSPLANTATION (BONE MARROW TRANSPLANTATION)

General aspects

HSCT is increasingly used in the treatment of haematological conditions, neoplasms and some genetic defects (Table 35.5). It involves

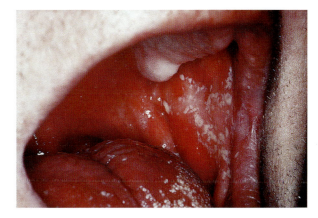

Fig. 35.3 Thrush.

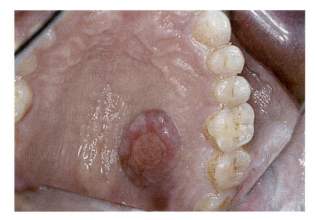

Fig. 35.4 Kaposi sarcoma in a renal transplant patient with diabetic nephrosclerosis.

stem cells of myeloid, erythroid, megakaryocyte, lymphoid and macrophage origins. The cells are either autologous or allogeneic and obtained from bone marrow (BMT), peripheral blood, or banked cryopreserved umbilical cord or fetal liver blood. Most transplants are

Table 35.5 *Main indications for haemopoietic stem-cell transplantation (HSCT)*

Indications	Examples
Lymphoproliferative disease	Leukaemias
	Lymphomas
	Myelomatosis
Solid tumours	Breast cancers
	Colon cancers
	Ewing sarcoma
	Germinal cell tumours
	Gliomas
	Lung cancers
	Melanomas
	Ovarian carcinomas
	Renal carcinomas
	Sarcomas
Non-malignant diseases	Aplastic anaemia
	Autoimmune diseases
	Fanconi syndrome
	Immunodeficiencies
	Inborn errors of metabolism
	Thalassaemia

Table 35.6 *Donor cells used in haemopoietic stem-cell transplantation (HSCT)*

Donor	Comments
Autologous	Best for HSCT in non-malignant disease – no graft-versus-host disease (GVHD). In malignant disease, there is a risk of re-introducing malignant cells
Sibling: syngeneic (identical twin)	Best: no GVHD
Sibling: human leukocyte antigen (HLA)-matched	Minimal GVHD
Unrelated donor: HLA-matched	Some GVHD

made between HLA-identical siblings, though other family members, or matched volunteers, may be used (Table 35.6).

General management

Patients destined for HSCT must first be profoundly immunosuppressed to reduce the chances of graft rejection by 'conditioning', often with cyclophosphamide, plus total body irradiation (TBI) or busulfan ('reduced intensity conditioning'). All conditioning regimens are toxic but those using reduced intensity conditioning have lower morbidity and mortality.

The donor cells are then mixed with heparin and infused intravenously in order to colonize the recipient's marrow; over the next 2–4 weeks, they start to produce blood cells. Throughout this period and for the following 3 months, the patient is usually provided with an indwelling catheter to facilitate therapy and intravenous feeding. Recipients must also be treated with methotrexate, corticosteroids, ciclosporin, intravenous immunoglobulins, tacrolimus, sirolimus or alemtuzumab (anti-CD52 lymphocytes) for 6 months or more to prevent or ameliorate GVHD. Since patients are severely immunoincompetent until the donor marrow is fully functioning, they must also be isolated and protected from infections, and may require transfusions

of granulocytes, platelets or red cells, granulocyte colony-stimulating factors and antimicrobials.

Dental aspects

Oral mucositis is the most distressing complication of HSCT, seen in 30–50% of patients and particularly problematic after TBI. Mucositis may also be a predictor of gastrointestinal toxicity and the onset of hepatic veno-occlusive disease. Mucositis is also an important driver of health-care costs; patients use more antibiotics and analgesics, have more days of fever, and stay in the hospital longer. Less common orofacial complications include infections (which usually develop within the first month of the transplant), sinusitis, parotitis, oral pain or bleeding. GVHD presents with lichenoid reactions or xerostomia. Ulceration may be drug-induced (e.g. by everolimus). Ciclosporin may cause gingival swelling, and this and other immunosuppressants have resulted in lip and occasionally oral carcinomas, Kaposi sarcoma or lymphomas.

A meticulous pre-transplant oral assessment is required and dental treatment should be undertaken with particular attention to establishing optimal oral hygiene and eradicating sources of potential infection. Dental treatment should be completed before transplant and elective dental care is best deferred for 6 months after transplant not least because there is temporarily a bleeding tendency and immune defect since patients become thrombocytopenic and leukopenic. If surgical treatment is needed during that period, antibiotic prophylaxis is probably warranted. Local anaesthetic (LA) is satisfactory. Conscious sedation can be given if needed. General anaesthesia (GA) must always be given in hospital.

Consideration must also be given to the implications of immunosuppressive therapy, bleeding tendencies, infection and veno-occlusive liver disease.

GRAFT-VERSUS-HOST DISEASE

General aspects

Graft-versus-host disease (GVHD) is a serious complication of transplantation; it is seen mainly after HSCT but can occasionally follow solid organ transplants, especially liver and small bowel transplantation. Allogeneic T lymphocytes recognize host major histocompatibility complex (MHC) antigens (HLA mainly) and, even in HLA-identical individuals, may recognize minor non-MHC histocompatibility antigens (mHag). Such activated T cells secrete cytokines (IL-2, IFNγ) and tumour necrosis factor alpha [TNFα], causing a 'cytokine storm', exaggerated by the release of bacterial lipopolysaccharides from the gastrointestinal tract that has been damaged by TBI.

The overall HSCT survival rate is 42% but patients with progressive chronic GVHD have only a 10% survival rate. GVHD affects a number of tissues, including mucosae, and may be acute or chronic.

Acute GVHD involves the skin, liver and gut with a distinctive syndrome of fever, dermatitis, hepatitis and enteritis within 100 days of HSCT. The overall grade of acute GVHD predicts outcome, with the highest rates of mortality in those with severe (grade IV) GVHD. Response to treatment also predicts outcome in grades II–IV GVHD. Patients with no response or with progression have a mortality rate as high as 75%, compared with 20–25% in those with a complete response.

Chronic GVHD also affects skin, liver and gut but is a more diverse syndrome and develops after day 100. Chronic GVHD may arise as an extension of acute GVHD but may also start *de novo* or may emerge after a quiescent interval. The immunopathogenesis of chronic GVHD is, in part, Th2 lymphocyte-mediated, resulting in a syndrome of immunodeficiency and autoimmunity. Chronic GVHD mortality rates are higher in patients with extensive disease, progressive-type onset, thrombocytopenia and HLA-non-identical marrow donors.

Clinical features

Acute GVHD may initially cause a pruritic or painful red to violaceous rash, typically first on the palms and soles, cheeks, neck, ears and upper trunk, but sometimes progressing to cover the whole body. Liver involvement causes asymptomatic rises in serum bilirubin, alanine aminotransferase (ALT), aspartate aminotransferase (AST) and alkaline phosphatase (similar to cholestatic jaundice). Gastrointestinal involvement affects the distal small bowel and colon, causing diarrhoea, bleeding, cramping pain and ileus. Other findings include a greater risk of infectious and non-infectious pneumonia, sterile effusions, haemorrhagic cystitis, thrombocytopenia, anaemia and haemolytic–uraemic syndrome (HUS; thrombotic microangiopathy).

Chronic GVHD resembles systemic progressive sclerosis, systemic lupus erythematosus, lichen planus, Sjögren syndrome, eosinophilic fasciitis, rheumatoid arthritis and primary biliary cirrhosis. It can lead to skin and mucosal lichenoid lesions or sclerodermatous thickening, sometimes causing contractures and limitation of joint mobility. Oral effects mimic Sjögren syndrome (Ch. 18) with hyposalivation and decreases in salivary immunoglobulin A and antioxidants. Oral and gastrointestinal manifestations include dysphagia and increasing pain. Ocular manifestations include symptoms of burning, irritation, photophobia and pain from lack of tears. Pulmonary manifestations include obstructive lung disease with wheezing, dyspnoea and chronic cough unresponsive to bronchodilators. Neuromuscular manifestations include weakness, neuropathic pain and muscle cramps, and sometimes myasthenia gravis or polymyositis.

General management

Most patients undergoing HSCT are given systemic prophylaxis for GVHD with ciclosporin or tacrolimus in combination with methotrexate and/or prednisolone (prednisone). There are no reliable strategies known specifically to prevent GVHD but several systemic agents, such as corticosteroids, cyclophosphamide, azathioprine, methotrexate, ciclosporin, tacrolimus and mycophenolate mofetil, may be beneficial; strategies under investigation include sirolimus, thalidomide, clofazimine, pentostatin, hydroxychloroquine, photopheresis therapy, anti-TNF and rituximab.

Acute GVHD is treated with intravenous methotrexate for up to 14 days. Subsequent dose-tapering or switching to an oral agent is continued over several weeks to months. *Chronic GVHD* is treated with oral prednisolone alone or in combination with ciclosporin. If the response is positive, it is continued, tapering off over 6–9 months.

Dental aspects

Oral aspects may be encountered in addition to those discussed above in relation to HSCT. Oral GVHD may be associated with mucositis, hyposalivation, higher caries risk, altered taste, candidosis, herpes infections, lichenoid lesions, progressive systemic sclerosis-like changes, oral pain and oral cancer.

Other transplant complications may include a bleeding tendency, various adverse drug effects, such as adrenal suppression, and drug-induced gingival overgrowth, which is dose-related and thus more common in those on higher doses of ciclosporin (i.e. heart, liver and lung transplant patients), in arterial hypertension (an adverse effect of immunosuppressives) and in diabetes mellitus (caused by some immunosuppressive medications such as corticosteroids).

TRANSPLANTATION AND TISSUE ENGINEERING OF CRANIOFACIAL STRUCTURES

Craniofacial tissue replantation or transplantation to treat congenital anomalies, trauma and diseases is in its infancy. Tissue engineering also promises the regeneration or *de novo* formation of dental, oral and craniofacial structures. Most craniofacial structures are derivatives of mesenchymal cells, and mesenchymal stem cells have been isolated from the dental pulp, deciduous teeth and periodontium. Several craniofacial structures, such as calvarial bone, the mandibular condyle and subcutaneous adipose tissue, have been engineered from mesenchymal stem cells, growth factor and/or gene therapy approaches.

TOOTH TRANSPLANTATION

Autotransplantation of teeth is useful, has many indications in dentistry and has been used for decades. Transplanted teeth can survive for an average of 6 years but some survive for 4 decades. Immature teeth survive best as donor teeth, and the shorter time out of the mouth, the better the success. Transplanted teeth may, however, develop replacement resorption or ankylosis. Cryopreservation of teeth creates new possibilities (e.g. when autotransplantation is needed, but the recipient site is too small and orthodontic treatment is needed to gain space for the transplant). Biological tooth replacement using stem cells is experimental at present.

The molecular control of key processes in tooth development, such as initiation, morphogenesis and cytodifferentiation, is being increasingly better understood and already bioengineered tooth tissues can be regenerated at the site of previously lost teeth.

SALIVARY GLANDS TRANSPLANTATION

Transplantation of the major salivary glands has been used successfully to provide substitute lubrication in severely dry eyes, significantly improving Schirmer's test, tear break-up time, rose Bengal staining and symptoms. Long-term graft survival is around 70%. However, the surgery is fairly complex and, in over one-third of eyes with a viable graft, salivary epiphora results, which is independent of gustatory stimuli. Since the salivary tear film is substantially hypo-osmolar, microcystic epithelial oedema can result and subsequent corneal transplantation can be unsuccessful.

Transplantation of minor salivary glands is a promising new treatment option – as the procedure is simple with minimal surgical risks, the grafts remain viable in over 90% and they seem to be capable of sustaining a basal secretion for up to at least 36 months. Prospective controlled studies are needed to establish the long-term gland survival and to characterize the salivary tear film and its impact on the eye.

Salivary gland regeneration and gene transfer to salivary glands are currently experimental only.

JAW TRANSPLANTATION

There is potential for regeneration within the bony tissues of the craniofacial region, and guided tissue regeneration and distraction osteogenesis (Ch. 16) are already in widespread use.

In Germany, in 2004, a patient who lost his mandible in radical cancer surgery had a functional jawbone created using bone stem cells. Three-dimensional computed tomography (CT) and computer-aided design techniques were used to create a titanium mesh cage to replace the jaw defect; this was filled with bone mineral blocks and infiltrated with recombinant human bone morphogenetic protein (BMP) and liquid bone marrow containing the patient's stem cells. This transplant was implanted into the latissimus dorsi muscle and, 7 weeks later, transplanted as a bone–muscle free flap to repair the mandibular defect. *In vivo* skeletal scintigraphy showed bone remodelling and mineralization inside the transplant both before and after transplantation. CT provided evidence of new bone formation. Postoperatively, the patient's mastication and aesthetics improved.

FACE TRANSPLANTATION

By 2013, almost a score of composite tissue allotransplants of the face had been reported.

Self as donor ('face replantation')

The first account of a procedure to replace all or part of a person's face was in the second century BC, when an Indian surgeon, Sushruta, used autografted skin in rhinoplasty. The world's first full-face *replant* operation was in 1994, also in India, on 9-year-old Sandeep Kaur, whose face was ripped off when her hair was caught in a thresher. In 1997, a similar operation was reported from Australia, when a person's face and scalp were torn off in an accident, and successfully reattached.

Partial face transplantation

The world's first partial face *transplant* operation was in France in 2005. A triangle of central facial tissue from a brain-dead woman was grafted on to a 38-year-old woman whose nose, lips, chin and adjacent cheeks had been amputated. Bone-marrow graft and immunosuppression with thymoglobulin, tacrolimus, mycophenolate mofetil and prednisolone (prednisone) were used; they were well tolerated and there were no surgical complications. Mild rejection at day 20 responded to prednisolone. Rejection episodes on days 18 and 214 were similarly reversed. Anatomical and psychological integration and recovery of sensation were good. Sensitivity to light touch, heat and cold were normal by 6 months. Motor recovery and labial contact allowing complete mouth closure was achieved by 10 months. At 18 months, the patient was satisfied with the functional and aesthetic results.

In April 2006, in China, a similar transplant of the cheek, upper lip and nose was reported. In 2008, a patient in France received the world's first successful almost full-face transplant as treatment for neurofibromatosis. In 2009, there were reports of two similar transplants in the USA and two in France (one of the French patients died from cardiac arrest).

Full-face transplant

In 2010, the first full-face transplant was performed in Spain on a man injured in a shooting accident, and the French media reported another full-face transplant, including lacrimal ducts and eyelids. In 2011, a full-face transplant was performed in Boston and a successful face transplant was reported from Forth Worth, Texas. In 2012, one of the longest and most extensive facial transplants ever was carried out in Baltimore. In the same year, three successful full-face transplants were reported from Turkey.

FURTHER READING

Buxton, P.G., Cobourne, M.T., 2007. Regenerative approaches in the craniofacial region: manipulating cellular progenitors for oro-facial repair. Oral Dis. 13, 452.
Cross, D., et al., 2013. Developments in autotransplantation of teeth. Surgeon 11, 49.
da Fonseca, M.A., Hongs, C., 2008. An overview of chronic oral graft-vs-host disease following pediatric hematopoietic stem cell transplantation. Pediatr. Dent. 30, 98.
Devauchelle, B., et al., 2006. First human face allograft: early report. Lancet 368, 203.
Duailibi, S.E., et al., 2008. Bioengineered dental tissues grown in the rat jaw. J. Dent. Res. 87, 745.
Dubernard, J.-M., Devauchelle, B., 2008. Face transplantation. Lancet 372, 603.
Dubernard, J.M., et al., 2007. Outcomes 18 months after the first human partial face transplantation. N. Engl. J. Med. 357, 2451.
Filipovich, A.H., 2008. Diagnosis and manifestations of chronic graft-versus-host disease. Best Pract. Res. Clin. Haematol. 21, 251.
Geerling, G., Sieg, P., 2008. Transplantation of the major salivary glands. Dev. Ophthalmol. 41, 255.
Geerling, G., et al., 2008. Minor salivary gland transplantation. Dev. Ophthalmol. 41, 243.
Goldman, K.E., 2006. Dental management of patients with bone marrow and solid organ transplantation. Dent. Clin. North Am. 50 (4), 659. viii.
Gordon, C.R., et al., 2009. The world's experience with facial transplantation: what have we learned thus far? Ann. Plast. Surg. 63 (5), 572.
Guggenheimer, J., et al., 2003. Dental management of the (solid) organ transplant patient. Oral Surg. Oral Med. Oral Pathol. Oral Radiol. Endod. 95, 383.
Guo, S., et al., 2008. Human facial allotransplantation: a 2-year follow-up study. Lancet 372, 631.
Ikeda, E., Tsuji, T., 2008. Growing bioengineered teeth from single cells: potential for dental regenerative medicine. Expert Opin. Biol. Ther. 8, 735.
Ivanovski, S., et al., 2006. Stem cells in the periodontal ligament. Oral Dis. 12, 358.
Kagami, H., et al., 2008. Restoring the function of salivary glands. Oral Dis. 14, 15.
Lantieri, L., et al., 2008. Repair of the lower and middle parts of the face by composite tissue allotransplantation in a patient with massive plexiform neurofibroma: a 1-year follow-up study. Lancet 372, 639.
Lew, J., Smith, J.A., 2007. Mucosal graft-vs-host disease. Oral Dis. 13, 519.
Little, J.W., et al., 2008. Dental Management of the Medically Compromised Patient, seventh ed. Mosby, St Louis.
Mao, J.J., et al., 2006. Craniofacial tissue engineering by stem cells. J. Dent. Res. 85, 966.
Maria, O.M., et al., 2007. Cells from bone marrow that evolve into oral tissues and their clinical applications. Oral Dis. 13, 11.
McLoon, L.K., et al., 2007. Myogenic precursor cells in craniofacial muscles. Oral Dis. 13, 134.
Niederhagen, B., et al., 2003. Location and sanitation of dental foci in liver transplantation. Transpl. Int. 16, 173.

Petti, S., et al., 2013. Orofacial disease in solid organ and hematopoietic stem cell transplant recipients. Oral Dis. 19 (1), 18. doi:10.1111/j.1601-0825.2012.01925.x. Epub 2012 Mar 28

Sartaj, R., Sharpe, P., 2006. Biological tooth replacement. J. Anat. 209, 503.

Scully, C., et al., 2007. Special Care in Dentistry: Handbook of Oral Healthcare. Churchill Livingstone/Elsevier, Edinburgh.

Shanmugarajah, K., et al., 2011. Clinical outcomes of facial transplantation: a review. Int. J. Surg. 9 (8), 600.

Siemionow, M., et al., 2009. Near-total human face transplantation for a severely disfigured patient in the USA. Lancet 374 (9685), 203.

Sloan, A.J., Smith, A.J., 2007. Stem cells and the dental pulp: potential roles in dentine regeneration and repair. Oral Dis. 13, 151.

Sun, H.-Y., Singh, N., 2011. Opportunistic Infection-associated immune reconstitution syndrome in transplant recipients. Clin. Infect. Dis. 53 (2), 168.

Temmerman, L., et al., 2006. Tooth transplantation and cryopreservation: state of the art. Am. J. Orthod. Dentofacial Orthop. 129, 691.

Warnke, P.H., 2006. Repair of a human face by allotransplantation. Lancet 368, 181.

Warnke, P.H., et al., 2004. Growth and transplantation of a custom vascularised bone graft in a man. Lancet 364, 766.

Warnke, P.H., et al., 2006. Man as living bioreactor: fate of an exogenously prepared customized tissue-engineered mandible. Biomaterials 27, 3163.

Westbrook, S.D., et al., 2003. Adult hemopoietic stem cell transplantation. J. Am. Dent. Assoc. 134, 1224.

Yelick, P.C., Vacanti, J.P., 2006. Bioengineered teeth from tooth bud cells. Dent. Clin. North Am. 50, 191.

Zollner-Schwetz, I., et al., 2008. Oral and intestinal Candida colonization in patients undergoing hematopoietic stem-cell transplantation. J. Infect. Dis. 198, 150.

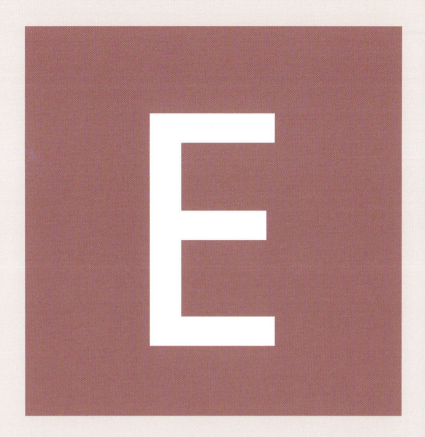

Appendix

Causes of disease are genetic (inherited) or acquired – which can be environmental (from trauma, infection, chemicals or irradiation) or related to lifestyle (e.g. lack of exercise, poor diet, habits – tobacco, alcohol, drugs, betel and others). Many diseases result from an interaction of several of these factors.

GENERAL HEALTH PROMOTION

Since disease arises from the interactions of negative genetic, environmental and lifestyle factors, it follows that it may be prevented by avoiding or minimizing these factors – as summarized in Table 36.1 and Figure 36.1. Already the effects of genetic diseases like haemophilia can be minimized by providing the missing protein (blood clotting factor VIII) and, in the future, genetic manipulation may be more widely possible ('gene therapy'). The term 'lifestyle' refers to how individuals live their life and how they handle problems and interpersonal relations – 'the unique way in which individuals try to realise their fictional final goal and meet or avoid the three main tasks of life: work, community, love' (Adler). Lifestyle choices are crucial. Apart from improving or maintaining good health by avoiding contracting infections, including sexually shared infections (SSIs; Ch. 32), the three most important measures are to take regular exercise, eat a healthy diet, and avoid substance dependence and other deleterious habits.

EXERCISE

When exercise is combined with a proper diet, weight can be controlled and obesity – a major risk factor for many diseases – prevented. In contrast, physical inactivity often occurs together with an unhealthy diet, contributing to obesity, diabetes, heart disease and cancer.

There are real health benefits from exercise, ranging from protecting against cardiac disease (hypertension, atheroma and coronary artery disease) to reducing the chances of cancer and Alzheimer disease. In addition, exercise can: increase stamina; improve brain function; reduce stress (by releasing endorphins), depression and anxiety; control weight; build and maintain healthy bones, muscles and joints; and reduce the risk of developing diabetes.

To achieve health benefits, enough regular, moderately intense physical activity to burn an extra 200 calories daily is needed at the very least. At a minimum, this means about 30 minutes of activity daily – such as a brisk walk.

There are at least ten scientifically proven reasons for taking regular exercise, as follows:

1. *Exercise helps minimize obesity.* Exercise, by burning calories, helps minimize obesity (Ch. 27). Men who are obese are more likely than non-obese men to die from cancer of the colon, rectum or prostate; obese women are more likely to die from cancer of the gallbladder, breast, uterus, cervix or ovaries. Other health problems that stem from obesity include diabetes, ischaemic heart disease (IHD), hypertension, metabolic syndrome, stroke, gallbladder disease, liver disease, osteoarthritis,

gout, sleep apnoea, menstrual irregularities and infertility in women, and psychosocial effects.

2. *Exercise helps increase levels of HDL or 'good' cholesterol.* Levels of high-density lipoproteins (HDL), when low, and low-density lipoproteins (LDL), when high, predict a risk for IHD. Exercise helps increase HDL and lower LDL levels and, by strengthening the heart and lowering blood pressure, protects against atheroma, myocardial infarcts and strokes (Ch. 5).

3. *Exercise helps lower high blood pressure.* Hypertension can be reduced by exercise. Blood pressure levels predict the risk for coronary heart disease and stroke. Physical activity also reduces obesity, which is associated with hypertension (Ch. 5).

4. *Exercise helps promote healthy blood sugar levels.* High blood sugar levels in diabetes, a risk factor for coronary heart disease, can be lowered by exercise (Ch. 6).

5. *Exercise helps improve the metabolic syndrome.* The metabolic syndrome (syndrome X or insulin resistance syndrome) is a cluster of abdominal obesity (excess body fat around the waist), insulin resistance (causing high blood sugar) and increased blood pressure, which increases the risk for diabetes, heart disease and stroke (Ch. 23). Having just one of these factors contributes to the risk of serious disease and, in combination, the risk is even greater. Exercise improves these factors.

6. *Exercise helps build muscle strength.* By building or preserving muscle mass and strength, and improving the ability to use calories, exercise helps reduce body fat. By increasing muscle strength and endurance, and improving flexibility and posture, regular exercise also helps prevent back pain. Exercise helps build muscle but this benefit fades if exercise stops for any reason, so *regular* exercise is needed.

Table 36.1 *Prevention of disease*

Environmental		Lifestyle	
Trauma	Avoid alcohol use, accidents, aggression and dangerous environments, activities and sports	Exercise	Take regular daily exercise for a minimum of 30 min
Infections	Avoid needlestick injuries and use latex protection (condoms, gloves, rubber dam). Be vaccinated	Diet	Eat a balanced diet with five portions of fruit/vegetables daily, minimize sugar and avoid food fads
Chemical	Label and take care with toxic agents and avoid communicable diseases	Substance dependence	Abstain if possible from use of tobacco, alcohol, recreational drugs and betel
Irradiation	Minimize exposure (to sun, X-rays, lasers, damaging lights, etc.) and use safety measures such as protective eyewear and screens		

Environment

Health and safety at work

Vehicle and road safety

Body protection in sports

Lifestyle

Exercise regularly

Eat more vegetables and fruit; fewer calories

Tobacco abstinence

Alcohol and other drugs of abuse abstinence

Prevent infections (immunization: hygiene: avoid contact)

Sleep hygiene

Sun avoidance

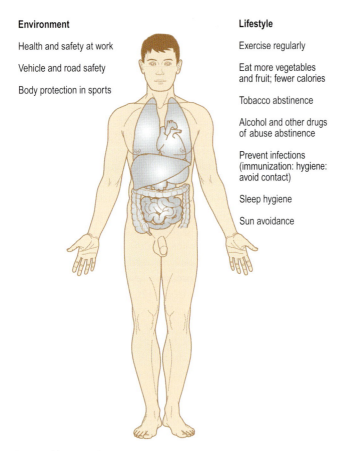

Fig. 36.1 Health promotion.

7. *Exercise helps promote bone density*. Regular exercise from a young age can increase bone density and help avoid or minimize osteoporosis (Ch. 16).
8. *Exercise helps improve mobility*. People who exercise regularly have been shown to be more mobile and independent compared with those having a sedentary lifestyle (Ch. 25).
9. *Exercise helps the immune system*. Exercise helps the immune system combat infections. The mechanism is unclear. In contrast, when exercise is performed without food intake, and is too continuous, prolonged or of high intensity (as in athletes), immune function can be depressed.
10. *Exercise helps improve mood*. People who exercise regularly have been shown to be generally happier and less liable to depression compared with those having a sedentary lifestyle (Ch. 10).

DIET

The keys to a healthy diet are eating the right amount of food for the activity undertaken *and* eating a range of foods to ensure a balanced diet. This includes: fruit and vegetables; wholegrain bread, pasta and rice; some protein-rich foods such as meat, fish, eggs and lentils; and some dairy foods. The diet must also be low in fat (especially saturated fat), salt and sugar. Generous amounts of vegetables and fruit daily appear to protect against cancers of stomach, colon and lung, and possibly against cancers of the mouth, larynx, cervix, bladder and breast. Carbohydrates as wholegrain unrefined products may help protect against colon cancer, diverticulitis and caries. A high-fibre diet may also offer some protection against hypertension and IHD. Minimizing the intake of saturated fats (especially those from dairy sources) and partially halogenated vegetable fats may lower the risk of IHD and some cancers. Ready meals,

convenience foods and takeaways are often high in added salt, sugar or fat, and should only be eaten in moderation. See the US Department of Agriculture's food guidance system (http://www.choosemyplate.gov; accessed 30 September 2013).

CALORIES

A calorie is the amount of energy required to heat 1 g of water to 1°C; however, because this is a small energy quantity, it more common to use the kilocalorie or Calorie – equivalent to 1000 calories. Energy is usually expressed either in kilojoules or in kilocalories. These two units – joules and calories – are directly related. To convert one to the other, the number of calories multiplied by 4.186 gives the number of joules; or the number of kilocalories multiplied by 4.186 gives the number of kilojoules.

ELEMENTS (MINERALS) AND TRACE ELEMENTS

Iron (Fe) is an important component of haemoglobin. Sodium (Na), potassium (K), calcium (Ca) and phosphorus (P) are needed in large quantities to take part in physiological reactions such as nerve impulse transmission or to form bones and teeth. Trace elements vital to good health include iodine (I), which is necessary for thyroxine, and fluoride (F), which helps to protect against caries.

VITAMINS

See Chapter 27.

SUBSTANCE DEPENDENCE

Substance dependence is defined as self-administration without any medical indication and despite adverse medical and social consequences, and in a manner that deviates from the cultural norm and is harmful. This applies to tobacco, alcohol and a range of drugs of abuse (Ch. 34).

TOBACCO

Nicotine is absorbed readily from tobacco smoke in the lungs; it is one of the most heavily used addictive drugs, and is highly addictive (Ch. 34). Cigarette smoking is a major hazard to health and promotes many diseases (Box 36.1). Smoking cessation should be gradual because withdrawal is less severe in those who quit gradually. Aids include nicotine chewing gum or patches, or drugs.

ALCOHOL

Alcohol is damaging to health and high in calories, so cutting down can help control weight. Women can drink up to 2–3 units of alcohol a day and men up to 3–4 units a day without significant risk to their health (Ch. 34). A unit is half a pint of standard strength beer, lager or cider, or a pub measure of spirit. A glass of wine is about 2 units and alcopops are about 1.5 units.

DRUG ABUSE

Use of illegal drugs can cause dry mouth, bruxism, dilated pupils, tachycardia, aggression, talkativeness, tachypnoea and hallucinations, leading to hyperpyrexia, seizures, arrhythmias and collapse (Ch. 34).

Box 36.1 *Health problems from tobacco*

- Cigarette smoking is particularly linked to atherosclerotic heart disease, cancers of the lung, oesophagus, mouth and bladder, and chronic obstructive pulmonary disease
- Carbon monoxide in the smoke increases the risk of cardiovascular disease
- Tobacco use is a major cause of stroke and leading cause of death
- Smokers metabolize some other drugs more rapidly and require, for example, higher doses of benzodiazepines than non-smokers
- Women who smoke generally have an earlier menopause. If women smokers also take oral contraceptives, they are more prone to cardiovascular and cerebrovascular diseases than are other smokers; this is especially true for women older than 30
- Pregnant women who smoke cigarettes run a greater risk of having stillborn or premature infants, or infants with a low birth weight
- Children of women who smoked while pregnant have a raised risk for developing conduct disorders
- Second-hand smoke (passive smoking) causes lung cancer in adults and greatly increases the risk of respiratory illnesses in children and sudden infant death
- Tobacco use can also damage oral health and cause:

  oral cancer

  keratosis

  periodontal disease, particularly necrotizing gingivitis

  Implant failure

  dry socket

  candidosis

  dry mouth (xerostomia)

  halitosis

  staining of teeth

High doses can cause mood swings and psychoses, including hallucinations and paranoia, and can give rise to respiratory failure and death. Intravenous use of illegal drugs can also easily lead to infections, including SSIs, viral hepatitis and HIV/AIDS.

USEFUL WEBSITES

(Accessed 8 July 2013)
Department of Health: Tobacco. <http://webarchive.nationalarchives.gov.uk/+/www.dh.gov.uk/en/Publichealth/Healthimprovement/Tobacco/index.htm>.
National Institutes of Health. <http://health.nih.gov/category/WellnessLifestyle>.
Partners in Information Access for the Public Health Workforce. <http://phpartners.org/hpro.html>.
Patient.co.uk: Health promotion/lifestyle. <http://www.patient.co.uk/showdoc/16/>.

This chapter includes synopses of many relevant conditions; if a specific condition is not located here, please see index, as it may be elsewhere in the book. For eponymous medical signs, see also http://en.wikipedia.org/wiki/List_of_eponymous_medical_signs (accessed 30 September 2013).

Abrikossof tumour. Granular cell tumour.

Adamantiades syndrome. Behçet syndrome.

Addison disease. Autoimmune hypoadrenocorticism (Ch. 6).

Adie's (Holmes–Adie) pupil. A benign condition in which one pupil is dilated and reacts only very slowly to light or convergence.

Albers–Schonberg disease. Osteopetrosis.

Albright syndrome (McCune–Albright syndrome). Polyostotic fibrous dysplasia with skin pigmentation and an endocrine abnormality (usually precocious puberty in girls; Ch. 16).

Allgrove syndrome. Autosomal recessive condition due to chromosome 12 mutation. Achalasia of cardia, adrenal insufficiency, alacrima (triple A syndrome) plus hyposalivation.

Alstrom syndrome. Congenital nerve deafness and retinitis pigmentosa.

Apert syndrome. Craniofacial synostosis with craniosynostosis, facial dysmorphology, hands and feet defects, and learning disability.

Argyll Robinson pupils. Small, irregular, unequal pupils that fail to react to light but do react to accommodation. Caused by neurosyphilis and other diseases.

Arnold–Chiari syndrome. A congenital malformation in which the brainstem and the cerebellum are longer than normal and protrude into the spinal cord.

Ascher syndrome. Congenital double lip with blepharochalasis (redundant eyelids) and thyroid goitre.

Asperger syndrome. A form of autism.

Avellis syndrome. Unilateral paralysis of the larynx and palate.

Battle's sign. Bruising over the mastoid bone, a sign of basilar skull fracture.

Becker syndrome. Severe muscular dystrophy resulting in progressive weakness of limb and breathing muscles, almost exclusively in boys.

Beckwith–Wiedemann syndrome. Congenital gigantism, omphalocoele or umbilical hernia.

Beeson's signs. Myalgia, facial oedema and fever in trichinosis.

Behçet syndrome. The triad of oral aphthous ulcers, genital ulceration and uveitis.

Bell palsy. A common lower motor neuron facial palsy, caused by inflammation in the stylomastoid canal (Ch. 13).

Bence Jones protein. Overproduction of gamma-globulins in myelomatosis, particularly of immunoglobulin light chains that spill over into the urine (Bence Jones proteinuria; Ch. 8).

Berardinelli–Seip syndrome. An autosomal recessive form of generalized lipodystrophy.

Biemond syndrome. Congenital obesity and hypogonadism.

Binder syndrome. Congenital maxillonasal dysplasia, and absent or hypoplastic frontal sinuses.

Blackfan–Diamond syndrome. Congenital red cell aplasia.

Block–Sulzberger disease (incontinentia pigmenti). Congenital hyperpigmented skin lesions, skeletal defects, learning disability and hypodontia.

Bloom syndrome. Congenital telangiectasia, depigmentation, short stature and susceptibility to oral carcinoma.

Boeck syndrome. Sarcoidosis (Ch. 15).

Book syndrome. Autosomal dominant disorder of palm and sole hyperhidrosis, hypodontia and premature whitening of hair.

Bourneville disease (epiloia, tuberous sclerosis). Autosomal dominant phakomatosis including fibromas at the nail bases (subungual fibromas), hamartomas in the brain, kidneys and heart, and nodules in the nasolabial folds (adenoma sebaceum) (Ch. 13).

Briquet syndrome. Somatisation (Ch. 10).

Brugada syndrome. A genetic disease characterized by abnormal ECG and a risk of sudden cardiac death (Ch. 5).

Bruton syndrome. Sex-linked agammaglobulinaemia, cervical lymph node enlargement, oral ulceration, recurrent sinusitis and absent tonsils.

Burkitt lymphoma. (Ch. 8).

Byar–Jurkiewicz syndrome. Gingival fibromatosis, hypertrichosis, giant fibroadenomas of the breast and kyphosis.

Cannon disease. Congenital white sponge naevus.

Carabelli cusp. Congenital additional palatal cusp on upper molars.

Carney syndrome. Autosomal dominant multisystem disorder of myxomas and lentigos.

Carpenter syndrome. Autosomal recessive acrocephalopolysyndactyly type II.

Castleman disease (angiolymphoid hyperplasia). Nodal lymphoproliferation that may progress to a malignant vascular tumour or lymphoma. Sometimes associated with paraneoplastic pemphigus.

CATCH22. *C*ardiac abnormality, *a*bnormal facies, *T*-cell deficit (due to thymic hypoplasia), *c*left palate and *h*ypocalcaemia (due to hypoparathyroidism). A chromosome *22* defect (DiGeorge syndrome).

Charles Bonnet syndrome. Visual hallucinations arising in people who have eye conditions such as age-related macular degeneration, cataract, glaucoma or diabetic eye disease.

Chediak–Higashi syndrome. Congenital immune defect in which neutrophils have large inclusions.

Christmas disease. Deficiency of blood clotting factor IX (Ch. 8).

Chvostek sign. Tapping the skin over the facial nerve elicits involuntary twitching of the upper lip or ipsilateral side of face – seen in hypoparathyroidism (Ch. 6).

Clutton joints. Syphilitic neuropathic joints.

Cockayne syndrome. Premature ageing, dwarfism, deafness and neuropathy.

Coffin–Lowry syndrome. Congenital osteocartilaginous anomalies and learning disability.

Coffin–Siris syndrome. Congenital defective neutrophil function, susceptibility to infection and skin pigmentation.

Costen syndrome. Outmoded term relating to patients with facial pain, otalgia and possible occlusal abnormalities.

Cowden syndrome. Congenital multiple hamartoma syndrome, with oral papillomatosis and risk of breast and thyroid cancer.

Coxsackie virus. Named after Coxsackie in New York State. Coxsackie viruses can cause herpangina, hand, foot and mouth disease, and other illnesses.

CREST syndrome. *C*alcinosis, *R*aynaud disease, *O*esophageal involvement, *s*clerodactyly and *t*elangiectasia (see Scleroderma; Ch. 18).

Crohn disease. Chronic inflammatory idiopathic granulomatous disorder of the ileum or any part of the gastrointestinal tract, including the mouth (Ch. 7).

Cronkhite–Canada syndrome. Hypogeusia is the dominant initial symptom, followed by diarrhoea and ectodermal changes (alopecia, nail dystrophy, and skin and buccal melanotic hyperpigmentation).

Cross syndrome. Athetosis, learning disability, gingival fibromatosis and hypopigmentation.

Crouzon syndrome. Autosomal dominant premature fusion of cranial sutures, mid-face hypoplasia and proptosis.

Curry–Jones syndrome. Unilateral coronal synostosis and microphthalmia, plagiocephaly, craniofacial asymmetry, iris coloboma, broad thumbs, hand syndactyly, foot polydactyly, erosive skin lesions, gastrointestinal abnormalities and developmental delay.

Cushing syndrome. Moon face with buffalo hump, hirsutism and hypertension due to an pituitary adenoma producing adrenocorticotropic hormone (ACTH; Ch. 6).

Danon disease. Rare genetic condition causing muscular dystrophy, cardiomyopathy and learning problems.

Darier disease (Darier–White disease). Autosomal dominant skin disorder with follicular hyperkeratosis and sometimes white oral papules.

Destombes–Rosai–Dorfman syndrome. Rosai–Dorfman syndrome (see below).

DiGeorge syndrome. Congenital immunodeficiency with hypoplasia of thymus and parathyroids, characteristic facies with down-slanting palpebral fissures and ocular and nasal anomalies, and cardiac, thyroid and parathyroid defects due to a third and fourth branchial arch defect related to a chromosome 22 anomaly (CATCH 22 syndrome – see above) (Ch. 20).

Down syndrome (trisomy 21). Chromosomal anomaly causing learning disability, short stature, brachycephaly, mid-face retrusion and upward-sloping palpebral fissures (mongoloid slant; Ch. 28).

Duhring disease. Dermatitis herpetiformis.

Duncan disease. Rare sex-linked lymphoproliferative syndrome, characterized by severe Epstein–Barr virus mononucleosis, immunoblastic sarcoma or lymphoma.

Eagle syndrome. Elongated styloid process associated with dysphagia and pain on chewing, and on turning the head towards the affected side.

ECHO viruses. *E*nteric *c*ytopathogenic *h*uman *o*rphan viruses.

Ehlers–Danlos syndrome. Congenital disorders of collagen characterized by joint hyperflexibility, hyperextensible skin, bleeding and bruising, and mitral incompetence (Ch. 16).

Ellis–van Creveld syndrome (chondroectodermal dysplasia). Congenital polydactyly, dwarfism, ectodermal dysplasia; hypodontia and hypoplastic teeth; multiple fraena.

Epstein–Barr virus. Herpesvirus implicated in infectious mononucleosis, hairy leukoplakia, nasopharyngeal carcinoma and some lymphomas.

Epstein pearls. Small cysts due to persistence of epithelial rests in the alveolar ridge.

Fabry disease (angiokeratoma corporis diffusum universale). X-linked recessive error of glycosphingolipid metabolism with skin angiokeratomas, hypertension, fever, renal disease and risk of myocardial infarction.

Fallot tetralogy. Combination of ventricular septal defect (VSD) and pulmonary stenosis, with aorta 'overriding' (sitting 'astride') the VSD and with right ventricular hypertrophy.

Fanconi anaemia. Rare autosomal recessive syndrome of congenital anaemia, congenital skeletal defects (e.g. abnormal radii), hyperpigmentation and pancytopenia; associated with abnormal susceptibility to oral or other head and neck carcinomas and leukaemia at an early age (Ch. 8).

Felty syndrome. Rheumatoid arthritis and neutropenia.

Fitzgerald–Gardner syndrome. Gardner syndrome (see below).

Fordyce disease (Fordyce spots). Congenital ectopic sebaceous glands seen mainly in the buccal mucosa or lips.

Freeman–Sheldon syndrome. Rare form of multiple congenital contracture syndrome (arthrogryposis).

Frey syndrome. Skin gustatory sweating and flushing after trauma to skin over a salivary gland, due to crossover of sympathetic and parasympathetic innervation to the gland and skin.

Friedreich ataxia. Inherited progressive central nervous sytem damage causing features ranging from muscle weakness and speech problems to heart disease. Usually an autosomal recessive trait, leading to degeneration of many spinal cord tracts extending to the brainstem, and thus severe ataxia, loss of reflexes and secondary deformities. Degenerative heart disease with arrhythmias may be associated.

Froehlich syndrome. Congenital obesity, hypogonadism, and risk of learning disability and open bite.

Gardner syndrome. Autosomal dominant syndrome of intestinal polyposis, bony abnormalities, soft-tissue tumours, multiple osteomas, fibromas and pigmented lesions of fundus of eye.

Garré osteomyelitis. Proliferative periostitis.

Gasserian ganglion. Trigeminal ganglion.

Gaucher disease. Inherited defect of lysosomal glucocerebrosidase – most common in Ashkenazi Jews, and causing skeletal defects, hepatosplenomegaly, anaemia and thrombocytopenia.

Gilles de la Tourette syndrome. A familial early-onset syndrome, seen mainly in males, of chronic motor tics involving the head and neck especially and associated with compulsive vocal tics and sometimes swearing (coprolalia). Tongue-thrusting and lip-smacking are common and sometimes regarded as lewd (copropraxia). Many of those affected have obsessive–compulsive tendencies or attention-deficit hyperactivity, but intelligence is usually normal. Temporomandibular or other oral pain may result and self-mutilation, such as tongue- and lip-biting, may be associated. The dopamine receptor blocker haloperidol is usually effective; pimozide and/or clonidine may also be used. Drugs used to treat the syndrome may cause xerostomia or tardive dyskinesia. Interactions of these drugs with general anaesthetic agents, other central nervous system depressants and atropine means that dental treatment is best carried out under local analgesia.

Glossopharyngeal neuralgia. Severe pain in the posterior tongue, fauces, pharynx and sometimes beneath the angle of the mandible.

Goldenhar syndrome. Variant of congenital hemifacial microsomia, with microtia (small ears), macrostomia, agenesis of mandibular ramus and condyle, vertebral abnormalities and epibulbar dermoids.

Goltz syndrome (focal dermal hypoplasia). X-linked disorder with multiple mesenchymal defects, skin lesions, oral warts and dental defects.

Gorham disease. Rare osteolysis without sex, race or age predilection, affecting bones. Jaw is the main location; histology mostly shows haemangioma-like proliferation.

Gorlin–Goltz syndrome (Gorlin syndrome; multiple basal cell naevi syndrome). Autosomal dominant trait, with multiple basal cell carcinomas, odontogenic keratocysts, and vertebral and rib anomalies.

Graves disease. Hyperthyroidism with ophthalmopathy and exophthalmos (Ch. 6).

Grinspan syndrome. Lichen planus, diabetes and hypertension (probably due to lichenoid reactions to antihypertensive and antidiabetic drugs).

Guillain–Barré syndrome. Acute infective polyneuritis; facial palsy may be seen.

Hailey–Hailey disease. Autosomal dominant benign familial pemphigus presenting in second or third decade with skin and oral blisters and vegetations.

Hajdu–Cheney syndrome. Ulcerating lesions on the palms of the hands and soles of the feet, with softening and destruction of bones (acro-osteolysis).

Hallermann–Streiff syndrome. Congenital cranial anomalies, micro-ophthalmia, cataracts, mandibular hypoplasia and abnormal temporomandibular joint.

Hand–Schuller–Christian disease. Langerhans histiocytosis causing skull lesions, exophthalmos and diabetes insipidus (Ch. 8).

Hansen disease. Leprosy.

Heck disease. Focal epithelial hyperplasia. Caused by human papillomavirus 13 or 32, and seen especially in various ethnic groups such as American Native Indians and Inuits.

Heerfordt syndrome (uveoparotid fever). Sarcoidosis associated with lacrimal and salivary swelling, uveitis, fever and sometimes facial palsy (Ch. 15).

Henoch–Schönlein purpura. Allergic purpura, typically following streptococcal infection.

Hermansky–Pudlak syndrome. Congenital albinism and bleeding tendency.

Hirschsprung disease. Congenital aganglionic megacolon.

Hodgkin disease. Nearly one-half of all lymphomas are Hodgkin disease, which can affect any age group, particularly males in middle age (Ch. 8).

Horner syndrome. Usually unilateral miosis (pupil constriction); ptosis (drooping of the upper eyelid); loss of sweating of the ipsilateral face; enophthalmos (retruded eyeball). Caused by interruption of sympathetic nerve fibres peripherally (e.g. as a result of trauma to the neck, or lung cancer infiltrating the superior cervical sympathetic ganglion; Ch. 13).

Horton cephalgia. Migrainous neuralgia.

Hunter syndrome. A mucopolysaccharidosis.

Hunterian chancre. Syphilitic primary chancre.

Hurler syndrome (Hurler–Scheie syndrome). Congenital mucopolysaccharidosis causing growth failure, learning disability, large head, frontal bossing, hypertelorism, coarse facial features (gargoylism) and mandibular radiolucencies (Ch. 23).

Hutchinson–Gilford syndrome (progeria). See Werner syndrome.

Hutchinson teeth. Screwdriver-shaped incisor teeth in congenital syphilis.

Hutchinson triad. Hutchinson teeth, interstitial keratitis and deafness.

Immerslund–Grasbeck syndrome. Congenital vitamin B_{12} deficiency.

Jackson–Lawler syndrome. A type of pachyonychia in congenital syphilis with no oral leukoplakia, but neonatal teeth and early loss of secondary teeth.

Jadassohn–Lewandowsky syndrome. Pachyonychia congenita.

Jones syndrome. See Curry–Jones syndrome.

Kallmann syndrome. Hypogonadotropin eunuchoidism (Ch. 6).

Kaposi sarcoma. Malignant neoplasm of endothelial cells caused by human herpesvirus 8 (KSHV or KS herpesvirus), seen mainly in AIDS, immunosuppressed patients, elderly Jews and those of Mediterranean or Middle Eastern origin (Ch. 20).

Kartagener syndrome. Congenital dextrocardia, immunodeficiency and sinusitis.

Kawasaki disease (mucocutaneous lymph node syndrome). Idiopathic disorder with fever, lymphadenopathy, desquamation of hand and feet, cheilitis and cardiac lesions.

Kearns–Sayre syndrome. A mitochondrial cardiomyopathy.

Kikuchi–Fujimoto disease. A self-limiting lymphadenopathy that can be confused histologically and clinically with lymphoma or systemic lupus erythematosus.

Kimura disease. A chronic inflammatory disorder, mostly in males, causing a painless, slowly enlarging, soft-tissue mass, lymphadenopathy and peripheral eosinophilia.

Kindler syndrome. Autosomal recessive skin disorder with blistering, photosensitivity, progressive poikiloderma and diffuse cutaneous atrophy.

Klinefelter syndrome. A chromosomal abnormality affecting men and causing hypogonadism.

Klippel–Feil anomalad. Congenital association of cervical vertebrae fusion with short neck, low-lying posterior hairline, syringomyelia and other neurological anomalies, and sometimes unilateral renal agenesis and cardiac anomalies.

Koplik spots. Small white spots on the buccal mucosa in measles prodrome.

Kostmann syndrome. Autosomal recessive defect in neutrophil numbers. In contrast to normals, CD64+ (FC γ RI receptor) is expressed on neutrophils but CD16+ (FC γ RIII receptor) is expression decreased.

Kuttner tumour. Immunoglobulin G4 syndrome.

Kveim test. Outdated skin test for sarcoidosis using antigen from the lymph nodes or spleen of human sarcoidosis patients, injected intracutaneously.

Laband syndrome (Zimmermann–Laband syndrome). Hereditary gingival fibromatosis with skeletal anomalies and large digits.

Langerhans cell histiocytoses (histiocytosis X). Rare tumours arising from dendritic intraepithelial antigen-presenting cells (Langerhans cells; Ch. 8).

Larsen syndrome. Autosomal recessive condition, consisting of cleft palate, flattened facies, multiple congenital dislocations and deformities of feet.

Laugier–Hunziker–Baran syndrome. A rare, acquired, benign hyperpigmentation of the lips, oral mucosa and nails.

Laurence–Moon–Biedl syndrome. Congenital retinitis pigmentosa, obesity, polydactyly, learning disability and blindness.

Leigh disease. A progressive neurodegenerative disorder related to respiratory chain deficiency and a mitochondrial defect.

Lesch–Nyhan syndrome. Congenital defect of purine metabolism causing learning disability, choreoathetoid cerebral palsy and self-mutilation.

Letterer–Siwe disease. Rapidly progressive disseminated form of Langerhans histiocytosis, often fatal because of pancytopenia and multisystem disease (Ch. 8).

Lewar disease. Pulse granuloma.

Löfgren syndrome. Acute benign form of sarcoidosis, with erythema nodosum and bilateral hilar lymphadenopathy (Ch. 15).

Lowe syndrome (cerebrohepatorenal syndrome). Congenital hypotonia and flexion contractures.

Ludwig angina. Infection of sublingual and submandibular fascial spaces.

Lyme disease. *Borrelia burgdorferi* infection from deer ticks, causing rashes, fever, arthopathy and facial palsy. First recognized in Lyme, Connecticut, USA.

Madelung disease. Benign symmetrical lipomatosis.

Maffucci syndrome. Multiple enchondromas, haemangiomas (often in the tongue) and risk of malignant chondrosarcomas.

MAGIC syndrome. *M*outh *a*nd *g*enital ulcers and *i*nterstitial *c*hondritis – a variant of Behçet syndrome.

Mallory–Weiss syndrome. Mucosal gastric tear near the oesophageal/stomach junction causing bleeding.

Mantoux test. Skin test for delayed-type hypersensitivity reaction to bacillus Calmette–Guérin (BCG; for tuberculosis).

Marcus Gunn syndrome. Jaw-winking syndrome (eyelid winks during chewing), with ptosis.

Marfan syndrome. Autosomal dominant condition in which patient is tall and thin, and has arachnodactyly (long, thin, spider-like hands) (Ch. 16).

Marie–Sainton syndrome. Cleidocranial dysplasia.

Maroteaux–Lamy syndrome. A mucopolysaccharidosis.

Meig syndrome. Ascites, pleural effusion and benign ovarian tumour.

Melkersson–Rosenthal syndrome. Facial swelling similar to that in Crohn disease or orofacial granulomatosis, with facial palsy and fissured tongue.

Mendelson syndrome. Inhalation of gastric contents causing pulmonary oedema.

Ménière disease. Labyrinthine dysfunction with vertigo, tinnitus and sensorineural hearing loss, nausea and sometimes nystagmus. Betahistine and cinnarizine are helpful but phenothiazines, prochlorperazine or thiethylperazine may be required.

Miescher cheilitis. Oligosymptomatic orofacial granulomatosis or Crohn disease affecting the lip alone.

Migrainous neuralgia (cluster headaches; histamine cephalgia; Sluder headaches). Pain in the head and face, defined by the International Headache Society as unilateral, excruciatingly severe attacks of pain in the ocular, frontal and temporal areas, recurring in separate bouts with daily or almost daily attacks for weeks or months, usually with ipsilateral lacrimation, conjunctival injection, photophobia and nasal stuffiness and/or rhinorrhoea.

Mikulicz disease. Salivary gland and lacrimal gland swelling often related to Sjögren syndrome or immunoglobulin G4 syndrome.

Mikulicz syndrome. Salivary gland and lacrimal gland swelling related to malignant disease.

Mikulicz ulcer. Minor aphthous ulceration.

Miller syndrome. Autosomal recessive post-axial acrofacial dysostosis.

Moebius syndrome. Congenital anomaly involving multiple cranial nerves, mainly the abducens (VI) and facial (VII), often associated with limb anomalies.

Moon molars. Hypoplastic molars from congenital syphilis.

Morquio syndrome. A mucopolysaccharidosis (Ch. 23).

Munchausen syndrome. The fabrication of stories by the patient, with the aim of receiving operative intervention (Ch. 10).

Murray–Puretic–Drescher syndrome (juvenile hyaline fibromatosis). Autosomal recessive disease characterized by large cutaneous nodules, especially around the head and neck, joint contractures, gingival swelling and osteolytic lesions.

Nager syndrome. Acrofacial dysostosis.

Nelson syndrome. Hyperpigmentation caused by overproduction of adrenocorticotropic hormone in response to adrenalectomy – used for breast cancer (Ch. 6).

Neumann bipolar aphthosis. The association of recurrent aphthae with genital ulceration; this is probably emerging Behçet syndrome.

Nikolsky sign. Blistering, or the extension of a blister, on gentle pressure (seen in pemphigus and pemphigoid; Ch. 11).

Noonan syndrome. Congenital short stature and webbed neck, sometimes with cardiac anomalies, pulmonary stenosis and cherubism.

Ollier syndrome. Multiple enchondromas.

Osler–Rendu–Weber disease (hereditary haemorrhagic telangiectasia; HHT). Autosomal dominant disorder where telangiectases are present orally and periorally, in the nose and gastrointestinal tract, and occasionally on the palms (Ch. 8).

Paget disease. Disease of bone (Ch. 16).

Pallister Hall syndrome. Autosomal dominant disease due to mutations in the *GLI3* gene and neonatally lethal.

Papillon–Lefèvre syndrome. Congenital defect in cathepsin C, causing palmoplantar hyperkeratosis, juvenile periodontitis that affects both dentitions, and immunodeficiency.

Parrot nodes. Frontal bossing in congenital syphilis.

Parry–Romberg syndrome. Hemifacial atrophy.

Patterson–Brown-Kelly syndrome (Plummer–Vinson syndrome). Dysphagia (due to post-cricoid candida web), microcytic hypochromic anaemia, koilonychia and angular cheilitis (Ch. 8).

Paul–Bunnell test (Paul–Bunnell–Davidsohn). Serological test for heterophile antibodies in infectious mononucleosis (glandular fever).

Peutz–Jegher syndrome. Autosomal dominant condition of circumoral melanosis and intestinal polyposis.

Pfeiffer syndrome. Craniosynostosis.

Pierre Robin sequence. Congenital micrognathia, cleft palate and glossoptosis.

Pindborg tumour. Calcifying epithelial odontogenic tumour.

Plummer–Vinson syndrome. See Patterson–Brown-Kelly syndrome.

Pospischill–Feyrter aphthae. Palatal ulceration in neonates.

Prader–Willi syndrome. Congenital obesity, hypogonadism, learning disability, diabetes and dental defects.

Quincke oedema. Angioedema.

Ramon syndrome. Cherubism, arthritis, epilepsy, gingival fibromatosis and learning disability.

Ramsay Hunt syndrome. Lower motor neuron facial palsy with vesicles in ipsilateral pharynx, external auditory canal, and face – due to herpes zoster of geniculate ganglion of seventh nerve.

Rapp–Hodgkin syndrome. Ectodermal dysplasia, kinky hair, cleft lip/palate, popliteal pterygium and ectrodactyly.

Raynaud syndrome. Vascular spasm in response to cooling, seen in the digits in connective tissue disorders (Ch. 18).

Reiter disease. Association of arthritis, urethritis, balanitis and conjunctivitis, found mainly in men with sexually shared infection and human leukocyte antigen (HLA)-B27.

Rett syndrome. Congenital bruxism and hand-wringing, often with learning disability.

Reye syndrome. Rare serious illness affecting brain and liver, occurring in children after viral infection and treated with aspirin.

Reynolds syndrome. A rare autoimmune disease, consisting of the combination of primary biliary cirrhosis and progressive systemic sclerosis.

Rieger syndrome. Congenital ocular anomalies, iridal hypoplasia, glaucoma, maxillary hypoplasia and dental hypoplasia with oligodontia and microdontia.

Riley–Day syndrome. Inherited familial dysautonomia, seen particularly in Ashkenazi Jews. Sympathetic dysfunction, enlarged salivary glands, sialorrhoea and self-mutilation.

Robinow syndrome. Fetal facies syndrome: a rare autosomal syndrome of short stature, characteristic facial dysmorphism, genital hypoplasia and mesomelic brachymelia.

Romberg syndrome (Parry–Romberg syndrome; hemifacial atrophy). Progressive atrophy of half the face, associated with contralateral Jacksonian epilepsy and trigeminal neuralgia.

Rosai–Dorfman syndrome (sinus histiocytosis with massive lymphadenopathy or Destombes–Rosai–Dorfman syndrome). A benign histiocytic proliferative disorder that primarily affects lymph nodes.

Rothmund–Thomson syndrome. Congenital poikiloderma, hypogonadism, dwarfism, cataracts and microdontia.

Rubinstein–Taybi syndrome (broad thumb–great toe syndrome). Short stature, small head, prominent beaked nose, down-slanting eyes, developmental delay, and broad, sometimes angulated thumbs and first toes. Undescended testes occur in males. Other variable features include congenital heart disease, kidney abnormalities, and eye and hearing problems.

Rud syndrome. Recessive disorder marked by ichthyosis, hypogonadism, learning disability, epilepsy and dwarfism.

Rutherfurd syndrome. Corneal dystrophy, gingival fibromatosis and delayed tooth eruption.

Ruvalcaba–Myhre–Smith syndrome. Congenital macrocephaly, learning disability, intestinal polyps, pigmented macules on penis, tongue polyps.

Sabin–Feldman test. Serological test for toxoplasmosis.

Saethre–Chotzen syndrome. Autosomal dominant craniosynostosis with mutations in TWIST gene (7p21), cleft palate and disturbances of the facial skeleton and extremities.

Sanfilippo syndrome. A mucopolysaccharidosis.

SAPHO syndrome. *S*ynovitis, *a*cne, *p*ustulosis, *h*yperostosis and *o*steitis.

Scheie syndrome. A mucopolysaccharidosis (Ch. 23).

Schmidt syndrome. Congenital hypoadrenocorticism, hypoparathyroidism, diabetes and malabsorption, with candidosis.

Seckel syndrome. Congenital microcephaly, learning disability, zygomatic and mandibular hypoplasia.

Shprintzen syndrome. Velocardiofacial syndrome.

Shwachman–Diamond syndrome. Rare disorder affecting the pancreas, bone marrow – with neutropenia and thrombocytopenia – and skeletal defects.

Sipple syndrome. Multiple endocrine neoplasia type 3 (MEN 3; sometimes called 2b) affecting several endocrine glands with multiple mucosal neuromas, phaeochromocytoma and medullary thyroid carcinoma (Ch. 6).

Sjögren syndrome. Hyposalivation and keratoconjunctivitis sicca (i.e. dry mouth and dry eyes; Ch. 18).

Sjögren–Larsson syndrome. Congenital ichthyosis, learning disability, cerebral palsy and indifference to pain.

Sluder syndrome. Migrainous neuralgia.

Sly syndrome. A mucopolysaccharidosis.

Smith–Lemli–Opitz syndrome. Congenital short stature, learning disability, syndactyly, urogenital and maxillary anomalies.

SSS syndrome (silent sinus syndrome). A rare entity of unilateral enophthalmos and hypoglobus secondary to thinning of the maxillary sinus roof in the absence of sinonasal inflammatory disease.

Stevens–Johnson syndrome. Severe erythema multiforme (Ch. 11).

Stickler syndrome. Collagenopathy affecting collagens II and IX, causing a distinctive facial appearance, eye abnormalities, hearing loss and joint problems.

Still disease. Juvenile rheumatoid arthritis.

Sturge–Weber syndrome (encephalotrigeminal angiomatosis). Congenital hamartomatous angioma of face (naevus flammeus), oral mucosa and underlying bone (with hemihypertrophy of bone and accelerated eruption of associated teeth), extending intracranially to cause convulsions, and contralateral hemiplegia and intracerebral calcifications, and sometimes learning disability.

Sutton's ulcers. Major aphthae.

Sweet syndrome. Acute neutrophilic dermatosis; red mucosal lesions and aphthae.

Takayasu disease. Pulseless aorta and large arteries.

Thibierge–Weissenbach syndrome. CREST syndrome – scleroderma with calcinosis and ischaemia.

Treacher Collins syndrome (mandibulofacial dysostosis). Autosomal dominant defect in first branchial arch with downward-sloping (antimongoloid slant) palpebral fissures, hypoplastic malar, mandibular retrognathia, deformed pinnas, hypoplastic sinuses, colobomas in outer third of the eye, middle and inner ear hypoplasia (deafness).

Trotter syndrome. Acquired unilateral deafness, pain in mandibular (third) division of trigeminal nerve, ipsilateral palatal immobility, and trismus due to invasion of nasopharynx and trigeminal nerve, by a malignant tumour. Pterygopalatine fossa syndrome is a similar condition where first and second divisions of trigeminal nerve are affected.

Turner teeth. Hypoplastic tooth due to damage to the developing tooth germ.

Tzanck cells. Abnormal squamous cells in pemphigus or herpetic infections

Urbach–Wiethe disease. Lipoid proteinosis.

Van der Woude syndrome. Cleft lip or palate with lip pits and hypodontia.

Vincent disease (acute ulcerative gingivitis). Non-contagious anaerobic infection with overwhelming proliferation of *Borrelia vincentii* and fusiform bacteria. Predisposing factors include smoking, viral respiratory infections and immune defects such as in HIV/AIDS.

von Hippel–Lindau disease. Autosomal dominant condition with café-au-lait spots, retinal angiomatosis, central nervous system haemangioblastomas, phaeochromocytomas, pancreatic neuroendocrine tumours and renal cancer.

von Recklinghausen disease. Multiple neurofibromas with skin pigmentation, skeletal abnormalities and central nervous system involvement (Ch. 13).

von Willebrand disease. Common bleeding disorder caused by defective blood clotting factor VIII and platelet dysfunction (Ch. 8).

Waardenburg syndrome. Congenital heterochromia iridis (differently coloured eyes), deafness and white forelock, with prognathism. Specific associated genes are members of the homeobox family that regulate the transcription of other genes: Waardenburg type 1 with PAX3; Waardenburg type 2 with MITF, 3q14.1; and Waardenburg type 3 with PAX3, 2q35.

Waldeyer ring. Lymphoid tissue surrounding the entrance to the oropharynx (tonsils and adenoids).

Warthin tumour. A benign salivary gland neoplasm – adenolymphoma or papillary cystadenoma lymphomatosum.

Wegener granulomatosis. Idiopathic disseminated malignant granulomatous disorder that may affect lungs, kidneys and mouth, sometimes related to *Staphylococcus aureus* (Ch. 8).

Weil disease. Leptospirosis.

Werner syndrome. Congenital alopecia, dwarfism, senility, early atherosclerosis, delayed tooth eruption and mandibular hypoplasia.

Whipple disease. A bacterial infection with *Tropheryma whippelii*, which affects primarily middle-aged white men.

Williams syndrome. Genetic disorder of cognitive impairment (usually mild learning disability), unique personality characteristics, distinctive ('elfin') facial features and cardiovascular disease (elastin arteriopathy).

Wilson disease. Hepatolenticular degeneration.

Wiskott–Aldrich syndrome. X-linked recessive immunodeficiency with thrombocytopenia, eczema, infections and lymphoreticular malignancies (Ch. 20).

Witkop disease. Hereditary benign intraepithelial dyskeratosis – seen mainly in parts of the USA.

Yersiniosis. Infection with *Yersinia pseudotuberculosis*.

Zimmermann–Laband syndrome. See Laband syndrome.

Zinsser–Engman–Cole syndrome. Rare syndrome of skin pigmentation, oral leukoplakia, nail dystrophy, pancytopenia and predisposition to malignancy.

Zollinger–Ellison syndrome. Intractable peptic ulcers, high gastric acidity and gastrin-secreting, non-beta islet cell tumours (nesidioblastomas), usually of the pancreas, but sometimes duodenum (Ch. 7).

USEFUL WEBSITES

(Accessed 11 June 2013)
all-acronyms.com. <http://www.all-acronyms.com/cat/7>.

FURTHER READING

Scully, C., et al., 2009. A marathon of eponyms. 1. Albers–Schonberg disease (osteopetrosis). Oral Dis. 15, 246.

Scully, C., et al., 2009. A marathon of eponyms. 2. Bell palsy (idiopathic facial palsy). Oral Dis. 15, 307.

Scully, C., et al., 2009. A marathon of eponyms. 3. Crouzon syndrome. Oral Dis. 15, 367.

Scully, C., et al., 2009. A marathon of eponyms. 4. Down syndrome. Oral Dis. 15, 434.

Scully, C., et al., 2009. A marathon of eponyms. 5. Ehlers–Danlos syndrome. Oral Dis. 15, 517.

Scully, C., et al., 2009. A marathon of eponyms. 6. Frey syndrome (gustatory sweating). Oral Dis. 15, 608.

Scully, C., et al., 2009. A marathon of eponyms. 7. Gorlin–Goltz syndrome (naevoid basal cell carcinoma syndrome). Oral Dis. 16, 117.

Scully, C., et al., 2010. A marathon of eponyms. 8. Hodgkin disease or lymphoma. Oral Dis. 16, 217.

Scully, C., et al., 2010. A marathon of eponyms. 9. Imerslund–Grasbeck syndrome (juvenile pernicious anaemia). Oral Dis. 16, 219.

Scully, C., et al., 2010. A marathon of eponyms. 10. Jadassohn-Lewandowsky syndrome (pachyonychia congenita). Oral Dis. 16, 310.

Scully, C., et al., 2010. A marathon of eponyms. 11. Kaposi sarcoma. Oral Dis. 16, 402.

Scully, C., et al., 2010. A marathon of eponyms. 12. Ludwig angina. Oral Dis. 16, 496.

Scully, C., et al., 2010. A marathon of eponyms. 13. Melkersson–Rosenthal syndrome. Oral Dis. 16, 707.

Scully, C., et al., 2010. A marathon of eponyms. 14. Noonan syndrome. Oral Dis. 16, 839.

Scully, C., et al., 2011. A marathon of eponyms. 15. Osler–Rendu–Weber disease. Oral Dis. 17, 125.

Scully, C., et al., 2011. A marathon of eponyms. 16. Paget disease of bone. Oral Dis. 17, 238.

Scully, C., et al., 2011. A marathon of eponyms. 17. Quincke oedema (angioedema). Oral Dis. 17, 342.

Scully, C., et al., 2011. A marathon of eponyms. 18. Robin sequence. Oral Dis. 17, 443.

Scully, C., et al., 2011. A marathon of eponyms. 19. Sjögren syndrome. Oral Dis. 17, 538.

Scully, C., et al., 2011. A marathon of eponyms. 20. Treacher Collins syndrome. Oral Dis. 17, 619.

Scully, C., et al., 2011. A marathon of eponyms. 21. Urbach–Wiethe disease. Oral Dis. 17, 729.

Scully, C., et al., 2012. A marathon of eponyms. 22. Virchow node. Oral Dis. 18, 107.

Scully, C., et al., 2012. A marathon of eponyms. 23. Wegener granulomatosis. Oral Dis. 18, 214.

Scully, C., et al., 2012. A marathon of eponyms. 24. Xmas (Christmas) disease. Oral Dis. 18 (3), 315. doi:10.1111/j.1601-0825.2009.01556.x.

Scully, C., et al., 2012. A marathon of eponyms. 25. Yersiniosis. Oral Dis. 18 (4), 417. doi:10.1111/j.1601-0825.2009.01557.x.

Scully, C., et al., 2012. A marathon of eponyms. 26. Zinsser–Cole–Engelmann syndrome. Oral Dis. 18 (5), 522. doi:10.1111/j.1601-0825.2009.01558.x.

Index